Sixth Edition

Manipal Manual of Surgery

As per the latest CBME Guidelines | Competency Based Undergraduate Curriculum for the Indian Medical Graduate

Volume 1

Book Shaped by the Students

Read in Over 20 Countries

The Iconic Textbook now in 2 Volumes

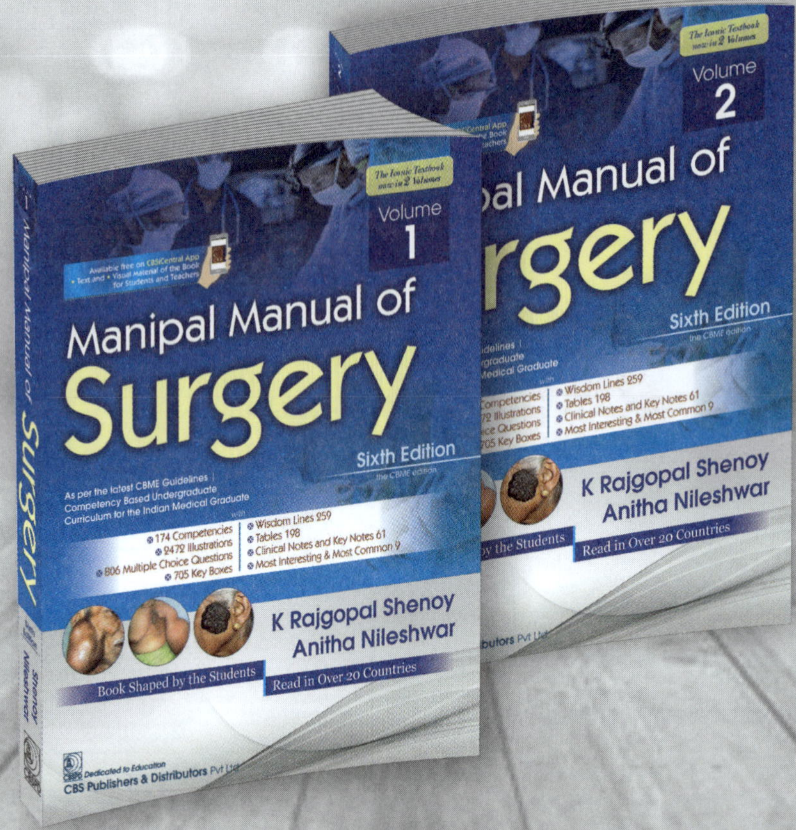

Other CBS Titles by the Same Authors

- *Manipal Manual of Clinical Methods in Surgery*
- *Manipal Manual of Instruments*, Second edition
- *Manipal Manual of Surgery with Clinical Methods for Dental Students*, Fourth edition

Sixth Edition

Manipal Manual of Surgery

As per the latest CBME Guidelines | Competency Based Undergraduate Curriculum for the Indian Medical Graduate

Volume 1

Chief Editor

K Rajgopal Shenoy MBBS, MS, FRCS (Glasgow)
Professor
Department of Surgery
Former Associate Dean–Academics and Head of the Department
Kasturba Medical College, and
Consultant Surgeon, Kasturba Hospital, Manipal 576104
Karnataka, India
Manipal Academy of Higher Education (MAHE)
email: kallyarajgopalshenoy@gmail.com

Coeditor

Anitha Shenoy (Nileshwar) MBBS, MD, FRCA
Professor and Former Head
Department of Anaesthesiology
Kasturba Medical College, and
Consultant Anaesthesiologist, Kasturba Hospital, Manipal 576104
Karnataka, India
Manipal Academy of Higher Education (MAHE)
email: anitharshenoy@gmail.com

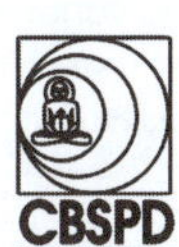

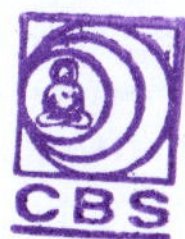

CBS Publishers & Distributors Pvt Ltd
New Delhi • Bengaluru • Chennai • Kochi • Kolkata • Lucknow • Mumbai
Hyderabad • Jharkhand • Nagpur • Patna • Pune • Uttarakhand

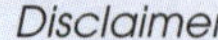

Disclaimer

Science and technology are constantly changing fields. New information, research and experience broaden the scope of knowledge. The editors and contributors have tried their best in giving information available to them while preparing the material for this book. Although, all efforts have been made to ensure optimum accuracy of the material, yet it is quite possible some errors might have been left uncorrected. The editors, the contributors, the publisher and the printer will not be held responsible for any inadvertent errors or inaccuracies.

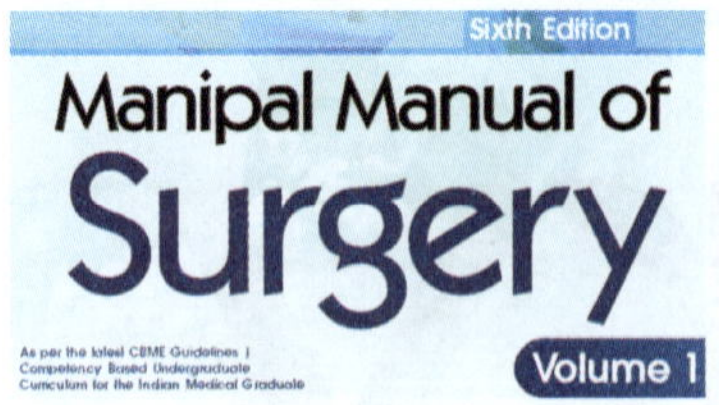

Book Shaped by the Students

Read in Over 20 Countries

ISBN: 978-93-54660-25-2

the CBME edition

Sixth Edition: 2023
Reprint: 2024
First Edition: 2000
Reprint: 2001, 2002, 2003, 2004
Second Edition: 2005
Reprint: 2006, 2007, 2008, 2009
Third Edition: 2010
Reprint: 2011, 2012
Fourth Edition: 2014
Reprint: 2016, 2017, 2019
Fifth Edition: 2020

Published by Satish Kumar Jain and produced by Varun Jain for

CBS Publishers & Distributors Pvt Ltd
4819/XI Prahlad Street, 24 Ansari Road, Daryaganj, New Delhi 110 002, India.
Ph: 011-23289259, 23266838 Website: www.cbspd.com
e-mail: delhi@cbspd.com

Corporate Office: 204 FIE, Industrial Area, Patparganj, Delhi 110 092
Ph: 011-49344934 Fax: 011-49344935 e-mail: publishing@cbspd.com; publicity@cbspd.com

Branches

- **Bengaluru:** Seema House 2975, 17th Cross, K.R. Road, Banasankari 2nd Stage, Bengaluru 560 070, Karnataka, India
  Ph: +91-80-26771678/79 Fax: +91-80-26771680 e-mail: bangalore@cbspd.com
- **Chennai:** 7, Subbaraya Street, Shenoy Nagar, Chennai 600 030, Tamil Nadu, India
  Ph: +91-44-26680620, 26681266 Fax: +91-44-42032115 e-mail: chennai@cbspd.com
- **Kochi:** 42/1325, 1326, Power House Road, Opp KSEB, Ernakulum, Kochi 682 018, Kerala, India
  Ph: +91-484-4059061-65,67 Fax: +91-484-4059065 e-mail: kochi@cbspd.com
- **Kolkata:** 147, Hind Ceramics Compound, 1st Floor, Nilgunj Road, Belghoria, Kolkata-700056, West Bengal, India
  Ph: 033-25633055/56 e-mail: kolkata@cbspd.com
- **Lucknow:** Basement, Khushnuma Complex, 7 Meerabai Marg (Behind Jawahar Bhawan), Lucknow-226001, UP, India
  Ph: +0522-4000032 e-mail: tiwari.lucknow@cbspd.com
- **Mumbai:** PWD Shed, Gala no 25/26, Ramchandra Bhatt Marg, Next to JJ Hospital Gate no. 2, Opp. Union Bank of India, Noorbaug, Mumbai-400009, Maharashtra, India
  Ph: +91-22-66661880/89 e-mail: mumbai@cbspd.com

Representatives

• **Hyderabad**	0-9885175004	• **Jharkhand**	0-9811541605	• **Nagpur**	0-8692091830
• **Patna**	0-9334159340	• **Pune**	0-9664372571	• **Uttarakhand**	0-9716462459

Printed at: Magic International Pvt. Ltd., Greater Noida, UP, India

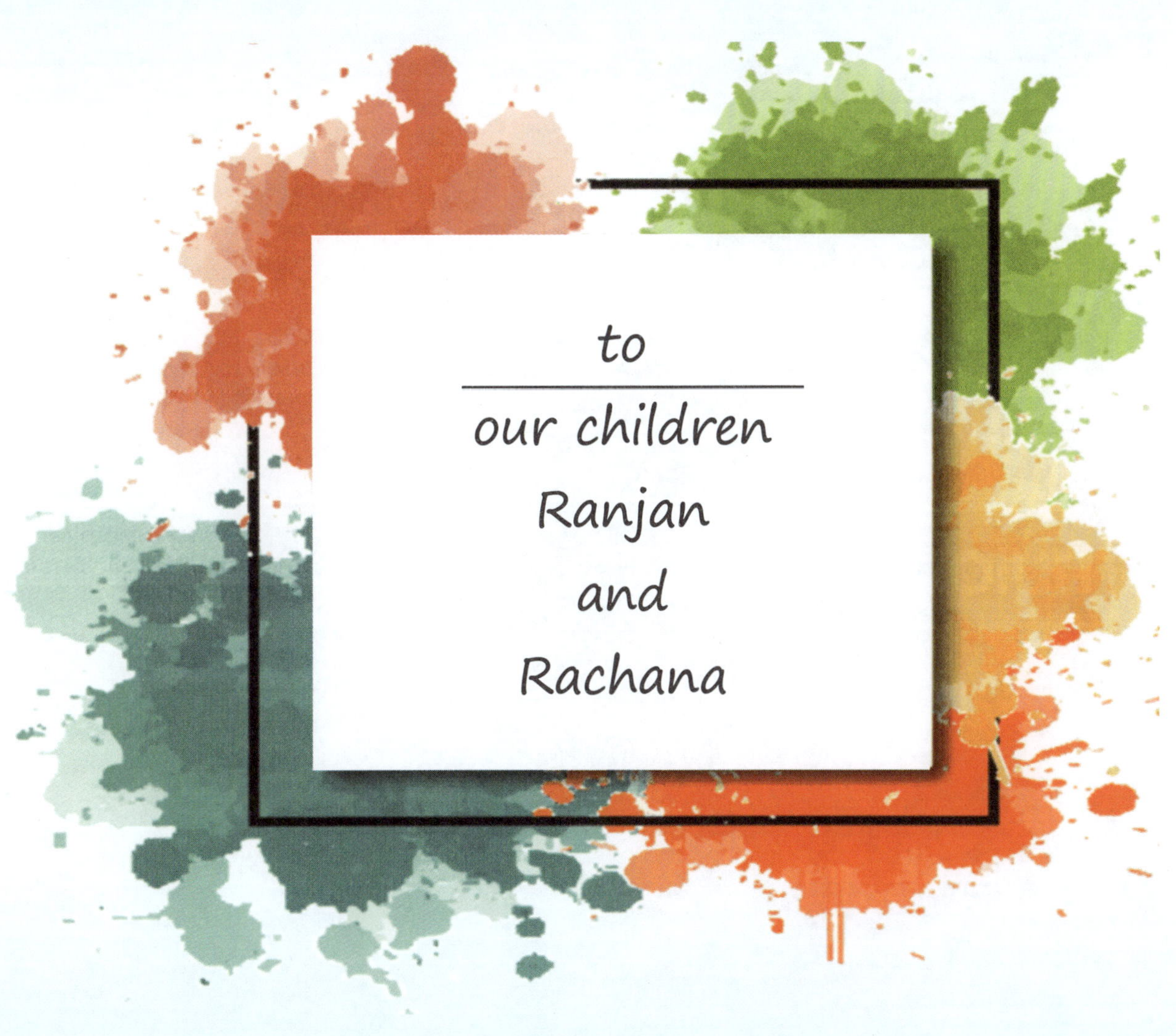

to

our children
Ranjan
and
Rachana

Forewords

I am extremely happy to write the foreword to this edition of *Manipal Manual of Surgery*.

Having close association with Dr Rajgopal Shenoy for over 30 years, I am fully aware of his extraordinary ability as a teacher and as a skilful surgeon. His additional qualities of being a brilliant scholar and a prolific writer makes him unique. Dr Shenoy is respected as one of the great teachers in the country. Many years of hard work and dedication is visible in the content of the books, he has authored. The new editions being released on regular intervals is the proof of the popularity.

The clinical photographs are of high quality and the summary of each chapter being highlighted makes the revision study easier for the students nearer to examinations.

The latest edition is sure to have more information with the latest advances which obviously will be of value to the student community at large both in India and abroad. National Medical Commission has brought out few changes in the curriculum with emphasis on Competency Based Medical Education (CBME). Authors have incorporated most of these competencies in this edition which will further help the students in preparing for studies and enhance their knowledge.

As the current President of the Association of Surgeons of India, I have no hesitation in recommending the book for both the undergraduate and postgraduate students in surgery and I wish Dr Rajgopal Shenoy all the best in his sincere efforts to spread the knowledge.

Prof Siddesh G

President, Association of Surgeons of India

Senior Consultant and Director, SIGMA Hospital, Mysore

Former Professor and Head, Department of Surgery, JSS Medical College, Mysore

The sixth edition of *Manipal Manual of Surgery* edited by Dr K Rajgopal Shenoy is a welcome book which is meant for both the undergraduate and postgraduate students. A very popular book in general surgery, liked by both undergraduate and postgraduate students, and even the faculty members because of the easy language, well-explained text and a number of tables, diagrams and photographs. The book is really a pleasant read. The authors in the latest edition have tried to revamp the book to include the newer scenarios included in the Competency Based Medical Education (CBME) recommended by National Medical Commission and National Board of Examinations. The MCQs given after the chapters are very helpful in answering the multiple choice questions in examinations and will also be helpful in OSCE. I will especially recommend this book to the students before they take their examinations, whether theory or practical, as this book provides a lot of quotes and mnemonics that the student can use as memory-aids. The author has extensive teaching experience of more than 35 years. During the covid pandemic, he was associated with many teaching activities and participated in hundreds of clinical teaching program. I even like the paper which is used for this book as it is just very comfortable to read, handle, does not tear and is also lightweight. The colours used in the book are very soothing. This book is comprehensive, fully updated as per the recent needs and easy to assimilate. So, I recommend this book be kept as a personal copy by all undergraduate and postgraduate students, practitioners, and even the faculty members. This book must be available in all medical libraries both in India as well as overseas.

Prof Ajay K Khanna

MS, FRCS, FAMS, FACS, FICS, FACRSI, FMAS, FCLS, FRSTMH, FAIS, FUICC, FFIM, FUWAI, MNAMS, DSc, MBA, PDCR

Former Head, Department of Surgery, Institute of Medical Sciences, Banaras Hindu University, Varanasi, India

We are living in an ocean of knowledge but which drop is useful to us is a big question. Dr K Rajgopal Shenoy is a teacher par excellence and I have known him for the last so many years. He took the challenge to collect all the pearls and compiled them in the form of *Manipal Manual of Surgery* which is undoubtedly one of the most favourite books read by medical undergraduates internationally.

Sixth edition of the book has been revamped to meet the requirements of competency based medical education recently promoted by the NMC curriculum complemented with simple language, diagrams and photographs. I am sure that the sixth edition will provide great learning experience for both the undergraduates and "aide-memoire" for surgical postgraduates. I convey my best wishes for the latest edition and happy reading for all the students.

Prof Sanjay Jain
Professor of Surgery
Gandhi Medical College, Bhopal
Vice-President, Association of Surgeons of India

This edition of *Manipal Manual of Surgery* by Prof Rajgopal Shenoy is the first surgical manual to be brought out in India based on Competency Based Medical Education (CBME) introduced by the NMC in 2019 in Indian medical curriculum. It is a welcome addition to the textbooks in the vast discipline of surgery. Written in a clear and lucid style by the master of the subject, it is full of illustrations and would certainly serve as a very valuable textbook for the students, teachers of surgery and practicing surgeons. It is an outstanding and remarkable contribution by Prof Shenoy, with his rich experience of 36 years in teaching undergraduate and postgraduate students.

Prof K Balaji Singh
MS, FRCS (G), FIAGES, FALS
Dean–Students, Professor and Head, Department of General Surgery,
Sri Ramachandra Medical College and Research Institute
Sri Ramachandra Institute of Higher Education and Research, Porur, Chennai

Preface to the Sixth Edition

It gives us great pleasure to write the preface to the sixth edition of *Manipal Manual of Surgery* (MMS). As we complete 35 years of teaching in a single institute, we find our role as teacher and clinician very satisfying. I never imagined in 2000, when we brought out the first edition 'Millenium edition', that it will be accepted by the students. Thank you, my dear students for your support.

When we look back, we realize that many changes have been incorporated in the previous five editions. The necessity of the sixth edition arose because of introduction of Competency Based Medical Education (CBME) by National Medical Commission. The aim of the CBME is that the teachers should be able to assess the students for whatever is taught. Assessment can be done during theory classes, small group teachings, student-directed learning, etc. Learning objectives are included within the theory topic itself, eventhough they are not written separately. In the new curriculum, a few topics have been deleted from the older curriculum and a few have been added. However, we have not deleted those topics from our book because we want students to get a thorough knowledge about the subject and secure very good marks.

We also have introduced in the beginning of the book a new section called 'Principles of Surgery' which deals with ethics, communication, conduct, consent, research, audit, medicolegal aspects, biomedical waste disposal and many other important topics. We want you to understand the subject rather than just study by rote. We want you to be able to write essay and short answers properly rather than being able to answer only MCQs. The subject is vast and to incorporate all these changes is extremely difficult. We are aware that additional knowledge is required for students to appear for qualifying examinations for postgraduation—NEET specialty exams. Knowledge may also help you in preparing for foreign entrance examinations. In spite of so many changes in the new book, very few additional pages have been added because we have deleted unnecessary and outdated information and obsolete surgeries.

Keeping all these things in mind, we have prepared the sixth edition and we call it as CBME edition. Most of the competencies have been given the specific numbers for your quick reference. Clinical competencies have not been given any number because it will be dealt by your teachers when they take bedside clinics. Clinics are learnt bedside, not 'bookside'. The more clinical cases you see, the better clinician you will become. However, a wide range of clinical topics are discussed, including clinical methods, with excellent quality photographs which will help in your university clinical examination also.

I am also proud to say that very senior, internationally famous Prof Desarda MP from Pune himself contributed his repair, popularly called as Desarda repair for hernia, in my book. At the same time, another surgeon of repute, young Prof Amith Kumar Jain from Bengaluru, himself wrote his original work on diabetic foot in detail in this edition. Our aim is also to popularise Indian authors' work.

In the last two years, the world has seen COVID pandemic all over the world. It has affected teaching very badly. However, Association of Surgeons of India, Learning General Surgery, National PG Clinics, White Army and many other platforms provided extensive online discussions. I am proud today that I was part of these discussions. The knowledge that I gained from this has also been incorporated in this edition. Bringing a new edition with changes was also a challenge to the publishers due to nonavailability of quality paper and the cost of the book also. This was one of the reasons for bringing out the book in 2 volumes. Hope you will take advantage of the 2 volumes—ease of carrying and using it as and when required. We wish and pray that the Sixth Edition (CBME edition) will be of immense benefit to all of you. Read well, look at the figures properly, make use of the flowcharts, practice drawing the line diagrams—you will definitely be successful and will grow to become a good compassionate doctor. Wish you all the best.

Enjoy reading *Manipal Manual of Surgery*, sixth edition.

K Rajgopal Shenoy
kallyarajgopalshenoy@gmail.com

Anitha Shenoy (Nileshwar)
anitharshenoy@gmail.com

Preface to the First Edition

I developed interest in surgery and teaching due to my eminent teachers (role models) in my undergraduate days at Government Medical College, Bellary (1977–1983) and postgraduate days at Kasturba Medical College, Mangalore (1983–1986). Kasturba Medical College, Manipal, gave me enough opportunities, encouragement, and confidence to develop interest in teaching. The genesis of the manual is attributed to the tremendous response to my lecture notes in surgery. The book has been named as a manual as it is complete, comprehensive, precise and simple.

Manipal Manual of Surgery is written, keeping in mind the time constraint and vastness of the subject, that the student has to face before an examination. Reference books are not essential to learn basic facts of surgery. The standard books are undoubtedly necessary to gain in-depth knowledge as well as understanding of the subject. Every student should refer to them whenever necessary. This manual is best utilized as a revision and handbook that gives precise facts in a clear, concise way that makes a student feel that surgery is after all not an insurmountable obstacle to pass the final MBBS examination.

One may wonder what is the necessity of another book when you have so many established books in the market? With the voluminous advances in surgery the **textbooks have virtually become jungles** where students get lost. I have made this book simple, easily understandable with flow charts, tables and key boxes. The manual covers the text, clinics and coloured photographs. Relevant clinical cases kept for clinical examination are discussed similar to bedside clinics. At the same time, some important and illustrative clinical problems discussed in this manual are actual case reports. Speciality topics which are written by senior faculty members of our institution add glory to the book. We have tried to shed light through the jungles so that one can come out safely.

I call this as a complete book in surgery, but do not believe in including orthopaedics in it because it is a subject that has developed as a separate speciality. By merely adding some more pages the purpose will not be served when good orthopaedics books are available in the market. The *viva voce* examination is a unique section which helps in reducing your ***anxiety*** before you appear for viva.

I take this opportunity to express my gratitude to all the staff from the department of surgery and specialities who have helped me in one or more ways in the outcome of the book. I should make a special mention of Prof U Santosh Pai who has been a constant source of inspiration to me while I was preparing this manual. It is him who gave me an appropriate title for this book. My wife, Dr Anitha, not only contributed anaesthesiology topics but also helped me in editing this manual.

My close friend and classmate, Dr L Ramachandra, Associate Professor in the department of surgery who has helped me in editing many chapters and has given me valuable suggestions. Dr Gopinath Pai, Dr Sreedharan. Dr Shashidhar Matta (Assistant Professor), Dr Shashikumar, (Urologist), Dr Gautham Prakash, Dr Divya Shenoy, Dr Juliana Samuel, Dr Krishnamurthy, Dr Anand Nadkarni (Interns) also have contributed to the completion of the book.

I sincerely thank Mr Umesh Acharya from dental college for drawing simple and beautiful diagrams, Mr Parashuram Bhat and Kiran from photography section for the coloured photographs. **I believe that students should spend more time in looking at those simple line diagrams and photographs which can often illustrate more than the text.**

I thank Prof KP Rao, Dept of Printing, MIT, Manipal, for timely help, guidance, and encouragement given to me during the preparation of the computer prints Ms Shailashree (Supriya Computers, Udupi), Mr Ganesh (Ganesh Computers, Udupi), and Ms Vatsala (MAHE, Manipal), for helping me in the first phase of the computer work. The final work has been completed by Mr Dharmvir of CBS Publishers & Distributors, New Delhi. He has done an excellent job and I am very grateful to him.

I greatly appreciate the constant support and encouragement given to me by Mr SK Jain, Managing Director, Late Mr BR Sharma of CBS Publishers & Distributors, New Delhi and Mr VK Jain, Production Director, deserves special thanks for the excellent production of the book.

I sincerely hope that this *Manual* will be useful to you. Any criticisms, and contributions to this book are welcome. **I wish all my dear students the very best. Do enjoy reading this book.**

K Rajgopal Shenoy

Acknowledgements

CHAPTERS

Anitha Shenoy (Nileshwar)
Professor and Former Head, Department of Anaesthesiology
KMC, Manipal
• Haemorrhage • Shock • Acid–Base Balance
• Fluid and Electrolytes • Anaesthesiology
• Blunt Abdominal Trauma • Perioperative Care

Ashok Godhi
Former Principal, Professor, Department of Surgery
JNMC, KLE University, Belgaum, Karnataka
• Communication and Counselling

Ganesh Kamath
Professor and Head, Department of Cardiothoracic Surgery
KMC, Manipal
• Chest Injuries and Cardiothoracic Surgery

NC Sreekumar
Professor and Head
Department of Plastic Surgery and Burns
KMC, Manipal
• Burns

K Laxman
Senior Consultant Surgeon
Bengaluru
• Research in Surgery

SS Prasad
Former Professor, Department of Surgery
KMC, Manipal
• Liver Transplantation • Metabolic Response to Injury

Chandrakanth Shetty
Former Professor, Department of Radiodiagnosis and Imaging
KMC, Manipal
• Principles of Radiology

Raja A
Former Professor and Head, Department of Neurosurgery
KMC, Manipal
• Neurosurgery

B Srinivas Pai
Professor, Department of Surgery, SDMM College, Dharwad
• Carcinoma Breast

GG Laxman Prabhu
Professor and Head, Department of Urology
KMC, Mangalore
• Urology

Sunilkrishna M
Professor
KMC, Manipal
• Surgical Audit, Laparoscopic Surgery, CBME Titles

Ananth Pai
Professor, Medical Oncology
KMC, Manipal
• Chemotherapy Concepts and Principles

Joseph Thomas
Associate Professor
Department of Plastic Surgery and Burns
KMC, Manipal
• Burns, Tendon Injuries

CONTRIBUTED TOPICS

Desarda Mohan Phulchand
Professor, Senior Consultant, Pune
• Desarda Repair of Hernia

Rajgopal KV
Professor, Department of Radiology and Imaging
KMC, Manipal
• Imaging

Prakashini K
Professor and Head, Department of Radiology and Imaging
KMC, Manipal
• Imaging

Amit Kumar Jain
Consultant and Head, Amit Jain's Institute of Diabetic Foot
Brindavan Areion Hospital, Bengaluru
• Diabetic Ulcer Foot

Donald Fernandes
Former Professor and Head, Department of Radiation Oncology
KMC, Manipal
• Principles of Radiotherapy

Mahesh Gopa Setty
Consultant Transplant Surgeon, Bengaluru
- Small Intestine Transplantation

Ashwini Mahopatra
Professor of PTCD
KMC, Manipal
- Tuberculous Lymphadenitis

HV Shivaram
Consultant Surgeon, Aster Hospital, Bengaluru
- Management of Massive Ventral Hernia and Bariatric Surgery

Aravind Bisnoi
Professor and Consultant, CVTS
KMC, Manipal
- Vascular Injuries

Rajesh Nair
Associate Professor, Department of Neurosurgery
KMC, Manipal
- Head Injuries

Avinash R Odugoudar
Former Assistant Professor, Department of Urology
KMC, Manipal
- Urology

Vikram Palimar
Professor and Head, Department of Forensic Medicine
KMC, Manipal
- Medicolegal Aspects in Surgery

Krishna Kalyan Reddy
Assistant Professor
KMC, Manipal
- Operative Surgery, Accessories

Authors are Indebted to the following Colleagues/ assistants and postgraduate students

Prof. Amit Jain
Professor, SRRMC, Bengaluru
Pictures, Flowcharts, Algorithms, Corrections

Meera Gopal
Editing the book with utmost care and passion

Poojitha Yella, Srividya S Rao, Anaparti Rasagna
Contributed and edited antibiotics, sutures, needles, tissue engineering, day case/care surgery and many other topics

Adithi Rao (Junior Resident)
Correcting scripts and editing

We wish to acknowledge the valuable support provided by the following

Dr Ramdas Pai, Chancellor, Manipal Academy of Higher Education (MAHE), Mrs Vasanthi Pai, Trustee, MAHE Trust, Manipal, and Dr Ranjan Pai, CEO, MEMG, for giving us the opportunity to grow in this prestigious institution of eminence from postgraduate degree till date (almost 40 years).

Prof HS Ballal, Pro-Chancellor, MAHE, for providing constant encouragement and Dr Sharath Rao, Dean, KMC, Manipal, for everlasting support. We are thankful to the following faculty of the Department of Surgery who have directly and indirectly helped MMS, 6th edition. Dr BV Dinesh, Head of the Department of Surgery, Dr Ramchandra L, former HOD, Dr Bharath SV, Dr Vijayendra K, Dr Kirtan, Dr Kshama Hegde, Dr Ranjini Karthik and Prof Kanthilatha Pai from Department of Pathology.

A big thanks to the fabulous team at CBS Publishers & Distributors, Mr SK Jain CMD, Mr Varun Jain Director, Mr YN Arjuna Senior Vice President—Publishing, Editorial and Publicity, Mrs Ritu Chawla General Manager—Production, and their team Mr Tarun Rajput DTP operator, Mr Sanju Designer, Mr Surendra Jha and Mr Prasenjit Paul Copyeditors.

K Rajgopal Shenoy

Anitha Shenoy (Nileshwar)

Contents

VOLUME 2

SECTION VI: *VIVA VOCE* EXAMINATION

Competencies

Competency Based Undergraduate Curriculum for the Indian Medical Graduate

Code	*Competency*	*Chapter*	*Page no*
SU1.1	Describe basic concepts of homeostasis. Enumerate the metabolic changes in injury and their mediators.	15	52
SU1.3	Describe basic concepts of perioperative care.	6, 20	19, 92
SU3.1	Describe the indications and appropriate use of blood and blood products and complications of blood transfusion.	18	72
SU4.1	Elicit document and present history in a case of burns and perform physical examination. Describe pathophysiology of burns.	32	277
SU4.2	Describe clinical features, diagnose type and extent of burns and plan appropriate treatment.	32	278
SU4.3	Discuss the medicolegal aspects in burn injuries.	32	286
SU5.1	Describe normal wound healing and factors affecting healing.	21	100, 103
SU5.3	Differentiate the various types of wounds, plan and observe management of wounds.	21	99
SU5.4	Describe medicolegal aspects of wound healing and gunshot wounds.	54	985
SU6.1	Define and describe the aetiology and pathogenesis of surgical infections.	22, 24, 25	109, 138, 148
SU6.2	Enumerate prophylactic and therapeutic antibiotics. Plan appropriate management.	12	44
SU7.1	Describe the planning and conduct of surgical audit.	4	14
SU7.2	Describe the principles and steps of clinical research in general surgery.	5	16
SU8.1	Describe the principles of ethics as it pertains to general surgery.	3	10
SU9.1	Choose appropriate biochemical, microbiological, pathological, imaging investigations and interpret the investigative data in a surgical patient.	9, 19	30, 78
SU9.2	Biological basis for early detection of cancer and multidisciplinary approach in management of cancer.	66	1215
SU9.2.1	Describe the basis for early detection of cancer with colorectal tumorogenesis as an example.	66	1215
SU9.2.2	Define the "screening".	66	1215
SU9.2.3	Enumerate the cancers which are amenable for screening.	66	1215
SU9.2.4	Classify the criteria for screening.	66	1215
SU9.2.5	List the advantages and disadvantages of screening.	66	1215
SU9.2.6	Describe the need for a multidisciplinary team in management of cancer.	66	1215
SU9.2.7	List the composition of the multidisciplinary team.	66	1215
SU9.2.8	Enumerate the advantages and disadvantages of a multidisciplinary team.	66	1215
SU10.2	Describe the steps of obtaining informed consent for laparoscopic hernioplasty in a simulated environment.	2	9
SU11.2.1	Enumerate the indications of general anaesthesia.	64	1165
SU11.2.2	Describe the various techniques of general anaesthesia.	64	1166
SU11.2.3	Describe advantages and complications of regional anaesthesia.	64	1173
SU11.2.4	Enumerate the types of regional anaesthesia.	64	1173
SU11.2.5	Enumerate the indications of regional anaesthesia.	64	1173
SU11.2.6	Describe indications, advantages, complications of local anaesthesia.	64	1174
SU11.2.7	Describe the drugs used in general, regional and local anaesthesia.	64	1183
SU11.4	Enumerate the indications and principles of day care general surgery.	13	47
SU11.5	Describe principles of providing postoperative pain relief and management of chronic pain.	7	22

Code	Competency	Chapter	Page no
SU11.6	Describe principles of safe general surgery.	14	50
SU12.1	Enumerate the causes and consequences of malnutrition in the surgical patients.	11	38
SU12.2	Describe and discuss the methods of estimation and replacement of the fluid and electrolyte requirements in the surgical patient.	20	85
SU13.1	Describe the immunological basis of organ transplantation.	65	1191
SU13.2.1	Describe the principles of immunosuppresive therapy.	65	1194, 1201
SU13.2.2	Enumerate indications, describe surgical principles, management of organ transplantation.	65	1193, 1195
SU13.3	Discuss legal and ethical issues concerning organ donation.	65	1201
SU14.1	Describe aseptic techniques, sterilization and disinfection.	10	34
SU14.3	Describe the materials and methods used for surgical wound closure and anastomosis (sutures, knots, and needles).	70	1269, 1295
SU15.1	Describe classification of hospital waste and appropriate methods of biomedical waste disposal.	8	27
SU17.1	Describe pathophysiology of shock, types of shock and principles of resuscitation including fluid replacement and monitoring.	17	59
SU17.1	Describe the principles of first aid to trauma patients.	54	980
SU17.2	Describe clinical features of shock with appropriate treatment.	17	59
SU17.3	Describe principles in management of mass casualities.	54	986
SU17.4	Describe pathophysiology, mechanism of head injuries.	63	1152
SU17.5	Describe clinical features for neurological assessment and GCS in head injuries.	63	1155
SU17.6	Choose appropriate investigations and discuss the principles of management of head injuries.	63	1156
SU17.7	Describe the clinical features of soft tissue injuries. Chose appropriate investigations and discuss the principles of management.	54	1000
SU17.8	Describe the pathophysiology of chest injuries.	62	1125
SU17.9	Describe clinical features and management principles of chest injuries.	62	1125
SU19.1	Describe the etiology and classification of cleft lip and palate.	35	371
SU19.2	Describe the principles of reconstruction of cleft lip and palate.	35	372
SU20.1	Describe etiopathogenesis of oral cancer symptoms and signs of oropharyngeal cancer.	35	349, 355
SU20.2	Enumerate the appropriate investigations and discuss the principles of treatment.	35	351
SU21.1	Describe surgical anatomy of the salivary glands, pathology and clinical presentation of disorders of salivary glands.	36	377
SU21.2	Enumerate the appropriate investigations and describe the principles of treatment of disorders of salivary glands.	36	377
SU22.1	Describe the applied anatomy and physiology of thyroid.	37	394
SU22.2	Describe the etiopathogenesis of thyroidal swellings.	37	402
SU22.4	Describe the clinical features, classification and principles of management of thyroid cancer.	37	414
SU22.5	Describe the applied anatomy of parathyroid.	38	437
SU22.6	Describe and discuss the clinical features of hypo- and hyperparathyroidism and the principles of their management.	38	438
SU23.1	Describe applied anatomy of adrenal glands.	38	446
SU23.2	Describe the aetiology, clinical features and principles of management of disorders of adrenal gland.	38	447
SU23.3	Describe the clinical features, principles of investigation and management of adrenal tumours.	38	448
SU24.1.3	Describe the types, etiopathogenesis, clinical features, investigations and management of chronic pancreatitis. Also the various surgical modalities available for treatment of chronic pancreatitis.	42	633
SU24.2	Describe the anatomy of the pancreas. Describe the clinical features, principles of investigation, prognosis and management of pancreatic exocrine tumours.	42	615
SU24.3	Describe the principles of investigation and management of pancreatic endocrine tumors.	42	644
SU25.1	Describe applied anatomy and appropriate investigations for breast disease.	39	455
SU25.2	Describe the etiopathogenesis, clinical features and principles of management of benign breast disease including infections of the breast.	39	458

Code	Competency	Chapter	Page no
SU25.3	Describe the etiopathogenesis, clinical features, investigations and principles of treatment of benign and malignant tumours of breast.	39	465, 471, 472
SU26.1	Outline the role of surgery in the management of coronary heart disease, valvular heart diseases and congenital heart diseases.	62	1143
SU26.3	Describe the clinical features of mediastinal diseases and the principles of management.	62	1136
SU26.4	Describe the etiology, pathogenesis, clinical features of tumours of lung and the principles of management.	62	1140
SU26.11	Describe the post-splenectomy sepsis— prophylaxis.	44	716
SU27.1	Describe the etiopathogenesis, clinical features, investigations and principles of treatment of occlusive arterial disease.	27	176
SU27.3	Describe clinical features, investigations and principles of management of vasospastic disorders.	28	206
SU27.4	Describe the type of gangrene and principles of amputation.	28, 70	207, 1281
SU27.5	Describe the applied anatomy of venous system of lower limb.	30	230
SU27.6	Describe the pathophysiology, clinical features, investigations and principles of management of DVT and varicose veins.	30	232, 240
SU27.7	Describe pathophysiology, clinical features, investigations and principles of management of lymphedema, lymphangitis and lymphomas.	29	212
SU28.1	Describe the applied anatomy of biliary system. Describe the clinical features, investigations and principles of management of diseases of biliary system.	42	601
SU28.1	Describe the clinical features, principles of investigation, prognosis and management of pancreatitis.	42	646
SU28.1.1	Describe the clinical features, investigations and principles of management of splenic injuries.	44	703
SU28.1.1,2,3,9,10:	Describe applied anatomy of abdominal wall and its weaknesses in pathophysiology of abdominal hernias.	52	932
SU28.1.4	Describe clinical presentation, examination findings, and role of radiological investigations in diagnosis and management of hernia.	52	937
SU28.1.5	Describe complications of abdominal hernias.	52	944
SU28.1.6	Describe general principles of management of abdominal wall hernias and the basic operative approach.	52	941
SU28.1.11	Describe differential diagnosis of inguinal and inguinoscrotal swellings.	52	939
SU28.1.15	Describe anatomy, pathophysiology, required investigations for diagnosis of femoral hernia and the surgical techniques in management of femoral hernia.	52	949
SU28.1.16	Describe classification of ventral hernias and clinical presentation and indications for surgical management of various ventral hernias.	52	955
SU28.1.17	Describe special hernias—spigelian, lumbar, obturator, perineal, sciatic and paranormal hernias and etiology, clinical presentation, various surgical approaches and techniques in their management.	52	961
SU28.3.1	Describe applied anatomy and physiology of peritoneum.	45	719
SU28.3.2	Describe the causes, clinical features, investigations, management and complications of localised and generalised peritonitis.	45	720
SU28.3.3	Summarize the tubercular peritonitis, spontaneous bacterial peritonitis, pneumococcal peritonitis, familial mediterranean fever (periodic peritonitis).	45, 46	736, 758
SU28.4.1	Etiopathogenesis of intraperitoneal abscess.	45	732
SU28.4.3 and SU28.4.4	Define and classify mesenteric cyst. Pathology, clinical features, differential diagnosis, investigations and management of mesenteric cyst.	45	744
SU28.4.6	Describe etiology, clinical features, differential diagnosis and management of retroperitoneal fibrosis.	45	745
SU28.4.7	Describe classification, clinical features, investigation to make diagnosis and management of retroperitoneal tumours.	45	746
SU28.5	Describe etiopathogenesis, clinical features, investigations, principles of management and complications of GERD and Barrett's oesophagus.	40	514
SU28.5	Describe surgical anatomy of oesophagus.	40	511

Code	Competency	Chapter	Page no
SU28.15.2	Describe etiology, pathogenesis, clinical symptoms and signs of acute appendicitis.	51	916
SU28.15.3	Describe complications and principles of management of acute appendicitis.	51	919
SU28.15.4	Describe the differential diagnosis of appendicitis in children, adult, and elderly individuals.	51	920
SU28.15.5	Describe management of appendicular mass.	51	923
SU28.15.6	Describe surgical management and postoperative complications of acute appendicitis.	51	927
SU28.15.7	Describe components, advantages and disadvantages of scoring systems applied in diagnosis of acute appendicitis.	51	920
SU28.15.8	Describe tumours of appendix and clinical features, management of them.	51	928
SU28.15.9	Demonstrate the signs of acute appendicitis.	51	918
SU28.16.1	Describe applied anatomy including congenital anomalies of the rectum and anal canal.	49	861
SU28.16.2	Describe clinical presentation, diagnosis and management of imperforate anus and other congenital anorectal malformations.	48	851
SU28.17.2	Describe investigations for diseases of the rectum including those used for staging of carcinoma rectum.	49	867
SU28.17.3	Describe etiology, clinical features and management of rectal prolapse.	49	877
SU28.17.5	Describe pathology, clinical features, diagnosis and principles of treatment of carcinoma rectum.	49	864
SU28.17.7	Describe aetiology and management of anal incontinence.	49	882
SU28.17.8	Describe aetiopathogenesis, clinical features and management of anal fissure.	49	893
SU28.17.9	Describe aetiology, clinical features, non-surgical management and surgeries for hemorrhoidal disease.	49	884
SU28.17.10	Describe aetiology, types, clinical features, complications of anorectal suppurative diseases.	49	889
SU28.17.11	Describe aetiopathogenesis, clinical features and management of fistula *in ano*.	49	890
SU28.17.12	Describe aetiopathogenesis, clinical features, diagnosis and management of carcinoma of anal canal.	49	897
SU29.1	Describe the causes, investigations and principles of management of haematuria.	56, 61	1029, 1114
SU29.2	Describe the clinical features, investigations and principles of management of congenital anomalies of genitourinary system.	57	1039
SU29.3	Describe the clinical features, investigations and principles of management of urinary tract infections.	61	1118
SU29.4	Describe the clinical features, investigations and principles of management of hydronephrosis.	57	1047
SU29.5	Describe the clinical features, investigations and principles of management of renal calculi.	57	1042
SU29.6	Describe the clinical features, investigations and principles of management of renal tumours.	57	1054
SU29.7	Describe the principles of management of acute and chronic retention of urine.	58	1077
SU29.8	Describe the clinical features, investigations and principles of management of bladder cancer.	58	1065
SU29.9	Describe the clinical features, investigations and principles of management of disorders of the prostate.	59	1081
SU29.11	Describe the clinical features, investigations and management of urethral strictures.	58	1072
SU30.1	Describe the clinical features, investigations and principles of management of phimosis, paraphimosis and carcinoma penis.	60	1092
SU30.2	Describe the applied anatomy, clinical features, investigations and principles of management of undescended testis.	60	1098
SU30.3	Describe applied anatomy, clinical features, investigations, principles of management of epididymo-orchitis.	60	1100
SU30.4	Describe applied anatomy, clinical features, investigations and principles of management of varicocele.	60	1103
SU30.5	Describe applied anatomy, clinical features, investigations and principles of management of hydrocoele.	60	1099
SU30.6	Describe applied anatomy, clinical features, investigations and principles of management of testicular tumours.	60	1105

Volume 1

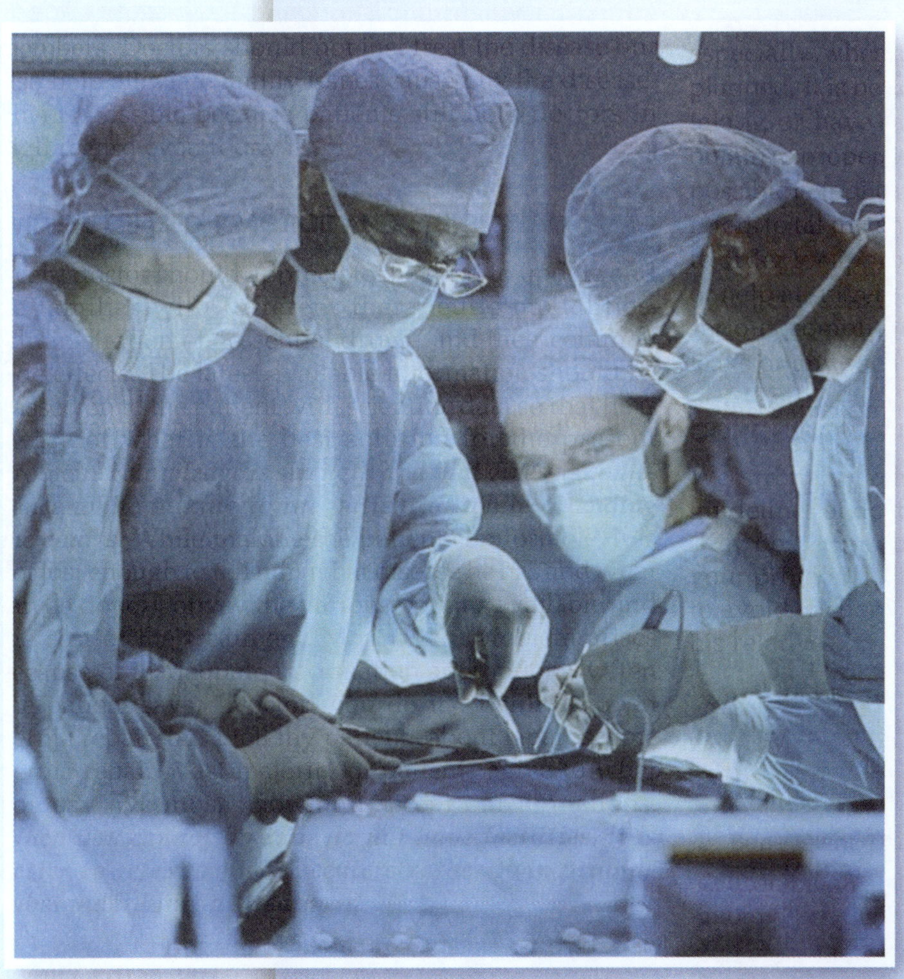

Basic Principles of Surgery
General Surgery
Gastrointestinal Surgery

Section

I

Basic Principles of Surgery

CHAPTER

1

Doctor–Patient Relationship

- Attitude
- Benevolence
- Communication, continued learning, competency, counselling, consent
- Dignity and diversity
- Evidence-based practice and ethics
- Family physician
- Get help

Referring to the work of physicians, *Dr Elmer Hess, a former President of the American Medical Association*, once wrote: "There is no greater reward in our profession than the knowledge that God has entrusted us with the physical care of His people. The Almighty has reserved for Himself the power to create life, but He has **assigned to a few of us the responsibility of keeping in good repair the bodies in which this life is sustained"**. Accordingly, reverence for human life and individual dignity is both the hallmark of a good physician and the key to truly beneficial advances in medicine.

INTRODUCTION

What prompted me to select this topic to be written and published? The answer lies in the observation that litigations against doctors are becoming common. Doctors are being targeted often because of complications that happened during their treatment of patients. Expectations from the patients are high and the reasons for litigations are many. Patients expect that doctors provide a complete and even miraculous cure. They may feel that the hospital has charged exorbitant fees even though the patient did not get cured, developed complications or died. Patients are aware of consumer courts. Many lawyers are ready to support their clients and get them compensation. All these are facts. Complications are known to occur in spite of the best treatment. ***The main factor often missing in this entire scenario is the vital doctor–patient relationship***. This article highlights the importance of a good rapport between the doctor and the patient. The following points are important not only to maintain doctor–patient relationship but also to decrease friction between the patient and the doctor.

ATTITUDE

Attitude of a doctor towards the patient is the first step that builds a rapport between the two. Four important principles of ethics which every doctor should follow and will help develop good doctor–patient relationship are: ***1. Always do good (beneficence) to the patient, 2. Do no harm (non-maleficence) to the patient, 3. Respect autonomy of the patient (confidentiality), and 4. Do justice*** (Key Box 1.1). When the patient is in pain and is suffering, identify the condition properly, treat it and console him. Rather than treat them like customers at a hotel or a shop, a humanitarian approach to make them comfortable would be much more appropriate and help build a good relationship. If we do not know a procedure, it is better to admit that I do not do this procedure, and refer to a person who does it rather attempting and causing complications (harm). Not disclosing patient details with the public or unknown people is important (autonomy) although there may be some exceptions such as some communicable diseases. While triaging, in a busy emergency department, urgent resuscitation and treatment should be given to those who are likely to survive and be useful to family and society rather than those who are unlikely to survive. Here religion, caste, relatives, political influence should not decide your actions. (Kindly refer to Chapter 3: Ethics in General Surgery for more details).

Key Box 1.1

Principle of Ethics

- Beneficence
- Non-maleficence
- Autonomy
- Justice

More details in Chapter 3

BENEVOLENT

A doctor should be gentle while receiving the patient and then examining the patient. He should have empathy and understanding toward the patient. That does not mean that he should shed tears. The doctor should be kindhearted, gracious, considerate, and compassionate. While suturing the wounds and while removing sutures or while applying large dressings for leg wounds or such other procedures, extreme care and empathy should be shown. Very often, these are done by junior surgeons/residents who have to be clearly told about these aspects.

COMMUNICATION, CONTINUED LEARNING, COMPETENCY, COUNSELLING, CONSENT

The doctor–patient relationship starts from the first visit of the patient to the doctor. Develop a good rapport with the patient. The first impression is the best impression. Good communication skills impress. Do not negate patient's views even after you convince effectively. If we look back to 20–30 years ago, our family physicians did not even have MBBS degree, leave alone specialization and super specialization. They were ready to listen to the patient, do home visits, attend midnight calls and accept whatever money that was given to them. Doctors were looked upon as Gods and patients accepted both success and failure. ***Their success was largely because of good communication skills.*** The world is changing at a great speed and moving ahead.

Communication alone does not heal, and good medical care is needed. Medicine is changing. We cannot sit idle without updating our knowledge. ***With continuous medical education (CME), theoretical knowledge can be updated. One can improve skills by attending conferences, attending workshops and thus attain competency.*** Patients also feel happy that the doctor has attended many conferences all over the world and has improved his knowledge.

Always explain to the patient what you are doing, why you are doing and what possible complications can happen. These have to be told in a language that the patient understands and get his signature. This is called informed consent. At surgery, do what is required for the patient. Do not do an additional procedure for an incidental finding for which you have not taken consent

Key Box 1.2

5Cs for Doctor–Patient Relationship

- Communication
- Continued learning
- Competency
- Consent
- Counselling

(Key Box 1.2). Every major surgery can have complications/morbidity and mortality. The patient must be counselled before surgery (Figs 1.1. and 1.2). Counselling and consent are given in more detail in the next chapter.

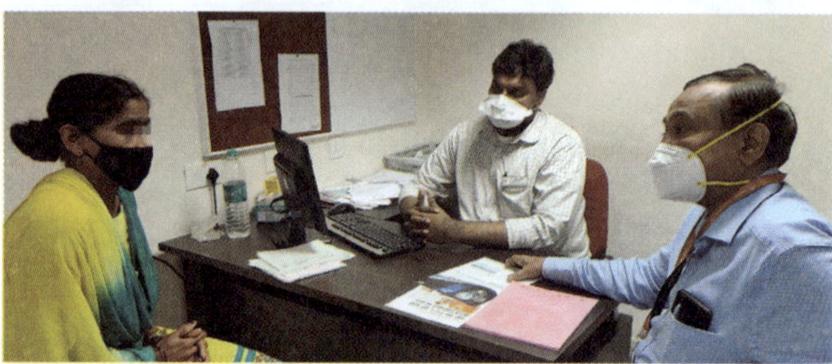

Fig. 1.1: The patient is being briefed about her illness, why and what type of surgery will be done, possible alternatives for surgery and complications related to surgery

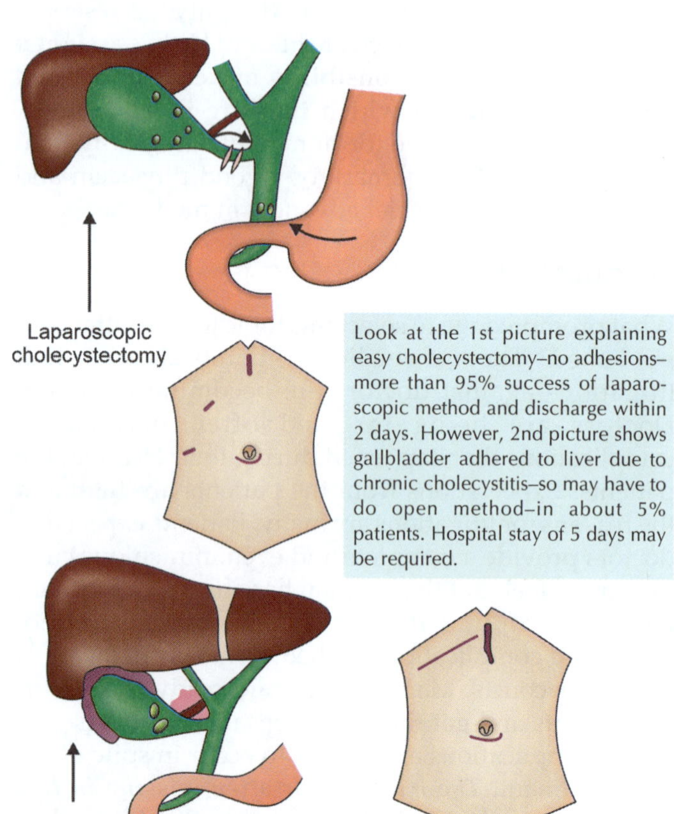

Fig. 1.2: Illustration of how simple sketches can be used to explain procedures to patients

DIGNITY AND DIVERSITY

India is a country with multiple languages and many cultures. Diversity is our strength. The doctor should be sensitive to these cultural differences while treating the patients. Appreciate and respect their culture. Do not discourage discussions. Maintain their dignity. Our deeds should not have any deleterious effect on the body or mind. Understand the patient behaviour in the background of their culture, occupation, habits and family circumstances. Often, in India, the disease may trigger problems at home or a fight between family members. Doctors should not just treat the disease but also help alleviate family issues caused by the disease. This is possible because patients still hold doctors in high regard even today.

EVIDENCE-BASED PRACTICE AND ETHICS

Every doctor should appreciate the need to update and be familiar with different therapeutic modalities, administration of "essential drugs" and their common side effects. The latest available information should be passed on to the patient with scientific data so that he is aware of what is the best solution for the present problem. ***Knowledge is strength and that gives us confidence while talking to the patient or while attending the courts.*** While making the patient comfortable, it is not just enough to tell him what disease he has and what can be done. Convey the various options available and the cost of the treatment. Most often, problem arises because of inadequate information and options. Often the patient says, "Doctor, you do it". I still do open hernia repair, but I tell my patients about laparoscopic hernia repair. Vast majority of patients agree to what you say. We must know and accept our limitations. ***When you cannot do it or do not have facilities, it is better to refer to higher centers rather than provide substandard initial treatment.***

FAMILY PHYSICIAN

In the present times, a surgeon or a physician cannot truly become a family physician because of specialization. However, we can have all the characteristics of a family physician. To name a few: Patient listening, maintaining a smile even at the late-night clinic, enquiring about the patient's professional life, family life adds a personal touch to the practice of medicine. The aim of a medical college teacher is to help the student do the MBBS degree course, i.e. to become ***competent to practice preventive, promotive, curative and rehabilitative medicine with respect to the commonly encountered health problems in a patient and in community.*** Most of the doctors achieve this and become successful in practice.

GET HELP

'Call for help' is an important step in today's practice, especially when a complicated surgical procedure is planned. It is better to inform the patient when you are taking or have taken a colleague's help. It is vital to obtain a proper informed consent after explaining all possible complications to the patient. 'Call for help' also refers to taking another opinion to arrive at a diagnosis, to order for appropriate investigations, to take decision or help at surgery and also to manage some unexpected serious complications such as bleeding, anastomotic leaks or any such events.

CONCLUSION

We strongly believe that if you follow these simple guidelines of doctor–patient relationship of ABCDEFG (Key Box 1.3), you will not only achieve higher goals in your profession and be successful, but will also be able to avoid frictions, abuses and attacks by the patient or his relatives.

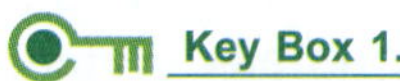

Key Box 1.3

ABCDEFG of Doctor–Patient Relationship

A: Attitude

B: Benevolent

C: Communication, continued learning, competency, informed consent

D: Dignity and diversity

E: Evidence-based science

F: Family physician

G: Get help

Wish you all the best, my dear students! I wish you a bright future.

CHAPTER

2

Communication and Counselling

CHANGING SCENARIO AND THE NEED FOR COUNSELLING

Health care has been witnessing phenomenal changes in the recent years. In the past, the doctors planned and administered the treatment, the outcome of which was willingly accepted by the patients; a paternalistic attitude was prevalent among the doctors. In choosing the doctors and the hospitals, the patients had very few options. Illiteracy was rampant and patients were generally ignorant about the diseases.

This scenario has been progressively changing in the last few decades. People have become more educated; the media has played its role in mass health education; the common man has some general knowledge about common diseases. Doctors, corporate hospitals and nursing homes have proliferated and patients have the option of selecting the doctors and hospitals of their choice. Doctors have retracted from the paternalistic roles; patients have to participate in the decision-making process. The phenomenal growth of medical science, astounding technological advances, increasing health care costs, improving awareness, rising expectations of the patients, and most importantly the Consumer Protection Act have brought into sharp focus the importance of communication and counselling in the medical practice.

Counselling means exchange of ideas to reach a conclusion (Webster). There is hardly any place for counselling while eliciting patients' history; a formal consent is required for physical examination, especially the internal examination, viz. digital rectal examination and per vaginal examination. It is at the end of physical examination that the counselling skills become increasingly important in explaining the diagnostic dilemma, accuracy of lab reports, treatment options, outcome, complications and costs (Key Box 2.1).

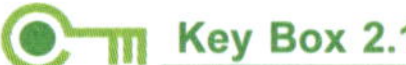

Key Box 2.1

Aims of Counselling

- Explain medical details of the disease
  - Diagnostic dilemma
  - Lab reports and their accuracy
  - Treatment options
  - Complications
  - Outcome
  - Cost
- Address psychosocial, emotional and spiritual issues
- Obtain consent

Explain Medical Details of the Disease

Diagnostic dilemma: The patients often expect that every disease should be accurately diagnosed in the first visit; in simple disease it is possible, but not in complicated ones and if this is made known to them, their mind is prepared to accept subsequent changes in the diagnosis. When the final diagnosis is less serious than the first, the patients are happy to accept it; but if it is more serious, the patients are unhappy and tend to lose faith in the doctor. The intensity of these undesirable effects of change in the diagnosis can be minimized by proper counselling, e.g. benign-looking breast lump turns out to be malignant in the histopathological report.

Accuracy of investigation and their complications: Many patients believe that it is possible to prove the diagnosis by lab tests and that more expensive tests are more accurate; counselling should remove this misconception; lab tests are not 100% sensitive and specific. Patients with simple curable diseases do not pose much problem, but those with serious and life-threatening or incurable diseases often demand foolproof lab diagnosis and such a proof is not always possible to secure. In the absence of such a proof and when the lab test reports are conflicting, counselling becomes increasingly difficult, e.g. disagreement between the pathologists about the presence or absence of cancer in the specimen. Counselling should also include a brief mention about the anticipated complications of investigations, e.g. allergic reaction to IV contrast agent.

Treatment options and their complications: That the patient has to participate in the planning and execution of the treatment has become an accepted norm. The doctor has to offer treatment options, discuss the merits and demerits of each of them and then decide to administer it. Possible complications and their approximate incidence should be discussed, e.g. recurrent laryngeal nerve palsy in thyroid surgery.

Outcome: It is a fond desire of many patients that every disease is completely curable. Many diseases, disabilities and deaths are not totally preventable by the most modern medicine. Discussion about the outcome of treatment is especially important in surgical patients because operation is an event which has no parallel in non-surgical branches of medicine; and any adverse postoperative outcome is almost always attributed to surgery. In search of cure for incurable diseases, the patients keep changing doctors and hospitals spending their resources until they are told and convinced that the cure is unachievable. Patients' ability to cope with the disease and accept the outcome of treatment improves if it is told to them before executing the treatment what is the anticipated outcome—palliation or cure.

Cost: It is better to overestimate the cost than to underestimate it and to express it as a range than as a finite figure, unless it is a package.

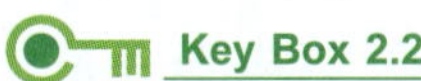

Key Box 2.2

Patient issues that may need attention

- **Psychosocial, emotional and spiritual issues:** Anxiety, illness, ability to function/earn, lifespan, social status
- **Fear:** Pain, disability, deformity, disfigurement, death
- **Worry:** Cost, family
- **Shy:** Genital/sexual problem
- **Embarrassment:** Previous treatment by some other doctor, ask for the second opinion
- **Patients' preferences**, e.g. CPR in case of cardiac arrest

Address psychosocial, emotional and spiritual issues: Anxiety, fear, worry, shyness, embarrassment, religious and cultural issues, and patients' preferences are addressed on individual basis (Key Box 2.2). Patients' mental make-up and will power have significant bearing on the management of the patients.

Methods of Counselling

There is no single best method suitable for all patients on all occasions. Counselling is individualized and personalized. Verbal counselling is the most common method. Showing charts and diagrams is an easy and effective way of convincing. Giving patient education material for reading or showing videos are other methods. Showing other patients being treated for similar disease is quite helpful. The patients' family physician can be used for counselling because he has a better rapport with the patient than the specialist. If there are a number of patients with the same/similar condition/disease (e.g. maternity hospitals or cancer hospitals), group counselling is useful. Complex situations (e.g. living donor liver transplantations) need the services of counselling experts. Speaking the patients' language and having good vocabulary and communication skills makes the job easier (Key Box 2.3).

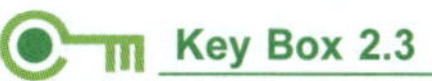

Key Box 2.3

Methods of Counselling

- Verbal counselling
- Diagrams, charts, illustrations
- Printed literature for patient education
- Patient education video
- Show similar patients treated/being treated
- Using the patient's family doctor for counselling
- Group counselling
- Counselling experts

Factors Influencing Counselling

There are many factors influencing the counselling. Patients' background, literacy, level of understanding and trust in the doctor are the most important factors. Suspicious and indecisive mind of the patient is an obstacle. Patients' perceptions of doctor's honesty, trustworthiness, dependability and intentions have their own measure of impact on counselling. Nature of illness, whether simple to diagnose and treat with assured successful outcome, or a complex disease, difficult to diagnose and treat with a guarded prognosis, or a fatal, incurable disease have an important bearing on counselling (Key Box 2.4).

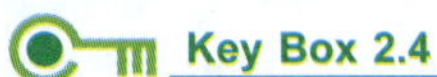
Key Box 2.4

Factors Influencing Counselling

- **Diseases:** Curable, incurable, fatal
- **Patients' perception about the doctors**
  - Knowledge, competence and attitudes
  - Ethical, honest, trustworthy
  - Compassionate, empathetic
  - Cheating, exploiting, indifferent
- **Patients and relatives**
  - Trusting and faithful
  - Illiterate, ignorant
  - Educated, knowledgeable
  - Suspicious and doubting
  - Indecisive and procrastinating

PATIENTS' RIGHTS

Patients' rights are supreme and should be respected; right to refuse the plan of treatment, right to information, to have second opinion, to change the doctor and the hospital in the middle of treatment. The doctor need not feel embarrassed. The Consumer Protection Act has given another right—right to file a suit in the consumer forum. Many consumer cases against doctors are avoidable, if every patient is counselled properly and more importantly the counselling notes are documented and authenticated by the doctor, patient/patient's relative and a witness. Some hospitals have adopted video recording of the counselling as a foolproof method of documenting (Key Box 2.5).

Counselling and the percentage: In medicine, nothing is 100%. This should be used liberally while counselling, e.g. 10% conversion rate in laparoscopic cholecystectomy; 50–60% 5-year survival in cancer patient; 90–95% cure rate in hernia repair; 5–10% recurrence rate after fistulectomy; 50–60% chance of saving a diabetic foot.

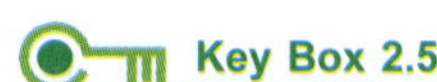
Key Box 2.5

Patients' Rights and Counselling

Right to

- Refuse treatment
- Have second opinion
- Change the doctor/hospital in the middle of the treatment

Respect their rights

- Do not embarrass/insult the patient
- Document

Truth and counselling: In a hurry/enthusiasm to convince the patient, one is often tempted to overstep and overstate the positives and understate the negatives. It is always better to tell the truth, because ***truth is constant, consistent and durable, and hence truth need not be remembered*** (Key Box 2.6).

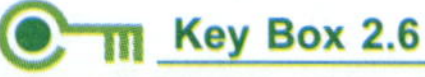
Key Box 2.6

Truth and Counselling

- Tell the truth, the whole truth, nothing but the truth
- Truth is constant, consistent and durable
- Truth need not be remembered
- Bitter truth can be made more palatable
- When the whole truth is not known, tell what is known for sure

Do's and don'ts: Do repeat, reinforce counselling at the appropriate time.

Don't argue, confront, quarrel, give false assurances, guarantee 100% results, make adverse remarks about other doctors, give opinions or sensitive information on phone.

Quality of counselling and its effects: Patients are in a state of physical, psychological, financial and emotional distress. Counselling should more or less address all these issues; it should be cautious, careful, convincing, re-assuring and consoling. It strengthens the faith and improves reputation of the doctors and hospitals; establishes rapport, builds relationship, reduces complaints, consumer cases, assaults and vandalism. Substandard counselling is done carelessly, is indifferent, confusing and intimidating; it results in loss of faith and reputation of the doctors and hospitals, suspicion in doctor's intentions, arguments and quarrels, assaults, ransacking, complaints and consumer cases (Fig. 2.1).

Counselling triangle: While counselling, the doctor should be acutely aware of the presence of others and place himself in three different places—his own place, in the patient's place and the place of the relatives and look and listen to himself.

Consent: Consent form is an important documentary evidence in the consumer forum. Printed consent form which is usually signed by the patient/relative at the time of admission, giving blanket consent for all tests and treatment is a weak evidence. Consent taken after counselling notes are documented is strong evidence and can save the doctors from many consumer cases.

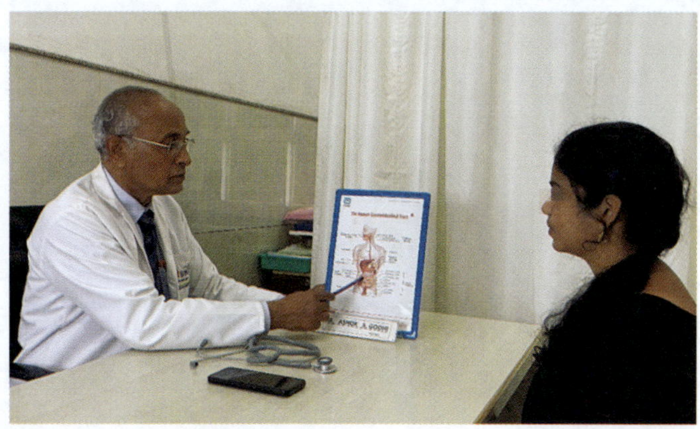

Fig. 2.1: Dr Ashok Godhi explaining and counselling with the help of a picture

Communication and counselling skills are put to acid test by worst situation such as when the treatment results in a severe adverse outcome due to most unanticipated rare complication, e.g. death due to drug reaction. A successful counselling will convince, console and calm the agitated and aggrieved relatives who understand the human limitations of the doctors and the uncertainties of the medical science. Conversely, unsuccessful counselling can result in an extremely unhappy patient even if the treatment of a complicated disease was successful and the team of doctors were extremely happy about the outcome.

Counselling is an art more than science. As much a share of success of a doctor in the practice of medicine goes to communication and counselling skills as his medical knowledge and technical skills.

Competency

SU10.2: Describe the steps of obtaining informed consent for laparoscopic hernioplasty in a simulated environment.

For medical simulation, a healthy person is trained and asked to act as a patient. He is trained to mention a few symptoms and signs. In a similar manner, he will be told about a surgical procedure and its complications, etc. Simulation helps in educating trainees/undergraduates so that their communication skills/performance will improve when they see the real patient.

I have given one example of informed consent for a patient undergoing laparoscopic hernioplasty. Every surgery should have separate consent form. Remember that the relevant procedure has to be explained in patient's own language or in a language that the patient understands. The patient should not only sign the consent form but also consent for HIV testing, blood transfusion and anaesthesia.

The steps of obtaining informed consent are as follows:

1. The consultant surgeon will explain about the disease, why surgery is needed and what type of surgery is planned (open or laparoscopic) and its complications.
2. He/she will allow the patient to ask any questions and clarify his/her doublts, if any.
3. The patient, once satisfied, will need to sign on the consent form for surgery. One witness will also need to sign on the consent form.
4. The consent form is then counter-signed by the surgical consultant and indicate his name, date and time.
5. Consultant anaesthetist explains the type of anaesthesia (regional or general anaesthesia) and possible complications related to anaesthesia. The patient will then need to consent for administration of anaesthesia. This form also needs a witness signature and the consultant anaesthetist's signature, name, date and time.

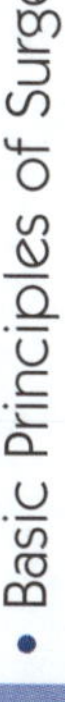

CHAPTER

3

Ethics in General Surgery

Competency

SU8.1: Describe the principles of ethics as it pertains to general surgery.

INTRODUCTION

Ethics in surgery is not something new. It has existed since ancient times. It existed during Hippocrates (460–c.370 BC) period also. During Hippocrates period, physicians were told to follow strict discipline, professionalism, and rigorous practice. Generally, they are advised to not harm people and if possible, help. Some code of conduct and morals existed even in ancient kingdom ruled by kings all over the world. We should know that surgery may cure a patient of his disease or surgery may save his life but surgery can also cause disfigurement, disability or even result in more problems due to complications.

Definition: Ethics is the discipline concerned with what is morally good and bad, or right and wrong. Surgery always deals with action and it is related to the body. Thus it is more relevant today because the field of medicine has developed rapidly. There are wide range of investigations available and many of them are costly also. Developments in surgery have been rapid with advent of new technologies. These add quality to life and at the same time, a kind of glamour and sophistication to surgery itself. A treating surgeon often needs to decide how much he should disclose about the nature of the disease to the patient or his relatives. He may also be in a dilemma as to what investigation to order, and how long and to what extent should he provide treatment, for example, how many days to prolong life of a patient who is terminally ill and has advanced malignancy (Fig. 3.1). This chapter discusses in brief about ethics pertaining to general surgery.

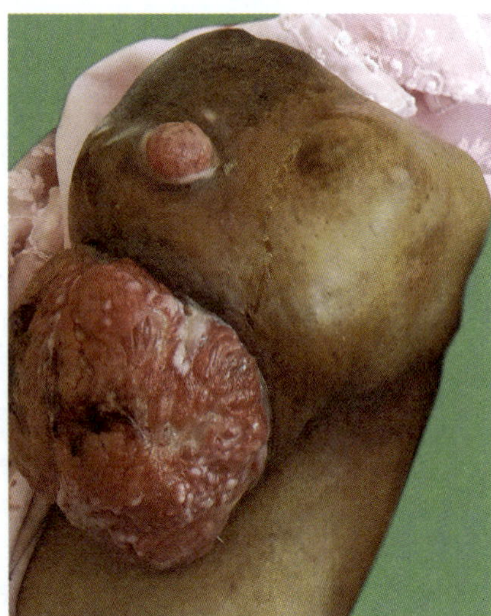

Fig. 3.1: Fungating carcinoma breast with bleeding

PRINCIPLES OF ETHICS

The four main ethical principles are: 1. Beneficence, 2. Non-maleficence, 3. Autonomy and 4. Justice. Some alteration of these are not uncommon depending upon the location, hospital practices and considering religion and race. The first two can be traced back to the time of Hippocrates "to help and do no harm", while the latter two evolved later. Let us look at each one of them with examples.

1. **Beneficence:** This means, as surgeons, we have an obligation to treat patients who are suffering, possibly due to pain or any wounds, to relieve them of the pain or any such symptom. What will you do if a patient presents to you with a bleeding ulcer?

   Irrespective of the paying capacity of the patient, his race or religion, it is our duty to stop that bleeding, make him comfortable and then proceed to do what needs to be done.

2. **Non-maleficence:** One should not practice evil or do harm, often stated in Latin as ***Primum non nocere.*** This means surgeons also have an obligation not to harm the patient. Even though no surgeon would intentionally harm any patient, his surgery or investigations ordered also should not cause harm. For example, a patient with metastatic stage 4 disease of carcinoma rectum with secondaries in the liver and ascites presented with intestinal obstruction. The patient had a past history of myocardial infarction 2 months prior and was on medications. The surgeon decided to do colostomy to relieve obstruction. However, the patient died in the postoperative period due to leakage of ascitic fluid from incision site, sepsis and cardiac failure. There was an expert available in the hospital who could have done stenting to relieve obstruction. The surgeon did not inform him nor did he take his suggestions. The surgeon can be held responsible for causing harm to the patient when he could have managed the situation without surgery.

3. **Autonomy:** Every adult human being in sound mind has a right to decide what shall be done with his own body. He or she has a right to know what disease he/she is having. The surgeon should give all the information about the disease, treatment plans and complications. Without this information, trust never develops between patient and the doctor. He has the right to give consent for treatment or refuse treatment even after the facts have been explained. However, if the patient is unconscious, mentally disabled, is an infant or a child, he/she will not be able to take decisions. A patient with hypotension and shock with altered sensorium due to gas gangrene has a risk of loss of limb and loss of life. He may not be in a position to understand. In such situations, the details, pros and cons must be explained to the relatives, and proceed with amputation/debridement after getting the consent from patient's legal representative. However, if the surgeon feels that a few hours of resuscitation can improve his mental status, he can wait for a few hours till he regains normal mental status and get consent from the patient.

   Informed consent: Informed consent is a process of taking consent from the patient/legal guardian for undergoing any procedure after the procedure is explained in detail to the patient in his own language or a language that he understands (Key Box 3.1).

> **Key Box 3.1**
>
> **Informed Consent**
>
> - Firstly, the patient should be made comfortable during counselling and he should be able to comprehend what is being explained.
> - The doctor must explain about the condition of the patient and the type of treatment planned, in the presence of a witness.
> - This must be explained in the patient's own language, taking the help of a translator as necessary.
> - The patient's understanding improves with the use of simple diagrams to explain.
> - A written informed consent must be taken either from the patient or legal representative, if the patient cannot sign or is minor. The form must have details of the patient, procedure, expected complications, date and time of taking consent.
> - The patient, the doctor and the witness must sign on the consent form acknowledging the explanation and giving consent to the procedure.
> - Only the procedure documented in the consent form should be performed. If another lesion is encountered as a surprise finding during surgery, it should not be excised. Example: During cholecystectomy, the surgeon finds a 5 cm cyst in the liver. It was asymptomatic. If prior consent is not taken, it should not be removed.

Informed consent in emergency situations: Example: A patient is unconscious due to head injury following road traffic accident but has life-threatening bleeding from a ruptured spleen. In this situation, the treating surgeon should apply the first two ethical principles: Beneficence and non-maleficence, and operate. Who can give consent in this situation? The patient's legal representative (spouse, son, guardian, etc.) can give consent. On some occasions, no relative is present and the patient is brought in by police personnel. In this situation, the Medical Superintendent of the hospital can give his consent to do surgery in order to stop the haemorrhage by splenectomy/ splenorrhaphy.

Truth telling: A valuable bond develops between the patient and the doctor when the truth has been conveyed to the patient. For example, the patient has gallstone disease with symptoms. The surgeon must not only explain to the patient about the disease and the need for surgery but also the type of surgery, complications and difficulties that can be expected in the given patient. Any other alternate treatment options available as per guidelines issued by the speciality societies—such as Association of Surgeons of India or American Society of Surgeons, etc. must also be mentioned. For example, laparoscopic cholecystectomy is the surgery of choice but laparoscopic facilities are not available in a rural set-up, the patient must be informed about advantages of the laparoscopic procedure, non-availability of those facilities in that rural set-up and about the facilities available at a nearby place.

In a few countries including India, when a patient is diagnosed to have cancer or some serious disease, the son or daughters often request that the treating doctors not reveal the facts about the disease or chances of survival to the patient directly. Culturally, this is acceptable in a society where a senior member takes the decision. However, legally this is not. To get around the problem, the patient can be asked whether it is acceptable to him, if further treatment plans are discussed with his son, daughter or brother, who will take decisions on his behalf. This is acceptable, if the patient agrees to it.

Confidentiality: Surgeons must not discuss the disease or patient condition to anyone without permission from the patient. However, other health care professionals who may be required to treat such patients for various medical reasons or for scientific studies, can be informed. Such situations are also implied that the patient has been told about this. However, when there is any doubt regarding presence of communicable diseases such as HIV or hepatitis B, or even COVID infections, one must inform people who are connected with the patient to protect others from acquiring infection from the patient.

4. **Justice:** It is a fair, equitable and appropriate treatment of persons. Several issues govern this. It depends upon hospital resources and the time we give each patient. Is it the same for patients with and without insurance, paying and nonpaying patients? Another example is when a physician prescribes an expensive drug, it may benefit him and there may be another drug which is equally good and cheap but does not benefit him.

LIFE AND DEATH

- As of now, euthanasia, intentional killing of a person, is rejected as unlawful malpractice. The patient may be terminally ill but conscious and well-oriented. The use of analgesic medications to the point of causing death may be considered as an intention to kill. Here, the surgeon or palliative medicine experts may have to prove their innocence.
- Patients who are brain-dead or have seriously damaged brain, once certified by concerned specialists, are taken off ventilatory support and are allowed to die. However, the patient's family or relatives have to be briefed about his condition and have to be informed that the decision is taken by a group of specialists.

Examples

1. A patient with cirrhosis of liver with encephalopathy is slowly recovering but has a massive variceal bleeding. The patient is not consenting for banding therapy when explained by the doctors. If the varices are not banded, he may die or have serious consequences but the patient does not consent. How does one proceed in this situation? Beneficence and autonomy have conflicts. If you follow the rules of autonomy, you should not proceed. If you follow the rules of beneficence, you should proceed with banding. Now look at his mental status. He is a bit drowsy and has encephalopathy. He is not capable of understanding what the doctors are explaining. So now beneficence takes precedence. The specialist should go ahead with banding after explaining the procedure, advantages and risks involved to the patient's relatives.
2. A 65-year-old retired banker was diagnosed to have a 6 cm tumor in the liver, a hepatocellular carcinoma and a big and suspicious nodule in the lung probably metastasis. He was advised to undergo surgery for the liver tumor followed by other modalities of treatment including chemotherapy and removal of lung lesion, etc. The patient said he does not want to undergo surgery as he is scared that he may die of complications and that he would resort to alternative medicines. What should be done now? It is his autonomy, he has taken this decision in spite of knowing about the disease and probable survival. So, we should not force him to undergo surgery. However, if he comes with pain/discomfort/any other complications later, it is our duty to give him the best palliation. We can also suggest that he seek a second opinion. **Jehovah's witness patients refuse blood transfusion even when they know that their life could be in danger.** This group is a sect of Christianity. Here autonomy comes into the picture, not justice.
3. A 70-year-old man undergoes total gastrectomy followed by esophagojejunostomy for carcinoma stomach. He was a smoker with COPD, diabetes, also had myocardial infarction a few months back and was on treatment. He developed multiorgan failure on day 6 due to pneumonia and deteriorated very fast. He was intubated and he went into coma by day 14 and no improvement was seen till day 21. How to

proceed in such cases? This is the time to discuss patient's condition with his family and explain to them about his condition, whether his lung condition is reversible, take them into confidence and discontinue the treatment.

4. A 75-year-old lady was brought with bleeding per rectum of 8 months duration and jaundice of 1 month duration. It was treated as hemorrhoids for a few months. Rectal examination, biopsy and later MRI revealed advanced carcinoma rectum infiltrating the anal sphincter. She also had multiple metastasis in both lobes of liver. Relatives of many patients insist that diagnosis should not be told to the patient. How do we proceed? Call the patient and ask her whether her disease and best plan of action can be explained to her son/representative and whether she would consent for that.
5. A 35-year-old lady underwent hysterectomy for excessive bleeding. She was discharged after 5 days. However, she returned after 4 weeks with abdominal pain, distension and high-grade fever. CECT scan revealed foreign body—a left-over mop in the peritoneal cavity. The patient underwent exploration and the mop was removed. She did well and was discharged. What should the surgeon tell the patient? He has to tell the truth. That mop was left behind by mistake. One can also apologise to the patient. The expenses of the second operation or surgeon's fees can also be waived off by the hospital authorities and some amount of compensation can be given to the patient. Here is a situation of harm caused to the patient inadvertently by not following certain guidelines/check lists to prevent them.
6. During COVID-19, an 85-year-old, otherwise fit patient in Nagpur whose saturation was 60%, who required an oxygen bed told the doctors in the hospital to give that oxygen bed to a 35-year-old patient who was also having 60% saturation since there was only one oxygen bed available. It was a great sacrifice. However, if you face this situation in real life in emergency department, what should be your decision? Decision cannot be based on wealth of the patient, influence from the authorities or influence from politicians. A 35-year-old patient has a longer life. He may be the only bread-earning member of his family. He may have the responsibility of looking after his parents. So, he has a definite edge over the 85-year-old man/woman. So, this is fair decision and justice to resuscitate the 35-year-old man.
7. An advanced case of liver cell failure, portal hypertension, uncontrolled ascites (Fig. 3.2), with large obstructed ulcerated irreducible hernia with sepsis for surgery—surgery was done to relieve pain, fungation and ulceration—only as palliation. All the details about the risks were explained to the patient. Surgery was done after consent was obtained. He died on the 3rd postoperative day of sepsis, hypotension and shock.

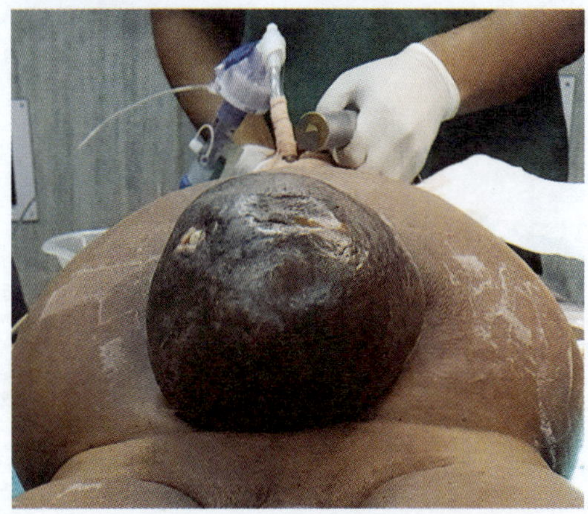

Fig. 3.2: Tense ascites with obstructed umbilical hernia

CONCLUSIONS

If you follow guidelines of ABCDEFG of doctor–patient relationship which is given in Chapter 1 and principles of ethics given in this chapter, it is a great service to the humanity. You will give your best to your patients. You will also uphold the virtues and values of medical education and ethics.

FURTHER READING

Rev Col Bras Cir-. 2020 Jun 15; 47: 2020. Surgical ethics: a framework for surgeons, patients, and society.

CHAPTER

4

Surgical Audit

- Types
- Audit cycle
- What to audit?
- What makes a good audit topic?
- What is not an audit?
- Steps of audit

Competency

SU7.1: Describe the planning and conduct of surgical audit.

INTRODUCTION

Surgical audit can be defined as the systematic unbiased review of surgical practice with the objective of recognizing deficiencies and improving standards of care. It involves critical analysis by peers and any lapses or deficiencies detected during the course of the treatment of the patient are listed. An audit should aim at improving the standards laid down in the respective departments. It should also aim at studying morbidity and mortality. An audit is helpful in studying not only the quality of services provided by the department but is also useful to the individual surgeon to keep track of his/her own personal outcome data. Contributing to a clinical database ensures that a surgeon's own performance is monitored continuously. It should be compared to national data to ensure the accepted standards are achieved.

Example 1: National database of laparoscopic cholecystectomy shows that in about 3–4% of cases, laparoscopic surgery needs to be converted to open surgery. However, if a surgeon's own data records show more than 10% conversion rate, he needs to audit and find out the reason behind this high failure rate. Thus, an audit helps improve treatment policies, standard of care and may be more economical.

Example 2: A hospital may have set certain standards for thyroidectomy such as "identification of the recurrent laryngeal nerve (RLN) should be done in all cases and that is the best method to avoid injuries to this nerve". Audit of recurrent laryngeal nerve paralysis after total thyroidectomy would include a careful check of the operative notes to see how many surgeons identified the RLN at surgery and how many did not.

TYPES

Essentially, two types of audit may be encountered: **National audits and local/hospital audits**. Both are designed to improve the quality of care. National audits should be driven by needs identified during the local and hospital-based audits that are closest to the patient. Recently an audit of treatment given to COVID-19 patients was done to check whether all the guidelines given by the government were followed. Topics for hospital-based audits are often identified at the departmental morbidity and mortality meetings, where issues related to patient care are discussed. Tuberculosis is a notifiable disease and it is a national issue. So, hospitals can audit these types of cases. After report from the local hospitals, a national audit can be designed to be completed by the local audit department and surgical teams.

Audit can also be categorised and used to study different aspects of patient care. For example, an audit of smoking behaviours of patients can be categorised into: (a) *Structure of care*: Refers to the resources required, e.g. the availability of a smoking cessation clinic in a locality. (b) *Process of care*: Refers to the actions and decisions taken by practitioners together with users, e.g. waiting times for an appointment at the smoking cessation clinic. (c) *Outcome of care*: Measures the physical or behaviour response to an intervention, e.g. the number of smokers who quit smoking for 1 year.

AUDIT CYCLE

Important steps of audit cycle (audit process) are as follows:

1. Define the audit question in a multidisciplinary team.
2. Identify the evidence and current standards or guidelines.
3. Design the audit to measure performance against agreed standards based on strong evidence. One needs to seek advice and ensure that institutions have agreed to undertake the audit.
4. Define an agreeable timeline.
5. Conduct the audit.
6. Analyse results and compare performance against agreed standards.
7. Undertake gap analysis:
   a. If all standards are reached, reaudit after an agreed interval.
   b. If there is a need for improvement, identify possible interventions such as training and agree with the involved parties.
   c. Implement the changes.
8. Allow sufficient time for changes to be included in the new guidelines.
9. Reaudit, analyse and discuss whether the practice has improved.

WHAT TO AUDIT?

Surgeons can decide about the topics based on the need/requirement. It is a good idea to find out the common surgical procedures done in the hospital and select a topic related to the procedures. Some examples are given below.

- Simple questions with straightforward outcomes: *Example:* Did all patients receive antibiotic prophylaxis prior to surgical incision?
- Simple measurements and interventions: Are all patients appropriately assessed for possibility of deep vein thrombosis (DVT) risks and received appropriate prophylaxis during their hospital stay? How many lymph nodes are removed after modified radical mastectomy performed for carcinoma breast or hemicolectomy for carcinoma colon.
- Audit anything that you are not certain about: Fluid requirements in acute pancreatitis or non-operative management of splenic injuries, etc.

WHAT MAKES A GOOD AUDIT TOPIC?

- Priorities in your hospital/department: *For example:* Diabetic ulcer on the leg is common not only in our hospital but also in India and it is a relevant topic.
- A topic in an area of medicine that interests you and you may choose the topic.
- Re-audits of previous projects: If there is a previous audit that was never re-audited and the loop was not closed, then this is a good audit.

WHAT IS NOT AN AUDIT?

1. Comparison of treatment or interventions: *Example:* Comparing antibiotics followed by drainage versus antibiotics without drainage for breast abscess.
2. Outcomes of novel treatment: *Example:* Results of endoscopic cystogastrostomy.
3. Outcomes of novel service: *Example:* Role of CECT scan in nutrition.
4. Pure research or service evaluation: *Example:* Finding a new technique for hernia repair.
5. Census work

All these are considered original research work and not an audit.

STEPS OF AUDIT

The audit process is divided into five official steps and the cycle is only considered complete if all steps are performed. The five steps of audit cycle are as follows:

Step 1: Define the standard to be reviewed—American College or Royal College guidelines, or in sepsis—Surviving Sepsis Campaign 2021 guidelines, etc. It is important to consider local policies also.

Step 2: Decide what data to be collected? Who will be collecting the data and is it retrospective or prospective?

Step 3: Compare standard current practice with the actual performance data collected from the department. Evaluate how well the standards were met and if not, identify reasons for this.

Step 4: Recommend a change, if required, agree to the changes and then implement. *Example:* After an audit from the hospital, it is found that when clindamycin was used, ulcers healed faster in diabetic patients.

Step 5: Close the audit cycle loop—once the suggested change is implemented, one cycle of audit is closed.

CHAPTER

5

Principles and Steps of Clinical Research in General Surgery

- Principles of clinical research
- Steps of clinical research
- Secondary research

Competency

SU7.2: Describe the principles and steps of clinical research in general surgery.

INTRODUCTION

The dictionary defines research as "the systematic investigation into and study of materials and sources in order to establish facts and reach new conclusions". The keywords in this definition are: (1) 'Systematic investigation' meaning an orderly and methodical investigation; (2) 'Establish facts' meaning that you are collecting new data, and (3) 'Reach new conclusions' meaning that you are adding to the already existing knowledge.

Clinical research is research in the field of health sciences particularly clinical sciences. The National Cancer Institute defines clinical research as follows: "Research in which people, or data or samples of tissue from people, are studied to understand health and disease. Clinical research helps find new and better ways to detect, diagnose, treat, and prevent disease. Types of clinical research include clinical trials, which test new treatments for a disease, and natural history studies, which collect health information to understand how a disease develops and progresses over time".

We live in the era of evidenced-based surgery. Society at large expects us to practice scientific surgery. As long ago as 1853, Ruskin described the concept of science as follows: "The work of science is to substitute facts for appearances and demonstrations for impressions". Any field, including surgery, can claim to be scientific only when the body of its knowledge is backed by reliable and honest data that is collected and analysed in good research studies. Thus it is essential that practicing clinicians understand the principles that underlie scientific studies and comprehend the methodology used in research projects. Further, understanding and undertaking research projects bring with it several advantages to the practicing clinician. These include (1) gaining the respect of his/her fellow clinicians, (2) better recognition in society, and (3) getting better respect and compliance from his/her patients. Also, various organisations are making it mandatory for its members to have research publications before they can progress in their careers.

PRINCIPLES OF CLINICAL RESEARCH

Clinical research is governed by several important principles. Some of these principles are highlighted hereunder.

1. **Ethical conduct:** The utmost importance must be given to ethical conduct in carrying out clinical research. The researcher must exercise total honesty and integrity. The significant qualities of an ethical researcher was laid out by Salter and has been listed in Key Box 5.1

   The researcher must always have in mind the physical and emotional comfort of the subject of clinical research. The ethical principle of "do no harm" must be the primary principle while undertaking research.

Key Box 5.1

Qualities of a Good Researcher (after Salter)

Integrity	Inquisitive
Intelligence	Innovative
Ingenuity	Industrious
Initiative	Incisive

2. **Usefulness to society:** Clinical research must address common clinical problems. It should try and answer the controversies or difficult questions that a clinician faces in everyday practice. It would be incorrect to undertake research only for the sake of research and publishing papers.
3. **Propriety:** The researcher must always show propriety in whatever he/she does. This takes several forms including financial regularity, communication with his colleagues and his subjects, proper maintenance of records and transparency in sharing data with others.
4. **Address biases:** The researcher must be careful to make sure that biases or prejudices do not compromise the conclusions that are drawn from the data. Several kinds of biases exist. The important ones are: (1) Selection bias where the subjects in each of the study groups are chosen in such a manner that the results may be skewed; (2) Observer bias where the person tabulating the end result may skew the results deliberately or even unwittingly; and (3) Confounding factor/s where an intervention or a condition other than the one being studied may influence the outcome.

STEPS OF CLINICAL RESEARCH

Clinical research is undertaken in a systematic manner involving several steps. These steps are summarised in Fig. 5.1.

Step 1. Recognise a clinical problem and carry out a literature search to understand what is known thus far about the subject. Once this is determined, one can go about asking a research question. An example of a common clinical question would be whether a drain has to be used after a cholecystectomy or not.

Step 2. Asking the correct research question and putting forth a sensible hypothesis is an important step in research. One talks of the 'null hypothesis' in research.

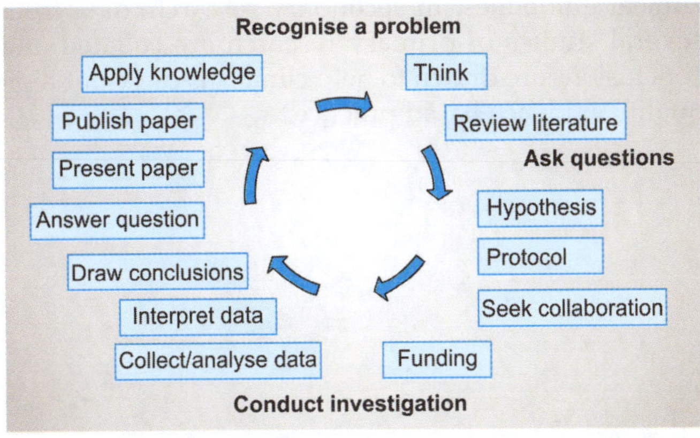

Fig. 5.1: Basic steps in clinical research

This essentially means that the researcher starts by saying that the intervention proposed does not have an influence on the outcome. If the data proves otherwise, then a conclusion is drawn that the intervention is indeed helpful. Continuing the above example, the null hypothesis would be that the use of a drain would not be useful after cholecystectomy.

Step 3. Draw up a protocol. A protocol is a detailed document that describes several aspects of the study including the aim of the study with the research question, the methods that are being used to answer this question and all the administrative issues that go with the study. The protocol is required to make sure that the researcher and his colleagues know exactly what is to be done. The steps described in the protocol are never violated. The important components of a protocol are listed below:

*3a. **A Title*** that adequately describes the study and does enough to arouse the curiosity of the reader.

*3b. **Summary*** of the project. This is required to be submitted for various approvals that are required before the study is undertaken.

*3c. **Rationale*** of the study which describes the logic behind undertaking the study, leading up to why a particular research question had to be asked.

*3d. **Objectives*** of the study—lay down the research questions in detail and explain the outcomes that are going to be measured to get answers.

*3e. **Methods*** section of the protocol is the most important part that describes in detail what is going to be done. This has several subsections as under:

3e1. Subjects involved: Describes the characteristics of the group of patients who are going to be studied

3e2. Sample size: Explains the number of patients in the groups being studied. The sample size is important to determine the 'power' of the study and whether the conclusions of the study can be applied to all the patients at large, or not.

3e3. Study design: Study design is the pre-eminent component of a research project. A detailed explanation of the various kinds of studies is outside the purview of this chapter. Only the very basic principles involved will be explained. Choosing the appropriate study design for a given research question is important. The value of the research project and the conclusions drawn therefrom depend on the choice of a proper study design.

Anecdotal experiences reported as case reports or small numbers of patients (series) are of limited value because the information from these studies cannot be realistically extrapolated to a population in general.

Retrospective studies collect data from patients who have already been treated or operated on. These studies are not as valuable as prospective studies because the methodology used is not standardized, there may be several data points that may be missing, and the interventions may vary from one patient to another.

Prospective studies are a lot more reliable because the methods employed, the interventions undertaken, the tests done and the collection of data are all well controlled. The researcher can implement further safeguards against biases in the form of randomisation and blinding. *Randomisation* is a process where the researcher has no role in assigning the patients to the various study groups. The allocation is generally done through computer generated numbers. This process eliminates selection bias. Blinding is a process where the observer who measures the outcomes of the study is not aware of the intervention that has been undertaken in the study subject. Blinding eliminates observer bias.

The randomised controlled trial (RCT) is perhaps the highest form of unbiased scientific study. Conclusions drawn from an RCT are rated to have the highest scientific value. However, it is not easy to conduct an RCT with sufficient numbers of patients particularly in surgical disciplines.

3e4. Interventions involve a detailed description of the tests and procedures that are going to be undertaken on the patients. These may be biochemical or radiological tests. It also includes interventions in the form of administration of the study drug or an operative procedure. In the example taken, one may consider measuring pain through regular Visual Analogue Scale (VAS) scores, get a chest X-ray to rule out atelectasis and an abdominal ultrasound to detect collections.

3e5. Outcome measurements describe the endpoints that are going to be measured in the study. Defining the endpoints and determining the correct metrics to measure them form an important part of the protocol. In the cholecystectomy example, one can consider postoperative pain, incidence of subhepatic collections, length of stay in hospital, postoperative infection, incidence of atelectasis as possible and points of the study.

Step 4. Obtain the necessary permissions from the regulatory authorities/bodies. Armed with the protocol, the researchers start with getting clearance from the head of the unit/the head of the department and the medical administrator. The protocol will then be scrutinized by the scientific and ethical committees of the institution. Once cleared by these committees, the study has to be registered with an authority like the Clinical Trial Registry of India.

Step 5. Conduct the study with honesty and diligence and collect data.

Step 6. Analyse the data using the previously decided set of statistical methods.

Step 7. Draw conclusions based on the analysis of the data collected.

Step 8. Share the results and conclusions of the study either in the form of a presentation read at a conference or paper published in a good journal. It is quite possible that the results of this study are so significant that one might have to change ones' clinical practice based on the study. In the example given above, many studies have shown that using a drain after a routine cholecystectomy is actually not required at all.

SECONDARY RESEARCH

The processes described so far are considered to be primary research. There is another form of research called secondary research. Examples of secondary research include systematic reviews, meta-analysis and clinical guidelines. In secondary research, data from several studies of primary research are collated and conclusions are drawn to help clinicians carry out high quality evidence-based practice.

CHAPTER

6

Perioperative Care

Competency

SU1.3: Describe basic concepts of perioperative care.

The perioperative period is a term used to describe the three distinct phases of any surgical procedure, which include the preoperative phase, the intraoperative phase, and the postoperative phase.

PREOPERATIVE CARE

Every patient presenting for surgery must be optimally prepared before surgery to ensure best possible outcome of surgery. Optimisation is done based on the urgency of surgery, nature of the disease and presence of other comorbidities.

Elective Surgery

There is sufficient time available for evaluation and preparation of patients presenting for elective surgery. Preoperative evaluation will consist of detailed history, physical examination and investigations based on the findings. There is no 'routine' investigation. All investigations must be tailored to the patient and the surgery. A patient with no other comorbidity and minimum change in his homeostasis may require no further preparation, whereas some will require considerable preparation.

Examples:

- A patient may have pre-existing conditions unrelated to surgery such as asthma, chronic obstructive pulmonary disease, hypertension or diabetes. They must be thoroughly evaluated and their condition optimized prior to surgery. Smoking should be stopped at least 4 weeks before surgery. Patients with respiratory conditions and those presenting for major thoracic or abdominal surgery may be advised incentive spirometry and respiratory exercises to improve their breathing ability.
- A patient with thyrotoxicosis must be made euthyroid before thyroidectomy, a patient with phaeochromocytoma must have the hypertension well under control before surgery.
- *Nutrition:* Nutritional support may be considered for patients who are severely malnourished. Examples may be carcinoma esophagus, achalasia cardia or a few cases of intestinal fistulae. These patients should receive seven or more days of enteral or parenteral nutrition prior to surgery. Enteral nutrition has a number of advantages such as preservation of gut mucosa, decreased leakage of gut bacterial antigens, reduction of inflammation, maintenance of immune function and decreased hyperglycemia. Healing after surgery is improved with better nutrition.
- Patients with coagulopathies or bleeding disorders may be at increased risk for bleeding. They may require perioperative transfusion of blood products. Anti-platelet drugs should be stopped 7 days before the procedure unless they need to be continued. Low dose aspirin, however, is usually continued. Refer to Key Box 6.1.

Key Box 6.1

Elective Surgery

1. Optimise pre-existing conditions: Control of diabetes, hypertension, bronchial asthma
2. Functional status to be normal while operating on thyroid and adrenals
3. Nutritional support
4. Tailor investigations to the patient's condition and surgery

Emergency Surgery

These surgeries can be broadly classified further into surgeries for trauma and non-trauma.

- **Urgent surgery:** There is usually some time available for optimization of these patients, say a few hours, before surgery. For example, acute appendicitis, intestinal obstruction, obstructed hernia, blunt abdominal trauma. This time is utilized to treat them with intravenous fluids to optimize blood volume, correct electrolyte imbalance, administer antibiotics, bronchodilators if asthmatic and to obtain investigations done such as echocardiogram. Most of abdominal emergency cases need to have a nasogastric tube inserted and urinary bladder catheterized.
- **Emergency surgery:** Occasionally, some surgeries are absolutely emergent and no time should be wasted to optimize these patients. In these patients, evaluation, resuscitation, surgery and optimization happen simultaneously. *Examples:* Life-threatening conditions such as a patient with uncontrolled bleeding after polytrauma, limb-threatening conditions such as vascular injury.

Patient Preparation (Key Box 6.2)

Preoperative care also includes preparing the part for surgery, marking the site and side and obtaining **informed consent (Follow WHO checklist)**. Consent is taken after explaining to the patient, the nature of surgery, anticipated outcome, possible complications and postoperative course, possible need of postoperative intensive care and even mortality (as applicable in those cases) in his own language. A witness to the process of obtaining consent must also sign on this document along with the patient and the surgeon.

- In addition, the patient must be referred to the anaesthetist (pre-anaesthesia checkup) who will once again evaluate the patient from his/her perspective, obtain additional investigations as necessary and take informed consent.
- All patients are kept fasting for solids and milk for at least 6 hours and to clear fluids for at least two hours prior to surgery. This is done to minimize the risk of vomiting and pulmonary aspiration of regurgitated gastric contents during anesthesia which can lead to aspiration pneumonia.
- Instructions regarding premedication, investigations (as required on the morning of surgery) and other regular medications as prescribed by the anaesthetist must be followed (Refer to Chapter 64 on Anaesthesia for further details).

Key Box 6.2

Preparation of the Patient

1. Informed consent and signature
2. Clipping of the hair just before surgery
3. Mark the site—especially small lumps in the breast, hernias, benign lumps
4. Nil per oral 6 hours for solids, and 2 hours for liquids
5. Follow anaesthesia orders. Give drugs prescribed by anaesthetist

INTRAOPERATIVE CARE (Fig. 6.1)

The intraoperative period is the most stressful part of surgery and is the combined responsibility of the surgeon, the anesthetist, nurses and the entire surgical team.

- On the day of surgery, the patient is wheeled into the operation theatre, where his identity, surgery, site and side, availability of blood products (as necessary), fasting status and consent are once again checked before beginning anesthesia. Antibiotics are given within 30 minutes to an hour before commencement of surgery.
- Once anaesthesia has been given, the anaesthetist monitors the vitals of the patient while the surgeon concentrates on the surgery. The maintenance of depth of anaesthesia, administration of intravenous fluids, blood products, analgesics, and maintenance of physiology of the patient is the responsibility of the anaesthetist.
- The surgeon undertakes the surgery with aseptic precautions, with an effort to minimize blood loss, tissue damage and in a reasonable period of time. Once surgery is done, the incision is closed after careful count of the gauzes and instruments (done by the nurse) so that nothing is left behind unintentionally inside the patient's body.
- Upon completion of surgery and emergence from anaesthesia, the patient is shifted to the postanesthetic care unit for further observation. The patient can then be shifted to the ward after fulfilling discharge criteria (hemodynamically stable with adequate oxygenation, fully conscious, is able to void if not catheterized and is pain free). The patients are shifted to high dependency units, if they have undergone major surgery but are stable postoperatively. If the patient needs postoperative mechanical ventilation or is hemodynamically unstable, then he is shifted to the intensive care unit for further management.

POSTOPERATIVE CARE (Fig. 6.2)

Upon arrival in the recovery area, the surgeon and the anaesthetist explain to the recovery nurse in charge of the patient about the surgery, intraoperative events and give instructions for postoperative care (Key Box 6.3).

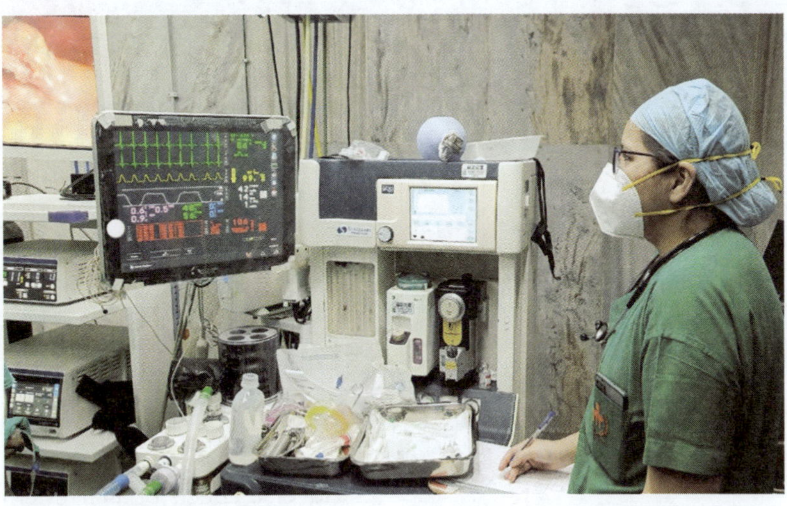

Fig. 6.1: Intraoperative care with monitoring vitals

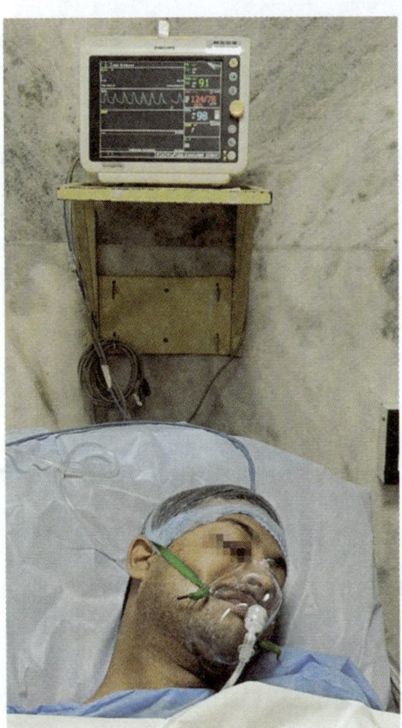

Fig. 6.2: Postoperative care with monitoring of vitals

Key Box 6.3

Postoperative Care

1. Vitals: Airway, breathing, circulation and disposition
2. Analgesia
3. Fluid and electrolyte balance: Intake/output chart
4. Thromboprophylaxis—mobilisation of legs
5. Nutrition
6. Antibiotics

- **ABCD:** Monitoring and restoration to normal physiology and function of organs [(A—airway, B—breathing, C—circulation and D—disposition (consciousness)]. The patients are monitored closely and appropriate management done till their vitals are normal.
- **Pain relief:** Adequate analgesia is important in the postoperative period. This may include intravenous paracetamol, opioids, nonsteroidal anti-inflammatory drugs or regional analgesia depending on the nature of the pain and severity.
- **Fluid and electrolyte balance:** The patients are monitored closely postoperatively to ensure their fluid and electrolyte status is normal. An intake-output chart is maintained for all patients who have undergone major surgery. Their fluid input (including blood products) is matched with output (urine, blood loss and any other excessive secretions). In the early postoperative period, one must remember that antidiuretic hormone (ADH) is released which results in conserving of water. Aldosterone secretion increases leading to reabsorption of sodium and potassium secretion.
- **Bowel movements:** Patients who undergo laparotomy have paralytic ileus, so it is common not to have bowel movement for 2 to 3 days. Once bowel sounds are heard, the patient is given sips of water followed by soft diet.
- **Leg movements,** both passive and active are done, to minimize thromboembolic complications. They are also prescribed thromboprophylaxis depending upon the nature of the surgery.
- **Nutrition:** Patients who undergo gastrectomy, esophageal surgeries and surgeries on intestines, may require parenteral nutrition for a few days. Enteral nutrition is resumed as early as possible.
- **Preventing infection:** In all contaminated and dirty cases, antibiotics have to be continued for a period of 5 to 7 days. In cases of sepsis and septic shock, they have to be continued for 14 days.
- Once the patients are stable, they are discharged home with instructions for home care and follow-up.

CHAPTER

7

Pain Management

- The pain pathway
- Assessment of pain
- Routes of administration of analgesia
- Adverse effects of analgesic medication
- Chronic pain
- Adjuncts

Competency

SU11.5: Describe principles of providing postoperative pain relief and management of chronic pain.

INTRODUCTION

Pain is a sensation of discomfort associated with injury. It can be acute or chronic. Acute pain (nociception) is associated with tissue damage and an inflammatory response, it is self-limiting and of short duration. Often it does not involve neural tissue. Chronic pain, however, persists long after the tissue damage is treated. Chronic pain, on the other hand, is the pain which persists even after 3 months of surgical illness. In surgical patients, it can be due to postoperative pain, malignancies or diseases such as chronic pancreatitis.

PRINCIPLES OF PROVIDING POSTOPERATIVE PAIN RELIEF

One of the main fears patients have about surgery is the postoperative pain and it is only humane that this is relieved. In addition, pain has adverse effects on various systems of the body such as tachycardia, hypertension, arrhythmias and rarely even myocardial ischaemia and infarction. The patients may not breathe properly leading to retained secretions because of inadequate cough, atelectasis, pneumonia and respiratory failure. The hypertension can precipitate bleeding, e.g. after thyroidectomy.

Pain relief can be given in many ways but it must be tailored to the patient since pain medications have adverse effects and hence, safety must be ensured at all times. The pain prescription must contain clear instructions regarding the name of the drug, dose, route, frequency, monitoring required, treatment for known side effects such as for nausea and vomiting and when to call the duty doctor.

THE PAIN PATHWAY

Postoperative pain varies with the patient's tolerance to pain, type of surgery, anaesthetic and the site, and extent of incisions given. The pain may be somatic, visceral or both. It is important to understand how pain is transmitted and appreciated by the body to treat it effectively (Fig. 7.1).

Pain is produced in the injured tissue due to the release of prostaglandins, serotonin, substance P and acetylcholine which stimulate the peripheral nociceptors (transduction). These stimulate the peripheral nerve supplying the area and the impulses are transmitted through it to the dorsal horn of the spinal cord (transmission). These impulses then travel through the ascending tracts to the thalamus (transmission) and the sensory cortex where the pain is perceived (perception). The perception of pain can be inhibited by stimulating the descending inhibitory pathway and release of inhibitory neurotransmitters such as GABA, glycine, opioid peptides and norepinephrine (modulation). Generally, acute postsurgical pain can be controlled by addressing each component of this pain pathway and hence it is called **multimodal approach to pain control**.

Transduction is reduced by local anaesthetic infiltration (e.g. bupivacaine) and the use of nonsteroidal anti-inflammatory drugs (Key Box 7.1). Transmission through peripheral nerves can be blocked by nerve blocks (transverse abdominis pain block for abdominal surgery). Transmission through the spinal cord to

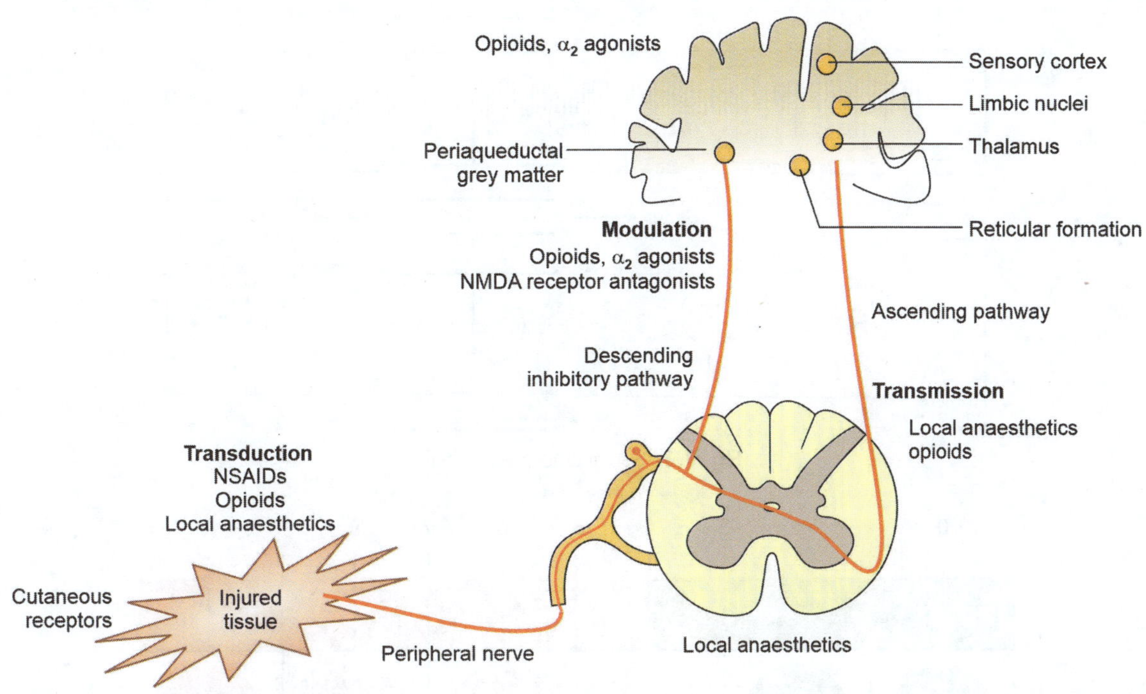

Fig. 7.1: Pain pathway, mechanisms of pain and medications that can be given to block each of these components

Key Box 7.1

Pain Mechanisms and Medications

Mechanism	Medications
Transduction	Local anaesthetic infiltration, NSAIDs
Transmission	Local anaesthetics (nerve blocks, epidural)
Perception	Opioids, alpha2 agonists
Modulation	Opioids, alpha2 agonists, NMDA receptor antagonists

ascending pathways can be inhibited using epidural analgesia. Opioids (morphine, fentanyl, tramadol, nalbuphine) reduce perception. They also have a modulating effect on pain perception through their effects on the μ receptors in the brain as well as spinal cord.

ASSESSMENT OF PAIN

- Pain is totally a subjective phenomenon. The patient knows by his experience about nature of the pain and other related features. *Example*: Any severe pain in the abdomen results in vomiting. Thus, one can deduce that the pain is severe. Each person may respond differently to the pain. When a patient says he has pain, he probably has pain and must be believed. He can simply rate it as none, mild, moderate or severe.
- **Numerical rating score (NRS):** In this, whenever the patient has pain, he can be asked to rate the pain on a scale numbering from 0 to 10, where 0 means no pain and 10 represents the most severe pain they can imagine (Fig. 7.2). The patient can then be followed up using the same scale to gauge whether severity of the pain has changed or whether the analgesia provided is sufficient. Pain score <3 is acceptable.

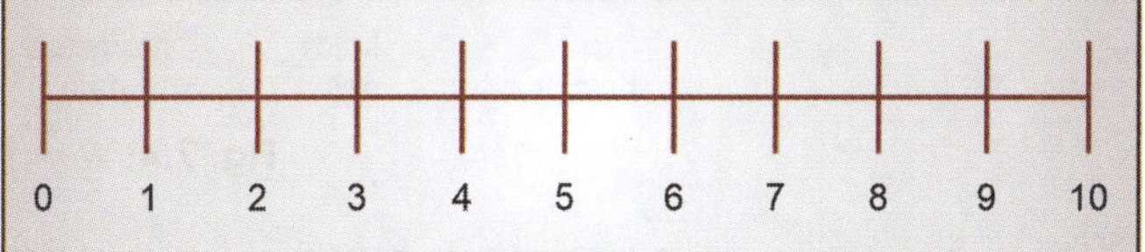

Fig. 7.2: Numerical rating scale

NRS of 10: Very severe pain: Ureteric colic, mesenteric ischaemia or dissecting aneurysms, etc.

NRS 4–6: Moderate pain, e.g. acute cholecystitis or appendicitis

NRS 2–3: Dull aching pain, e.g. hepatomegaly or splenomegaly

- **Visual analogue scale (VAS):** In this, the patient is shown a 10 cm long scale, where one end represents no pain and the other end (10 cm) represents very severe pain (Fig. 7.3). However, unlike the NRS, the patient is not shown any number in between and the patient slides a rider across the scale to point out the level of his pain. The numbers are present on a continuous scale on the side facing the investigator and can be in fractions also.
- **Wong-Baker FACES scale:** This scale consists of a series of faces, where one end has a happy face representing no pain and the other end, a face

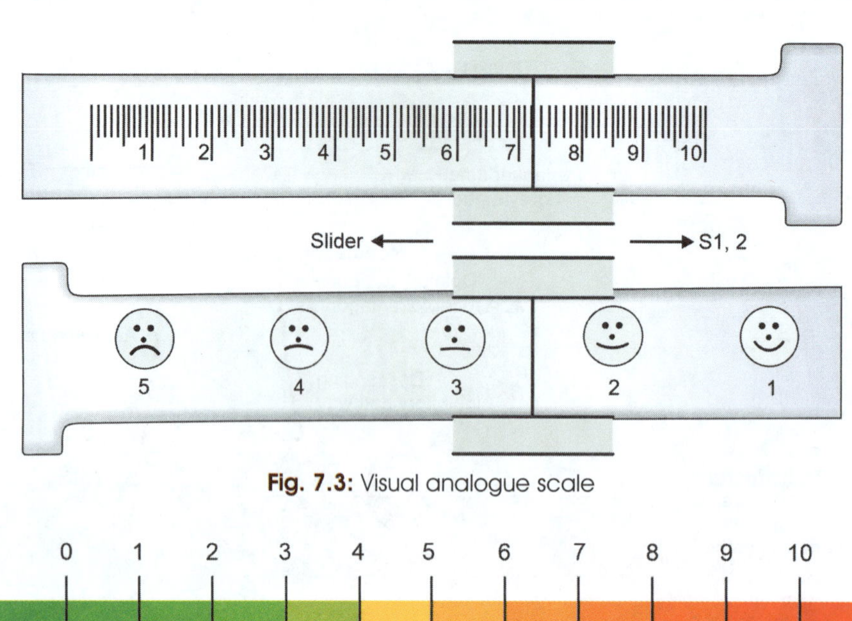

Fig. 7.3: Visual analogue scale

Fig. 7.4: Wong-Baker FACES scale

depicting severe pain (Fig. 7.4). This is particularly useful for older children.

ROUTES OF ADMINISTRATION OF ANALGESIA

Pain medications can be given by various routes.

Oral route: This route is a common method of providing postoperative analgesia for day care surgeries. A combination of a mild opioid such as codeine or tramadol along with paracetamol gives good pain relief for superficial surgeries such as hernia repair or breast lumpectomy. The oral route can be used only after the patient is able to take orally after surgery and thus would not be feasible in the immediate postoperative period after surgery on the bowel, etc. It is also not suitable for patients who are still sedated, not regained their ability to swallow and are at risk of aspiration. They may also have postoperative nausea and vomiting.

Intramuscular route: Regular injections of intramuscular opioids used to be given for postoperative pain relief. Although the analgesia might last longer than intermittent intravenous opioids, repeated intramuscular injections are not pleasant and must be avoided.

Subcutaneous route: To avoid the pain of repeated intramuscular injections, a cannula can be inserted subcutaneously, usually in the deltoid region and the intermittent injections can be given subcutaneously through this cannula. However, absorption of the medications can be unreliable.

Intravenous route: For patients who have undergone major surgery and are in-patients, postoperative analgesia is given very commonly by the intravenous route. This may be given intermittently on a regular and 'as required' basis by the nurse. A continuous infusion is better for the immediate postoperative period for a patient who has undergone major surgeries. These patients must be closely observed for any complications including respiratory depression and hypotension.

Epidural analgesia: This involves insertion of a thin plastic catheter into the epidural space before surgery. Infusion of dilute solution of local anaesthetic (0.25% bupivacaine or 0.2% ropivacaine) either alone or in combination with an opioid (usually fentanyl at 2 µg/cc) provides excellent analgesia. The patient is not drowsy, is more comfortable and outcomes are better.

Patient-controlled analgesia (PCA): This method is by far the most preferred and safest of the different approaches. By definition, the patient himself/herself administers the medication when he/she thinks pain

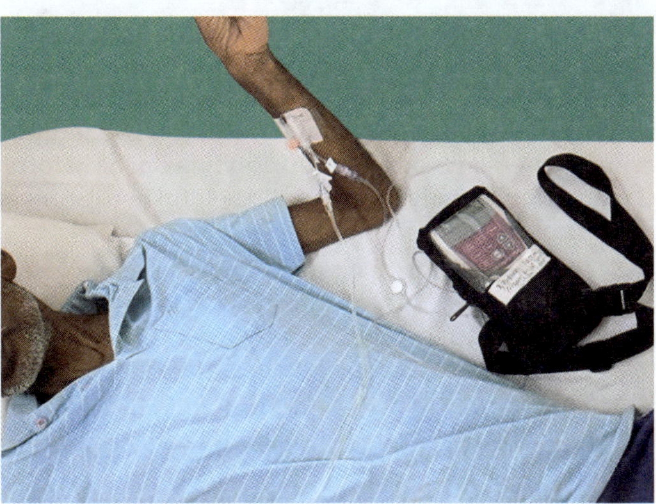

Fig. 7.5: Patient with PCA in our hospital

relief is required. This can be used for either intravenous route or the epidural route, although the drugs and dosages will differ with the route. This requires an electronic pump which can be programmed by the pain nurse or the anaesthetist. They can set the amount of **bolus** of the drug to be delivered, the minimum mandatory interval before which another bolus cannot be given (**lock-out period**) and the **hourly maximum dose**. The pump is fitted with a trigger button, which when pressed will deliver the drug to the patient. **To ensure safety, only the patient is allowed to press the button** and no one else (nurse, parent, relative, etc. not allowed). Thus, if a patient has been administered a bolus, unless he is awake enough to press the button, he would not get another dose. This increases safety (Fig. 7.5).

ADVERSE EFFECTS OF ANALGESIC MEDICATIONS

Provision of analgesia after surgery is humane and a necessity. However, it has to be titrated to the patient. The type of analgesia given to a patient will vary with the surgical procedure, patient consent, presence of comorbidities and facilities available at the hospital. Superficial and key-hole surgeries are associated with less pain compared to open major body cavity surgeries. A multimodal approach helps in reducing the amount of each medication and adds safety and efficacy to the treatment.

The patient must be monitored closely for any adverse effects due to these medications. Common adverse effects attributable to opioids are respiratory depression, hypotension and bradycardia. Epidural narcotics can produce pruritus as well. Local anaesthetics when given epidurally can cause hypotension and urinary retention. The patients must be monitored closely postoperatively and documented.

CHRONIC PAIN

When pain persists beyond three months of injury, it is termed chronic pain. While, in acute pain, the injured tissue is the source of pain; in chronic pain, the injured tissue might have 'healed' but the pain persists. This is due to plasticity of the spinal neurons and a phenomenon called wind-up. In this situation, an impulse that is normally painless also can become painful. Features of chronic pain include hyperaesthesia, hyperalgesia (increased sensitivity to touch and pain) and allodynia (stimuli that are not normally painful are sensed as painful). It can be debilitating and can affect health-related quality of life.

Types of Chronic Pain (Key Box 7.2)

1. **Neuropathic pain:** This type of pain is burning or shooting in nature. It can occur due to irritation of a nerve or due to entrapment of nerves. Diabetic neuropathy in the foot can produce neuropathic pain with tingling and numbness. Chronic groin pain after inguinal hernioplasty and mesh repair is not uncommon (10 to 15%). It may be due to ilioinguinal or genitofemoral nerve irritation or entrapment by mesh fibrosis or sutures. Thus, when performing mesh removal after a previous Lichtenstein repair, it is recommended to remove as much of the mesh as possible (preferably all mesh material) together with triple neurectomy anterior to the annulus, i.e. outside of the abdominal cavity without dissection behind the transversalis fascia.
2. **Nociceptive pain:** A nociceptor (pain receptor) is a sensory neuron that sends pain signals to the spinal cord and the brain as a result of damaging or potentially damaging stimuli. This pain occurs due to actual tissue injury, e.g. burns or bruises. These receptors are present in the skin and in the central nervous system. As a result of stimuli, the cutaneous nociceptors are activated leading to ***exaggerated*** response in the dorsal horn of the spinal cord.
3. **Psychogenic pain:** This is due to depression. This depression will add to any illness resulting in chronic pain.

Key Box 7.2

Types of Chronic Pain

1. Neuropathic pain
2. Nociceptive pain
3. Psychogenic pain
4. Musculoskeletal pain
5. Inflammatory pain
6. Mechanical pain

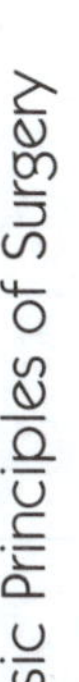

4. **Musculoskeletal pain:** This occurs due to excessive activity of muscles or consequent to injury to muscles or ligaments, e.g. back pain, myofascial pain.
5. **Inflammatory pain:** Autoimmune disorders such as rheumatoid arthritis or gout can be associated with joint pains as they get involved due to the disease.
6. **Mechanical pain:** Pain experienced by patients with malignant conditions is often due to expanding malignancy and involves stretch or compression of surrounding tissues, nerves, blood vessels or bone.

Management of Chronic Pain

Patient evaluation: A thorough history must be taken regarding the onset, characteristics, site, side, severity, etc. of the pain and associated symptoms. Unlike acute pain, it is important to also note how much this pain is interfering with the patient's daily activities. Structured questionnaires (McGill Pain Questionnaire) are available to document all aspects of this assessment. A detailed physical examination, especially neurologic examination must be done.

Treatment

This includes pharmacologic, nonpharmacologic, adjunct therapies and interventional treatments when they do not respond adequately to these.

Pharmacologic Treatment of Chronic Pain

The WHO has advised Step-Ladder pattern for the use of medications to treat chronic pain.

The WHO three-step analgesic ladder states as follows:
Step 1 (mild pain with NRS 1–4): Treated with acetaminophen and adjuvants as required.

Step 2 (moderate pain with NRS 5–6): Milder analgesics such as hydrocodone, oxycodone, tramadol, nonopioid analgesics and adjuvants can be used.

Step 3. In patients with severe pain (NRS 7–10), strong opioids such as morphine and fentanyl can be used in addition to those mentioned above. Morphine is usually given in the form of tablets or liquid every 4 or 6 hours. Slow release-enteric coated morphine is also available. Nausea and constipation are common complications. Morphine can also be given subcutaneously, if pain is severe.

First-line therapy for musculoskeletal pain includes nonsteroidal anti-inflammatory drugs and paracetamol. NSAIDs act by inhibiting the enzyme cyclooxygenase (COX), thereby blocking the production of prostaglandins. They may be contraindicated in patients with stomach ulcers and renal dysfunction. Adjunctive therapy includes capsaicin cream or lignocaine.

First-line drug for neuropathic pain is gabapentin or pregabalin. They prevent the reabsorption of neurotransmitters called **serotonin** and **norepinephrine**. They also reduce spontaneous neuronal activity. The addition of antidepressants such as amitriptyline can be helpful. Carbamazepine may be especially helpful in trigeminal neuralgia.

Second-line drugs include opioids. In more severe cases—example: Pain of chronic pancreatitis—oral preparations of morphine can be used. Fentanyl and buprenorphine cutaneous patches are also available. When patients have neuropathic and nociceptive elements, tapentadol can be used. It is an opioid with norepinephrine reuptake inhibition. Side effects of opioids such as constipation are less with this drug. However, the benefit of pain relief must be weighed against the possible side effects such as dependence, constipation, respiratory depression, etc. For this reason, adjunctive therapies must be tried first and opioids must be used with caution in patients, particularly with non-malignant conditions.

Nonpharmacological options include heat and cold therapy, relaxation therapy, ultrasound stimulation, acupuncture, physical therapy, occupational therapy, and TENS units. Interventional techniques such as epidural steroid injections, radiofrequency nerve ablations, nerve blocks and trigger point injections can be used to treat chronic pain. Transcutaneous nerve stimulators and acupuncture increase the levels of endorphin production in the central nervous system. In trigeminal neuralgia, nerve decompression is a better option by doing craniotomy than percutaneous coagulation of the ganglion.

ADJUNCTS

- **Neurolysis:** It refers to division of neural fibres, e.g. coeliac plexus blocks with alcohol in pancreatic cancer and gastric cancer.
- Anti-oestrogen drug such as tamoxifen 20 mg tablet in carcinoma breast and anti-androgen cyproterone 50/100 mg tablets in carcinoma prostate for disseminated metastasis are used. They also relieve bony pain. Both these drugs are antipituitary also, avoiding pituitary ablation surgery.
- **Infusion of diamorphine:** Various routes can be used: Intravenous, subcutaneous, intrathecal or epidural.

Pain is a symptom when acute and borders on to disease when chronic. If acute pain is well-addressed, the likelihood of chronic pain is much reduced. If chronic pain occurs, prompt treatment may be sought so that healing can be faster. Good pain relief will be taken as a blessing.

CHAPTER

8

Biohazard Disposal/ Biomedical Waste Management

- Hazards associated with biomedical waste (BMW)
- Steps of BMW management
- Segregation of biomedical waste
- BMW rules in India

Competency

SU15.1: Describe classification of hospital waste and appropriate methods of biomedical waste disposal.

INTRODUCTION

Biohazard or biomedical waste (BMW) refers to hazardous waste generated in the hospital during the diagnosis or treatment of patients, or in research laboratories, including experimental activities. Broadly, this generated waste falls into two categories—general waste (non-hazardous solid waste, 80%) and biomedical waste (20%). Biomedical waste includes infectious waste (10%) and chemical/radioactive waste (5%). Infectious waste can be from viruses, toxins, blood products, etc. Examples of chemical waste include solutions used in biochemistry labs or chemicals used for sterilization/ disinfection in operation theatres. Radioactive materials are used in the radionuclear department for isotope scanning or for treating diseases (e.g. thyroid disorders).

HAZARDS ASSOCIATED WITH BIOMEDICAL WASTE

- The WHO issued a statement in 2020 mentioning that due to improper methods of medical waste disposal, 21 million hepatitis B cases, 2 million hepatitis C cases, and 2,60,000 HIV cases had occurred.
- Broadly, biomedical waste can be classified as follows:
  1. **Infectious waste:** Example: Badly infected wounds in the leg or wounds in the perineum. Dangerous pathogens may cause dangerous infections in treating doctors or nurses. A few examples are given in Key Box 8.1.
  2. **Chemical waste:** These can produce corrosive and physical injuries.
  3. **Pharmaceutical waste:** A few drugs, such as nicotine, warfarin and epinephrine, can be acutely toxic. Cytotoxic drugs can cause mutations and can be teratogenic. A few drugs can be carcinogenic.
  4. **Radioactive waste:** These can produce genetic changes and tissue destruction.

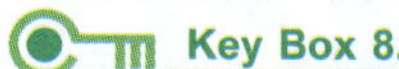

Key Box 8.1

Sources of Infectious Waste

- Cultures of infectious agents from laboratories
- Waste from surgeries and autopsies
- Waste originating from infected patients in isolation wards, e.g. feces and urine in cholera
- Waste having come in contact with infected hemodialysis patients (e.g. dialysis tubes, filters, disposable towels, gloves, aprons, etc.)

STEPS OF BMW MANAGEMENT

1. Identify points of waste generation—wards, OPDs, operation theatres, etc.
2. Segregate (at the point of generation) into the appropriate colour-coded containers.
3. Transport to the central collection point.
4. Apply barcode and sticker. This is as per the changes implemented in 2015.
5. Weigh the BMW to help approximate the amount generated. For example, in a 1000-bedded hospital, 1 bed may produce 500 g of BMW. Thus, all the waste in all different coloured containers are weighed.
6. Transport by a vehicle to the final treatment plant with a GPS system to track the vehicle and ensure proper disposal of the BMW. Treatment and/or disposal of waste should be done within 48 hours of generation.

Please note: Liquid BMW is collected from a separate line from all points and then joined together and collected in the effluent treatment plant (ETP). About 500 ml of HYPO is put in the sump to disinfect the liquid. Every month, a sample from this sump is sent to the pollution board for analysis to determine the efficacy of the system.

SEGREGATION OF BIOMEDICAL WASTE

According to BMW guidelines (2016), segregation should be done with containers of four different colours. Each container is designated for a particular waste category (Figs 8.1 and 8.2)

1. **Yellow:** Human tissues—pathology specimens, sponges, cotton, dressing materials, any item soaked with blood, sanitary pads, body fluids, tissue paper, masks, caps, bedding materials, expired drugs, cytotoxic drugs, discarded drugs, infected aspirated fluid from the body, liquids from floor washings or from laboratories. A separate sticker **-C-** is put for cytotoxic materials. Stickers are also put for COVID materials (Fig. 8.3).
2. **Red:** Disposable plastic materials that can be recycled—wastes generated from gloves, tubes, catheters, urine bags, etc.
3. **Black:** Paper, packing material, wrappers, glove covers, etc. These can be recycled.
4. **White:** Sharp objects—blades, scalpels, syringes with needles, suture material needles, etc.
5. **Blue:** Glass materials—broken ampules, discarded materials from labs or wards, metallic body implants.

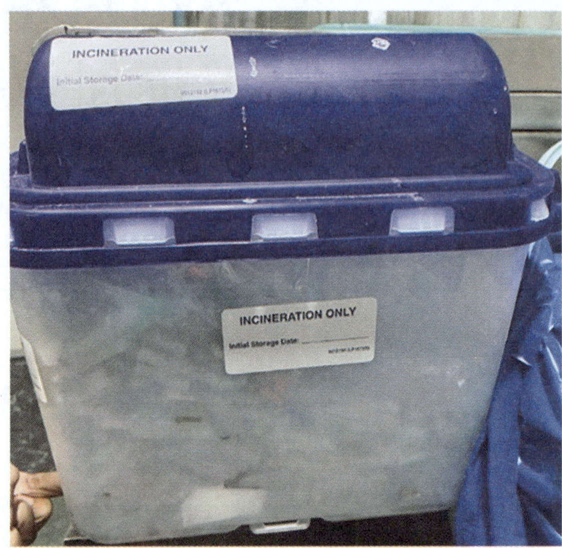

Fig. 8.1: Waste for incineration

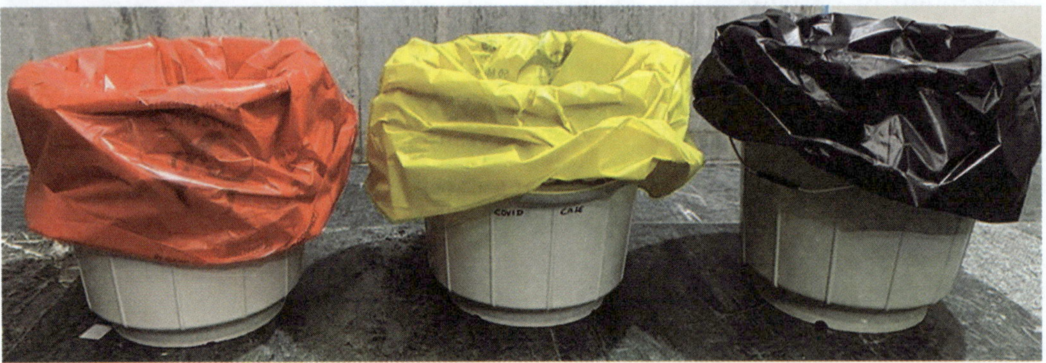

Fig. 8.2: Collection of biomedical wastes in different containers

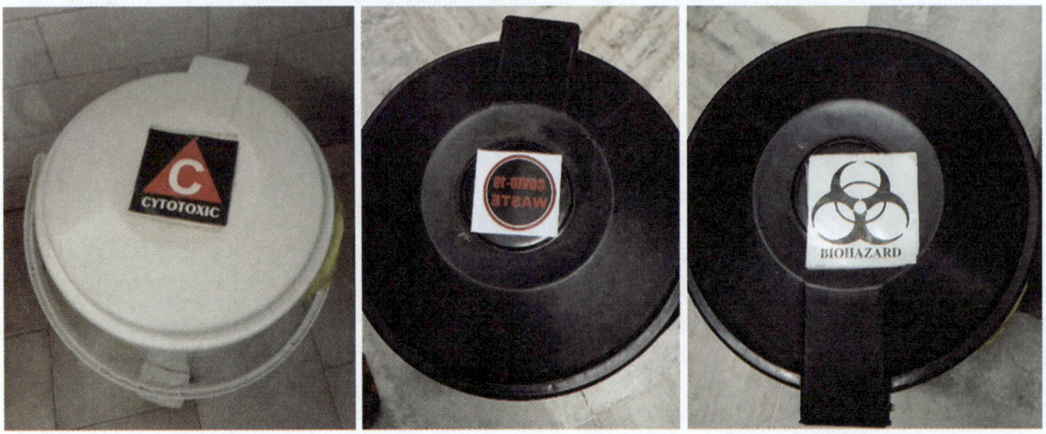

Fig. 8.3: Stickers indicating cytotoxic, COVID, and biohazard wastes

BMW RULES IN INDIA

The Ministry of Environment and Forests formulated a BMW rule in 1998 that had classified waste and segregated them into colour-coded containers. The new BMW guidelines (2016, with amendments added in 2018 and 2019) describe the following:

1. Every hospital should have a final disposal and recycling unit and a common biomedical waste treatment facility (CBMWTF).
2. Only if there is no CBMWTF within 75 km can a hospital create its own disposal facility.
3. Hospitals should have a biomedical committee that meets once in 6 months and submits an annual report to licensing authorities.
4. Doctors, nurses, and all healthcare workers should be educated about BMW management services.
5. Hospital committees should inspect the waste disposal area and functioning of the unit.
6. If required, audits can be done with CCTV cameras.

CHAPTER

9

Investigation and Interpretation

Competency

SU9.1: Choose appropriate biochemical, microbiological, pathological, imaging investigations and interpret the investigative data in a surgical patient.

Refer to the chapter on radiology for details about radiological investigations and interpretations.

INTRODUCTION

When a surgical patient is investigated for a disease, many investigations are done. Often many of them may not help either in the diagnosis or in the treatment (Key Box 9.1). **Ultrasound examination is the most common non-invasive and simple preliminary investigation in abdominal conditions, breast, thyroid or any cystic swellings. It has been called extension of surgeon's hand or extension of clinical examination**. To avoid unnecessary investigations, proper history taking including co-existing diseases such as diabetes, hypertension, allergy, etc. followed by a thorough clinical examination must be done first. Once a working diagnosis is made, relevant investigations are ordered. One should then see the results, interpret and give appropriate treatment. As you read further lines, you will get a better understanding. This topic deals with only a few examples, but students are expected to apply these principles to every disease. I have given four examples to highlight the importance of the investigations.

Key Box 9.1

Important Points to Remember

1. Investigations can be broadly classified as investigations that help in the diagnosis (to be done first), investigations that help in detecting spread of the disease (metastatic work-up in malignancies), and investigations to assess the fitness of the patient for surgery.
2. When you order investigations, ask yourself whether this investigation is necessary and will this patient benefit from this investigation?
3. Think twice before you order any invasive investigations that can be associated with serious complications. One example: Colonic perforation during colonoscopy. If you need to establish the diagnosis to prove tuberculosis/carcinoma, colonoscopy is certainly indicated. However, colonoscopy is not recommended for a patient with a 7-days history of constipation.
4. Need to know the side effects: *Example:* CECT scan. Exposure of the patient to CECT scan is equivalent to 200 chest X-rays and contrast used can give rise to renal failure.
5. Junior surgeons and postgraduates especially, who order investigations must also see the reports and try interpretation. If you have requested for MRI foot for diabetic foot, there is no need to obtain X-rays of the foot.

EXAMPLES

Example 1. Carbuncle (multiple hair follicle infections) over the nape of the neck

- This is a common problem in diabetic patients. Firstly, haematological investigations are ordered. Normal white cell count ranges between 4500 and 11000 cells per microliter. If white cell count is elevated, it indicates significant infection.
- Two important biochemical investigations which are obtained in a diabetic patient are fasting blood sugar—FBS, and post-prandial blood sugar—PPBS and creatinine. If blood sugars are high (FBS more than 150 mg/dl and PPBS more than 200 mg/dl), the patient has to be treated for diabetes. If serum creatinine is high, it indicates renal damage, and one has to be careful in selecting antibiotics—better to avoid gentamicin, amikacin, etc.

- If doubtful of the diagnosis, ultrasound imaging can be requested to confirm the diagnosis. An abscess will appear hypoechoic.
- Aspiration of pus seen at the ultrasound imaging is sent for culture and sensitivity.
- It is usually caused by *Staphylococcus aureus*, and it responds to cloxacillin or clindamycin. If patient has toxicity, we may have to start vancomycin.
- Once abscess is drained (Fig. 9.1), the tissue is sent for microbiological examination again. The wall of the abscess cavity or tissue can also be sent to pathology depending upon the nature of the abscess. Then look at the histopathology report and plan further treatment, if necessary.
- Thus, in this patient haematological investigations such as haemoglobin, total count including differential count of neutrophils, blood sugar and creatinine, imaging (may not be required in all), pus culture sensitivity are important.

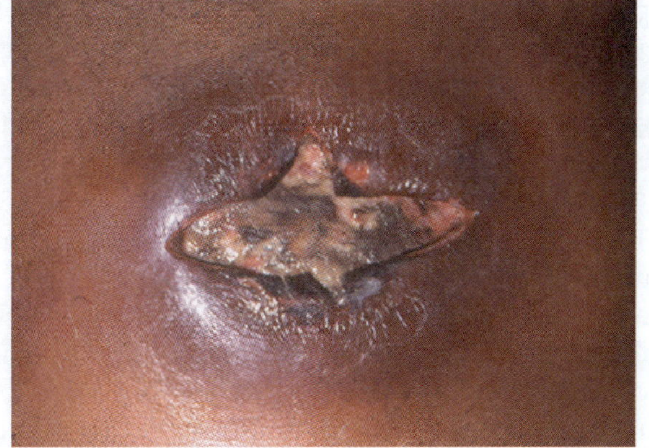

Fig. 9.1: Carbuncle on the back is incised by cruciate incision. Slough is removed. The pus is sent for culture sensitivity

Example 2. Toxic multinodular goitre

- Haematological investigations are ordered. 4,500 to 11,000 WBCs per microliter (4.5 to 11.0 × 10^9/l) is normal white blood cells count or leucocyte count.
- If leucocyte counts are low (4,000 cells/µl), it indicates leukopenia. It may be side effect of drugs used to control toxicity. *Example:* Carbimazole, in this case.
- Thyroid hormone levels: T_3 and T_4 levels are elevated suggesting thyrotoxicosis. Usually, T_4 toxicosis is common. When these hormones are elevated, thyroid-stimulating hormone (TSH) is very low due to feedback mechanism. In Hashimoto's thyroiditis or in cases of hypothyroidism, TSH is elevated but T_3 and T_4 are usually low. Hence, they need thyroid hormone supplementation.
- Ultrasound imaging is the first investigation. Look for nodules, nature of nodules, suggestion of malignancy (details are given in thyroid chapter).
- Ultrasound-guided FNAC is not done in toxic nodules but is routine in all thyroid swellings to rule out malignancy. If any mitotic figures or microcalcifications are present it will suggest malignancy.
- In large goitres, vital structrues such as trachea, esophagus, internal jugular vein and common carotid arteries are displaced or infiltrated as in malignant goitres. To identify these anatomical structures and to avoid injuries to these strictures, CECT scan can also be done.
- A few other investigations are done to assess fitness of the patient, to control comorbidity, if any, in this patient. Cardiac status—echocardiogram to know the ejection fraction, and if necessary, coronary angiogram in cases of myocardial ischemia.

Example 3. Obstructive jaundice: As you can see here, sclera are stained with bilirubin—deep yellow coloured almost with greenish tinge due to biliverdin deposition. Following investigations are done and interpretations are given below. The patient had carcinoma head of the pancreas with palpable gallbladder (Fig. 9.2).

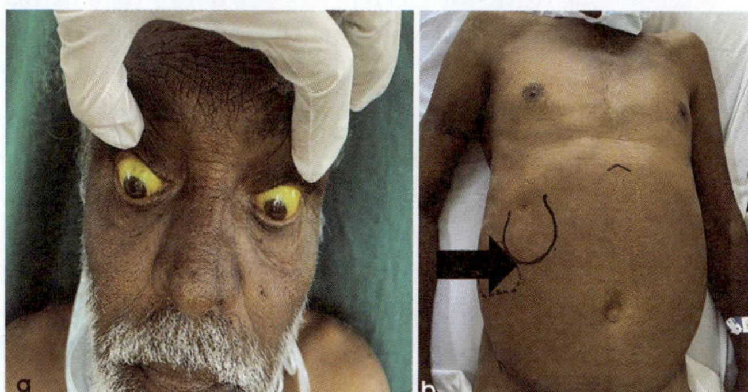

Fig. 9.2: (a) Deep yellow sclera; (b) Palpable gallbladder

- Liver function test: Bilirubin, alanine transaminase (ALT), aspartate transaminase (AST), alkaline phosphatase (ALP), albumin and total protein, gamma-glutamyl transferase (GGT), L-lactate dehydrogenase (LD), prothrombin time (PT).
  a. Normal bilirubin levels are 0.2 to 0.6 mg/dl. Elevation beyond 2 mg/dl will be visible in the sclera. Very high values are often found in obstructive jaundice. If more than 50% of the total bilirubin is direct bilirubin, it is obstructive in origin. If more than 50% is indirect, it could be hemolytic jaundice.
  b. ALT and AST levels are elevated in hepatitis because they represent hepatocellular damage.
  c. ALP is elevated when there is obstruction to the biliary tree—classically in a patient with obstructive jaundice. (More details in Chapter 42, page 616).

d. Albumin is synthesised only in the liver. Hence low levels of albumin is a feature of chronic liver disease or chronic malnutrition.

e. GGT: The main role of GGT is helping the liver in metabolising drugs or toxins. High levels of GGT are seen in liver diseases including chronic alcoholic liver damage and fatty liver.

f. LDH: Normal levels: 140 units per litre (U/L) to 280 U/L. Increased levels are seen in high tumour burden cases which means tumour is spreading. It can also be seen in benign conditions with increased tissue breakdown.

g. INR and prothrombin time will be prolonged.

- Culture and sensitivity: If patient has high grade fever with chills and rigors, it indicates cholangitis— send blood for culture and sensitivity. Invariably gram-negative organisms dominate along with other organisms.
- Imaging: When ultrasound probe is kept in the right hypochondrium, one can see dilated biliary radicles—which is the first indication of distal obstruction. If gallbladder is also enlarged, it will suggest lower bile duct obstruction.
- CT scan is done not only to confirm ultrasound findings but also to know the resectability by demonstrating plane between superior mesenteric vein/superior mesenteric artery—if it shows hypodense lesions, they suggest secondaries in the liver.
- Tumour markers such as CEA (carcinoembryonic antigen) and CA 19-9 were normal. Details about tumour markers are given in the respective topics such as gallbladder cancer, pancreatic head cancer and carcinoma colon, etc.
- One example of a typical patient with obstructive jaundice has been given here.

Total bilirubin (serum)	(H) 20.94 mg/dl
Direct bilirubin (serum)	(H) >17 mg/dl
Total protein (serum)	6.40 g/dl
Albumin (serum)	3.50 g/dl
Globulin	2.90 g/dl
Aspartate transaminase (AST) (serum)	(H) 51 IU/L
Alanine transaminase (ALT) (serum)	32.0 IU/L
Alkaline phosphatase (ALP) (serum)	(H) 568 U/L

- If you see this report of a jaundice patient, direct bilirubin is more than 50% of total bilirubin with very high values of alkaline phosphatase—it suggests obstructive jaundice.
- Tumour markers in this patient done were: CEA: 3.0 ng/ml and CA 19-9: 21 U/ml. These are done to find out or to get the clue about possibility of gallbladder cancer or carcinoma head of the pancreas.

Example 4. Carcinoma breast

- Initial triple assessment is done: Clinical examination, mammogram and tru-cut biopsy are done and carcinoma is confirmed.
- Then metastatic work-up: If chest X-ray shows cannon ball metastasis, it is a stage 4 disease.
- CT-PET scan is done to look for metastasis all over the body depending upon staging and grading of the tumours, etc. (details are given later).
- Core needle biopsy is subjected for immunohistochemistry. It is required to plan appropriate chemotherapy or hormonal therapy or therapy with newer agents including trastuzumab. Details of IHC are given below.

IMMUNOHISTOCHEMISTRY (IHC)

Immunohistochemistry, also known as IHC, is an important diagnostic modality in the work-up of cancers. It is widely applied in the field of oncopathology to detect the presence of specific antigens on the tumour cell, that help in confirmation of cancers and their subtyping. It is useful in identifying the cell type and origin of a metastasis to find the site of the primary tumour. IHC is also widely used to predict the response to therapy in various tumours, i.e. carcinoma of breast.

The technique involves fixing tumour tissue using a chemical such as formaldehyde which stabilises the structural properties of tissue. The tissue is then incubated with an appropriate primary antibody against specific tumour antigens/proteins, followed by a secondary antibody that is conjugated with a dye or enzyme. The binding of antigen on tumour with the antibody brings about a color reaction which is then visualized under microscope.

The panel of immunohistochemical antibodies available is substantial that are used as diagnostic, prognostic and predictive biomarkers. Following are some examples of commonly used IHC antibodies:

- Estrogen receptor (ER) (Figs 9.3 and 9.4), progesterone receptor (PR), Her 2 and Ki 67 (proliferation marker) in breast cancers for subtyping and predicting response to therapy.
- Cytokeratin 7 and cytokeratin 20 in the work-up of metastasis of unknown origin.
- CD15 and CD30 in Hodgkin's lymphoma (Fig. 9.5).
- CD19, 20 for B cell lymphomas, CD3 for T cell lymphoma.
- CD117 for gastrointestinal stromal tumours.
- CD99 and FLI 1 for Ewing's sarcoma.
- Melanoma: S100
- Vascular: CD31, CD34
- Colorectum: Cytokeratin

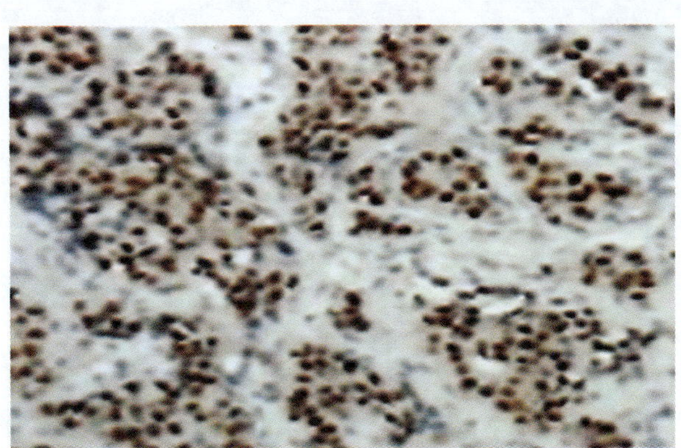

Fig. 9.3: Positive staining for oestrogen receptor (seen as brown nuclear positivity in tumour cells of breast cancer) helps to predict response to tamoxifen therapy

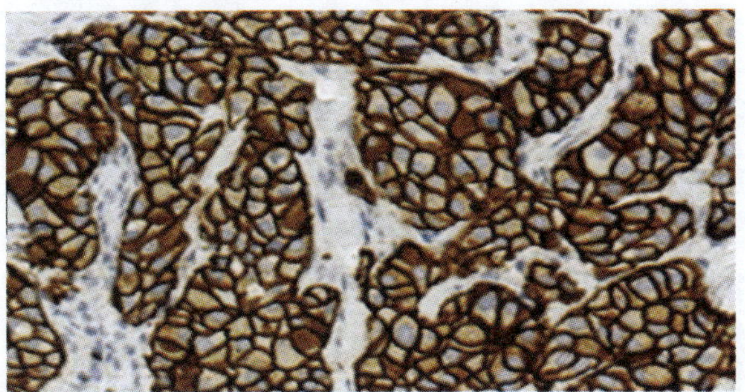

Fig. 9.4: Positive staining for Her2 (seen as strong brown membranous positivity in tumor cells of breast cancer) helps to predict response to targeted therapy with Trastuzumab (*Courtesy:* Dr Kanthilatha Pai, HOD pathology, KMC Manipal for contributing IHC slides and write up.)

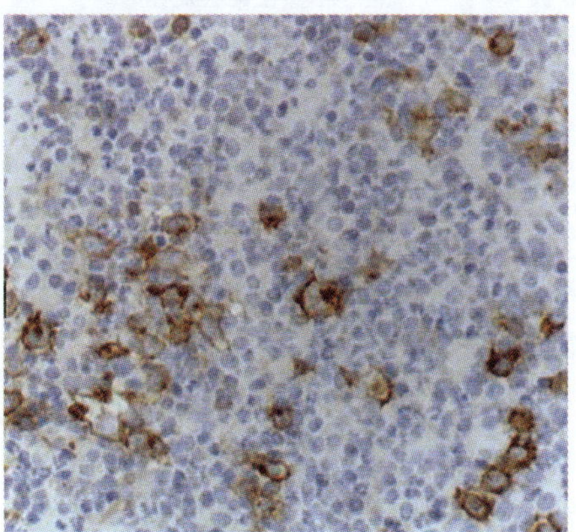

Fig. 9.5: Positively staining with CD30 of Reed-Sternberg cells helps to confirm diagnosis of Hodgkin's lymphoma

- Ovary: CA125, CK20
- Prostate: PSA
- GIST: CD117
- Thus, immunohistochemical stains can detect all types of tumours and can confirm malignancy. **S100 and actin stains** can be used to identify the **myoepithelial cell layer** in a duct or gland.
- IHC may also help in selecting a treatment and making prognostic predictions. Examples: Carcinoma of the breast is assessed for oestrogen receptor, progesterone receptor, and HER2 status.
- IHC can also detect infections such as cytomegalovirus (CMV), Epstein-Barr virus (EBV), etc. and detect an abnormal accumulation of **proteins** or **amyloid.**

Please note: *Abdominal investigations and interpretations require theoretical knowledge of both surgical and radiological investigations. One example of how to arrive at the diagnosis is given below. As you read the entire textbook you will be in a better position to understand this aspect.*

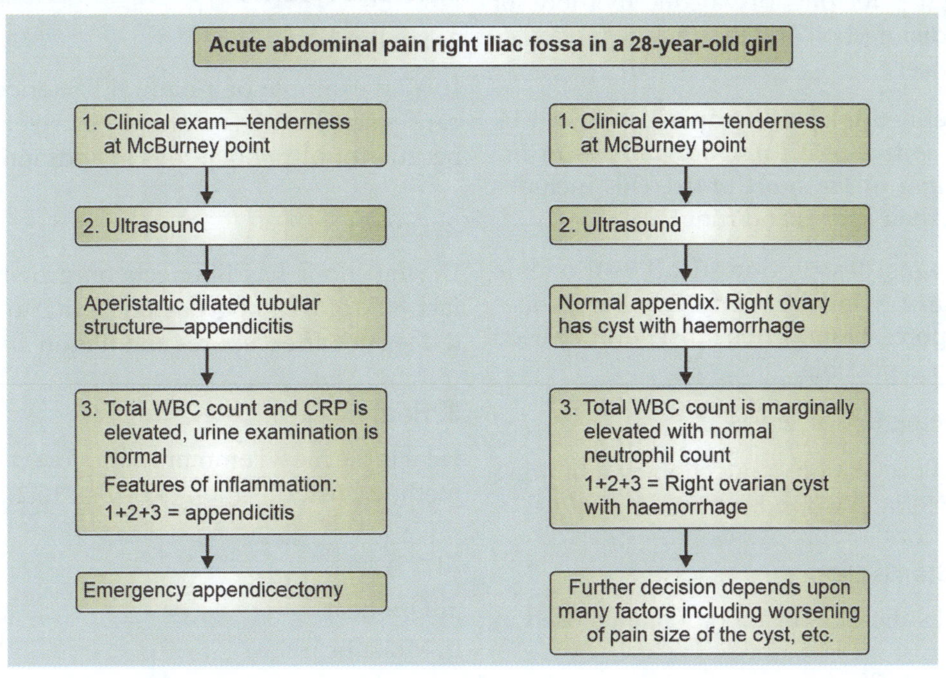

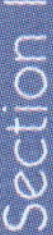

CHAPTER

10

Asepsis, Sterilization and Disinfection

- Sterilization
- Disinfection
- Physical agents
- Chemical agents

Competency

SU14.1: Describe aseptic techniques, sterilization and disinfection.

SURGICAL PATIENT

In spite of scientific advances in understanding pathogenesis of various diseases and better understanding of pharmacotherapy, infection remains the 'number one' enemy for surgeons. So, every attempt should be made to minimise the infection rates in the ward, hospital and in the operation theatre. Joseph Lister called infective agents as disease dust and introduced carbolic acid spray as an antiseptic agent. Hence, ***Joseph Lister is called the father of modern surgery.*** This chapter deals with fundamental principles of various methods of sterilisation and disinfection and their usage in day-to-day clinical practice.

Sterilisation is defined as a process by which an article, object or surface is free of ***all microorganisms in the vegetative form and in the spore state.*** This includes viruses, bacteria, their spores and fungi.

Disinfection means destruction of all pathogenic organisms capable of giving rise to infection. Rarely does this process kill spores. Disinfection must never be used when sterilisation is possible.

Asepsis means being free of sepsis.

Antisepsis means prevention of infection by inhibiting the growth of bacteria in wounds or tissues.

Agents Used in Sterilisation

Key Box 10.1 gives the classification of agents used in sterilisation.

Key Box 10.1

Classification

Physical agents	Chemical agents
1. Sunlight	1. Alcohol
2. Drying	2. Aldehyde
3. Heat	3. Dye
• Dry heat	4. Halogens
• Moist heat	5. Phenols and cresols
4. Filtration	6. Gases
5. Radiation	7. Surface-active agents
	8. Metallic salts

PHYSICAL AGENTS

1. Sunlight

It is an example of a natural bactericidal agent which causes sterilisation of tank water, rivers, etc. It is mainly because of ultraviolet rays in addition to heat rays.

2. Drying

Drying in air has ill-effects on growth of bacteria. In fact, 80% of weight of bacteria is due to water. However, it does not affect spores and it is an ***unreliable*** method.

3. Heat

Heat is the most commonly employed and most reliable method of sterilisation (Key Box 10.2).

Two Types

I. Dry heat

II. Moist heat

Key Box 10.2

Heat

- Most reliable
- Rapid method of sterilisation
- No harmful residue

I. Dry Heat

This method of heat kills the organisms by protein denaturation and oxidative damage.

Types

a. **Red heat:** Inoculating loop or wires, tip of forceps and needles are held in the flame of a Bunsen burner till they become red hot.

b. **Flaming:** Glass slides, scalpels and mouths of culture tubes are passed through Bunsen flame a few times.

c. **Incineration:** This is used to destroy soiled dressings, bedding, bandages, etc.

d. **Hot air oven** is the most widely used method of sterilisation by dry heat (Key Box 10.3).
   - Temperature required is 160°C for one hour or 180°C for 20 minutes.
   - Glassware, forceps, scissors, scalpel glass syringe can be sterilized. Materials like oils, greases, dry powder, etc. can also be sterilized by this method.

Key Box 10.3

Hot Air Oven

- Glass syringes, test tubes, pipettes
- Metal forceps, scissors, scalpels
- Oil, jelly, powder
- Swab sticks

Sterilisation control—indicators

1. Spores of nontoxigenic strain of *Clostridium tetani*
2. Browne's tube
3. Thermocouples.

II. Moist Heat

This method of heat kills organisms by coagulation and denaturation of their proteins.

In case of spores, steam condenses on it, increases its water content, causes hydrolysis and breakdown of the bacterial protein.

Types

A. At temperature below 100°C

a. **Pasteurisation:** Temperature of 63°C for 30 minutes (holder method) or 72°C for 15 to 20 seconds (flash method), followed by cooling quickly to 13°C or lower. Mycobacteria, brucellae and salmonellae are destroyed by this method but spores are not destroyed.

b. **Inspissation:** Serum or egg media (Lowenstein-Jensen media) are sterilized in the inspissator at 80–85°C for half an hour on three consecutive days.

c. **Vaccine bath:** Vaccines of nonsporing bacteria are sterilised in special vaccine baths at 60°C for one hour.

B. At 100°C

a. **Boiling** (temperature 100°C): Vegetative bacteria are killed at 100°C but sporing bacteria require considerable time for boiling. Hence, boiling is not recommended for sterilising instruments.

b. **Tyndallisation:** Steam at 100°C for 20 minutes on three consecutive days. It is used for sterilisation of egg, serum or sugar containing media.

c. **Autoclaving or steam under pressure** (temperature above 100°C): This is the most popular method.

Principle: Water boils when its vapour pressure equals that of surrounding atmosphere. When pressure inside a closed vessel increases, the temperature at which water boils also increases. When steam comes into contact with cooler surface, it condenses to water and gives up its latent heat to that surface. Condensed water ensures moist conditions for killing the microbes present. All the air must be removed from autoclave chamber before autoclaving.

Temperature employed: Sterilisation is carried out between 108°C and 147°C. Commonly, temperature of 121°C at 15 lb pressure for 15 minutes is used (Key Box 1.5).

- Thus dressings, instruments, laboratory-ware, media can be sterilised with autoclaving. However, it is not suitable for bottled fluids.

Sterilisation control: Spores of *Bacillus stearothumophilus* are used as test organism.

- Chemical indicators: Browne's tubes
- Thermocouples
- Autoclave tapes.

4. Filtration

It is used to get rid of microorganisms from heat labile liquids and substances such as sugars and urea, which are used for preparation of media. Hence, it is useful for antibiotic solutions, sera and carbohydrate solutions used in the preparation of culture medium. Different types of filter include earthenware filters, asbestos filters, sintered glass filters, membrane filters, etc.

5. Radiation

a. **Nonionising radiation:** Low energy type, for example:
   1. *Infrared radiation:* Used for mass sterilisation of syringes.
   2. *Ultraviolet radiation:* This can be used to disinfect hospital ward, operation theatre, viral laboratory, etc.

b. **Ionising radiation:** X-rays, gamma rays are examples. They have high penetration power and highly lethal to all cells including bacteria. ***Gamma radiation is used to sterilise plastic tubes, catheters, syringes, culture plates, etc.*** This method is also known as ***cold sterilisation,*** as there is no appreciable increase in the temperature.

CHEMICAL AGENTS

Chemical agents act by protein coagulation and disruption of cell membrane. They are mainly used for disinfection rather than sterilisation.

Disinfectants are antimicrobial agents used to kill potentially infectious agents present on inanimate object, e.g. surfaces, water, etc.

Chemical disinfectants which can be safely applied to skin or mucous membrane and are used to prevent infection by inhibiting the growth of bacteria are called *antiseptics.*

1. Alcohols

Ethyl alcohol (ethanol) and isopropyl alcohol are commonly used. They rapidly kill bacteria, including tubercle bacilli, but they have no action on spores and viruses. They are used in concentration of 60–70% in water as skin antiseptics before a surgical incision.

- ***Isopropyl alcohol*** is better than ethanol because it is fat solvent, more bactericidal and less volatile. Hence, it is used to disinfect clinical ***thermometers.***
- Methyl alcohol is effective against fungal spores. However, it is ***toxic*** and inflammable and hence, not used.

2. Aldehydes

They are bactericidal and sporicidal.

a. ***Formaldehyde (HCHO):*** This is used to preserve anatomical specimen. It is an irritant, water-soluble gas.
   - Formaldehyde gas is used to fumigate wards, sick rooms, etc.

b. ***Glutaraldehyde:*** It is effective against ***tubercle bacilli, fungi and viruses.*** It is less irritant than formaldehyde.
   - This is used to sterilise cystoscopes, bronchoscopes, endotracheal tubes and metal instruments, which are heat-sensitive.
   - 2% buffered solution is used.
   - It has no deleterious effect on cement or lenses of instrument.
   - Commercially available as 'Cidex'.

3. Dyes

- They are aniline dyes (Key Box 10.4) and acridines which are used as skin and wound antiseptics. Acriflavine, proflavine are the examples for acridine dyes.
- They act against gram-positive and gram-negative organisms. They are little, if at all, affected by presence of pus.
- Whenever a cavity has to be packed or a tie over dressing to be applied following skin grafting, gauze soaked in acriflavine can be used.

Key Box 10.4

Aniline Dyes

- Brilliant green, malachite green, crystal violet
- More active against gram-positive organisms
- Pus inhibits their activity

4. Halogens

Iodine is a bactericidal agent with moderate activity on spores. It is also active against tubercle bacillus. Iodine is used almost exclusively as a skin disinfectant (antiseptic).

- Mixtures of iodine with surface-active agents that act as carrier for iodine are known as ***iodophores.*** Betadine is an example of this. This is also active against fungi, trichomonas.
- When chlorine or hypochlorites are added to water, the chlorine reacts with water to form hypochlorous acid. It is a strong oxidizing agent and effective disinfectant.
- Chlorine and hypochlorite solution (EUSOL) also are other examples.

5. Phenols and Cresols

These are obtained by distillation of coal between temperatures of 170°C and 270°C. They cause cell membrane damage.

- Phenol (carbolic acid) was introduced first by Lister, father of antiseptic surgery. It is a powerful microbicidal substance. It is bactericidal at a concentration of 1%.
- Lysol, cresols, chlorhexidine are also phenols. Chlorhexidine (hibitane) is nontoxic, skin antiseptic, active against gram-positive and also gram-negative organisms and moderately active against mycobacteria.

6. Gases (Vapour-Phase Disinfectants)

a. ***Ethylene oxide:*** It is a highly inflammable, colourless gas. Hence, it is mixed with inert gases such as carbon dioxide or nitrogen so that its explosive tendency is eliminated. It is highly lethal to all kinds of microbes including spores and tubercle bacilli.

- It is used for sterilising heart-lung equipment, books, clothing, glass, plastic, etc. Thus routinely used catheters such as Foley's catheters, Ryle's tube, etc. are sterilised by ethylene oxide gas.

b. ***Formaldehyde gas:*** Used for fumigation of operation theatres and rooms, often after doing septic case.

c. ***Betapropiolactone:*** It is also used for fumigating purposes. It is also active against viruses.

7. Surface-active Agents

Substances that alter energy relationships at interfaces leading to reduction of surface or interfacial tension are known as surface-active agents or surfactants. They are used as wetting agents, detergents, etc.

- The most commonly used preparations are cationic surface-active agents. They are bactericidal. They have no action on spores, tubercle bacilli, etc. Commercially available preparation include cetrimide (cetavlon). They are most active in alkaline pH. *Pseudomonas aeruginosa* is particularly resistant to these compounds.
- Soaps are also active against gram-positive and gram-negative organisms.

8. Metallic Salts

The salts of silver, copper and mercury are used as disinfectants. Mercurochrome is less toxic and is used as mild antiseptic.

Clinically it is used in the treatment of skin grafted ulcers after the graft has taken up well.

- Few examples of sterilization are given in Key Box 10.5

Key Box 10.5

Quick Revision of Sterilization of Commonly Used Instruments in the Operation Theatre

- Surgeon's knife (scalpel) : Glutaraldehyde
- Forceps, retractors, etc. : Hot air oven
- Foley's catheter : Gas sterilisation (ethylene oxide)
- Glass syringes : Hot air oven
- Operation theatre : Formaldehyde gas
- Clinical thermometer : Isopropyl alcohol

TESTING OF DISINFECTANTS

1. ***Rideal-Walker test:*** Phenol is taken as standard disinfectant. Suspension of typhoid bacilli is subjected to the action of varying concentrations of phenol and the disinfectant to be tested and compared with phenol.
2. ***Chick-Martin test:*** Disinfectant acts in presence of organic matter.

CHAPTER

11

Nutrition in Surgical Patients

Competency

SU12.1: Enumerate the causes and consequences of malnutrition in the surgical patients.

Introduction

The goal of nutritional support in the surgical patient is to prevent or reverse the catabolic effects of disease or injury and to ensure that their nutritional requirements are met using the most suitable route with minimal complications. The ultimate validation for nutritional support should be improvement in clinical outcome and restoration of function.

Pearls of Wisdom

Nutrition is an important component of the care of the surgical or critically ill patient. Malnutrition can be fatal. Overnutrition can also be harmful. Provision of services of a physician, dietician, microbiologist and good nursing care are vital to patient recovery.

CAUSES OF MALNUTRITION

1. Patient is not able to swallow/eat: Carcinoma oesophagus, carcinoma stomach
2. Anastomotic breakdown: Leak after Whipple's pancreaticoduodenectomy, after colonic or intestinal resections
3. Enterocutaneous fistula
4. Small gut syndrome
5. Debilitating diseases: Crohn's disease, intestinal tuberculosis, advanced malignancies

CONSEQUENCES OF MALNUTRITION OR PATHOPHYSIOLOGY OF GASTROINTESTINAL (GI) FAILURE

Autocannibalism: When gastrointestinal tract (GIT) fails or during starvation, the existing energy stores are consumed to supply energy. Glycogen stored in the liver undergoes glycogenolysis and gets depleted in 24 to 48 hours. Normal physiological functions of the organs of an average adult at rest [Basal metabolic rate (BMR)/ Resting energy expenditure (REE)] need about 20 kcal/ kg/day. Therefore, when GIT fails, the fat in the adipose tissue and protein in the muscles and viscera are mobilised and metabolised to supply and sustain REE. This is called autocannibalism (eating one's own tissues to survive). It weakens the muscles (e.g. respiratory and cardiac muscles), viscera (liver, kidneys, etc.) and immune system, resulting in increased morbidity and mortality (Fig. 11.1).

Patients receiving intravenous (IV) fluids are semi-starving: 500 ml of 5% dextrose containing 25 g of dextrose provides about 100 kcal (each gram of carbohydrate provides about 4 kcal), and, therefore, an adult kept nil by mouth (NBM) and receiving 4–5 bottles of 5% dextrose/day gets about 400–500 kcal. The balance amount of REE (for a 50 kg individual, REE = 50 × 25 = 1250 kcal; 1250 – 500 = 750 kcal) comes from glycogen for 24 to 48 hours and thereafter from autocannibalism which is detrimental.

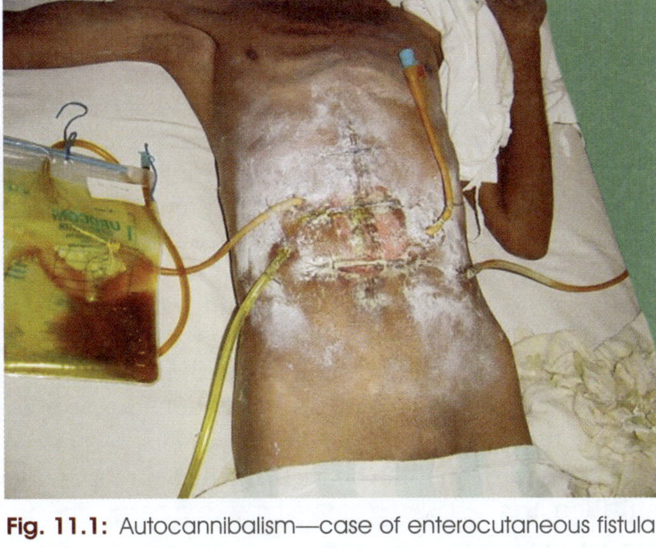

Fig. 11.1: Autocannibalism—case of enterocutaneous fistula

Fasting in healthy persons versus fasting in patients: When resting healthy persons are fasting, the metabolic rate drops to basal level. Although critically ill patients who are kept nil by mouth (NBM) are also resting, their basal metabolic rate is accelerated (hypermetabolic), and their REE is increased proportionate to the level of stress due to injury or illness.

PATIENT EVALUATION

Every patient admitted to the hospital must have their nutritional status assessed to determine the severity of nutrient deficiencies or excess and to predict the nutritional requirements.

A thorough history

- History of unintentional weight loss: Weight loss is an important indicator of nutritional status. A recent history of 20% weight loss indicates mild, 20 to 40% moderate, and more than 40% severe undernutrition. Body mass index (BMI) is another easily calculated indicator. Mid-arm circumference and triceps skin fold thickness are anthropometric indices that are useful. Low serum albumin (3–3.5 g%—mild, 2–3 g%—moderate, and <2 g%—severe undernutrition) is not a sensitive indicator because of the long half-life and a large pool size. Prealbumin, retinol-binding protein and transferrin have shorter half-lives, smaller pool size and are more sensitive indicators.
- History of chronic illness
- Dietary habits and any recent changes
- Medication intake

A complete physical examination

- Assess loss of muscle and adipose tissues by anthropometric techniques such as skin fold thickness and midarm circumference.
- Skin and hair changes
- Neuromuscular functions
- Any organ dysfunction

Biochemical determinants

- Albumin and prealbumin levels
- Transferrin levels
- Creatinine excretion
- Total lymphocyte count (assess immunologic function)

ESTIMATING ENERGY REQUIREMENTS

Several equations can be used to calculate the energy requirement for a given individual. The most widely accepted equation is the Harris-Benedict equation that estimates the resting energy expenditure (REE) or the basal metabolic rate (BMR).

In a normal resting physiological state, the BMR for men and women is as follows.

Men:

BMR = 66.5 + (13.75 × weight in kg) + (5.003 × height in cm) – (6.775 × age in years)

Women:

BMR = 655.1 + (9.563 × weight in kg) + (1.850 × height in cm) – (4.676 × age in years)

Use of simple formulae such as 25–30 kcal/kg/day to provide nutrients is also acceptable. Another method is by using indirect calorimetry and calculation of nitrogen balance. As surgical patients undergo physiological stresses, the value thus derived needs to be multiplied by a stress factor to calculate accurate energy requirements. For practical purposes, it is easier to remember that the adult REE is 20 kcal/kg/day and it increases to 25, 30, and 40 kcal/kg/day in mild, moderate and severe stress.

Condition	Stress factor
Moderate malnutrition	
Minor elective surgery	1.1
Mild stress	
Major elective surgery	1.2
Moderate stress	
Skeletal trauma	1.4
Severe stress	
Head injury	1.6
Severe burns	2

For example, a 55-year-old man, with a weight of 60 kg and a height of 170 cm, is undergoing major GI surgery, then his basal caloric requirement is 30 × 60 kg = 1800 kcal. A stress factor of 1.2 can be added for elective major surgery, it becomes 2160, or roughly 2200 kcal.

How much nutrition to be given: Sixty per cent of the total calories should come from carbohydrates and 40% from fats. These calories are nonprotein calories. Calories obtained from proteins should not be taken into account for calculating the energy needs because they are building blocks in tissue repair and are not meant for burning for calories. The protein requirement of the resting adult is 0.8 g/kg/day, and it increases to 1.1, 1.5, and 2.1 g/kg/day in mild, moderate and severe stress. Recommended daily allowances of vitamins, minerals and trace elements are added to the formulations. The daily intake and output of fluids should also be calculated and balanced.

PERIOPERATIVE NUTRITIONAL SUPPORT

- Preoperative assessment of nutritional status must be done in patients undergoing elective surgery and nutritional support provided in those who are not able to take it volitionally. Nutritional support is given to meet energy requirements for essential metabolic processes and tissue repair, and to meet substrate requirements for protein synthesis. A healthy adult can withstand semistarvation (receiving IV fluids only) for about 4 to 5 days without ill-effects. Beyond this period, they need nutritional support in order to prevent the adverse effects of autocannibalism. Many patients are nutritionally depleted at the time of admission and will need nutritional support much earlier.
- Cells can perform their function only when they get nutrients and oxygen. When the nutrients are metabolised in the cells, the tissues get energy to perform their physiological functions. Gastrointestinal system (GIT) is the source of supply of nutrients (energy) to all the tissues. It has to supply nutrients on a day-to-day basis because the body has limited expendable reserves (stores). Lack of nutrients results in energy crisis.
- In critical care units, priority is given to treatment of hypoxia, haemorrhage, haemodynamic instability, fluid, electrolyte, acid–base imbalance, and sepsis. These deserve their priority, but hyponutrition and the consequent energy crisis should not be ignored.
- In healthy, non-malnourished patients undergoing elective surgery, the insult to metabolism begins when the patient is kept NPO from midnight in anticipation of surgery. In cases of GI surgeries, this might be followed by a fasting period in the postoperative period also, leading to a starvation period of more than 24 hours. This can strain the starvation response, and must be prevented for best outcomes. Recent enhanced recovery after surgery (ERAS) protocols allow liquid intake up to 2 hours before surgery, encourage carbohydrate loading preoperatively which help in dampening the metabolic insult. In malnourished patients, although a total correction of malnutrition before elective surgery may not be possible, some form of preoperative intervention can be impactful in selected patients. A few factors to be considered are the indication for the surgery, whether elective or emergency (should not risk delaying the surgery to optimise the patient nutritionally in case of life-threatening conditions), the patient's level of malnutrition, likelihood of it responding to preoperative nutrition and the available options for supplementation.

A few criteria that can be used to initiate preoperative nutrition are:

- BMI <18 kg/m^2
- Unintentional weight loss of more than 10% of body weight in 6 months.
- Serum albumin <3 g/dl
- If patient is expected to be unable to meet caloric requirements for more than 7 days perioperatively.
- Catabolic diseases

ROLE OF IMMUNONUTRITION

- Patients undergoing elective surgery benefit from preoperative initiation of immunonutrition as injury induced by surgery leads to significant suppression of immune function. It must be initiated 5–7 days preoperatively for optimum benefit. Patients who may benefit include severely malnourished patients undergoing major oncologic GI surgery, head and neck surgery, patients with severe trauma or burns. Studies have shown that their administration is associated with reduced rates of infection and other complications, and shorter length of hospital stay.

The nutrients that have been proven to cause improvement in immune functions include:

- Arginine: Supports T lymphocytes; provides substrate for generation of nitric oxide
- Glutamine
- Omega-3 polyunsaturated fatty acids: Promotes synthesis of favourable prostaglandins; decreases production of inflammatory cytokines, etc.

ROUTE OF ADMINISTRATION OF NUTRITION

ENTERAL NUTRITION

It is paradoxical that sick patients who need to eat more to meet the increased metabolic demands are often unable to eat. They have anorexia, nausea, vomiting and altered sensorium. Oral feeding is impossible in patients with faciomaxillary injuries or those on ventilators. In many of them, the intestines are functioning. Enteral route is best for providing nutrition. Hence the dictum, **"When the gut is working, use it"**.

- **Enteral access:** Following are the routes to introduce nutrients into the GIT (Table 11.1):
  - *Nasogastric feeding* (Fig. 11.3): When the stomach emptying is normal and swallowing is impossible or contraindicated, nasogastric feeding (Ryle's tube) provides nutrition.
  - *Nasojejunal feeding* (Fig. 11.4): In gastric stasis, feeding can be given through a nasojejunal (NJ) feeding tube introduced either blindly, under radiologic or endoscopic guidance to place its tip in the jejunum (postpyloric).
  - *Feeding gastrostomy:* By open method or by percutaneous endoscopic gastrostomy (PEG) when RT or NJ tube insertion is impossible.
  - *Percutaneous endoscopic gastrostomy (PEG):* With the help of an endoscope, a gastrostomy tube is placed in a retrograde manner and brought out through a skin incision. It is technically very easy and can be done under local anaesthesia. It has replaced feeding gastrostomies (open method). It is popular nowadays (Fig. 11.2). Complications include colonic perforation, sepsis, bleeding, wound infection, etc.
  - *Feeding jejunostomy:* After major/complex operative procedures on the oesophagus, stomach and pancreas, a feeding jejunostomy is frequently established.
- **What to feed:** A number of preparations are commercially available but most cost-effective ones are the blenderised kitchen feeds. Enteral feeds are hyperosmolar and provide 1.2 to 2.0 kcal/ml.
  - *Polymeric feeds:* These are commonly prepared in the kitchen. Liquid and powder preparations are commercially produced. These contain polysaccharides, polypeptides and oils. Soups of dal, vegetables and chicken are examples of polymeric feeds.
  - *Elemental feeds:* These are predigested *in vitro* and contain oligosaccharides, oligopeptides and medium and long chain triglycerides (MCT and LCT). They are useful in patients with irritable bowel disease and short bowel.
  - *Modular feeds:* Contain monosaccharides, amino acids and fatty acids.
  - *Disease-specific feeds:* The composition of the feeds needs to be altered in certain disease states. Renal failure—low protein, low/no electrolytes; hepatic failure—more branched chain amino acids (BCAA) and less aromatic amino acids; respiratory failure—more fats (55% cal) and less carbohydrates.
- **How to feed:** The feeds can be gravitated, injected with a syringe or pumped into the tubes either continuously or intermittently. Start with 50 ml every 2 hours on the first day and if tolerated, increase gradually to 200 ml every 2 hours until the target is reached.

Table 11.1 Feeding methods (Figs 11.3 and 11.4)

Ryle's tube (RT) feeding	Gastrostomy	Feeding jejunostomy
Easy, quick, cheap method Indicated in stroke, comatose patients, etc. Chances of aspiration are high. Hence, 30° propped up position is recommended	Indicated when RT cannot be passed, e.g. inoperable carcinoma oesophagus, stricture Malecot's catheter is introduced into the stomach and kept in place using a purse string suture (Stamm's gastrostomy)	Indicated after major oesophageal surgeries, high duodenal fistulae A Ryle's tube is introduced into the jejunum under vision (during surgery) and kept in place using a purse string suture

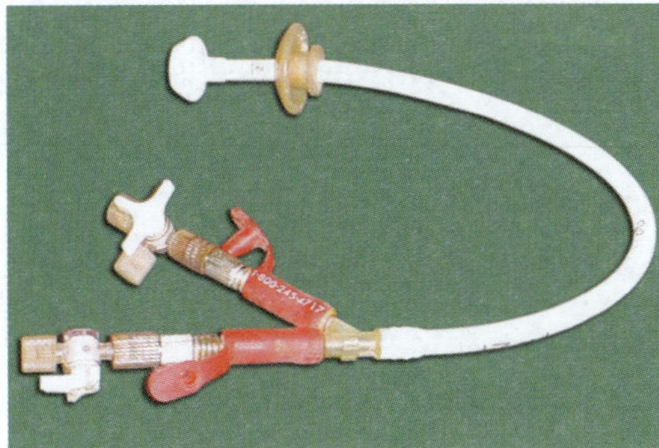

Fig. 11.2: Percutaneous endoscopic gastrostomy tube

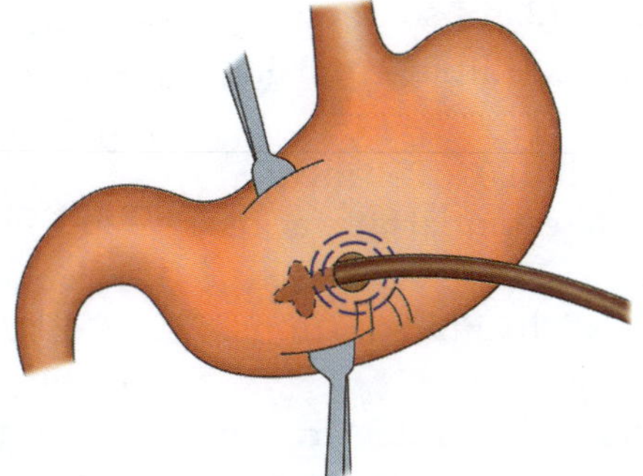

Fig. 11.3: Feeding gastrostomy

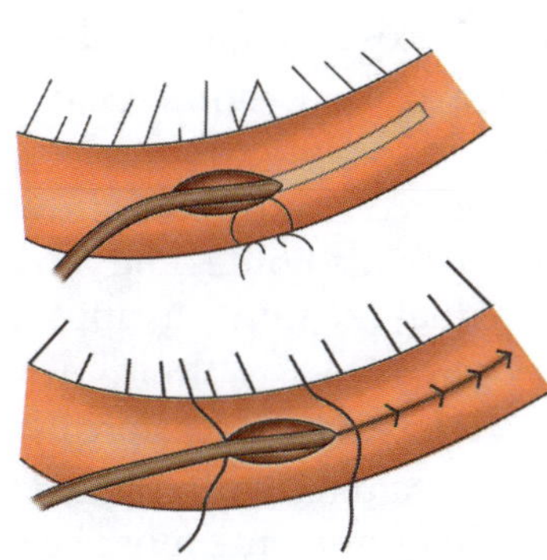

Fig. 11.4: Feeding jejunostomy

Advantages of enteral nutrition:

1. **The integrity of gut mucosa depends on provision of nutrients into the gut lumen.** If the fasting period exceeds more than a few hours, the gut mucosal cells start disintegrating and the villi get destroyed. This may permit the intestinal bacteria to enter the circulation leading to sepsis. Translocation of bacteria from the intestines into the circulation has been identified as the **'motor of multiorgan failure'**.
2. Use of natural route of nutrition requires less nursing supervision.
3. Infection rate is lower with enteral nutrition.
4. Greater insulin response is seen with enteral nutrition.
5. There is a lower tendency to retain salt and water.
6. Enteral nutrition is cheaper.

Complications of enteral nutrition: Nausea, vomiting, abdominal distension and diarrhoea are common. However, intractable diarrhoea should be investigated for *Clostridium difficile* infection. Electrolyte imbalance, hyperosmolar coma, refeeding syndrome and aspiration are other problems. Mechanical complications include tube clogging, displacement, leak and erosion.

PARENTERAL NUTRITION

When enteral nutrition is not possible for more than a few days, parenteral nutrition (PN) may need to be considered. When all nutrition is done by the parenteral route, it is termed total parenteral nutrition. Partial parenteral nutrition may be given to supplement inadequate enteral nutrition.

Parenteral nutrition (PN) to GI failure is like dialysis to renal failure and ventilator support to respiratory failure. When enteral feeding is not possible, parenteral nutrition should be given. Prolonged ileus, intestinal obstruction, malabsorption, short gut, inflammatory bowel disease, high output intestinal fistulae are some common indications for PN (Fig. 11.5).

PN formulations are marketed as:

1. Dextrose + amino acid solutions (2 in 1 solution)
2. Dextrose + amino acid solution + lipid emulsion (3 in 1 solution)
   - Lipid emulsions are available in 100 to 250 ml bags or glass bottles and contain the essential fatty acids that are milky in appearance.
   - Insulin is commonly added to PN solutions. Heparin is occasionally added.
   - Vitamins may be added to the solutions. Electrolyte requirements must be calculated separately on a daily basis.

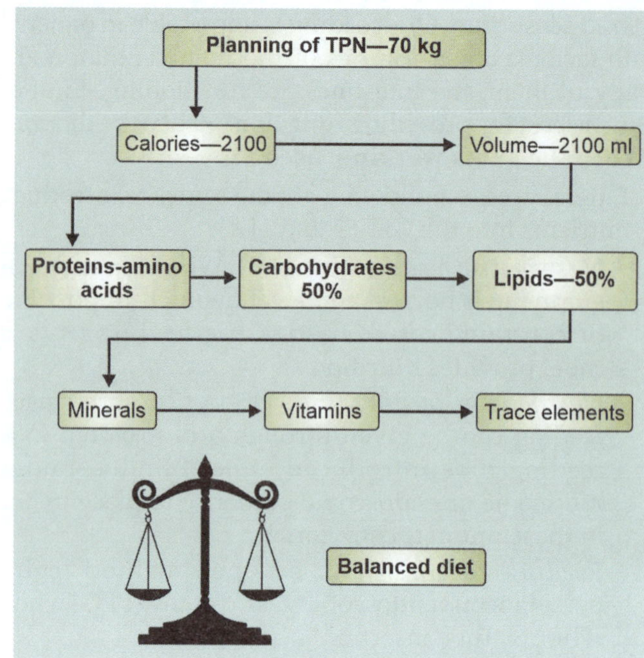

Fig. 11.5: Planning of total parenteral nutrition (TPN)

Electrolyte Requirements

The daily requirements of various electrolytes are given below.

Electrolyte	mmol/kg/day
Sodium	1–2
Potassium	1
Calcium	5–10
Magnesium	5–10

Vitamins are given separately. One ampule of water-soluble vitamins must be infused daily, over a period of time exceeding 30 minutes to avoid urinary loss. Folic acid, vitamins B_{12}, K, A and D need to be given once a week. Trace elements are given weekly to patients on long-term PN.

The choice of volume and composition of TPN solution must be based on the patient's metabolic requirement, clinical status and laboratory parameters. TPN orders should be reviewed each day, so that changes in electrolytes or acid–base balance can be addressed appropriately without wasting costly TPN solutions.

Routes of Administration

1. **Peripheral vein:** Solutions with less than 800 mOsm/L may be administered through a peripheral vein. This is suitable for short-term PN.
2. **Central vein:** Either internal jugular or subclavian vein is cannulated. PN solutions with higher osmolality must be given through a central vein.

3. **Peripherally inserted central vein catheter:** This also may be used for short-term purposes.
4. **Subcutaneously implanted central vein catheter** ports are especially suitable for long-term, domestic or ambulatory PN.

Pearls of Wisdom

The central venous access should be dedicated to PN and should not be used for administration of drugs or other fluids. This line should be handled with strict asepsis to prevent bacterial growth.

Methods of Administration

The solutions can be gravitated but the rate of infusion is better controlled, if given through pumps. Smaller volumes are given initially and is gradually increased to reach the target volume/day. Absolute aseptic precautions are observed while handling the catheters and the PN formulations, since central vein catheter infection is a dangerous complication. Central vein catheter should be used exclusively for administering PN solutions and should not be used for any other purpose.

Monitoring during PN

Aim

1. To identify excess or deficiency of individual nutrients.
2. To identify complications.

Daily: Blood sugar, serum electrolytes, blood urea and serum creatinine.

Biweekly: Liver function tests, coagulation profile, complete haemogram.

Merits of PN: Assured delivery of nutrients, accurate and rapid correction of fluid, electrolyte and acid–base imbalances but it is complicated and expensive.

Complications of PN

1. **Technical complications:** Injury to subclavian/carotid artery, brachial plexus, haemo- or pneumothorax.
2. **Catheter-related:** Central line sepsis is the most dangerous, at times, life-threatening and yet, preventable complication and its incidence is a measure of patient safety. It may not be possible to control sepsis with antibiotics alone without removing the central catheter. Thrombosis and catheter clogging are other problems.
3. **Gut mucosal atrophy:** Patients on total parenteral nutrition develop atrophy of the intestinal mucosa which loses its barrier function and becomes permeable to bacteria. The consequent bacterial translocation leads to sepsis and multiorgan dysfunction syndrome (MODS). This is not seen in patients on partial PN supplemented with EN.
4. **Cholestasis:** Some patients on long-term TPN develop cholestasis, jaundice and gallstones which resolve on starting oral/EN.
5. **Fluid, electrolyte and acid–base imbalances** are common.

CHAPTER

12

Prophylactic and Therapeutic Antibiotics in Surgery

- Antibiotic prophylaxis
- Choice of antibiotic
- Therapeutic antibiotics
- Classification of antibiotics

Competency

SU6.2: Enumerate prophylactic and therapeutic antibiotics. Plan appropriate management.

INTRODUCTION

Antibiotics are indicated for use in a surgical patient either to prevent infection (**prophylactic**) or to treat an established infection (**therapeutic**). **Empirical** antibiotics means antibiotics which are used to treat clinically suspected infections till culture and sensitivity reports are available. Before the days of antibiotics almost every surgery was infected, and the mortality rates were very high. The discovery of penicillin in 1928 by Sir Alexander Fleming changed the world of medicine. Every patient who undergoes in-patient surgery will have prophylactic antibiotics. Prophylactic antibiotics depend upon the type of most probable organisms which may colonise after a particular surgery. One example is the use of gentamicin for potential contamination that can happen during division of the cystic duct during laparoscopic cholecystectomy.

Common Organisms in Surgical Site Infections

- *Staphylococcus aureus*
- *Staphylococcus epidermidis*
- Aerobic streptococci
- Anaerobic cocci

ANTIBIOTIC PROPHYLAXIS

Prophylactic antibiotics are most used to prevent infection of the surgical site.

It is important to note that only infection of the surgical incision is prevented, and it does not prevent other nosocomial infections.

Antibiotic prophylaxis is indicated in clean contaminated and contaminated operations. In clean surgeries, antibiotics are only indicated in case of prosthetic implants such as orthopaedic surgeries. Other clean surgeries such as breast or hernia operations, evidence has shown that antibiotic prophylaxis is not required.

Most of the surgical site infections are caused by endogenous gram-positive cocci that reside on the skin of the patient. Infection from exogenous sources such as health care workers or cross-contamination from other patients reflects poor hospital standards and strict action should be taken to prevent such infections.

Antibiotics must be administered preoperatively, 1 hour before the skin incision is made, in order to attain maximum blood and tissue concentrations before bacterial growth can become established. However, vancomycin and levofloxacin, if these drugs are used for prophylaxis, have to be administered within 120 minutes of the procedural incision due to longer administration times. In case of long duration surgeries, or in surgeries with excessive blood loss, a repeat dosing will be required, usually at 4 hourly intervals, to maintain the desired tissue levels.

Unnecessary prolonged usage of prophylactic antibiotics is potentially harmful and increases the risk of other nosocomial infections.

Everyone should know commonly used antibiotics, mechanism of action and their coverage (Table 12.1).

Table 12.1 Commonly used antibiotics, mechanism of action and their coverage

Antibiotic class	Mechanism of action	Coverage
Penicillin	Inhibit cell wall synthesis	Gram-positive
Aminopenicillin, e.g. ampicillin, amoxicillin	Inhibit cell wall synthesis	Staphylococci, streptococci, *E. coli*, Proteus
1st gen cephalosporins, e.g. cefazolin, cephalexin	Inhibit cell wall synthesis	Gram-positive, few gram-negative
2nd gen cephalosporins, e.g. cephotetan, cefoxitin	Inhibit cell wall synthesis	Gram-positive, few gram-negative and anaerobes
3rd gen cephalosporins, e.g. ceftriaxone, cefaperazone, ceftazidime	Inhibit cell wall synthesis	Gram-negative predominantly. Ceftazidime is also active against Pseudomonas
4th gen cephalosporins, e.g. cefepime	Inhibit cell wall synthesis	Gram-negative and few gram-positive
Aminopenicillin with beta lactamase inhibitors, e.g. piperacillin tazobactam	Inhibit cell wall synthesis	Gram-positive, gram-negative and anaerobic
Carbapenems, e.g. ertapenem, imipenem meropenem	Inhibit cell wall synthesis	Gram-positive, gram-negative, and anaerobic anti-pseudomonal
Fluoroquinolones, e.g. ciprofloxacin, levofloxacin	Inhibit bacterial DNA synthesis by inhibiting DNA gyrase	Gram-negative anti-pseudomonal
Aminoglycosides, e.g. gentamicin, amikacin	Inhibit bacterial protein synthesis by binding to 30S ribosomal subunit	Gram-negative anti-pseudomonal
Lincosamide, e.g. clindamycin	Inhibit bacterial protein synthesis by binding to 50S ribosomal subunit	Gram-positive, anaerobic, active against MRSA
Glycopeptides, e.g. vamcomycin	Inhibit cell wall synthesis	Gram-positive. Active against MRSA
Antimetabolites, e.g. trimethoprim-sulphamethoxazole	Interfere with bacterial folic acid synthesis	Gram-positive, negative. Active against MRSA
Nitroimidazole, e.g metronidazole	Cause DNA damage	Anaerobic

Choice of Antibiotic

As most of the SSIs are caused by gram-positive cocci like *Staphylococcus aureus*, coagulase negative Staphylococcus, etc., prophylactic antibiotics directed against these are used for clean and clean contaminated cases such as elective biliary and gastric surgeries (Key Box 12.1). The recommended antibiotic is a first-generation cephalosporin such as cefazolin. An alternative in patients with penicillin allergy is clindamycin. In cases which require a gram-negative or anaerobic coverage, either a second-generation cephalosporin can be used, or a first-generation cephalosporin with metronidazole is another choice.

In cases of emergencies, such as necrotising soft tissue infections that require debridement or perforation peritonitis with gross intra-abdominal contamination that require exploratory laparotomy, the antibiotic used for prophylaxis is continued as the therapeutic drug even after the surgery. It is better to use the term empirical antibiotics than prophylactic antibiotics in this type of situation. Once the culture sensitivity pattern is available, antibiotics are changed accordingly.

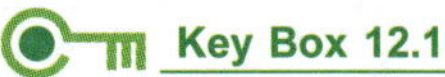

Prophylactic Antibiotics

- The antibiotic should have a narrow spectrum of coverage of the relevant organisms that are prevalent in causing surgical site infection—which depends on the site and type of surgery.
- The same antibiotic should not be a part of the therapeutic regimens for infection as it may lead to induction of resistance.
- Should be administered 1 hour before surgery and should be stopped within 24 hours after surgery—ideally single dose.
- Should be safe.

THERAPEUTIC ANTIBIOTICS

In cases of established infection, the use of antibiotics is therapeutic, to eradicate the organism causing the infection. To choose appropriate antibiotics, it is important to identify the causative organism and determine its sensitivity pattern, to tailor treatment and avoid the emergence of resistant strains.

It should be kept in mind that antibiotic treatment does not replace surgical treatment, and it is just an adjunct to proper surgical drainage and eradication of infection. In a case of simple peritonitis—example acute appendicitis without shock, antibiotics are given for 5 to 7 days. However, in cases of peritonitis and shock due to appendicular perforations, antibiotics may have to be given for 10 to 14 days. More details are given in the Chapter 45 on peritonitis.

Antibiotic therapy can be started empirically as soon as a diagnosis of surgical infection is made, and the choice of antibiotic depends on the most common organisms suspected to cause the infection (Key Box 12.2). Prior to starting empirical antibiotics, it is important to collect pus or tissue samples from the wound, to be sent for cultures, so that the organism can be identified, sensitivity pattern can be obtained, and accordingly we can modify the choice of antibiotic, if necessary.

Key Box 12.2

Therapeutic Antibiotics

- Choose appropriate antibiotics based on culture and sensitivity pattern of the organism.
- Avoid overdosing and inappropriate combinations.
- Educate patients to avoid self-prescribing antibiotics.
- Stop treatment with antibiotics as soon as infection subsides.
- Adopt antibiotic stewardship programmes in hospitals and increase awareness among all doctors.

There are two approaches to choosing therapeutic antibiotics—**narrow-spectrum** coverage, which treats a known infection when the sensitivity pattern of the organism is available; or **broad-spectrum** coverage, when the organism is not known and complete gram-positive, gram-negative, and anaerobic coverage is required, e.g. in patients with perforation peritonitis, we can start a 3rd generation cephalosporin such as cefoperazone along with metronidazole. *Examples:* **Cefazolin, vancomycin, and gentamicin**. For patients receiving cefazolin, 2 g is the current recommended dose except for patients weighing greater than or equal to 120 kg, who should receive 3 g.

Once the sensitivity pattern of the organism is available, then the antibiotic treatment can be de-escalated, if the patient is improving. If there is no clinical response to antibiotics, then a thorough review of the patient must be done, as there might be an underlying persistent infection that might need to be drained surgically, or a new infection might have developed.

Please note: The various infections and their treatment have been given in the respective chapters. For example, breast abscess—antibiotics MRSA, etc. in Chapter 39 on breast. In the same fashion, details about antibiotics can be got from other chapters such as skin, peritonitis, intestinal obstruction, etc.

Some common infections, causative organisms and antibiotic treatment are given in Table 12.2.

Table 12.2 Common infections, organisms, antibiotics and treatment plan

Disease	Organisms	Antibiotics	Treatment
1. Boil/carbuncle/breast abscess/parotid abscess	*Staphylococcus aureus*	Cloxacillin, clindamycin, vancomycin	Antibiotics, incision and drainage/excision
2. Necrotising fasciitis	Streptococci, *Staphylococcus aureus*, gram-negative organisms	Cephalosporins Amikacin	Antibiotics and early aggressive debridement
3. Intra-abdominal perforations/ infections/peritonitis	Enterococci, gram-negative organisms, anaerobic organisms streptococci, *Staphylococcus aureus*	Cephalosporins Amikacin Metronidazole	Treatment of the source of infection—suturing, removal of organ or drainage of pus
4. Severe sepsis/peritonitis	Enterococci, gram-negative organisms, anaerobic organisms, streptococci, *Staphylococcus aureus*	Piperacillin and tazobactam combination with metronidazole	Treatment of the source of infection—suturing, removal of organ or drainage of pus
5. Gas gangrene	Clostridial organisms	Vancomycin and tazobactam or a carbapenem or ceftriaxone with metronidazole. Penicillin and clindamycin are the other drugs	Early antibiotics Emergency debridement Hyperbaric oxygen

CHAPTER

13

Day Case/Care Surgery

- Types of care
- Type of surgery facilities
- Selection criteria
- Preoperative assessment
- Perioperative management
- Discharge

Competency

SU11.4: Enumerate the indications and principles of day care general surgery.

INTRODUCTION

Day care surgery is a term applied to performing a surgical procedure as a day case. This provides advantages to both patients and healthcare providers. It causes less disruption to the patient's daily situation and contributes to financial savings to the hospital. It is an integral component of healthcare delivery in resource-rich countries, whereas in resource-poor countries, it is on the rising trend due to increasing popularity. There should be a team comprising of surgeon, anaesthetist, floor managers, operational managers and nursing staff.

- In India day case/care surgery is gaining popularity in cities. However, more than 70–80% population is in rural India. Most of these patients come late to the hospital and often they are illiterate. Hence the day case surgery is currently limited to urban patients in India.

Definitions

- Day surgery: Admitted and discharged within the 12-hour day.
- Overnight stay: 23-hour admission with early morning discharge.
- Short-stay surgery: Admission of up to 72 hours.

Indications for Day Care Surgery

- Hernia surgeries
- Cataract surgeries
- Excision of lumps, excision of foreign body
- Parotidectomy
- Laparoscopic surgeries such as cholecystectomy

TYPES OF CARE

A. **Office-based care:** The investigations and ambulatory interventions are performed on an outpatient basis, providing ready access to patients. The disadvantage is that vey few procedures performed under local anaesthesia are included in this. Procedures that need general anaesthesia are not performed as this requires additional equipment and healthcare personnel.

B. **Stand-alone day care surgery:** The surgeries in this care are performed in an isolated facility, either on a remote site or in the campus of a parent hospital. Procedures are limited to those performed under local anaesthesia, regional anaesthesia or minor procedures under general anaesthesia. This is to avoid overnight admissions which need to be transferred to the parent hospital, which may be some distance away.

TYPE OF SURGERY FACILITIES

A. **Self-contained integrated day:** These are well-equipped hospitals having reception area, operation theatres and postoperative ward. Many surgeries can be performed here including laparoscopic cholecystectomies, laparoscopic hernia surgeries, etc.

There should be a good cooperation between all persons involved in the day case surgery. Patients should be able to understand the instructions given to him by the consultant. He should be able to come back to the hospital in case of any complications.

B. **Integrated day and short-stay surgery facilities:** Here day care and short-stay surgery are feasible, where challenging procedures or day surgery on a less fit patient can be considered.

SELECTION CRITERIA

A. Medical Criteria

1. **Age:** Physiological health of the patients is more important than the chronological age. There is no upper age limit.
2. **Comorbidity:** American Society of Anesthesiologists (ASA) classification is traditionally used to evaluate the patients (Table 13.1).

   ASA 1 and 2 patients are confined to the stand-alone units, whereas ASA 3 patients are suitable for hospital-integrated units. Patients with hypertension are considered for day surgery when blood pressure is below 180/110 mmHg. Patients with significant respiratory and cardiac disease have to be reviewed by anaesthetist before being accepted for day surgery.
3. **Obesity:** Obesity is defined as body mass index of more than 30 kg/m^2. Traditionally, guidelines towards obese patients were conservative due to the fear of complications. The course of these patients is uneventful, although there is increased risk for non-serious intraoperative and postoperative respiratory complications. Complications of morbid obesity such as sleep apnoea, hypertension and congestive cardiac failure should be managed preoperatively with an experienced team.
4. **Epilepsy:** Patients with controlled epilepsy on medications should be managed as normal patients. It is important not to omit the medications in the pre-operative medications. Patients with poorly controlled epilepsy on medications should be managed pre-operatively with a medical team.
5. **Diabetes:** The incidence of diabetes is on the increasing trend worldwide. An HbA1c of 8.5% indicates a good control. Patients with well-controlled type 1 and 2 diabetes mellitus can be considered for day surgery. The complications of diabetes such as renal disease, cardiovascular disease should be evaluated pre-operatively by an experienced team. These patients should not be given oral hypoglycemic agents. Also, they should be operated first rather than late in the evening. If the patient is on afternoon or evening lists or undergoing a complex surgery, he can be managed with the help of a diabetic team or the anaesthetist.
6. **Anticoagulants:** Preoperative risk assessment with a cardiologist is important in managing patients on anticoagulation when it is felt that surgery will require its discontinuation. Patients are often on anticoagulation due to atrial fibrillation, venous thromboembolism, or a prosthetic heart valve. Patients may be receiving anticoagulants following stenting or coronary artery bypass graft. A few drugs may have to be stopped for 7 days before surgery. One such example is clopidogrel.
7. **Smoking:** Patient should stop smoking at least 48 hours before surgery. Substance abuse patients are not the candidates for day case/care surgery.

Table 13.1 The American Society of Anesthesiologists (ASA) physical status classification

ASA 1	A normal healthy patient
ASA 2	A patient with mild systemic disease
ASA 3	A patient with severe systemic disease
ASA 4	A patient with severe systemic disease that is a constant threat to life
ASA 5	A moribund patient who is not expected to survive without the operation

B. Social Criteria

A patient accompanied by a responsible adult is the key to a safe and comfortable discharge. A travel time of less than one hour is considered ideal although the comfort of the journey is more important. The means of contacting the hospital, if a complication occurs, is an important aspect of a safe discharge. As mentioned earlier, due to these reasons, many of our patients will not get the benefit of day case/surgery.

C. Surgical Criteria

An operating time of 2 hours in duration is considered safe as a day surgery. Suitable control of pain and the ability to eat and drink a reasonable amount is the main requirement. Venous thromboembolism risk assessment is important in patients undergoing complex surgery.

PREOPERATIVE ASSESSMENT

The preoperative assessment of the patient is best done by an anaesthetist who specializes in day surgery. It should be done early in the pathway to allow time to optimise health problems before surgery. All patients should be considered for day surgery unless proven otherwise. Relevant investigations are conducted to assess the fitness of the patient for surgery. Informed and written consent is taken after informing the patient about admission, operation, and discharge.

PERIOPERATIVE MANAGEMENT

- **Scheduling:** Day surgeries are preferably planned in the morning to make monitoring and early discharge of the patient feasible. If there is a list in the afternoon, local and regional anaesthesia cases are planned for later in the day. Mixing of day case and complex inpatient cases is not recommended.
- **Anaesthesia and analgesia:** Multimodal analgesia is required to make a day case surgery successful. It is started in the preoperative period with paracetamol and non-steroidal anti-inflammatory drugs. Intra-operative anaesthesia is maintained by any of the inhalational agents. The anaesthetist rather than the drugs used matter more. Total intravenous anaesthesia (TIVA) offers the advantage of reduced postoperative nausea and vomiting. Short-acting agents are preferred whenever feasible. When morphine is used, it is given in minimal doses to reduce postoperative nausea and vomiting. Local anaesthetic such as bupivacaine when injected into the wounds helps prolong the effect of analgesia. Postoperative monitoring of pain is important and further doses of analgesia should be given accordingly to make the patient comfortable and fit for discharge on the same day.
- **Postoperative complications:** The complications of day surgery are like that of inpatient surgery. However, since day surgery patients are discharged on the same day, monitoring in the immediate postoperative period is important. Reactionary hemorrhage is uncommon but important in cases such as tonsillectomy and laparoscopic procedures. Slow bleeding and hypovolaemia can be dangerous. In India such surgeries can be done only if patient understands the complications and also he has the facility to call for ambulance and reach the hospital quickly. Covert haemorrhage is a danger in laparoscopic procedures and it might manifest as delayed recovery or uncontrollable abdominal pain. High index of suspicion is required in such patients and timely intervention is vital. Postoperative nausea and vomiting is not uncommon and needs to be managed to facilitate same day discharge.

DISCHARGE

Discharge criteria are important in assessing a patients fitness for discharge which is done by a trained day surgery nurse. Postoperative review by a surgeon is important but the discharge should not be delayed by failure of their timely attendance. There must be a care-taker person to look after the patient once he or she gets discharged after the surgery. He should be able to provide some simple basic care such as pain relief tablets or even to dress a small ooze from the suture line. He should available for the next 24 hours to the patient soon after the surgery.

Discharge Criteria

1. Just before discharge, look at the operated sites. *Example:* Hernial site at groin, oral cavity as in tonsillectomy. If any degree of suspicion arises, observe them more carefully for another few hours. If any oozing or bleeders are identified within 6–8 hours means better to stop the bleeding and delay discharge.
2. Look at the vitals: Pulse rate, breathing, blood pressure. Only when they are stable, discharge can be considered.
3. Talk to the patient and ask him to obey a few commands such as showing the tongue, identifying relatives or hospital. Simple leading question is—where are you now? Do you have any pain? Can you tolerate this pain?
4. A few common side effects of anaesthetics such as nausea or vomiting are present or not, if present should be minimal. Such patient tolerates liquid and semi-solid food.
5. A contact number should be given to the patient in case of any emergency.

REFERENCES

1. Bailey and Love's short practise of surgery, 27th edition.
2. McWhinnie D, Jackson I, Smith I, Skues M. Patient safety in the ambulatory pathway. British Association of Day Surgery Handbook Series. London: BADS, 2013.

CHAPTER

14

Principles of Safe General Surgery

Competency

SU11.6: Describe principles of safe general surgery.

INTRODUCTION

Since the last three decades, tremendous growth has been seen in a number of surgeries performed. World has also seen advances in all medical fields including surgery. Minimal access surgery is one of the major changes which happened in these 30 years and has been accepted very well by surgeons and patients. In fact, surgeon's aim is not only to operate but also operate with minimal morbidity and least mortality. Minimal access surgery or laparoscopic surgery is one example of such developments. It is also important that many such skilled surgeries require training. In a few cases, learning curve is long. An attempt to do surgery may land with complications, compromising patient's safety. Legal issues are also becoming more common in the last 3 decades. Thus, safe practise of general surgery aims to achieve maximum success. It will also decrease litigations for surgeons. Let us look at those principles.

WHO SURGICAL SAFETY CHECKLIST (2008)

World Health Organisation (WHO) in 2008 released a checklist consisting of 19 items. If one follows this system, one can decrease number of deaths/blunders/complications related to surgery. Worldwide a large number of deaths or errors occur in the operating table which results in mortality. It is a simple checklist to implement. Many centres in the world have used this and have reduced the complications related to instruments or adverse events which occur in the hospital before or during or after conduct of a surgical procedure. **Dr Makary,** Professor of Surgery, Johns Hopkins University School of Medicine, is the creator of The Surgery Checklist (Fig. 14.1).

Surgery is basically a teamwork. If the entire team consisting of surgeon, anaesthetist and nursing staff know about the patient disease, problems, if any, including allergy, indication for surgery, possible complications and recovery in the postoperative period, many of the complications could have been avoided.

Every surgery has a critical event. Before proceeding, the surgeon can discuss this with his colleagues/other surgeons and go ahead. Classical example: Before ligation and division of cystic duct in cases of difficult cholecystectomy. A wrong decision at this stage can have serious consequences of division of CBD and associated with serious complications and mortality also.

In Western countries, the consultant who examines the patient may not be the operating surgeon. Often appointments are given and patient comes to the hospital on the day of surgery. Surgeon comes to OT, he will see a few CT scans or reports and operate. He might have been busy also. Because of this, wrong side of the patient has been operated many a time. Wrong side breast lump has been removed. Due to communication errors between nursing staff and surgeons, nurses may not be well prepared for an unexpected emergency which necessitates additional set of instruments, e.g. vascular injury. If a prior intimation is given to them, such situations can be avoided. This can happen anywhere and hence, WHO advises the use of checklist.

Sign in means checking before induction of anaesthesia, time out means before skin incision and sign out means before the patient leaves the operating room. These principles help in avoiding operating on

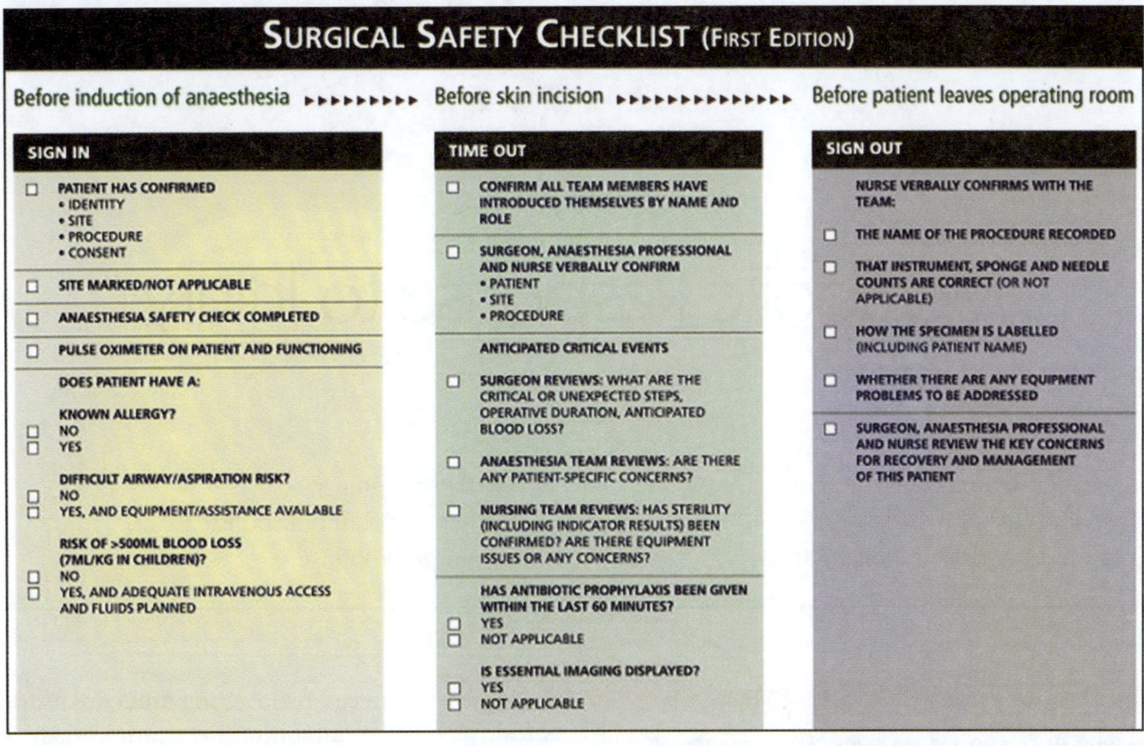

SURGICAL SAFETY CHECKLIST (FIRST EDITION)

Before induction of anaesthesia ▸▸▸▸▸▸▸▸▸ Before skin incision ▸▸▸▸▸▸▸▸▸▸▸▸▸▸ Before patient leaves operating room

SIGN IN

☐ PATIENT HAS CONFIRMED
- IDENTITY
- SITE
- PROCEDURE
- CONSENT

☐ SITE MARKED/NOT APPLICABLE

☐ ANAESTHESIA SAFETY CHECK COMPLETED

☐ PULSE OXIMETER ON PATIENT AND FUNCTIONING

DOES PATIENT HAVE A:

KNOWN ALLERGY?
☐ NO
☐ YES

DIFFICULT AIRWAY/ASPIRATION RISK?
☐ NO
☐ YES, AND EQUIPMENT/ASSISTANCE AVAILABLE

RISK OF >500ML BLOOD LOSS (7ML/KG IN CHILDREN)?
☐ NO
☐ YES, AND ADEQUATE INTRAVENOUS ACCESS AND FLUIDS PLANNED

TIME OUT

☐ CONFIRM ALL TEAM MEMBERS HAVE INTRODUCED THEMSELVES BY NAME AND ROLE

☐ SURGEON, ANAESTHESIA PROFESSIONAL AND NURSE VERBALLY CONFIRM
- PATIENT
- SITE
- PROCEDURE

ANTICIPATED CRITICAL EVENTS

☐ SURGEON REVIEWS: WHAT ARE THE CRITICAL OR UNEXPECTED STEPS, OPERATIVE DURATION, ANTICIPATED BLOOD LOSS?

☐ ANAESTHESIA TEAM REVIEWS: ARE THERE ANY PATIENT-SPECIFIC CONCERNS?

☐ NURSING TEAM REVIEWS: HAS STERILITY (INCLUDING INDICATOR RESULTS) BEEN CONFIRMED? ARE THERE EQUIPMENT ISSUES OR ANY CONCERNS?

HAS ANTIBIOTIC PROPHYLAXIS BEEN GIVEN WITHIN THE LAST 60 MINUTES?
☐ YES
☐ NOT APPLICABLE

IS ESSENTIAL IMAGING DISPLAYED?
☐ YES
☐ NOT APPLICABLE

SIGN OUT

NURSE VERBALLY CONFIRMS WITH THE TEAM:

☐ THE NAME OF THE PROCEDURE RECORDED

☐ THAT INSTRUMENT, SPONGE AND NEEDLE COUNTS ARE CORRECT (OR NOT APPLICABLE)

☐ HOW THE SPECIMEN IS LABELLED (INCLUDING PATIENT NAME)

☐ WHETHER THERE ARE ANY EQUIPMENT PROBLEMS TO BE ADDRESSED

☐ SURGEON, ANAESTHESIA PROFESSIONAL AND NURSE REVIEW THE KEY CONCERNS FOR RECOVERY AND MANAGEMENT OF THIS PATIENT

Fig. 14.1: Surgical safety checklist (Reproduced with permission of the World Health Organization, wholibdoc.who.int/publications/2009/9789241598590_eng_ Checklist.pdf")

wrong patients, wrong side, wrong procedure. Anticipating major events such as vascular injuries or excessive bleeding, etc. are also part of the checklist. It also helps in better coordination between operating surgeons, anaesthetists, and nurses. Simple checklists will avoid such gross blunders or errors. Counting mops and needles are also part of this. The list can be modified depending upon the local hospital policies and practises. Modification of this checklist, a single 5-step approach, advocated by the National Patient Safety Agency (NPSA) for all patients in England and Wales undergoing surgical procedures is given below.

Five Steps to Safer Surgery

A simple 5-step approach, *"Five Steps to Safer Surgery"* is a surgical safety checklist. It involves briefing, sign-in, timeout, sign-out and debriefing.

1. **Briefing:** Before the procedure starts. A briefing about the patient, what is the disease, who is doing the surgery, who are assisting, what is the plan and what are the possible complications, is there possibility of excessive blood loss. Please note safety list is not about discussing complications of surgery with the patient but briefing to the team. One example is carcinoma parotid with doubtful infiltration of facial nerve. Here a nurse is requested to keep nerve stimulator ready, anaesthesia consultant is informed that muscle relaxants must be avoided and a plastic surgery team is informed in advance to ensure their availability.
2. **Sign in:** Before induction of anaesthesia, reconfirm whether consent is taken or not, presence of allergy, anticipated blood loss, anaesthesia machine and drugs. Check the side of marking specially when lesions are small—breast lumps, lymph nodes.
3. **Time out:** Stop for a moment before starting incision. Again, confirm patient identity, surgical site infection bundle, thromboprophylaxis, antibiotics or any adverse events which can happen—may be all these are already discussed but check again.
4. **Sign out:** At the end of the procedure, check sponge count, needle and sharp count, check position of tubes and tourniquets. Discuss possible complications with doctors as well as nurses in the team.
5. **Debriefing:** At the end of the procedure, discuss again about what has been done and what should not have been done. *Example:* Why did I injure internal jugular vein in thyroidectomy? Why did the creation of pneumoperitoneum take a long time? Was there any instrument failure? Should anything else be improved? This is done with a view to improve care of patients in the future.

REFERENCE

Ann R Coll Surg Engl. 2011 Oct; 93(7): 501–503.

CHAPTER

15

Metabolic Response to Injury

- Energy expenditure
- Changes in skeletal muscle
- Changes in liver protein metabolism
- Response to injury
  - Neuroendocrine response
  - Immune response

Competency

SU1.1: Describe basic concepts of homeostasis. Enumerate the metabolic changes in injury and their mediators.

'Homeostasis' is a state of dynamic equilibrium, wherein the body maintains its key physiological variables within a predefined range through feedback mechanisms. As opposed to its literal meaning suggestive of 'stagnancy', homeostasis allows a wide range of continuous changes of body parameters within their physiological limits, letting various compensatory mechanisms to act in case of any deviation from normalcy. Sir David Cuthbertson (1942) proposed that human beings respond to injuries in two distinct phases of hypermetabolic state, namely the 'ebb phase' and the 'flow phase'. The 'ebb phase' begins immediately following an event of stress such as burns, trauma, surgery or critical illness and lasts for 24–48 hours. Generally, hemodynamic disturbances like hypotension is seen in this phase, hence it aims to conserve circulating fluid volume and energy, and is characterised by reductions in basal metabolic rate (BMR), cardiac output, oxygen consumption; lactic acidosis and glucose intolerance. The renin–angiotensin cascade is an important component of the 'ebb phase'. The hormones responsible are the adrenal hormones (i.e. catecholamines, cortisol and aldosterone). The 'flow phase' follows the 'ebb phase,' lasts for days to weeks depending on the severity of injury and is concerned with recovery and repair following the initial injury. It is a catabolic (breakdown) phase that prevents further tissue damage and protects critical organ function. The catecholamines (adrenaline) are mainly responsible for the increased energy production and consumption. This is followed by an anabolic (synthetic) phase, the onset of which is again based on the injury severity. The transition happens about 3–8 days after an uncomplicated elective surgery but may take several weeks after sepsis or severe trauma. Clinically it coincides with the oral intake of fluids, soft diet and diuresis and may last for several months, during which it replaces body protein and fat stores, normalizing the positive nitrogen balance after the metabolic response to stress is stopped. The following issues are important aspects of the metabolic response to stress.

ENERGY EXPENDITURE

During stress, energy expenditure **increases by 15–25%** due to:

- Central thermodysregulation caused by pro-inflammatory cytokines.
- Increased sympathetic activity.
- Increased lactate production in ischaemic areas which in turn gets metabolised by the energy consuming **Cori cycle.**
- Increased cardiac output.
- Increased protein turnover.

The clinical importance is the awareness of increase in this energy expenditure in order to determine metabolic and nutritional support for the patient.

CHANGES IN SKELETAL MUSCLE

During the catabolic phase of stress response, increased protein turnover is seen. There is muscle wasting due to:

- Increased muscle protein degradation
- Decreased muscle protein synthesis.

This results in the release of amino acids, **mainly alanine and glutamine,** which are used by the liver and immune system for the synthesis of proteins, such as acute phase proteins and cytokines. Although all types of muscles contain proteins, proteins from skeletal and smooth muscles (in that order) are preferentially catabolised compared to those from cardiac muscles. **The main pathways which govern protein catabolism in skeletal muscles are:**

- ATP-dependent ubiquitin proteasome pathway
- Lysosomal cathepsin
- Calcium calpain pathway

However, in the critically ill, the amino acids released by protein catabolism in muscle cannot be used for protein resynthesis. A negative nitrogen balance occurs and if adequate nutritional support is not provided, rapid loss of muscle tissue occurs resulting in dependence on mechanical ventilation and inadequate healing. Hence, exaggerated skeletal muscle catabolism results in asthenia, increased fatigability, poor quality of life, and increased morbidity and mortality. Another physiological defect in such conditions is impaired excitation–contraction coupling at the level of the sarcolemma and sarcoplasmic reticulum. This condition has been termed 'critical illness myopathy.'

CHANGES IN LIVER PROTEIN METABOLISM

Normally, the liver synthesises two types of proteins:

1. Structural proteins
2. Export proteins, e.g. albumin.

Based on response to stress, the proteins synthesised by liver can be divided into:

1. Positive acute phase reactants, e.g. fibrinogen, C-reactive proteins (CRP) and ceruloplasmin.
2. Negative acute phase reactants, e.g. albumin.

As the name suggests, they increase and decrease respectively in response to stress.

Clinical significance: In response to IL-6, 'acute phase response' occurs which is characterized by production of acute phase proteins by the liver that act as inflammatory mediators, anti-proteinases and scavengers in tissue repairs. In this phase, there is granulocytosis, increase in serum concentrations of CRP and ceruloplasmin, decrease in serum concentrations of albumin and transferrin, changes in serum concentrations of divalent cations (copper increases; zinc and iron decrease). Hence, investigating for these laboratory parameters might suggest an underlying inflammatory process, especially when anticipated after an event of stress.

Special note on albumin: Albumin is the major protein synthesised by liver. Hypoalbuminemia is commonly associated with malnutrition and severe stress/sepsis. It is tempting to presume that a fall in albumin level during stress is due to diversion of its synthesis by the liver towards synthesis of positive acute phase reactants instead. This might not be true. The serum level of albumin is governed by its rates of synthesis and transcapillary escape. During stress, the transcapillary escape rate of albumin increases about 3 times. This is because of increased microvascular permeability, which results in hypoalbuminemia during stress/sepsis.

Insulin resistance: After an event of stress, like a major surgery, stress hormones including glucagon, catecholamines, growth hormone and cortisol are secreted and inflammatory reaction is generated by cytokines all of which enhance the action of insulin, due to which amino acids, free fatty acids and glucose are released into the bloodstream from various tissues. The body also switches from glucose to fat for substrate metabolism. This results in stress-hyperglycemia and an insulin resistant state, particularly in critically ill patients with sepsis. One of the clinical implications here is to infuse insulin to normalize the glucose level and good glycemic control will improve the outcome of critically ill patients.

RESPONSE TO INJURY

Introduction

The ultimate aim of the response of the body to injury is to maintain the 'milieu interieur'—a stable internal environment that allows biological processes to proceed despite varying external environmental conditions. It depends upon the severity of the injury and can be considered under the following headings:

- Neuroendocrine response
- Immunological response
- Metabolic response

Neuroendocrine Response (Fig. 15.1)

One of the earliest pathways to get activated following injury is the 'neuroendocrine pathway'. The neuroendocrine pathway starts with nociceptive receptors and involves the spinal cord, thalamus, hypothalamus, and pituitary. Stimulation of the hypothalamus is a key event in the pathway and results in:

- Release of corticotrophin-releasing hormone (CRH), which triggers the release of ACTH from the anterior pituitary. ACTH acts on the adrenals to increase the secretion of cortisol and aldosterone. The levels of TSH, FSH, LH may increase or decrease.

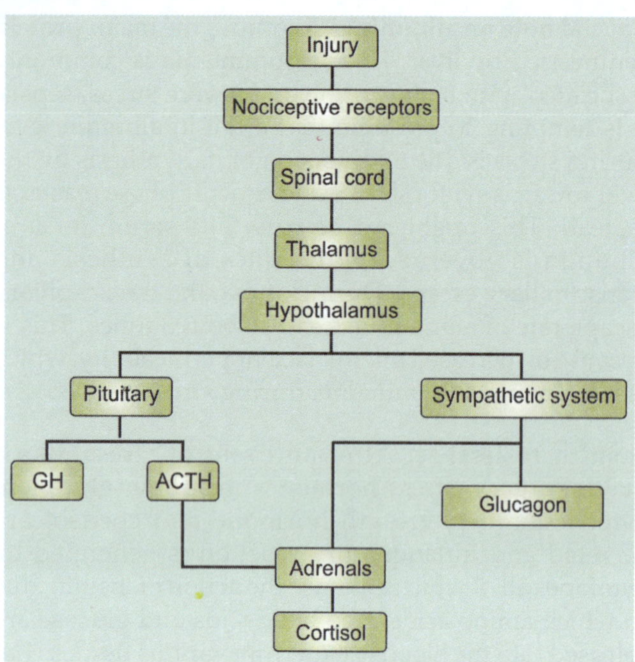

Fig. 15.1: Neuroendocrine response

- Hypothalamic activation of the sympathetic nervous system, causes the release of adrenaline from the adrenal medulla and noradrenaline from nerve terminals.
- Increased release of growth hormone and glucagon.
- Posterior pituitary hormone arginine vasopressin level increases.

To summarise, the levels of ACTH, cortisol, growth hormone, adrenaline, and glucagon are increased following injury, mainly because of activation of the neuroendocrine pathway.

Immune Response (Fig. 15.2)

The immune system of the body may be subdivided into the:

- **Innate immune system,** which mainly includes macrophages.
- **Adaptive immune system,** which includes T and B lymphocytes.

Immune responses are mediated by protein signalling compounds called 'cytokines.' The immune response to injury includes a proinflammatory and an anti-inflammatory response.

The initial response to injury is **proinflammatory**, which leads to:

- **Pyrexia,** due to action of proinflammatory cytokines on the hypothalamus
- **Propagation** of the hypothalamic stress response
- **Proteolysis** in skeletal muscle
- **Production** of acute-phase proteins in liver

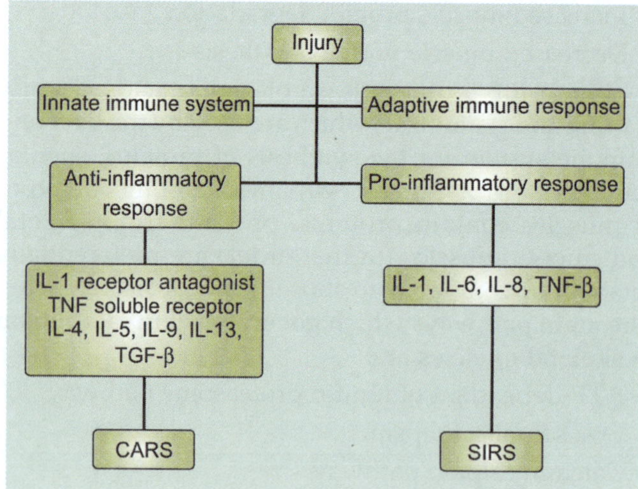

Fig. 15.2: Immune response

The proinflammatory cytokines are interleukin-1 (IL-1), tumour necrosis factor-α, interleukin-6 (IL-6), and interleukin-8 (IL-8). Following this, to control a robust proinflammatory response, endogenous anti-inflammatory mediators take action to check a potentially exaggerated inflammatory and immune response. *Example:* IL-4, IL-5, IL-9, IL-13, IL-10, IL-1 receptor antagonist, soluble tumour necrosis receptors and transforming growth factor-β are released into circulation to counteract the proinflammatory cytokines, thereby developing Th2-type counter-inflammatory response. There is a delicate balance between the proinflammatory and anti-inflammatory immune responses. Unopposed proinflammatory response leads to 'systemic immune response syndrome' (SIRS). On the other hand, exaggerated anti-inflammatory response results in "compensatory anti-inflammatory response syndrome (CARS)" or "counter-inflammatory response syndrome". Excessive or prolonged elaboration of either of them may result in sepsis and/or death.

Note on the stress response to surgery: Although in an evolutionary perspective, the stress response allows an injured animal to survive better by catabolizing stored body fuels, the latest argument errs on the notion that it is unnecessary in the current surgical practice and the potential deleterious effects of an unopposed response has already been discussed. The body's response to surgical stress *per se* is essentially the same as to other stressors like trauma, but a few specific factors affecting surgical response are noteworthy:

- **Age:** As the age increases, the hormonal response in the postoperative period lasts longer.
- **Nutrition and diet:** Perioperative nutritional support, particularly the degree of diet has an effect on metabolic response to surgery.

- **Surgical method:** Pneumoperitoneum CO_2 insufflation can cause both local and systemic effects, thereby altering the metabolic response to surgery. Cytokine synthesis from mesothelial cells was also found to be less after laparoscopy as compared to open surgery.
- **Operative stress:** Surgical trauma/stress is an important factor determining the magnitude of inflammatory and metabolic response to surgery.
- Intraoperative and postoperative thermoregulation and the factors determining them like anaesthetic drugs, open body cavities, age, etc. influence the metabolic response to surgery.
- **Type of anaesthesia:** The ability of anaesthetic agents and neural blockade to modify the metabolic and neuroendocrine response has been enthusiastically studied. For example, regional anaesthesia with local anaesthetics, particularly epidural blockade is known to have many beneficial effects such as reduced thromboembolic event, pulmonary, cardiac and gastrointestinal postoperative complications, thereby modifying the metabolic response to surgery.

Summary of response to injury has been given in Key Box 15.1.

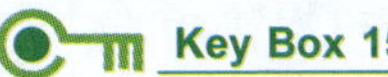

Key Box 15.1

Points to Remember

Hormones whose levels rise following injury:
- ACTH
- GH
- Glucagon
- Cortisol
- Adrenaline

Hormones whose levels fall following injury:
- Insulin
- Thyroid hormones
- Testosterone

Proinflammatory cytokines:
- IL-1
- IL-6
- IL-8
- TNF-α

Anti-inflammatory cytokines:
- IL-4
- IL-5
- IL-9
- IL-13
- TNF-β

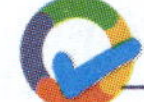

Multiple Choice Questions

1. Which hormone level does not rise during injury?
A. ACTH
B. Adrenaline
C. Glucagon
D. Thyroxine

2. Albumin level decreases during stress because of:
A. Decreased production
B. Decreased intake
C. Liver failure
D. Increased microvascular permeability

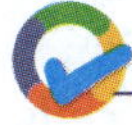

Answers

1. D **2.** A

CHAPTER

16

Tissue Engineering and Stem Cell Therapy

- Step 1: Choosing cell sources
- Step 2: Further differentiation
- Step 3: Scaffolds
- Step 4: Seeding
- Step 5: Implantation
- Applications
- Issues and concerns

INTRODUCTION

Tissue engineering is a relatively new field but also a mine of unfulfilled potential for treating various diseases. Tissue engineering aims to generate cells/tissues in laboratories that mimic human tissues as much as possible because most human tissues hardly show any regenerative capacity, so the only way to repair any loss or damage acquired would be to replace it and hope for ideal outcomes.

This process is broadly divided into two methods:

- ***In vitro***: Cells and the scaffold carrying them (as required) are developed outside the body and implanted thereafter.
- ***In vivo***: Cellular or cell-free scaffolds are implanted into the body and promote regeneration and repair by ingrowing into the body's cells.

Tissue engineering is relevant for surgeons through the myriad of possibilities that it offers, ranging from acting as models for testing therapeutic efficacy to scaffolds for reconstructing or replacing areas with extensive skin or soft tissue loss, cartilage loss, and blood vessels, cardiac muscle, valves, hollow viscera, and pancreatic islets. Future prospects may include solid organ replacement.

Biological sciences, material sciences, and engineering contribute to different aspects of the research and development of stem cells, ideal scaffolds, and conducive environments.

Sources of cells for tissue engineering include fully differentiated somatic cells and stem cells.

STEP 1: CHOOSING CELL SOURCES

Somatic Cells

Fully differentiated cells from normal tissues are grown *in vitro* and are developed on a scaffold. These cells can be obtained from the recipient by tissue biopsy (autologous cells) or from unrelated donors (allogenic cells). Examples include autologous chondrocyte implantation for areas of deficient cartilage and smooth muscle with uroepithelial cells for bladder wall reconstruction. Autologous cells carry the advantage of no risk of immune-mediated rejection. Allogenic cells carry the disadvantages of needing immunosuppression and limited *in vitro* proliferative ability, making it impractical for larger volumes.

Stem Cells

These are undifferentiated cells with the unique ability of infinite cell division and hence constant renewal. If stimulated with appropriate growth factors, they can also differentiate into specialised cell lines. These features make stem cells the most attractive option for regenerative therapies.

They are classified depending on where they are derived from, namely embryonic stem cells, fetal stem cells, adult or somatic stem cells, and induced pluripotent stem cells.

a. **Somatic stem cells:** In adults, there exists reserve of stem cells (especially in rapidly proliferating systems) to provide replacements at the end of their functional lifespans or during damage or disease. These cells are especially predominant in the gastrointestinal epithelium and bone marrow. However, they can differentiate into a limited number of cell types and hence are 'multipotent'.

Examples include hematopoietic stem cells (mainly in hematological malignancies), mesenchymal stem cells (mainly for tissue engineering), and neural stem cells.

b. **Mesenchymal stem and stromal cells (MSCs):** Mesenchymal stem cells or stromal cells resemble fibroblasts and are obtained from bone marrow, adipose tissue, or the umbilical cord.

These cells have the ability to adhere to plastic surfaces and display certain cell surface markers. They are typically used for their ability to differentiate into mesodermal-derived cells, such as osteoblasts, chondrocytes, adipocytes, and myocytes.

They can also express growth factors and hence have both trophic and immunomodulatory properties.

They are usually obtained by bone marrow aspiration from the iliac crest or by liposuction, following which they are cultured *in vitro* or are differentiated into desired cell types by the addition of growth factors. The ease of obtaining these cells has made them an attractive option, especially for treating burns and repairing cartilage.

c. **Embryonic stem cells:** These are obtained from the inner cell mass of blastocysts using unused embryos created at the time of *in vitro* fertilization. These cells are totipotent and give rise to all the cells of the body. They have a superior proliferative ability, but their development has given rise to several ethical issues. There are strict guidelines in place for their development, and the dominant view in most countries is that their potential therapeutic benefits outweigh their ethical concerns. However, these cells are allogenic and have the problem of rejection. Advances in nuclear transfer have paved the way for developing pluripotent stem cells designed for the recipient.

d. **Fetal stem cells:** These are obtained from the tissues of fetuses that have been aborted. They are also pluripotent. Uses include cell therapy in diabetes mellitus, spinal cord injuries, neurological disorders, etc. However, they are also associated with several ethical issues.

e. **Induced pluripotent stem cells (iPSCs):** This is based on the principle that certain adult cells can be reprogrammed to become pluripotent stem cells by manipulating their genetic structure. This is achieved by transferring specialized transcription factors (e.g. OSKM reprogramming factors, Yamanaka factors) via viruses to the cells of interest. This breakthrough comes with several advantages.

First, it overcomes any ethical concerns associated with embryonic stem cells. Second, it overcomes the risk of rejection, as the cells obtained from the recipient can themselves be reprogrammed and used for therapy. Third, a tissue bank of iPSCs from volunteer donors can be created.

However, the problem associated with the use of potentially oncogenic viruses is a disadvantage. Current research has focused on overcoming these issues with the use of non-retroviral vectors and virus-free transfer options. Newer advances in CRISPR-Cas9 gene editing have also helped tailor iPSCs for disease research.

f. **Endothelial progenitor cells:** They express surface markers found in peripheral blood and are involved in the development of vessels and blood cells.

STEP 2: FURTHER DIFFERENTIATION

Current research aims at the most ideal environment that stem cells need to finally differentiate into cells and tissues of interest. Efforts are currently focused on creating an environment as close to the normal development process as possible. The growth factors, matrices, and scaffolds used for various tissue types differ; however, they usually follow the same sequence of initial differentiation of iPSCs into either of the three lineages of ectoderm, mesoderm, or endoderm, followed by further differentiation, both of which are done *in vitro*. They are used only after they are fully phenotyped and assessed for functionality.

STEP 3: SCAFFOLDS

Scaffolds, which are physical support systems for stem cells and their progeny, mimic the extracellular matrix (ECM). They function just like the ECM does, allowing cells to attach, providing necessary signals, and aiding growth, migration, and nutrition, and are biocompatible and non-immunogenic. Rigid and semirigid porous scaffolds, into which stem cells are seeded, are used. Scaffolds can be natural or artificial.

Natural Scaffolds

Human tissues and organs are processed using detergents to remove cells, and the ECM left behind is used. This is especially useful when the target tissue being regenerated has a complex structure, such as complex solid organs. These whole organs needed for engineering are obtained from cadavers. Hence, their disadvantage lies in their limited availability.

Artificial Scaffolds

There is a wide assortment of artificial scaffolds available, and they are ideally biocompatible, bioresorbable, and biodegradable. They are made from both natural and synthetic materials, such as polysaccharides, collagen, fibrin, polyglycolide, graphene, ceramics, glasses, etc. The development of these scaffolds has been furthered by the use of 3D printing and electrospinning technology. They are usually porous and hydrophilic. Composite scaffolds and 'smart scaffolds' that respond to physical stresses are also being developed.

Scaffolds are commonly used to restore vascular integrity and are now advanced to include angiogenic growth factors as well.

STEP 4: SEEDING

Cells are typically incorporated into the scaffolds *in vitro*. Techniques include static cell seeding, dynamic cell seeding (uses rotation), magnetic cell seeding (uses supramagnetic microbeads binding to cells), photo-polymerized systems using UV light, vacuum seeding, and bioreactor perfusion systems.

STEP 5: IMPLANTATION

The efficacy of the engineered tissue ultimately depends on how well it integrates into the host tissue and reproduces its functions. Hence, an integral part of developing these tissues is postproduction testing in similar stressful environments that are subjected to in the body to ultimately ensure successful outcomes.

APPLICATIONS

1. Embryonic stem cells programmed to develop into retinal pigment epithelium cells to treat age-related macular degeneration (experimental). iPSCs have also been used for the same.
2. Somatic cell nuclear transfer to produce beta pancreatic cells from stem cells (experimental).
3. Hematopoietic stem cells for bone marrow transplant in hematological malignancies.
4. Adult stem cells for ischemic heart failure (trials).
5. Stem cells for perianal fistulas (trials).
6. MSCs for graft vs host disease (trials).

ISSUES AND CONCERNS

1. Safety concerns: Development of malignancy is an issue with using pluripotent stem cells, and rigorous post-development purification and assessment is needed to ensure that all cells are differentiated. To reduce the effects of oncogenic viruses, viral vectors that do not integrate into the genome and non-viral vectors can be used.
2. Infection transmission: Adequate screening is a must.
3. Need for immunosuppression.
4. Risk of rejection.
5. Side effects of immunosuppression.
6. Inadequate data as the entire field still in its early stages of development.
7. Ethical issues.
8. Cost of development.

REFERENCES

1. Williams N, O'Connell P, McCaskie A. Bailey and Love's Short Practice of Surgery. 27th ed. CRC Press, pp. 33–41, 2018.
2. Townsend C, Beauchamp R, Evers B, Mattox K, Sabiston D. Sabiston Textbook of Surgery. 21st ed. Elsevier, pp. 150–156, 2021.
3. Sultana N, Bandyopadhyay-Ghosh S, Soon C. Tissue Engineering Strategies for Organ Regeneration. CRC Press, 2020.

CHAPTER

17

Shock and Haemorrhage

Shock
- Hypovolaemic
- Cardiogenic
- Distributive (septic, anaphylactic, neurogenic, acute adrenal insufficiency)
- Obstructive (tension pneumothorax, cardiac tamponade)

Haemorrhage
- Classification
- Pathophysiology
- Management

Indicators of fluid responsiveness
- Central venous pressure
- IVC collapsibility index
- Passive leg raising

Competency

SU17.1: Describe pathophysiology of shock, types of shock and principles of resuscitation including fluid replacement and monitoring.

SU17.2: Describe clinical features of shock with appropriate treatment.

SHOCK

Definition

Shock is defined as an acute failure of the circulatory system to supply blood in **sufficient quantities** or under **sufficient pressure to the tissues**. It is a syndrome characterised by **hypoperfusion and severe dysfunction of vital organs.**

Pathophysiology

Whenever there is hypoperfusion due to any reason, the body tries to compensate by releasing massive amounts of catecholamines (fight or flight response). This causes progressive vasoconstriction of cutaneous, muscular and visceral circulation in an attempt to preserve blood flow to the vital organs, the heart, brain and the kidneys. The heart rate increases resulting in an increase in cardiac output. Thus, in most cases, tachycardia is the earliest sign of shock. The peripheral vascular resistance also increases due to the catecholamine release which in turn causes the diastolic blood pressure to rise and helps to maintain organ perfusion.

These compensatory mechanisms are effective in the early stages and are limited. In later stages, other vasoactive hormones such as histamine, bradykinin, β endorphins and other cytokines are also released. The hypoperfusion results in deprivation of oxygen and essential substrates at the cellular level causing a shift to anaerobic metabolism and development of lactic acidosis. With prolongation of shock, there is inadequate ATP production and the cells begin to lose their normal integrity. The electrical gradient across the cell membrane gets lost, the cell swells up eventually causing cellular death.

Types of Shock

- Hypovolaemic shock: Loss of fluids or blood (haemorrhagic shock)
- Cardiogenic shock
- Distributive shock: Septic shock, anaphylactic shock, neurogenic shock
- Obstructive shock: Tension pneumothorax, cardiac tamponade, massive pulmonary embolism

Clinical Features

Fast and feeble pulse, cold and clammy peripheries, and reduced urine output are prominent features of a person in shock. Depending on the stage of shock, the patient may be lethargic, confused, restless, delirious or even unconscious. The patient may develop tachypnea as a response to hypoxia (due to hypoperfusion of tissues) and lactic acidosis. The patient can show features specific to the cause of shock (bleeding in haemorrhagic shock, myocardial infarction in cardiogenic shock). Severe shock may progress to cardiac arrest.

Diagnosis

Shock is mainly diagnosed by the clinical features. The patient will manifest with hypotension, tachycardia, tachypnea, obtundation or abnormal mental status, cold, clammy extremities, mottled skin, oliguria, metabolic acidosis, and hyperlactatemia. History and physical examination will lead to the diagnosis of shock and the cause of shock. Arterial blood gas showing a base deficit or high lactate values can reliably help in the diagnosis of shock.

General Principles of Resuscitation

The diagnosis and treatment of shock is always concurrent and treatment at any point must not be delayed due to any ongoing test/investigation for a good outcome. **Monitoring** should include clinical examination as well as with a pulse oximeter, non-invasive blood pressure and electrocardiogram.

The basic management principle is to ensure better perfusion and oxygen delivery to the tissues. **Assess ABC** (airway, breathing and circulation).

Assess airway: A patient in shock could be obtunded or even unconscious. Secure airway, if the patient is unable to maintain his airway. Give oxygen.

Assess breathing: If the patient is apnoeic or is tachypneic and is not maintaining adequate gas exchange, one may need to initiate mechanical ventilation.

Assess circulation: Circulation is inadequate in shock. The priority of resuscitation is to restore perfusion. Obtain two large bore peripheral intravenous access (18 or 16 G). Begin resuscitation with rapid infusion of 500 ml to a litre of Ringer lactate or isotonic saline. Continue resuscitation with intravenous fluids, blood products or both as necessary and appropriate for the cause of shock to restore perfusion.

In haemorrhagic shock, after the initial litre of intravenous fluid, packed cell volume, fresh frozen plasma and platelets will be needed to replace lost blood volume. Type specific blood is preferred but in an emergency, O–ve packed cells can be given. If the facility is available, it is wiser to activate massive transfusion protocol (MTP) for more appropriate usage of blood products. A patient in hypovolaemic shock due to loss of fluids (as in severe diarrhoea) will require fluid replacement but may not need blood products to be transfused. Timely resuscitation in the initial phases includes infusion of appropriate quantity of isotonic electrolyte solutions and blood. Definitive control of haemorrhage and restoration of adequate circulating volume are the primary goals of management in haemorrhagic shock.

A patient in septic shock and anaphylactic shock will also require intravenous fluids. However, a patient in cardiogenic shock will require infusion of vasopressors and inotropes. They are often given diuretics to prevent or treat pulmonary congestion. A patient in obstructive shock will need urgent relief of this obstruction. This can be done easily for tension pneumothorax (needle thoracostomy) and for cardiac tamponade (pericardiocentesis). However, it is more difficult to treat massive pulmonary embolism.

End-points of Resuscitation

The initial end-points of resuscitation (to be achieved within a few hours) are a heart rate of < 100/min, blood pressure of 90/60 mmHg and an oxygen saturation of 93–95%. As perfusion improves, one must aim for normalising homeostasis. The final end-point of resuscitation is a normal base deficit (eliminate metabolic acidosis). This should be achieved within 12–24 hours of admission.

Specific Treatment

Specific treatment for different types of shock depends on the cause and is given in the appropriate section.

HAEMORRHAGE

CLASSIFICATION

I. Depending on Nature of the Vessel Involved

A. *Arterial haemorrhage:* The blood jets out and is bright red in colour. Pulsation of the artery may be seen. It can be easily controlled, as it is visible.

B. *Venous haemorrhage:* The blood does not jet out but oozes. It is dark red in colour. It is non-pulsatile, and difficult to control because the vein gets retracted.

C. *Capillary haemorrhage:* The blood does not jet out but oozes out slowly. The blood is red in colour. It becomes significant, if there are bleeding tendencies.

II. Depending on the Timing of Haemorrhage

A. *Primary haemorrhage:* This occurs at the time of surgery.

B. *Reactionary haemorrhage:* This occurs within 6–12 hours of surgery. The usual causes are hypertension in the postoperative period, violent sneezing, coughing, or retching. For example, the superior thyroid artery may bleed after thyroidectomy, if the ligature slips; hence, it is better to ***ligate it twice***.

C. *Secondary haemorrhage:* This occurs within 5–7 days of surgery. It is due to infection which eats away the suture material, causing sloughing of vessel wall (e.g. bleeding within 5–7 days of surgery for haemorrhoids).

III. Depending on the Duration of Haemorrhage

A. *Acute haemorrhage*: This occurs suddenly (e.g. oesophageal variceal bleeding due to portal hypertension).

B. *Chronic haemorrhage:* This occurs over a period of time (e.g. haemorrhoids/piles, chronic duodenal ulcer, tuberculous ulcer of the ileum, diverticular disease of the colon).

IV. Depending on the Nature of Bleeding

A. *External haemorrhage*/revealed haemorrhage (e.g. epistaxis, haematemesis).

B. *Internal haemorrhage*/concealed haemorrhage (e.g. splenic rupture following injury, ruptured ectopic gestation, liver laceration following injury).

Clinical Notes

A patient who had undergone subtotal thyroidectomy for toxic goitre was shifted to the postoperative intensive care unit. Within 10 minutes, the nurse came to inform the surgeon that 450 ml of blood was collected in the 'Redivac' suction bottle. The dressing was opened and there was no large collection of blood in the surgical wound. The presence of a large haematoma was thus ruled out. The blood pressure (BP), which was previously under control, had shot up to 210/110 mmHg postoperatively, possibly due to pain. Careful monitoring and treatment reduced the BP to 140/90 mmHg. After 24 hours, the drainage was only 100 ml. The incision did not need re-exploration. This case illustrates reactionary haemorrhage due to hypertension.

PATHOPHYSIOLOGY OF HAEMORRHAGIC SHOCK

A loss of >30–40% blood volume results in a fall in blood pressure, and gross hypoperfusion of the tissues and vital organs, leading to haemorrhagic shock. Haemorrhagic shock can be classified as follows (American College of Surgeons) depending on the amount of blood lost and clinical features:

Classification of Haemorrhagic Shock

Class I

- When blood loss is <750 ml (<15% of blood volume), it can be called *mild haemorrhage*.
- 60–70% of blood volume is present in the low-pressure venous system (capacitance vessels). 10% of the blood volume is present in the splanchnic circulation.
- When there is blood loss, peripheral venoconstriction takes place, which compensates for the loss of blood volume by shifting some blood into the central circulation. Some amount of blood volume correction also occurs due to withdrawal of fluid from the interstitial spaces.
- Apart from mild tachycardia and thirst, there may be no other symptoms or signs suggesting hypovolaemia. The blood pressure, urine output, and mentation are all normal.

Class II

- Loss of 750–1500 ml (15–30% of blood volume) results in *moderate shock*.
- Peripheral venoconstriction may not be sufficient to maintain circulation. Hence, adrenaline and noradrenaline (endogenous catecholamines) released from the sympathoadrenal system cause powerful vasoconstriction of both arteries and veins.
- Increased secretion of ADH causes retention of water and salt. Thirst increases.
- Clinically, the patient shows a heart rate of 100–120 beats/minute and an elevated diastolic pressure. The systolic pressure may remain normal.
- Urine output is reduced to about 0.5 ml/kg/h and the capillary refill time is more than the normal 2 seconds. Extremities may look pale and the patient is confused and thirsty.

Class III

- Loss of 1500–2000 ml (30–40% of blood volume) produces Class III shock. All the signs and symptoms seen in Class II haemorrhagic shock get worse.
- The patient's systolic and diastolic blood pressures fall and the heart rate increases to around 120 beats/minute. The pulse is thready.
- The respiratory rate increases to > 20/minute. Urine output drops to 10–20 ml/hour. The patient appears pale and is aggressive, drowsy, or confused.

Class IV

- A blood loss of >2000 ml (>40% of blood volume) results in Class IV shock. The peripheries are cold and ashen.
- The pulse is thready and >120/minute. The blood pressures are very low or unrecordable.
- The patient may be moribund.
- If persistent, other organs may get damaged:

- Mucosal ulcerations, upper GI bleeding, absorption of bacteria and toxins, **bacterial translocation,** and bacteraemia
- *Liver:* Reduced clearance of toxins
- *Kidney:* **Acute renal failure**
- *Heart:* **Myocardial ischaemia**, depression
- *Lungs:* Loss of surfactant, increased alveolo-capillary permeability, interstitial oedema, and increased arteriovenous shunting result in **acute lung injury** (ALI).

- **Multiorgan failure** consequent to haemorrhagic shock is associated with a high mortality rate.
- Early diagnosis of bleeding and appropriate management is crucial to improve survival and outcome.

MANAGEMENT OF HAEMORRHAGIC SHOCK

I. Treatment—General Measures

- Hospitalisation
- A patient in haemorrhagic shock needs immediate resuscitation to prevent or minimise damage to the vital organs and tissues. Resuscitation and control of haemorrhage should happen simultaneously.
- **O-M-IV:** First, provide oxygen, attach a monitor to record vitals (heart rate, blood pressure, respiratory rate, and oxygen saturation) and obtain two large bore intravenous access.
- Remember **O-M-IV** for all critically ill patients: O for **o**xygen, M for **m**onitor, and IV for **i**ntra**v**enous access. Blood sample for investigations, blood grouping, and cross-matching should be sent at this stage.
- Care of all critically ill patients begins with **A** (airway), **B** (breathing), and **C** (circulation).
- **Airway and breathing:** Oxygen should be administered by face mask to all patients who are in shock, but are conscious and are able to maintain their airway. If unconscious, endotracheal intubation and ventilation with oxygen may be necessary.

Circulation

- **Haemorrhage control (*see* below)**
- Resuscitation and haemorrhage control must happen simultaneously.
- **Two large peripheral lines (18 or 16 G)** are preferred for initial resuscitation. Intravenous fluids, preferably at 40–42°C (crystalloids—Ringer lactate, or plasmalyte) are infused rapidly to restore volume.
- Send blood sample for investigations, blood grouping, and cross-matching.
- **Dextrose containing solutions are not recommended.** Infusion of large amounts of isotonic saline may cause hyperchloraemic acidosis and is not recommended.
- Insertion of central lines is not recommended (unless done by skilled personnel), as it takes much longer to insert, requires expertise, and may be associated with complications.
- External jugular venous access is another option for quick transfusion of large amounts of fluids and blood products.
- If a peripheral intravenous access is not available, an **intraosseous needle** may be inserted to infuse fluids into the bone marrow (Fig. 17.1). All infusions that can be given intravenously can also be given intraosseously.

Intraosseous Cannulation

- The bone marrow of long bones is in direct communication with the vascular tree and hence, anything injected into the bone marrow will reach circulation. Thus, when intravenous access is not available and access to the circulation is required in an emergency as in major trauma, burns, circulatory arrest, intraosseous needles can provide rapid and life-saving access to the circulation. This is most often performed in children but can be done in adults also in emergency circumstances.
  - **Contraindications:** Fracture of the long bone being punctured, previous puncture of the same bone either at the same site or another site on the same bone, infection at the site, burn at entry site and inability to locate landmarks.
  - **Sites:** Intraosseous puncture is most commonly made at the upper end of tibia, one finger-breadth below the tibial tuberosity on the medial surface. The other sites are lower end of femur, lower end of radius, manubrium sternum, iliac bone and the calcaneus.
  - **Needle:** A large bore needle is required. A bone marrow aspiration needle with a guide such as Jamshidi needle is best suited for this procedure. Several others such as Sur-Fast intraosseous needle, Sussmane-Raszynski needle or the EZ-IO can be used. If these are not available, any large bore needle with stylet can be used for this purpose.

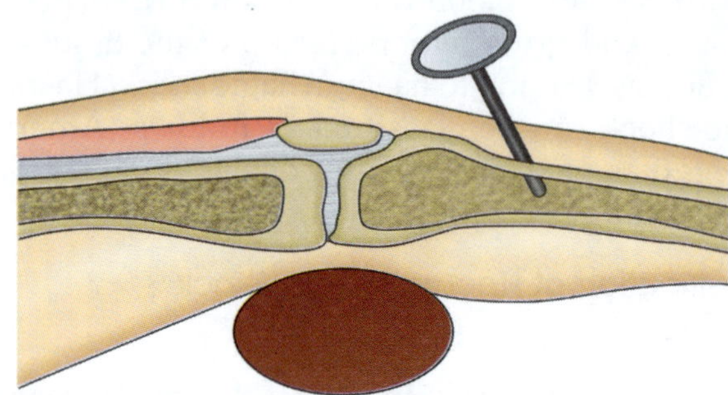

Fig. 17.1: Intraosseous cannulation

- **Procedure:** The limb to be used must be stabilized using a pillow or roll. Under aseptic precautions, the skin over the puncture site is anaesthetized using 2 ml of local anaesthetic. The bone is held steady with the nondominant hand and the needle held in the palm of the dominant hand such that the needle, wrist and elbow are in the same straight line. The bone is punctured with a rotatory movement through the skin and then the bone. Loss of resistance indicates entry of the needle into the marrow. Care must be taken not to penetrate the opposite surface of the bone. The operator must be careful and not place his hand in the needle path. The marrow may or may not be aspirated from the needle. A 10 ml syringe containing saline is connected to the needle. If the saline can be injected freely and without any extravasation, an infusion of saline or Ringer lactate can be commenced through the needle. A free flow of this solution may be obtained but may need to be injected, if there is resistance. Anything that can be given intravenously can also be given by the intraosseous route.
- Care must be taken to check the correct position of the needle. Puncture of the opposite surface of the bone must be avoided to prevent leakage of fluid through that hole into the tissues. The limb must be observed closely for any swelling due to extravasation. An intravenous access must be secured as soon as possible and the intraosseous line removed. Generally, an intraosseous line is removed in a few hours' time but it can be used up to 48 hours.
- **Complications:** Infections at the site of insertion such as cellulitis, osteomyelitis can occur due to poor aseptic technique. Extravasation of fluid and compartment syndrome can occur, if not carefully watched. Fracture of the bone can also occur if excessive force is applied during insertion.

- The American College of Surgeons classification of haemorrhagic shock (as given above) may be used as a quick guide to gauge the amount of blood loss. If the patient is tachycardic (heart rate >120/min) and hypotensive (systolic blood pressure is <90 mmHg), the patient has Class III shock or higher and has lost >30–40% blood volume.
- Remember that the numbers given above are a rough guide. The actual clinical presentation may change with comorbid illnesses, other injuries, or concurrent medications.
- If infusion of 1–2 litres (in an adult) of Ringer lactate has not been successful in returning the vitals to normal values, the patient may have lost a large amount of blood and may be having ongoing bleeding. Such patients require transfusion of blood products (packed cells and fresh frozen plasma).
- It may be necessary to activate **massive transfusion protocol** (when available at the hospital), if the patient is bleeding profusely. Replacing the lost volume and controlling haemorrhage is important to restore perfusion and prevent tissue damage.
- Most blood banks do not issue whole blood (as it is uneconomical for a scarce commodity), and provide component therapy. In an actively bleeding patient who is in hypovolaemic shock, the ratio of **packed cells : fresh frozen plasma : platelets would be 1:1:1.**
- Generally, **typed and cross-matched blood is given**. However, if the shock is severe and the patient is in Class IV shock, O –ve blood may be given as a life-saving measure. Subsequently, cross-matching needs to be done before giving type-specific blood.
- In cases where the haemostasis is not yet achieved, volume infusion should be controlled to maintain systolic BP at 80–90 mmHg till the bleeding can be stopped. This is called *'hypotensive fluid resuscitation' or 'permissive hypotension'.*
- Use of a fibrinolytic agent like tranexamic acid 1 g stat and then 8th hourly is advised to reduce bleeding.
- Once bleeding is controlled, infuse sufficient volume to allow blood pressure to reach normal levels as soon as possible (***first phase of resuscitation***).
- **The second phase of resuscitation** involves continuation of fluid therapy to ensure the base deficit is eliminated. This is important to ensure that the microcirculation is normal. This should happen within 12–24 hours (the earlier, the better).
- All through the resuscitation, it is important to maintain patient's body temperature (by using warm air blowers, keep him covered). Hypothermia impairs coagulation, increases bleeding, depresses respiration and circulation, and increases the chances of infection.
- Use of inotropes and vasoconstrictors is not indicated, as they may harm tissue perfusion.
- However, if inotropes have been started as a life-saving measure, an attempt should be made to wean them as soon as the volume status is corrected and the patient is stable.

II. Treatment—Specific Measures

Control Haemorrhage

1. Pressure and packing

- This is the method of choice to stop bleeding when the bleeding site is accessible.
- Packing using roller gauze with or without adrenaline to control bleeding from the nose and scalp.

- Pressure packing the middle thyroid vein during thyroidectomy and the lumbar veins during lumbar sympathectomy.
- A Sengstaken tube is used to control bleeding from oesophageal varices—internal tamponade.

2. Position and rest

- Elevation of the leg controls bleeding from varicose veins.
- Elevation of the head-end reduces venous bleeding in thyroidectomy—**anti-Trendelenburg position**.
- Sedation to relieve anxiety—midazolam in titrated doses of 1–2 mg intravenously may be given. This may help control blood pressure and the consequent bleeding.

3. Tourniquets

Indications

- Reduction of fractures
- Repair of tendons
- Repair of nerves
- When a bloodless field is desired during surgery

Contraindications: Patient with peripheral vascular disease. (The arterial disease may be aggravated due to thrombosis resulting in gangrene.)

Types:

- Pneumatic cuffs with a pressure gauge
- Rubber bandage

Precautions:

- ***Too loose*** a tourniquet does not serve the purpose.
- ***Too tight***: Arterial thrombosis may occur, which may result in gangrene.
- ***Too long*** (duration of application): Gangrene of the limb.

Application of a tourniquet to control bleeding is not advised unless pressure bandaging has not been helpful because of possible ischaemia of the limb. Hence, if applied, the time of application must be noted down. Deflate as soon as possible within 45–60 minutes.

Complications

- Ischaemia and gangrene
- Tourniquet nerve palsy[1]

4. Surgical methods to control haemorrhage

- Application of **artery forceps** (Spencer Wells forceps) to control bleeding from veins, arteries and capillaries.
- Application of **ligatures** for bleeding vessels.
- **Cauterisation** (diathermy).
- Application of **bone wax** (**Horsley's wax,** which is bee's wax in almond oil) to control bleeding from cut edges of bones.
- **Silver clips** are used to control bleeding from cerebral vessels ***(Cushing's clip)***.
- **Surgical procedure:** Laparotomy and **splenectomy** for splenic rupture, hysterectomy for uncontrollable postpartum haemorrhage, laparotomy for control of bleeding from ruptured ectopic pregnancy.

HYPOVOLAEMIC SHOCK

- Loss of blood—haemorrhagic shock
- Loss of plasma—as in burns shock
- Loss of fluid—dehydration as in gastroenteritis

Features (Key Box 17.1)

The primary problem is a decrease in preload. The decreased preload causes a decrease in stroke volume. Clinical features depend on the degree of hypovolaemia, and are similar to those of haemorrhagic shock. Severe (Class III or IV) shock results in tachycardia, low blood pressure, and decreased urine output.

The peripheries are cold and the patient may be confused or moribund (*see* Pathophysiology of haemorrhagic shock).

Treatment

- Replace the lost blood volume.
- The primary goal is to restore tissue perfusion and oxygenation as early as possible.
- ***Crystalloids:*** If crystalloids are used to replace blood loss, 1.5–2 times the lost volume need to be given. Ringer lactate is the crystalloid of choice. Large volumes of saline infusion may cause hyperchloraemic metabolic acidosis. 5% dextrose is not used to expand the intravascular volume, as it is hypotonic once dextrose metabolises.
- ***Colloids:*** When colloids are used to replace lost blood volume, a volume equal to the lost volume may be given. However, they are not preferred.

Key Box 17.1

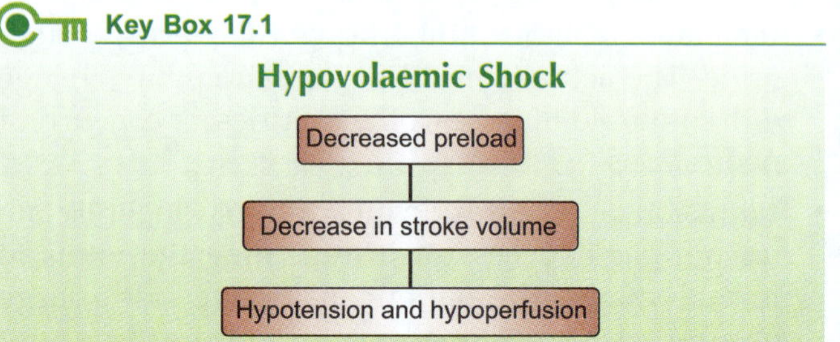

[1]In MS examination, a candidate was asked to examine a case of radial nerve palsy. The patient had an injury to the wrist 4 months prior. The cut flexor tendons had been sutured. The candidate could not correlate the radial nerve palsy to the injury at the wrist. He failed! It was a case of tourniquet palsy.

- Crystalloids are preferred during the initial phase of resuscitation. If a large volume of blood is lost, transfuse blood products. Please refer to the management of hamorrhagic shock described earlier in this chapter.

CARDIOGENIC SHOCK

The blood flow is reduced because of an intrinsic problem in the heart muscle or its valves. A massive myocardial infarction may damage the cardiac muscle so that there is not much healthy muscle to pump blood effectively. Any damage (especially acute) to the valves may also reduce the forward cardiac output, resulting in cardiogenic shock.

Features

- The primary problem is a decrease in contractility of the heart. The decreased contractility causes a decrease in stroke volume.
- Left ventricular pressures rise as forward cardiac output reduces. The sympathetic nervous system is activated, resulting in increased systemic vascular resistance.
- Clinically, the patient presents with tachycardia, low blood pressure, and decreased urine output.
- The jugular venous pulse may be raised, and an S3 or S4 gallop may be present.
- The lung fields may show bilateral extensive crepitations due to pulmonary oedema.
- The peripheries are cold, and the patient may be confused or moribund.

Treatment

- The primary goal is to **improve cardiac muscle function**.
- Oxygenation can be improved by administering oxygen, either by a face mask or by endotracheal intubation and ventilation as necessary.
- **Inotropes** improve cardiac muscle contractility.
- **Vasodilators** such as nitroglycerine may dilate the coronary arteries and peripheral vessels, and improve tissue perfusion. Lowering systemic vascular resistance reduces impedance to forward cardiac output (afterload). However, the patient must be monitored closely to avoid excessive reductions in blood pressure.
- **Intra-aortic balloon pump** or ventricular assist devices may be used to augment cardiac output.
- If hypotension continues to be refractory, revascularisation (surgical or interventional) or valve replacement may be considered on an emergency basis.

DISTRIBUTIVE SHOCK

In distributive shock, the afterload is excessively reduced, thereby affecting circulation. Distributive shock may occur in the following situations:

- Septic shock
- Anaphylactic shock
- Neurogenic shock
- Acute adrenal insufficiency

Septic Shock

Pathophysiology

- Sepsis is the response of the host to bacteraemia/ endotoxaemia.
- It may be produced by gram-negative or gram-positive bacteria, viruses, fungi, or even protozoal infections.
- Severe sepsis may result in persistent hypotension despite adequate fluid resuscitation.
- Local inflammation and substances (especially endotoxin) released from organisms activate neutrophils, monocytes, and tissue macrophages. **This results in a cascade of proinflammatory and anti-inflammatory cytokines and other mediators, such as IL-1, IL-8, IL-10, TNF-α, prostaglandin E1, endogenous corticosteroids, and catecholamines.**
- This results in cellular chemotaxis, endothelial injury, and activation of the coagulation cascade (Key Box 17.2).

Features

- These substances produce **low systemic vascular resistance (peripheral vasodilatation)** and ventricular dysfunction, resulting in persistent hypotension.
- **Generalised tissue hypoperfusion** may persist despite adequate fluid resuscitation and improvement in cardiac output and blood pressures. This is due to abnormalities in regional and microcirculatory blood flow. These abnormalities may lead to **cellular dysfunction, lactic acidosis (anaerobic metabolism), and ultimately, multiorgan failure.**
- Early phases of septic shock may produce evidence of volume depletion, such as dry mucous membranes and cool, clammy skin.

Key Box 17.2

Disturbance of Procoagulant–Anticoagulant Balance

- Inflammatory response in sepsis activates tissue factor which in turn activates coagulation
- Fibrinogen is converted to fibrin
- Lowered levels of natural anticoagulants such as protein C, protein S and antithrombin III

Procoagulant—anticoagulant imbalance → diffuse microvascular thrombi

- After resuscitation with fluids, however, the clinical picture is typically more consistent with that of **hyperdynamic shock.** Features include tachycardia, bounding pulses with a widened pulse pressure, a hyperdynamic precordium on palpation, and warm extremities.
- Signs of possible infection depend on the source of sepsis. These may include fever, localised erythema or tenderness, consolidation on chest examination, abdominal tenderness, guarding, rigidity, and meningismus.
- Signs of **end-organ hypoperfusion** include tachypnoea, cyanosis, mottling of the skin, digital ischaemia, oliguria, abdominal tenderness, and altered mental status.
- Often, a definitive diagnosis cannot be made on the basis of initial clinical features; hence, empirical treatment for several possible conditions should be commenced.

Treatment

- **Removal of the septic focus is an essential step,** and is a priority in the treatment of septic shock (e.g. resection of gangrenous bowels, closure of perforation, appendicectomy).
- Early **empirical antibiotic therapy** should be administered to treat the precipitating infection. This must be given within the first hour of arrival.
- **Supportive care:** Oxygenation and, if necessary, endotracheal intubation and mechanical ventilation should be administered.
- **Intravenous fluids:** Restoration of intravascular filling pressures must be done using crystalloids, colloids, and blood as necessary. **Crystalloids, such as isotonic saline** or **Ringer's lactate,** may be used. Large amount may be required, which may contribute to tissue oedema. Colloids restore intravascular volume faster and remain longer in the central circulation. However, they are expensive and often used in patients with a high-risk of pulmonary oedema (due to cardiac dysfunction) who may not tolerate large volume of fluids. Avoid hetastarch, as it may increase the risk of renal injury and mortality. If the patient is anaemic, **blood transfusions** may be required to raise haemoglobin levels to 8–10 g%.
- **Vasoactive agents,** such as norepinephrine, may be used to produce vasoconstriction and raise the systemic vascular resistance to normal. Dopamine, dobutamine, or adrenaline may need to be added. Vasopressin infusion may be useful in patients with refractory shock. All these potent drugs are given as infusions under careful and continuous monitoring of blood pressure, as well as cardiac filling pressures (central venous pressures).

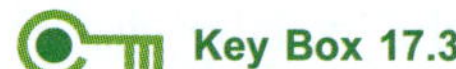

Key Box 17.3

Summary of Septic Shock

- Early diagnosis of septic shock
- Empirical antibiotics initially
- Appropriate antibiotics after culture and sensitivity testing
- Ultrasonography, CT scan, and chest X-ray are key investigations
- **Treatment of source of infection**
  - Pneumonia
  - Drainage of pus
  - Closure of perforation
  - Resection of gangrene
- Early and aggressive resuscitation, supportive care and close monitoring in intensive care unit (ICU).

Pearls of Wisdom

Measure and monitor serum lactate. The aim is to eliminate lactic acidosis with fluid resuscitation and better perfusion.

Clinical Notes

- A 54-year-old lady was admitted to the casualty with low blood pressure and dyspnoea since one day. She had a history of fever, vomiting, and diarrhoea since 3–4 days, and was treated in a local nursing home. When she got worse, was referred to our hospital. In spite of fluid therapy, profound hypotension persisted, and within half an hour of arrival to the casualty, she suffered a cardiopulmonary arrest.
- Her trachea was immediately intubated, cardiopulmonary resuscitation (CPR) was given, and she was shifted to the intensive care unit for further management. She required high doses of dopamine, adrenaline, and noradrenaline to maintain blood pressure. A blood gas analysis showed severe metabolic acidosis (pH = 7.02, $PaCO_2$ = 35 mmHg, and HCO_3^- = 12 mmol/L).
- Considering the history, a diagnosis of septic shock was made when she continued to have hypotension even after her central venous pressures were normal. Peritoneal dialysis was done, as she was in oliguric renal failure. Haemodialysis was not possible, as she was hypotensive and on inotropes. A search for a septic focus was initiated. Ultrasound abdomen showed a dilated kidney and an obstructed urinary system.
- A DJ-stenting of the ureter, which was done to relieve the obstruction, drained pus. Once the pus was drained, appropriate antibiotics were given, and with continued cardiorespiratory support, she showed steady improvement. She was gradually weaned off the ventilator and inotropes, and was discharged from the hospital five

weeks later. At discharge, she was fully conscious, stable, ambulant, and very grateful to the medical fraternity.

☞ This case illustrates the importance of resuscitation, cardiorespiratory support, removal of the septic focus, and antibiotics in the treatment of septic shock.

Anaphylactic Shock

Features

It occurs on exposure to an allergen that the patient is sensitive to. It may be pollen, foodstuffs, preservatives in the food, or a medication. Anaphylactic shock that occurs in the hospital is usually due to some drug allergy (e.g. to penicillin). Latex allergy is also being increasingly recognised.

The reaction may be in the form of **mild rashes,** with or without **bronchospasm,** or a full blown anaphylactic shock, wherein the patient presents with rashes, **generalised oedema** (including laryngeal oedema), **bronchospasm** and **hypotension,** and if not treated in time, cardiac arrest.

Treatment

I. Primary

- Oxygen and, if necessary, endotracheal intubation and ventilation.
- Adrenaline, 0.5–1 mg IM or 50–100 µg IV boluses, as necessary, to maintain blood pressure.
- Intravenous fluids—isotonic saline or Ringer lactate
- Leg-end elevation of bed.

II. Secondary

- Chlorpheniramine maleate
- Hydrocortisone 100 mg intravenously

If facilities exist, take a 10 ml sample of blood to analyse for serum tryptase levels. If raised, it confirms anaphylactic reaction.

Neurogenic Shock

Causes: High spinal cord injury, vasovagal shock.

Features: Hypotension without tachycardia (more often bradycardia) that may deteriorate to cause shock and cardiac arrest.

Treatment: Intravenous fluids, inotropes, and vagolytics, as necessary.

Acute Adrenal Insufficiency

Risk Factors (Key Box 17.4)

Adrenal crisis occurs, if the adrenal gland is deteriorating, as in:

Key Box 17.4

Risk Factors for Adrenal Crisis

- Infection
- Trauma or surgery
- Adrenal gland or pituitary gland injury
- Premature termination of treatment with steroids such as prednisolone or hydrocortisone.

- Primary adrenal insufficiency (Addison's disease)
- Secondary adrenal insufficiency (pituitary gland injury, compression)
- Inadequately treated adrenal insufficiency.

Features

- Headache, profound weakness, fatigue, slow and lethargic movement, joint pain.
- Nausea, vomiting, abdominal pain, high fever and chills.
- Low blood pressure, dehydration, rapid heart and respiratory rates, confusion or coma.

Treatment

- Care of airway, breathing, and circulation
- Intravenous fluids
- Hydrocortisone 100 mg intravenously every 6 h to provide mineralocorticoid activity
- Treat the precipitating factor
- Antibiotics as necessary

OBSTRUCTIVE SHOCK

In obstructive shock, there is impedance to either inflow or outflow of blood into or out of the heart. It may be due to cardiac tamponade or due to tension pneumothorax.

Cardiac Tamponade

In **cardiac tamponade**, the pericardium is filled with blood or fluid, which hampers venous filling as well as outflow. Therefore, the cardiac output reduces drastically, even to zero. It is a medical emergency. Prompt recognition and treatment can save lives.

Causes

- Injury to the heart due to trauma
- Perforation of vena cava or atrial walls during cannulation or intracardiac procedures
- Rupture of ventricular or aortic aneurysm
- Postoperatively after cardiac surgery

Pericarditis can lead to accumulation of fluid in the pericardial sac. This pericardial effusion tends to occur more slowly but can produce cardiac tamponade when there is large amount of fluid accumulation. It can be due to infections (bacterial or fungal), inflammatory causes (uraemia, systemic lupus erythematosus, rheumatoid arthritis), cancer or certain medications.

Features

- The filling pressures of the left-sided and right-sided chambers equalise.
- **Beck's triad:** Low blood pressure, muffled heart sounds and distended neck veins.
- The patients also have pulsus paradoxus where there is at least a 10% decrease in systolic blood pressure with inspiration.
- This can lead to cardiac arrest.

Treatment

- This is a life-threatening condition and must be treated immediately, especially when acute.
- **Pericardiocentesis:** Drain the pericardial cavity using a wide bore needle, attached to a syringe. It is inserted from the subcostal area, under the xiphoid process, pointing towards the left shoulder with continuous aspiration (Fig. 17.2). Use of ultrasound to perform this procedure under vision improves safety and is recommended.
- Decompression of the pericardial cavity allows venous filling of the heart and forward flow. Blood pressure improves immediately.
- Monitor electrocardiogram during this procedure. Watch for arrhythmias that can occur, if the needle stimulates the myocardium.

Tension Pneumothorax

Causes

- Lung injury due to trauma
- Ventilator-induced barotrauma
- Rupture of emphysematous bullae in a patient with chronic obstructive pulmonary disease.

Features

- Profound cyanosis, distended neck veins
- Tachypnoea, dyspnoea, or respiratory arrest
- No air entry on the side of pneumothorax, hyper-resonance to percussion
- Tachycardia, hypotension, and cardiac arrest

Treatment

- A wide (large) bore needle/cannula (needle thoracostomy) must be inserted into the pleural cavity to drain the air. Traditionally, it was advised that the needle should be inserted in the midclavicular line in the 2nd intercostal space on the affected side (Fig. 17.3).
- However, in adults diagnosed to have a tension pneumothorax, the current Advanced Trauma Life Support (ATLS) guidelines advise that the needle is inserted in the 5th intercostal space in the mid-axillary line.
- This is followed by tube thoracostomy.

Pearls of Wisdom

A massive pulmonary embolus is a differential diagnosis for obstructive shock.

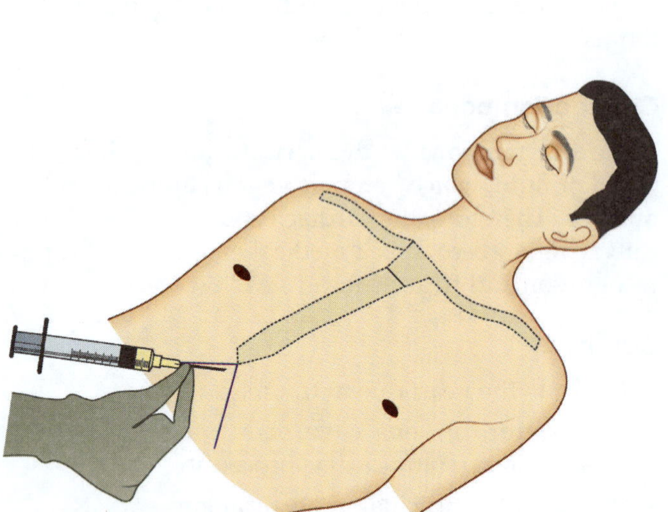

Fig. 17.2: Pericardiocentesis

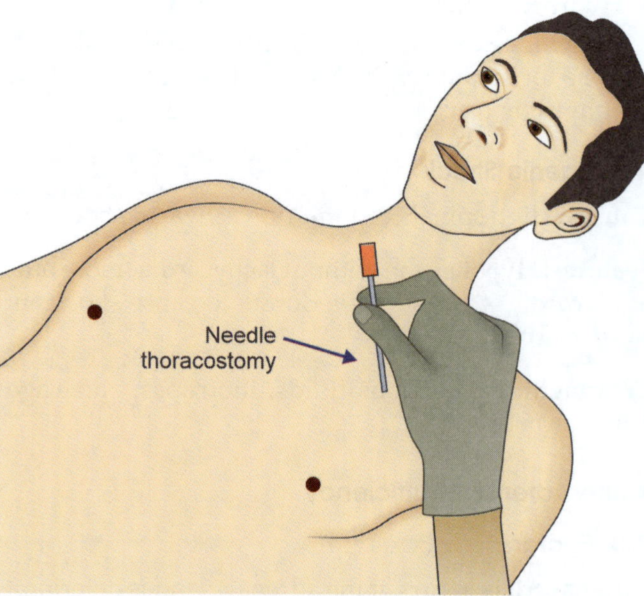

Fig. 17.3: Needle thoracocentesis

INDICATORS OF FLUID RESPONSIVENESS

Measurement of CVP has been used traditionally as an indicator of fluid responsiveness. The newer ones include pulse pressure variation, systolic pressure variation, stroke volume variation, inferior vena caval diameter and passive leg raising.

CENTRAL VENOUS PRESSURE (CVP)

- Pressure in the intrathoracic great veins is called central venous pressure.
- It is the same as right atrial pressure.
- Normal CVP is 2–6 mmHg in a person breathing spontaneously. It is higher (8–12 mmHg) in a patient who is receiving mechanical ventilation.
- CVP is used as a surrogate measure of blood volume. A low CVP suggests hypovolaemia.
- In shock, measurement of CVP is useful for planning proper fluid management. Thus, it is desirable to monitor CVP while treating patients in shock.
- However, it must be remembered that CVP may also be affected by contractility of the right ventricle, changes in intrathoracic and intrapericardial pressures. Thus, a high CVP does not always indicate hypervolaemia. In such situations, other means of fluid responsiveness such as pulse pressure variation or systolic pressure variation, measurement of inferior vena caval diameter can be used.

Method

- The internal jugular vein (IJV) or subclavian vein are preferred routes of accessing the central veins (Key Box 17.5).
- A 16-cm long IV catheter is introduced into the central vein with the patient supine, head down, and neck rotated to the opposite side (Fig. 17.4). Head down position helps in engorging the vein. Ultrasound guidance to cannulation is now considered the standard of care. Seldinger's technique is employed, and the catheter is advanced up to the junction of the superior vena cava and the right atrium (corresponding externally to the manubrium sterni).
- Aspirate through the lumen to check for free flow of blood into the connecting tube.

Key Box 17.5

Access to Right Heart/Great Veins

- Internal jugular vein
- Subclavian vein
- Median cubital vein
- External jugular vein

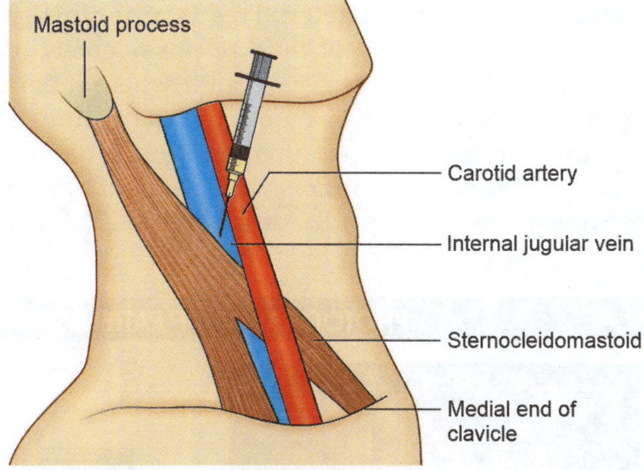

Fig. 17.4: Right internal jugular vein cannulation

- The tube is connected to an electronic pressure transducer. The 'zero reference point' must be at the **midaxillary level,** if the patient is in **supine position,** or at the **manubriosternal joint,** if he is in the semi-reclining position (45°). If the facility for using an electronic transducer is not available, a saline manometer may be used.
- CVP must be measured at end-expiration when the influence of intrathoracic pressure on CVP is minimum.

Uses

1. If CVP is low, venous return should be supplemented by IV infusion, as in cases of hypovolaemic shock.
2. When CVP is high, further infusion of fluids may result in pulmonary oedema.
3. In cardiogenic shock, CVP may be normal or high, and it is affected by the reduced ventricular contractility. In such situations, therefore, it may not accurately reflect intravascular volume.

Complications

1. Pneumothorax
2. Accidental carotid artery puncture
3. Haematoma in the neck
4. Bleeding
5. Air embolism
6. Infection

Dynamic indicators of fluid responsiveness such as stroke volume variation, systolic pressure variation and pulse pressure variation measure the changes in stroke volume, systolic pressure or pulse pressure respectively with changes in intrathoracic pressure. A variation more than 10–13% indicates fluid responsiveness (the patient's haemodynamic parameters will respond to volume infusion). This parameter is useful when patients are being mechanically ventilated with a tidal volume of at least 8 ml/kg body weight.

Inferior vena cava diameter: This is a noninvasive method of measurement of fluid responsiveness. It is measured using ultrasound at a point where it enters the right atrium. Using M mode, the maximum and minimum diameter are measured. If the IVC diameter is <10 mm, the patient requires volume and if >25 mm, the patient is reasonably full. A variability >25% in IVC diameter with respiration (IVC collapsibility index) also indicates fluid responsiveness.

Passive leg raising: By about 30° will result in increased venous return. An improvement in haemodynamics with this reversible manoeuvre suggests need for volume replacement.

PHOTOGRAPHS OF PATIENTS WITH SEPTIC SHOCK (Figs 17.5 to 17.10)

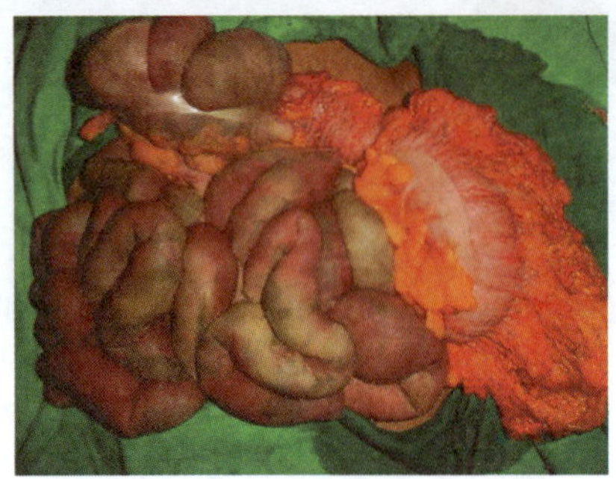

Fig. 17.5: Extensive gangrene

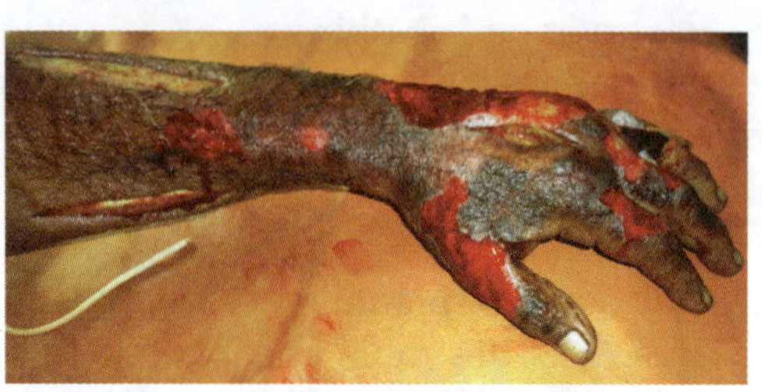

Fig. 17.6: Necrotising fasciitis of upper limb

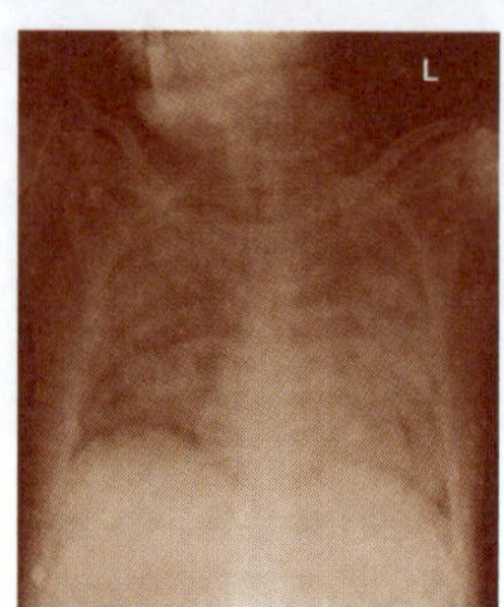

Fig. 17.7: Chest X-ray in septic shock patient

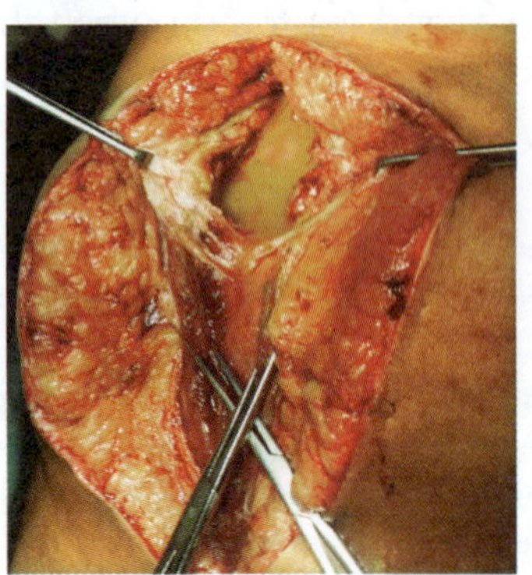

Fig. 17.8: Faecal peritonitis

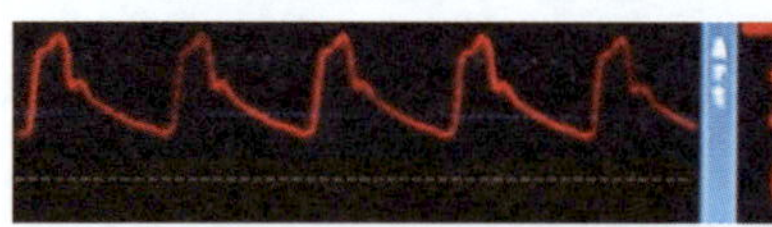

Fig. 17.9A: Intra-arterial blood pressure monitoring

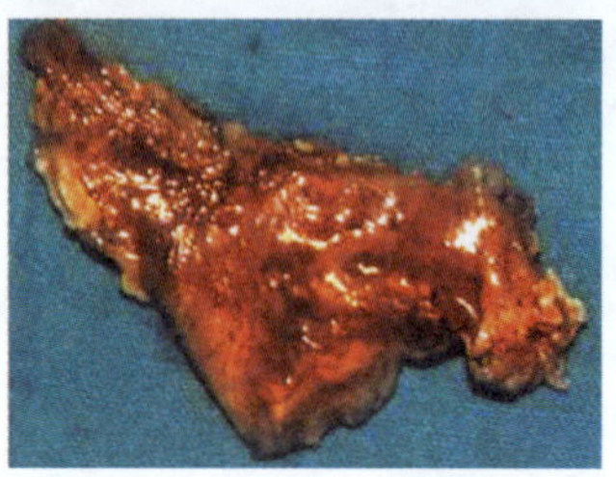

Fig. 17.9B: Pancreatic necrosis—necrosectomy specimen

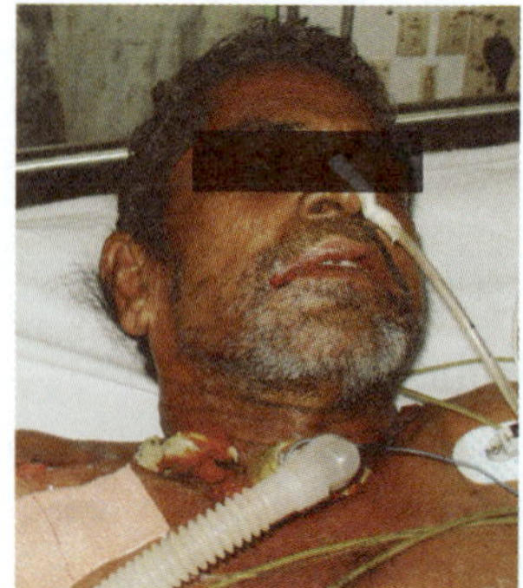

Fig. 17.10: Septic shock patient recovering

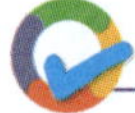

Multiple Choice Questions

1. Which of the following medications is least preferred in the initial management of haemorrhagic shock?

A. Oxygen B. Ringer lactate
C. Packed cells D. Vasopressors

2. Which of the following solutions is best suited in the initial management of hypovolaemic shock?

A. Normal saline
B. Ringer lactate
C. Hydroxyethyl starch
D. Albumin

3. Characteristic features of septic shock include the following *except*:

A. Hypotension B. Tachycardia
C. Oliguria D. Alkalosis

4. Hyperbaric oxygen is helpful in the following conditions *except*:

A. Carbon monoxide poisoning
B. Gas gangrene
C. Decompression sickness
D. Before chemotherapy

5. Regarding central venous pressure:
A. Right internal jugular vein is the route of choice
B. CVP is a reliable indicator of blood volume status
C. CVP remains constant with respiration
D. CVP is low in tension pneumothorax

6. The following is NOT a feature of cardiac tamponade:
A. Tachycardia B. Hypertension
C. Muffled heart sounds D. High CVP

7. Which of the following is a good indicator of fluid responsiveness in a spontaneously breathing patient:
A. Stroke volume variation
B. Inferior vena caval diameter
C. Systolic blood pressure
D. Heart rate

8. During haemorrhage, if the systolic blood pressure is normal but diastolic blood pressure is high, the patient may be in Class ______ shock.
A. I B. II
C. III D. IV

9. In haemorrhagic shock, if the patient has lost 30–40% blood volume, he is in Class ______ shock.
A. I B. II
C. III D. IV

10. Tension pneumothorax is a reason for which of the following types of shock?
A. Hypovolaemic shock B. Obstructive shock
C. Distributive shock D. Septic shock

11. The drug of choice in anaphylactic shock is:
A. Adrenaline B. Histamine
C. Promethazine D. Chlorpheniramine

12. The 'zero reference point' for arterial pressure transducers in seated patients should be at the:
A. Level of the nipple
B. Level of the manubriosternal junction
C. Level of the xiphoid process
D. Level of the radial artery

13. The central venous pressure is high in which type of shock?
A. Hypovolaemic shock
B. Anaphylactic shock
C. Septic shock
D. Obstructive shock

14. Translocation of bacteria from which organ may lead to multiorgan failure (and thus, this organ is called 'motor of multiorgan failure')?
A. Kidney B. Brain
C. Gut D. Liver

15. The route of choice for administering adrenaline in anaphylactic shock is:
A. Intramuscular B. Intravenous
C. Subcutaneous D. Inhalational

16. Which is the blood product of choice in bleeding patients with a fibrinogen concentration of <100 mg/L?
A. Packed cells B. Fresh-frozen plasma
C. Platelets D. Cryoprecipitate

17. Beck's triad is a feature of:
A. Cardiac tamponade
B. Tension pneumothorax
C. Pulmonary thromboembolism
D. Massive myocardial infarction

18. The following is NOT a feature of tension pneumothorax:
A. Reduced breath sounds
B. Dullness on percussion
C. Low blood pressure
D. Hypoxia

19. Intra-aortic balloon pump is used in which type of shock:
A. Hypovolaemic shock
B. Obstructive shock
C. Cardiogenic shock
D. Septic shock

Answers

1. D	**2.** B	**3.** D	**4.** A	**5.** B	**6.** B	**7.** B	**8.** B	**9.** C	**10.** B
11. A	**12.** B	**13.** D	**14.** C	**15.** B	**16.** D	**17.** A	**18.** B	**19.** C	

CHAPTER

18

Blood Transfusion

- Blood transfusion
- Blood products
- Complications of blood transfusion
- Autologous transfusion
- Bleeding disorders
- Hyperbaric oxygen

Competency

SU3.1: Describe the Indications and appropriate use of blood and blood products and complications of blood transfusion.

BLOOD TRANSFUSION

Administration of whole blood or its components into a patient is often necessary for various reasons. Since the only available source of blood is by voluntary human donation, which is scarce, whole blood is separated into its components, namely packed red blood cells, fresh frozen plasma, platelets, and cryoprecipitate. Some coagulation factors may be isolated and separately stored (e.g. factor VIII for administration into haemophiliacs). Packed red cells are the most common blood products used. Their transfusion increases the oxygen carrying capacity of blood. Transfusion of one unit of packed cells raises haemoglobin by approximately 1 g% in an adult.

Indications for Blood Transfusion (Key Box 18.1)

I. Packed red cells are used to replace acute and major blood loss in:
   - Haemorrhagic shock
   - Major surgery—open heart surgery, gastrectomy
   - Extensive burns

Key Box 18.1

Guidelines: When to Transfuse

- Haemoglobin <7 g%: Transfusion of red cells is likely to be associated with reduced mortality.
- Haemoglobin 7–10 g%: The decision to transfuse blood should be taken, only if there are clinical symptoms and signs due to anaemia.
- Haemoglobin >10 g%: Transfusion is not indicated.

II. Packed red cells are also used to treat anaemia due to:
   - Extensive burns
   - Chronic blood loss—haemorrhoids, bleeding disorders, chronic duodenal ulcer, etc.
   - Inadequate production—malignancies, nutritional anaemia

III. Platelet concentrates are administered to replace platelets in thrombocytopaenia. Fresh frozen plasma is given to replace plasma volume as well as Vit K dependent coagulation factors unresponsive to vitamin K replacement (e.g. liver disease, to reverse effects of warfarin). Cryoprecipitate is used to replace fibrinogen in patients with disseminated intravascular coagulation.

IV. Whole fresh blood administration is described in massive trauma with heavy blood loss, the rationale being that the patient rapidly loses all components of blood, so all components need to be replaced. Thus, it makes sense to administer whole blood, rather than individual components. However, many blood banks are reluctant to allow whole blood transfusion. This is to ensure that the donated blood can be optimally utilised. In such cases, red blood cells, fresh frozen plasma, and platelets are given in a 1:1:1 ratio.

BLOOD PRODUCTS

Packed Red Blood Cells (PRBC)

When whole blood is centrifuged, red blood cells settle down and the platelet-rich plasma remains supernatant.

The plasma is transferred to another bag, while preservative is added to red cells and the bag is sealed. Each bag of packed cells contains approximately 250–300 ml with a red cell concentration of 70%. Red cell transfusion is required for patients whose haemoglobin is <7 g% (e.g. patients undergoing chemotherapy, major surgery, delivery, trauma, grossly anaemic neonates and infants, sickle cell anaemia—especially in sickle cell crisis). Each unit of packed cells should increase haemoglobin by 1 g% and haematocrit by 3%.

The red cells may be leucodepleted (white blood cells removed) for use in patients requiring multiple transfusions to prevent development of antibodies to leukocytes or in those who are known to react to leucocytes.

The rate of blood or blood product administration depends on the quantity and speed at which it is lost from the body. Slow transfusion is indicated in those with cardiac disease, renal dysfunction, severe chronic anaemia, and in paediatric patients.

In semi-emergent situations (e.g. treatment of low haemoglobin in patients awaiting surgery or delivery), each bag of packed cells may be transfused slowly. The initial 25 ml may be given slowly to check whether the patient tolerates it. Thereafter, it can be transfused at a rate of 3–4 ml/kg/h (approximately 1.5 h for a bag of red cells). The red cells must be transfused within 4 hours of removing it from the refrigerator, as bacterial growth may be promoted after that.

In emergent situations, red cells may be transfused much faster in order to keep up with the loss. When large amounts are transfused in a short period (*see* section on massive transfusion), the effects of other components, such as citrate, become significant.

Packed red blood cells must be both ABO and Rh compatible unless the patient has life-threatening massive bleeding, in which case O –ve packed cells may be transfused.

Platelets

The bag containing platelet-rich plasma is again centrifuged to express off the plasma so that the bag with the remaining platelets can be sealed off. Each unit (50 mL) should contain at least 5.5×10^{10} platelets (platelet concentrate), and each unit should elevate the platelet count by 5–10,000 cells/mm^3 in a 70 kg person. Platelets may be transfused prophylactically or for therapeutic purposes.

Prophylactic platelet transfusion may be done when the platelet count is <10,000 cells/mm^3 in oncology patients. In patients who are at high risk of alloimmunisation (e.g. leukaemia), the threshold for platelet transfusion is even lower at 5000 cells/mm^3, whereas in patients with clinical instability, the threshold may be raised to 20,000 cells/mm^3. Patients who need to undergo major surgery or require invasive procedures, such as spinal anaesthesia, liver biopsy, etc. generally need their platelet count elevated to >50,000 cells/mm^3. However, patients requiring surgery in critical areas, such as neurosurgery or ophthalmic surgery, will need their platelet count raised to >1,00,000 cells/mm^3.

Therapeutic platelet transfusion is required in patients who are known to be thrombocytopenic and are actively bleeding (platelet count <50,000 cells/mm^3). The dose of platelets may be calculated as follows: One unit of platelets (60 ml) for every 10 kg body weight.

Platelets must be transfused within 4 hours of commencing the infusion. ABO compatibility is not required for platelets. Filters of 170–260 μ must be used to transfuse platelets as with other blood components.

Fresh Frozen Plasma (FFP)

The remaining plasma (200–230 ml) may be stored in a frozen form (called fresh frozen plasma) at –18°C for one year. It needs to be thawed over half an hour before use.

Fresh frozen plasma transfusion is indicated in patients with prolonged INR >1.5 who are bleeding or require surgery. FFP provides coagulation factors to those who are actively bleeding and those on warfarin. It is administered in a dose of 10–20 ml/kg body weight, and must be ABO compatible. FFP must be transfused as soon as possible after thawing, and definitely within 24 hours. A hanging unit must be transfused within 6 hours of commencement of transfusion due to risk of bacterial contamination.

Cryoprecipitate

FFP may be further treated to produce cryoprecipitate, which is rich in fibrinogen. Transfusion of cryoprecipitate (each bag contains 20 ml) is indicated in patients with fibrinogen levels <1 g% (e.g. disseminated intravascular coagulation (DIC)). The dose is 0.2 units/kg body weight, but usually 10 units are transfused initially and repeated as necessary.

Important points to remember before transfusing blood products

- Always obtain informed consent from patients or immediate relatives (in emergent situations) prior to the transfusion.
- Recheck the patient's blood group and that of the donor blood, preferably along with one other qualified person, to ensure that the correct bag is being transfused to the patient. The patient's hospital number and the blood bag number should also be checked. Both people must sign on the transfusion report.

- Visually check the blood bag for any obvious abnormalities, such as very dark blood or visible clots, and if present, do not transfuse, and return it to the blood bank. Check the date of collection and date of expiry before transfusion. The storage shelf-life of red blood cells depends on the preservative added (Key Box 18.2).
- Watch for any transfusion reactions.

Key Box 18.2

Storage of Blood

Preservative	RBC survival (days)
ACD (acid-citrate-dextrose)	21
CPD (citrate-phosphate-dextrose)	28
CPDA (citrate-phosphate-dextrose-adenine)	35
SAGM (saline-adenine-glucose-mannitol)	35

Whole blood transfusion is not advisable for routine use and is also not available from blood banks. However, there is some evidence in the literature that fresh whole blood transfusion may be helpful in patients with massive trauma, as all blood components are replaced simultaneously to match the loss. However, this is difficult practically, as the blood products still need to be screened for various antigens and infections.

Other blood products available are fibrinogen concentrate (high risk of hepatitis), factor VIII and factor IX concentrates (for use in haemophilia and Christmas disease, respectively) and factor VII concentrate (for use in disseminated intravascular coagulation—DIC).

COMPLICATIONS OF BLOOD TRANSFUSION

IMMUNE COMPLICATIONS

Haemolytic Reactions

Major (ABO) Incompatibility Reaction

- This is the result of mismatched blood transfusion.
- The majority of cases are due to technical errors, such as sampling, labelling, dispatching.
- This causes intravascular haemolysis.

Clinical features

- Haematuria
- Pain in the loins (bilateral)
- Fever with chills and rigors
- Oliguria due to products of mismatched blood transfusion blocking the renal tubules. It results in acute renal *tubular necrosis.*

Treatment

- Stop the blood transfusion. Send the blood bag to the blood bank and recheck.
- Repeat coagulation profile.
- IV fluids, monitor urine output, check urine for Hb.
- Diuresis with furosemide 20–40 mg IV or injection mannitol 20% 100 ml IV to flush the kidney.
- If renal failure does occur, haemodialysis may be required.
- If haemodynamically unstable, cardiovascular support may be required.

Minor Incompatibility Reaction

- Occurs due to extravascular haemolysis.
- Usually mild, occurs at 2–21 days.
- Occurs due to antibodies to minor antigens.
- Malaise, jaundice, and fever.
- Treatment is supportive.

Nonhaemolytic Reactions

Febrile Reaction

- Occurs due to sensitisation to WBCs or platelets
- Increased temperature—no haemolysis
- Use of 20–40 mm filter or leucocyte-depleted blood may prevent it.

Allergic Reaction

- Occurs due to allergy to plasma products.
- Manifests as chills, rigors, and rashes all over.
- Often subsides with antihistamines, such as chlorpheniramine maleate 10 mg IV.

Transfusion-related Acute Lung Injury (TRALI)

It is a rare complication, that occurs within 6 hours of a transfusion due to the presence of antileucocyte antibodies in the transfused plasma, which cause the patient's white cells to aggregate in the pulmonary circulation. This leads to degranulation of leucocytes, causing increased capillary permeability and non-cardiogenic pulmonary oedema. Symptoms may vary from mild dyspnoea to full blown acute respiratory distress syndrome. Proper supportive therapy will see that it resolves within 24–48 hours.

Congestive Cardiac Failure (CCF)

CCF may occur, if whole blood is transfused rapidly, especially in patients with chronic anaemia due to circulatory overload.

Treatment

- Slow transfusion, injection furosemide 20 mg IV.
- Packed cell transfusion is the choice in these patients.

INFECTIOUS COMPLICATIONS

Serum hepatitis, *AIDS, malaria, and syphilis* are dangerous infectious diseases that may be transmitted from one patient to another through blood transfusion. The danger is increased in cases of multiple transfusions and in emergency situations. ***"Prevention is better than cure".*** Hence, it is mandatory to screen the blood for these diseases before transfusion.

OTHER COMPLICATIONS

Citrate toxicity (causing hypocalcaemia), dilutional coagulopathy (thrombocytopenia and dilution of clotting factors) can occur especially in massive tranfusion.

MASSIVE BLOOD TRANSFUSION

Definition: Massive blood transfusion has been defined as follows:

- Replacement of >1 blood volume (or >10 units of packed cells) in 24 hours.
- Half the patient's blood volume in 6 hours.
- >4 RBC units in one hour with ongoing need for transfusion, or
- 500 ml over 5 min with haemodynamic instability and need for transfusion.

Massive blood loss may occur with trauma, postpartum haemorrhage, or during major surgeries.

Massive transfusion protocol: In patients with massive bleeding who are expected to require massive transfusion, the blood bank should be intimated to activate massive transfusion protocol (MTP). A blood sample must be sent for cross-matching with an initial request for 2 units of red blood cells. After this, if MTP is requested, the blood bank releases blood products in different 'boxes' (Table 18.1).

The blood products are obtained box by box as necessary. If the bleeding stops, the blood bank should be intimated immediately, so that MTP can be terminated. If bleeding continues, boxes three and four are alternately requested for. In such patients, regular and half hourly measurements of acid–base status, haemoglobin, platelets, prothrombin time (PT), activated partial thromboplastin time (aPTT), fibrinogen, and serum calcium are required with an aim to normalise their values. The use of thromboelastography or Rotem allows visualisation of the process of clot formation and helps identify specific defects. This is now being made available as 'point-of-care' testing.

Table 18.1 Release of blood products on activation of MTP

Box	PRBC	FFP	Platelet	Cryoprecipitate
One	2	2	–	–
Two	4	4	1 adult	–
Three	4	4	–	3
Four	4	4	1 adult	

Disseminated Intravascular Coagulation (DIC)

- It occurs in massive blood transfusion, wherein all factors of coagulation are consumed, resulting in a bleeding disorder (consumption coagulopathy).
- It produces severe afibrinogenemia.
- It is treated by replacement with fibrinogen (cryoprecipitate) and other clotting factors.

AUTOLOGOUS TRANSFUSION

This concept originated to avoid transfusion reactions that may develop when homologous blood is used.

- Here, the patient's own blood is used.

Types of Autologous Transfusion

1. **Predeposit:** 2–5 units of blood may be donated over 2–4 weeks before elective surgery.
2. **Preoperative haemodilution:** For cases like surgery for thyrotoxicosis or abdominopelvic resection, wherein one can expect 1–2 units of blood loss. Just before surgery, 1–2 units of blood are removed, stored in blood bags and serially numbered. Normovolaemia is ensured by infusing 2–3 times the volume drawn with crystalloids. The blood drawn is retransfused in the reverse order after the procedure (the last bag first and the first bag containing higher haematocrit is given last).
3. **Blood salvage:** Blood which is lost during surgery is collected, mixed with anticoagulant solution, washed, and reinfused. This may be done, if the surgery does not involve severe infection, bowel resection, or malignancy, and does not contain materials such as bone cement.

Advantage: All the risks involved with blood transfusion are avoided.

Disadvantages

- May not be acceptable to the patient.
- Requires sophisticated equipment.

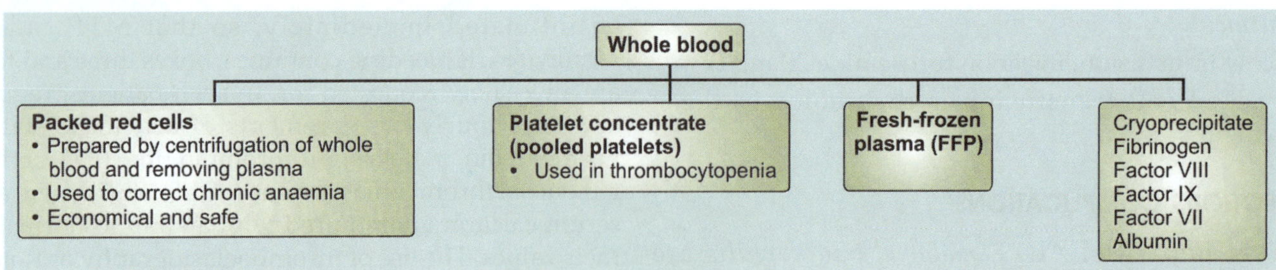

Fig. 18.1: Blood products

Blood Products

Figure 18.1 depicts blood products.

Pearls of Wisdom

Packed cells and fresh frozen plasma transfusion should not be used to treat malnutrition.

Tranexamic acid is very useful as an antifibrinolytic agent to reduce blood loss.

BLEEDING DISORDERS

Haemophilia

This is the most common bleeding disorder, which occurs due to an X-linked genetic disorder of coagulation.

Types

1. **Haemophilia A:** This results from a reduction of factor VIII (anti-haemophilic factor) and is carried by a recessive gene.
2. **Haemophilia B:** This results due to deficiency of factor IX.

Haemophilia A

- 'Excessive, unusual and unexpected bleeding' during surgery could be due to haemophilia 'A'. This must be confirmed with laboratory tests.
- A haemophilic patient's daughters will be carriers, but all sons will be normal.
- Thus, a carrier woman has 50% chance of producing a haemophiliac male or a female carrier.
- The level of coagulation factor VIII in the blood may be <1% of that in a normal individual.

Clinical Features

1. Bleeding into joints (haemarthrosis)

- Large joints, such as knees, elbows, ankles, and wrists are affected.
- Spontaneous bleeding is common. It may also occur due to minor trauma.
- Repeated bleeding may result in permanent damage to the articular surfaces, resulting in deformity of the joints.

Table 18.2 Blood changes in haemophilia A and von Willebrand's disease

	Haemophilia 'A'	von Willebrand's disease
Bleeding time	Normal	↑
Prothrombin time	Normal	Normal
VIII: C	↓↓↓	↓
vWF	Normal	↓

2. Bleeding into muscles

- Calf muscle and psoas muscle haematomas are common, resulting in contraction and fibrosis of muscle, muscle pain, and weakness of the limb.
- Intramuscular injections should be avoided.

Investigations (Table 18.2)

Treatment

- Administration of factor VIII concentrate by intravenous infusion is the treatment whenever there is bleeding.
- It should be given twice daily, since it has a half-life of 12 hours.
- Any major surgical procedure should be carried out only after raising factor VIII:C levels to 100% pre-operatively, and it should be maintained >50% until healing occurs.
- Synthetic vasopressin (DDAVP) produces a rise in factor VIII:C.

Causes of Death

- Cerebral haemorrhage used to be the most common cause of death in haemophiliacs. However, HIV infection seems to be the most common cause of death today.
- Hepatocellular carcinoma and cirrhosis due to HIV and HCV also are the other causes (due to repeated blood transfusions).

Haemophilia B (Christmas Disease)

- **Incidence:** One in 30,000 males. The inheritance and clinical features are identical to haemophilia A.
- It is caused by a deficiency of factor IX.
- Treatment is with factor IX concentrates.

von Willebrand's Disease (vWD)

- In vWD, there is defective platelet function and factor VIII:C deficiency due to a deficiency or abnormality of vWF.
- Epistaxis, menorrhagia, and bleeding following minor trauma or surgery are common.
- Haemarthrosis is rare.
- Treatment is similar to mild haemophilia. DDAVP, IV infusion of factor VIII:C or vWF is required before surgery.

A clinical haematologist must be consulted to help optimise a patient with bleeding disorders for surgery.

HYPERBARIC OXYGEN

Hyperbaric oxygen is administered to patients when their own haemoglobin is unable to carry adequate oxygen or when hyperoxia is required. Hyperbaric O_2 is administered using either a monoplace (single patient) or multiplace compression chamber.

Indications

1. **Carbon monoxide poisoning:** Hyperbaric O_2 at 2–3 atm is given to increase the O_2 dissolved in plasma (5–6 ml/dl at 3 atm, whereas it is 0.3 ml/dl at 1 atm) which is sufficient to meet the O_2 requirement of the body, even in the absence of normal haemoglobin (severe CO poisoning).
2. Infections such as **gas gangrene:** Hyperoxia suppresses the growth of anaerobic organisms.
3. Cancer therapy to potentiate radiotherapy
4. Arterial insufficiency
5. **Decompression sickness and air embolism:** Hyperbaric oxygen reduces the size of air bubbles, and rapidly eliminates nitrogen from the air bubbles.

Contraindications

Untreated pneumothorax: May expand with hyperbaric O_2, resulting in life-threatening tension pneumothorax.

Multiple Choice Questions

1. Which of the following statements about packed red cells is true?

A. It has a haematocrit of 35%
B. The volume in one adult bag is 500 mL
C. Shelf-life is 35 days with CPDA solution
D. It contains no plasma

2. Haemolytic reactions due to mismatched blood transfusion include the following *except*:

A. Haematuria
B. Pain in the loins
C. Fever with chills and rigors
D. Diuresis

3. Which of the following is decreased in disseminated intravascular coagulation?

A. Prothrombin time
B. Partial thromboplastin time
C. Bleeding time
D. Platelets

4. The following are true in haemophilia *except*:

A. Prothrombin time is unaffected
B. Partial thromboplastin time is unaffected
C. Platelet count is unaffected
D. Bleeding time is unaffected

5. The following are true about blood products *except*:

A. Fresh-frozen plasma is given in severe liver failure
B. Cryoprecipitate is not used during massive transfusion
C. Fibrinogen has a high risk of hepatitis
D. Factor VIII is used in haemophilia

6. The following are true about platelet transfusion *except*:

A. They remain viable for 3–5 days
B. Each unit will raise platelet count by 5–10,000 cells/mm^3
C. Platelets must be ABO compatible
D. Platelets may be low after heparin

Answers

1. C **2.** D **3.** D **4.** C **5.** B **6.** C

CHAPTER

19

Acid–Base Balance

- Basic definitions
- Henderson-Hasselbalch equation
- Regulation of acid–base balance
- Acid–base disorders
- Rapid interpretation of an ABG report

Competency

SU9.1: Choose appropriate biochemical, microbiological, pathological, imaging investigations and interpret the investigative data in a surgical patient.

Please note: Here you can study the interpretation of ABG.

INTRODUCTION

Human blood has a hydrogen ion concentration [H^+] of 35 to 45 nmol/L and it is essential that its concentration is maintained within this narrow range. Hydrogen ions are nothing but protons which can bind to proteins and alter their characteristics. All the enzymes present in the body are proteins and an alteration in these enzyme systems can change the homeostatic mechanisms of the body. Hence, a disturbance in acid–base balance can result in malfunction of the various organ systems.

BASIC DEFINITIONS

What is pH?

pH notation is a more common method of expressing the hydrogen ion concentration. It is defined as the negative logarithm to base 10 of the [H^+] expressed in mol/L. pH of blood = 7.4.

What is an acid? What is a base? What is a buffer?

- An **acid** is a substance that dissociates in water to produce H^+.
- A **base** is a substance that accepts H^+.
- A **buffer** is a combination of a weak acid and its conjugate base. By combining with a strong acid or a strong base, they produce the corresponding salt and a weak acid or a weak base, respectively.

  For example: A weak acid, such as carbonic acid with its conjugate base, sodium bicarbonate, is called the bicarbonate/carbonic acid buffer system. When a strong acid, such as hydrochloric acid, is added to the solution, it combines with the weak alkali (sodium bicarbonate) to form sodium chloride and carbonic acid. When a strong base, such as sodium hydroxide is added, it combines with the weak acid (carbonic acid) to form sodium carbonate and water. Thus, a strong acid and a strong base are converted into a weak acid and a weak base by the bicarbonate/carbonic acid buffer system.

The hydrogen ion concentration of blood is maintained within narrow limits because of the presence of buffers in the body. **These natural buffers are of two types: Extracellular and intracellular.**

- The extracellular buffers are bicarbonate/carbonic acid buffer system, phosphate buffer system and plasma proteins. The intracellular buffers are haemoglobin and other proteins.
- The most important buffer system in the body is the bicarbonate–carbonic acid buffer system. This is because of the ability of the body to maintain or alter the concentrations of its two components separately. The concentration of carbonic acid is regulated by respiration wherein the excess carbonic acid is eliminated as carbon dioxide by the lungs. The bicarbonate concentration is independently regulated by the kidneys.

THE HENDERSON AND HENDERSON-HASSELBALCH EQUATIONS

The hydrogen ion concentration is proportional to the concentration of buffer systems of the body. The hydrogen ion concentration, carbonic acid levels and the bicarbonate levels of blood are related according to the following equation:

$$[H^+]\ (\text{nmol/L}) = K \times \frac{H_2CO_3(\text{mmol/L})}{HCO_3^-(\text{mmol/L})}$$

where K = constant. This equation is called the Henderson equation.

The amount of carbonic acid in the blood is directly proportional to the partial pressure of carbon dioxide in the blood. Thus, the carbonic acid concentration is a product of the partial pressure of carbon dioxide in blood and its solubility coefficient.

$[H_2CO_3] = \alpha\ PCO_2$, where α = solubility coefficient of carbon dioxide in blood and PCO_2 is the partial pressure of carbon dioxide in blood.

α = 0.03 ml/mmHg/100 ml blood and normal PCO_2 = 40 mmHg

$[H_2CO_3] = \alpha\ PCO_2 = 0.03 \times 40 = 1.2$ ml/dl.

K = 800 for the carbonic acid/bicarbonate buffer system. The normal bicarbonate level of blood is 24 mmol/L.

$$[H^+]\ (\text{nmol/L}) = \frac{800 \times 1.2}{24} = 40\ \text{nmol / L}$$

The Henderson equation can also be written as follows.

$$[H^+]\ (\text{nmol/L}) = K \times \frac{\alpha\ PCO_2\ (\text{mmHg})}{HCO_3^-}$$

From this equation, it is evident that the hydrogen ion concentration increases when the PCO_2 increases or when the $[HCO_3^-]$ levels decrease. Similarly, a decrease in hydrogen ion concentration occurs when the PCO_2 decreases or when the $[HCO_3^-]$ levels increase.

When expressed in logarithmic form, the Henderson equation is written as follows:

$$pH = pK_a + \log \frac{[HCO_3^-]}{[H_2CO_3^-]}$$

This logarithmic version of Henderson equation is called the Henderson-Hasselbalch equation.

The pK_a (negative logarithm of the constant K) of the carbonic acid/bicarbonate buffer system is 6.1.

$$\begin{aligned} pH &= 6.1 + \log 24/1.2 \\ &= 6.1 + \log 20 = 6.1 + 1.3 = 7.4 \end{aligned}$$

It is important to appreciate that the $[H^+]$ and pH are inversely related. When the $[H^+]$ rises, the pH decreases and vice versa.

REGULATION OF ACID–BASE BALANCE

The normal pH of blood is 7.35–7.45. Acidosis is defined as a pH less than 7.35. Conversely, when the pH is more than 7.45, alkalosis is said to exist. Acidosis and alkalosis are of two types each—respiratory and metabolic.

An increase in carbon dioxide (CO_2) levels increases the plasma $[H^+]$ and decreases the pH (respiratory acidosis). Similarly, a decrease in plasma carbon dioxide levels reduces the $[H^+]$ and increases the pH (respiratory alkalosis). A decrease in $[HCO_3^-]$ reduces the pH and is called metabolic acidosis. Similarly, an increase in $[HCO_3^-]$ increases the pH and produces metabolic alkalosis.

The pH is regulated in the human body mainly by two organs: The **respiratory system** and the **renal system**.

The arterial carbon dioxide levels are regulated by the respiratory system. Any increase in carbon dioxide levels stimulates the respiratory centre in the medulla thus augmenting respiration, alveolar ventilation and elimination of extra CO_2 levels. A decrease in CO_2 levels may reduce the stimulus to breathe and cause hypoventilation. This response is limited by hypoxia as the hypoxic drive stimulates the patient to maintain respiration. Respiratory response to changes in CO_2 level occurs very fast.

The plasma bicarbonate levels are regulated by the kidneys. Any decrease in $[HCO_3^-]$ stimulates the kidneys to retain and synthesise bicarbonate. High $[HCO_3^-]$ results in elimination of more bicarbonate in urine. In general, the pulmonary response to a change in acid–base status is faster and occurs immediately. However, renal regulation takes time, a few hours to days. Kidneys filter and reabsorb all the bicarbonate in the urine. When necessary, kidneys can also produce extra bicarbonate through the glutamine pathway.

ACID–BASE DISORDERS

When an acid–base disorder occurs, the initial disturbance that occurs is termed the primary disorder. The body attempts to normalise the pH by certain compensatory mechanisms resulting in a secondary disorder, e.g. primary metabolic acidosis results in an increase in hydrogen ions and a consequent decrease in bicarbonate ions. To compensate for this, the patient hyperventilates and reduces the arterial carbon dioxide levels, thus moving the pH back to normal (compensatory respiratory alkalosis).

Thus, there are four primary disorders and four secondary disorders (Key Box 19.1).

Key Box 19.1

Primary Disorder	Secondary Disorder
Respiratory acidosis	Metabolic alkalosis
Respiratory alkalosis	Metabolic acidosis
Metabolic acidosis	Respiratory alkalosis
Metabolic alkalosis	Respiratory acidosis

RESPIRATORY ACIDOSIS

Causes

This disorder occurs when the patient's ability to maintain minute ventilation is compromised. This may be acute or chronic in origin. The causes may be classified as follows:

- **Central nervous system:** Central nervous system depression due to trauma, tumour, infections, ischaemia or drug overdose. Spinal cord injuries, especially cervical or high thoracic, can cause respiratory muscle paralysis.
- Peripheral nervous and muscular systems: Guillain-Barré syndrome, tetanus, organophosphorus poisoning, poliomyelitis, myasthenia gravis.
- Primary pulmonary disease: Asthma, chronic obstructive pulmonary disease, acute respiratory distress syndrome, pneumonia.
- Loss of chest wall integrity: Flail chest.

Clinical Features

- The features of the underlying problem predominate the clinical picture.
- If acute, hypoxia and hypercarbia result in tachycardia, hypertension, arrhythmias, confusion, drowsiness and coma. The hypoxia, if untreated, can be fatal.
- If gradual in onset, as in chronic obstructive pulmonary disease (COPD), the patient's kidneys may compensate by retaining bicarbonate resulting in compensatory metabolic alkalosis. Arterial blood gas analysis in these patients typically shows low PaO_2, high $PaCO_2$, high bicarbonate levels and a near-normal pH.

Treatment

- Treat the cause.
- Maintenance of oxygenation and ventilation using mechanical ventilatory support till recovery of the primary problem occurs.

RESPIRATORY ALKALOSIS

This occurs due to an increase in minute ventilation. This increase can be sustained only in abnormal conditions. This may be acute or chronic in origin.

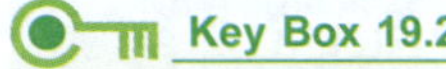

Key Box 19.2

Hyperventilation

- Head injury
- Hydrogen ions (metabolic acidosis)
- Hyperpyrexia
- Hysteria
- High altitudes

Causes (Key Box 19.2)

- Supratentorial lesions: Head injury
- Fever
- Pain
- Anxiety, hysterical hyperventilation
- High altitudes
- It may also occur secondarily as a compensation to primary metabolic acidosis.

Features

- Usually features of the underlying disease predominate the picture.
- Acute severe hypocarbia ($PaCO_2$ <20 mmHg) may cause cerebral vasoconstriction, reduced cerebral blood flow, confusion, seizures and tetany.
- The alkalosis and consequent hypokalaemia can also cause cardiac arrhythmias.

METABOLIC ACIDOSIS

Causes

This is associated with a decrease in bicarbonate ions due to one of two reasons:

1. **Overproduction or retention of non-volatile acids in the body**, as in:
   - Diabetic ketoacidosis
   - Lactic acidosis
   - Salicylate poisoning, methanol poisoning
   - Renal failure
2. **Loss of bicarbonate ions from the body as in**
   - Diarrhoea
   - Intestinal fistulae

Features

- Usually features of the underlying disease predominate the picture.
- Hypotension, reduced cardiac output
- Hyperventilation—rapid, deep respirations
- Deep, gasping type of respiration seen in diabetic ketoacidosis is called **Kussmaul's respiration**.
- Hyperkalaemia, arrhythmias
- Lethargy, coma

Metabolic acidosis can be of high anion gap or normal anion gap type.

Anion Gap

The law of electroneutrality states that the total number of positive charges must be equal to the total number of negative charges in the body fluids. Thus, cations (positively charged ions such as sodium and potassium) must produce a charge exactly balanced by anions. However, the concentrations of only sodium, potassium, chloride and bicarbonate ions are routinely measured in clinical practice. The number of the measured cations (Na^+) exceeds the sum of measured anions (Cl^- and HCO_3^-) producing a 'deficit' called the 'anion gap' (Fig. 19.1). The normal anion gap is 9–14 mmol/l. This gap is due to the presence of unmeasured anions in the body.

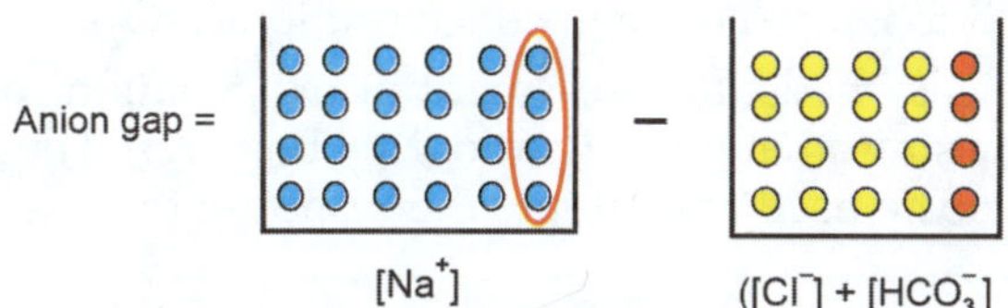

Fig. 19.1: Normal anion gap. The main cation is sodium (shown as blue circles) and the main anions are chloride ions (yellow circles) and bicarbonate (red circles).

Since the extracellular concentrations of potassium is small, it is often ignored in the calculation of anion gap.

Anion gap may be used to distinguish the cause of metabolic acidosis.

Causes of high anion gap acidosis: MUDPILES (methanol, uraemia, diabetic ketoacidosis, paracetamol/propylene glycol, iron/isoniazid, lactic acidosis, ethylene glycol, salicylate poisoning).

- **Anion gap is increased (>14 mmol/L) in metabolic acidosis due to an increase in fixed acid load.** These acids react with the bicarbonate ions in the plasma lowering its concentration. This results in high anion gap metabolic acidosis (HAGMA) (Fig. 19.2).

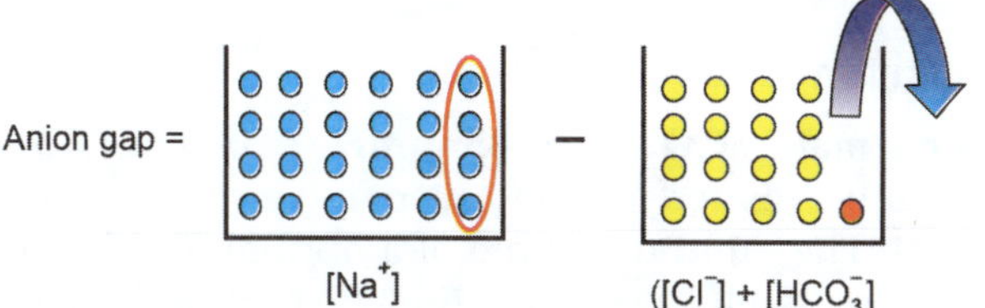

Fig. 19.2: Illustration of high anion gap acidosis. Note the loss of bicarbonate ions (red circles)

Causes of normal anion gap acidosis: Diarrhoea, isotonic saline infusion, early renal failure, renal tubular acidosis, ureteroenterostomy.

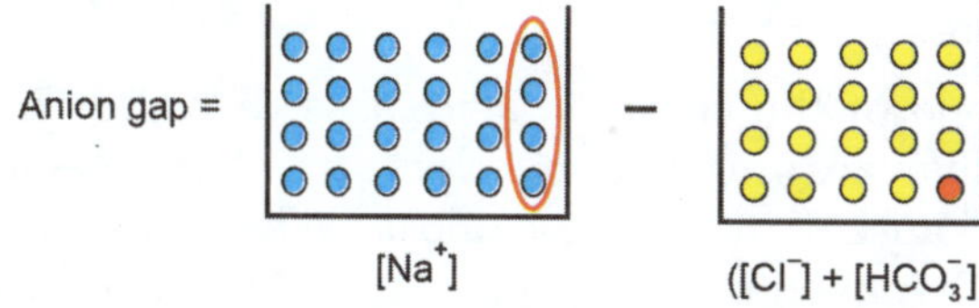

Fig. 19.3: Normal anion gap metabolic acidosis. Note the loss of bicarbonate ions (red circles) and their replacement with chloride (yellow circles)

- **Anion gap remains unchanged in metabolic acidosis due to loss of bicarbonate ions** as the lost bicarbonate ions are replaced by chloride ions. There is no change in the measured anion concentration and thus, the anion gap remains normal (Fig. 19.3). This type of metabolic acidosis is also called **'hyperchloraemic metabolic acidosis'**. Example: Diarrhoea, renal tubular acidosis.
- **Corrected anion gap:** The anion gap (AG) can be falsely low in hypoalbuminaemia, a common clinical condition in the critically ill. Adjust anion gap for albumin as given below:

  Adjusted AG = Observed AG + 2.5 × [4.5 – measured albumin (g/dl)]

Treatment

- Identify the cause and treat.
- Ensure adequate ventilation.
- If pH <7.1 and the patient is unstable, may administer sodium bicarbonate. The chances of life-threatening arrhythmias are reduced when pH is >7.2.

  Bicarbonate required (mmol/L) =

  15 – measured [HCO_3^-] × 0.6 × Body wt (kg)

(Each ml of 8.4% $NaHCO_3$ solution contains 1 mmol of HCO_3. Each ml of 7.5% $NaHCO_3$ solution contains 0.9 mmol of HCO_3^-).

Half the calculated dose of bicarbonate should be given slowly and should be followed up with repeat blood pH measurements as required.

METABOLIC ALKALOSIS

Causes

This may be either due to loss of acid from the body or retention of bicarbonate. It may be due to:

- Loss of gastric hydrochloric acid as in vomiting, prolonged nasogastric drainage.
- Retention of bicarbonate in exchange for loss of chloride ions as in diarrhoea.
- Excessive loss of H^+ from kidneys in exchange for K^+ in severe hypokalaemia.
- Primary or secondary hyperaldosteronism.
- Excessive exogenous administration of alkali, e.g. indiscriminate use of $NaHCO_3$, antacid abuse.

Features

It is one of the common acid–base disorders in the intensive care unit. The underlying problem gives a clue to the cause of metabolic alkalosis. When severe, it can cause hypoventilation and seizures. Associated hypokalaemia can cause arrhythmias and contribute to difficulty in weaning patients off a ventilator.

Treatment

- Treat the primary problem.
- Most of the metabolic alkaloses are 'chloride-responsive'. Administration of saline and correction of potassium deficits reduce the alkalosis.
- Chloride deficit (mmol)
  = 0.2 × Body weight (kg) × (100 – serum Cl^-)
- The calculated deficit can be replaced over 24 hours using 0.9% saline (contains 154 mmol/L of chloride)
- Chloride unresponsive alkalosis may be due to hypokalaemia or hypomagnesemia. Treat them.

COMBINED DISORDERS

In some clinical situations, patients can have combined disorders. HAGMA and NAGMA can co-exist (Fig. 19.4). Similarly, metabolic acidosis and alkalosis can be present in the patient at the same time (Fig. 19.5). Hence, whenever a patient presents with HAGMA, check whether there is a co-existing disorder.

A 'gap-gap analysis' helps in identifying whether HAGMA is associated with other disorders.

Gap-Gap
= (12 – measured anion gap)/24 – measured HCO_3^-)

If the ratio is 1, infer that the patient has HAGMA.

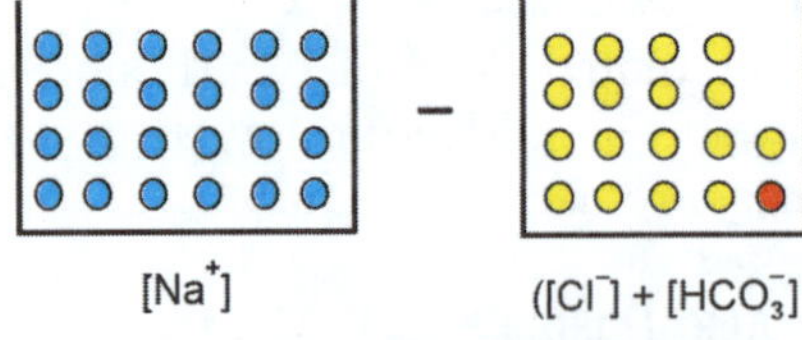

Fig. 19.4: A combination of HAGMA and NAGMA. Bicarbonate ions are lost producing HAGMA but some of them are replaced by chloride ions (NAGMA).

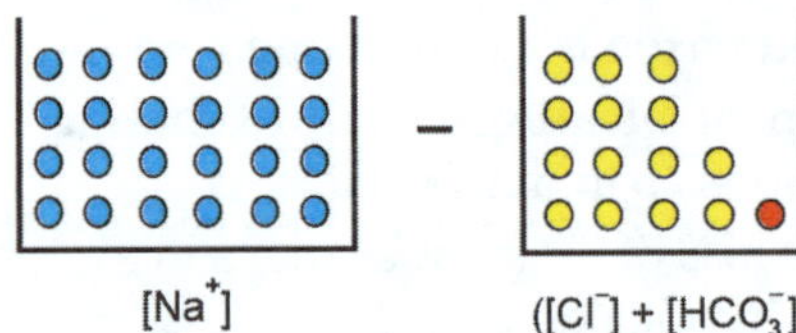

Fig. 19.5: In this case, bicarbonate ions are lost producing HAGMA but the patient has lost chloride ions as well (excessive vomiting).

If <1, there is co-existing NAGMA with HAGMA.

If >1, there is co-existing HAGMA and metabolic alkalosis.

RAPID INTERPRETATION OF AN ABG REPORT

Analysis and conclusion of arterial blood gas (ABG) report must always be done in conjunction with history and clinical examination. ABG analysis is done to assess:

1. **Oxygenation status**
2. **Ventilatory status**
3. **Acid–base status**

Oxygenation

The partial pressure of oxygen in arterial blood (PaO_2) of a normal, healthy, young adult is usually 90–100 mmHg. While assessing oxygenation, the PaO_2 must always be related to ispired oxygen concentration (FIO_2).

An easy bedside assessment of oxygenation can be made using a PaO_2/FIO_2 ratio (Key Box 19.3). The ratio can also be used to evaluate the response to therapy.

Key Box 19.3

PaO_2/FIO_2 ratio	Status of oxygenation
≥500	Normal
250–500	Adequate
100–250	Poor
<100	Critical

A pulse oximeter is helpful to assess whether the patient's oxygenation is life-threatening or not. A saturation of 98–100% may be reassuring. However, early changes in the oxygenation status may be missed, if one relies on a pulse oximetry and the patient is breathing high concentrations of oxygen. This is because of the sigmoid shape of the oxygen dissociation curve where the SaO_2 will be 99–100%, whether the PaO_2 is 100 mmHg or 500 mmHg. **Hence, an arterial blood gas analysis must always be obtained whenever a doubt exists about the** oxygenation status of the patient.

Ventilation

The **normal $PaCO_2$ is 35–45 mmHg.** The $PaCO_2$ must always be related to the alveolar ventilation of the patient. The minute volume of a normal healthy adult at rest would be 100 ml/kg/min. Sixty to sixty-five per cent of this actually ventilates the alveoli, the rest is dead space ventilation.

If the alveolar ventilation decreases (either due to a decrease in minute volume or an increase in dead space ventilation), the arterial $PaCO_2$ will rise. On the other hand, the arterial $PaCO_2$ may remain normal but the patient's minute volume may have increased.

Do not assume that the patient must be well when the $PaCO_2$ is normal. A clinical examination of the patient is necessary to rule out respiratory distress (dyspnoea, tachypnoea, active accessory muscles of respiration, tracheal tug, flaring of alae nasi, etc.). The patient may not be able to sustain this increased levels of ventilation for a prolonged period of time, is likely to get exhausted and may require mechanical ventilatory support.

Acid–Base Status

The assessment of acid–base status must be done in three steps and in the following order.

a. *Assess the pH first:* Normal pH—7.35 to 7.45. If the pH is less than 7.35, the patient has acidosis and if it is more than 7.45, the patient is alkalotic. The direction of change in pH shows the primary disorder. This is because the compensatory mechanisms never overshoot the requirement of reaching the normal pH.

b. *Assess the $PaCO_2$ next:* Is the $PaCO_2$ normal? The normal $PaCO_2$ is 35–45 mmHg. If the pH is abnormal but the $PaCO_2$ normal, it suggests a metabolic disorder. However, the body usually tries to compensate for a change in pH. The respiratory compensation is early and fast.

   If the changes in pH and $PaCO_2$ are in opposite directions (one is increased and the other decreased), the primary disorder is respiratory. If the changes in pH and $PaCO_2$ are in the same direction (both are increased or decreased), the primary disorder is metabolic.

For example, **if the pH is 7.2 and the $PaCO_2$ is 60 mmHg**, the decrease in pH suggests acidosis. The $PaCO_2$ has moved in the opposite direction (increased) and suggests respiratory acidosis. Similarly, if the pH is alkalotic and the $PaCO_2$ is low, it suggests primary respiratory alkalosis.

A change in $PaCO_2$ also changes the serum bicarbonate concentration (Key Box 19.4).

Key Box 19.4

Condition	PCO_2	$[HCO_3^-]$
Acute respiratory acidosis	10 mmHg↑	↑1 mmol/L
Acute respiratory alkalosis	10 mmHg↓	↓2 mmol/L
Chronic respiratory alkalosis and acidosis	10 mmHg↓	↓5 mmol/L

Key Box 19.5

Metabolic acidosis: Expected $\Delta PaCO_2 = 1.2 \times \Delta[HCO_3^-]$

Metabolic alkalosis: Expected $\Delta PaCO_2 = 0.7 \times \Delta[HCO_3^-]$

Metabolic disorders: Changes in serum bicarbonate concentration is accompanied by compensatory changes in $PaCO_2$ (Key Box 19.5).

As described previously, whenever metabolic acidosis is present, calculate anion gap to help diagnose the type of metabolic acidosis (high anion gap or normal anion gap). Similarly, when a patient has metabolic alkalosis, assess whether it is chloride responsive or unresponsive type and treat accordingly.

It must be remembered that these are general guidelines applicable to patients who are breathing spontaneously. These are useful for rapid bedside assessment of acid–base status. Occasionally, the patients can present with different combinations of acid–base disorders such as a mixed respiratory and metabolic alkalosis, or a mixed respiratory and metabolic acidosis.

In critically ill patients with multiorgan failure such as renal and respiratory abnormalities and receiving mechanical ventilation, the physiology can be very complicated. Mixed disorders are common in such patients and a more detailed analysis as described previously may be required.

Clinical Notes

1. A 30-year-old man was admitted to the ICU with history of consumption of organophosphorus poisoning 4 hours ago. On admission, he is drowsy, breathing 60% oxygen by face mask and has a bradycardia. A blood gas analysis taken half an hour later shows a PaO_2 = 100 mmHg, $PaCO_2$ = 60 mmHg and a pH of 7.24.

Analysis

Oxygenation: The PaO_2 on 60% oxygen should have been about 300 mmHg. The PaO_2/FIO_2 ratio in this patient is 100/0.6 = 167. Thus, although the PaO_2 is adequate to sustain life, the patient's oxygenation status is poor.

Ventilation: Raised $PaCO_2$ suggests respiratory acidosis.

Acid–base status: The pH shows acidosis. The pH has decreased, whereas the $PaCO_2$ has increased. Hence, the patient has primary, uncompensated respiratory acidosis.

2. A 60-year-old man, a known diabetic since the last 15 years is admitted with diabetic ketoacidosis. He required endotracheal intubation and ventilation with 60% oxygen. An arterial blood gas analysis shows the following:

   PaO_2 = 60 mmHg, $PaCO_2$ = 28 mmHg, pH = 7.14 and $[HCO_3^-]$ = 12 mmol/l

Analysis

Oxygenation: The PaO_2 on 60% oxygen should have been about 300 mmHg. The PaO_2/FIO_2 ratio in this patient is 60/0.6 = 100. Thus, although the PaO_2 is just adequate to sustain life, the patient's oxygenation is poor.

Ventilation: Low $PaCO_2$ suggests respiratory alkalosis.

Acid–base status: The pH shows acidosis. The pH has decreased, whereas the $PaCO_2$ has also decreased. Hence, it is not respiratory acidosis and must be metabolic. The bicarbonate levels are far below normal and suggests a primary metabolic acidosis. The low $PaCO_2$ suggests secondary respiratory alkalosis. The patient has primary metabolic acidosis with partial compensation.

3. A 65-year-old man with a 40-year history of smoking, posted for elective herniorrhaphy was sent to the pre-anaesthetic clinic for evaluation. Since, he gave history of poor exercise tolerance as evidenced by breathlessness even on mild exertion, and clinical examination revealed presence of COPD, an arterial blood gas analysis was done while the patient breathed room air. The report showed a PaO_2 = 55 mmHg, $PaCO_2$ = 60 mmHg, pH = 7.34 and $[HCO_3^-]$ = 30 mmol/l.

Analysis

Oxygenation: The PaO_2/FIO_2 ratio is 55/0.21 = 262. Thus, although the PaO_2/FIO_2 ratio seems adequate, the actual PaO_2 is less than 60 mmHg and suggests hypoxaemia.

Ventilation: High $PaCO_2$ suggests respiratory acidosis.

Acid–base status: The pH shows acidosis. The pH has decreased, whereas the $PaCO_2$ is high. Hence, it is respiratory acidosis. The bicarbonate levels are high which suggests metabolic alkalosis. Since, the pH is acidotic but near normal, the patient must be having primary respiratory acidosis with compensatory metabolic alkalosis. He has fully compensated respiratory acidosis. This picture of chronic hypoxaemia and hypercarbia is typical of patients suffering from severe chronic obstructive pulmonary disease.

Multiple Choice Questions

1. The normal hydrogen ion concentration of plasma is ______ nmol/L.

A. 30 B. 40
C. 50 D. 60

2. The most important buffer system in the plasma is:

A. Phosphate buffer system
B. Ammonia buffer system
C. Proteins
D. Bicarbonate-carbonic acid buffer system

3. pH is the negative logarithm to the base 10 of hydrogen ion concentration expressed in ______.

A. mol/L B. mmol/L
C. nmol/L D. µmol/L

4. The solubility coefficient of carbon dioxide in plasma is ______ ml/mmHg/dl.

A. 0.3 B. 0.03
C. 0.003 D. 3

5. The following is true in primary metabolic acidosis with secondary respiratory alkalosis:

A. pH and PCO_2 are decreased
B. pH decreases but $PaCO_2$ increases
C. pH and $PaCO_2$ are increased
D. pH increases but $PaCO_2$ decreases

6. The following is one of the causes of metabolic acidosis with increased anion gap:

A. Diarrhoea B. Intestinal fistula
C. Pancreatic fistula D. Diabetic ketoacidosis

7. The following equation represents the nonlogarithmic form of acid–base equation:

A. Harrison B. Henderson
C. Hutchinson D. Hanson

8. The following may be a cause of respiratory alkalosis:

A. Morphine overdose
B. Chronic obstructive pulmonary disease
C. Salicylate poisoning
D. Curare poisoning

9. Following are true for albumin *except:*

A. First line of treatment in hypovolaemic shock
B. Does not carry risk of transfusion hepatitis
C. Used in nephrotic syndrome
D. It should not be used to treat malnutrition

10. Metabolic acidosis with normal anion gap is also called:

A. Hyperchloraemic acidosis
B. Hyperkalaemic acidosis
C. Hypernatraemic acidosis
D. Hypercalcaemic acidosis

Answers

1. B **2.** D **3.** A **4.** B **5.** A **6.** D **7.** B **8.** C **9.** A **10.** A

CHAPTER

20

Fluids and Electrolytes

- Physiology of fluids
- Water regulation
- Disturbances of volume
- Regulation of sodium concentration
- Disturbances in concentration
- Disturbance in composition of body fluids
- Perioperative fluid therapy
- Types of intravenous fluids

Competency

SU12.2: Describe and discuss the methods of estimation and replacement of the fluid and electrolyte requirements in the surgical patient.

A good understanding of the physiology of fluids and electrolytes is fundamental to the practice of surgery. Most surgical conditions are associated with changes in this balance and it is only appropriate that these are identified and treated effectively.

NORMAL PHYSIOLOGY

The human body consists of about 50–70% liquids and 30–50% solids by weight. The liquid portion varies with age, sex and body habitus. The variation is the result of individual differences in the fat content of the body which contains very little water. Hence, thin individuals have greater total body water (TBW) content as compared to obese individuals. Similarly, the TBW is about 50% in women and 60% in men. Neonates have up to 80% TBW. Of this total body water, intracellular water constitutes 40% of body weight (2/3rd of TBW) and the extracellular portion, 20% of body weight (1/3rd of TBW). The interstitial fluid and plasma portions of extracellular fluid constitute 15% and 5% of body weight, respectively (Fig. 20.1).

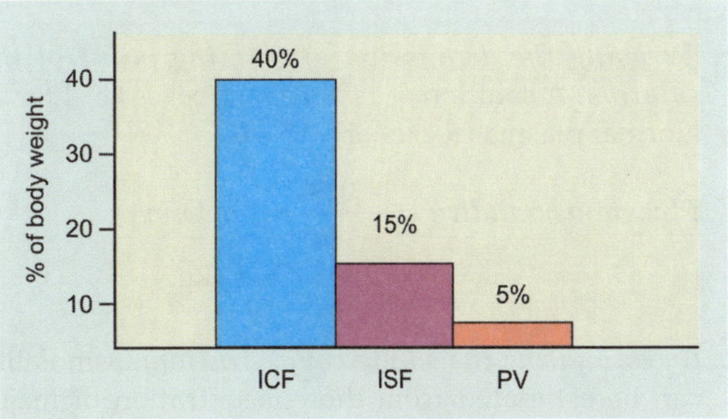

Fig. 20.1: Relation of various fluid compartments to body weight. ICF—intracellular fluid; ISF—interstitial fluid; PV—plasma volume

Table 20.1 Composition of body fluids

Composition	Intracellular (mmol/L)	Extracellular (mmol/L)
Cations		
Sodium	10	140
Potassium	150	4
Calcium	2	2.5
Magnesium	20	1.5
Anions		
Chlorides	10	111
Bicarbonate	10	25
Sulphate	70	1.5
Phosphates	45	1

Composition of Body Fluids

These fluid compartments are separated by semipermeable membranes allowing their fluid composition to be maintained within distinct limits. Table 20.1 shows the composition of the intracellular and extracellular fluid compartments. The composition of the intracellular compartments may vary according to the tissue, e.g. fat contains very little water.

The tonicity of plasma is determined by the solutes, sodium and its corresponding anions, chlorides and bicarbonate, together with substances such as glucose, urea and proteins. These particles are osmotically active and hence, tonicity is described in terms of osmolality (mOsm/kg H_2O).

Osmolarity is concentration of a solution in terms of osmoles (or mosmoles) of **solute per litre of solution** (solute + water). **Osmolality** is concentration of a solution in terms of **osmoles (or mosmoles) per kilogram of solvent**. Osmolality is independent of the temperature of the solution and volume of the solute. Hence, osmolality is the preferred term in clinical practice.

Osmolarity: Osmoles per litre
Osmolality: Osmoles per kilogram

Osmolality of a solution can be measured in two ways:

1. ***By using the depression of freezing point of the solution:*** A solution of 1 Osm/kg freezes at –1.86°C. Normal plasma freezes at –0.54°C.

$$\textit{Plasma osmolality} = \frac{-0.54}{-1.86} \times 10^3 \text{ mOsm/kg} = 290 \text{ mOsm/kg}$$

2. ***By estimating the solute concentration:*** Osmolality can be estimated from the concentration of major solutes of plasma.

$$\text{Osmolality} = 2 \times [\text{Na}^+] \text{ mmol/L} + \frac{[\text{Glucose (mg\%)}]}{18} + \frac{[\text{Blood urea (mg\%)}]}{6}$$

Example: If a patient's sodium concentration is 140 mmol/L, blood glucose concentration is 180 mg% and blood urea is 30 mg%, his plasma osmolality can be calculated as follows:

$$\text{Osmolality} = 2 \times [140] + \frac{180}{18} + \frac{30}{6} = 280 + 10 + 5 = 295 \text{ mOsm/kg}$$

From the equation, it is evident that sodium contributes the most to the osmolality of plasma.

A change in osmolality is usually due to changes in sodium. The normal range of plasma osmolality is 285–300 mOsm/kg.

Plasma Colloidal Osmotic Pressure

The plasma proteins normally do not pass out of the capillaries into the interstitium. These raise the plasma osmotic pressure above that of the interstitial fluid by an amount referred to as colloidal osmotic pressure (plasma oncotic pressure). The normal plasma colloidal osmotic pressure is 25 mmHg. Albumin is responsible for 75% of this oncotic pressure.

The body has mechanisms to regulate and maintain the volume of fluids, their concentration and composition within narrow limits to maintain homeostasis. Hence, a systematic assessment of fluid status of a patient involves the assessment of body fluid volume, its concentration and its composition in that order.

WATER REGULATION (Regulation of Volume)

The primary methods of body water regulation are:

1. ***Regulating the volume of liquid ingested:*** When the extracellular fluid volume reduces, the thirst centre in the hypothalamus is stimulated which encourages the person to ingest more water.
2. ***Regulating the volume of urine excreted:*** This is regulated by plasma antidiuretic hormone (ADH). A reduction in plasma volume releases ADH from the posterior pituitary which in turn acts on the ADH receptors in the collecting tubules of the kidney. This results in increased reabsorption of water and reduced production of urine. ADH release may also be stimulated by increased plasma osmolality and angiotensin.

DISTURBANCES OF VOLUME

A decrease in the circulating volume is called hypovolaemia and an increase, hypervolaemia.

HYPOVOLAEMIA

This is common in surgical patients. The assessment of acute loss of blood volume is detailed in Chapter 12. The reduction in blood volume due to loss of water can be in the following ways:

a. Gut—vomiting, diarrhoea, fistulae
b. Skin and lungs—0.5 ml/kg/h normally, increases by 12% for every 1°C rise in body temperature.
c. Sequestration of fluid in third space refers to noncontributory fluid space that is unavailable to the circulatory system.

Assessment of Dehydration

This is a clinical assessment based upon:

1. **History:** Severity and duration of loss of fluid.

Table 20.2	Assessment of dehydration	
Degree of dehydration	**Loss of body weight (%)**	**Clinical features**
Mild	5	Reduced skin turgor, sunken eyes, dry mucous membranes
Moderate	10	Oliguria, hypotension and tachycardia in addition to the above
Severe	15	Profound oliguria and compromised cardiovascular function

2. **Examination:** Thirst, dryness of mucosa, loss of skin turgor, orthostatic hypotension, tachycardia, reduced jugular venous pressures and decreased urine output in the presence of normal renal function. Dehydration can be classified as given in Table 20.2.

Laboratory Assessment

Haemoconcentration leads to falsely elevated haemoglobin, packed cell volume estimations and increased blood urea concentration. The kidneys reabsorb more water than usual leading to increased urine osmolality (>650 mOsm/kg).

HYPERVOLAEMIA

Causes

1. Excessive infusion of intravenous fluids.
2. Retention of water in abnormal conditions, such as cardiac, renal and hepatic failure.
3. Absorption of irrigation fluid as during transurethral resection of prostate using distilled water.

Diagnosis

- History and physical examination can lead to the cause.
- Physical examination: Distended neck veins, pedal oedema, body weight gain.
- Circulatory overload:
  - Hypertension, tachycardia, pulmonary oedema
  - Confusion, restlessness, convulsions and coma.

The development of these signs depends on the rate and volume of fluid overload, renal function and cardiovascular reserve.

Management

1. Treat the cause
2. Restriction of water and salt
3. Diuretics (or dialysis, if necessary) to remove excess water.

REGULATION OF SODIUM CONCENTRATION

Water constitutes the major component of all body fluids but the composition varies with the fluid compartment. The most abundant cation of extracellular fluid is sodium and is the prime determinant of ECF volume. Ninety per cent of the ECF osmolality is due to sodium.

The human body has no known mechanism to regulate sodium intake. The body regulates sodium output by:

- Regulating glomerular filtration rate
- Regulating plasma aldosterone levels

Addition or loss of water produces a change in the concentration of the solute. The quantity of solute relative to the volume of water is thereby increased (ECF is concentrated) or decreased (ECF is diluted) with loss or addition of water, respectively. Changes in concentration are generally changes in water balance rather than changes in sodium regulation. Since the changes in volume and concentration are interdependent and the changes in water content are not easily measured, an estimate of the fluid volume and concentration is usually made by using the measured sodium levels and serum osmolality.

DISTURBANCES IN CONCENTRATION

HYPONATRAEMIA

Hyponatraemia is defined as a sodium level less than 135 mmol/L. It may occur as a result of water retention, sodium loss, or both. True hyponatraemia is always associated with low plasma osmolality. It may be associated with expanded, contracted or a normal extracellular volume.

Causes

Assessment of hyponatraemia should begin with an estimation of the extracellular fluid volume (clinically and if necessary, using central venous catheters). Thus, true hyponatraemia can be of three types: Hypervolaemic hyponatraemia, hypovolaemic hyponatraemia and normovolaemic hyponatraemia (Fig. 20.2).

I. Hypervolaemic Hyponatraemia

Hypervolaemic hyponatraemia may be associated with clinical features of hypervolaemia, such as oedema. Acute hypervolaemia (e.g. TURP syndrome—acute absorption of hypotonic fluids into the intravascular compartment) may result in cerebral oedema and pulmonary oedema. As plasma osmolality decreases, water moves from the extracellular space into the cells

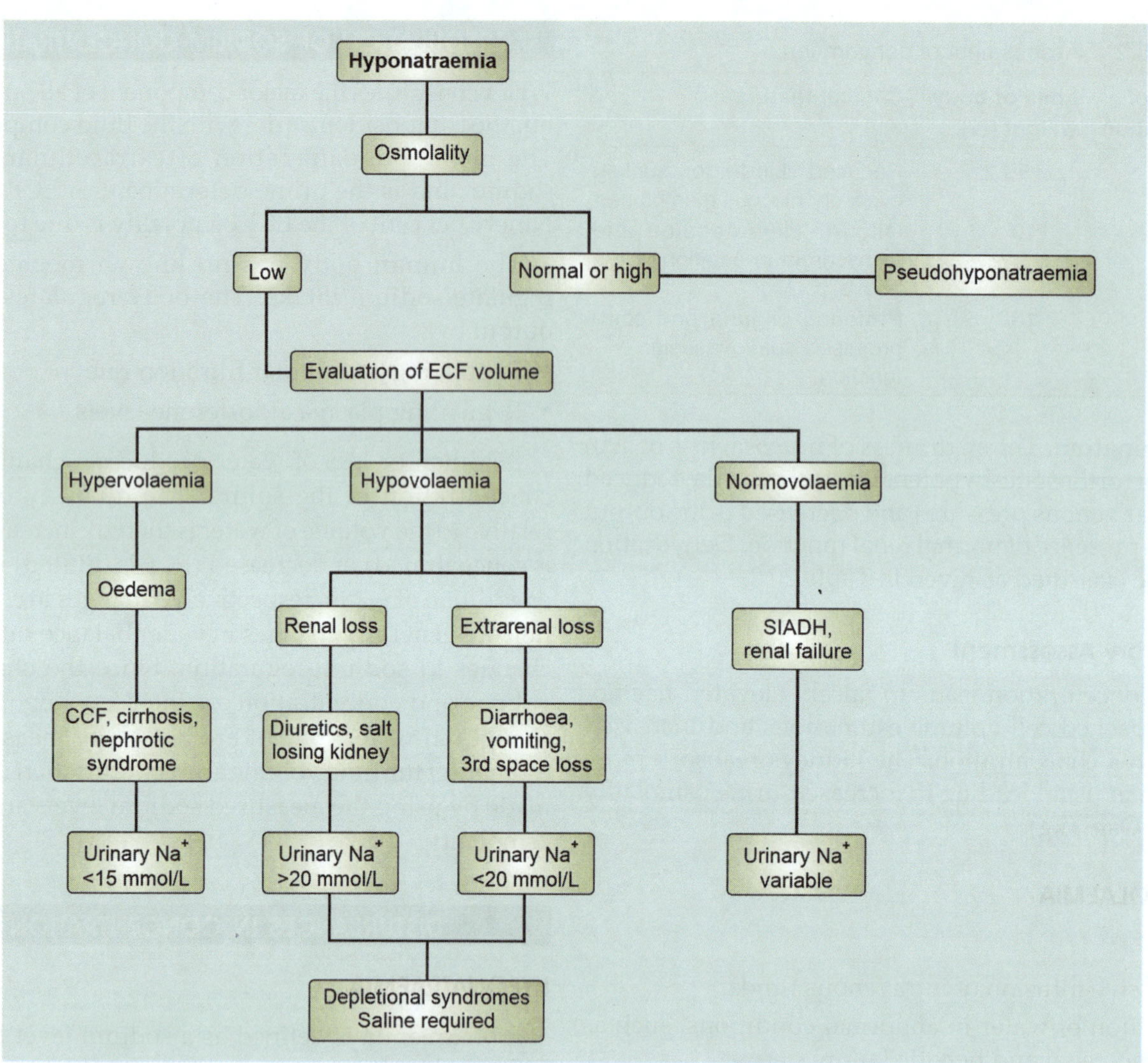

Fig. 20.2: Evaluation of hyponatraemia

leading to oedema. The expansion of brain cells is responsible for the symptomatology of water intoxication: Nausea, vomiting, lethargy, confusion, restlessness, etc. If severe ([Na^+] <100 mmol/L), it can result in seizures and coma. Chronic hypervolaemia as in congestive cardiac failure, cirrhosis and nephrotic syndrome may manifest with pedal oedema and elevated jugular venous pressures until decompensation occurs. The urinary sodium concentration is less than 15 mmol/L.

Treatment

Acute hyponatraemia (duration <72 h) can be safely corrected more quickly than chronic hyponatraemia. The following factors must be evaluated: Patient's volume status, duration and magnitude of the hyponatraemia and the degree and severity of clinical symptoms.

Fluid restriction, diuretics and correction of the underlying condition may be adequate in most cases. A combination of intravenous normal saline and diuresis with a loop diuretic (e.g. frusemide) also elevates serum sodium concentration.

Acute symptomatic hyponatraemia is a medical emergency. It should be treated with hypertonic saline (1.6% or 3%). Concomitant use of loop diuretics increases free water excretion and also decreases the risks of fluid overload.

The sodium concentration must be corrected to relieve symptoms and to a concentration of 125 mmol/L. Patients who are acutely symptomatic, the treatment goal is to increase the serum sodium by approximately 1–2 mEq/L/h until the neurologic symptoms subside. The correction should be slow and over a period of 12–24 hours with frequent checks of sodium concentration (every 2–4 h) to avoid overcorrection.

Avoid an absolute increase in serum sodium of more than 15–20 mEq/L in a 24-hour period. If sodium correction is undertaken too rapidly, the resulting osmolality changes in the extracellular fluid can cause central pontine myelinolysis. This condition is serious and can be irreversible.

The following equation can aid in the estimation of a sodium deficit to help determine the rate of saline infusion:

Calculated sodium deficit = (140 – current serum Na^+) × (body weight in kg) × 0.6

A litre of normal saline (0.9%) contains 154 mEq sodium chloride (NaCl) and 3% saline 500 mEq NaCl. In chronic severe hyponatraemia (i.e. serum sodium <115 mEq/L), the rate of correction should be slow and should not exceed 0.5–1.0 mEq/L/h, with a total increase not to exceed 10 mEq/L/day.

II. Hypovolaemic Hyponatraemia

Hypovolaemia corrected inappropriately with hypotonic fluids such as 5% dextrose may result in hyponatraemia. The hypovolaemia may be due to renal causes such as diuresis or a salt-losing kidney. The urinary concentration of sodium is more than 20 mmol/L in these patients. Extrarenal loss of volume as in diarrhoea, vomiting or 3rd space loss may result in urinary concentration less than 20 mmol/L. All these are termed depletional syndromes and require saline infusion.

Treatment

Based upon the volume status, administer isotonic saline to patients with hypotonic hyponatremia who are hypovolaemic to re-expand the contracted intravascular volume.

III. Normovolaemic Hyponatraemia

Occasionally, hyponatraemia may exist with normovolaemia. In such situations, the plasma osmolality must be estimated. If it is low, renal failure or the syndrome of inappropriate ADH secretion (SIADH) may be considered.

Treatment

For patients who have hypotonic hyponatraemia and are normovolaemic (euvolaemic), asymptomatic, and mildly hyponatraemic, water restriction (1 L/day) is generally the treatment of choice. For instance, a fluid restriction to 1 L/day is enough to raise the serum sodium in most patients. This approach is recommended for patients with asymptomatic SIADH. Pharmacological agents can be used in some cases of more refractory SIADH, allowing more liberal fluid intake. Demeclocycline is the drug of choice to increase the diluting capacity of the kidneys by achieving vasopressin antagonism and a functional diabetes insipidus.

Pseudohyponatraemia

Occasionally, the hyponatraemia is only an apparent one due to the accumulation of other solutes such as glucose, urea, plasma proteins or lipids. The plasma osmolality is either high or normal in these patients. Such hyponatraemia is called pseudohyponatraemia.

Serum osmolality is governed by contributions from all molecules in the body that cannot easily move between the intracellular and extracellular spaces. Sodium is the most abundant electrolyte but glucose, urea, plasma proteins and lipids are also important. Normally, their concentrations are small and contribute to the plasma osmolality only to a small extent. However, when the concentrations of these molecules increase to very high levels, the relative concentration of sodium in unit volume of serum may reduce. The actual amount of sodium is normal in these patients and hence the term pseudohyponatraemia. High blood sugar level or uraemia leads to higher plasma osmolality but high plasma protein or lipid levels is associated with normal plasma osmolality.

Treatment

The treatment of pseudohyponatraemia mainly involves treatment of the cause and supportive therapy.

HYPERNATRAEMIA

Hypernatraemia is defined as a plasma sodium concentration of more than 150 mmol/L and may result from pure water loss, hypotonic fluid loss or salt gain.

Causes of Hypernatraemia

I. *Pure water depletion*

1. Extrarenal loss	Failure of water intake (coma, elderly, postoperative patients) Mucocutaneous loss—fever
2. Renal loss	Diabetes insipidus, chronic renal failure

II. *Hypotonic fluid loss*

1. Extrarenal loss	Gastrointestinal (vomiting, diarrhoea) Excessive sweating
2. Renal loss	Osmotic diuresis (glucose, urea, mannitol)
3. Salt gain	Iatrogenic (sodium bicarbonate, hypertonic saline), salt ingestion steroid excess

The hypertonicity of plasma leads to cellular dehydration. Clinical evidence of dehydration may not be apparent until 10–15% of body weight has been lost. Rehydration should be slow to prevent cerebral oedema.

The diagnosis can be established by measuring plasma and urine osmolalities and urine output.

- Uosm > Posm and ↓ urine output → Extrarenal causes (e.g. diarrhoea, fistulae)
- Uosm > Posm and ↑ urine output → Osmotic diuresis
- Uosm < Posm and ↑ urine output →↑ ADH or renal response to ADH.

Treatment

1. Administration of water orally/nasogastric tube
2. Administration of IV fluid—5% dextrose or 0.45% saline
3. Change in serum sodium should not be more than 1–2 mmol/L/h. Rapid rehydration can cause cerebral oedema.

DISTURBANCES IN COMPOSITION OF BODY FLUIDS

POTASSIUM BALANCE

The normal potassium level is 3.5–5.5 mmol/L. Hypokalaemia and hyperkalaemia are two clinically important disturbances.

Hypokalaemia (Key Box 20.1)

This is defined as a plasma concentration of potassium less than 3.5 mmol/L.

Symptoms

- Anorexia, nausea
- Muscle weakness, paralytic ileus
- Altered cardiac conduction: Delayed repolarisation, reduced height of 'T' wave, presence of 'U' wave, wide QRS complexes and arrhythmias.

Management

- Diagnosis and treatment of the cause
- Repletion of body stores
- Potassium supplements, in the form of milk, fruit juice, tender coconut water.

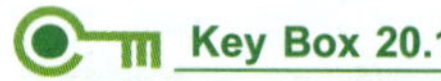
Key Box 20.1

Causes of Hypokalaemia

- Reduced intake
- Tissue redistribution: Insulin therapy, alkalaemia, β_2 adrenergic agonists, familial periodic paralysis
- Increased loss: Gastrointestinal losses—diarrhoea, vomiting, fistulae
- Renal causes: Diuretics, renal artery stenosis, diuretic phase of renal failure

- Syrup potassium chloride orally—15 ml contains 20 mmol of potassium.
- If the patient cannot take orally or the hypokalaemia is severe, intravenous potassium chloride is usually given at a rate of 0.2 mmol/kg/h. If there are life-threatening arrhythmias, it may be given at a rate not exceeding 0.5 mmol/kg/h under electrocardiographic monitoring and serial measurements.

Hyperkalaemia

This is defined as a plasma concentration of potassium more than 5.5 mmol/l.

Clinical Features

- Vague muscle weakness, flaccid paralysis

Electrocardiographic Changes

- Tall, peaked 'T' waves with shortened QT interval (6–7 mmol/l)
- Wide QRS complex, widening and then loss of 'P' wave (8–10 mmol/l)
- Wide QRS complex, merge into 'T' waves (sine wave pattern)
- Ventricular fibrillation (K^+ >10 mmol/l)

Treatment of Hyperkalaemia

1. Calcium gluconate (10%): 10–30 ml.
2. Sodium bicarbonate: 1–2 mmol/kg over 10–15 minutes.
3. 100 ml of 50% dextrose with 10–12 units of insulin over 15–20 minutes.
4. Hyperventilation
5. Salbutamol nebulisation
6. Calcium exchange resins
7. Peritoneal or haemodialysis

Clinical Notes

A 21-year-old lady was found to be collapsed as she was feeding her 15-day-old baby in the nephrology ward. On arrival, the cardiac arrest response team found her to have ventricular tachycardia without pulse. Cardiopulmonary resuscitation was given and she was shifted to the intensive care unit after return of spontaneous circulation. Investigations showed that her potassium level was 1.6 mmol/L. She had been admitted to the nephrology unit for postpartum acute renal failure. She had been dialysed three times following which she had gone into the diuretic phase of recovery from acute renal failure. She was putting out about 5 litres of urine per day in the last two days. Her hypokalaemia was corrected over 2–3 days. She recovered completely and could be discharged from the ward in 5 days time.

MAGNESIUM

It is the second most abundant intracellular cation. The normal serum magnesium concentration is 0.7–1 mmol/L. Most of it is present in the muscle and bone. Only about 1% is intravascular. Consequently, the serum concentration does not reflect body stores.

Role of magnesium in the body: Magnesium is required for the functioning of most enzyme systems including Na, K-ATPase, for synthesis of proteins, DNA, RNA, and parathormone. It also prevents influx of calcium into the cell.

Magnesium is a muscle relaxant and produces vasodilatation, cardiac depression, bronchodilatation and tocolysis.

Hypomagnesaemia

Serum concentration <0.7 mmol/L.

Causes

- Inadequate intake as in prolonged starvation or malabsorption, inappropriate fluid therapy.
- Excessive losses through nasogastric drainage, diarrhoea or diuresis.
- Redistribution as with insulin infusion or massive transfusion.

Clinical Features

- Predominantly neurological or neuromuscular abnormalities—muscular weakness, cramps
- Anorexia, lethargy and weight loss
- Hyperirritability, hyperexcitability, muscle spasms, stridor, tetany and convulsions
- Hypertension, pulmonary oedema
- Prolonged PR and QT intervals, ST depression and flattening of T waves
- Supraventricular and ventricular tachyarrhythmias
- Features of hypokalaemia and hypocalcaemia can also be seen.

Treatment

Magnesium sulphate is available as 50% (500 mg/ml) solution. Each ml contains 2 mmol of magnesium. In hypomagnaesemia, 8 mmol can be diluted in 50 ml of 5% dextrose or 0.9% saline and given over 30 minutes. If the patient has life-threatening arrhythmias, such as pulseless ventricular tachycardia due to hypomagnesaemia (torsade de pointes), and is unresponsive to defibrillation and epinephrine, it can be given as a bolus of 2 g.

Hypermagnesaemia

Most common cause: Iatrogenic.

Clinical Uses of Magnesium

- Antiarrhythmic agent for ventricular arrhythmias (torsade de pointes)
- As an antihypertensive, particularly for pre-eclampsia and eclampsia
- As an anticonvulsant
- As a bronchodilator

Clinical features of hypermagnesaemia depend on plasma concentration

- 4–5 mmol/L—muscle weakness and loss of tendon reflexes
- 6–7.5 mmol/L—respiratory arrest
- 10 mmol/L—cardiac arrest.

Hence, when patients are administered magnesium in large doses or as prolonged infusions, their ankle jerks must be monitored. If found sluggish, further doses or the infusion must be stopped.

CALCIUM

- Calcium is the most abundant mineral in the body. Ninety-nine per cent is deposited in the skeleton. In addition, calcium ions are important for the control of muscular and neural activities, in blood clotting, as cofactors for enzymatic reactions and as second messengers.
- Calcium homeostasis reflects a balance between reserves in the bone, rate of absorption across the digestive tract, and rate of loss from the kidneys.
- The hormones parathyroid hormone (PTH), vitamin D and calcitonin maintain calcium homeostasis in the ECF. Parathyroid hormone and vitamin D raise Ca^{2+} concentrations and calcitonin lowers it.
- Calcium absorption from the digestive tract and reabsorption along the distal convoluted tubule are stimulated by PTH from the parathyroid glands and calcitriol from the kidneys. The average daily requirement of calcium in an adult is 0.8–1.2 g/day.
- Half the serum calcium is bound to albumin and as albumin levels become low, this bound fraction is lower leading to a low total serum calcium concentration.
- Hence, the serum calcium level should be related to the albumin levels and corrected as follows:
- Corrected calcium (mg/dl) = measured total Ca (mg/dl) + 0.8 (4.0 – serum albumin [g/dl])
- Free ionic calcium is important for the electrical activity of the nerves and muscles and is more reliable (Normal: 1.0–1.4 mmol/L).

Hypercalcaemia (Key Box 20.2)

Hypercalcaemia exists when the Ca^{2+} concentration of the ECF is above 11 mg%.

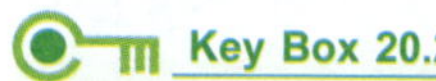

Key Box 20.2

Causes of Hypercalcaemia

- Hyperparathyroidism
- Malignant cancers of the breast, lung, kidney or bone marrow

Features

Severe hypercalcaemia (12–13 mg%) causes symptoms, such as fatigue, confusion, cardiac arrhythmias, and calcification of the kidneys and soft tissues throughout the body (moans, stones and groans).

Hypocalcaemia (Key Box 20.3)

Hypocalcaemia exists when calcium level is <9 mg%. mmol/L).

Key Box 20.3

Causes of Hypocalcaemia

- Hypoparathyroidism
- Vitamin D deficiency
- Chronic renal failure

Features

Muscle spasms, stridor, generalised convulsions, myocardial depression, cardiac arrhythmia and osteoporosis.

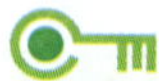

Competency

SU1.3: Describe basic concepts of perioperative care.

PERIOPERATIVE FLUID THERAPY

A patient undergoing surgery needs intravenous fluids to replace volume deficit acquired during starvation, normal maintenance for the duration of surgery and volume lost during surgery. Depending on the extent of dissection, fluid accumulates in these tissues in the form of oedema (third space losses). In addition, blood loss also needs to be replaced.

Perioperative fluid therapy in a patient whose body homeostasis is normal.

The replacement is as follows:

1. **Fluid requirement during starvation:**
   - Patients awaiting anaesthesia and surgery are kept fasting for at least two hours for clear fluids. This could be longer in patients requiring bowel surgeries.
   - People need fluids to cover insensible losses (through skin and respiratory tract) and urine output. This is 1–1.5 ml/kg/h.
   - The volume deficit that occurs due to fasting before surgery is replaced. The current fasting guidelines allow patients to drink clear fluids up to 2 hours prior to surgery. Hence, the patients should not be dehydrated.
   - If there are any signs of hypovolaemia due to vomiting, diarrhea, bowel preparation or any other cause, the patient may need to be administered additional fluids.
2. **Maintenance requirement:** The average daily requirement of water for an average-sized adult is 2000 ml. In general, a volume of 25–30 ml/kg/day meets the daily maintenance needs. This is calculated as 1–1.5 ml/kg/h. The maintenance fluids are given to cover insensible losses and urine output as mentioned before.
3. **Third space losses:**
   - The third space refers to accumulation of fluid in spaces that are not in continuity with plasma.
   - During surgery, there could be loss of fluid into interstitial space leading to oedema. It is difficult to quantify how much fluid seeps into the third space during surgery but it is proportional to the extent of dissection during surgery. It was believed that the third space losses could be as much as 4, 6, or 8 ml/kg/h for surgeries with minimal, moderate or large amount of dissection.
   - This is currently considered as an overestimation. Excessive fluid administration can lead to loss of endothelial glycocalyx and oedema. Inadequate fluid therapy can give rise to hypoperfusion, renal failure and organ dysfunction.
   - The current opinion is that maintenance fluids should be given as described earlier and fluids boluses of 250 ml must be given as required by monitoring the haemodynamic effects.
   - When in doubt, passive leg raising can increase venous return and help in decision-making.
   - Usually, urine output is measured during major surgery and an output of 0.5–1 ml/kg/h is desired. However, intraoperative urine output has no correlation to the incidence of postoperative renal failure and hence should not be used as a guide to intraoperative fluid therapy.
   - In complicated and extensive surgeries or in patients with compromised cardiac status or renal failure, more sophisticated monitoring techniques such as central venous pressure, stroke volume variation or inferior vena caval diameter measurements may be required.

4. Blood loss is replaced by compatible blood transfusion (homologous or autologous), if the haematocrit falls below 25%. Blood loss is replaced with an equal amount of colloids or 2–3 times the volume with crystalloids, if the haematocrit is >25% in an otherwise healthy individual. Crystalloids are electrolyte solutions that distribute themselves throughout the body water and hence, a larger volume needs to be given.

Perioperative Fluid Therapy in Patients with Disturbed Fluid Balance

Derangements of fluid therapy can be classified as:

a. Disturbances of volume
b. Disturbances of concentration
c. Disturbances of composition.

In the evaluation of a patient with a suspected problem in fluid and electrolyte or acid–base balance, careful sequential analysis of the volume, concentration and composition must be done in that order. This must be followed by appropriate therapy (as described earlier in this chapter). Also refer to Chapter 17 for management of shock.

TYPES OF INTRAVENOUS FLUIDS (Table 20.3)

These can be broadly divided into three groups: Crystalloids, colloids and special purpose solutions.

Crystalloids

These are essentially solutions of electrolytes in water, e.g. Ringer lactate. Some also contain dextrose, e.g. dextrose saline, 5% dextrose and paediatric maintenance solutions. They vary in the content of different electrolytes.

Ringer lactate:

- This is also called a balanced salt solution as this is a solution of electrolytes in water, with a composition very similar to extracellular fluid.

Table 20.3 Intravenous fluids

Solution	pH	Osmolarity (mOsm/l)	[Na⁺]	[K⁺]	[Ca⁺⁺]	[Cl]	Other components
Plasma	7.4	291	140	4	2.5	103	Many others
Ringer lactate	6.75	273	130	4	2.7	109	Lactate as bicarbonate
Isotonic saline	5.5	308	154	–	–	154	–
Plasmalyte	7.4	295	140	5	0	98	[Mg⁺⁺] 2
5% dextrose	4.5	253	–	–	–	–	Dextrose 5 g/L

- This is the solution of choice to replace third space losses. Ringer lactate does not provide any calories.
- It has a pH of 6.5. It contains Na^+ 131 mmol/L, K^+ 5 mmol/L, Ca^{++} 2 mmol/L, chloride 111 mmol/L and lactate 29 mmol/L (lactate gets converted to bicarbonate in the body).
- It has an osmolarity of around 270–278 mOsm/L and hence is marginally hypo-osmolar.

Normal saline:

- Normal saline is a misnomer; it is ideally called isotonic saline or 0.9% saline.
- It contains 154 mmol each of sodium and chloride per litre of solution. It has a pH of 5.
- Its osmolarity is 308 mOsm/L. This does not provide any energy.
- Isotonic saline may be used as replacement solution. However, large amounts of isotonic saline infusion can cause hyperchloraemic metabolic acidosis.

5% dextrose:

- Each 100 ml contains 5 g of dextrose. It has a pH of 4. One litre of 5% dextrose will provide 200 kcal of energy.
- It may be used to replace insensible free water loss. Once the dextrose is metabolised, only water remains. Hence, it is called a hypotonic solution.
- It may be used to dilute inotropes, vasopressors, inodilators, sodium nitroprusside, aminophylline, etc.
- It may be used as part of glucose-insulin-potassium solution.

Newer solutions:

- Ringer's acetate is similar to Ringer lactate but the lactate has been replaced by acetate. The lactate in Ringer lactate can cause confusion during serum lactate measurements in sepsis. This is avoided by using acetate.
- Plasmalyte is a crystalloid where the amount of chloride has been further reduced and calcium has been replaced with magnesium. It also has gluconate and acetate instead of lactate.
- The newer solutions are increasingly being used especially in critically ill patients and when large amounts need to be given.

Colloids

- Colloids are suspensions of large molecules in solution, usually in saline.
- Unlike the ions in crystalloids, such as saline or Ringer lactate, these molecules cannot cross the cell membrane. They remain in the intravascular compartment

for a longer period and hence become effective plasma expanders.
- These are used to restore blood volume in emergency situations, e.g. polytrauma with severe haemorrhage, massive GI bleed and shock.

1. Albumin

- It is available as 5 and 20%.
- It is prepared from pooled human plasma. Since it is pasteurised at 60°C for 10 hours, the chances of transmission of diseases is very low. It is also tested using nuclear acid test (NAT) to detect hepatitis B and C viruses as well as HIV1.
- 5% albumin is used as a plasma expander. 20% albumin can be used to replace lost albumin in severe hypoalbuminaemia in addition to plasma expansion.

Indications

- Can be used as a plasma expander to treat shock.
- Used in severe burns—acute severe hypoalbuminaemia.
- Used in nephrotic syndrome.

Contraindications

- Heart failure
- Severe anaemia

2. Gelatins

- Good plasma expander.
- They are of two types: Urea-linked gelatin (Haemaccel) and succinylated gelatin (Gelofusine).
- Plasma expansion lasts for 4–6 hours.
- Severe reactions including anaphylaxis can occur with urea-linked gelatin but less with succinylated gelatin.

3. Dextran 40

- Reduces viscosity and red cell sludging.
- Used to maintain patency of microvascular free flaps by reducing thrombosis.
- May affect renal function and coagulation.

4. Hydroxyethyl Starch (HES)

- Derived from starch.
- Hydroxyethyl radicals are substituted onto the carbon atoms of glucose molecules.
- The effects depend on the molecular weight, molar substitution and the C2–C6 ratio.
- HES solutions are classified as high (>450 kDa), medium (130–200 kDa) and low (<130 kDa) molecular weight starches.
- The term substitution is used to represent the number of hydroxyethyl residues per 10 glucose subunits. Accordingly, they may be highly substituted (molar substitution 0.62–0.75), medium (0.5–0.6) or low (<0.4).
- Thus HES 130/0.4 means the molecular weight is 130 kDa and the molar substitution is 0.4.
- HES with a molar substitution of 0.7 is called hetastarch, 0.6 is hexastarch, 0.5 is pentastarch, and 0.4 is tetrastarch.

Adverse Effects

- HES may interfere with coagulation.
- Incidence of severe reactions (1:16,000).
- Use in shock is associated with increased risk of renal injury and mortality and hence, must be avoided.
- Although initial studies showed that adverse effects are less with lower molecular weight and lower substitution HES 130/0.4 (tetrastarch), doubts have been raised about the safety of tetrastarch. Consequently, the European Medicine Agency has recommended its withdrawal from the market.

Special Purpose Solutions

Sodium bicarbonate: It is available as 7.5% (0.9 mEq/ml) and 8.4% (1 mEq/ml) of sodium bicarbonate.

Uses:

- As an alkalinising agent
- To treat metabolic acidosis
- To treat hyperkalaemia
- Forced alkaline diuresis

Disadvantages:

- Increased sodium load
- Alkalosis with a shift of oxygen dissociation curve to the left (increased affinity of haemoglobin to O_2, reducing its unloading)
- Increased intracranial pressure and intraventricular haemorrhages in neonates
- Circulatory overload leading to cardiac failure
- Carbon dioxide load leading to respiratory failure

Mannitol (10 and 20%):

- It is an osmotic diuretic. Mannitol expands intravascular volume initially by drawing fluid from the interstitium. This is followed by diuresis.
- Its main use is to reduce intracranial pressure by producing diuresis.
- It is also used to reduce intraocular pressure. It should be used with caution in patients with cardiac failure, renal failure, etc.

Hypertonic saline (1.6, 3, and 5%): These solutions are available to treat hyponatraemia.

Multiple Choice Questions

1. The following electrolyte contributes most to the osmolality of plasma:

A. Sodium B. Potassium
C. Magnesium D. Calcium

2. The normal plasma osmolality is ______ mOsm/kg.

A. 190 B. 290
C. 160 D. 260

3. Plasma osmolality is determined in the laboratory using:

A. Freezing point B. Boiling point
C. Saturation point D. Isoelectric point

4. The second major intracellular cation is:

A. Sodium B. Potassium
C. Calcium D. Magnesium

5. In chronic hyponatraemia, the sodium concentration should be increased at a rate not exceeding ______ mmol/Ll/h.

A. 1 B. 5
C. 10 D. 15

6. The following is one of the drugs used to treat hyperkalaemia:

A. Digoxin B. Magnesium sulphate
C. Atropine D. Insulin

7. Tall 'T' wave in the electrocardiogram is a feature of:

A. Hypokalaemia B. Hyperkalaemia
C. Hypocalcaemia D. Hypercalcaemia

8. Rapid infusion of the following fluid can cause intraventricular haemorrhage in neonates:

A. 5% dextrose
B. 8.4% sodium bicarbonate
C. 0.9% saline
D. Ringer lactate

9. The following colloid is often used to reduce plasma viscosity:

A. Dextran 40
B. Hetastarch
C. Gelatin
D. Albumin

10. Hypercalcaemia may be seen in the following conditions *except:*

A. Hyperparathyroidism
B. Malignant cancers of the breast and lung
C. Vitamin D toxicity
D. Chronic renal failure

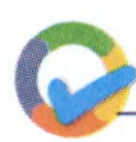

Answers

1. A **2.** B **3.** A **4.** D **5.** A **6.** D **7.** B **8.** B **9.** A **10.** D

Section

II

General Surgery

CHAPTER

21

Wound, Keloid and Hypertrophic Scar

- Types of wounds: Classification
- General principles of management of open wounds
- Components of wound healing
- Hyperbaric oxygen
- Negative pressure assisted wound closure
- Factors affecting wound healing
- Compartment syndrome
- Hypertrophic scar and keloid
- Healing of specialised tissues
- Classification of surgical wounds

Competency

SU5.3: Differentiate the various types of wounds, plan and observe management of wounds.

Definition: A discontinuity or break in the surface epithelium.

TYPES OF WOUNDS: CLASSIFICATION

I. Simple vs Complex

- **Simple wounds:** Involve only skin.
- **Complex wounds:** Involve underlying nerves, vessels and tendons.

II. Closed vs Open Wounds

IIa. Closed wounds

- Contusion
- Abrasion
- Haematoma

Contusions: These can be a minor soft tissue injury without a break in the skin, or a major injury such as when being run over by a vehicle. Generally, they produce discolouration of the skin due to a collection of blood underneath it.

Abrasions: In these wounds, the epidermis of the skin is scraped away. These wounds are painful because they expose dermal nerve endings. They require cleaning, antibiotics, and proper dressings.

Haematomas: These refer to a collection of blood usually following injury. These may occur spontaneously in patients who have bleeding tendencies like haemophilia. Depending on the site, they may be subcutaneous, intramuscular, intra-articular, or even subperiosteal. A knee joint haematoma may need to be aspirated followed by application of a compression bandage. Small haematomas are usually absorbed and may get infected if they are not.

IIb. Open wounds

- Incised
- Lacerated
- Penetrating
- Crushed

Incised wounds: These are caused by sharp objects, such as a knife, blade, or glass. They have a sharp edge and are usually less contaminated. They are ideally treated by primary suturing, which results in a neat and clean scar.

Lacerated wounds: These are caused by blunt injury, such as a fall on a stone or a road traffic accident (RTA). The edges are jagged. The injury may either involve only skin and subcutaneous tissue or deeper structures as well. Due to the blunt nature of the trauma, there is crushing of the tissue which may result in a haematoma, bruising, or even necrosis. These wounds are treated by wound excision and primary suturing provided they are performed within six hours of the injury.

Penetrating wounds: These are not uncommon. Stab injuries of the abdomen are a very notorious example. These may look like an innocent injury with a small 1–2 cm cut, but internal organs like the intestines, liver, spleen, or mesenteric blood vessels might also be damaged. All penetrating wounds of the abdomen should be admitted and observed for at least 24 hours. Layer by layer exploration and repair is recommended, but may not always be possible due to the oblique track of the injury.

Crushed wounds: These are caused by blunt trauma due to RTAs, wall collapses, earthquakes or industrial accidents. These wounds are dangerous as they may cause severe haemorrhage, death of the tissues, and/or crushing of blood vessels. These patients are more prone to gas gangrene and tetanus. Adequate treatment involves a thorough debridement to remove all dead and necrotic tissue.

III. Tidy vs Untidy Wounds

IIIa. Tidy wounds: Incised, clean, healthy tissue, seldom associated with tissue loss (Key Box 21.1).

IIIb. Untidy wounds: Crushed/avulsed, contaminated, devitalised tissues, often associated with tissue loss.

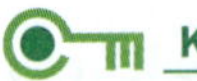
Key Box 21.1

Repair in Tidy Wound

- Nerves: Fascicular repair under magnification (loupe or microscope) using 8–0 or 10–0 monofilament nylon
- Artery: To be repaired by using 6–0 prolene
- Tendon repaired by monofilament nonabsorbable suture (polypropylene 3–0 or 4–0)
- Skin loss: Skin flap/skin graft

IV. Acute vs Chronic Wounds

IVa. Acute wounds: Stab wounds, RTAs, and blast injuries.

IVb. Chronic wounds: Leg ulcers and pressure sores.

General Principles of Open Wound Management

(Fig. 21.1)

- Admission or observation in the hospital.
- Monitoring of vitals.
- Systemic antibiotics depending on the extent of wound contamination.
- Injection tetanus toxoid for prophylaxis against tetanus.
- Treatment of the wound by cleaning, dressing, or suturing.

Healing of the Wound

Healing by primary intention occurs in clean, incised wounds (e.g. surgical incisions) wherein there is only a potential space between the edges. It produces a clean, neat, thin scar.

Healing by secondary intention occurs in infected wounds or in those with skin loss. It produces an ugly scar.

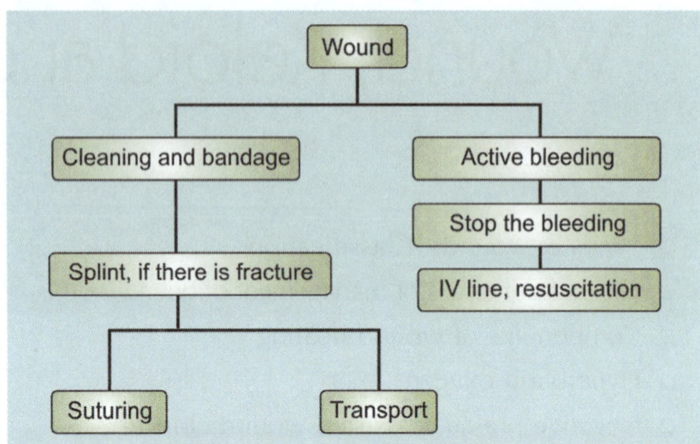

Fig. 21.1: Wound management

COMPONENTS OF WOUND HEALING

(Table 21.1, Figs 21.2 to 21.5)

Competency

SU5.1: Describe normal wound healing and factors affecting healing.

I. Inflammatory (Lag) Phase

- Injury results in the release of inflammatory mediators, mainly histamine from platelets, mast cells and granulocytes. This results in increased capillary permeability.
- Later, kinins and prostaglandins play a chemotactic role for white blood cells and fibroblasts.
- In the first 48 hours, polymorphonuclear (PMN) leucocytes dominate and play the role of scavengers by removing dead and necrotic tissue (Fig. 21.6).

II. Proliferative (Collagen) Phase

- Between days 3–5, PMN leukocytes diminish in number, and monocytes, which play the role of specialised scavengers, increase.
- By day 5 or 6, **fibroblasts** appear, proliferate, and eventually give rise to a protocollagen, which is converted into collagen in the presence of protocollagen hydroxylase. O_2, ferrous ions and ascorbic acid are necessary for this step.

$$\text{Protocollagen} \xrightarrow[\text{hydroxylation}]{\text{Protocollagen hydroxylase}} \text{Collagen}$$

(Oxygen, Fe^{++}, vitamin C)

Section II • General Surgery

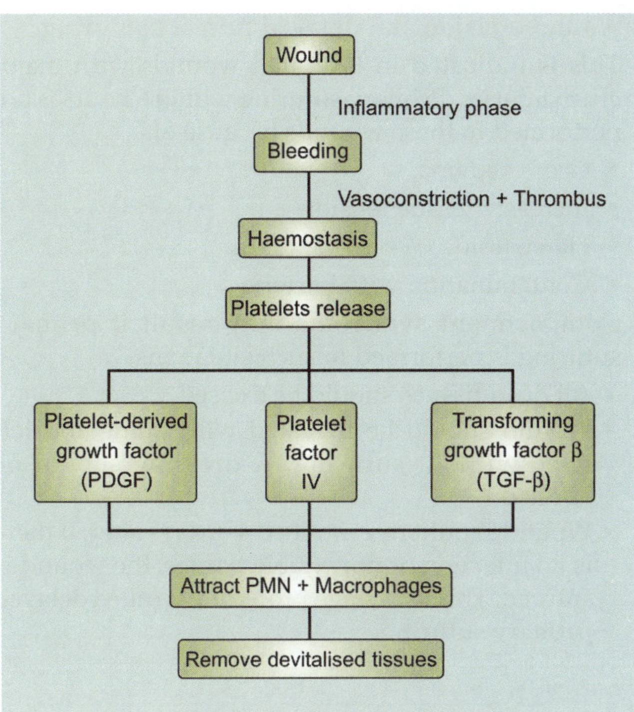

Fig. 21.2: Inflammatory and proliferative phases

- Fibroplasia and capillary budding give rise to granulation tissue.
- Ground substance and mucopolysaccharides (proteoglycans) are secreted by fibroblasts, and help in the binding of collagen fibres. Thus, a wound is composed of **Fibre** + **Gel** + **Fluid system** (resembles Iron rods + Cement + Water used for a concrete slab).
- **Epithelialisation** occurs mainly from the edges of the wound through cell migration and multiplication. This is mainly brought about by marginal basal cells. The entire wound is re-epithelialised within 48 hours. When there is a wound with skin loss, skin appendages also help in epithelialisation. Slowly, the skin surface gets keratinised.

III. Remodelling (Maturation) Phase

- It occurs between days 5 and 14.
- It is brought about by myofibroblasts (specialised fibroblasts with contractile elements). It is nature's way of reducing the size of the defect to aid in wound healing.
- Wound contraction readily occurs in areas of loose skin like the back and gluteal region, and is greatly reduced in wounds over the tibia (shin) or malleolar surface. **Corticosteroids, irradiation, and chemotherapy delay wound contraction.**
- **Connective tissue formation:** Formation of granulation tissue is the most important and fundamental step in wound healing. (It can be compared to concrete slab laying.)

IV. Phase of Scar Formation

- Fibroplasia and laying of collagen increases
- Vascularity reduces (devascularisation)
- Epithelialisation continues
- Ingrowth of lymphatics and nerve fibres takes place
- Remodelling of collagen takes place with cicatrisation, resulting in a scar.

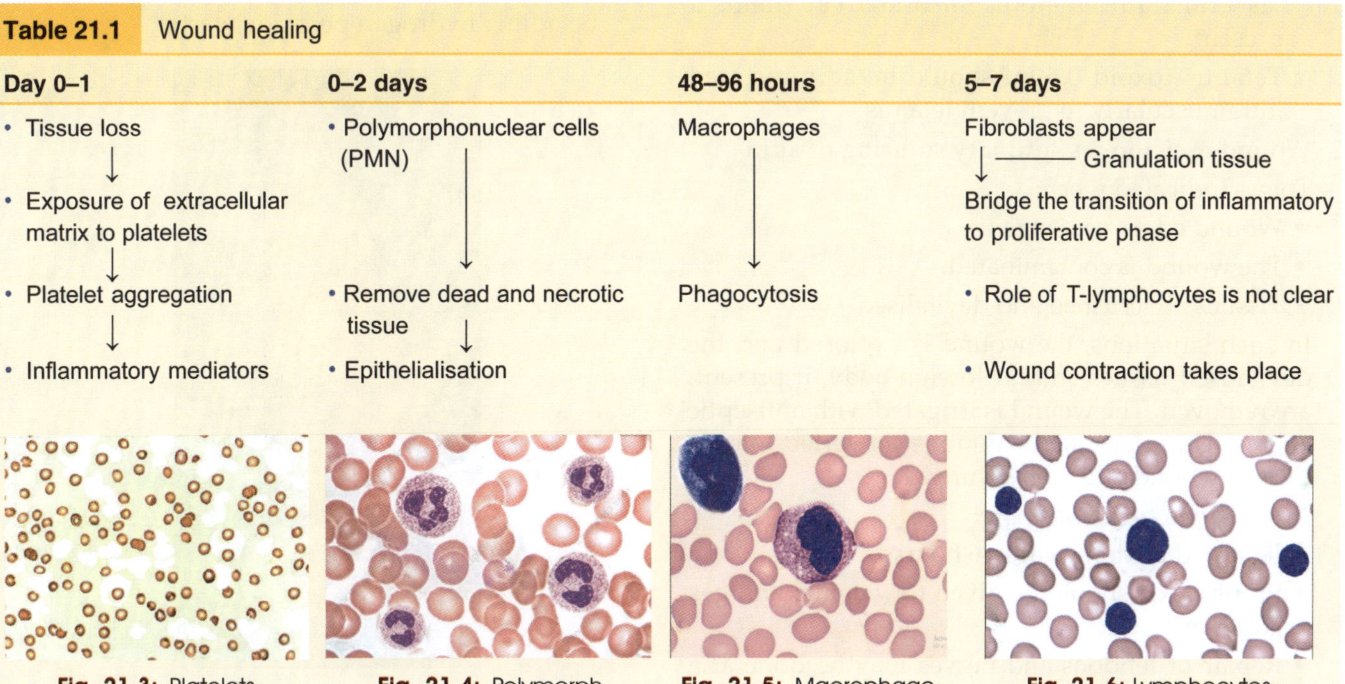

Table 21.1 Wound healing

Day 0–1	0–2 days	48–96 hours	5–7 days
• Tissue loss ↓	• Polymorphonuclear cells (PMN) ↓	Macrophages ↓	Fibroblasts appear ↓ —— Granulation tissue
• Exposure of extracellular matrix to platelets ↓			Bridge the transition of inflammatory to proliferative phase
• Platelet aggregation ↓	• Remove dead and necrotic tissue ↓	Phagocytosis	• Role of T-lymphocytes is not clear
• Inflammatory mediators	• Epithelialisation		• Wound contraction takes place

Fig. 21.3: Platelets **Fig. 21.4:** Polymorph **Fig. 21.5:** Macrophage **Fig. 21.6:** Lymphocytes

Complications of Wound Healing

1. **Infection:** It is the most important complication and results in delayed wound healing. Majority of bacteria are endogenous. Depending upon pus/culture-sensitivity report, appropriate antibiotics are given.
2. **Ugly scar:** It is the result of infections.
3. **Keloid** and hypertrophic scar (*see* page 106)
4. **Incisional hernia** and wound dehiscence
5. **Pigmentation** of the skin
6. **Marjolin's ulcer** (*see* page 242).

WOUND CLOSURE OR WOUND SUTURING

1. **Primary suturing:** Wound suturing within a few (ideally 6) hours following an injury.

   Primary suturing can be done provided:
   - The wound was incised or cut with a sharp object, such as a knife or razor blade.
   - There is minimal injury to surrounding structures.
   - There is no wound infection. If a wound is sutured in the presence of infection, the suture material is eaten away (digested) by organisms, which results in wound gaping.

   Precautions to be taken:
   - If any foreign body is present, it should be removed.
   - Any associated injuries to blood vessels, nerves, or tendons should be recognised and repaired.
   - Wounds over the abdomen may have associated visceral injuries—look for and treat them, if present.
   - Tetanus toxoid 0.5 ml should be administered intramuscularly to prevent tetanus.
2. **Wound excision and primary suturing of skin**

   This is indicated when:
   - Wound edges are jagged.
   - The wound is contaminated.
   - Tissues are crushed and devitalised.

   In such situations, the wound is explored and the devitalised tissues and/or foreign body, if present, are removed. The wound is irrigated with antiseptic agents. Thus, lacerated wound is converted into an incised wound and then sutured.

   Precautions to be taken are:
   - It should be done within 6 hours.
   - Prophylaxis should be given for tetanus and gas gangrene.
   - Repair of tendons and nerves may be done at a later date if there is excessive contamination.
3. **Wound excision and delayed primary suturing**

   This is indicated in lacerated wounds with major crush injuries. Primary suturing within 6 hours is not performed in these wounds because of:
   - Gross oedema
   - Increased tissue tension
   - Haematoma
   - Contamination with bacteria

   Compartment syndrome may result if primary suturing is performed in such situations.
   - All dead tissues should be excised
   - Wound should be irrigated with saline and left open without suturing. A dressing should be applied.
   - Wound should re-examined 4–6 days later. If there is no infection or non-viable tissues, the wound is sutured. This two-stage procedure is called **delayed primary suturing.**

Pearls of Wisdom

Saline is increasingly being used to wash wounds as H_2O_2 and betadine may cause more damage.

Wound with skin loss (Fig. 21.7): It may occur after surgical procedures or accidents, etc.

Principles of debridement
- Ideally done under general anaesthesia
- Assess the extent of injury/tissue loss
- Control bleeding
- Excision of devitalised tissue, ideally using scissors
- Good saline wash/irrigation is better than betadine/hydrogen peroxide wash.

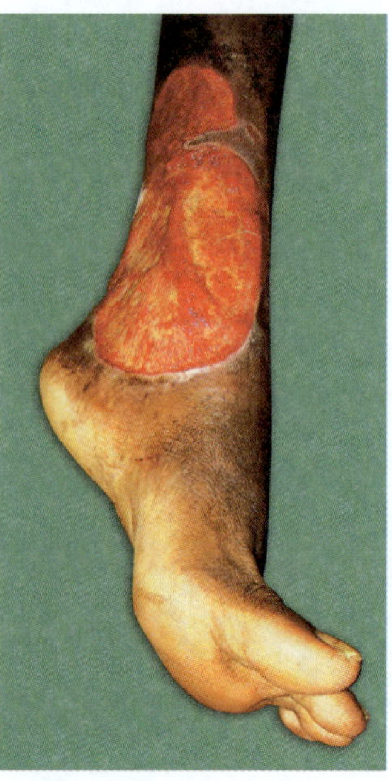

Fig. 21.7: Wound with skin loss

Pearls of Wisdom

Aim is to convert an untidy wound into a tidy wound.

Complications of skin loss

- Secondary wound infection.
- The underlying structures like tendons and nerves are in danger.
- Diabetic patients may develop septicaemia.
- Deformity and disability may occur at a later date.

Hence, skin grafting should be done as soon as possible.

4. Secondary suturing

Postoperatively, sutures may give way due to persistent discharge of pus caused by severe infections. In such cases, 7–14 days later (after controlling infection), the skin is freed from the edge of the wound and the granulation tissue and skin are approximated. This type of suturing is called secondary suturing.

CHARACTERISTICS OF AN IDEAL WOUND DRESSING

- Creates a moist environment
- Removes excess exudates
- Prevents desiccation
- Allows gaseous exchange
- Impermeable to microorganisms
- Thermally insulating
- Prevents particulate contamination
- Provides mechanical protection
- Non-toxic
- Non-traumatic
- Easy to use and cost-effective

Types of dressings:

- Non-adherent fabrics
- Absorptive: Gauze, foams
- Occlusive:
  - Nonbiologic: Films, hydrocolloids, alginates, hydrogels
  - Biological: Homografts, xenografts
- Creams and ointments: Antibacterial, enzymatic

HYPERBARIC OXYGEN (HBO)

- HBO uses oxygen as a drug and a hyperbaric chamber as a tool for elevating oxygen concentration to the target area.
- Transcutaneous oxygen pressure ($TcPO_2$) is used to assess wound oxygenation (<35 mmHg is significant).
- The rationale for HBO treatment is that tissue hypoxia or ischaemia results in impaired wound healing.
- Patients who benefit from HBO are those with marked hypoxic wounds.
- HBO therapy involves inhalation of 100% oxygen at a pressure 1.9–2.5 times the atmospheric pressure for 90–120 min. Oxygenation may be up to 10 times higher than usual.
- Treatment is given once daily, 5–6 times/week.
- Complications include middle ear barotrauma, pneumothorax, seizures, and respiratory distress syndrome.
- Contraindications for HBO include pneumothorax, and treatment with doxorubicin, bleomycin or disulfiram.

NEGATIVE PRESSURE ASSISTED WOUND CLOSURE

- This technique can be used to treat acute and chronic wounds (*see* page 171).
- It may lead to a reduction in oedema, an increase in local blood flow, and stimulation of granulation tissue.
- Its exact mechanism is unknown. However, it is believed that this technique leads to wound healing by removing exudates while keeping the wound moist.
- It stimulates endothelial proliferation and angiogenesis and causes increased cellular proliferation and a higher microvessel density.
- It also alters wound fluid composition by removing proteinases and inflammatory cytokines, and increases the speed of healing.
- It causes significant improvements in cost-effectiveness and a decreased length of hospital stay.
- It is particularly beneficial for large wounds.

FACTORS AFFECTING WOUND HEALING

General Factors

Competency

SU5.1: Describe normal wound healing and factors affecting healing.

1. **Age:** Wounds heal faster in children. In old age, wound healing is delayed because dermal collagen content decreases with aging. In addition, collagen fibres in elderly patients show distorted architecture and organisation.
2. **Debilitation** results in malnutrition. Wound healing is delayed probably because of vitamin C deficiency. Following injury, vitamin C deficiency can occur after 3–4 weeks. Vitamin C is necessary for the synthesis and maintenance of collagen. **Zinc deficiency is known to delay the healing of pilonidal sinus**. Zinc deficiency is rare—it occurs in large burns, severe polytrauma, and hepatic cirrhosis.

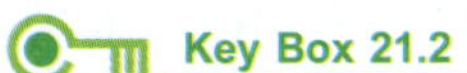

Key Box 21.2

Diabetes and Wound Healing Factors

Tissue hypoxia due to atherosclerosis
Thickened basement membrane →↓ tissue perfusion
Trauma—repetitive due to neuropathy
Tissue metabolism is increased—relative hypoxia
Total failure of defence mechanism
Observe **5 Ts**

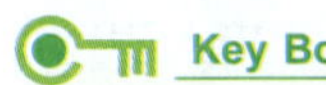

Key Box 21.3

Chemotherapeutic Drugs

- Decrease mesenchymal cell proliferation
- Reduce number of platelets
- Reduce inflammatory cells
- Reduce growth factors
- Decrease wound breaking strength

3. **In diabetic patients**, wound healing is delayed because of several factors such as **microangiopathy, atherosclerosis, decreased phagocytic activity**, proliferation of bacteria due to high blood sugar, etc. (Key Box 21.2). Also, a poor immune response is seen in diabetic patients.
4. **Jaundiced** and **uraemic** patients have poor wound healing because fibroblastic repair is delayed.
5. **Cytotoxic** drugs such as doxorubicin and **malignancy delay healing** (Key Box 21.3).
6. **Systemic infection/inflammation:** Infection/inflammation in some part of the body delays wound healing.
7. **Corticosteroids,** if given early, may delay wound healing because of their anti-inflammatory properties. However, they do not interfere once healing is established.
8. **Malnutrition:** This results in delayed wound healing including intestinal anastomotic leakage and wound dehiscence.

Pearls of Wisdom

Albumin levels must be <2 g/dL to have an effect on wound healing.

Local Factors

1. **Poor blood supply:** Wounds over the knee or shin heal very slowly, but wounds on the face heal fast.
2. **Local infection:** Organisms eat away the suture material, destroy granulation tissue, and cause slough and purulent discharge. If the bacterial count exceeds 10^5 organisms/mg tissue or if any β-haemolytic streptococci are present, the **wound will not heal**.

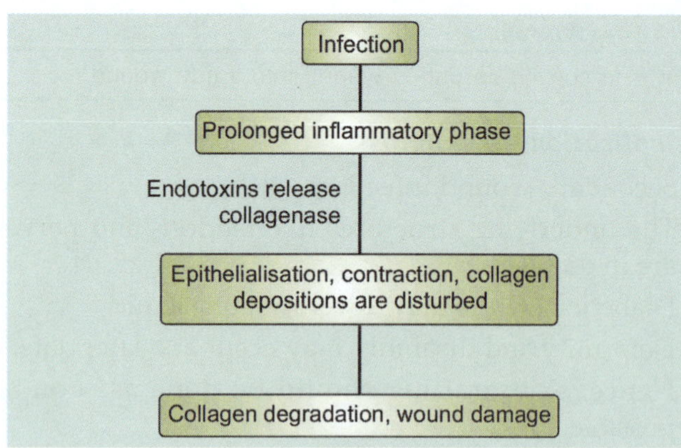

Collagen synthesis is reduced and collagenolysis is increased. Antibiotics should be given immediately or within 2 hours to prevent infection.

3. **Haematoma** precipitates infection.
4. **Faulty technique** of wound closure.
5. **Tension** while suturing.
6. **Hypoxia:** This may reduce the killing property of macrophages and the production of fibroblasts. If contamination occurs, the tissue oxygen level decreases.
   - Collagen synthesis is affected in cases of hypoxia. In anaemic patients, wound healing is delayed because of decreased angiogenesis and decreased collagen production.
   - Smoking causes vasoconstriction and elevated carbon monoxide levels.
7. **Ionising radiation:** It causes endothelial cell injury with endarteritis and results in atrophy and fibrosis.
8. **Foreign body** prevents healing because it precipitates infection.

COMPARTMENT SYNDROME

- Typically occurs in closed lower limb injuries.
- Following trauma, an inflammatory reaction results in gross oedema of the region.
- These occur in tight, divided compartments in the leg that contain nerves and vessels.

Definition

It is a serious condition characterised by increased pressure in one of the compartments of the body (e.g. lower limb in case of fracture leg), resulting in ischaemia of the tissues. In the lower limb, vessels, nerves and muscles are enclosed by tight unyielding fascia. This is the reason why even small amount of blood within a compartment can give rise to compartment syndrome.

Types

- Acute: Following trauma—especially fractures of long bones of the lower limb

- Chronic: Due to repeated injury to the muscles of the leg—may be induced by exercise.

Pathogenesis

Following trauma to the leg, damage to the blood vessels results in ischaemia to the muscles, which in turn results in an inflammatory reaction that leads to diffuse oedema of the tissues. This is aggravated by bleeding within the compartment, resulting in compartment syndrome. Factors precipitating compartment syndrome include crush injuries, plaster cast applications, tight compression bandages, anticoagulants, burns, etc.

Clinical Features

- Severe pain in the leg, disproportionate to the severity of the trauma.
- Sensory disturbances due to nerve compression.
- Pain, pallor, pulselessness, paraesthesia (Fig. 21.8), and paralysis are other features which may occur within 12 hours of the onset of compartment syndrome.
- Painful passive stretching of the limb is characteristic of compartment syndrome.

Measurement of Compartmental Pressure

- It is measured by introducing a transducer catheter within 5 cm of the injury zone.
- Compartment pressure >30 mmHg of the diastolic blood pressure is suggestive of increased compartmental pressure and is an indication for urgent fasciotomy.

Treatment

- The lower leg has four compartments: Anterior, lateral, superficial posterior, and deep posterior. The fasciotomy of the lower leg can be done with either a single incision or two incisions (lateral and medial).

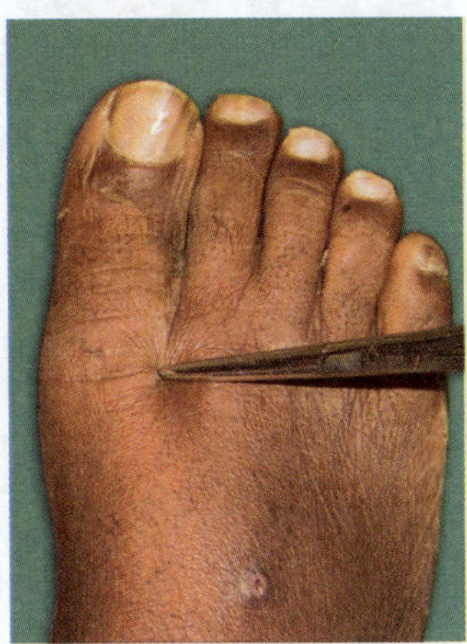

Fig. 21.8: Paraesthesia between first and second toes

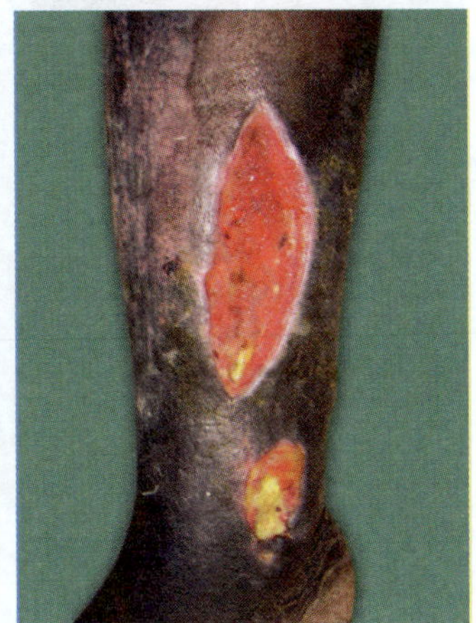

Fig. 21.9: Fasciotomy

- The two-incision technique is more common. The lateral incision (Fig. 21.9) is made longitudinally, approximately 2 cm anterior to the fibular shaft. The medial incision is made longitudinally, 1–2 cm posterior to the subcutaneous posteromedial border of the tibia.
- The incisions are made 8 cm long. After incising the deep fascia, the muscles bulge out. The soleus muscle must be detached from the tibia to decompress the deep flexor compartment.
- The most important aim is to preserve the blood supply by relieving the compression on the posterior tibial and peroneal arteries.

Complications

- Infections
- Gangrene requiring amputation.

HYPERTROPHIC SCAR AND KELOID

- As the name suggests, there is hypertrophy of mature fibroblasts (excessive collagen) in hypertrophic scars. Blood vessels are minimal in this condition.
- However, in keloids, proliferation of immature fibroblasts with immature blood vessels are found. These two conditions represent variations in the normal process of wound healing (Table 21.2).
- Keloids are **very common in Africans** and are least common in Caucasians (Key Boxes 21.4 and 21.5).
- A keloid is **not a true tumour,** but has a marked tendency for **local recurrence** after excision.
- Keloids take the shape of a butterfly over the sternum, which is its most common site of occurrence. It is extremely difficult to treat keloids over the sternum.

Key Box 21.4

Types of Scar

- Atrophic
- Hypertrophic
- Keloid

Key Box 21.5

Aetiology of Keloid

- **K**ey factors: Surgery, burns, vaccinations
- **E**levated levels of growth factor (more of type 'B' collagen)
- **L**aceration or abrasion
- **O**ver the sternum (incision)
- **I**nheritance and injection
- **D**eep pigmented skin (Blacks)

Remember as **KELOID**

Table 21.2 Comparison of hypertrophic scar and keloid (Figs 21.10 to 21.12)

Hypertrophic scar	Keloid
General features	
• It occurs from a prolonged inflammatory phase of wound healing. It never gets worse after 6 months • Itching is not usually present. If present, it is not severe • Nontender • Not vascular • Does not extend beyond the boundary of the original incision or wound. It rises above skin	• It continues to get worse even after 1 year and up to a few years • Severe itching is present • Margin is tender • Vascular, red, erythematous (immature blood vessels) • Extends to normal tissues, has **claw-like** process. Hence the name
Precipitating factors	
• Scar crossing normal skin creases • Over sternum, over joints • Young persons	• Black race • Tuberculosis patients • Incision over the sternum, ear lobe • Equal in both sexes • Hereditary and familial • Vaccination sites, injection sites, incision sites, piercing sites
Natural history	
• May become small	• Does not become small
Complications	
• Do not occur	• Ulceration, infection
Treatment	
• It is often not necessary • Stocking, armlets, gloves • Elastic bandage may help • Excision can be done • Silicone application • Topical retinoids	• It is difficult. Injection of steroid preparation such as triamcinolone acetate (Kanacort) into the lesion (intralesional) has been found to be extremely useful. It flattens the keloid. **Intrakeloidal excision** and skin grafting are to be tried last. Recurrence is common. Care should be taken **not to extend** the incision onto the normal surrounding tissues. • Silicone application • Topical retinoids

Pearls of Wisdom

Any form of excision has high chance of recurrence

We once had a patient who had undergone wide excision and grafting 6 times for a sternal keloid. The jaw and sites of vaccination are other common sites for keloids (Figs 21.10–21.12, Key Box 21.6).

Pearls of Wisdom

Collagen bundles are virtually absent in keloids. It is extremely difficult to treat a keloid.

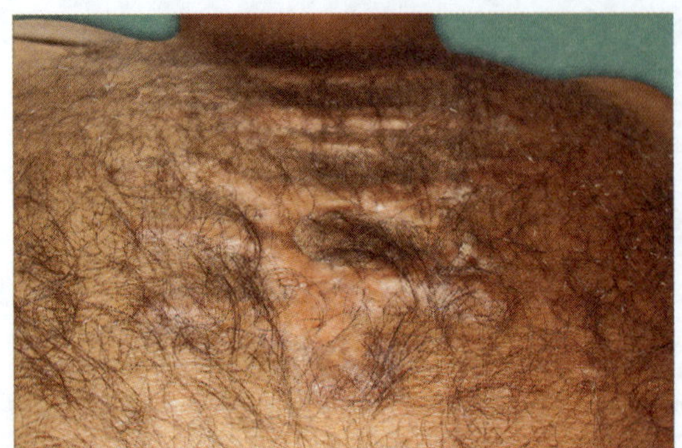

Fig. 21.10: Recurrent keloid over the sternum. Excision attempted three times

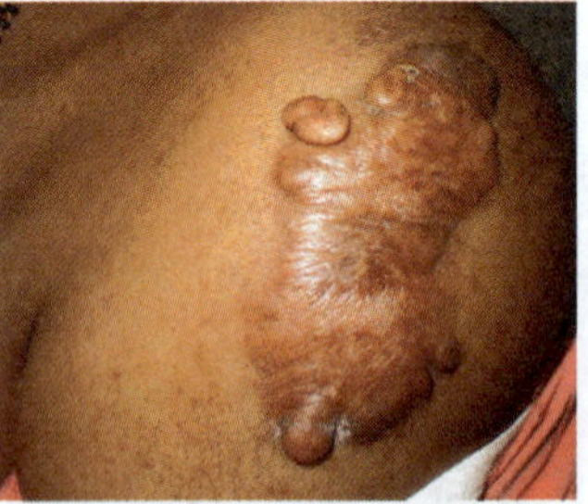

Fig. 21.11: Keloid over vaccination site

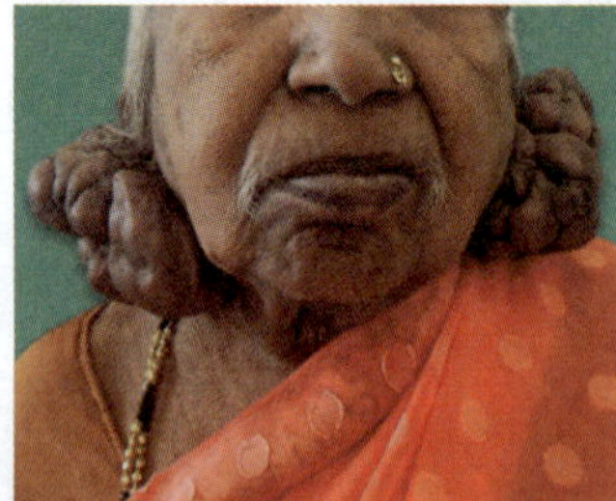

Fig. 21.12: Extensive keloid of the ear (*Courtesy:* Dr BP Suresh, Subbaiah Institute of Medical Sciences Shivamogga)

Key Box 21.6

Keloid Sites

High chances	Least chances
Skin of ear lobe	Eyelid
Presternal	Genitalia
Deltoid	Palm, sole
Upper back	Across joint

What is a Contracture?

When a scar crosses joints or flexion creases, a tight 'web' may form which is referred to as a contracture (*see* Chapter 32: Burns and Skin Grafting for more details).

MISCELLANEOUS

Healing of Specialised Tissues (Key Box 21.7)

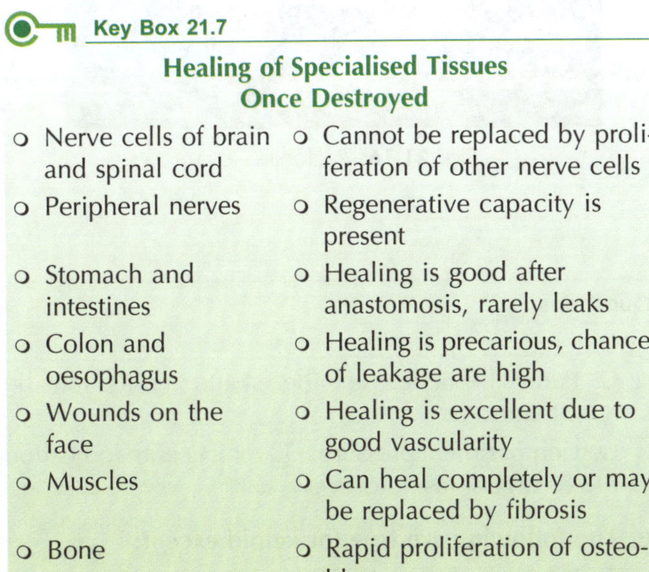

Key Box 21.7

Healing of Specialised Tissues Once Destroyed

Nerve cells of brain and spinal cord	Cannot be replaced by proliferation of other nerve cells
Peripheral nerves	Regenerative capacity is present
Stomach and intestines	Healing is good after anastomosis, rarely leaks
Colon and oesophagus	Healing is precarious, chances of leakage are high
Wounds on the face	Healing is excellent due to good vascularity
Muscles	Can heal completely or may be replaced by fibrosis
Bone	Rapid proliferation of osteoblasts

SURGICAL WOUNDS

Surgical wounds may be classified depending upon their nature (Table 21.3, Figs 21.13–21.16).

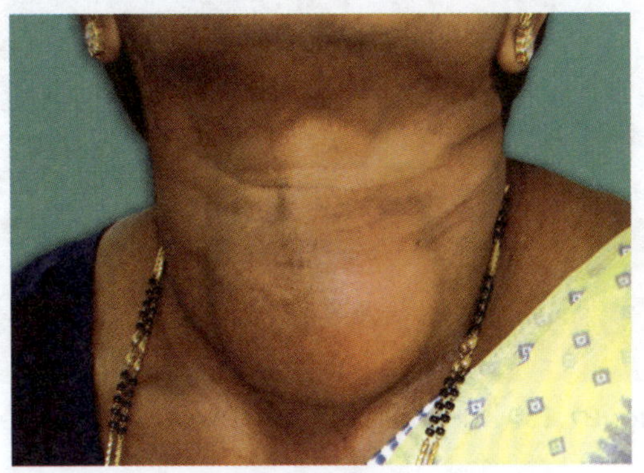

Fig. 21.13: Excision of neck swelling—clean

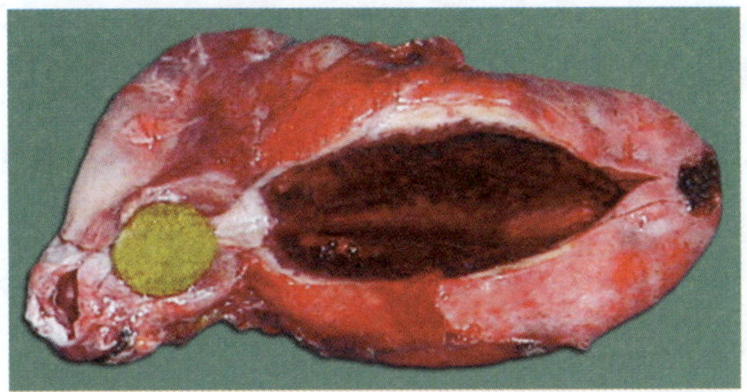

Fig. 21.14: Cholecystectomy—clean contaminated

Table 21.3 Classification of surgical wounds

Wounds class	Definition	Examples of typical procedures	Wound infection rate (%)	Usual organism
Clean (Fig. 21.13)	• Nontraumatic • Elective surgery • Gastrointestinal, respiratory or genitourinary tract not entered.	• Mastectomy • Vascular procedures	2	*Staphylococcus aureus*
Clean contaminated (Fig. 21.14)	• Respiratory, genitourinary or gastrointestinal tracts entered but minimal contamination	• Gastrectomy • Hysterectomy • Cholecystectomy	<10	Related to viscus entered
Contaminated (Fig. 21.15)	• Open, fresh, traumatic wounds • Uncontrolled spillage from an unprepared viscus • Minor break in sterile technique	• Ruptured appendix • Resection of unprepared bowel	20	Depends on underlying cause
Dirty (Fig. 21.16)	• Open, traumatic dirty wounds • Traumatic perforated viscus • Pus in the operative field	• Resection of gangrene	30–70	Depends on underlying cause

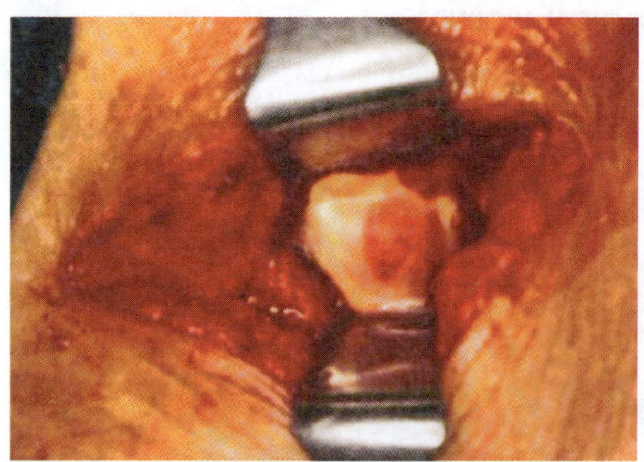

Fig. 21.15: Appendicular abscess—contaminated

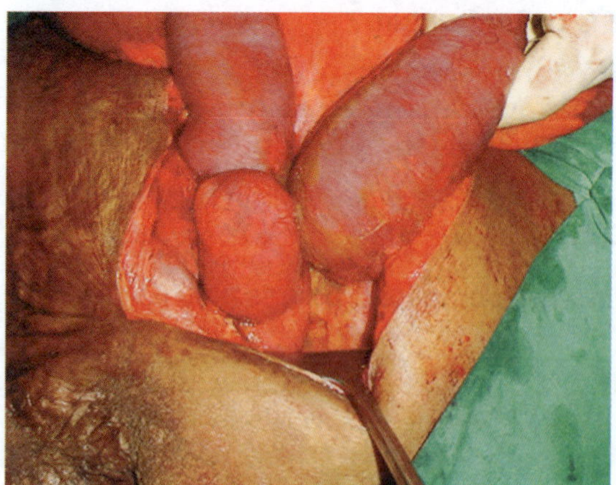

Fig. 21.16: Peritonitis—dirty

Multiple Choice Questions

1. **Platelet aggregation occurs in which phase of wound healing?**
   A. Inflammatory phase B. Proliferative phase
   C. Remodelling phase D. Scar formation phase
2. **A chronic scar can change into:**
   A. Martorell's ulcer B. Marjolin's ulcer
   C. Meleney's ulcer D. Malignant melanoma
3. **The ideal solution for washing wounds is:**
   A. Saline B. Betadine
   C. Hydrogen peroxide D. Eusol
4. **The following are true for wound healing *except*:**
   A. Vitamin C is necessary for the synthesis of collagen
   B. Diabetic patients have decreased phagocytic activity
   C. Once healing is established, corticosteroids may be given
   D. Poor wound healing in jaundiced patients is due to poor functioning of macrophages
5. **The following are true for compartment syndrome *except*:**
   A. It usually occurs in the lower limbs
   B. The most prone site is the posterior compartment
   C. Paraesthesia between the 1st and 2nd toe may be a feature
   D. Compartment pressure >30 mmHg is an indication for urgent fasciotomy
6. **The following are true for keloid *except*:**
   A. It extends into normal skin
   B. It continues to become worse even after several years
   C. It does not give rise to itching
   D. It often recurs after excision
7. **The following are true for hypertrophic scar *except*:**
   A. It does not extend into normal skin
   B. It does give rise to itching
   C. It becomes worse even after 2 years
   D. It is more common in Africans
8. **The following are true for keloid *except*:**
   A. Sternum is one of the common sites
   B. Collagen bundles are present
   C. Intrakeloidal injections may be used to treat it
   D. Deeply pigmented skin is more vulnerable for its formation

Answers

1. A **2.** B **3.** A **4.** D **5.** B **6.** C **7.** C **8.** B

CHAPTER

22

Acute Infections, Sinuses, Fistula and Surgical Site Infections

Competency

SU6.1: Define and describe the aetiology and pathogenesis of surgical infections.

INTRODUCTION

Ever since surgery evolved as a speciality, infection and haemorrhage have been two well-known enemies of surgeons. Although many newer antibiotics have come into existence, infection still dominates and is a major cause of morbidity and mortality in patients with 'benign disease.' This is the sad outcome of disease complications. Hence, it is important to effectively diagnose and treat infections as early as possible. Common surgical infections and their details are given below.

CELLULITIS

Cellulitis is a spreading subcutaneous inflammation caused by ***haemolytic** Streptococci **that produce hyaluronidase and streptokinase.*** This leads to spreading of inflammatory exudates in the subcutaneous and fascial planes, resulting in a gross swelling of the affected part. Cellulitis spreads quickly in areas of loose subcutaneous tissue, such as the scrotum, or in areas of loose connective and interstitial tissue, such as the face and forearm.

Sources of Infection

- Injury—minor or major
- Graze/scratch/abrasion
- Snakebite, scorpion bite, etc.

Precipitating Factors

- Diabetes
- Low resistance of an individual

Common Sites

- Lower limbs
- Face and neck
- Scrotum

Clinical Features (Fig. 22.1)

The affected part shows evidence of inflammation such as redness, itching, and a diffuse swelling. Skin is stretched and shiny. Pain, fever, and toxaemia follow later. It is differentiated from an abscess by the features mentioned in Key Box 22.1.

In untreated cases, suppuration, sloughing, and gangrene may occur.

Treatment

- Bed rest with legs elevated to reduce oedema of legs.

Key Box 22.1

Cellulitis	Abscess
No edge (diffuse swelling)	Well-circumscribed, has an edge
No limit	Limit is present
No pus	Pus is present
No fluctuation	Fluctuation is positive

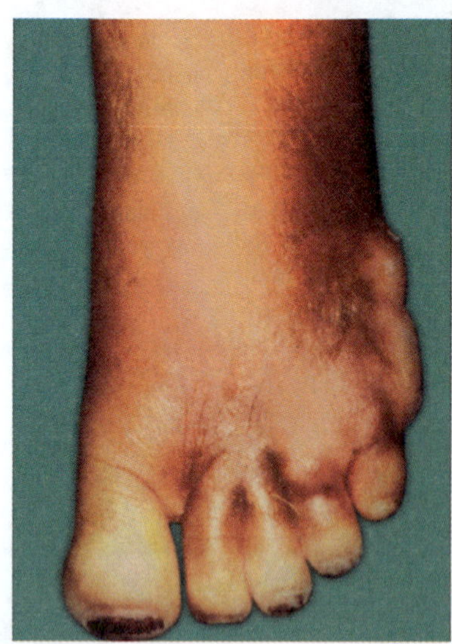

Fig. 22.1: Cellulitis of the foot with abscess

- Glycerine $MgSO_4$ dressing—reduces oedema of the part by osmotic effect.
- Diabetes mellitus, if present, is treated with injection **insulin** given **subcutaneously.**
- Appropriate antibiotics such as injection cephalosporins have to be given.
- Amoxycillin clavulanate potassium 25–40 mg/kg/day every 12 hours for 5–7 days depending on the severity of the condition.
- Antisnake venom is given in cases of snakebite.

Complications

1. Cellulitis may turn into an **abscess** which needs to be drained.
2. **Necrotising fasciitis:** Certain highly invasive strains of *Streptococcus pyogenes* may cause extensive necrosis of the skin and subcutaneous tissues, resulting in necrotising fasciitis. This is treated by debridement and skin grafting (*see* page 284) (Fig. 22.2).

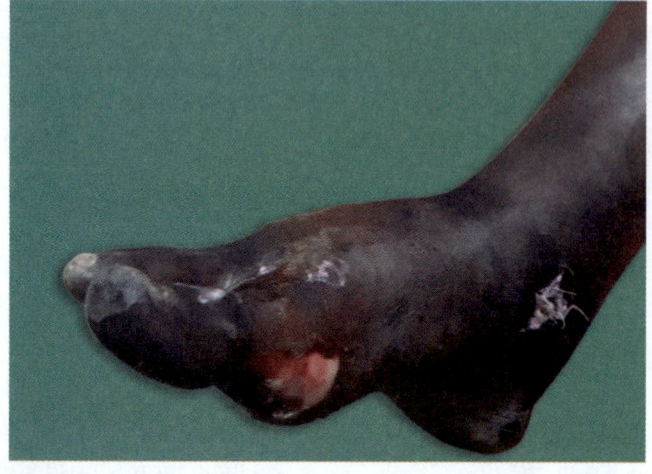

Fig. 22.2: Extensive cellulitis and necrotising fasciitis with gangrene

3. **Toxaemia and septicaemia:** *Streptococcal toxic shock syndrome* may result if exotoxins are produced by the organisms.
4. Cellulitis may precipitate **ketoacidosis** in patients with diabetes mellitus.

LUDWIG'S ANGINA

It refers to cellulitis of the submental and submandibular regions combined with inflammatory oedema of the mouth. Virulent streptococcal organisms are responsible for infection surrounding the submandibular region. Anaerobes also play a major role (Key Box 22.2).

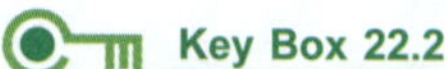

Key Box 22.2

Precipitating Factors

Caries tooth
Cancer of the oral cavity
Calculi in the submandibular gland
Chemotherapy
Cachexia
Chronic disease—diabetes *Observe 6 Cs*

Clinical Features

- Elderly patients presenting with diffuse swelling in the submandibular and submental regions (brawny oedema).
- Oedema of the floor of the mouth, which pushes the tongue upwards and results in difficulty swallowing.
- High grade fever with toxicity.
- **Putrid halitosis** is characteristic of this condition.

Treatment

- Rest and hospitalisation.
- Appropriate antibiotics.
- Intravenous fluids (to correct dehydration) and Ryle's tube feeding.
- If it does not respond to conservative treatment, surgical intervention is recommended.

Surgery (Decompression)

Under general anaesthesia, a 5–6 cm curved incision is made below the mandible in the submandibular region over the most prominent part of the swelling. The submandibular gland is mobilised, the mylohyoid muscle is divided, and the pus is drained. ***Even if pus is not found, the oedematous fluid comes out, which greatly improves the condition of the patient.*** The wound is closed with loose sutures after irrigating the cavity with antiseptic agents, and a drainage tube is kept in place.

Complications

1. Mediastinitis and septicaemia
2. Swelling of the tissues in the floor of the mouth results in elevation of the tongue, as the infection is contained by the mylohyoid. This leads to upper airway obstruction and oedema of the glottis, resulting in stridor.

LYMPHANGITIS

- It is also a nonsuppurative, poorly localised infection caused by streptococci, staphylococci, or clostridia.
- It presents as red painful streaks over the affected lymphatics.
- **Filarial infection** is a common cause of lymphangitis in coastal India (*see* page 216).
- **High grade fever, chills and rigors,** and features of systemic inflammatory response syndrome (SIRS) are common.
- **Tender, painful lymph nodes** in the groin are characteristic of lower limb lymphangitis.

Treatment

- Rest, elevation, $MgSO_4$, local dressing, antibiotics, anti-inflammatory drugs.
- Anti-filarial treatment in appropriate cases.

ABSCESS

An abscess is a localised collection of pus (dead, dying neutrophils and proteinaceous exudate).

CLASSIFICATION

1. **Pyogenic abscess:** It is the commonest form of an abscess. It can be subcutaneous, deep, or can occur within viscera such as the liver or kidney. In this chapter, pyogenic abscess refers to soft tissue abscess.
2. **Pyaemic abscess:** Occurs due to circulation of pyaemic emboli in the blood (pyaemia).
3. **Cold abscess:** Usually refers to tubercular abscess due to involvement of either lymph nodes or spine.

PYOGENIC ABSCESS

It is usually produced by ***staphylococcal infections.*** The organisms enter the soft tissue through an external wound (minor or major). It can also be due to cellulitis or haematogenous spread from a distant focus such as tonsillitis or caries tooth.

Pathophysiology

- Following injury, there is inflammation of the part brought about by the organism such as *Staphylococcus.* Pathological events are summarised in Fig. 22.3.
- The end-result is the production of pus composed of dead leukocytes, bacteria, and necrotic tissue. The area around the abscess is encircled by fibrin products and it is infiltrated with leukocytes and bacteria. It is called a **pyogenic membrane.**

Symptoms

The patient feels ill and complains of **throbbing pain** at the site, which occurs due to pressure of the pus on the nerve endings. Fever, with or without chills and rigors, may be present.

Signs

1. **Calor–heat:** The affected part is warmer due to local rise of temperature.
2. **Rubor–redness:** It is due to inflammation resulting in hyperaemia.
3. **Dolor–pain:** An abscess is extremely tender.
4. **Tumour–swelling:** It consists of pus. It is tensely cystic with surrounding brawny oedema.

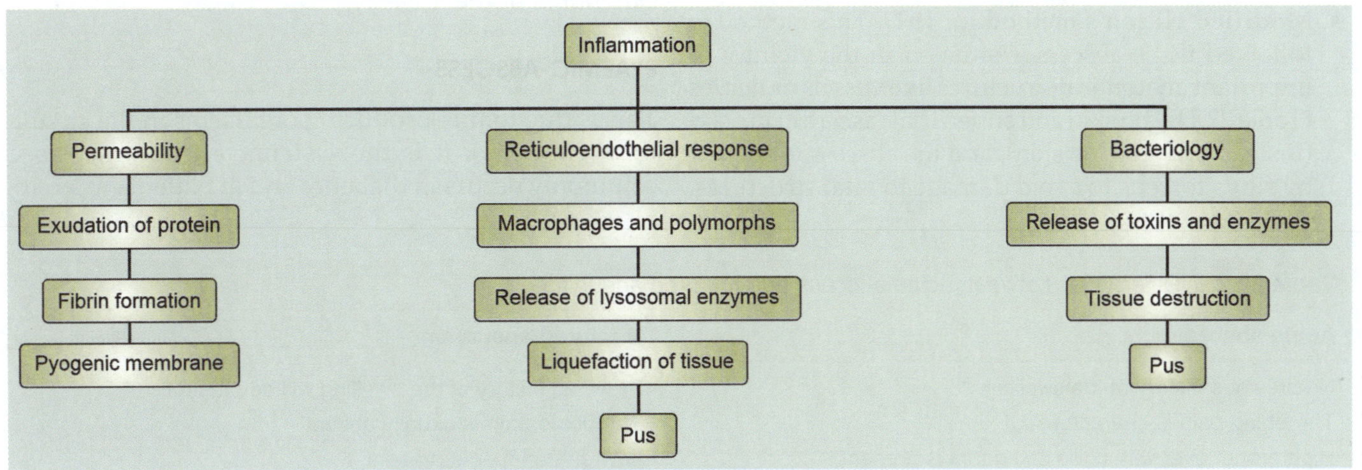

Fig. 22.3: Pathological events during inflammation

5. **Loss of function:** The function of the part is impaired, due to pain.
6. **Fluctuation:** It may be elicited. However, in a deep-seated abscess (e.g. breast abscess), it may be negative.
   - Untreated abscess tends to point spontaneously along the area of least resistance to the nearest epithelial surface, e.g. skin, gut, oral cavity.
   - However, deep-seated abscess such as breast abscess may cause much tissue destruction before pointing.

Treatment

Incision and drainage (I&D) under general anaesthesia. General anaesthesia is preferred because in the presence of infection, local anaesthesia may not act and it would be difficult to break all the loculi of an abscess without causing pain.

Procedure

- A **stab** incision is made over the most prominent (pointing) part of the abscess. The pus which comes out is collected and sent for culture and sensitivity. A sinus forceps or a finger is introduced within the abscess cavity and all the loculi are broken down. Fresh oozing of the pus is an indication that the procedure is complete. The abscess cavity is irrigated with saline or a mild antiseptic agent like iodine solution.
- The cavity, if large, may need to be packed with roller gauze dipped in iodine solution, which is removed 1–2 days later. Roller gauze packing prevents premature closure of the skin, thereby facilitating healing from the depth of the cavity through granulation tissue formation. With appropriate antibiotics and proper dressings, the wound heals within 5–7 days.
- Antibiotic of choice is cloxacillin for staphylococcal abscess. Dosage: 500 mg 6th hourly for 5–7 days.
- **Modified Hilton's method** for I&D. This method is followed if the abscess is situated in the vicinity of important anatomical structures like vessels or nerves (Table 22.1). The skin and superficial fascia are incised (instead of a stab incision), and the abscess is opened by sinus forceps to avoid damage to vital structures.

Table 22.1 Relationship of nerves or vessels with an abscess

Site	Anatomical structure
Axilla	→ Axillary vessels
Neck	→ Subclavian vessels and brachial plexus
Parotid region	→ Facial nerve
Midpalmar space	→ Median nerve

Differential Diagnosis

1. **Ruptured aneurysm** may present as a subcutaneous abscess with pain, redness, local rise of temperature, and sometimes even leukocytosis. Ruptured vertebral artery aneurysm in the posterior triangle and popliteal artery aneurysm in the popliteal fossa have been incised, mistaking them for an abscess (Table 22.2).

   Caution: When in doubt, aspirate with a wide bore needle before incising an abscess.

Pearls of Wisdom

Before incising an abscess/swelling, look for **T**emperature and **T**enderness, **A**uscultate and **A**spirate.
"Remember as **TATA**"

2. **Soft tissue sarcoma** in the thigh may be confused for a deep-seated abscess. However, throbbing pain, high grade fever with chills and rigors, and short duration of the swelling clinches the diagnosis of an abscess.

Antibioma

It is an antibiotic-induced swelling (oma). Once an abscess is formed, antibiotics seldom effect a cure but the partially sterilise the pus. Antibiotics also produce fibrosis, resulting in thickening of the abscess wall. Clinically, this may result in a **hard lump**.

Common sites of antibioma are the **breast, thigh, and ischiorectal fossa**. Antibioma in the breast may mimic carcinoma of the breast.

PYAEMIC ABSCESS

This is due to pus-producing organisms in the circulation (pyaemia). It is the systemic effect of sepsis. It commonly occurs in diabetics and in patients receiving

Table 22.2 Differences between acute abscess and ruptured aneurysm

Acute abscess	Ruptured aneurysm
No previous history of the swelling	Previous history of the swelling will be present
Throbbing pain is characteristic	Throbbing pain is usually absent
High grade fever with chills and rigors is present	Low grade fever is present
Extremely tender	Tender

chemotherapy and/or radiotherapy. Pyaemic abscess is characterised by the following features:

- They are multiple
- They are deep-seated
- There is minimal tenderness
- There is no local rise of temperature

Hence, it is called nonreactive abscess to differentiate it from pyogenic abscess. This is treated by multiple incisions over the abscess site and drainage (like a pyogenic abscess) with antibiotic cover.

Leptospirosis is a zoonosis caused by infected urine of cattle, dogs or rats. It causes severe myalgia/myositis of thigh muscles and thus can be confused for pyaemic abscesses. High grade fever is also a feature. When in doubt ask for ultrasound. Severe form of leptospirosis is called as Weil's disease. It can cause multiorgan failure and death.

COLD ABSCESS

- Even though this is a chronic abscess due to a chronic disease (tuberculosis), for the completeness of the chapter on abscess and for the convenience of reading, it is discussed here.
- Cold abscess refers to an abscess that has no signs of inflammation. Usually, it is due to tuberculosis, e.g. following tubercular lymphadenitis or due to tuberculosis of spine. However, other chronic diseases like leprosy, actinomycosis, and Madura foot also produce abscesses that are 'cold' in nature (Key Box 22.3). In this chapter, cold abscess due to cervical tubercular lymphadenitis is discussed.

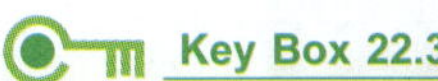
Key Box 22.3

Cold Abscess—Causes

- Tuberculosis (main cause)
- Actinomycosis
- Leprosy
- Madura foot

CERVICAL TUBERCULOUS LYMPHADENITIS

- It is the most common form of extrapulmonary tuberculosis.
- Tuberculous infections of the cervical lymph nodes—often termed **scrofula** and **king's evil**—are typically caused by tuberculous mycobacteria, but may also be caused by non-tuberculous mycobacteria.
- It is seen in endemic areas and in immunocompromised individuals.
- Lymph node tuberculosis constitutes 20–40% of extrapulmonary tuberculosis. It is more common in children and women, and in Asians and Pacific islanders.
- The disease may be caused by *Mycobacterium tuberculosis*, atypical mycobacteria, or *Mycobacterium bovis*.

Aetiopathogenesis

- In 80% of the cases, mycobacteria pass through tonsillar crypts and affect the tonsillar node or jugulodigastric group of nodes in the anterior triangle of the neck.
- In 20% of the cases, lymph nodes in the posterior triangle are affected due to adenoid involvement.
- Rarely, infection can spread from tuberculosis of the apex of the lung. Organisms directly penetrate Sibson's fascia (suprapleural membrane) and may cause enlargement of supraclavicular node.
- Other lymph nodes in the neck, such as the preauricular and submandibular nodes, may also be affected.
- Tuberculous bacilli survive within macrophages, and release a toxin called *tuberculosis necrotising toxin* (TNT), which causes host cell death.
- In general, the incidences of lymphadenopathy at various sites are shown in Fig. 22.4.

Pathological Types

- **Caseating type:** Most common type seen in young adults.
- **Hyperplastic type:** Lymph nodes show marked degree of lymphoid hyperplasia. Least caseation is seen in patients with good body resistance.
- **Atrophic type:** Seen in elderly patients. Lymphoid tissue undergoes degeneration. Glands are small with early caseation. A few lymph nodes may show scattered calcifications.

Clinical Features

- Common in the age group of 11–30 years.
- HIV-immunocompromised disease is a strong risk factor for developing tuberculous infections.

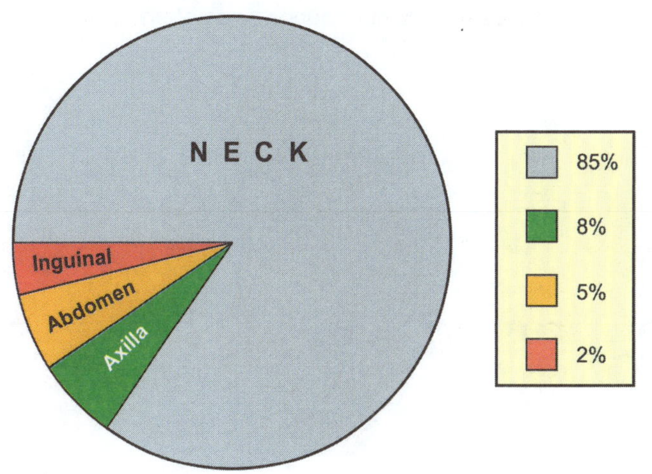

Fig. 22.4: Incidence of lymph node tuberculosis

- Tuberculous lymphadenitis presents as a gradually increasing painless swelling of one or more lymph nodes and lasts from a few weeks to a few months. Multiple sites may be involved.
- Systemic symptoms such as chills, fever, weight loss, fatigue, and night sweats are common, especially in those with extensive disease. Seen in about 40% of patients.
- In tuberculosis, interleukin-1(IL-1) and interleukin-6 (IL-6) are released, resulting in high-grade fever. However, this effect is somewhat counteracted by cortisol levels (which are also increased), resulting in low-grade fever.

Stages of Tuberculous (TB) Lymphadenitis

1. Stage of Lymphadenitis (Fig. 22.5)

- Common in young adults between 20 and 30 years of age.
- Upper anterior deep cervical nodes are enlarged.
- Nontender, discrete, mobile, firm lymph nodes are palpable.

2. Stage of Periadenitis/Stage of Matting (Fig. 22.6)

- Results due to capsular involvement
- Nodes move together—matting
- Firm, nontender
- Matting is pathognomonic of tuberculosis
- Other rare causes of matting are chronic lymphadenitis and anaplastic variety of lymphoma.

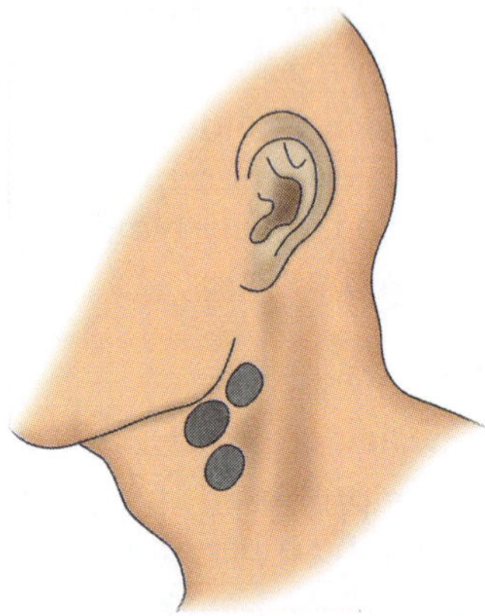

Fig. 22.5: TB lymphadenitis—discrete nodes

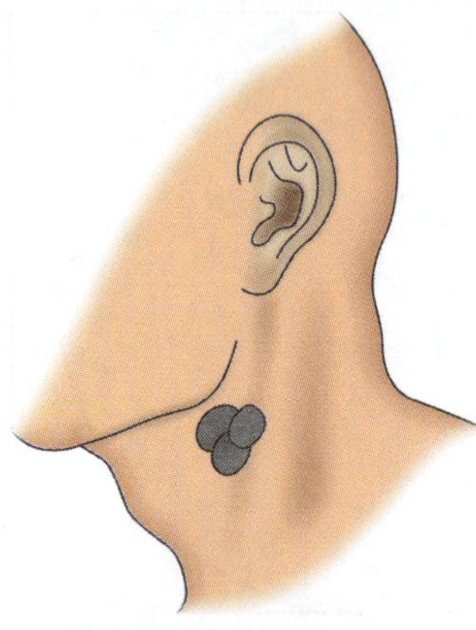

Fig. 22.6: TB lymphadenitis—matted nodes

3. Stage of Cold Abscess (Figs 22.7–22.11)

It occurs due to caseating necrosis of the lymph nodes, which results in a fluctuant swelling in the neck. Clinical features of a cold abscess in the neck are:

- No local rise of temperature, tenderness, or redness

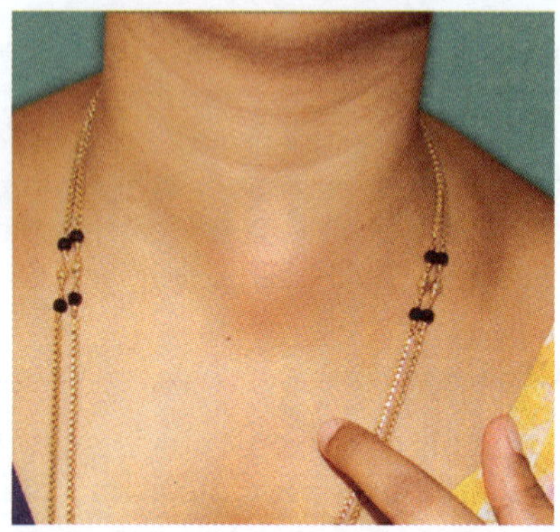

Fig. 22.7: Cold abscess in the midline above suprasternal notch—another common site

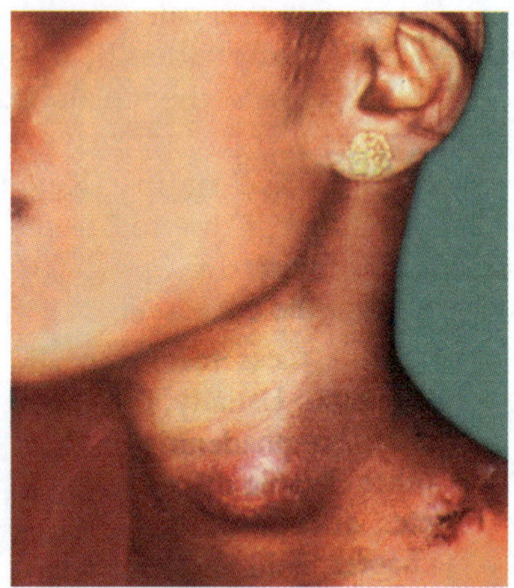

Fig. 22.8: TB lymphadenitis—cold abscess

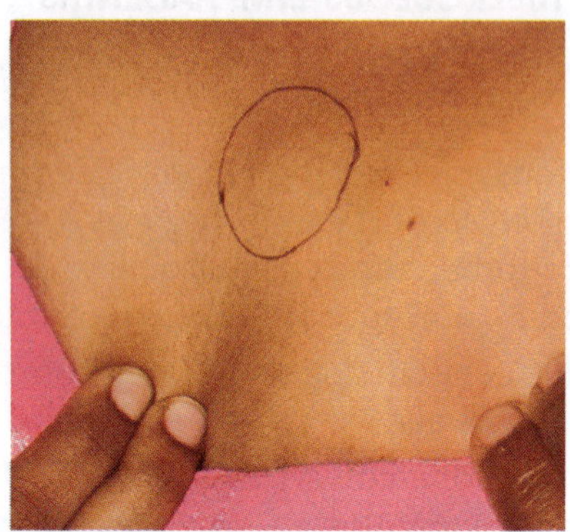

Fig. 22.9: Cold abscess in the second intercostal space

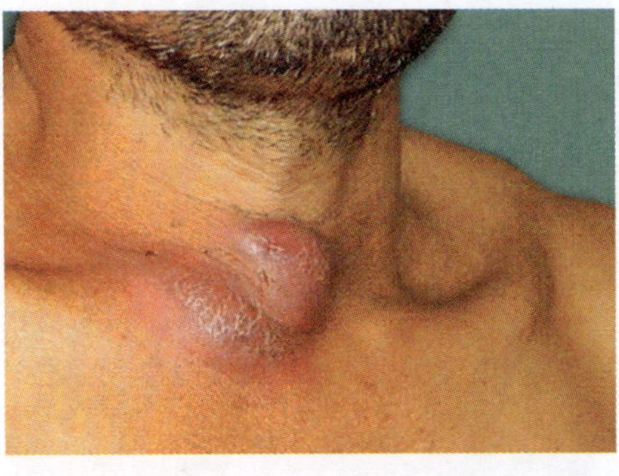

Fig. 22.10: Cold abscess of the right sternoclavicular joint

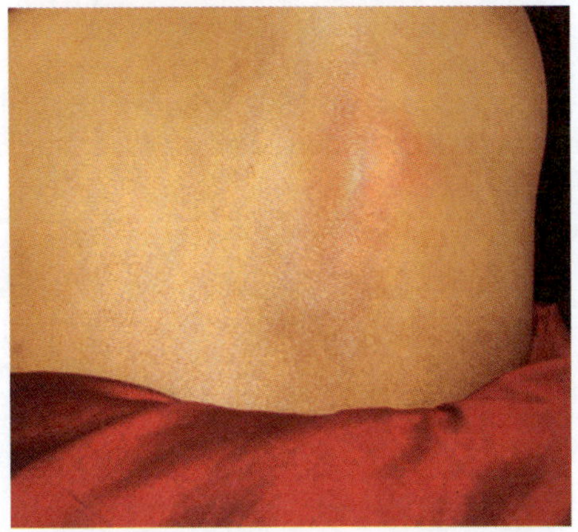

Fig. 22.11: Cold abscess in the paravertebral region secondary to tuberculosis of spine

- Soft, cystic, fluctuant, transillumination—negative swelling.
- It becomes less prominent on sternocleidomastoid contraction test, indicating that it is deep to the deep fascia.

Pearls of Wisdom

Multiple, matted, mobile lymph nodes are characteristic of tuberculosis.

Differential Diagnosis

Branchial cyst may be confused for cold abscess in the anterior triangle. Cold abscess is of a shorter duration and may present with other lymph nodes in the neck. Branchial cyst, being a congenital swelling, is of a longer duration.

Treatment of Cold Abscess (Figs 22.12A and B)

- **Nondependent aspiration** using a wide bore needle to avoid a persistent sinus.
- A wide bore needle is preferred because the caseous material is thick.
- Incision and drainage should not be done as it causes persistent tuberculous sinus.
- Antituberculous treatment is administered.

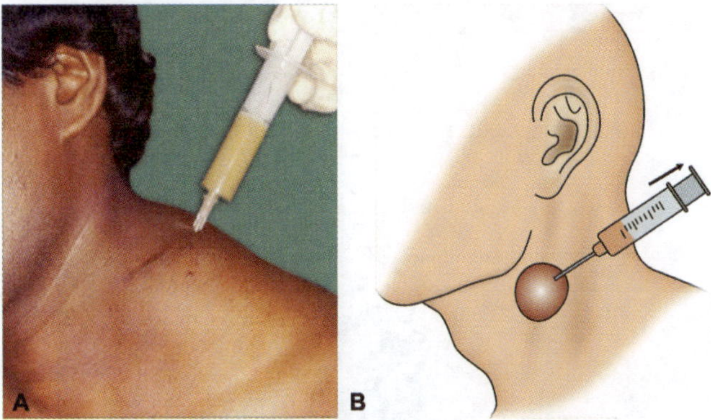

Fig. 22.12A and B: Nondependent aspiration

4. Stage of Collar Stud Abscess (Figs 22.13 and 22.14)

It results when a cold abscess deep to the deep fascia ruptures through the deep fascia and forms another swelling, which is fluctuant, in the subcutaneous plane. Cross fluctuation test may be positive. It is treated like a cold abscess.

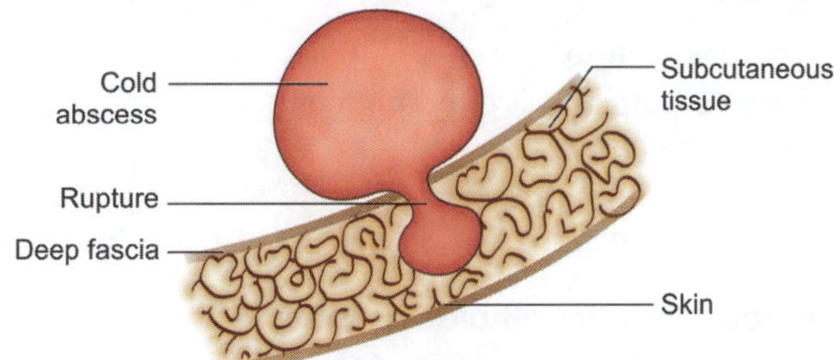

Fig. 22.13: Collar stud abscess

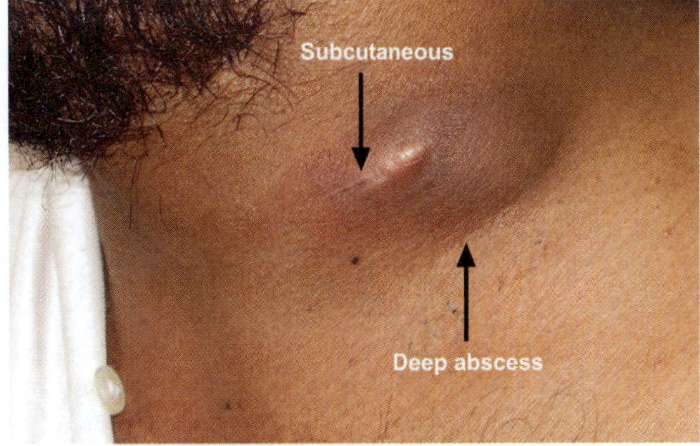

Fig. 22.14: Collar stud abscess

5. Stage of Sinus (Fig. 22.15)

- A sinus is a blind tract leading from the surface down into the tissues.
- It occurs when a collar stud abscess ruptures through the skin.
- In India, tubercular sinus is the most common sinus in the neck.

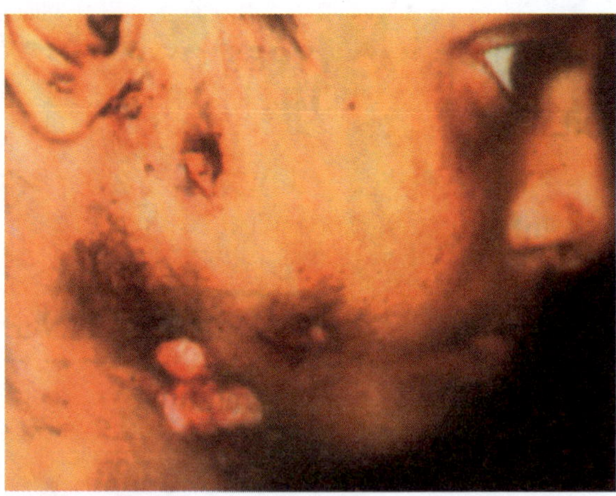

Fig. 22.15: Multiple tubercular sinuses in the neck and in front of the ear

- It is common in young females. There may be multiple sinuses.
- Tubercular sinuses have a wide opening.
- The sinus resembles an ulcer with an undermined edge.
- There is no induration.
- Surrounding skin is hyperpigmented and sometimes bluish in colour.
- A group of lymph nodes is usually palpable underneath the sinus.

Tuberculosis of Intrathoracic Nodes

- Occurs is about 25% of all TB lymphadenitis cases.
- Pressure on the bronchus gives rise to atelectasis and lung infection.
- Pressure on the oesophagus causes dysphagia and oesophagotracheal fistula (Fig. 22.16).
- Retroperitoneal nodes may give rise to chylous ascites and chyluria.
- HIV infection and lymph node TB (Key Box 22.4).

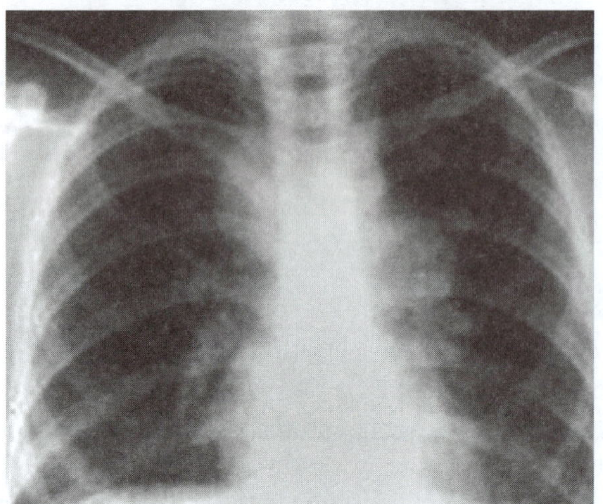

Fig. 22.16: Large mediastinal lymph nodes

Key Box 22.4

HIV Infection and Lymph Node Tuberculosis

- It is more common than lymphoma and sarcoma
- Patients are male and older
- Multiple sites are more commonly affected
- Disseminated disease (virulent) may be seen
- Nodes can be tender
- Weight loss is more common

TB-IRIS: Tuberculosis associated Immune Reconstitution Inflammatory Syndrome. This is seen in patients with tubercular lymphadenitis on retroviral therapy. It manifests as deterioration of a treated infection or as a new presentation of a previously subclinical infection. Thus, lymph nodes may persist or may become bigger.

- It occurs due to an antigenic response caused by the bactericidal action of antitubercular drugs.
- It needs only reassurance and anti-inflammatory drugs.
- A short course of steroids may be needed if pressure symptoms are present.
- However, if lymph nodes do not respond and are increasing, a biopsy should be done to rule out lymphoma.

Investigations

TB lymphadenitis is most commonly diagnosed by histopathology. Other investigations used for diagnosis are acid-fast bacilli (AFB) smear or Ziehl-Neelsen (ZN) staining and culture of lymph node material.

Collection of sample/material for examination may be done by either:

1. Fine needle aspiration, or
2. Excisional lymph node biopsy.

1. **Fine needle aspiration (FNA):** It is considered as the first line of evaluation of suspected tuberculous lymphadenopathy. FNA had good sensitivity and specificity (77% and 93%, respectively). Materials obtained should be tested for:
   a. AFB smear microscopy (ZN staining or fluorescence microscopy)
   b. Mycobacterial culture with drug susceptibility testing
   c. Cytology
   d. Nucleic acid amplification testing (Xpert MTB/RIF) and line probe assays.
2. **Excisional biopsy:** This allows for a larger sample to be collected and has a higher diagnostic yield than FNA. Because a sinus tract may form if an incisional biopsy is performed, excisional biopsy is preferred. Materials obtained should be tested for:
   a. AFB smear microscopy (ZN staining or fluorescence microscopy)

b. Mycobacterial culture with drug susceptibility testing

c. Histology: TB may be confirmed if **epithelioid cell granulomas** and caseation are seen. The chance of diagnosing TB is increased if multinucleated cells are present. In patients living with HIV, these typical granulomas are usually not found, as T cells (which are essential for their formation) are affected.

d. Nucleic acid amplification testing (Xpert MTB/RIF) and line probe assays.

- Histopathology findings of caseating granulomas, Langhans giant cells and foreign body giant cells are suggestive of TB.
- Nucleic acid amplification testing (NAAT)—CB-NAAT (cartridge-based NAAT)/Xpert MTB/RIF helps in both the diagnosis of TB and in detection of rifampicin resistance. NAAT identifies the complex nucleic acid of *Mycobacterium tuberculosis* but cannot assess the viability of the bacteria. It cannot be used for monitoring the response to the treatment as it identifies the complex nucleic acid of dead *Mycobacterium tuberculosis* bacilli as well.
- **Line probe assays** are molecular tests which make use of PCR to evaluate drug susceptibility to isoniazid, rifampicin, aminoglycosides, and fluoroquinolones.
- Mycobacterial culture is the gold standard for diagnosis. It also helps in performing drug susceptibility testing (DST) on MTB complex growth, which may be used for decision making by the treating physician/surgeon.
- **Tuberculin skin test (Mantoux test)** is a delayed type hypersensitivity reaction to antigens of *Mycobacterium tuberculosis*. The reagent used is protein purified derivative (PPD) which is injected intradermally. The induration is measured between 48 and 72 hours. An induration >10 mm is considered to be reactive and is suggestive of *M. tuberculosis* infection. However, it does not indicate active disease. A 5–9 mm induration is an intermediate response and may be attributed to BCG vaccination, *M. tuberculosis*, or atypical mycobacterial infections. **An induration <4 mm is considered negative**.
- **Interferon-gamma release assays (IGRAs)** may be used in place of Mantoux test for diagnosing TB infection.
- **Imaging:**

  a. Chest X-ray should be done in all patients suspected with lymph node tuberculosis, as lungs are the portal of entry for bacilli. It may show features suggestive of active pulmonary tuberculosis or apical fibrosis suggesting previous exposure to tuberculosis. Positive chest radiograph abnormalities are more commonly seen in patients living with HIV.

  b. HRCT scan of the thorax or abdomen may be done if mediastinal or abdominal lymphadenopathy is suspected.

  c. Ultrasound scanning of the suspected anatomical site may be done to confirm the lymph node swelling, abscess and also helps in guided FNA.

  d. EBUS (endobronchial ultrasound) helps in localising the mediastinal lymph node and in guiding transbronchial needle aspiration (FNA) of mediastinal lymph nodes (mediastinoscopy or CT-guided FNA/biopsy are preferred if mediastinal lymph nodes are not accessible through EBUS).

Definitions of Diagnosis (INDEX TB Guidelines)

Bacteriologically Confirmed LNTB Cases (Lymph Node TB)

A patient with symptoms and signs of LNTB who has at least one of the following:

- Positive microscopy for AFB on examination of lymph node fluid or tissue
- Positive culture of *Mycobacterium tuberculosis* from lymph node fluid or tissue
- Positive validated PCR-based test (such as Xpert MTB/RIF)

Clinically Diagnosed LNTB Case

A presumptive LNTB patient who undergoes diagnostic testing and has all of the following:

- Negative microscopy, negative culture, and negative PCR-based tests
- No other diagnosis to explain the clinical features
- Strongly suggestive evidence of LNTB by radiological findings, histopathological findings, or clinical course

TREATMENT

Antitubercular drugs are the cornerstone of treatment for LNTB.

Isoniazid (H), rifampicin (R), pyrazinamide (Z), ethambutol (E) and streptomycin (S) are the 1st line antitubercular drugs and are very important in treating drug-sensitive tuberculosis.

Regimen

IP (intensive phase) of 2 months of HRZE followed by CP (continuation phase) of 4 months of HRE in new cases (patients without a history of previous exposure to ATT).

TREATMENT OF DRUG-RESISTANT CASES

MDR-resistance to Rifampicin and Isoniazid

- IP (intensive phase): 6–9 months of kanamycin, levofloxacin, pyrazinamide (Z), ethambutol (E), cycloserine, and ethionamide.
- CP (continuation phase): 18 months of levofloxacin, ethambutol (E), cycloserine, and ethionamide.
- If sensitive to isoniazid and resistant to rifampicin, isoniazid can be added to the above regimen in both phases.
- If resistant to isoniazid and sensitive to rifampicin (isoniazid monoresistance), treat with:
  - IP: 3–6 months of kanamycin, levofloxacin, rifampicin (R), pyrazinamide (Z), ethambutol (E).
  - CP: 6 months of levofloxacin, rifampicin (R), pyrazinamide (Z), ethambutol (E).
  - Individual monoresistance should be treated according to drug sensitivity testing results.

HIV CO-INFECTION

In India, the most common opportunistic infection related to HIV is tuberculosis. Patients with latent tuberculosis are more prone to develop tuberculosis in their lifetime, if they become infected with HIV. Extrapulmonary tuberculosis is more common in patients living with HIV (PLHIV) than in non-HIV infected patients. HIV has been accepted by WHO as a defining criteria for clinical stage 4 disease diagnosis. Tuberculous lymphadenopathy often suggests disseminated tuberculosis in PLHIV. In PLHIV, lymph node enlargement is usually symmetrical and multiple. Significant mycobacterial load is often reported in PLHIV. Chest X-ray findings of pulmonary tuberculosis are a common association with tuberculous lymphadenitis in PLHIV. Response to treatment with antitubercular treatment is similar to HIV negative patients; however, recurrence and death are higher in PLHIV.

Incidence of Different Lymph Node Sites Involved

The cervical group of lymph nodes is the most common group of lymph nodes involved (63.3%), followed by the mediastinal lymph nodes (26.7%) and the axillary lymph nodes (8.3%).

Cervical and mediastinal lymph nodes together constitute around 70% of the cases of TBLN. Axillary, mesenteric, hepatic, periportal, and inguinal lymph nodes constitute the rest. In descending order, the incidence of involvement of lymph nodes are cervical (64.9%), axillary (27%), and mediastinal (8%) nodes.

TBLN may involve single or multiple sites. When all TB lymphadenopathies are analysed, the incidence is as follows: Only cervical nodes (63.6%), cervical + axillary + inguinal nodes (15.1%), only hilar nodes (6%), only inguinal nodes (3%), axillary + inguinal nodes (3%) and axillary + abdominal + hilar lymph nodes (3%).

Role of Surgery in Tuberculous Lymphadenitis

- **Biopsy:** Lymph node biopsy, wedge biopsy from the edge of the sinus.
- **Aspiration:** Non-dependent aspiration of cold abscess and pus should be sent for AFB staining, Ziehl-Neelsen (ZN) staining.
- **Excision of lymph nodes** if they persist in spite of antitubercular treatment.
- **Excision of sinus wall** along with the tract.

OTHER SPECIAL TYPES OF PYOGENIC INFECTIONS

BOIL (Key Boxes 22.5 and 22.6)

- This is also called a furuncle. It is a hair follicle infection caused by *Staphylococcus aureus* or a secondary infection of a sebaceous cyst.
- It starts with a painful indurated swelling with surrounding oedema. After about 1–2 days, softening occurs in the centre and a pustule develops which bursts spontaneously and discharges pus. Necrosis of subcutaneous tissues produces a greenish slough. Skin overlying the boil also undergoes necrosis. ***Hence, boil is included under acute infective gangrene.***

Key Box 22.5

Precipitating Factors	Common Locations
Scratching	Face and back of the neck
Diabetes	Axilla
Poor immunity	Gluteal region

Key Box 22.6

Facts about a Boil

Dangerous boil	: On the skin of face
Tender boil	: External auditory
Sweet boil	: Diabetic patients
Boil likes	: Oily skin
Blind boil or dull boil	: Subsides without suppuration

- Furuncle of the external auditory meatus is a very painful condition because of the rich nerve supply of the skin. Pain is also due to the dense adherence of the skin to the perichondrium (there is no subcutaneous tissue).

Treatment of Boil

Incision and drainage with excision of slough. Antibiotic cloxacillin is given. Diabetes, if present, is treated.

Complications of Boil

- Necrosis of the skin.
- Pyaemic abscess and septicaemia.
- **Cavernous sinus thrombosis** due to a boil on the face or a stye on the eyelid.

CARBUNCLE (Figs 22.17A and B)

- Name is derived from Latin: Carbunculus, a small coal.
- This is an **infective gangrene** of the subcutaneous tissue caused by ***Staphylococcus aureus*** (Key Box 22.7). It commonly occurs in **diabetic patients** Patients with poor immunity or those undergoing radiotherapy may also develop carbuncle.
- **Sites: Nape of the neck** is the most common site, followed by the back and shoulder region. The skin of these sites is coarse and has **poor vascularity**.
- Carbuncle can also occur in kidney.

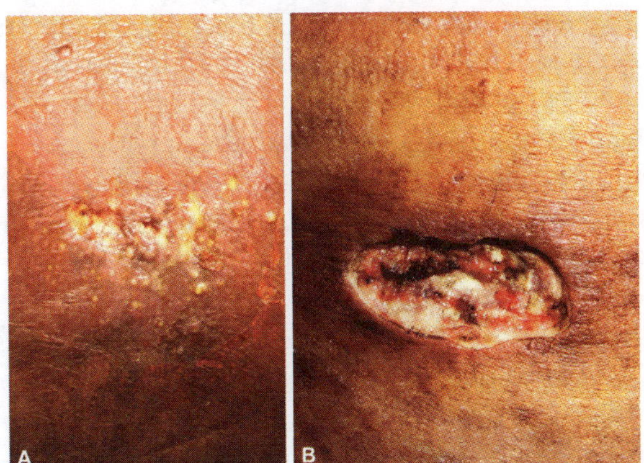

Fig. 22.17A and B: (A) Carbuncle of the back of neck—common site, sieve-like appearance, (B) after excision of the carbuncle—wound heals within 2 to 3 weeks. Some cases require split skin grafting

Key Box 22.7

Staphylococcal Infections of Surgical Importance

- Boil
- Carbuncle
- Breast abscess
- Parotitis
- Osteomyelitis

Pathology

The initial lesion is similar to a boil in the form of a hair follicle infection with perifolliculitis. Since the majority of patients are diabetic, infection takes a virulent course and results in subcutaneous fat necrosis, giving rise to multiple abscesses. These abscesses are **intercommunicating** and open to the exterior by multiple **sieve-like openings.** This appearance is described as **cribriform** appearance which is pathognomonic of a carbuncle.

Clinical Features

- Typically, the patient is a diabetic.
- Severe pain and swelling in the nape of the neck.
- Constitutional symptoms, such as fever with chills and rigors, are severe.
- Surface is red and angry-looking like **red hot coal.**
- Surrounding area is indurated.
- Later, skin over the centre of carbuncle softens and peripheral satellite vesicles appear, which rupture and discharge pus, giving rise to a **cribriform** appearance (Fig. 22.17A).
- The end result is the development of a large crateriform ulcer with central slough.

Complications

1. Worsening of diabetic status, resulting in diabetic ketoacidosis.
2. Extensive necrosis of the skin overlying the carbuncle. Hence, it is included under acute infective gangrene.
3. Septicaemia, toxaemia.

Treatment (Key Box 22.8)

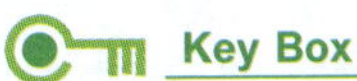

Key Box 22.8

Summary of Carbuncle

- Caused by **Cocci**
- Abscesses **Communicating**
- Red hot like **Coal**
- Appearance **Cribriform, Crateriform ulcer**
- Gangrene **Cutaneous** (subcutaneous)
- Drug of choice **Cloxacillin**
- Diabetes **Control**
- Incision **Cruciate**

Observe **8 Cs**

Pearls of Wisdom

Treatment of carbuncle is excision.

- Control diabetes, preferably with injectable **insulin.**
- Appropriate **parenteral antibiotics** are given till complete resolution occurs. Most strains of *Staphylococcus aureus* are sensitive to cloxacillin, flucloxacillin,

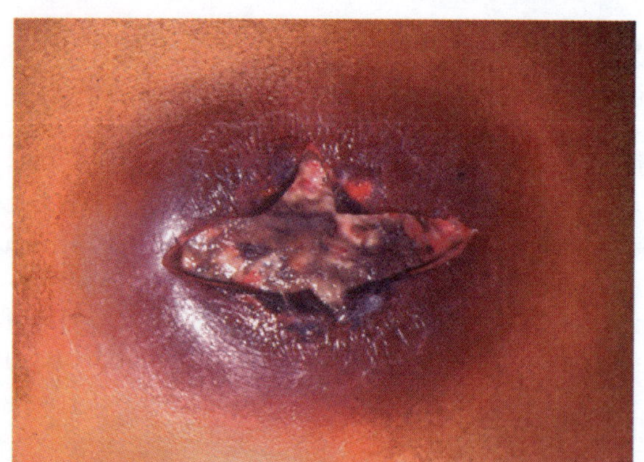

Fig. 22.18: Carbuncle with central slough. A cruciate incision should be given followed by excision

erythromycin, and some cephalosporins. However, ***methicillin-resistant Staphylococcus aureus (MRSA)*** bacteria are resistant to these drugs. They are sensitive only to the expensive drug **vancomycin,** which has to be given intravenously.

- Improve general health of the patient.
- If the carbuncle does not show any softening or shows evidence of healing, it is not incised and may be left open to the exterior. Alternatively, saline dressings may be applied to reduce oedema. Complete resolution may take place within 10–15 days.
- Surgery is required when there is pus (Fig. 22.18). A ***cruciate incision*** is preferred because of the multiple abscesses and extensive subcutaneous necrosis. Edges of the skin flap are excised, the pus is drained, loculi are broken down, slough is excised, and the ***cavity is irrigated with antiseptic agents.*** Like pyogenic abscess, wound heals with granulation tissue from the depth.

ERYSIPELAS

- It is an acute inflammation of the skin and subcutaneous tissue associated with severe lymphangitis. The causative organism is *Streptococcus pyogenes*. The precipitating factors are malnourishment, chronic diseases, etc. Thus, children and old people are commonly affected.
- Infection sets in after a small scratch or abrasion and spreads very rapidly, resulting in toxaemia. Sites: Face, eyelids, scrotum, and in infants, the umbilicus.

Clinical Features

- **Rose-pink** rash with a raised edge (on palpation) and a button hole consistency.
- **Vesicles** appear later and rarely become pustular.
- Oedema of the eyelids or scrotum, depending on the site.
- Features of ***toxaemia***
- When it occurs over the face, it involves the pinna because erysipelas is basically a ***cuticular lymphangitis***. This is described as ***Milian's ear sign positive,*** which is used to differentiate cellulitis of the face from facial erysipelas. In cellulitis of face, the pinna does not get involved because of the close adherence of the skin and cartilage.

Complications

1. Toxaemia and septicaemia
2. Gangrene of the skin and subcutaneous tissue
3. Lymphoedema of face and eyelids due to lymphatic obstruction and fibrosis

Treatment

Injection crystalline penicillin 10 lakh units 6th hourly IM/IV for 5–10 days.

CHRONIC ABSCESS

It occurs when the initial infective process or cause is not fully identified and properly treated.

Sites

Foot, hand, thigh, etc.

Causes

1. **Foreign bodies:** These are the most common causes of a chronic abscess. There is a typical history of a recurrent swelling discharging pus. Wooden pieces impacted in the thigh or in the foot are common. Infection of the synthetic mesh used in hernial repair is another example.
2. **Dead tissue:** As it occurs in diabetic patients.
3. **Pilonidal sinus:** This condition gives rise to recurrent abscesses. There is a typical history of pain and a swelling that ruptures and is followed by spontaneous recovery. However, the sinus persists.
4. **Chronic disease: Tuberculosis** is one of the causes. All features of cold abscess may be present but in an unusual location.

Clinical Notes

A 40-year-old female presented with swelling of the left thigh of 8 months duration. There were no signs of inflammation. FNAC was inconclusive. During surgery, a localised abscess with a thick wall and fleshy tissue was removed. The final report was tubercular abscess.

There was no evidence of tuberculosis anywhere in the body. Tuberculosis may present in different forms, as seen in this case. Detailed investigations were unable to reveal any evidence of pulmonary tuberculosis.

NECROTISING FASCIITIS

It is a spreading, destructive, invasive infection of the skin and soft tissues, which includes the deep fascia, but ***relatively spares muscle.***

Risk factors are given in Key Box 22.9.

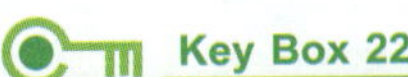

Key Box 22.9

Necrotising Fasciitis—Risk Factors

- Diabetes mellitus, malnutrition
- Obesity, corticosteroids
- Immune deficiency

Common Sites

It is common in the lower extremities. Other sites are the genitalia, groin, and lower abdomen. In these places, it is comparable or similar to gangrene and is called **Meleney's** gangrene.

Types and Microorganisms

- **Type I necrotising fasciitis : Polymicrobial:** It is due to a synergistic combination of anaerobes and coliforms or nongroup A streptococci— Very often, there is **no history of injury** when it occurs in the lower limbs.
- **Type II necrotising fasciitis** (Key Box 22.10): **Monomicrobial:** It is due to group A *β-haemolytic streptococci.* This has been referred to as flesh eating disease.
- **Type III necrotising fasciitis:** Gas gangrene due to clostridium (Chapter 3).
- **Type IV necrotising fasciitis (others):** Fungal (candida) and vibrio species-marine organisms.

Pathogenesis:

- Numerous cytokines, such as IL-1, IL-6, and TNF-α, are released due to inflammation caused by M proteins, which are produced by Streptococci.
- Streptococci also produce exotoxins, which destroy neutrophils. This results in the growth of bacteria, which in turn destroy the tissues.

Clinical Features

- Sudden pain in the affected area with gross swelling of the limbs (Figs 22.19–22.21).

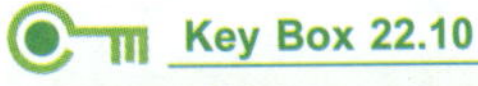

Key Box 22.10

Specific Features of Type II Necrotising Fasciitis

- Caused by *Streptococcus pyogenes*
- Occur in young healthy people
- Minor abrasions, laceration may be a precipitating factor
- Severe systemic illness with multiorgan failure—streptococcal toxic shock syndrome

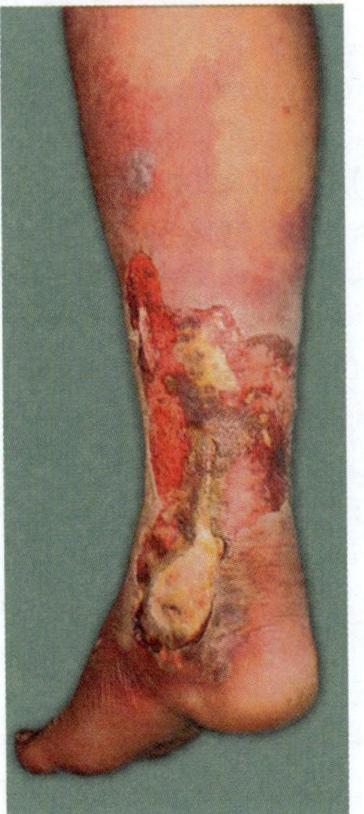

Fig. 22.19: Type II necrotising fasciitis in a healthy man. In spite of debridement and intensive care, he died of multiorgan failure

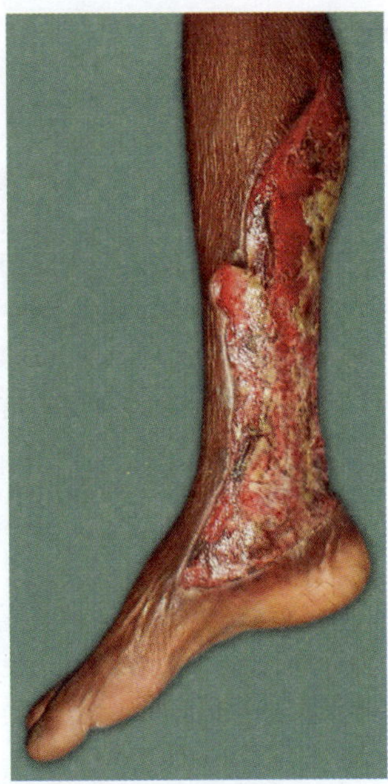

Fig. 22.20: This patient presented with features of cellulitis with renal failure. There were no precipitating factors. After debridement, recovery was complete

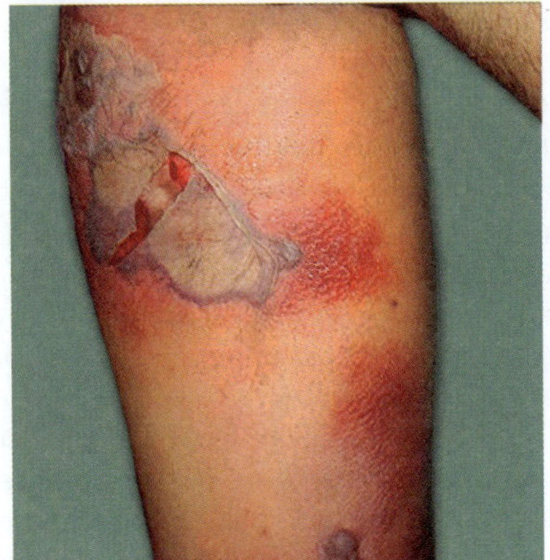

Fig. 22.21: Observe the skin changes in necrotising fasciitis

- The part is swollen, red, erythematous, and oedematous with skip lesions of skin necrosis and ulceration.
- ***Skin changes:*** Bronze hue, brawny induration, blebs, or crepitus are other important features. Very soon, skin patches and a dusky blue colour, followed by blebs and bullae appear.
- **Thrombosis of the nutrient artery** results in gangrene. Interestingly, muscles are spared.
- High degree fever, jaundice, and renal failure may occur soon in untreated cases.

Diagnosis

- Early diagnosis may be made by a scoring system proposed by Wong et al., which considers white cell count, CRP (C-reactive protein), haemoglobin, sodium, creatinine, and glucose levels. This system is called the **Laboratory Risk Indicator of Necrotising Fasciitis—LRINEC.**
- Full thickness biopsy taken at bedside may give the full diagnosis. Watery pus (**dishwater liquid**) is also characteristic.
- A high index of suspicion is required to diagnose necrotising fasciitis. When in doubt, one can do exploratory fasciotomy. Lack of resistance between normally adherent fascia to blunt dissection is diagnostic of necrotising fasciitis.
- **The finger test** is a bedside procedure done under local anaesthesia. A 2-cm incision is made and deepened to the deep fascia, at which level gentle probing with the index finger is applied. The presence of dishwater liquid and a lack of resistance are characteristic of necrotising fasciitis.

Treatment

Early, aggressive management with supportive and surgical treatment.

- Supportive treatment includes hospitalisation, adequate hydration, treatment of hypotension and broad-spectrum antibiotics.
- First and second generation cephalosporins are used to treat *Staphylococcus aureus*. However, in cases of resistant cases due to MRSA (methicillin resistant *Staphylococcus aureus*) ***vancomycin with carbapenem*** *may be urgently required.* Surgery should be performed as early as possible. Severe pain, colour changes in the skin, and drowsiness are indicators of sepsis. In such cases, do not wait for all reports and perform debridement on an emergency basis. This involves wide excision and generous debridement, followed by skin grafting after a few days or weeks. Debridement may have to be repeated till healthy tissue is encountered. Do not hesitate to amputate if the patient's life is in danger, because in a few patients, that is the only life-saving measure.
- **Type II cases (streptococcal):** High dose penicillins with clindamycin is the treatment of choice. **Clindamycin** has a special effect as it is a **potent suppressor of bacterial toxin synthesis.**
- **Intravenous immunoglobulin (IVIG)** has recently been described as a reasonable and desirable option for neutralizing streptococcal toxins.

ACUTE PYOMYOSITIS

Definition

Pyomyositis refers to a localised area of suppuration **within striated muscle**. It occurs after trauma (Key Box 22.11).

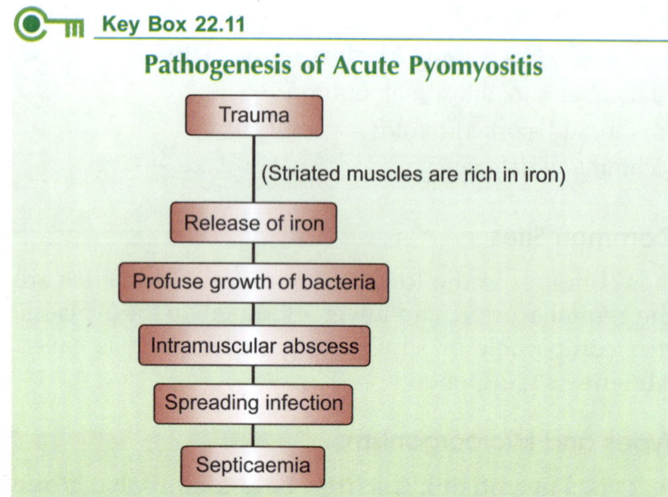

Clinical Features

- Classically, the quadriceps, gluteus, and shoulder and upper arm muscles are affected. Pain over the part, oedema, fever, and jaundice are common. Tenderness, induration, and muscle spasms are characteristic.
- **Renal failure follows soon.**

Investigations

- Sonographic-guided aspiration of pus followed by culture
- CT and MRI are ideal to determine the spread of the infection.
- Creatine kinase may go up to 50,000–2,00,000 units/L during the acute phase because of **rhabdomyolysis.**

Treatment

- Early diagnosis and early aggressive treatment
- Antibiotics
- Exploration—for diagnosis and treatment
- Wide excision of muscles and compartmental excision until viable tissues become visible (Figs 22.22 and 22.23).

Summary—Key Box 22.12.

NOSOCOMIAL INFECTIONS

- An ***acquired infection from the hospital is known as a nosocomial infection.***
- Infection may occur from the patient's own organisms (self-infection) or from external organisms.

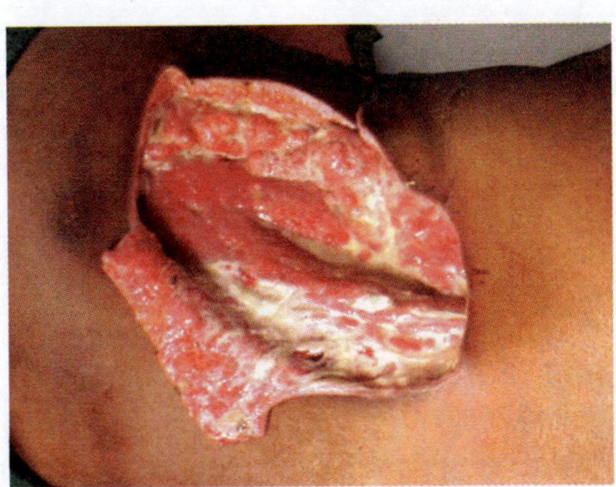

Fig. 22.22: Extensive pyomyositis affecting muscles of the back

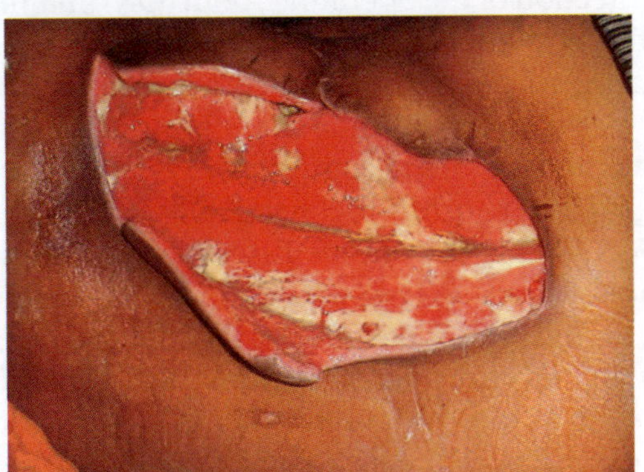

Fig. 22.23: Healing after 2 weeks

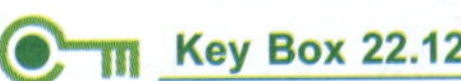

Key Box 22.12

Pyomyositis

- Trauma
- Transient bacteraemia
- Tropical countries
- Thigh muscles are affected
- Tender intramuscular abscess
- Tenderness, temperature, toxicity
- Total renal failure—rhabdomyolysis
- Treatment—early aggressive exploration and excision

Observe 8 Ts

- ***Surgical site infections (SSIs) are the third most frequently reported nosocomial infection,*** after pneumonia and catheter-related infections (including urinary tract infection).

SURGICAL SITE INFECTIONS (SSIs)

Definition

SSIs refer to infections of the tissues, organs, or spaces that have been exposed during invasive surgical procedures. They may be superficial, such as redness of a postoperative wound or a swollen local part. When associated with systemic inflammatory response syndrome (SIRS), it is called *sepsis*, and if it is associated with organ failure and requires inotropes, it is called *severe sepsis*. More details are given under septic shock (page 65).

When to Suspect SSIs?

- A postoperative patient with elevated temperature, tachycardia, tachypnoea, and an elevated white blood cell (WBC) count.
- The wound shows signs of inflammation such as rubor, colour, dolor, and tumour (swelling). These are the part of SIRS (systemic inflammatory response syndrome).
- Wound is tender with discharge.
- Microorganisms are identified in blood, pus, or urine.
- SIRS may be caused by variety of diseases, such as pancreatitis, polytrauma, malignancies, transfusion reactions, as well as infection.
- SIRS caused by an infection is known as sepsis. SIRS is mediated by the production of proinflammatory mediators, such as lipopolysaccharides (endotoxin) derived from gram-negative organisms and peptido-glycans from gram-positive organisms.

PIRO Classification Scheme

Predisposition: Advancing age or immunosuppression that may affect survival.

Insult (infection): It depends on the infecting organism or location of the disease.

Response: It refers to the development of SIRS, shock, elevated C-reactive protein, etc.

Organ dysfunction: Failure or dysfunction of organ(s).

Clinical Features

- **Superficial SSI:** The wound is tender, erythematous, and oedematous.
- **Deep incisional SSI:** Tenderness extends, and crepitus, vesicles, and/or bullae may be present.
- **Intra-cavitary SSI:** This depends on the system involved. A classical example is paralytic ileus continuing in abdominal infections.

Common Sources of Infections

Major surgical site infections present with systemic manifestations, whereas minor surgical site infections present with suture site discharge only.

In surgical wards, discharging wounds, infected urine, faeces, and sputum are sources of nosocomial infections.

Organisms

Staphylococcus aureus remains the most common SSI pathogen, followed by coagulase negative staphylococci, enterococci and *Escherichia coli.*

Risk factors for the development of SSIs are presented in Key Box 22.13.

Key Box 22.13

Risk Factors for Development of Surgical Site Infections

- **Patient-related** (*Remember as* **PATIENT**)
  - **P**eripheral vascular disease and smoking
  - **A**naemia
  - **T**rauma
  - **I**mmunosuppression including diabetes
  - **E**lderly (old age)
  - **N**utritional: Malnutrition
  - **T**oo much obesity
- **Local features** (*Remember as* **LOCAL**)
  - **L**ong (prolonged) surgical procedure
  - **O**xygenation is poor (hypoxia)
  - **C**ontamination of instruments and skin (poor skin preparation)
  - **A**ntibiotic prophylaxis is inadequate
  - **L**ocal tissue necrosis and low temperature (hypothermia)

Principles of Treatment of Established Surgical Site Infections

- **Antibiotics:** Empirical broad-spectrum antibiotics that cover all likely organisms must be started, and later switched to the appropriate antibiotic(s) as per the culture-sensitivity report.
- **Care of the wound:** Wound dressings
- Exploration of wound/peritoneal cavity, removal of source of sepsis, draining abscess cavity.

Pearls of Wisdom

What is the decisive period? It takes about 4 hours after surgery for the mobilisation of inflammatory, humoral, and cellular defences. This is the time when invading bacteria get established. Hence, prophylactic antibiotics should be given in this period.

Preventing Sources of SSIs

Surgical site infections may be largely prevented or reduced by an approach called the *surgical care bundle approach*. A **bundle** refers to a structured processes of **care** that improves patient outcomes. Surgeons may develop their own surgical care bundle for SSIs. This approach may be summarised by 6 Ss.

1. **Standardised antibiotic prophylaxis:** Antibiotics should be administered ideally 1 hour before the skin incision. It should be repeated every 3 hours if the surgery is prolonged.
2. **Skin is prepared by iodophors** (povidone iodine 10%) or chlorhexidine gluconate 4% in alcohol. Povidone iodine is safe, fast acting, and has broad-spectrum (with some sporicidal) activity. Preoperative ***hair removal (clipping) should be done immediately before any operation.***
3. **Sterile dressings** and proper wound care help protect the incision.
4. **Safe operating room:** Environmental cleaning and disinfection of the operating room (OR), maintenance of the ventilation system (the bacterial threshold limit for an empty OR is 35 CFU/m^3), and minimizing the OR traffic with continuous monitoring. SSI may be prevented by maintaining ***positive pressure*** in the operating rooms, mechanical ventilation, air-conditioning providing filtered air, maintaining temperature, etc. The surgeon and team ***should scrub for at least 3–5 minutes*** with 4% chlorhexidine gluconate. However, chlorhexidine ***alcohol-based 'fast rub'*** is more popular now. **OT attire and drapes:** Scrub suits, caps, masks, double gloves, and dedicated footwear are used as barriers. The life of a sterile glove is 3 hours. It should be changed if the surgery lasts > 3 hours.
5. **Showers and decolonization** with chlorhexidine gluconate 4% during the hospital stay.
6. **Screening for colonization** of the surgical site.

Bacterial factors

• Klebsiella	Surface capsule	Inhibit phagocytosis
• *Streptococcus pneumoniae*	Surface capsule	Inhibit phagocytosis
• Coagulase negative staphylococci	Slime, on the surface	
• Gram-negative bacteria	Endotoxins or lipopolysaccharide	
• Clostridia, streptococci	Powerful exotoxins	

Thus, good **surgical technique,** gentle tissue handling, perfect haemostasis, removal of dead tissues, and appropriate use of sutures, drains, and antibiotics play a major role in preventing SSI.

Pearls of Wisdom

Blood sugar level <200 mg/dl in the perioperative period is recommended to decrease morbidity and mortality.

A summary of prevention of SSIs is given in Fig. 22.24.

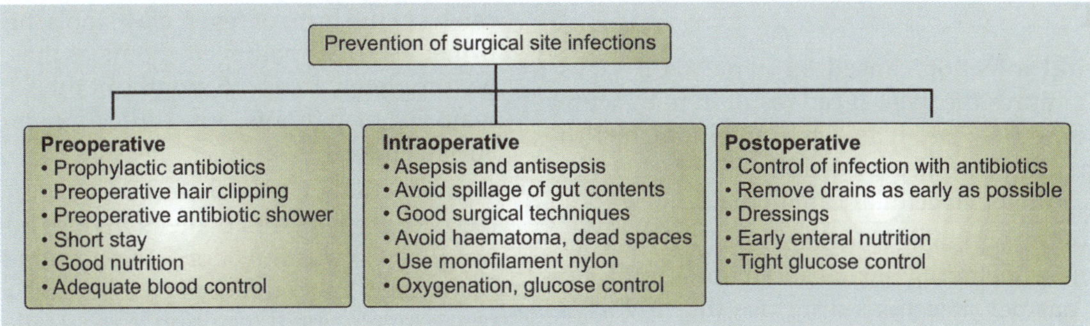

Fig. 22.24: Prevention of surgical site infections

Prevention of Hospital Infection

- Avoid unnecessary antibiotics to prevent the development of resistant organisms
- Autoclaving and sterilisation should be done optimally
- Proper ventilation of the wards
- Proper scrubbing before any procedure
- Proper disposal of urine, faeces, sputum
- Use of disinfectants
- Antibiotic prophylaxis (Key Box 22.14)

Key points regarding SSI are presented in Key Box 22.15.

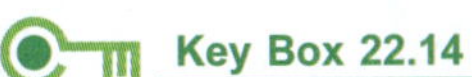
Key Box 22.14

Antimicrobial Prophylaxis

Operation	Likely pathogens
❍ Breast	*S. aureus*, coagulase-negative, staphylococci
❍ Appendicectomy	Gram-negative bacilli, anaerobes
❍ Biliary tract	Gram-negative bacilli, anaerobes
❍ Upper GI	Gram-negative bacilli, streptococci, oropharyngeal anaerobes (peptostreptococci)

Cefazolin is generally accepted as the antimicrobial agent of choice for clean-contaminated operations.

- ❍ **Dose:** 1–2 g/adult dose.
- ❍ **Timing:** No more than 30 minutes before skin is incised.

Prophylactic regimens

- ❍ **Vascular:** 3 doses of flucloxacillin with or without gentamicin, vancomycin.
- ❍ **Oesophagogastric:** 1 dose of 2nd generation cephalosporin and metronidazole.
- ❍ **Biliary:** One dose of 2nd generation of cephalosporin.
- ❍ **Small bowel:** 1 dose of 2nd generation of cephalosporin with metronidazole.
- ❍ **Appendix/colorectal:** 1 dose of 2nd generation of cephalosporin with metronidazole.

Key Box 22.15

Key Points in SSI

- ❍ SSI within 24 hours is caused by clostridia and streptococci
- ❍ SSI after 48 hours (5 days) is caused by gram-negative and other bacteria.
- ❍ Nasal carriers of *Staph. aureus* have ↑ risk of SSI.
- ❍ Prevention of SSI is by aseptic and antiseptic technique in OT as introduced by Lister, use of prophylactic antibiotics and patient's own ability to prevent infection.
- ❍ Skin to be prepared by germicidal antibiotics such as tincture of iodine, povidone iodine or chlorhexidine.
- ❍ The first dose of prophylactic antibiotics is given intravenously at the induction of anaesthesia.
- ❍ Monofilament sutures are better to decrease the SSI.

ASEPSIS AND ANTISEPSIS

Strictly speaking, they are equivalent and there is not much of a difference between them.

Asepsis refers to precautions taken before any surgical procedure to prevent against the development of infection. Some examples are: *wearing gloves, cleaning the patient's abdomen with iodine and spirit, sterilisation of instruments, and autoclaving.*

Antisepsis: It is defined as the practice of using antiseptics to eliminate disease-causing microorganisms. All surgical procedures today are performed only after taking aseptic precautions.

- Dressing of an already contaminated wound using carbolic acid, iodine.
- Broad-spectrum antibiotics are used in the presence of infection.
- Wearing a mask and cap in the operation theatre.

TRANSMISSIBLE VIRAL INFECTIONS

HEPATITIS B

- It is a viral infection caused by hepatitis B virus (HBV). It injures the liver. It can result in both acute and chronic disease. It is a major global health problem. Chronic disease results in death from cirrhosis and hepatocellular carcinoma.
- Method of transmission: Contact with blood or other body fluids, including sexual intercourse with an infected partner, injections-drug use that involves sharing needles, syringes. It can also occur with needle sticks or exposures to sharp instruments. It can also occur from tattooing, piercing
- Hepatitis B can be prevented by vaccines that are safe, available and effective.
- Symptoms: There can be febrile illness. It may last from a few days to several weeks. Jaundice, yellow urine, weakness, nausea, vomiting are other features. Abdominal pain is due to enlarged liver. A few patients with acute hepatitis can develop acute liver failure, which can lead to death.
- Diagnosis: It is done by detection of the hepatitis B surface antigen HBsAg.
- Methods of prevention: Prophylaxis by taking vaccine. In the hospitals, all blood donations should be tested for hepatitis B virus infections. Thus to avoid accidental transmission to people who receive blood products. This can happen more so in patients who require massive blood transfusions, urgent transfusions and multiple transfusions such as haemophilia cases, etc. All health care workers should not only wear double gloves but to avoid accidental pricks during suturing of tissues, or splashing of fluids during dental extractions etc.
- Treatment: Acute illness require treatment with paracetamol if fever is present. Otherwise no specific drugs are used. Tenofovir or entecavir—are the drugs to suppress hepatitis B virus.

HEPATITIS C

- Hepatitis C is caused by hepatitis C virus which belongs to RNA virus. There are many forms of hepatitis C—most common being type 1.
- Incubation period is an average of 45 days—however, it can be anywhere between 2 weeks and 12 weeks.
- Method of transmission: Almost similar in the lines of hepatitis B infections such as body fluids, injection drugs and needles, etc. Transmission does not occur via breast milk, kissing or coughing, sneezing, touching, etc.
- Initial presentation after the exposure of the virus is acute illness that lasts for the first 6 months which can be in the form of fever, clay stools, high coloured urine, loss of appetite, etc. Some of these cases may be completely free by 6 months of time. However, in majority of patients, viral infection progresses to chronic hepatitis stage.
- Complications: Cirrhosis and liver cancer: Both these can occur in hepatitis B infections also but in cases of hepatitis C virus infections, these complications can occur early. Very advanced patients can have multiple organ involvement resulting in renal failure, cerebral dysfunction ascites, etc. Intractable itching is also a feature.
- Diagnosis is established by demonstrating Anti-Hepatitis C Virus (HCV) antibodies. Like many other viral infections, they are demonstrated after about 12 weeks.
- Treatment: No specific treatment or drugs for this condition but symptomatic treatment is given. A few drugs have been used—they are *interferon,* and *ribavirin.*
- Prophylaxis: There is vaccine for hepatitis C. The best way is to use universal precautions such as using double glove, avoid prick injuries, avoid needle sharing, avoid direct exposure to blood and blood products and practise safe sex.

SINUSES AND FISTULAS

Sinus

- It is a blind track from the surface down into the tissues (Fig. 22.25). It is lined by granulation tissue. A few examples are listed below:
  1. *Congenital sinus:* Pre-auricular sinus, post-auricular sinus (Fig. 22.26).

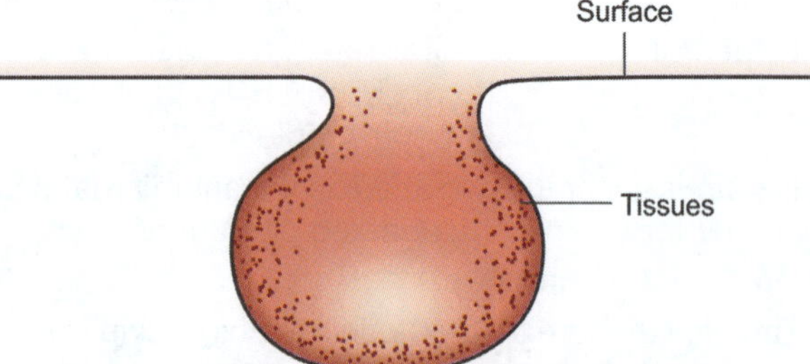

Fig. 22.25: Sinus (blind track)

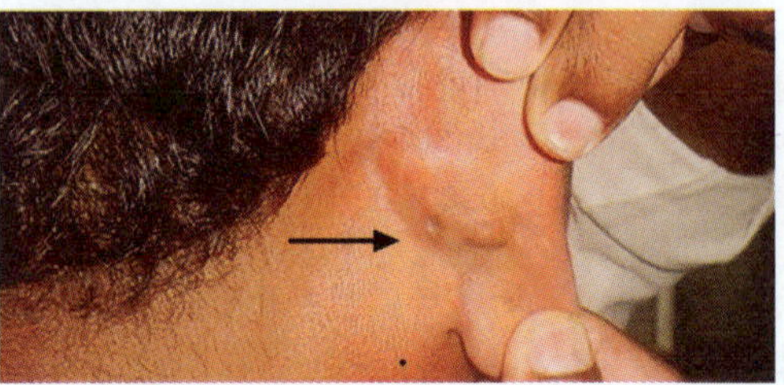

Fig. 22.26: Postauricular sinus

2. *Acquired sinus:*
   - *Median mental sinus* (*see* page 370): Results from a tooth abscess.
   - *Pilonidal sinus:* Occurs in the midline of the anal region (Fig. 22.27).
   - *Osteomyelitis:* Gives rise to a sinus that discharges pus ± bony spicules (Fig. 22.28).

- Most common sinus in the neck is due to tubercular lymphadenitis (Fig. 22.29). It discharges cheesy material. Skin surrounding the sinus shows bluish discolouration.

Fistula

It is an abnormal communication between the lumen of one viscus and the lumen of another (internal fistula) or a communication between a hollow viscus and the exterior, i.e. body surface (external fistula) (Fig. 22.30).

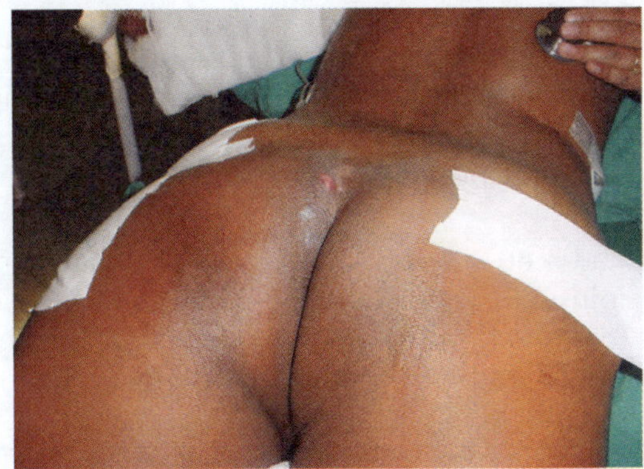

Fig. 22.27: A patient with pilonidal sinus positioned in jack-knife position for excision

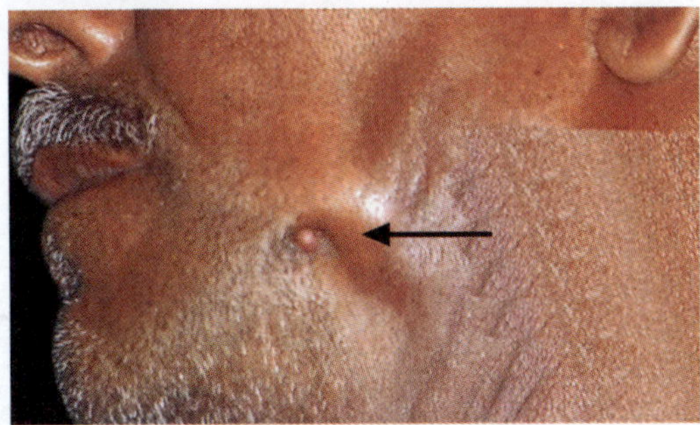

Fig. 22.28: Mandibular sinus due to badly infected caries teeth, osteomyelitis of mandible

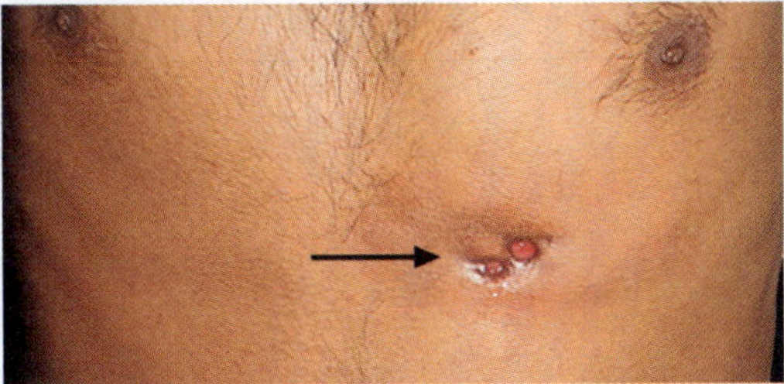

Fig. 22.29: Tuberculous sinuses in the chest wall. Observe that the edges of the sinuses are in flush with the skin

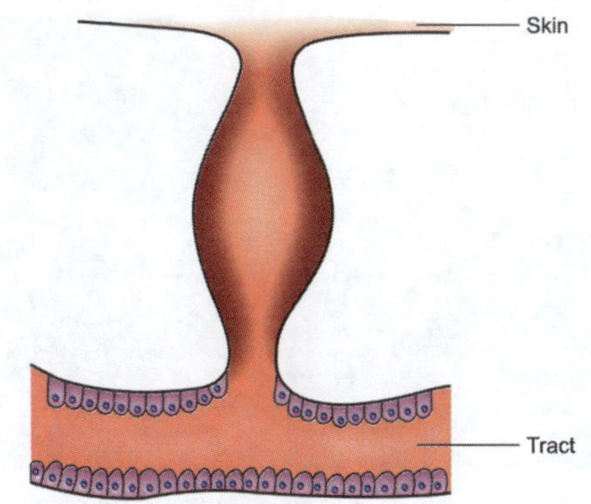

Fig. 22.30: Enterocutaneous fistula (communication)

Examples of Internal Fistulas

- Tracheo-oesophageal fistula
- Colovesical fistula

Examples of External Fistulas

- Orocutaneous fistula due to carcinoma of the oral cavity infiltrating the skin
- Branchial fistula (*see* page 328)
- Thyroglossal fistula (*see* page 324)
- Enterocutaneous fistula

Causes of Persistence of a Sinus or Fistula

1. Presence of foreign body
2. Persistent infection
3. Distal obstruction
4. Absence of rest
5. Epithelialisation of the track
6. Malignancy
7. Nondependent drainage, inadequate drainage
8. Dense fibrosis
9. Irradiation
10. Specific causes—tuberculosis, actinomycosis

Please refer to *Manipal Manual of Clinical Methods,* 1st edition, for clinical examination of a sinus or fistula.

Investigations

- Complete blood picture (**CBP**)—haemoglobin, total and differential count, erythrocyte sedimentation rate (**ESR**): **ESR** may be increased in tuberculosis. Increased total count suggests infection.
- Urine sugar, fasting blood sugar (**FBS**) and post-prandial blood sugar (**PPBS**) to rule out diabetes.
- **X-ray of the part:** To look for osteomyelitis of the mandible, toe, and any foreign body (Fig. 22.31).
- **X-ray kidney, ureter, bladder region (KUB), ultrasound abdomen:** Staghorn calculi in lumbar urinary fistula.

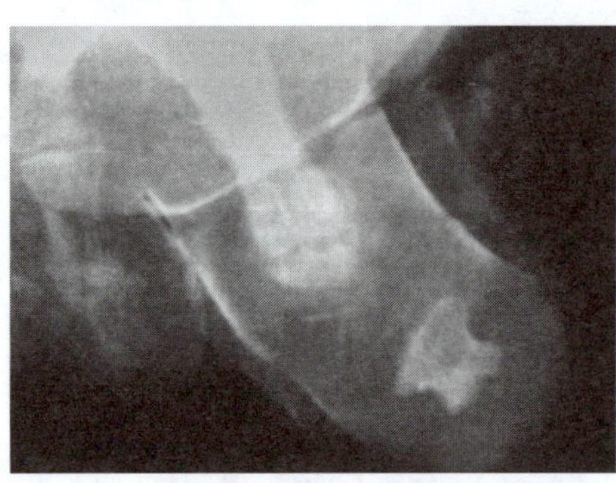

Fig. 22.31: Persisting sinus due to osteomyelitis of distal phalanx of great toe

- **Fistulography or sinusography** to determine the exact extent or origin of the sinus or fistula. A dye such as **lipiodol (poppy seed oil containing 40% iodine)** is used.
- **Biopsy from the edge of the sinus** is done if a specific aetiology is suspected (e.g. tuberculosis, malignancy).

Management (Key Box 22.16)

Following are a few examples:

- Sequestrectomy for osteomyelitis.
- Control of tuberculosis for tubercular sinus in the neck.
- Removal of the foreign body, if present (clinical notes)
- If the track is well formed and epithelialised, the entire track should be removed even if the disease is under control.

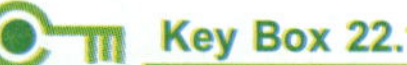

Key Box 22.16

Basic Principles

- Antibiotics
- Adequate rest
- Adequate excision
- Adequate drainage

Please note: Details regarding individual fistula and sinus have been discussed in their respective chapters.

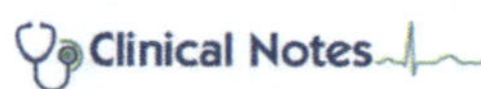

Clinical Notes

1. A patient who had undergone surgery for varicose veins had persistent seropurulent discharge from the inguinal incision. Initially, it was thought to be due to infection. The discharge persisted for a period of two months. The wound was explored. A gauze piece was found and removed. The wound healed well. Retrospective analysis of the surgery revealed slipping of the ligature applied to the long saphenous vein and several gauze pieces were used to control the bleeding point.
2. We had a 60-year-old man who had a small sinus in the loin with watery discharge. He had seen many doctors over many years. He was treated with antibiotics and antitubercular treatment without any relief. X-ray KUB revealed a staghorn calculus.

Multiple Choice Questions

1. Treatment of cold abscess is:

A. Excision
B. Incision and drainage
C. Marsupialisation
D. Nondependent aspiration

2. The following are true about tubercular sinuses in the neck *except*:

A. Usually multiple
B. Edge is bluish in colour
C. Induration is highly characteristic
D. Jugulodigastric nodes are commonly affected

3. The ideal treatment of a carbuncle is:

A. Drainage
B. Incision and drainage
C. Excision
D. Aspiration

4. The following are true about Ludwig's angina *except*:

A. It is caused by *Staphylococcus aureus*
B. Diffuse swelling in the submental and submandibular region is common
C. Putrid halitosis is common
D. It may also give rise to mediastinitis

5. The following are true about pyaemic abscess *except*:

A. They are usually multiple
B. They are deep to the deep fascia
C. The diagnostic feature is a high local rise in temperature
D. It occurs due to a pyaemic process

6. The following are true about carbuncles *except*:

A. Nape of the neck is the most common site
B. Cribriform appearance is diagnostic
C. Abscesses do not communicate with each other
D. Staphylococcus is the most common organism

7. The following are true about erysipelas *except*:

A. Rose pink rash is common
B. Cuticular lymphangitis is an important component
C. The pinna never gets affected in facial erysipelas
D. It is caused by *Streptococcus pyogenes*

8. Muscles are spared in which condition?

A. Gas gangrene
B. Necrotising fasciitis
C. Pyomyositis
D. Acute embolic gangrene

9. The following are features of necrotising fasciitis type II *except*:

A. It is monomicrobial—β-haemolytic streptococci
B. It may also occur in young, healthy individuals
C. The organism is not sensitive to clindamycin
D. It may give rise to toxic shock syndrome

10. Which of the following is true regarding prevention of surgical site infections?

A. Preoperative hair clipping should be done just prior to the surgical procedure
B. Skin is prepared by 20% povidone iodine
C. Blood sugar levels should be maintained within 200 mg/dl
D. Positive pressure ventilation at a temperature of 25°C is ideal

Answers

1. D **2.** C **3.** C **4.** A **5.** C **6.** C **7.** C **8.** B **9.** C **10.** A

CHAPTER

23

Tetanus and Gas Gangrene

- Tetanus
- A case report of neck rigidity
- Gas gangrene

TETANUS

Introduction

A nonimmunised, 18-year-old girl was admitted with moderate tetanus following a nail prick in her foot. In the hospital, she developed convulsions, laryngeal oedema, and cardiac arrest. She was resuscitated and shifted to the intensive care unit under an **anaesthesiologist's care**. Tracheostomy, ventilation, and paralysing agents were used. Unlike many others, she was lucky. She walked home after two months of stay in the intensive care unit after a lot of suffering and spending a lot of money. This happened in early 90s. Due to extensive immunisation programmes in the last few decades, tetanus has become a rare disease in India. Case history has been presented here to allow students to reflect on the following:

1. How important is immunisation to prevent tetanus?
2. How serious is this disorder?
3. Is it possible to save these patients if they are critically ill?

Definition

Tetanus is a serious disorder caused by toxin of the *Clostridium tetani* affecting nervous system, gives rise to muscle contraction of the neck, back and jaw muscles. It is popularly called lock jaw.

Aetiopathogenesis

It is caused by *Clostridium tetani*, an anaerobic spore-forming bacillus with terminal spores that have a drumstick-like appearance.

Pearls of Wisdom

Narcotic addicts who inject themselves beneath the skin at many sites are vulnerable—'Skin Poppers'.

Possible Routes of Infection

- **Umbilical cord (in neonates)**—seen in communities that practise cow dung application on the umbilical stump.
- Wound, as a complication of road traffic accidents where other aerobic organisms reduce oxygen tension in the wound, thereby facilitating growth of anaerobic *Clostridium tetani* (Key Box 23.1).
- **Minor injuries** with **rusted nails**, ear piercings, tattooing, injections, etc.
- Endogenous infection after **septic abortion** or **surgical operations** on the gastrointestinal tract.
- Tetanus due to infection acquired in the operation theatre.

  Thus, tetanus is a wound infection. **"No wound, no tetanus"** is true. Having entered the wound, the organisms multiply and produce powerful exotoxins which produce the disease. Thus, the organisms by themselves do not produce the disease. The toxins produced by the organisms are tetanospasmin (neurotoxin) and tetanolysin (haemolysin).
- **Tetanospasmin has affinity towards nervous tissues.** It reaches the central nervous system along the axons of motor nerve trunks. The toxin gets fixed to motor

Key Box 23.1

Wounds which are more Prone to Tetanus

Time—wound more than 6 hours old
Extensive contamination by soil, faeces, rust
Tissue devitalised or denervated
Animal or human bites
No less than 1 cm (more than 1 cm)
Ulcer or wound—deeper
Stellate wounds—burst type
Remember as **TETANUS**

cells of the anterior horn cells. The toxin, which is fixed to the motor end plate, acts in the following ways:

1. It **inhibits the release of cholinesterase,** leading to the accumulation of acetylcholine at the motor end plate. This causes tonic rigidity of limb, trunk, abdominal, and neck muscles.
2. It acts at the ***spinal level*** and causes reflex muscle contraction due to minor stimuli.

- **The toxin, once fixed to the nervous tissue, cannot be neutralised**. However, circulating toxins may be neutralised. The incubation period varies from a few days to months or years and is not important. The interval between the first symptom (dysphagia and stiffness of jaw) and reflex spasm is called the **period of onset**. If this is less than 48 hours, the prognosis is poor, whereas if it is more than 48 hours, the prognosis is better.
- **Tetanolysin** also contributes to pathogenesis of tetanus, but its action is not clear. It is a type of protein which is oxygen sensitive haemolysin.

Favourable Conditions for the Development of Tetanus

- No immunisation
- Foreign body
- Injury
- Improper sterilisation
- Devitalised tissues
- Anaerobic conditions

Special Types of Tetanus

1. **Tetanus neonatorum:** It occurs due to contamination of the umbilical cord in children born to non-immunised mothers. It usually manifests around 6–8 days of birth and is called **eighth day disease**. It carries almost 100% mortality.
2. **Local tetanus:** In this, muscle contraction occurs in the neighbourhood of the wound.
3. **Cephalic tetanus:** Usually occurs after a wound over the head and/or face. Cranial nerves, such as the facial and oculomotor nerves, may get **paralysed**. It carries a poor prognosis.
4. **Bulbar tetanus:** It involves the muscles of deglutition and respiration and is fatal.
5. **Latent tetanus:** It develops after a few months to years following a wound that might have been forgotten.
6. **Puerperal tetanus:** It occurs as a complication of abortion or puerperal sepsis.
7. **Postoperative tetanus:** It occurs due to improper sterilisation of instruments and carries 100% mortality. This type of tetanus should not occur in a modern operation theatre.
8. **Otitis tetanus:** It is due to chronic suppurative otitis media. In these cases, the wound is a tear in the tympanic membrane. It may occur in any age group, but is more common in children and young adults.

Clinical Features (Table 23.1)

- **Autonomic dysfunction:** Increased basal sympathetic tone, manifesting as tachycardia, bladder/bowel dysfunction, labile hypertension, pyrexia, pallor, sweating, and cyanosis of the digits.
- Episodes of bradycardia, low central venous pressure, and even cardiac arrest have been reported due to parasympathetic dysfunction.
- Complications include pneumonia, urinary tract infection, etc.

TREATMENT OF ESTABLISHED TETANUS

I. General management
II. Specific management

Table 23.1 Clinical features with differential diagnosis

Symptoms and signs	Differential diagnosis
• **Trismus** or **lock jaw,** occurs due to severe contraction of the masseter muscle, resulting in inability to open the mouth. It is the most common symptom of tetanus.	• Alveolar abscess or temporomandibular joint involvement
• **Dysphagia** occurs due to spasm of pharyngeal muscles.	• Tonsillitis
• **Neck rigidity**	• Meningitis
• **Rigidity of back muscles**	• Orthopaedic disorder
• **Risus sardonicus** due to spasm of facial and jaw muscles.	• Anxiety neurosis
• **Generalised convulsions** wherein every muscle is thrown into contraction, with severe clenching of teeth, arched back and extended limbs are described as opisthotonos (bow-like body; hence the name **dhanurvatha**).	• Epilepsy
• Mild temperature and tachycardia	• Sympathetic hyperactivity

I. General Management

- **Admission and isolation**[1] in a quiet room, to avoid even minor stimuli that may precipitate spasm (Fig. 23.1).
- **Wound care**—drainage of pus, excision of necrotic tissue, removal of any foreign body, and proper dressing. Exudate or pus may demonstrate gram-positive rods.
- **Inj. Tetanus toxoid** 0.5 ml intramuscularly (IM).
- **Antitetanus serum** (ATS) 50,000 units IM and 50,000 units slow intravenously (IV). This should be given only after giving a small subcutaneous test dose of serum diluted with ten times saline. It has become less popular due to the availability of human antitetanus globulin.
- **Human antitetanus globulin** 3000–4000 units intramuscular. It is better and safer than ATS, does not cause anaphylaxis, and does not require a test dose.
- **Inj. crystalline penicillin** 10 lakh units IM 6th hourly is the drug of choice against *Clostridium tetani*. It may have to be given for 7–10 days.
- **Metronidazole** 500 mg IV 8th hourly for 10 days. It is more effective than penicillin.
- After recovery, full immunisation with tetanus toxoid is required.

II. Specific Management

A. Mild Cases

- There is only tonic rigidity without spasm or dysphagia. These patients are managed by heavy sedation with a combination of drugs to prevent spasms or convulsions. The treatment method followed in our hospital is given in Table 23.2.
- **Benzodiazepines** and **morphine** act centrally to minimise the effects of tetanospasmin.
- **Chlorpromazine,** an α-receptor blocker, may decrease sympathetic activity. Other α-blockers like phenoxybenzamine and phentolamine have also been used.

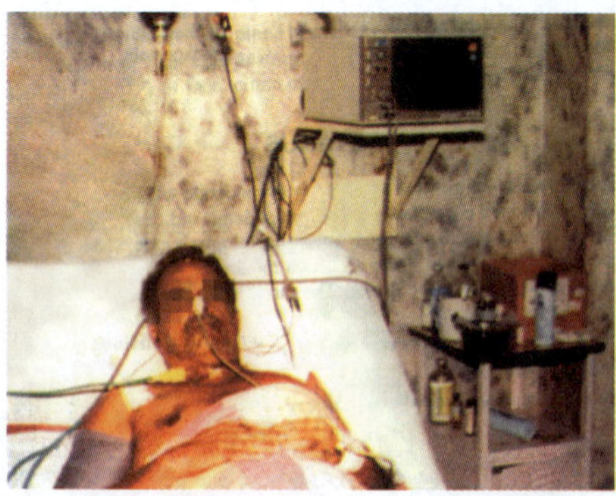

Fig. 23.1: Tetanus patient recovering in an intensive care unit

Table 23.2 Method of treatment

Drug	Dosage	Time
Chlorpromazine	50–100 mg	8 am, 2 pm, 8 pm and 2 am
Phenobarbitone	30–60 mg	10 am, 4 pm, 10 pm and 4 am
Diazepam	10–20 mg	12 noon, 6 pm, 12 midnight and 6 am

- These drugs are repeated in such a way that the patient receives some sedative every two hours. The dosage of the drugs is adjusted once every 2 or 3 days to get the maximum effect of sedation or muscle relaxation.
- Injection diazepam 10 mg, a tracheostomy set, and a resuscitation set with a laryngoscope and endotracheal tubes should be kept ready by the side of the patient.
- When high dose of diazepam is used, it can give rise to hyper-osmolarity and metabolic acidosis because of propylene glycol (vehicle). Midazolam is better.
- Labetalol has both alfa and beta blocking properties. It also can be used. Dose is: 0.25 mg to 1 mg/mt.

B. Seriously Ill Cases

- They have dysphagia and reflex spasms.
- A nasogastric tube is introduced for feeding purposes and to administer the drugs.
- Tracheostomy, if breathing difficulty arises.

C. Dangerously Ill Cases

This group includes patients with major cyanotic convulsions. In addition to continuing sedatives, these patients are paralysed with muscle relaxants (neuromuscular blocking agents) and are mechanically ventilated till they recover. The duration of required ventilatory support cannot be predicted. During this period, supportive therapy, such as adequate nutrition, bladder and bowel care, and frequent change of position to avoid bedsores, is required.

Magnesium sulphate may be used to treat autonomic complications and control spasms. It may be used alone or in combination with benzodiazepines. A loading dose of 5 g over 20 min is followed by infusion, the rate of which is titrated to control spasm as well as reduce muscle rigidity to a level acceptable by the patient for swallowing saliva, mouth care, and limb physiotherapy. Total abolition of muscle rigidity is not required and may lead to hypotonia.

[1]Isolation for tetanus has been misunderstood by surgeons. In many hospitals, tetanus patients are isolated in a remote corner of the hospital, well away from the reach of a skilled person. Many cases die due to convulsions and laryngeal spasm before they are intubated and resuscitated. The critically ill patients are admitted in an intensive care unit under the supervision of an anaesthesiologist's care in our institution (Fig. 3.1). Tetanus is not communicable from person to person.

Loss of patellar reflex may not be a valid indicator of hypermagnesaemia in all patients, as the reflex is sometimes masked by rigidity and tends to be lost early in elderly patients. The patients, therefore, should be monitored closely for ventilatory depression. Magnesium sulphate may not reduce the need for mechanical ventilation in patients with severe tetanus, but may help in reducing the requirement of other sedatives.

PROPHYLAXIS

1. ***Tetanus neonatorum*** may be prevented by administering two tetanus toxoid injections, **0.5 ml** IM, to the mother in the second trimester of pregnancy.
2. Infants and children are immunised with tetanus toxoid, diphtheria, and pertussis vaccine (DPT–triple antigen) at 6, 10, and 14 weeks of age, with a booster dose at 18 months 5 years, followed by 0.5 ml tetanus toxoid once every five years.
3. Immunised individuals who receive a provocative injury are administered a booster dose if they have not received one in the previous 5 years.

Tetanus may be **prevented by giving tetanus antitoxin** in the following situations: Wounds of head and/or face, penetrating wounds, wounds with contused and devitalised tissues and war wounds and road traffic accidents. 1,500 IU of antitoxin should be given subcutaneously or intramuscularly as early as possible. Treatment of wound is done. In severe wounds, the dose may be doubled.

Complications: Most of these may also be the causes of death.

1. **Aspiration** of pharyngeal contents into the lungs, resulting in aspiration pneumonia.
2. **Laryngeal spasm and respiratory arrest,** resulting in cardiac arrest.
3. **Autonomic disturbances,** resulting in cardiac arrhythmias: In some patients, **pacemaker insertion** may help if there is refractory bradycardia.

A Case Report of Neck Rigidity

Clinical Notes

A 48-year-old lady who had undergone vaginal hysterectomy 10 days prior was brought to our hospital as a case of 'tetanus.' On examination, she had neck rigidity and difficulty in mouth opening. Abdominal rigidity was mild. She appeared pale. Pallor was attributed to anaemia caused by 'dysfunctional uterine bleeding' (DUB), for which she was operated. She was diagnosed with postoperative tetanus and was started on treatment. The next day, she was unresponsive to commands. Laboratory reports, which had been sent the previous day, showed a total WBC count of 44,000 cells/mm^3 clinching the diagnosis of 'leukaemia.' Neck rigidity was due to leukaemic infiltrates in the meninges. Now you know the cause of uterine bleeding!!!

GAS GANGRENE

Definition: It is a highly fatal, rapidly spreading infection caused by clostridial organisms that results in myonecrosis.

- Gas produced by organisms consists of predominantly nitrogen, and others are hydrogen, carbon dioxide and oxygen. (*E. coli*, Klebsiella, Proteus, Candida, Bacteroides, Peptostreptococcus are a few other gas forming organisms.)
- Other names for gas gangrene are clostridial myositis, clostridial myonecrosis, infective gangrene of the muscles.

Aetiology

The disease is most commonly (60%) caused by *Clostridium perfringens* (*Clostridium welchii*). Other organisms include *Clostridium septicum, Clostridium oedematiens,* and *Clostridium histolyticum.* These are gram-positive, anaerobic, spore-forming bacilli.

MacLennan Anaerobic Wound Infection Types

1. Simple wound contamination—no invasion of underlying tissue
2. Anaerobic cellulitis—invades fascial planes with minimal toxins in muscles
3. Anaerobic myositis—muscle necrosis

Sources of Infection and Predisposing Factors

(Table 23.3)

Manured soil or cultivated soil, normal intestines.

Types of Gas Gangrene Infections

1. **Clostridial cellulitis:** In this condition, healthy muscles are not involved. It involves necrotic tissues and produces features of cellulitis such as tense, swollen parts with palpable crepitus. However, it is a mild infection and may be managed conservatively with antibiotics.
2. **Local type:** It refers to infection confined to a single muscle.
3. **Group type:** It refers to infection confined to a group of muscles in a single compartment. Such cases benefit from a compartmental excision.
4. **Massive type:** Gas gangrene involving the entire limb and requiring amputation.

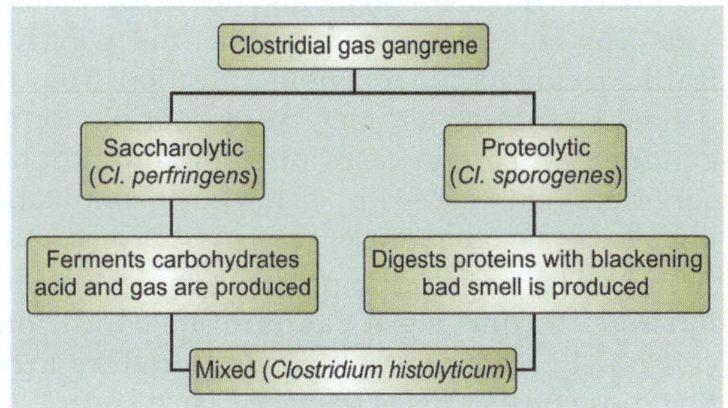

Table 23.3 Predisposing factors for the development of gas gangrene

Factors	Mechanism
Foreign body such as soil, clothing, bullets, glass pieces	Soil supplies calcium and silicic acid which causes tissue necrosis
Anoxia due to crushing of the arteries	Necrosis of the tissues results in proliferation of the organism
Dead and devitalised tissues	Anaerobic organisms multiply
Blood clots	Supplies calcium
Extravasated haemoglobin and myoglobin	Cease to carry oxygen

Table 23.4 Toxins and their effects

Toxins	Effects
1. Lecithinase (alphatoxin)—commonly found in *C. perfringens* type A strain	• Dermonecrosis Haemolysis Profound toxaemia
2. Beta toxin	• Necrosis of the tissues
3. Proteinase	• Breakdown of collagen fibres
4. Hyaluronidase	• Breaks the cement substance of the muscle cells—hyaluronic acid
5. Theta toxin	• Vascular injury and destroy leukocytes
6. Kappa toxin	• Destroy connective tissue and help speed necrosis

Risk Groups

- Patients who have had lower limb amputations performed for ischaemic gangrene (may develop infection from their own bowel organisms).
- High velocity gunshot wounds with perforation of a hollow viscus (military wounds).
- Immunocompromised patients.
- Trauma is postoperative—most common form of gas gangrene (70%).
- Patients with diabetes mellitus, blood vessel disease (atherosclerosis), or colon cancer.
- **Intravenous drug users and gas gangrene**: Repeated trauma of the needle due to intramuscular/deep injections, anaerobic environment facilitates development of gas gangrene in these patients. Clostridia can survive in heroin preparations.

Pathogenesis

- Gas gangrene develops in wounds that are heavily contaminated with soil or a foreign body, or in those associated with a laceration and devitalised muscle mass. This type of situation is common following road traffic accidents. Endogenous infection from the patient's faecal matter may be responsible for gas gangrene in certain cases of contamination of a surgical wound caused by below knee amputation done for some other cause.
- All these factors contribute to create low oxygen tension. Under these favourable conditions, clostridial organisms multiply and produce toxins that cause further tissue damage (Table 23.4).
- Once powerful toxins start acting, various pathological events, such as inflammation, oedema, muscle necrosis, and gangrene of the muscles, set in (Fig. 23.2).
- Features of SIRS (systemic inflammatory response syndrome) are present.

Refer to Key Box 23.2.

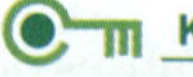
Key Box 23.2

Why Gas Gangrene Spreads Fast?

- Massive infection
- Gross injury
- Devitalised tissue
- Poor immunity
- Foreign body

Clinical Features (Table 23.5)

- Severe pain in the limb, swelling, fever, and toxicity.
- In untreated cases, the necrotic process continues and septicaemia, renal failure, peripheral circulatory failure, and death occur. Foamy liver is the condition wherein gas is produced in the liver as a part of septicaemia.

Systemic Complications

- Liver necrosis—jaundice
- Haemolytic anaemia
- Renal failure

Diagnosis

- In addition to clinical suspicion, an easy method of confirming the diagnosis is to examine the pus under microscopy after Giemsa staining.
- These organisms are gram-positive and spore-bearing.

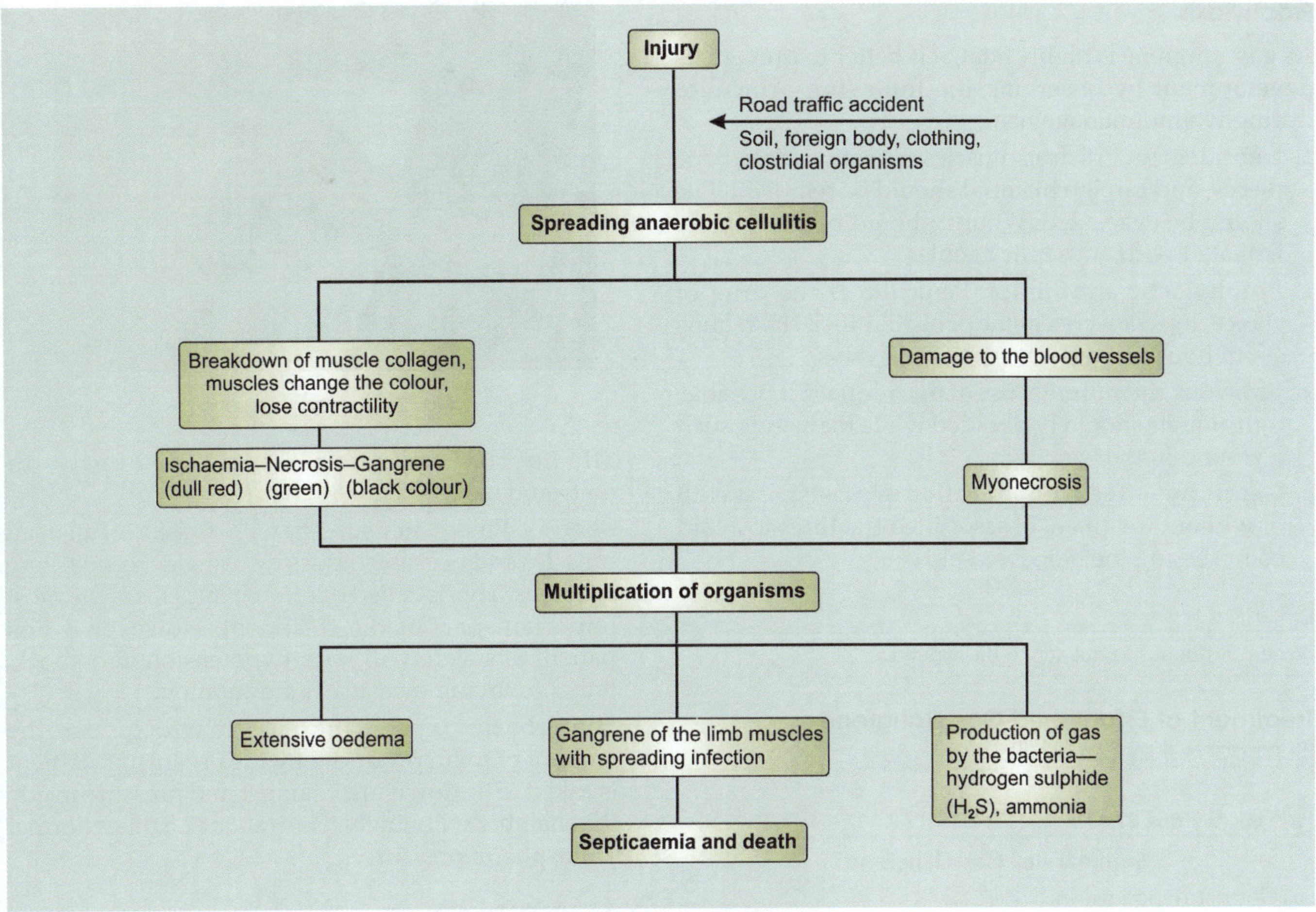

Injury

Road traffic accident

Soil, foreign body, clothing, clostridial organisms

Spreading anaerobic cellulitis

Breakdown of muscle collagen, muscles change the colour, lose contractility

Ischaemia–Necrosis–Gangrene (dull red) (green) (black colour)

Damage to the blood vessels

Myonecrosis

Multiplication of organisms

Extensive oedema

Gangrene of the limb muscles with spreading infection

Production of gas by the bacteria—hydrogen sulphide (H_2S), ammonia

Septicaemia and death

Fig. 23.2: Pathological changes

Table 23.5 Clinical features

Local features	**General features**
Severe pain and gross oedema of the wound	Anxious and alert
Sutured wound is under tension	Toxic and ill
Thin brownish fluid escapes which has **sickly sweet odour**	Rapid increase in the pulse rate
Palpable **crepitus**	Hypotension due to suppression of adrenals
Colour changes in the muscles	Vomiting
Skin becomes khaki-coloured due to haemolysis	Low grade fever

- Lecithinase test or Nagler's reaction: Many species of *Clostridium* produce lecithinase (*C. baratti, C. absonum, C. bifermantans, C. sordelli, and C. novyi*). But the alpha (α) toxin of *C. perfringens* has **phospholipase activity. It neutralises the Lecithin C activity which forms the basis for Nagler's reaction.**
- X-rays, computerized tomography (CT) scans and magnetic resonance imaging (MRI) scans: Will reveal gas and extent of tissue damage.

A few differences between clostridial myonecrosis and non-clostridial necrotising infections are given in Table 23.6.

Table 23.6

	Clostridial myonecrosis	**Nonclostridial necrotising infections**
• Exudate	Thin	Dishwater initially purulent later
• Erythema	Absent	Present—mild
• Muscle gangrene	Present	Absent
• Toxicity	Very rapid	Rapid
• Bullae	Haemorrhagic	Nonhaemorrhagic
• White blood cells in the discharge	Absent	Present

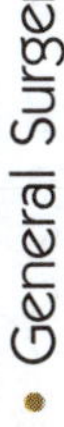

Prophylaxis

As gas gangrene is highly fatal, it is better to prevent its development by observing the following principles during wound management:

1. **Debridement:** All dead muscles, necrotic tissues, bone pieces, and foreign material should be removed. Pus should be evacuated. Wound should be thoroughly irrigated with antiseptic agents.
2. **Prophylactic antibiotics:** Penicillin is the drug of choice. Injection crystalline penicillin 10–20 lakh units 4–6th hourly should be given for 7 days.
3. **Judicious and minimal use of tourniquets:** If possible, tourniquets should be avoided while managing such a wound in the leg.
4. **Gentle but effective application of plaster cast** with or without treatment of associated fractures to avoid compressing the blood vessel.

Pearls of Wisdom

When in doubt, do not suture the wound.

Treatment of Established Gas Gangrene

(Summary—Key Box 23.3)

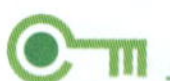

Key Box 23.3

Summary of Gas Gangrene

- Correct hypotension
- Control infection
- Treat dehydration
- Early debridement
- Administer hyperbaric oxygen
- Give blood transfusion
- Passive immunisation
- To save life, amputate

Principles of the treatment

The triad of gas gangrene treatment principles are: Antibiotics, debridement and hyperbaric oxygen therapy. Other treatment includes supportive treatment.

1. **Antibiotics** should be continued: Injection crystalline penicillin 10–20 lakh units 4–6th hourly should be given for 7 days. Systemic Inflammatory Response Syndrome (SIRS) can be caused by *Clostridium septicum*. It is treated by clindamycin 600–900 mg 8th hourly, vancomycin 1 g 12th hourly, or metronidazole 500 mg 8th hourly.
2. **Surgery:** Emergency surgery with excision of all dead muscles and necrotic tissues by using generous, long incisions. This is called debridement. This is the most important part of the treatment. However, when patient is severely ill with hypotension and shock, only life saving measure is amputation.
3. **Hyperbaric oxygen therapy:** It will reduce the amount of toxin produced by the organisms. Patient is asked to lie down in a chamber and pressure inside the chamber will slowly rise to about 2.5 times normal atmospheric pressure.

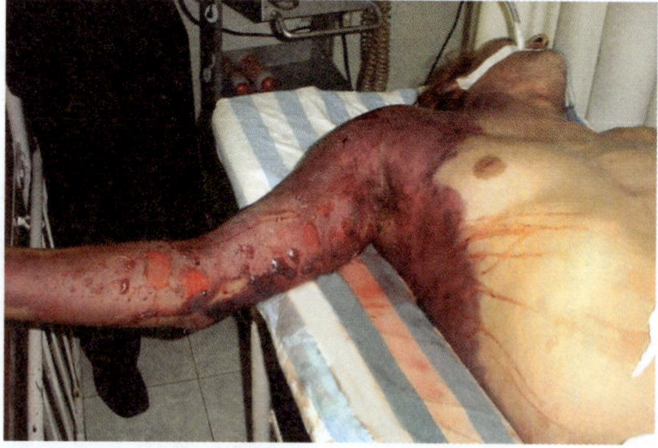

Fig. 23.3: Gas gangrene

Supportive Treatment

- Blood transfusions before, during and after surgery.
- Polyvalent anti-gas gangrene serum.

Clinical Notes

A 40-year-old gentleman presented to the hospital with massive gas gangrene involving his right upper limb, chest wall, abdominal wall, and back (Fig. 23.3). It started after an injury to his right elbow. The patient had initially received treatment at a local hospital. Due to lack of proper facilities, he was neither subjected to any surgical procedure nor given any resuscitation. When he came to our hospital, he was in septic shock.

It was too late when we saw the patient. He had severe hypotension and renal failure. Emergency resuscitation and debridement was done. However, within six hours of admission, he expired.

Multiple Choice Questions

1. Which of the following statements regarding tetanus is false?
   A. Exotoxins are produced by *Clostridium tetani*
   B. The toxin gets fixed to motor cells of anterior horn cells
   C. It stimulates the release of cholinesterase
   D. The period of onset is more important than the incubation period

2. Favourable conditions for the development of tetanus include all of the following *except*:
   A. Injury B. Foreign body
   C. Devitalised tissues D. Aerobic conditions

3. Hyperbaric oxygen may be used in all of the following conditions *except*:
   A. Gas gangrene
   B. Decompression sickness
   C. Carbon monoxide poisoning
   D. Necrotising fasciitis

4. The following facts are true regarding gas gangrene *except*:
   A. It is caused by *Clostridium welchii*
   B. Severe myonecrosis is a feature
   C. Brownish fluid has a foul odour
   D. Alpha toxin causes cell membrane damage

5. Positive Nagler reaction in gas gangrene is caused by:
   A. Lecithinase B. Beta toxin
   C. Proteinase D. Hyaluronidase

6. Sponge-like consistency of the part is typically seen in which condition?
   A. Necrotising fasciitis B. Diabetic leg ulcer
   C. Gas gangrene D. Pyomyositis

7. The following are true regarding *Clostridium welchii* *except*:
   A. Anaerobic B. Gram-positive
   C. Nonspore-bearing D. Produces toxins

8. The following are clinical features of gas gangrene *except*:
   A. Crepitus B. Khaki coloured skin
   C. Low grade fever D. Hypertension

9. The following are features of necrotising fasciitis type II *except*:
   A. It is monomicrobial—β-haemolytic streptococci
   B. It may also occur in young and healthy individuals
   C. Organism is *Clostridium perfringens*
   D. It may give rise to toxic shock syndrome

10. Which of the following is false regarding gas gangrene prevention?
   A. Antigas gangrene for risk groups
   B. Prophylactic antibiotics
   C. Blood sugar level should be maintained within 200 mg/dl
   D. Avoid tourniquets while operating on crushed wounds in the legs

Answers

1. C **2.** D **3.** D **4.** C **5.** A **6.** C **7.** C **8.** D **9.** C **10.** C

CHAPTER

24

Hand, Foot Infections and Tendon Transfer

- Paronychia
- Subcutaneous infections
- Acute lymphangitis of hand
- Terminal pulp space infections
- Apical subungual infection
- Web space infections
- Deep palmar abscess
- Acute suppurative tenosynovitis
- Mycetoma pedis
- Ingrowing toenail
- Tendon transfer

Competency

SU6.1: Define and describe the aetiology and pathogenesis of surgical infections.

INTRODUCTION

Hand infections are commonly encountered in manual labourers and are precipitated by injury, such as a thorn prick, cut injuries, etc. In 80–90% of cases, the causative organism is *Staphylococcus aureus* sensitive to cloxacillin. In the remaining cases, streptococci, gram-negative bacilli, or anaerobic organisms may play a role. Irrespective of the site of infection, oedema is commonly present on the dorsal aspect because of the following reasons:

- Lymphatics from the palmar aspect of the hand travel through the dorsal aspect to the corresponding lymph node.
- Presence of loose areolar tissue in the dorsum of the hand.
  - Hand infections may be severe in immunocompromised, systemically ill, and diabetic patients. It may spread rapidly and cause septicaemia and death.
  - It is unfortunate that in cases of gas gangrene and spreading infections, amputation may have to be done.

Pearls of Wisdom

Oedema is the chief cause of stiffness of the fingers. Hence, early physiotherapy should be encouraged.

Classification of Hand Infections (Table 24.1)

Table 24.1 Classification of hand infections

Superficial infections	Deep infections
1. Paronychia	1. Terminal pulp space infection
2. Subcutaneous infections	2. Apical subungual infection
3. Infection of dorsal space	3. Volar space infection
4. Acute lymphangitis	4. Web space infection
	5. Midpalmar space infection
	6. Tenosynovitis

SUPERFICIAL INFECTIONS

PARONYCHIA[1]

It refers to infection near the nail. It is the most common type of hand infection. There are two types—acute and chronic.

Acute Paronychia (Fig. 24.1)

- It occurs due to trimming of the nail or an ingrowing nail.
- Subcuticular infection starts in the lateral sulcus and ***spreads all around*** (paronychia means 'run around'). This is because the eponychium (skin overlying the nail base) is adherent to the nail base. Hence, the infection spreads beneath the nail base. The affected finger is painful. Throbbing pain suggests the pre-

[1]Paronychia—infection affects the base of nail.

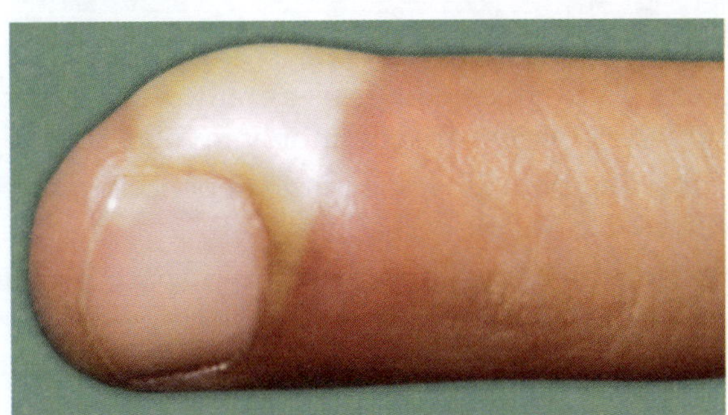

Fig. 24.1: Acute paronychia—very painful condition, can be treated very easily

sence of pus. Even collection of 0.5 ml of pus produces severe pain. Low grade fever may be present.

Treatment

- Early cases (before the formation of pus) may be managed by soaking, elevation, antibiotics, and immobilisation.
- After a digital block (with 5 ml of 2% *plain lignocaine* injected into the root of the digit), incision and drainage is done by incising the eponychium. ***Adrenaline should not be used for infiltration*** in the finger, penis, or ear lobule as these areas are supplied by end-arteries (no collateral circulation). Adrenaline is a vasoconstrictor and may cause gangrene. Pus is sent for culture and sensitivity. Antibiotics are given. Dressings are applied.

Chronic Paronychia[1]

- It is *not due to bacterial infection*, but due to **fungal infection**—moniliasis/Candida.
- It is common in women who wash clothes, utensils, etc. and constantly have wet fingers. As a result of this, fungal infection takes place. The infection is insidious in onset, chronic, and difficult to eradicate. It produces a dull nagging pain in the fingers. The eponychium is faintly pink and the nail is ridged.
- Antifungal agents such as nystatin or tolnaftate solution help the patient. Rubber gloves should be worn while using hands for washing.

SUBCUTAENOUS INFECTIONS (Figs 24.2–24.4)

1. **Intraepidermal abscess** (purulent blister): Cuts, pricks, and burns may cause this condition.
2. **Intradermal abscess:** This variety does not produce a dome-shaped elevation.
3. **Subcutaneous abscess:** This type of lesion is like that of cellulitis.

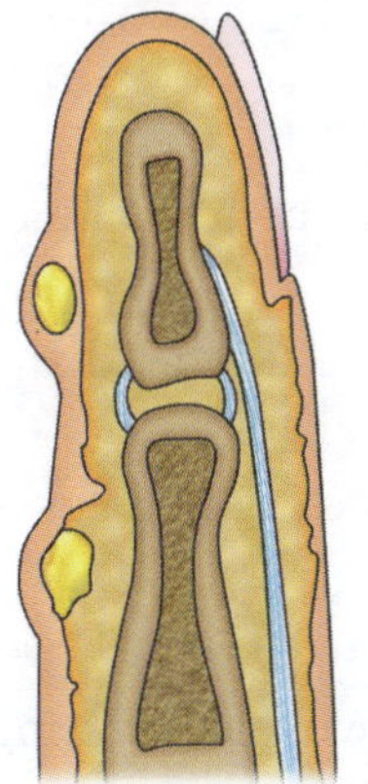
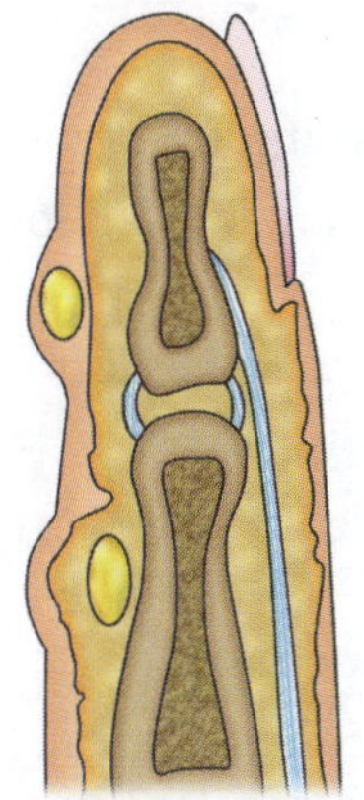
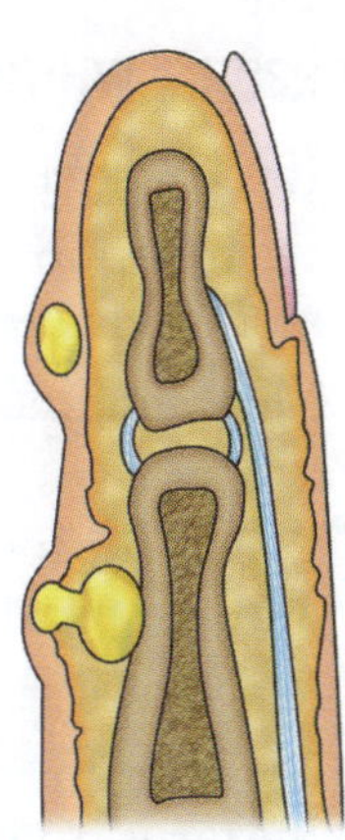

Figs 24.2 to 24.4: Intraepidermal abscess, intradermal abscess and subcutaneous abscess respectively **Fig. 24.4:** Collar-stud abscess also

4. **Collar-stud abscess:** It results when the epidermal component is connected to the dermal component.

Treatment

Incision and drainage under an antibiotic cover. Care should be taken to drain the deeper cavity.

ACUTE LYMPHANGITIS OF THE HAND

- It is caused by an injury, which may be a minor abrasion.
- The causative organism is **Streptococcus**.

Clinical Features

- Severe pain in the hand with fever, chills, and rigors.
- Gross oedema of dorsum of the hand.
- Red, hot streaks over the limb which indicate the route of lymphatics.
- Regional lymph nodes are swollen and tender.
  - Infection of little finger—epitrochlear nodes are enlarged.
  - Infection of ring and middle fingers—supraclavicular nodes are enlarged.
  - Infection of index and thumb fingers—axillary nodes are enlarged.

Treatment

- Injection crystalline penicillin 10 lakh units **IV** or **IM** for 5–7 days.
- Higher antibiotics may have to be used, depending on the response.

[1]Wet nails of women who wash dishes are vulnerable.

HERPETIC WHITLOW

- It is due to herpes simplex virus (HSV).
- Common in children, may follow herpetic gingivostomatitis.
- Most common viral infection of the hand—distal finger.
- Pain, pruritus, and vesicles are characteristics. Fever and lymphadenitis are present.
- It resolves spontaneously.
- The diagnosis is mainly clinical. However, culturing the virus from the vesicular fluid, assessing immunofluorescent serum antibody titres, or performing a Tzanck smear may confirm the diagnosis.
- Antivirals such as acyclovir or famciclovir are of some benefit if started within 48 hours.

DEEP INFECTIONS

INFECTION OF THE TERMINAL PULP SPACE (FELON)

This space commonly gets infected due to relatively deep prick injuries. It is the second most common infection of the hand, seen in about 25% of patients.

Anatomy of the Terminal Pulp Space

- It is a closed space, formed by the fusion of the distal flexion skin crease and the deep fascia attached to the periosteum of the distal phalanx, just distal to the insertion of flexor digitorum profundus. Each pulp space is subdivided by the presence of numerous septa which pass from the deep fascia to the periosteum. Thus, 15–20 small compartments are formed (Fig. 24.5).
- The digital artery, which is an **end-artery,** runs in this closed space (Fig. 24.6).

Clinical Features (Key Box 24.1)

- Injury to the affected finger is usually present. Thumb and index fingers are commonly involved.
- Throbbing pain is worse in the dependent position, with nocturnal exacerbations.
- An indurated, red, and tense pulp space is characteristic of this condition.
- Touch and movement worsen the pain.

Key Box 24.1

Terminal Pulp Space Infection—Felon

- **F**ingertip pulp abscess
- **E**xtremely painful
- **L**oss of normal resilience of pulp
- **O**steomyelitis of distal phalanx in untreated cases due to thrombosis of digital artery
- **N**o longer recommended **fish mouth** incision

Remember as **FELON**

Treatment

Incision and drainage under digital block—volar longitudinal incision.

Complications

1. If the pus is not released early, *thrombosis of the digital artery* takes place, *resulting in osteomyelitis and necrosis of the terminal phalanx,* which may result in shortening of the finger (Fig. 24.7).
2. Pyogenic arthritis of the distal interphalangeal joints.
3. Tenosynovitis secondary to pus, which requires regular physiotherapy to avoid the development of thickness.
4. Neuroma, which may be painful and cause discomfort.

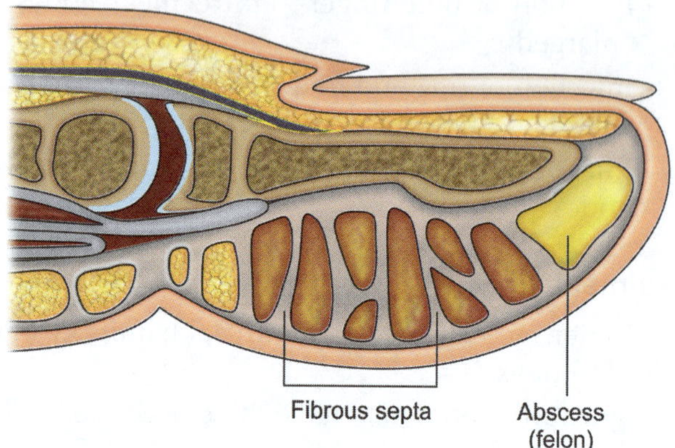

Fig. 24.5: Felon

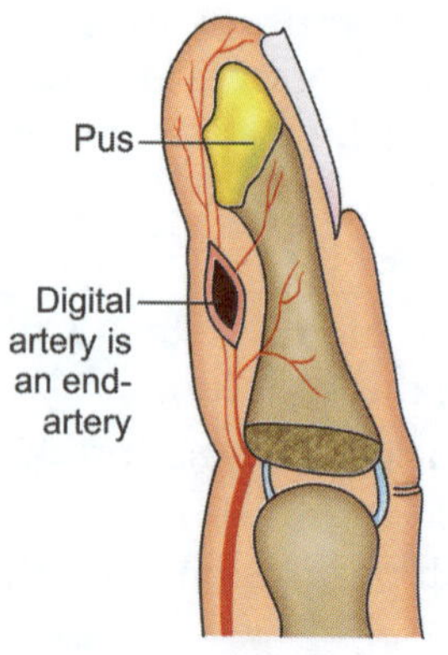

Fig. 24.6: Pulp space infection

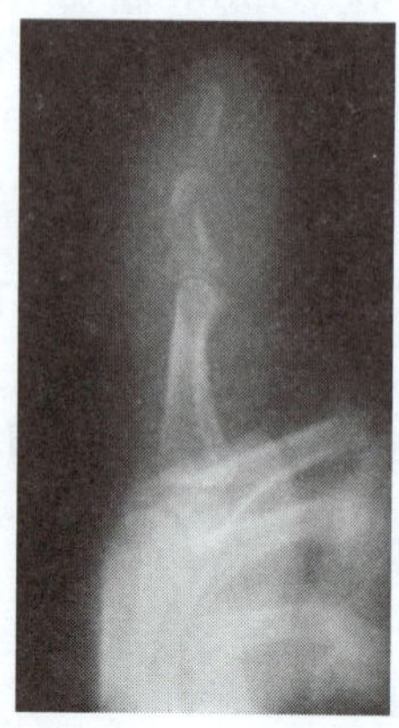

Fig. 24.7: Plain radiography of hand showing osteomyelitis of terminal phalanx

APICAL SUBUNGUAL INFECTION

- Infection is confined to the space between the distal quarter of the subungual epithelium and the periosteum of the distal phalanx. Penetration by a sharp object causes this condition. It often manifests as a tender yellow spot beneath the distal portion of the nail. Pain, redness, and minimal swelling are the features.
- Tenderness is maximum at the free edge of the nail. The pulp and distal parts of the fingers are relatively painless. It is treated by a "V" excision of a portion of the nail to open the abscess cavity under an antibiotic cover (Fig. 24.8).

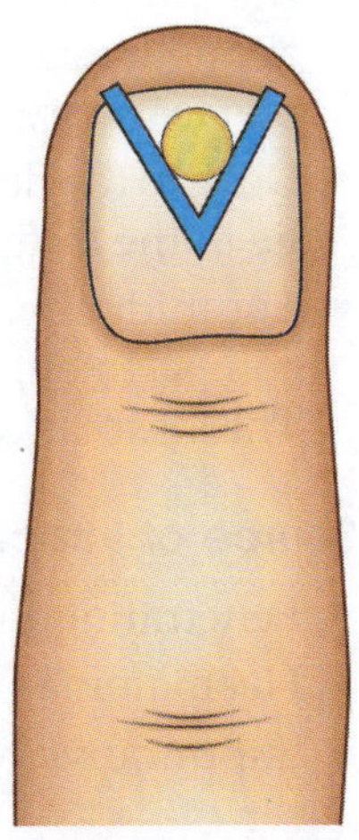

Fig. 24.8: "V" excision of the nail, for apical infection

MIDDLE AND PROXIMAL VOLAR SPACE INFECTIONS (Fig. 24.9)

- These spaces are loose in comparison to the terminal pulp spaces. They are filled with fibrofatty tissue.
- The middle volar space is closed, but proximally communicates with web space.
- The swelling is tender and indurated. The finger is held in flexion.
- It is treated by a transverse incision and drainage of the pus.

WEB SPACE INFECTIONS (Key Box 24.2)

Web spaces are the triangular spaces between the four divisions of the palmar aponeurosis. *There are 3 in number* (Fig. 24.10). The thumb has no palmar aponeurosis. They are filled with subcutaneous fat and are covered posteriorly by the metacarpal bones.

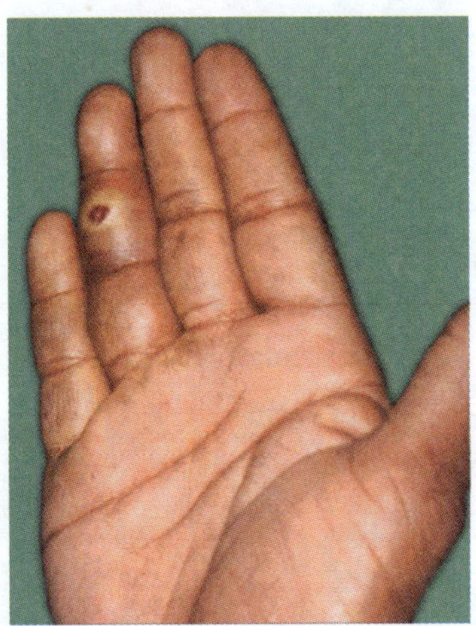

Fig. 24.9: Middle and proximal volar space infections

Key Box 24.2

Web Space Infections

- 3 web spaces
- Finger separation sign
- Gross oedema of dorsum
- Spread to other web space

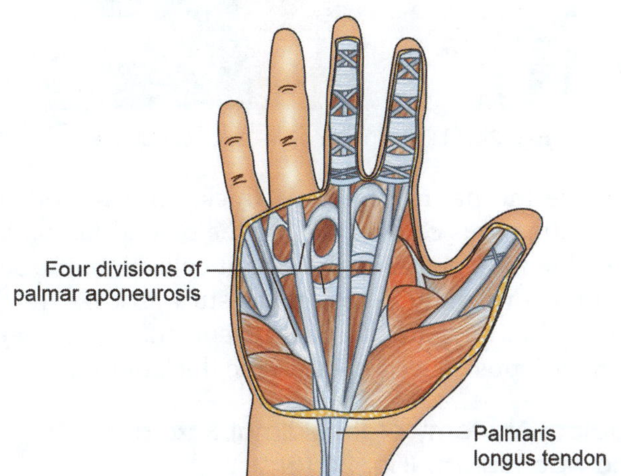

Fig. 24.10: Three web spaces

Causes of Web Space Infection

- Penetrating injuries
- Spread of a proximal volar space (palmar space) infection.
- Lumbrical canal infection—suppurating tenosynovitis.

Clinical Features

- Pain and swelling of the palm in the region of the web space.
- Extremely tender and hot swelling.
- **Finger separation sign:** Adjacent fingers are separated due to oedema.
- Gross oedema of the dorsum of the hand.
- If untreated, pus from one web space may spread to other web spaces and/or to the proximal volar space.

Treatment

Under anaesthesia, a transverse skin incision is made and the pus is drained (Fig. 24.11). The cavity is treated like any other abscess cavity. The skin edge is trimmed to leave a *diamond-shaped* opening behind for better drainage.

MIDPALMAR SPACE INFECTION/DEEP PALMAR ABSCESS

- Infection of the midpalmar space results in a deep palmar abscess.
- The midpalmar space is the space behind the palmar aponeurosis and in front of the metacarpal bones.

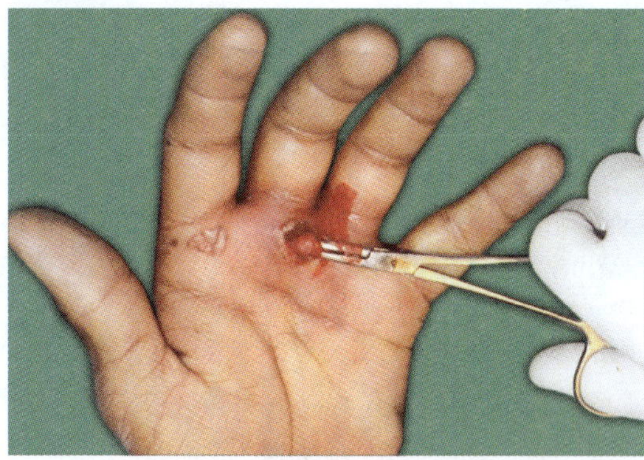

Fig. 24.11: Drainage of web space abscess

- Since the palmar fascia is thick, strong, and unyielding, pus collects deep to the palmar fascia. If it is due to penetrating injuries, it collects in the subcutaneous plane like a collar-stud abscess. In the centre of the palm, there is no subcutaneous tissue. Hence, pus collects beneath the thick dermis.

Surgical Anatomy of the Palmar Fascia and Aponeurosis (Fig. 24.12)

- The central, thick, fibrous part of the palmar fascia is the palmar aponeurosis.
- The palmar fascia covers the long flexors.
- The apex of the triangular palmar aponeurosis is continuous with the flexor retinaculum and the palmaris longus tendon.
- Distally, it forms 4 longitudinal digital bands that attach to the bases of the proximal phalanges.
- Two (medial and lateral) fibrous septa extend from the medial and lateral margins of the palmar aponeurosis. The septa are attached to 5th and 3rd metacarpals, respectively.
- Deep to the flexor tendons, digital arteries and nerves lie in the midpalmar space.
- The midpalmar space is continuous with the anterior compartment of the forearm *via* the carpal tunnel. This space is called the '**space of Parona**' (Fig. 24.13).

Source of Infection

- Penetrating injuries
- Haematoma
- Suppurative tenosynovitis

Clinical Features

- Obliteration of the *normal concavity of the palm*
- *Gross oedema* of the dorsum of the hand
- *Extreme tenderness* in the midpalmar space
- Fingers are held in *flexion* at the *metacarpophalangeal **(MP)*** joint because the palmar aponeurosis gets relaxed in this position. ***MP** joint movements are painful.*
- IP (interphalangeal) joint movements are not painful.

Pearls of Wisdom

Thus, swollen palm, oedema of the dorsum of the hand, flexed attitude of the MP joint, and separated fingers give the picture of a frog hand.

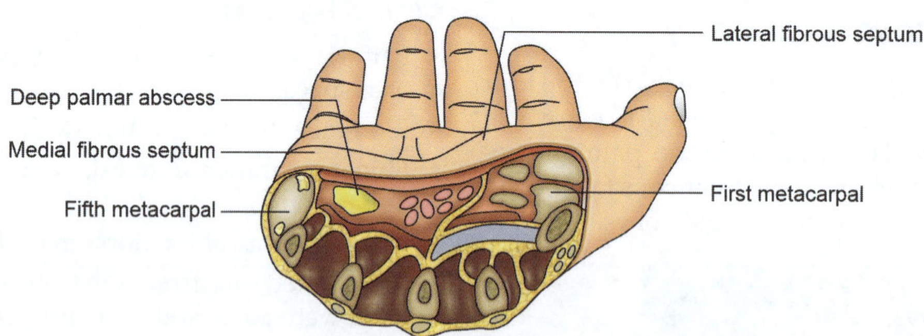

Fig. 24.12: Cross-section showing deep palmar space

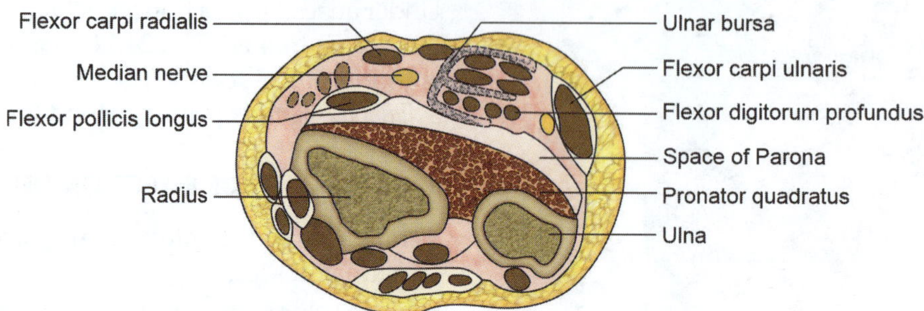

Fig. 24.13: Space of Parona and its relationship to other structures

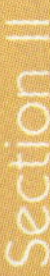

Treatment

- Under anaesthesia, a transverse crease incision is made until the palmar aponeurosis is seen, which is split *longitudinally* in the direction of the fibres *to avoid damage to the nerves and vessels.*
- The abscess cavity is treated as per the usual manner.

ACUTE SUPPURATIVE TENOSYNOVITIS[1]

Surgical Anatomy of the Flexor Tendon Sheath Arrangements (Fig. 24.14)

- The flexor tendon sheaths which enclose the tendons run along the entire length of the finger. In the palm, the medial tendons are enclosed by a common synovial pocket called the "ulnar bursa," whereas the lateral tendons are enclosed by the "radial bursa."
- These two bursae communicate in 75% of the cases. In 25% of the cases, the flexor tendon sheath of the thumb communicates with the radial bursa, and that of the little finger communicates with the ulnar bursa.
- Thus, infection flexor tendon sheaths may involve the entire hand.
- The flexor tendons sheaths extend from the base of the terminal phalanges to the heads of the metacarpal bones.

Clinical Features (Key Box 24.3, Figs 24.15 and 24.16)

- The patient gives a history of a pricking injury.
- Symmetrical, fusiform, painful enlargement of the fingers.
- Fixed, flexed fingers—***'Hook sign'***
- ***IP joint movements are very painful:*** Severe pain on passive finger extension.

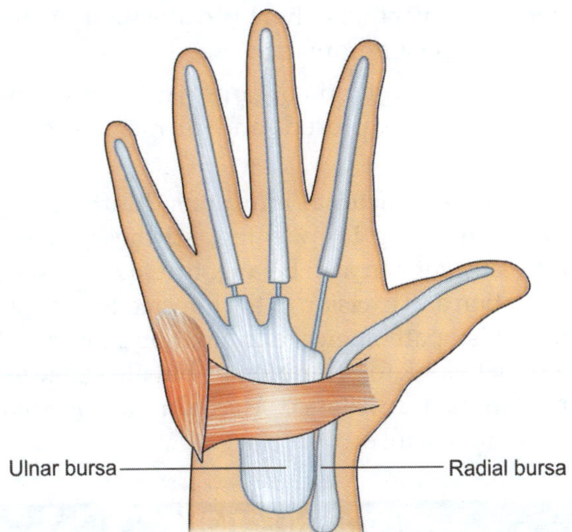

Fig. 24.14: Flexor tendon sheath arrangements

Key Box 24.3

Suppurating Tenosynovitis

- Sharp prick injuries
- Hook sign—bent finger
- IP joint movements painful
- MP joint movements need not be painful
- **'Kanavel's sign'**

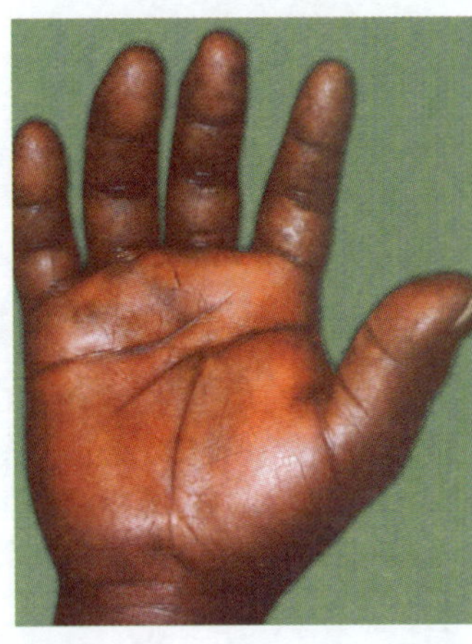

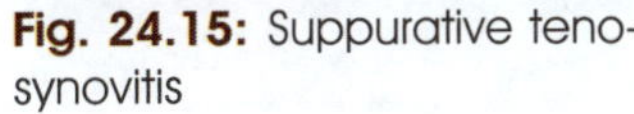

Fig. 24.15: Suppurative tenosynovitis

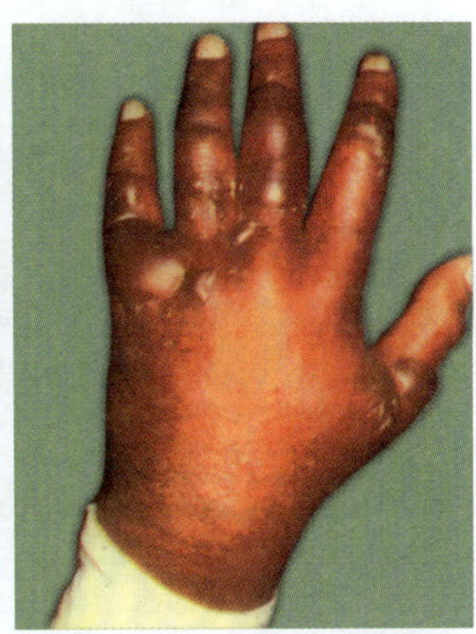

Fig. 24.16: Grossly swollen hand in a diabetic patient. It was looking dangerous, but responded to conservative line of treatment

- ***MP joint movements are not painful:*** This sign differentiates suppurating tenosynovitis from a deep palmar abscess.
- Similarly, when there is infection of the radial bursa, there is tenderness over the lateral side, over the flexor pollicis longus sheath.

Kanavel's Four Cardinal Signs of Flexor Tenosynovitis

1. The finger is held in flexion because this increases the volume of the synovial sheath and eases pain.
2. Symmetrical fusiform swelling of the entire finger.
3. Passive extension of the affected digit produces exquisite pain.
4. Maximum tenderness is at the proximal cul-de-sac of the synovial sheath of the index, middle, and ring fingers in the distal palm.

Treatment

- Under anaesthesia, multiple incisions may have to be given to decompress the flexor tendon sheaths to relieve tension and drain the pus, exudate, etc.
- The cavity is irrigated with antiseptic solution.

[1]Henry Hamilton Bailey lost his left index finger because of acute tenosynovitis.

- In severe cases, a small plastic catheter should be introduced into the synovial bursa and should exit by a counter-incision in the palm for antibiotic irrigation.
- Postoperatively, appropriate antibiotics should be given for about 2 weeks.
- The hand should be in an elevated position to reduce oedema.

Complications

1. Stiffness of the fingers
2. Suppurating arthritis of the joints
3. Osteomyelitis
4. Loss of tendon, digit
5. Spread of infection to space of Parona. It is the space deep to the flexor profundus and superficial to the pronator quadratus in the lower end of the forearm. Patients present with swelling of the forearm along with gross oedema of the hand. In addition to the treatment mentioned above, a separate incision may have to be given in the lower forearm for better drainage of pus.

GENERAL PRINCIPLES OF HAND INFECTION MANAGEMENT

- Early diagnosis and splinting.
- Early proper drainage
- Proper incision—preferably a crease incision
- Elevation of the hand to reduce oedema
- Pus culture and sensitivity
- Cloxacillin 500 mg 6th hourly and metronidazole 400 mg 8th hourly for 7–10 days. Higher antibiotics such as cephalosporins may have to be given.
- Physiotherapy to decrease stiffness of the fingers.
- Tetanus prophylaxis in high-risk patients.

Recommended Antibiotics

Staphylococcus aureus: First generation cephalosporins.

Anaerobics/*Escherichia coli*: Clindamycin or β-lactamase inhibitors, amoxicillin clavulanate potassium.

Herpetic Whitlow: Antivirals.

Position of Hand Functions (Fig. 24.17)

The hand is held as if holding a cup/glass, with the thumb in alignment with the forearm.

- Extension at wrist: 25°
- Flexion at metacarpophalangeal joint: 60°
- Flexion at interphalangeal joint: 10°
- Flexion at distal interphalangeal joint: 5°

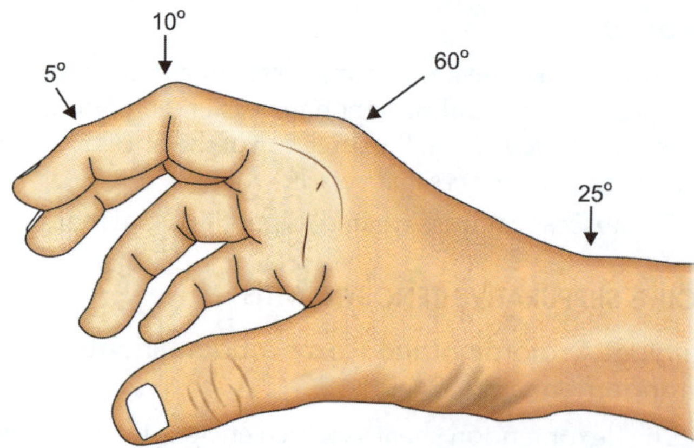

Fig. 24.17: Position of functions

OTHER HAND INFECTIONS

1. Compound palmar ganglion (*see* page 314).
2. Barber's pilonidal sinus (interdigital): It occurs due to repeated clipping by barbers.
3. ***Orf virus infections:*** It is also called ecthyma contagiosum, highly contagious pustular dermatitis due to parapoxvirus infection. It is endemic in sheep and goat herds worldwide. It is transmitted by direct contact. Lesions cannot only occur in hands but also in lips, ear nostrils, etc. Typically, it appears as an ulcerated nodule which is red in colour. It is self-limiting course, may take 1 to 2 months.
4. ***Milker's nodes:*** A viral disease transmitted by handling a cow's udder. Milker's nodules (pseudo cowpox) are harmless skin lesions most commonly seen in persons whose occupation regularly brings them into close contact with cattle. Lesions are multiple swellings with central ulceration. Like any other hand infections, there is oedema of the hands. Treatment is symptomatic.
5. ***Human bites:*** Common organism is Staphylococcus. The wound is explored, and proper treatment is given.
6. Atypical mycobacterial infections: It affects tendon sheaths resulting in swelling, stiffness, pain, and redness. Fever can also be a feature. Diagnosis is by exploration and excision of the infected tendon sheath lining. Histopathological examination should include not only to look for granulomas but also gene expert for Rifampicin resistance. *Mycobacterium marinum* is the common cause.

FOOT INFECTIONS

MYCETOMA PEDIS

Also called Madura Foot or Maduramycosis.

Definition: Mycetoma is a chronic, progressive and suppurative subcutaneous granulomatous infection characterized by painless swelling and draining sinus tracts, and purulent discharge. This type of process of swelling or becoming tumorous like phenomenon is described as tumefaction.

Types

1. **Bacterial mycetoma:** It is due to *Nocardia madurae* or Actinomyces. These organisms are normally present in the soil.
2. **Fungal mycetoma:** It is caused by *Madurella mycetoma*, etc.

Etiopathogenesis

- Male farmers between the 20 and 40 years of age are affected. Foot is the commonest site. Rarely it may involve the hands, back, or shoulders.
- Barefoot walking, which results in repeated minor trauma, implants the organisms within the subcutaneous tissue.
- Ultimate result is chronic granulomatous lesions of the foot involving the skin and subcutaneous tissues.
- The disease also involves deeper structures like bones, resulting in osteomyelitis.
- **Gross thickening of the subcutaneous tissue results in characteristic convexity (flattening) of the instep of the foot** (Fig. 24.18).

Clinical Features

- It starts as a **pale, painless, single nodule**. Later, multiple nodules develop and rupture, resulting in multiple sinuses.
- Chronic suppuration, **multiple sinuses**, and **sulphur granules** in the discharge are also characteristic of mycetoma pedis.

Diagnosis

- Sulphur granules in the discharge: Actinomycotic grains typically have Gram-negative centers with fine, branched Gram-positive filaments. In cases of eumycetomas, a mass of Gram-negative septate hyphae embedded in intercellular cement with wider filaments are found.

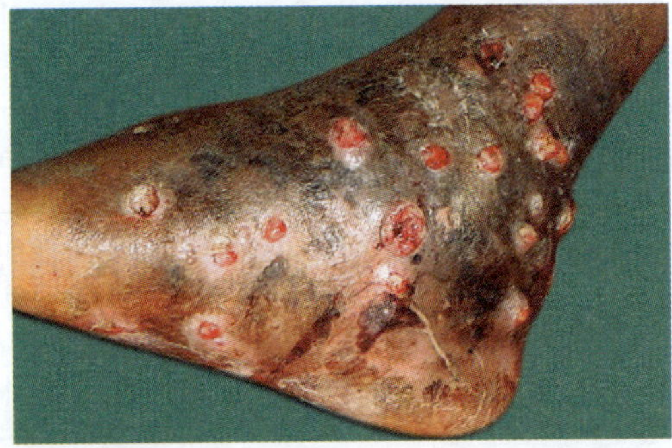

Fig. 24.18: Flattening of the foot (*Courtesy:* Prof Madakatti, Head, Department of Surgery, Karnataka Institute of Medical Sciences, Hubli, Karnataka)

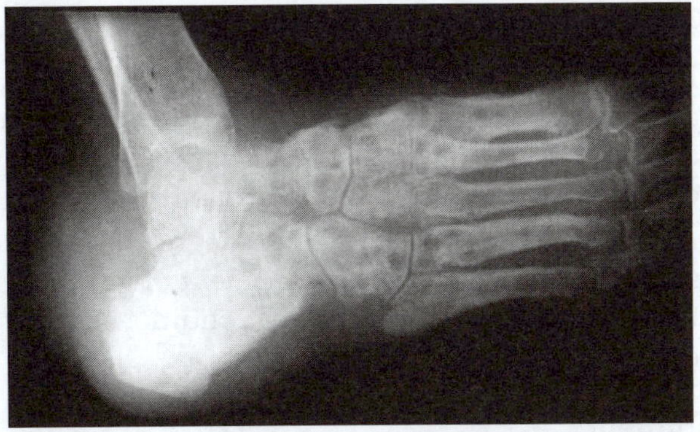

Fig. 24.19: Plain radiograph of the foot showing extensive rarefaction of the bones

- Plain radiograph of the foot (Fig. 24.19) may show soft tissue shadow, lytic lesions, periosteal reactions and sclerosis.
- CT/MRI: Dot in a circle sign is characteristic of mycetoma pedis. Done for assessment of bone and soft tissue involvement.
- FNAC: It can be taken when there is a mass like lesion. It can show the characteristic histopathologic changes such as polymorphous inflammatory cells intermixed with grains, neutrophils, lymphocytes, plasma cells, histiocytes, macrophages, and foreign body giant cells.
- Biopsy is important to determine the causative organism.

Treatment

- Broad-spectrum antibiotics to treat secondary infection along with **dapsone (drug of choice) 100 mg twice daily**. Treatment may have to be continued for 1–2 years.
- Fungal mycetoma may not respond to antibiotics and may be treated with ketoconazole.
- A combination of trimethoprim/sulfamethoxazole and rifampicin may also be tried.
- Amputation may be necessary in refractory cases to get rid of a deformed, diseased limb.

Mucocutaneous Splendore-Hoeppli Phenomenon

- It refers to the accumulation of eosinophilic material (asteroid-like) around microorganisms, known as 'asteroid bodies.'
- Fungal and bacterial infections may give rise to this (e.g. actinomycosis, candidiasis, etc.)
- This phenomenon results due to a localised immunological response to an antigen–antibody precipitate.

INGROWN TOENAIL (ONYCHOCRYPTOSIS)

- It is also described as an embedded toenail. The exact aetiology is not clear. However, a few patients have a family history of this condition. Excessive trimming of the nail may result in an ingrown toenail.
- As the nail grows inside, some degree of infection sets in, resulting in the development of granulation tissue which starts pouting. The condition is painful, disturbing, and unsightly.

Treatment

- **Conservative:** Dressing with antiseptic agents such as iodine. Copper sulphate may be applied to treat extra granulation tissue. Appropriate antibiotics are given.
- **Surgical:** Under local anaesthesia, a portion of the involved nail up to the base is removed, followed by application of phenol to the growing point of the nailbed at its base. It takes about 10–15 days for complete healing.
- **Zadik' s or Fowler' s operation:** The principle of this radical procedure is to expose the lateral spike and germinal matrix. This is achieved by incising the skin over the lateral margin and root of the nail.

MISCELLANEOUS

Pyogenic Granuloma (Fig. 24.20)

- It is not a true granuloma, but a capillary haemangioma
- It is due to trauma, not infection (pyogenic is a misnomer)
- It is smooth, red, and lobulated
- It may be painful
- It bleeds due to minor trauma
- In fingers, persistent irritation may result in excessive granulation tissue
- It may also occur in the oral cavity
- It is also known as 'pregnancy tumour' .

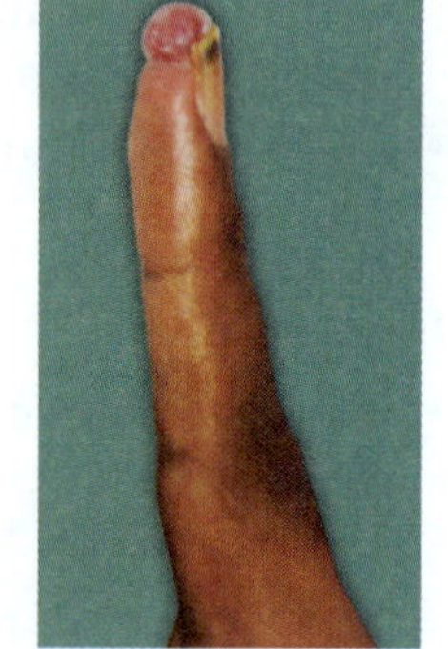

Fig. 24.20: Pyogenic granuloma

TENDON TRANSFER[1,2]

Tendon transfer surgeries are a highly useful form of reconstruction wherein the actions of lost or weakened neuromuscular action are supplemented or substituted by redirecting the action of other intact and relatively expendable musculo-tendinous units. Thus, certain actions and abilities that are deemed more important are reconstructed at the expense of others.

Several of these procedures have been described, developed, and popularized by Indian surgeons such as Paul Brand, Srinivasan, Fritchie, Antia among others. The surgical techniques and principles of tendon transfer underwent a lot of development under these illustrious surgeons especially for the treatment of nerve palsy from Hansen's disease which used to be endemic to certain parts of our country.

All tendon transfer surgeries follow certain principles which are paramount to the success of these highly sophisticated and technically demanding procedures. They require accurate realignment of the direction of force of the transferred musculotendinous unit as well preservation of transferred elements with minimal damage to the donor tissue. Success of the procedure also requires that both the surgeon and the patient understand the functional and aesthetic goals along with the limitations and expectations of surgery.

The basic principles of tendon transfer are as follows:

1. Supple joints prior to transfer: Prior to the procedure, the joint that the tendon transfer will move must be supple and have maximum x range of motion when moved passively.
2. Soft tissue equilibrium: The tissues through which the tendon transfer is negotiated must be healthy and free of any edema, inflammation or scar. These may hinder tendo-muscular glide and optimal wound healing following tendon transfer.
3. Donor of adequate excursion: The maximum linear movement of the transferred Musculo-Tendinous Unit (MTU) or its change in length on contracting or relaxing should be adequate to achieve the desired hand movement. The MTU chosen for transfer should ideally have an excursion similar that of the tendon which it is replacing.
4. Donor of adequate strength: The MTU to be transferred must be strong enough to achieve the desired movement, but at the same time, should not be too strong. A donor MTU that is too weak will have inadequate movement and function, while a donor that is too strong will result in imbalanced movement and inappropriate posture at rest. Thus, MTU chosen for transfer should ideally have strength similar that of the tendon which it is replacing.
5. Expendable donor: Use of a potential donor MTU for transfer, may result in some degree of weakness, loss of movement, or imbalance. These must not be more debilitating than the function it is replacing. Further, the choice of the donor MTU should preferably be those which have other MTUs that serve a since purpose or perform similar actions.
6. Straight line of pull: Tendon transfers are most effective if the MTU provides straight line of pull. Direction changes diminish the force that the transferred MTU is able to exert on its insertion.

However, change of direction may be required in a few cases and utilize pulleys to bring about this directional change.

7. Synergy: Muscle groups (finger flexors or wrist extensors) usually work together to perform a function or movement. MTU utilized for transfer must be synergistic to the function it is replacing with rare exceptions. Thus, extensors are not used to replace flexor actions and vice versa.
8. Single function per transfer: It is ideal to attempt achieving just single function out of a single MTU transfer. Every transfer will result in compromised strength and movement. There is an inherent tendency to lose at least one grade of power (MRC grade) when a tendon transfer is performed.

REFERENCES

1. Tendon Transfers Part I: Principles of Transfer and Transfers for Radial Nerve Palsy. Douglas M. Sammer, MD1 and Kevin C. Chung, MD, MS2.
2. Green's Operative Hand Surgery, 2-Volume Set, 8th Edition.

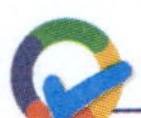

Multiple Choice Questions

1. Which of the following statements are false regarding paronychia?

A. It is caused by a fungal infection
B. It is a deep infection
C. It is the most common hand infection
D. Infection spreads beneath the eponychium

2. The following are true for terminal pulp space infection *except*:

A. It is called 'felon'
B. It may cause digital arterial thrombosis
C. Osteomyelitis of the distal phalanx will not occur due to extensive collaterals
D. Pyogenic arthritis may occur

3. The following are true for deep palmar abscess *except*:

A. It is an infection of the midpalmar space
B. Interphalangeal joint movements are very painful
C. Metacarpophalangeal joint movements are very painful
D. It communicates with the anterior compartment of the forearm

4. Kanavel's sign is:

A. Tenderness over the pulp space
B. Tenderness over the midpalmar space
C. Tenderness over the radial bursa
D. Tenderness over the ulnar bursa

5. Space of Parona refers to:

A. Space deep to the palmar aponeurosis
B. Space deep to the flexor digitorum superficialis
C. Space deep to the flexor profundus
D. Space deep to the flexor carpi ulnaris

6. The following are true for acute suppurating tenosynovitis *except*:

A. Finger is fixed and flexed
B. Interphalangeal joint movements are not painful
C. Metacarpophalangeal joint movements may be painful
D. Kanavel's sign may be positive

7. The characteristic feature of mycetoma pedis is:

A. The disease affects bones
B. It starts as a pale, painless, single nodule
C. It causes extensive rarefaction of the bone
D. There is convexity of the instep of the foot

8. The following are clinical features of mycetoma pedis *except*:

A. Crepitus
B. Multiple sinuses
C. Gross thickening of the subcutaneous tissues
D. Chronic nature

9. Pyogenic granuloma is due to:

A. Bacterial infection B. Viral infection
C. Fungal infection D. Trauma

10. The following are principles of hand infection management *except*:

A. Hand should be elevated
B. Early splinting
C. Tetanus prophylaxis in high-risk patient
D. Pencillin is the drug of choice

Answers

1. B 2. C 3. B 4. D 5. C 6. B 7. D 8. A 9. D 10. D

CHAPTER

25

Chronic Infectious Disease

- Actinomycosis
- Leprosy
- Deformities in leprosy
- Syphilis
- AIDS

Competency

SU6.1: Define and describe the aetiology and pathogenesis of surgical infections.

INTRODUCTION

Actinomycosis, leprosy, syphilis, and AIDS are the chronic diseases discussed in this chapter. Actinomycosis is a rare disease, leprosy and syphilis of more interest to dermatologists, and AIDS is an interesting topic to all clinicians. Hence, only relevant aspects of each of these diseases, as far as general surgeons are concerned, will be discussed here.

ACTINOMYCOSIS

Mycetoma are of two types. Eumycetoma is caused by fungi and actinomycosis is caused by bacteria. It predominantly occurs in the mycetoma belt that lies between the latitudes 15°S and 30°N, comprising countries such as Sudan, Somalia, India, Argentina, Mexico, etc.

Actinomycosis is caused by *Actinomyces israelii*, an anaerobic, gram-positive, branching, filamentous organism (ray fungus). It is normally present in the oral cavity, tonsillar crypts, and dental cavities. They become pathogenic in the presence of trauma. Other species include *A. neuri* and *A. neyeri*.

Three types of actinomycosis which are of interest to general surgeons are discussed here.

FACIOCERVICAL ACTINOMYCOSIS (50%)

- It is the most common manifestation of actinomycosis.
- It is common in patients with poor oral hygiene, bad caries tooth, etc.
- Diabetes mellitus, immunosuppression, local tissue damage secondary to radiation and neoplasia may precipitate actinomycosis.
- There is subacute or chronic inflammation for many months to years and a lumpy jaw (Key Box 25.1).
- Eventually, the cheek, mandible, jaws, and salivary glands are involved, resulting in suppuration. The most common site is the mandible.

Key Box 25.1

Differential Diagnosis

- Jaw tumour
- Osteomyelitis of jaw
- Malignancy of oral cavity

Clinical Features

Two patterns are identified:

1. Chronic slowly progressive inflammation resulting in an indurated mass.
   - **Extensive (marked) induration** of the lower jaw (mandible) and gums give the consistency of bone.
   - **Multiple subcutaneous nodules** over bluish skin covering the jaw.
   - The nodules rupture, resulting in ***multiple discharging sinuses***.
   - The discharge contains ***sulphur granules*** which contain gram-positive mycelia surrounded by gram-negative clubs.
2. Less commonly, it may present as an acute suppurative infection with rapid progression to abscess formation. This causes pain, trismus, dyspnoea, and dysphagia.
   - **Lymph nodes are not involved.** It spreads mainly by direct extension.

- **Triad of actinomycosis:** Subcutaneous mass, multiple sinuses, and seropurulent discharge.

ACTINOMYCOSIS OF THE THORAX AND LUNG (30%)

- It is common in children, and is caused by inhalation of ray fungus.
- Over a period of years, it produces actinomycosis of the lung with involvement of the pleura. Later, it also involves the chest wall, resulting in multiple discharging sinuses.
- There may be associated empyema and it may easily spread to the liver.

ACTINOMYCOSIS OF THE RIGHT ILIAC FOSSA AND LIVER (ABDOMINAL ACTINOMYCOSIS—20%)

- It commonly occurs after surgery when there is **mucosal injury** or discontinuity (e.g. after appendicectomy, after perforation of hollow viscus, neoplasia).
- The organisms which are normally present in the gut slowly migrate into the pericaecal tissue, then into the soft tissue and subcutaneous tissue, and produce subacute or chronic low-grade inflammation.
- No compromise of the bowel lumen.
- Once the portal venous radical gets involved, it spreads to the liver.

Clinical Features

- History of appendicectomy is present in almost all cases.
- 3–6 months later, fever and a swelling in the right iliac fossa appear.
- On examination, there is an indurated, nodular, and fixed mass in the right iliac fossa.
- Late stages produce multiple discharging sinuses, sometimes discharging faecal matter and sulphur granules. Unlike tuberculosis, the lymph nodes are not enlarged.

Differential Diagnosis

- Carcinoma caecum, Crohn's ileocolitis, pericolic abscess, etc.

Management of Actinomycosis in General

- It is a low-grade chronic disease and is difficult to eradicate.
- Inj. crystalline penicillin 10 lakh units once a day for 6 months–1 year. Tetracycline and lincomycin are alternatives. Amoxycillin 500 mg thrice daily may have to be given for 2–6 months.
- Sinuses in the jaw may have to be excised.
- Osteomyelitis has to be curetted out.
- Actinomycosis of the right iliac fossa may require a right hemicolectomy. Surgery is not easy. Often, there is extensive necrosis and abscess formation. Malignancy cannot be ruled out. If possible, resect. Otherwise, excise the fistulae, drain the abscesses, and administer IV antibiotics.

LEPROSY (HANSEN'S DISEASE)

- Leprosy is caused by *Mycobacterium leprae*, an acid-fast bacillus. Poverty, poor hygiene, and population (overcrowding) facilitate its spread.
- The disease is contracted in childhood or adolescence, but manifests after a latent period of 2–5 years.
- **Nasal secretions** are the main source of infection but *active ulcers and sweat* also contain lepra bacilli.
- Leprosy predominantly affects the **skin, upper respiratory tract (nasal cavity), and nerves**. Thus, characteristic lesions of leprosy include an anaesthetic patch of skin, or hypopigmented macule, thickened nerves, a deformed leonine face, and a collapsed nasal bridge.

Types (Table 25.1)

1. **Tuberculoid leprosy:** It occurs in patients with good immunity/strong tissue response.
2. **Lepromatous leprosy:** It occurs in patients with poor immunity/poor tissue response.
3. **Borderline leprosy:** It may be borderline lepromatous or borderline tuberculoid leprosy, depending on the immune response.

Table 25.1 Comparison of tuberculoid leprosy with lepromatous leprosy

	Tuberculoid leprosy	Lepromatous leprosy
1. Cell-mediated immunity	Strong	Low
2. Histology	Giant cells, epithelioid cells, histiocytes, lymphocytes are present. Bacilli are a few.	Bacilli distending the macrophages—'GLOBI'. Plenty of bacilli invading nerves, adnexa, sweat glands, etc.
3. Clinical	Localised. Anaesthetic, hypopigmented, raised skin patch. Early nerve damage, nerve thickening is a characteristic feature. Involvement of face and nose is not seen.	Generalised. Erythematous multiple macular rashes. Nerve involvement is usually not seen. Leonine facies, collapse of the bridge of the nose are characteristic.
4. Prognosis	Good	Not good

Diagnosis of Leprosy

1. **Skin biopsy:** A full-thickness biopsy is taken from the most active margin of the most active lesion and subjected to acid-fast staining. Skin smears may be taken from ears, elbows, and knees.
2. **PCR:** Polymerase chain reaction is used to detect *M. leprae* DNA.
   Note: No other blood test is available.

Treatment

1. **Lepromatous and borderline lepromatous leprosy (multibacillary disease)**
   - 3-drug regimen is the most ideal treatment.
     Dapsone 100 mg/day
     Clofazimine 50 mg/day
     Rifampicin 600 mg once monthly, supervised.
     Clofazimine 300 mg once monthly, supervised.
     } For a minimum period of 2 years. Skin smear should be negative.
2. **Tuberculoid and borderline tuberculoid leprosy (paucibacillary disease)**
   - Dapsone 100 mg daily
   - Rifampicin 600 mg once a month, supervised.
   } For a period of 6 months.

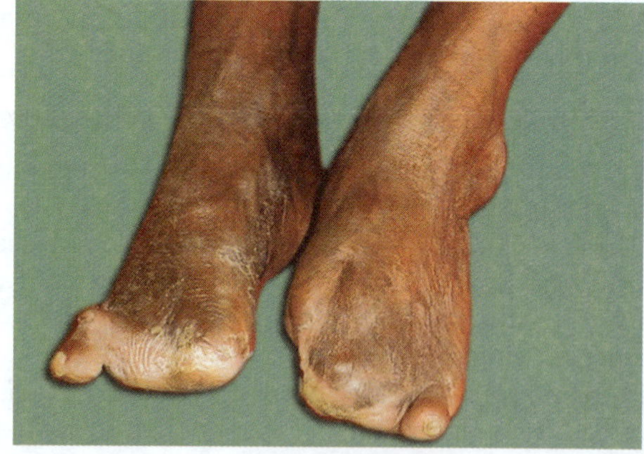

Fig. 25.2: Autoamputation of the toes in a case of leprosy

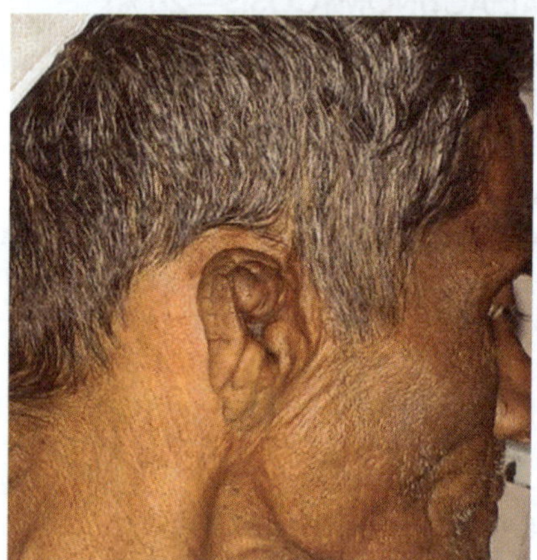

Leonine facies, collapse of the bridge of the nose are a few other features of lepromatous leprosy

Fig. 25.3: Observe deformed ear

DEFORMITIES IN LEPROSY

I. Primary Deformity (Figs 25.1 to 25.3)

They occur directly due to the disease.

- **Face:** It is involved in lepromatous leprosy and is described as 'leonine facies' with multiple nodules over the face, pigmentation, *loss of the lateral portion* of the eyebrows (madarosis), collapse of the nasal bridge due to destruction of nasal cartilages (warm and moist area), and paralysis of the facial nerve.
- **Hands:** Involvement of the ulnar nerve at the elbow and median nerve at the wrist gives rise to ***claw hand.***
- **Foot:** The posterior tibial nerve is involved at the ankle leading to clawing of the toes. Foot drop occurs when the lateral popliteal nerve below the knee joint is involved.

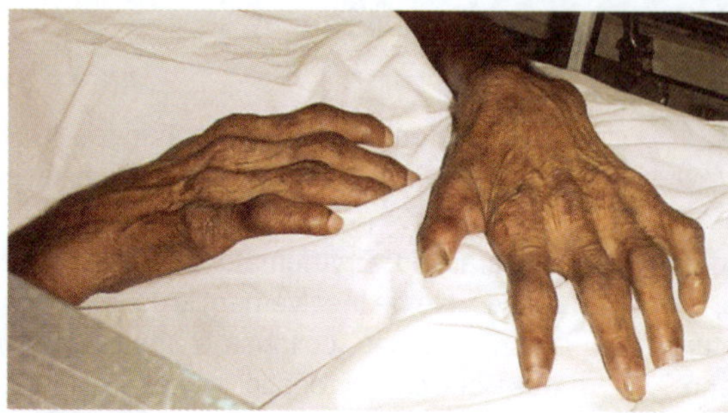

Fig. 25.1: Observe small muscle wasting in both the hands

Clinical Notes

MS exam case, KMC, Manipal (2004)

A 28-year-old lady complained of swelling in the posterior triangle of 8 months duration. The swelling was tender, a bit irregular, and had restricted mobility. 3 candidates offered nonspecific lymphadenitis as a diagnosis. Only one candidate thought of a nerve abscess. The clue was a thickened nerve above. It was a case of Hansen's disease (Fig. 25.4).

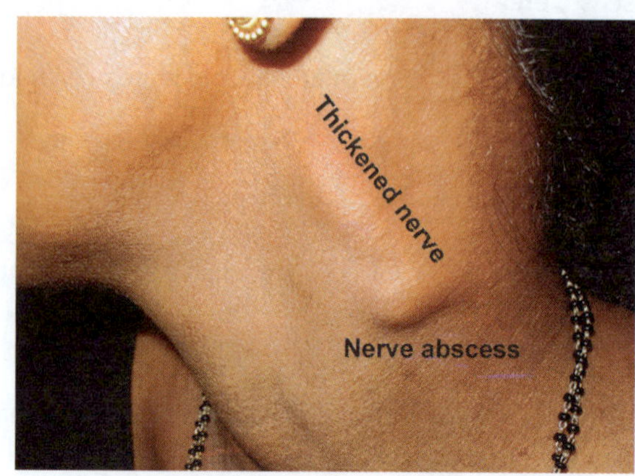

Fig. 25.4: Nerve abscess and thickened postauricular nerve

Section II • General Surgery

Ulnar Nerve Abscess (Key Box 25.2, Fig. 25.5) and Small Muscle Atrophy in the Hand (Fig. 25.6)

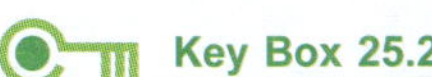 Key Box 25.2

Ulnar Nerve Abscess

- May be a part of pure neuritic leprosy.
- Presents as oval fluctuant swelling on the medial side of arm.
- Granuloma is common. Progression to abscess occurs in tuberculoid leprosy.
- **Schwann cell** is affected. Slowly whole endoneurial zone is occupied by endothelial cells.
- High resolution ultrasound can demonstrate echotexture of masses.
- MRI—with the post-gadolinium T_1W sequence—peripheral rim enhancement with central necrosis.
- Treatment: Incision, drainage, excision of granulomatous mass followed by treatment for leprosy.

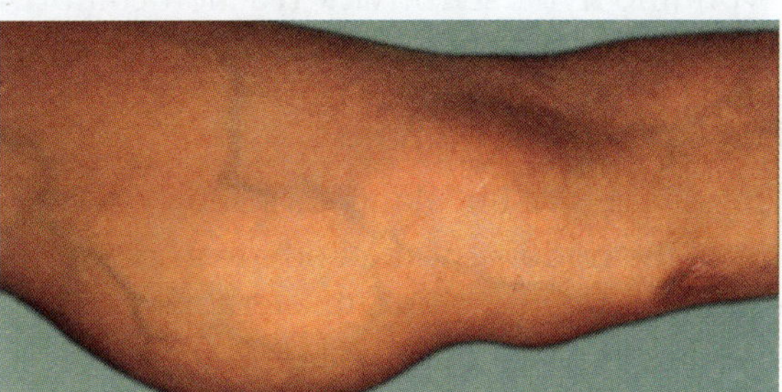

Fig. 25.5: Ulnar nerve abscess

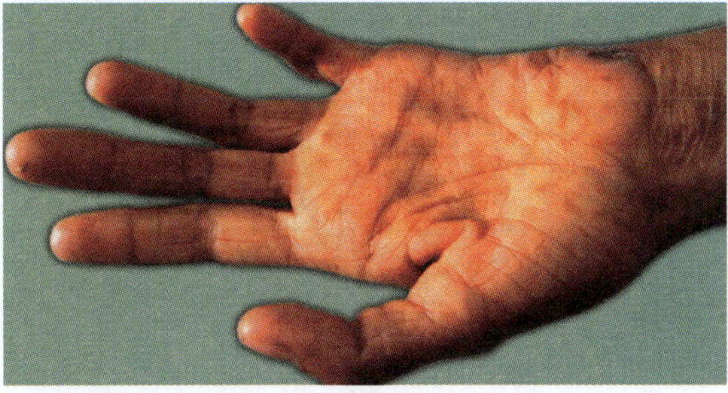

Fig. 25.6: Small muscles atrophy in the hand

Clinical Notes

A 33-year-old male presented to the outpatient department with inability to use his right hand for the last 6 months. He said he could not work or hold objects. Examination revealed small muscle atrophy, especially of the hypothenar and interossei muscles. A 2 cm 'skin ulcer' was also noticed. On careful questioning, he said he also had loss of sensation. Further examination revealed a 4-cm × 3-cm, firm, oval swelling on the medial side of his right arm, with some amount of fluctuation.

What is the diagnosis?

Ulnar nerve abscess (cold) secondary to leprosy. This is a case of pure neuritic leprosy with nerve abscess, an uncommon manifestation of *M. leprae*. No other peripheral nerve was involved.

Correction of Facial Deformities by Plastic Reconstruction

1. Prosthesis to correct the nose.
2. Lateral tarsorrhaphy to prevent exposure keratitis.
3. Temporalis muscle flap for the upper eyelid to prevent exposure keratitis.

Correction of Hand and Foot Deformities

- Claw hand may be corrected using the extensor carpi radialis brevis **(Paul Brand's procedure)**. Otherwise, the flexor digitorum superficialis may be used **(Bunnell's procedure)**.
- Foot drop may be corrected by using a tibialis posterior tendon transfer **(Ober's and Barr's procedure)**.

II. Secondary Deformities

Because of nerve involvement, sensations are impaired or lost. As a result, ulcers on the fingers, a deep, penetrating, *perforating* ulcer over sole of the foot, or even autoamputation of the toes may occur.

Treatment of Secondary Deformities

Nonhealing ulcer over the sole of foot is corrected with application of a POP (plaster of Paris) posterior slab off loading or nonweight-bearing cast. It takes off the pressure to help the ulcer heal. If the calcaneus is involved due to osteomyelitis, the bone has to be curetted out, followed by the application of regular dressings.

SYPHILIS: FRENCH DISEASE, GREAT POX

- This is a sexually transmitted disease caused by *Treponema pallidum*. It is a delicate spiral organism (spirochaete).
- Syphilis is infective only in its early stage. Early lesions are predominantly situated in moist areas, such as the genitalia and oral cavity.

Clinical Presentation

Key Box 25.3 describes congenital syphilis

I. Early syphilis

II. Late syphilis

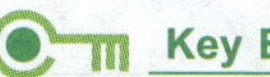 Key Box 25.3

Congenital Syphilis

Early

- Snuffles (rhinitis), epiphysitis, periostitis, osteochondritis.

Late

- **Hutchinson's triad**
  - Interstitial keratitis
  - 8th nerve deafness
  - Hutchinson's teeth

I. Early Syphilis

1. **Primary syphilis:** Classically, a genital chancre occurs in the penis or vulva after 3–4 weeks of sexual exposure.
   - The chancre is a shallow, indurated, painless ulcer called *Hunterian chancre* (Fig. 25.7). Associated inguinal nodes, which are shotty, multiple, and nontender clinch the diagnosis.
   - Extragenital chancres may occur over the lips, tongue, nipple, etc. They produce large enlargement of the corresponding lymph nodes. Chancres in the rectum and perianal region are common in homosexuals. They are painful and resemble anal fissures.

   Investigations

   Serological tests for syphilis

   A. **Nonspecific:** VDRL, Kahn, Meinicke, Wasserman
   B. **Specific treponemal antigen tests**
      - CFT—complement fixation test
      - TPHA—TP haemagglutination test
      - TPI—TP immobilisation test
      - FTA-Abs—fluorescent treponema antibody absorption test
      - Demonstration of *Treponema pallidum* in the clear exudate of the lesion by dark field microscopy confirms the diagnosis.
2. **Secondary syphilis:** It appears after 6–12 weeks of spirochaetaemia.
   - It is characterised by ***bilateral, symmetrical, coppery red rashes*** which are generalised. The *rash* is macular or papular, but *never vesicular.* Papules on moist sites such as the vulva and perineum enlarge to form condylomata lata—fleshy wart-like growths.
   - Small superficial ulcers in the mouth join to form ***snail track ulcers.***
   - Generalised lymphadenopathy involving the epitrochlear and occipital nodes may occur.
   - Moth-eaten alopecia, iritis, bone and joint pains.

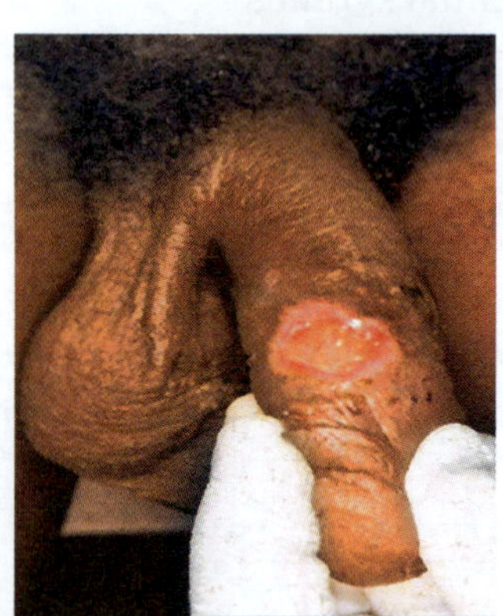
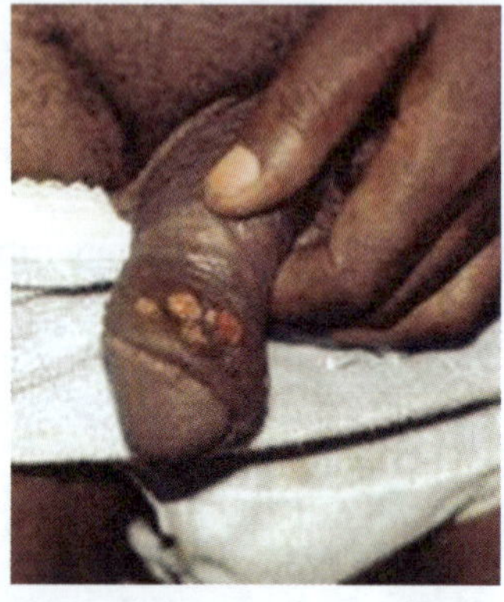

Fig. 25.7: Genital chancres

3. **Latent syphilis:** If secondary syphilis is not treated, it will develop into latent syphilis. There are no signs, but serum tests are positive.

II. Late Syphilis

It is also called tertiary syphilis. It basically affects vessels causing inflammatory reactions and the end result is as follows: 'Endarteritis obliterans' ! tissue necrosis ! ulcers or fibrosis.

This stage develops after 5–15 years of primary syphilis. It causes neurosyphilis and cardiovascular syphilis (aortitis).

Neurosyphilis includes general paresis and tabes dorsalis involving the posterior column and dorsal roots. It presents with sensory atonia, lancinating pain, and Argyll Robertson pupils.

A lesser form is a benign lesion called *gumma.* Gumma is a syphilitic hypersensitivity reaction comprising a granuloma with central necrosis and sloughing.

Clinical Features of Gumma

- Typically, it is a subcutaneous swelling.
- Affects the midline of the body (e.g. posterior one-third of the tongue, sternum, sternoclavicular joint).
- Edges are ***punched out*** if the gumma ulcerates.
- Floor contains ***wash leather slough.***
- On healing, it leaves a **silvery, tissue paper scar** (thin scar).

Pearls of Wisdom

Gumma may also involve the bone, testis, and liver (ovary is not involved).

Treatment

1. *Primary and secondary syphilis* are treated by Inj. procaine penicillin 2.4 MU in 1 ml stat. Doxycycline 100 mg BID is given for 21 days. Tetracycline 500 mg QID is also given.
2. *In tertiary/latent syphilis*: Inj. procaine penicillin 2.4 MU IM once a week for 3 weeks.
3. *In late syphilis:* Treatment is continued for 21 days. With the current effective treatment of syphilis, it is highly unusual to find late cases now.

AIDS AND THE GENERAL SURGEON

- **A**cquired **I**mmuno**d**eficiency **S**yndrome (**AIDS**) is the end stage of a progressive state of immunodeficiency.

  Causative organism: *Human immunodeficiency virus* (HIV).

- The details regarding the aetiopathogenesis and immunology of AIDS are discussed in medicine books. **Topics of surgical interest are discussed below.**

Prophylactic Measures to be adopted by Surgeons (Healthcare Workers) while Treating AIDS Patients (Universal Precautions) (Key Box 25.4)

I. In the Outpatient Department (OPD)

- Wear gloves[1] when examining any patient with an open wound.
- Wear gloves during proctoscopy or sigmoidoscopy.
- Use hand gloves and eye protection during flexible endoscopy.
- Use disposable instruments.
- Clean reusable instruments such as endoscopes with soap and water, and immerse them in glutaraldehyde.
- Do not perform any surgical procedure involving sharp instruments in the OPD.

Key Box 25.4

Summary of Universal Precautions to be taken in OT

Face mask to be worn
Avoid splashing on body: Be slow
Cover feet and legs: Shoe covers, boot
Extra glove: Double glove
Meticulous technique: Haemostasis, gentleness
Allow only required people
Spectacles: Protects from splash
Kidney tray: Use it to transfer sharps
Remember as **FACE MASK**

II. In the Operation Theatre

- Operating table is covered with a single sheet of polythene.
- The number of theatre personnel is reduced to minimum.
- Staff with abrasions or lacerations on their hands are not allowed inside the theatre.
- Staff who enter the theatre must wear shoe covers, gloves, disposable and water-resistant gowns, and eye protection.
- **Double gloves and eye protection** by staff directly involved in the operation (surgeon, assistant, scrub nurse) (Figs 25.8 to 25.10).
- **Surgical technique:**
  1. Avoid 'sharps' and needlestick injuries
  2. Preferably use scissors or diathermy instead of a scalpel
  3. Use **skin clips rather than skin sutures**
  4. Proper autoclaving after the surgery
  5. In the event of needlestick injury, allow the part to bleed and wash thoroughly under tap water.
  6. AZT—zidovudine, lamivudine and indinavir should be given to health workers following exposure of susceptible areas to infected material from AIDS patients.

RANGE OF SURGERY IN HIV-POSITIVE PATIENTS

I. **Anorectal disease** is the most frequent reason for surgical treatment in HIV-positive patients. This is common in homosexuals, in whom AIDS is also common. They have been grouped together as *"AIDS anus syndrome."* **Anorectal disease may be classified** into:

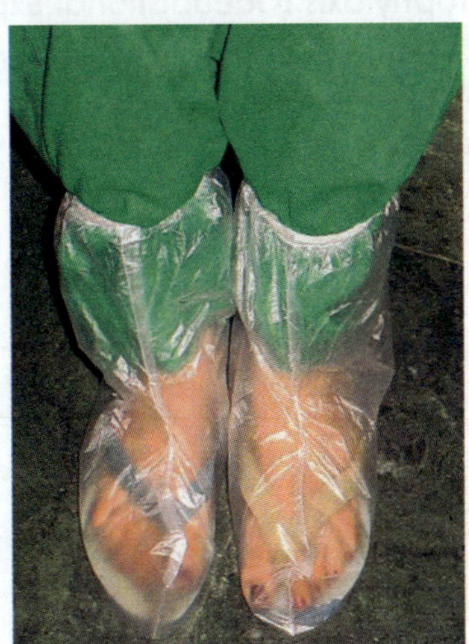

Fig. 25.8: Protection of feet

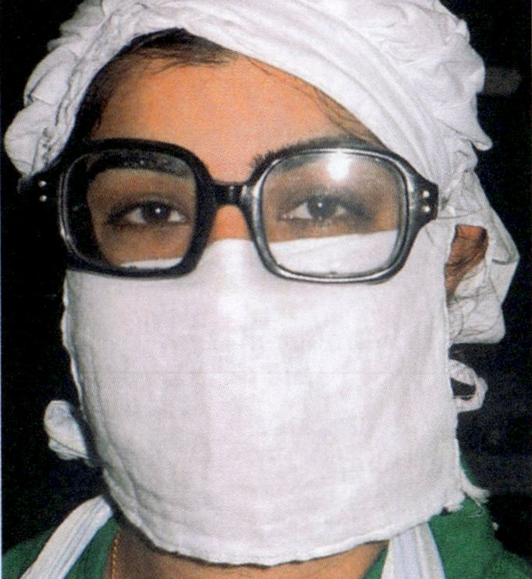

Fig. 25.9: Eye protection

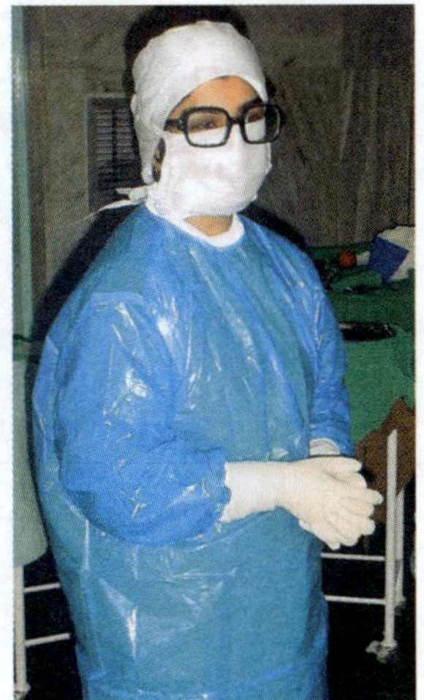

Fig. 25.10: Double glove

[1]Gloves were introduced by William Halsted to protect his nurse's hands from the harmful effects of carbolic acid (the nurse became his wife).

- Anal warts, diarrhoea
- Perianal sepsis—abscesses
- Anal ulceration, fissures
- Reduced sphincter tone and anal incontinence in homosexuals

II. **Abdominal pain:** This is due to a gastrointestinal opportunistic infection, usually caused by cytomegalovirus (CMV). It is a type of colitis and produces abdominal pain, cramps, loose stools, and blood and mucus in the stools, resulting in emaciation. Flexible sigmoidoscopy may reveal severe proctitis. Severe colitis may lead to acute toxic dilatation of the colon.
- Biliary tract infection by cryptosporidium may cause **acute cholecystitis**. AIDS-related sclerosing cholangitis may occur, resulting in right upper quadrant pain.
- **Abdominal lymphoma** with involvement of the liver and spleen may also cause abdominal pain.
- Severe abdominal pain may be due to **perforation** of the small or large bowel and should be treated as an emergency.
- **Appendicitis** is also common due to CMV infection.

III. **Lymphoma, Kaposi's sarcoma, etc.** They occur due to reduced cellular immunity because of:
- Immunosuppression used in organ transplantation
- Severe malnourishment
- HIV infection
- Lymphoproliferative disease (Key Box 25.5)
- Kaposi's sarcoma may affect the skin surface, gastrointestinal tract, lungs, etc. It presents as pigmented multifocal skin lesions.

Key Box 25.5

HIV-associated Lymphomas

1. Lymphomas in HIV patients—'B' symptoms and intra-abdominal and extranodal involvement including lung, bone marrow and liver are common.
2. HIV-associated lymphomas are ***Diffuse Large Cell*** (DLC) or Burkitt's lymphoma.
3. HIV-associated lymphomas present as ascites/pleural effusion, etc.
4. Treatment should be HAART (highly active anti-retroviral therapy) with standard chemotherapy and granulocyte-colony stimulating factor.

IV. **Oesophageal ulcers** may present as dysphagia and odynophagia. Endoscopy should be done using a glove and the scope should be washed thoroughly with soap and water and immersed in cetrimide solution for 15 minutes.

V. **Lymphadenopathy:** Very often, surgeons are called for lymph node biopsy to evaluate fever or generalised lymphadenopathy. All universal precautions must be observed in all patients.

Clinical Notes

A 23-year-old lady, carrying a 6-month-old child, presented to us with severe dysphagia and odynophagia. Endoscopy revealed extensive, unusual, oesophageal ulcers which prompted us to conduct a HIV test. It was positive. We called her husband and wanted to convey the message to him, but before we could, he said, 'I am HIV-positive, my wife is HIV-positive, and even my child is HIV-positive!!!'

Risk of HIV Transmission

- Risk of HIV transmission from patient to surgeon is very low but dangerous.
- Routine use of barriers (gloves and goggles), washing hands before and after examination of the patient, and careful handling of sharps and needles greatly reduce transmission of the disease.
- Post-exposure prophylaxis should begin immediately.
- Routes of exposure and incidence of HIV transmission:
  - Percutaneous—0.3%
  - Cutaneous— 0.09%
  - Mucus membrane—0.09%.

Post-Exposure Prophylaxis (Occupational Exposure)

1. Immediate decontamination of the injured area—washing the area with soap and water for cutaneous and percutaneous exposure. For punctured wounds, clean with alcohol-based agents. For infected eyes, irrigate with a copious amount of sterile water or saline.
2. Early reporting of exposure: Blood tests have to be done.
3. As soon as possible or within 2 hours, post-exposure prophylaxis should be done using the 3-drug regimen given below.

   Raltegravir 400 mg 3 times/day, tenofovir 300 mg/day and emtricitabine 200 mg/day.

Multiple Choice Questions

1. Which of the following statements about actinomycosis is false?

A. Sulphur granules are gram-positive mycelia surrounded by gram-positive clubs
B. *Actinomyces israelii* is an anaerobic organism
C. The organism has both bacterial and fungal characteristics
D. Multiple subcutaneous nodules over the jaw are characteristic

2. The following are true for treatment of actinomycosis *except*:

A. Crystalline penicillin is the drug of choice
B. Tetracyclines have no role in the treatment
C. Surgery may be required for abdominal actinomycosis
D. Ceftriaxone may be used for pulmonary actinomycosis

3. The following are features of tuberculoid leprosy *except*:

A. Bacilli are a few
B. Hypopigmented skin patches are seen
C. Nerve thickening is often a finding
D. Face and nose involvement is diagnostic of the condition

4. Hutchinson's triad does not include which of the following?

A. Interstitial keratitis
B. 8th nerve deafness
C. Chancre
D. Narrow-edged wide-spaced permanent incisors

5. Gummatous ulcer has all the following features *except*:

A. Commonly seen in the subcutaneous tissues
B. Floor has wash leather slough
C. Healing results in a hypertrophic scar
D. It has punched out edges

6. The following are features of secondary syphilis *except*:

A. Vesicles all over the body
B. Coppery red rashes
C. Snail track ulcers
D. Epitrochlear node enlargement

7. The characteristic feature of primary genital chancre in syphilis is:

A. It occurs 48 hours after sexual exposure
B. Multiple ulcers
C. Indurated ulcer with large, rubbery, inguinal nodes
D. Indurated, single, painless ulcer

8. The following are features of *Treponema pallidum* *except*:

A. It is a spirochaete
B. It is a gram-negative organism
C. It is visible by dark field illumination
D. It does not have a helical structure

9. The following are true for cytomegalovirus (CMV) infections, *except*:

A. It causes abdominal pain and colitis
B. It is related to chickenpox–herpesvirus
C. It may be transmitted by blood transfusion and organ transplantation
D. It is not transmitted to the child during pregnancy

10. The following may be HIV-associated lymphomas *except*:

A. B cell lymphoma
B. Diffuse large cell lymphoma
C. Burkitt's lymphoma
D. Hodgkin's lymphoma

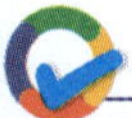

Answers

1. A **2.** B **3.** D **4.** C **5.** C **6.** A **7.** D **8.** D **9.** D **10.** D

CHAPTER

26

Differential Diagnosis of Leg Ulcer and Pressure Sore

- Clinical examination of an ulcer
- Management
- Wound dressings
- Traumatic ulcer
- Venous ulcer
- Trophic ulcer
- Tropical ulcer
- Post-thrombotic ulcer
- Rare ulcers
- Diabetic ulcer foot
- Amit Jain's classification for diabetic foot
- VAC
- Pressure sore
- Maggot therapy

INTRODUCTION

Leg ulcers are one of the important topics in surgery. They occur in children, adults, and the elderly. No age or sex is spared. Varying aetiological factors and the presence of complicated systemic diseases make the treatment of ulcers very difficult. Chronic ulcers in the elderly definitely cause considerable morbidity, and diabetic ulcer of the leg may cause life-threatening complications such as diabetic ketoacidosis and septicaemia. Hence, it is necessary to do a careful clinical examination of the ulcer to arrive at the diagnosis and plan the appropriate treatment.

Definition

An ulcer is a ***discontinuity of the skin or mucous membrane*** which occurs due to **microscopic death** of the tissues. Thus, ulcers may occur anywhere in the body (skin), oral cavity, penis (mucous membrane), duodenum, intestine, etc. In this chapter, lower limb ulcers will be discussed.

Classification

Ulcers may be classified based on the **pathology** or **clinical features**.

I. Pathological Classification (Key Box 26.1)

A. Nonspecific ulcers

1. **Traumatic:** This is the most common cause of leg ulcers. Trauma may be mechanical, physical due to burns or radiation, or chemical due to acids.
2. **Venous ulcers:** They include varicose ulcers and post-thrombotic ulcers, which may occur following deep vein thrombosis.
3. **Arterial ulcers:** Following are a few examples of arterial ulcers:
   - **Buerger's** disease—common
   - **Atherosclerotic** vascular disease—common
   - **Vasospastic** disorders such as Raynaud's disease—uncommon
   - **Martorell's ulcers** or hypertensive ulcers—rare
   - Patients with rheumatoid arthritis may develop leg or foot ulcers due to vasculitis.
4. **Neurogenic ulcer** (neuropathic ulcer, trophic ulcers)
   - Leprosy and diabetes are the common causes
   - Paraplegia, meningomyelocoele, posterior tibial nerve injury, and tabes dorsalis are other causes.

Key Box 26.1

Pathological Classification of Ulcer

A. Nonspecific ulcers

1. Traumatic	2. Venous
3. Arterial	4. Neurogenic—trophic
5. Tropical	6. Diabetic
7. Blood dyscrasias	

B. Specific ulcers

C. Malignant ulcers

5. **Tropical ulcer:** It is a rare ulcer due to malnutrition associated with infection caused by Vincent's organisms—*Borrelia vincentii* and Fusiforme organisms.
6. **Diabetic foot ulcer or diabetic leg ulcer.**
7. **Blood dyscrasias:** Sickle cell anaemia, thalassaemia, leukaemia, etc. may produce recurrent ulcerations over the leg.

B. Specific ulcers

These are due to a specific type of organism (e.g. tubercular ulcer, syphilitic ulcer, actinomycotic ulcer).

C. Malignant ulcers

These are squamous cell carcinoma, basal cell carcinoma, and malignant melanoma. Malignant ulcers are discussed in Chapter 31.

II. Clinical Classification (Table 26.1)

CLINICAL EXAMINATION OF AN ULCER

Inspection

1. Location of the ulcer

- Arterial ulcer: Tip of the toes,[1] dorsum of the foot.
- Long saphenous varicosity with ulcer: Medial side of the leg.
- Short saphenous varicosity with ulcer: Lateral side of the leg just above the lateral malleolus.
- Perforating ulcers: Over the sole at pressure points.
- Nonhealing ulcer: Over the shin and lateral malleolus.

2. Floor of the ulcer: This is the part of the ulcer which is exposed or seen.

- Red granulation tissue: Healing ulcer (Fig. 26.1)
- Necrotic tissue and slough: Spreading ulcer (Fig. 26.2)
- Pale, scanty granulation tissue: Tubercular[2] ulcer
- Wash-leather slough: Gummatous ulcer

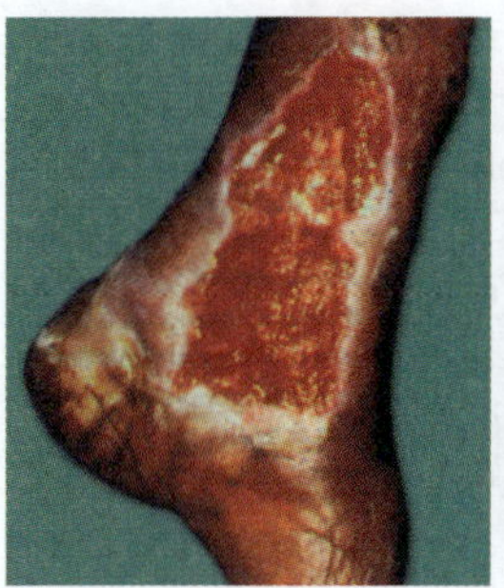

Fig. 26.1: Traumatic ulcer with red granulation tissue in the floor—typical healing ulcer

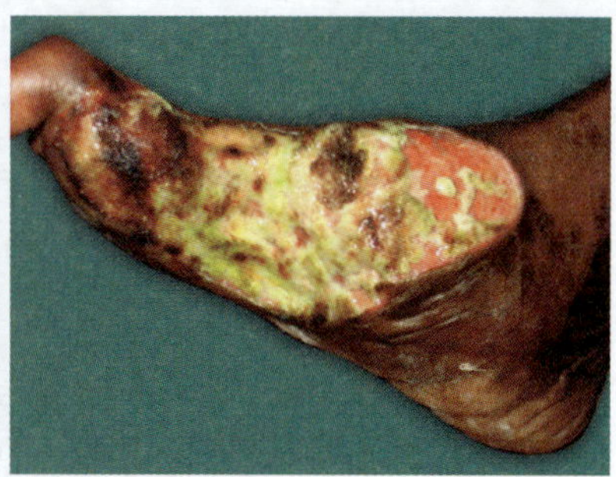

Fig. 26.2: Slough—dead soft tissue—typical spreading ulcer in a diabetic patient

- Part of the bone: Neuropathic ulcer
- Nodular: Epithelioma
- Black tissue: Malignant melanoma

3. Discharge from the ulcer

- Serous: Healing ulcer
- Purulent: Spreading ulcer
- Bloody: Malignant ulcer
- Discharge with bony spicules: Osteomyelitis
- Greenish: Pseudomonas infection

4. Edge: This is between the floor and the margin of the ulcer. ***The margin is the junction between the normal epithelium and the ulcer.*** It represents the **area of maximum cellular activity**. If destruction dominates, as in spreading ulcers, the edge is inflamed, oedematous and angry-looking (*stage of extension*). When an ulcer shows evidence of healing, the edge will be bluish due to granulation tissue covered by thin epithelium (*stage of transition*). In a healed ulcer, the outermost part of the edge is whitish due to fibrosis (*stage of repair*).

The types of ulcer edges are presented in Fig. 26.3.

- **Sloping edge** is seen in all **healing ulcers** such as traumatic ulcers and venous ulcers (Fig. 26.4).

Table 26.1 Clinical classification

A. Spreading	B. Callus	C. Healing
No granulation tissue	Pale granulation tissue	Red granulation tissue
Plenty of discharge	Serous discharge	Minimal serous discharge
Excessive slough	Slough present	Slough absent
Surrounding area inflamed and oedematous	Induration at the base, edge and surrounding area	Signs of inflammation are minimal
Purulent smell present	Smell can be present	Smell is absent

[1]When there is a block in the pipelines supplying water, distal houses suffer the maximum. Is it not?
[2]It is described as **apple jelly granulation tissue**.

- **Punched out edge** is seen in **gummatous ulcers** and **trophic ulcers**. Gummatous ulcers have punched out edges due to endarteritis obliterans caused by syphilitic organisms. Chronic, non-healing ulcers may also have punched out edges (Fig. 26.5).
- **Undermined edge** is seen in **tubercular** ulcers, probably due to more destruction of the subcutaneous tissues than the skin. The edge is classically thin and bluish in colour (Fig. 26.6).
- **Raised** (beaded) **edge** is seen in rodent ulcers or **basal cell carcinoma** (Fig. 26.7).
- **Everted** (rolled out) **edge** is diagnostic of **squamous cell carcinoma** (Fig. 26.8). The edge grows very rapidly and occupies the normal skin and, thus, becomes everted.

5. **Surrounding area**
   - Thick and pigmented: Varicose ulcer.
   - Thin and dark: Arterial ulcer.
   - Red and oedematous: Spreading ulcers like diabetic ulcer.
   - Scar around the ulcer: Marjolin's ulcer.

Palpation

1. **Edge:** Induration (hardness) of the edge is characteristic of squamous cell carcinoma. Some degree of induration may also be seen in chronic ulcers and long-standing varicose ulcers. Induration occurs due to extensive fibrosis. It is said to be a host defense mechanism. *Because of fibrosis, lymphatic spread is delayed.* Tenderness of the edge is characteristic of infected ulcers and arterial ulcers.
2. **Base:** *It is the area on which the ulcer rests.* Pick up the ulcer between the thumb and index finger to appreciate the tissues underneath. If the ulcer cannot be lifted up, the base cannot be made out. The base may be tendon, muscle, or bone, depending on the site of ulcer. ***Marked induration at the base is diagnostic of squamous cell carcinoma.*** Hunterian chancre is a benign ulcer and produces significant induration. Hence, it is also known as hard chancre (Key Box 26.2).

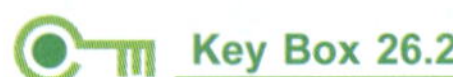
Key Box 26.2

Induration

- It means hardness
- Maximum induration: Squamous cell carcinoma
- Minimal induration: Malignant melanoma
- Brawny induration: Abscess
- Cyanotic induration: Chronic venous congestion as in varicose ulcer
- The base and the surrounding area should be examined for induration

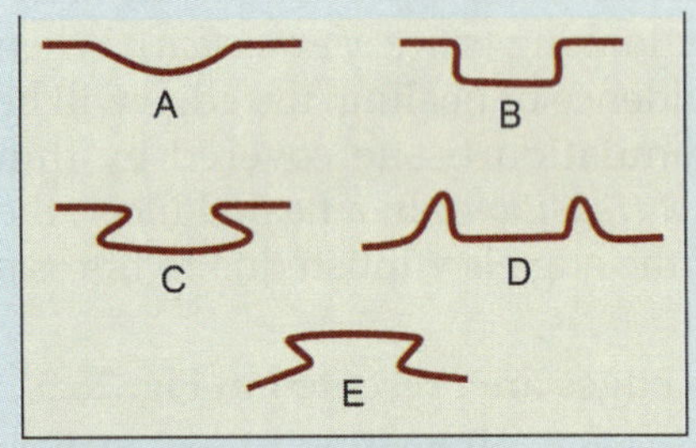

Fig. 26.3: Different types of edges of ulcer

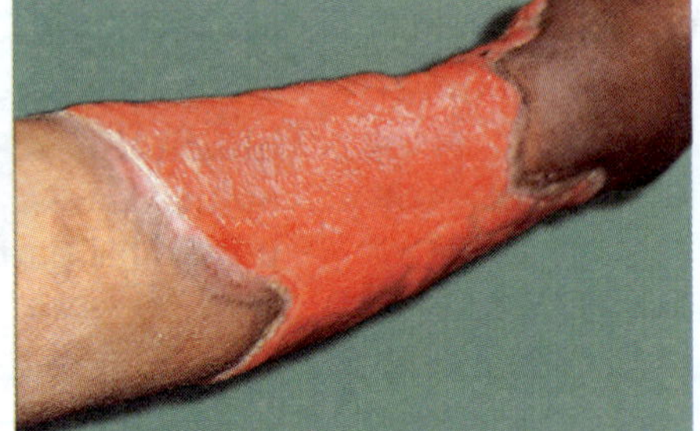
Fig. 26.4: Sloping edge

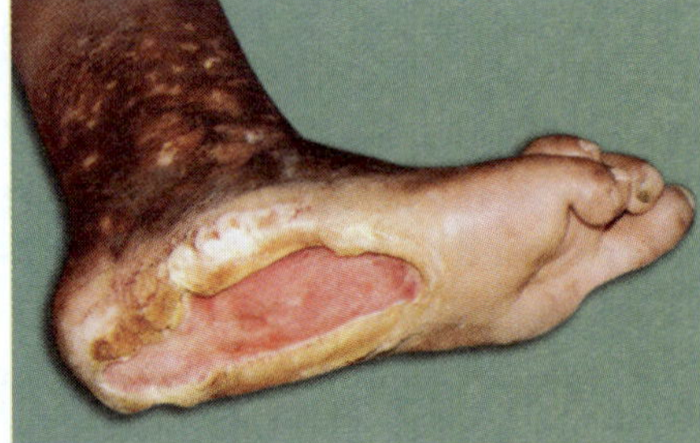
Fig. 26.5: Punched out edge—neuropathic ulcer (classically described for gummatous ulcer)

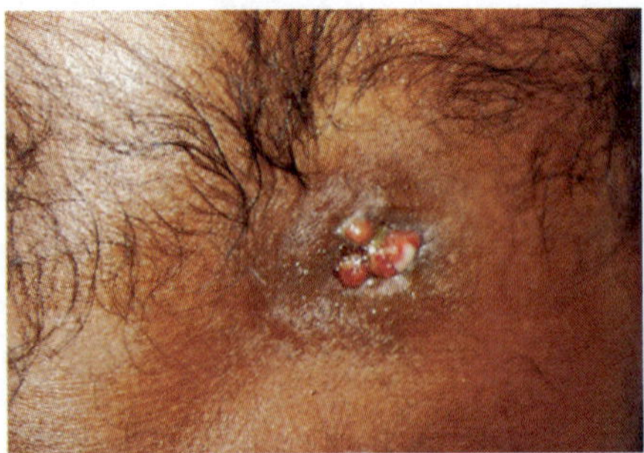
Fig. 26.6: Undermined edge—tubercular sinus/ulcer

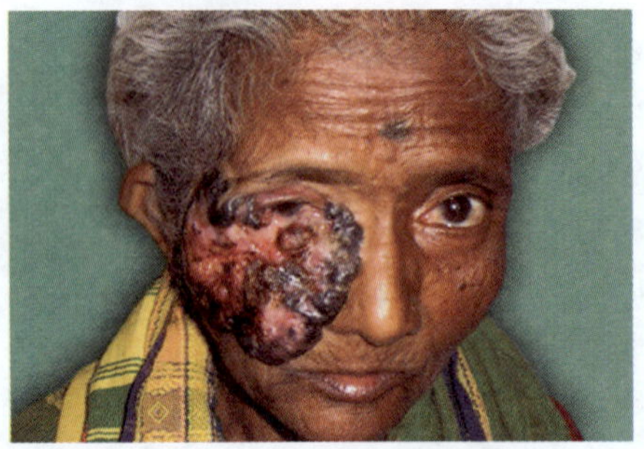
Fig. 26.7: Raised edge—basal cell carcinoma (*Courtesy:* Prof Vidyadhar Kinhal, Head, Surgery, VIMS, Bellary, Karnataka)

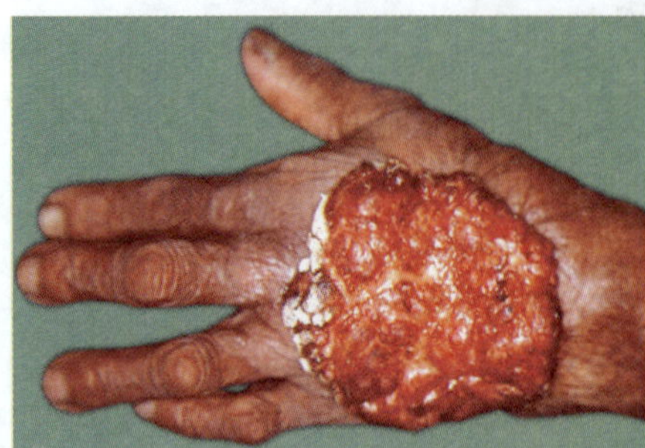
Fig. 26.8: Everted edge—squamous cell carcinoma

3. **Mobility:** A gentle attempt is made to move the ulcer to know its fixity to the underlying tissues. Malignant ulcers are usually fixed, whereas benign ulcers are not.
4. **Bleeding:** A malignant ulcer is friable, like a cauliflower. On gentle palpation, it bleeds. **Granulation tissue,** as present in a healing ulcer, also bleeds.[1]
5. **Surrounding area:** Thickening and induration is found in squamous cell carcinoma. Tenderness and pitting on pressure indicates spreading inflammation surrounding the ulcer.

Relevant Clinical Examination

1. **Regional lymph nodes**
   - Tender and enlarged: Acute secondary infection
   - Nontender and enlarged: Chronic infection
   - Nontender and hard: Squamous cell carcinoma
   - Nontender, large, firm, multiple: Malignant melanoma.
2. **Peripheral vessels:** Detailed examination of peripheral vessels is discussed under peripheral vascular disease. However, the dorsalis pedis, posterior tibial, popliteal, and femoral arteries should be palpated in cases of lower limb ulcers. Presence of weak pulses or absent pulses indicates peripheral vascular disease.
3. **Sensations:** Loss of vibration sense and loss of ankle jerk occur early in cases of diabetic neuropathy. Later, touch and pain are lost. ***Totally anaesthetic feet are characteristic of leprosy.***
4. **Function of the joint:** Movements of the involved joint are restricted either due to pain, involvement of the joint, or infiltration into the joint by malignant ulcers.
5. **Varicose veins:** If present, it is most probably a varicose ulcer. However, A-V fistulas may present as distal ulcers, with arterialisation of veins and a continuous murmur.

Systemic Examination

- **Central nervous system** (CNS) and spine in neuropathic ulcers. There may be gibbus, as in cases of TB spine, or an operated scar due to myelomeningocele, etc. *See* clinical notes.

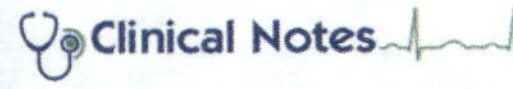

An 18-year-old girl with a nonhealing trophic ulcer was examined by a postgraduate student. He gave a diagnosis of trophic (neuropathic) ulcer due to leprosy as first diagnosis followed by polyneuropathy. He failed. It was a case of myelomeningocoele. The candidate had not examined the spine! The patient had an operated myelomeningocele.

- **Splenomegaly** in blood dyscrasias, such as in early stages of sickle cell anaemia.
- **Cardiovascular system** (CVS) may reveal a murmur, as in cases of arteriovenous fistula or features suggestive of cardiac diseases.

A summary of the clinical examination of an ulcer is given in Key Box 26.3.

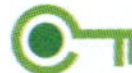

Key Box 26.3

Clinical Examination of an Ulcer

Inspection
- Location, size, shape, floor, edge, discharge, surrounding area

Palpation
- Tenderness, local rise of temperature, bleeding on touch, consistency of the ulcer, edge, surrounding area—oedema, mobility
- Regional lymph nodes
- Sensations
- Pulsations
- Function of the joint
- Systemic examination

Investigations

1. **Complete blood picture:** Hb%, TC, DC, ESR, peripheral smear.
   - Low Hb% is found in a chronic ulcer. It may be nutritional or due to frequent blood loss during dressings as in a diabetic ulcer.
   - High total count indicates infection.
   - Peripheral smear is done to rule out anaemia and sickle cell disease.
2. **Blood sugar estimation:** Both fasting and postprandial.
3. **Chest X-ray:** Many of these patients are smokers. They may have restricted pulmonary diseases.
4. **Pus** for culture/sensitivity.
5. **Doppler/duplex scan/lower limb angiography** in cases of arterial diseases and venous diseases. More details are given in the respective chapters.
6. **X-ray of the part:** It is done in look for osteomyelitis—common in diabetic ulcers.
7. MRI foot may be required to know the extent of the disease as in spreading ulcers or in chronic ulcers due to diabetes (rocker bottom foot) or due to Madura mycosis. In these type of cases, saving of foot becomes difficult. Amputation may be required.
8. **Biopsy:** Nonhealing/malignant ulcers.

[1]Granulation tissue is made up of capillaries and fibroblasts. Hence, it gives rise to fresh blood loss.

Treatment of Ulcers

It may be discussed under the following headings:

1. Treatment of spreading ulcers
2. Treatment of healing ulcers
3. Treatment of chronic ulcers
4. Treatment of the underlying disease

1. Treatment of Spreading Ulcers

- After obtaining pus culture/sensitivity report, appropriate antibiotics are given. Many solutions are available to treat the slough, such as hydrogen peroxide and **EUSol.**[1]
- Hydrogen peroxide (diluted), when poured over the wound, liberates nascent oxygen which bubbles out and helps in separating the slough. EUSol also separates the slough. ***Because there are reports that H_2O_2 and EUSol may cause more damage, they are no longer used.***
- Partially separated slough needs to be removed daily or on alternate days.
- **Excessive granulation tissue** or pouting granulation tissue (proud flesh) needs to be decapitated by excision or by the application of copper sulphate or silver nitrate solution.

By repeated dressings, the slough separates and the discharge minimizes, resulting in a healing ulcer with healthy red granulation tissue. Management thereafter is like that of a healing ulcer.

Table 26.2 presents the various ulcer dressings that are available today.

Table 26.2 Management classes of wound dressings, debridement agents and skin replacements currently available

Class	Composition	Characters/Functions	Commercial examples/ comments
1. Debriding agents • Hydrogen peroxide	H_2O_2 releases nascent oxygen which bubbles out and slough comes to surface.	Destroys anaerobic bacteria; heat generated causes vasoconstriction and haemostasis, frothing brings debris to the surface	Both these are not favoured today (EUSol is **E**dinburgh **U**niversity **Sol**ution)
• EUSol[1]	Hypochlorite solution	Mild debriding action	
2. Polymeric films	Plastic (polyurethane); semipermeable	Allows water vapour permeation; adhesive	Opsite; Tegaderm
3. Hydrocolloid dressings	Hydrophilic colloidal particles and adhesive. It is impermeable to fluids and bacteria	Absorbs fluid; necrotic tissue autolysis; little adherence; occlusive forms complex structures with water and aids in atraumatic removal of the dressing, hydrocol allows a high rate of evaporation without compromising wound hydration	Duoderm, Intrasite
4. Alginates	Polymer gel contains mannuronic acid and glucuronic acid—seaweed polymer that forms a gel when it absorbs fluid	Absorbs exudates; nonadherent, nonirritating, requires a cover dressing (permeable) Along with silver, antimicrobial action against MRSA and pseudomonas.	Algisorb, Sorbsan should not be used in presence of hepatic or renal impairment
5. Miscellaneous • Gauze • Tulles	Woven cotton fibres	Permeable with desiccation; debridement; painful removal	
6. Medicated dressings	Medications	Increased epithelialisation by 25–30%	Zinc oxide, Neomycin, Bacitracin, Zinc
• Impregnated gauzes	Fine mesh fabric (silicone, nylon) with dermal porcine collagens	Nonadherent; semipermeable	Biobrane II
7. Platelet-derived growth factor (PDGF) **8. Endothelial-derived growth factor (EDGF)**	Acts through tyrosine kinase receptor	Stimulates growth of cells and angiogenesis; increases granulation tissue; stimulation of repair—used when blood supply is good, classically neuropathic nonhealing ulcers of diabetics	Plemin, Regen-D Costly

[1]EUSol—Edinburgh University Solution (hypochlorite solution).

2. Treatment of Healing Ulcers

- Regular dressings for a few days with antiseptic creams (liquid iodine, zinc oxide, silver sulphadiazine, etc.).
- ***Swab to rule out the presence of Streptococcus haemolyticus, which is a contraindication for skin grafting.***
- If the ulcer is small, it heals on its own by epithelialisation from the cut edge.
- If the ulcer is large, a free split skin graft is applied as early as possible (Key Box 26.4).

Key Box 26.4

Advantages of Split Skin Graft

- Wound healing occurs fast
- Secondary infection is avoided because of early skin cover
- It prevents contractures
- It prevents Marjolin's ulcer—squamous cell carcinoma arising from scar tissues

3. Treatment of Chronic Ulcers

These are the ulcers which do not respond to conventional methods of treatment. Some special forms of treatment are available, but their efficacy is doubtful.

- Infrared radiation, short-wave therapy, and ultraviolet rays decrease the size of the ulcer.
- Amnion helps in epithelialisation.
- Chorion helps in the formation of granulation tissue (Fig. 26.9). These ulcers may ultimately require skin grafting.

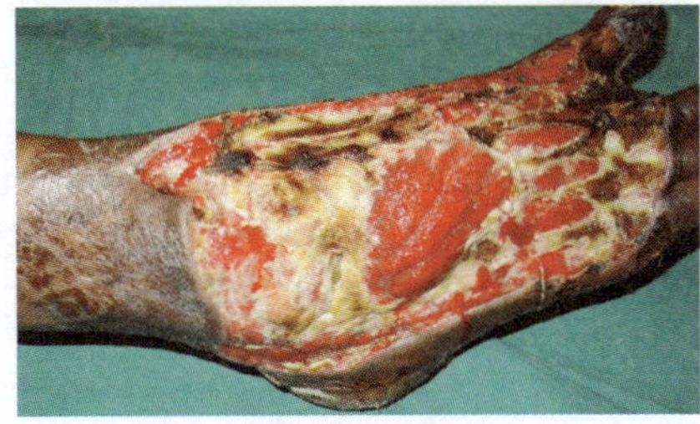

Fig. 26.9: Five days of usage of epidermal growth factor—granulation tissue started growing

4. Treatment of the Underlying Disease (vide infra)

Differential Diagnosis of Ulcers (Table 26.3)

Table 26.3 Causes of ulcer

Common causes	Uncommon causes	Rare causes
Varicose ulcer	Neurogenic ulcer	Martorell's ulcer
Arterial ulcer	Tropical ulcer	Bazin's disease
Diabetic ulcer	Post-thrombotic ulcer	
	Malignant skin ulcer	

TRAUMATIC ULCER (Fig. 26.10)

It may occur anywhere over the body. However, it is more common in areas where the skin is close to bony prominences (e.g. shin, malleoli), over which there are no muscles. They are usually single, very painful ulcers of healing type. With proper dressings and antibiotics, they usually heal within 5–7 days.

- **Footballer's ulcer** refers to a nonhealing ulcer over the shin due to direct trauma caused by a football. Sometimes, these ulcers may take a long time to heal. If not treated properly, they may become adherent to the bone.

VENOUS ULCER (Fig. 26.11)

- Occurs due to increased venous hydrostatic pressure
- Usually associated with varicose veins
- Located on the medial side of lower one-third of the leg in cases of long saphenous varicosity and on the lateral aspect of the leg in cases of short saphenous varicosity
- Shallow and superficial
- Never penetrates the deep fascia
- Usually painless, unless it is infected or causes periostitis tibia
- Shows evidence of healing
- Typically surrounded by pigmented skin

ARTERIAL/ISCHAEMIC ULCER (Fig. 26.12)

It is very painful and occurs in young patients with Buerger's disease or in elderly patients with atherosclerotic vascular disease. It commonly occurs on the tips of toes and fingers (Fig. 26.13). The ulcer is dry, deep,

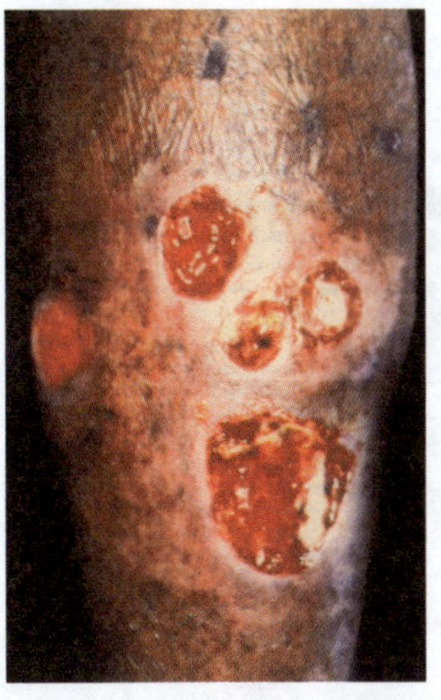

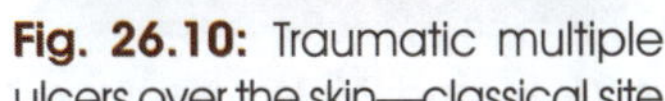

Fig. 26.10: Traumatic multiple ulcers over the skin—classical site

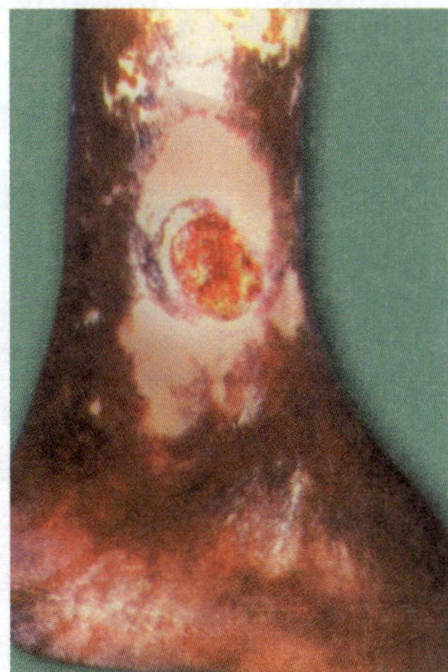

Fig. 26.11: Varicose ulcer—pigmentation is characteristic

Table 26.4 Differences between arterial and venous ulcers

	Arterial ulcer	Venous ulcer
Location	Tips of toes	Medial or lateral side of leg
Pain	Very painful	Absent
Number and shape	Many and irregular	Single and oval
Depth	Deep, penetrates deep fascia	Superficial, does not penetrate deep fascia
Pigmentation	Not a feature	Usually present
Nature of the vessels	Peripheral pulses are weak or absent; veins are not dilated	Peripheral pulses are normal; veins are dilated

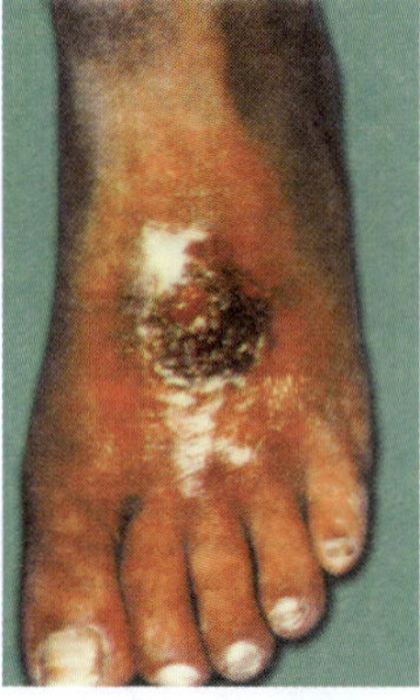

Fig. 26.12: Ischaemic ulcer on the dorsum of the foot—typical site

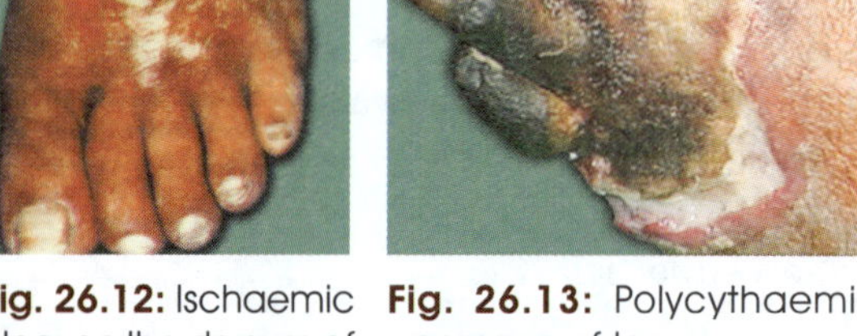

Fig. 26.13: Polycythaemia causing gangrene of toes

and penetrates the deep fascia. Evidence of chronic ischaemia in the rest of the foot clinches the diagnosis (Table 26.4 for differences between arterial and venous ulcers).

NEUROGENIC ULCER, NEUROPATHIC ULCER, TROPHIC ULCER (Figs 26.14 and 26.15)

- This type of ulcer develops in an anaesthetic limb, which may be caused by:
  - Diabetic neuropathy
  - Meningomyelocele
  - Leprosy
  - Alcoholic neuropathy
  - Nerve injuries
  - Transverse myelitis
- Trophic ulcers are caused by inadequate blood supply, malnutrition, and neurological deficits.
- The ulcer develops over pressure points such as beneath the heel, beneath the first and fifth metatarsals, and the gluteal region (decubitus ulcer). It develops as a callosity, gets infected, suppurates, and leaves a central hole that discharges pus. Slowly, it burrows deep inside and may involve the bone and cause osteomyelitis. Hence, it is also known as a **perforating ulcer**. End stage is Charcot's foot syndrome with varying degrees of bone and joint destruction and disorganization secondary to neuropathy, trauma, and changes in the bone metabolism.

Treatment

- **Immobilisation of the foot in a plaster of Paris** posterior slab with a walking boot almost cures the ulcer within 2–3 weeks, provided the primary disease (e.g. leprosy) is also controlled. If the ulcer is non-healing with slough, initial management should include de-sloughing agents and surgical removal of the slough. Limb which does not serve any purpose for walking necessitates amputation as in advanced cases of Charcot's foot.

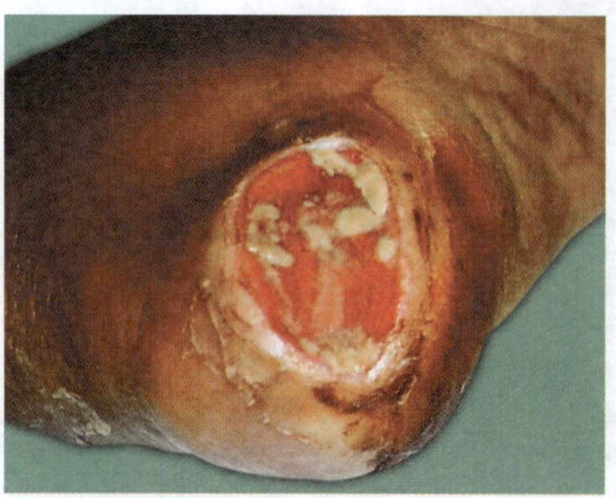

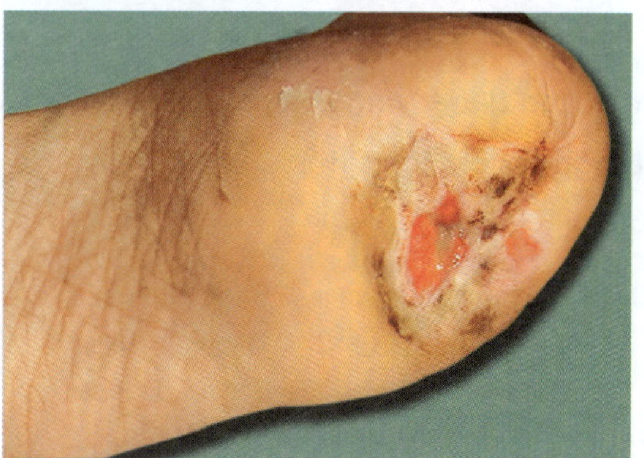

Figs 26.14 and 26.15: Neuropathic ulcer—classical site over the heel

TROPICAL ULCER

It occurs in tropical countries. The precipitating factors are:

- Malnutrition
- Humid zones
- Poor immunity
- Trauma or insect bite

The infection is caused by Vincent's organisms like bacteroides, *B. fusiformis,* and *Borrelia vincentii*. It starts as a pustule with extensive inflammation. The pustule bursts and the ulcer spreads rapidly and causes destruction of the surrounding tissue. Hence, it is also known as a **phagedenic ulcer.**[1] The edges are undermined, the floor contains slough, and there copious seropurulent discharge is present. Healing is delayed for up to a month. Metronidazole may be useful in bringing down the inflammation. Broad-spectrum antibiotics may also be required in cases of secondary infections. If healing takes place, it leaves behind a scar.

POST-THROMBOTIC ULCER

It occurs due to deep vein thrombosis. It may affect calf veins or may be due to femoral vein thrombosis. It is an example of a venous ulcer or a gravitational ulcer.

Precipitating Factors

- Accidents involving the lower leg
- Childbirth
- Abdominal operation.

Clinical Features

- Bursting pain in the limb
- Extensive induration of the leg or thigh depending on site of thrombosis
- Nonhealing with scanty granulation tissue
- Deep—always infiltrates the deep fascia
- Due to increased hydrostatic venous pressure, the part is significantly indurated (cyanotic induration), pigmented, and thickened with a rise in local temperature.
- The ulcer is not associated with superficial varicosity.
- **Homan's sign:** It is positive in calf vein thrombosis (pain in the calf region on forcible dorsiflexion of the foot with the knee extended).
- **Moses' sign:** Squeezing of the calf muscles from side to side produces pain. These two signs are positive in acute cases.

Treatment

- Rest and elevation of the leg
- Appropriate antibiotics
- Elastic crepe bandage

With conservative treatment for a few days to a few weeks, veins may recanalise and the ulcer may heal. The treatment is often very difficult (Chapter 30 on varicose veins).

RARE ULCERS[2]

MARTORELL'S ULCER

- Affects elderly patients over the age of 50 years.
- Commonly affects hypertensive patients (hence, the name **hypertensive ulcer)**.
- Atherosclerosis is also a precipitating factor, even though peripheral pulses are usually present.
- It occurs due to sudden **obliteration of end-arterioles** of the skin on the back or lateral side of the calf region.
- Severe pain
- Ischaemic patch of skin which develops into a deep, punched out, nonhealing ulcer.
- Delayed healing due to vascular insufficiency.

BAZIN'S ULCER

- Exclusively occurs in **young females** in the lower third of the leg and ankle region.
- Usually seen in **obese** patients who have thick ankles and an abnormal amount of subcutaneous fat.
- It begins with reddish-purplish nodules (hence, the name **erythrocyanosis frigida**) on the calves, which later rupture and produce a nonhealing ulcer.
- The aetiology of these ulcers is unclear. It may be due to **ischaemia of the lower leg** due to spasm of branches of the posterior tibial and peroneal arteries. These vessels are **abnormally sensitive to hot and cold weather,** similar to Raynaud's disease. In some cases, tubercular bacilli have been isolated, with ulcers responding to antitubercular treatment.
- These ulcers are managed conservatively.
- **Sympathectomy** may be beneficial in those patients who are hypersensitive to weather changes.

[1]Phagedenic (to eat). Rapidly spreading, ulcerative, destructive lesion. It can occur in the oral cavity and also over the penis.
[2]Students should not offer these ulcers as clinical diagnosis. They are rare ulcers, with rare clinical interest.

DIABETIC FOOT

"Diabetic foot is a complex disease with many complications and every effort should be made to understand and treat it in as simple way as possible"—Dr Amit Jain, Founder of Modern Diabetic Foot Surgery.

Diabetes is extremely common worldwide, is increasing day by day and it has various complications. Diabetic foot is a distressing, devastating complication of diabetes and is common neglected problem that can lead to amputation which can result in patient becoming handicap. The numerous problems (Amit Jain's categorization) associated with diabetic foot are listed in Key Box 26.5.

Key Box 26.5

Amit Jain's classification of problems of diabetic foot*

Categories of foot problems	*Type*	*Examples*
Category 1	Preponderant	Diabetes mellitus
Category 2	Current	Abscess, ulcer, gangrene, etc.
Category 3	Concurrent	Hypertension, heart disease, kidney disease, etc.
Category 4	Recurrent	Re-amputation, re-ulceration, re-admissions, etc.
Category 5	Subsequent	Mortality, major amputations, stump complications, etc.
Category 6	Supplement	Depression, loss of job, financial issues, etc.

- Various risk factors are given in Key Box 26.6.

Key Box 26.6

Risk Factors for Diabetic Ulcer Foot

- Male above 50 years
- DM of more than 10 years duration
- Blood glucose levels not controlled
- Peripheral neuropathy
- Abnormal structure of foot
- Peripheral vascular disease
- Smoking and hypertension
- Increased level of lipids
- Genetic factors

Diabetic foot is a triad that mainly consists of neuropathy, infection and ischemia.

1. **Neuropathy:**[1] It commonly manifests after about 10 years of diabetes though it can occur early if there is uncontrolled diabetes and it can be sensory, motor or autonomic. Neuropathy may be distal and diffuse with a stocking type of distribution. ***Nerve damage is due to the formation of sorbitol from sugar.*** Sorbitol causes demyelination of large fibres. New **arteriovenous communications** open beneath skin, diverting nutrient flow away from it. This ischaemic tissue is vulnerable to infection, causing nerve ischaemia. Loss of vibration sense and deep tendon reflexes occur early. Later, joint position, touch, pain, and temperature sensations are lost. As a result of this, a trophic ulcer develops. It progresses and may penetrate deeper and deeper. The patient is often unaware of this as he has no pain and he continues walking on it and ultimately the ulcer may get infected.
   - Diabetic neuropathy of the tibial nerve is dangerous. ***Clawing of the toes and hammer toe result due to the paralysis of intrinsic muscles of the foot.*** Sensation is absent over the entire sole due to involvement of the medial and lateral plantar nerves. These two factors predispose to the development of pressure sores over the plantar surface of the head of the metatarsals.
   - **Charcot's arthropathy (joints)** is a form of arthritis seen in neuropathic foot with good vascularity and it leads to severe deformity. Often midfoot bones and joints are affected.
   - **Autonomic neuropathy** leads to absence of sweating and gives rise to anhydrotic skin (Key Box 26.7).

Key Box 26.7

Diabetic Neuropathy

- Loss of vibration and touch
- Loss of pain and temperature
- Dead like feeling in the feet
- Sensation of walking on the 'sand'
- Susceptible for repeated trauma
- Nylon monofilament test is routinely used to test neuropathy by pressing in on the foot/sole

Pearls of Wisdom

Autosympathectomy is a feature of diabetic foot ulcers.

*If a patient has gone through any 5 problems, then the patient is said to have a "Diabetic Foot Storm" in his life. This term was recently coined by Amit Jain. Once he gets any 3 problems, he should be warned of diabetic foot storm and preventive strategies are advised including screening and education.

Professor of Surgery, Shri Raj Rajeshwari Medical College, Bengaluru

[1]Burning or tingling in plantar aspect of forefoot radiating to toes—**Morton's interdigital neuroma.**

- Various factors of neuropathy contribute to changes in the configuration of the foot and a change in gait. The foot becomes shorter and wider. The longitudinal arch becomes flat. New pressure points develop, resulting in ulcers in the foot (Key Box 26.8).

Key Box 26.8

Effects of Diabetic Neuropathy

- Loss of sensation
- Loss of sweating
- Loss of muscle strength
- Loss of curvature of foot
- Loss of normal joint position
- Loss of elasticity of skin

2. **Resistance to infection** is reduced in patients with diabetes mellitus. Patients with uncontrolled diabetes are more susceptible to infection. Even though leukocytosis occurs in diabetic patients with infection, the **phagocytic activity of the leukocytes is greatly reduced**.
   - **In ketoacidosis, granulocyte mobilisation is impaired** and chemotaxis is reduced. Thus, these patients are more susceptible to polymicrobial and fungal infections.
3. **Atherosclerosis:** Diabetic angiopathy involving major vessels results in ischaemia of the foot **(macroangiopathy)**. These patients have accelerated atherosclerosis. In addition, it also produces small vessel disease in the form of nonspecific thickening of the basement membrane (**microangiopathy**) (Key Box 26.9).

Key Box 26.9

Diabetes and Atherosclerosis

- 16% of diabetic patients have PVD (peripheral vascular diseases)
- Collateral circulation is reduced in diabetics
- Atherosclerotic plaque causes increased ulceration and cracking
- More severe the diabetes, more severe will be **peroneal occlusive disease**

Thus, neuropathy or microangiopathy singly or in combination with secondary infection favours the development of a diabetic ulcer. The ulcer forms due to minor trauma, such as from a thorn prick, trimming of the nail, or a shoe bite. It may also start as a callosity in the sole of the neuropathic foot. Hence, utmost care should be taken to protect the feet of patients with diabetes mellitus.

Different Sequence of Events in Diabetic Foot Patients (Fig. 26.16)

1. **Stage of cellulitis:** Following an injury or trivial trauma, redness can develop along with swelling and oedema of the leg.
2. **Stage of spreading cellulitis:** Cellulitis takes up a virulent course and spreads deeper and upwards along fascial planes. When infection is severe, necrotising fasciitis may occur with renal failure and septic shock.
3. **Stage of abscesses:** Secondary infection caused by mixed organisms along with anaerobes and non-clostridial gas-forming organisms produce multiple abscesses.
4. **Stage of gangrene:** Tense oedema and the existing vascular compromise produce ischaemia and gangrenous patches of skin, toes, etc. The gangrene can be wet gangrene or dry gangrene.
5. **Stage of osteomyelitis:** Infection involves deeper tissues like the bone, leading to osteomyelitis.
6. **Stage of septicaemia:** Some patient can present in emergency with septicemia. This is due to untreated cases of gangrene, abscess, cellulitis, etc. which can spread locally and systemically producing septicaemia and diabetic ketoacidosis.

Amit Jain's Staging for Cellulitis (Table 26.5)

This new staging system consists of 4 sequential progressive clinical stages of primary cellulitis and gives a corresponding treatment guide. This is extremely simple, easy to remember, practical staging that can be

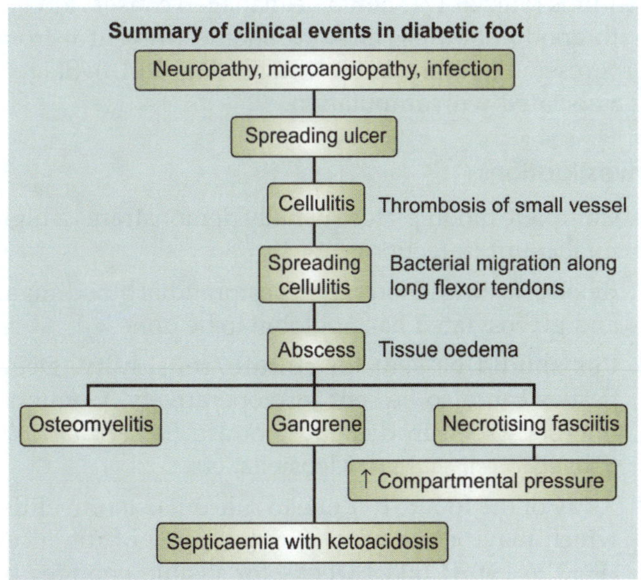

Fig. 26.16: Various stages of infection of the leg in diabetic patients. (Events need not follow the same order)

Table 26.5	Amit Jain's staging system for cellulitis	
Stage of cellulitis	**Clinical description**	**Treatment guideline**
Stage 1	Cellulitis without any abscess or necrosis	Broad spectrum antibiotics, limb elevation, and crepe bandage. Monitor the patient daily
Stage 2	Cellulitis with either localized abscess or skin necrosis	Requires some form of surgical intervention, like drainage of abscess or debridement.
Stage 3	Necrotizing fasciitis without myonecrosis	Extensive radical debridement of all the devitalized tissues/amputation based on extensiveness
Stage 4	Necrotizing fasciitis with myonecrosis	Radical debridement and some form of amputation is invariably performed at this stage

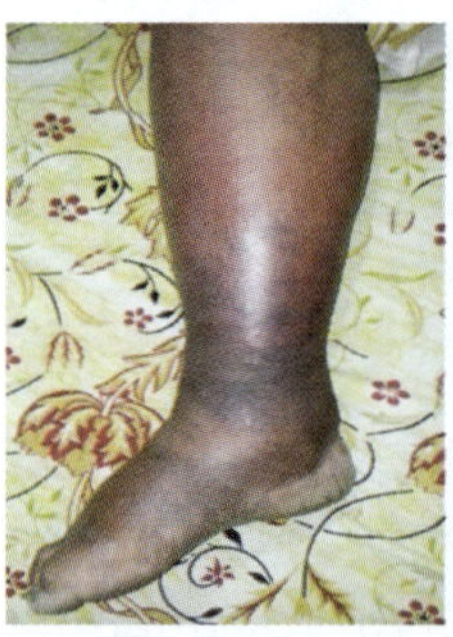

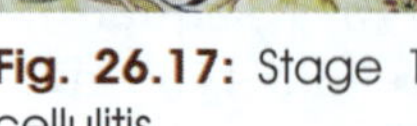

Fig. 26.17: Stage 1 cellulitis

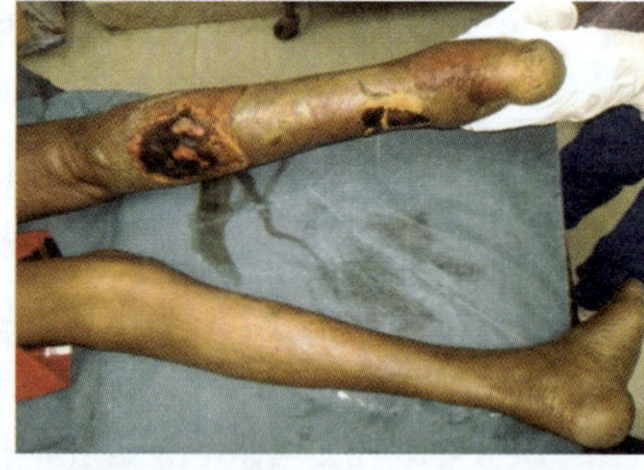

Fig. 26.18: Stage 3 wherein necrotizing fasciitis has occurred

used for extremities and also in nondiabetics. The stage 1 cellulitis (Fig. 26.17) should be managed conservatively with good antibiotics and one should prevent it from progressing to more serious stages (Fig. 26.18). Stage 4 is associated with amputation.

Investigations

1. Complete blood picture usually demonstrates a high total count (infection).
2. Blood—fasting blood sugar, postprandial blood sugar and glycosylated haemoglobin to be done.
3. Pus should be sent for culture/sensitivity. Deep tissues can also be sent intraoperatively. Common microbes seen in diabetic foot are *Escherichia coli, Staphylococcus aureus,* Klebsiella, etc.
4. X-ray of the foot to be done to rule out osteomyelitis, which may be the cause for chronicity of the ulcer (Fig. 26.19). It takes weeks for visible changes of osteomyelitis on radiograph. Today in all such doubtful cases, MRI of the foot/leg is done.

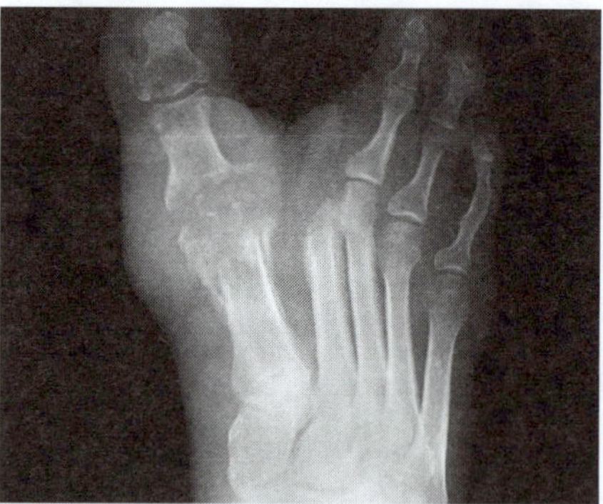

Fig. 26.19: Destruction of metatarsal bone and dislocation of metatarsal joint

5. Liver function test (LFT), ECG, chest X-ray, blood urea, and serum creatinine to be done as a routine (remember diabetes is a systemic disease).
6. Lower limb arterial duplex scan is an important investigation to check for the patency of vessels. It is useful investigation if foot pulses are not felt
   - Normally, the flow is laminar and triphasic
   - In patients with diabetic foot, the flow becomes turbulent and there is loss of diastolic forwards flow.
7. Hand held Doppler and measurement of ankle brachial index (ABI) is a bedside test. ABI of less than 0.9 indicates ischemia.

CT angiogram is done in case of ischemic ulcer not healing or presence of dry gangrene. If vessels are extensively calcified or if there is elevated creatinine, then MR angiogram can be considered. Often it is seen that below popliteal vessels are involved (Fig. 26.20).

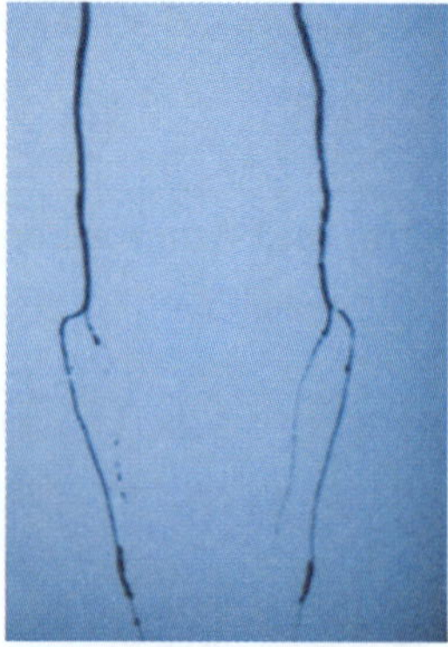

Fig. 26.20: Lower limb angiogram. Note the bilateral infrapopliteal arterial disease

DIABETIC FOOT CLASSIFICATION (see Key Box 26.10)

There are several classification for diabetic foot ulcer which is a common clinical focal pathology. The commonly used diabetic foot ulcer classification from West is Meggit-Wagner classification (Key Box 26.10). Another modern diabetic foot ulcer classification is Amit

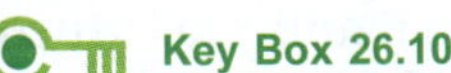

Key Box 26.10

Grading of Diabetic Ulcer Foot

Modified Wagner grading system of diabetic ulcer foot

Grade 0: No skin changes

Grade 1: Superficial ulcer

Grade 2: Ulcer extension

a. Involves ligament, tendon, joint capsule or fascia

b. No abscess, no osteomyelitis

Grade 3: Deep ulcer with abscess or osteomyelitis

Grade 4: Gangrene of the portion of forefoot

Grade 5: Extensive gangrene of foot

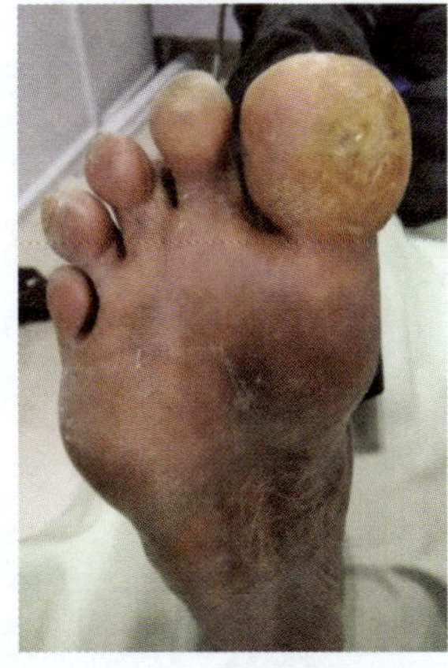

Fig. 26.21: Infected ulcer. This is class 3 diabetic foot ulcer (AJ S1A1C3)

Jain's ulcer classification (Key Box 26.11). This is a new original diabetic foot ulcer classification from India that divides ulcers into 3 types that are extremely easy to remember (Fig. 26.21). It also has an Amit Jain's ulcer scoring system that predictis amputation and a coding system (Amit Jain's SAC coding) to be used in lines of TNM system (Key Box 26.12).

Key Box 26.11

Amit Jain's diabetic foot ulcer classification

Class of diabetic foot ulcer	*Description*	*Causation*	*Examples*
Class 1	Simple ulcers	There is no intrinsic cause of non-healing	Trophic ulcers
Class 2	Complex ulcers	There is intrinsic cause of non-healing like bony or ischemia	Claw toe ulcers, ischemic ulcers, etc
Class 3	Complicated ulcers	These ulcers have underlying infection	Ulcers with osteomyelitis

Key Box 26.12

Amit Jain's SAC coding for diabetic foot ulcer

Size (S)	*Anatomical area involved (A)*	*Amit Jain's class of ulcer (C)*
S1–Less than 2 cm	A1–Forefoot	C1–Class 1
S2–2–4 cm	A2–Midfoot	C2–Class 2
S3–More than 4 cm	A3–Hindfoot	C3–Class 3

Amit Jain's Universal Classification for Diabetic Foot Complications

This is a new, simple, easy-to-remember, practical, open, complete, descriptive, modern diabetic foot classification which is also from India that includes almost all the complication of diabetic foot seen worldwide. It divides diabetic foot into 3 simple types (Table 26.6). It has a sequel (Amit Jain's surgical scoring system) that predicts major amputation and is governed by Amit Jain's law of classification which suggest using combination of classification like universal classification and surgical scoring, as a single classification cannot be made for diabetic foot complications that has many pathological entities.

Amit Jain's DIABETIC FOOT acronym covers all the lesions seen in this universal classification (Key Box 26.13)

Table 26.6 Amit Jain's universal classification for diabetic foot

Type of diabetic foot complication	Lesions
Type 1 diabetic foot complications [infective]	Cellulitis, abscess, wet gangrene, necrotizing fasciitis, etc.
Type 2 diabetic foot complications [noninfective] (Figs 26.22 and 26.23)	Trophic ulcers, dry gangrene, ischaemic ulcer, claw toe, hammer toe, charcot foot, diabetic bullae, etc.
Type 3 diabetic foot complications [mixed]	When type 2 complications get infected Classical examples—trophic ulcer with osteomyelitis, dry gangrene with secondary infection, etc.

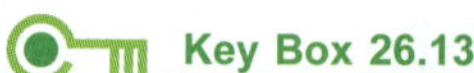

Key Box 26.13

Amit Jain's DIABETIC FOOT

Dry gangrene
Infective gangrene (Fig. 26.22)
Abscess (Fig. 26.23)
Bullosis diabeticorum
Erysipelas
Trophic ulcer
Ischemic ulcer
Cellulitis
Flesh eating bacterial disease, Fungal infections
Osteoarthropathy (Charcot foot)
Osteomyelitis
Toe deformities

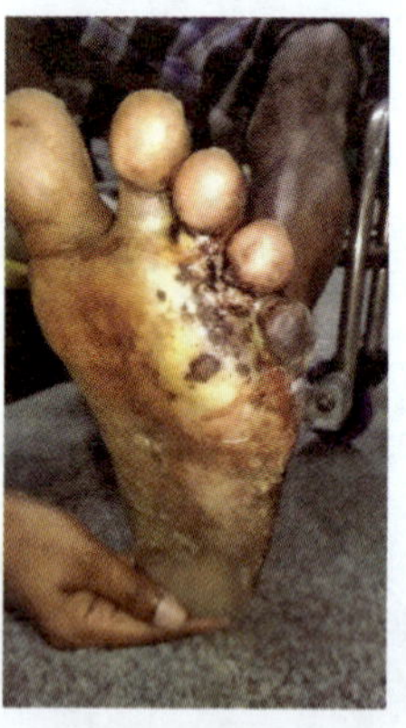

Fig. 26.22: Wet gangrene left foot. This is type 1 diabetic foot complication

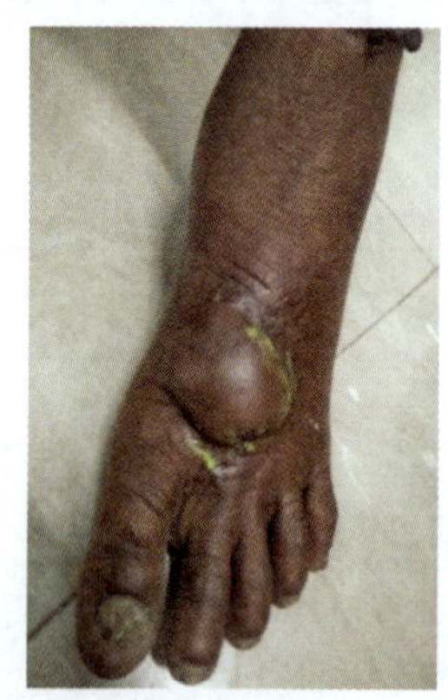

Fig. 26.23: Abscess. This is also type 1 diabetic foot complication

Treatment[1] of Diabetic Foot Ulcers

It may be discussed under the following headings:

- Control of diabetes
- Control of infection
- Local treatment of the ulcer—debridement
- Amit Jain's grading of debridement
- Various types of surgery for diabetic foot ulcer
- Care[2] of the patient as a whole
- Revascularisation of the foot
- Vacuum assisted closure (VAC) therapy
- Limited access dressing (LAD)

1. **Control of diabetes:** It is an important part of the treatment of diabetic foot ulcer. Diabetes precipitates infection, which worsens the diabetic status. These ulcers are better managed, at least in the initial period, with insulin rather than oral antidiabetic drugs alone. Inj. plain insulin is given 3–4 times/day depending on the requirement. With the availability of **glucometers** and the estimation of **GRBS**, the sliding scale method based on urine sugar estimation has become obsolete.
2. **Control of infection:** Commonly used empirical antibiotics are fluoroquinolones and cephalosporins. Often metronidazole is added if severe infection. Once the culture/sensitivity report is available, appropriate antibiotics should be started. Commonly, gram-positive, gram-negative, and/or anaerobic infections exist. Antibiotics may have to be continued for a long time based on the nature, type, and severity of infection. ***Presence of high-grade fever with chills and rigors suggests the development of multiple abscess pockets that need to be drained, rather than an indiscriminate change in antibiotics.*** If infection is not controlled properly, ketoacidosis may occur.
3. **Local treatment of diabetic foot ulcer:** Diabetic ulcer is a nonhealing ulcer. Hence the aim should be towards healing of that ulcer. Management of these ulcers involves debridement, dressings, using iodine solution in infections and offloading the ulcer. Once the ulcer is granulating well, then it can be allowed to heal on its own if small or one can do split skin grafting. One should avoid using povidone iodine or hydrogen peroxide on good granulating wound as they can delay wound healing.

   There are numerous modern wound dressing products available that can be used during the course of ulcer management like hydrogels, foams, hydrocolloid, alginates, etc. Hydrogels are commonly used nowadays and are also affordable. It provides moisture of wounds. Diabetic wounds heal very slowly or delayed healing (Fig. 26.24).

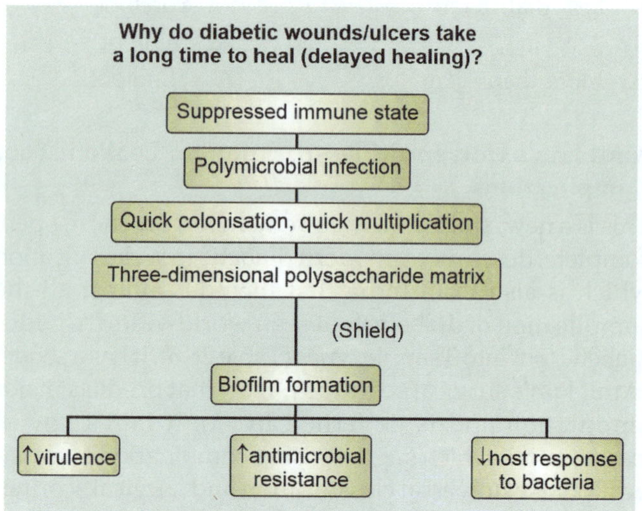

Fig. 26.24: Delayed healing of diabetic ulcers

[1]Even a small diabetic ulcer should be treated properly. Otherwise, a patient may have to 'pay through his foot' for it.
[2]This is an important aspect often forgotten by the treating physicians and surgeons.

Pearls of Wisdom

There are numerous products being launched yearly and one should be cautious in using them blindly. Remember, many patients are already in financial misery and one should avoid adding further financial burden through expensive products.

4. **Amit Jain's modified grading[1] for debridement** (Table 26.7): Debridement is an essential and key surgery to prevent the spread of infection. It is frequently performed for abscesses, infected ulcers, necrotizing fasciitis, etc. The new Amit Jain's grading system divides surgical debridement into 4 grades [G1–4] based on the tissues removed, extent of regions debrided [E1–3], and repetitions of debridement [R1, 2, 3,...] performed in the operation theatre. Debridement may be coded as GER (like TNM staging). This grading system is simple, easy, practical, reproducible, and applicable in day-to-day practice and may be used for upper extremities as well (Fig. 26.25).

Table 26.7 Amit Jain's modified grading for debridement

Grade of debridement [G]	Description	Modified coding
Grade 1	Removal of sloughs from the ulcer, callus removal, deroofing the large blisters/blebs, removal of desiccated tendons, etc.	G1
Grade 2	Removal of necrotic/unhealthy skin and subcutaneous tissue	G2
Grade 3	Removal of infected/necrotic skin, subcutaneous tissue along with either tendons/retinaculum/deep fascia	G3
Grade 4	Removal of infected/necrotic skin, subcutaneous tissue, tendon/retinaculum/deep fascia along with necrotic/infected muscle	G4
Extent of debridement [E]		
Only 1 site [foot/leg/thigh]		E1
2 Sites [foot + leg or leg + thigh]		E2
3 Sites [foot + leg + thigh]		E3
Repetition of debridement [R]		
Debridement not repeated		R0
Debridement repeated once		R1
Debridement repeated twice		R2
Debridement repeated thrice		R3
Debridement repeated ...		R ...

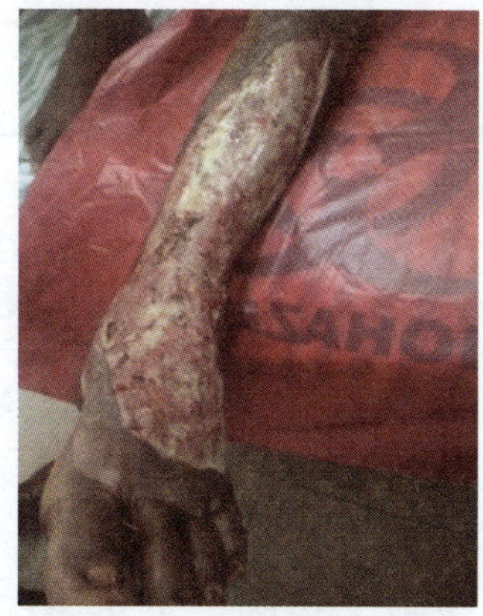

Fig. 26.25: Showing status post-debridement (Amit Jain's G3 E2 R0)

The other types of nonsurgical debridement are enzymatic debridement wherein papain urea is used, mechanical debridement and biological debridement wherein sterile maggots are used to remove necrotic tissue.

5. **Various types of surgery[2] for diabetic foot** (Table 26.8). Debridement is the commonly performed procedure. Amputation becomes necessary if tissues are destroyed or part is not salvageable. Always try to save limb as much as possible. There are different types of foot amputation (Table 26.9). Type 1 foot amputations are most commonly performed in clincal practice.

Table 26.8 Aim—to save the leg

Spreading ulcer with slough	Debridement
Healing ulcer	Skin grafting/flaps (reverse sural flap)
	Incision and drainage
Abscess	Disarticulate toe
Gangrene toe	Excision of metatarsal bones
Involvement of metatarsal bones	Forefoot amputation
Gangrene confined to toes	Multiple fasciotomy/decompression/debridement
Spreading cellulitis/necrotising fasciitis	Amputation below knee or above knee
Spreading cellulitis with gangrene Ischaemic limb	Revascularisation, infra-inguinal bypass

[1]This is a new classification and new grading system applied in diabetic foot. However, students are requested to verify the procedures with your senior faculty in the institution.

[2]Unfortunately in some patients, in an attempt to save the limb, all these surgeries will be done and at last, they may end up with amputation of the leg.

Table 26.9 Amit Jain's classification for foot amputation

Type of foot amputations	Description	Examples
Type 1 foot amputations	Simple	Toe amputation, transmetatarsal amputation
Type 2 foot amputations	Complex	Lisfranc, Chopart
Type 3 foot amputations	Complicated	Syme's amputation

All the amputations below malleoli are considered to be minor amputation, whereas amputation above malleoli are major amputations like below knee amputation. Amit Jain's destructive/amputation ladder (Fig. 26.26) provides various types of amputation available for extremity starting from distal to proximal most amputation (Key Box 26.14).

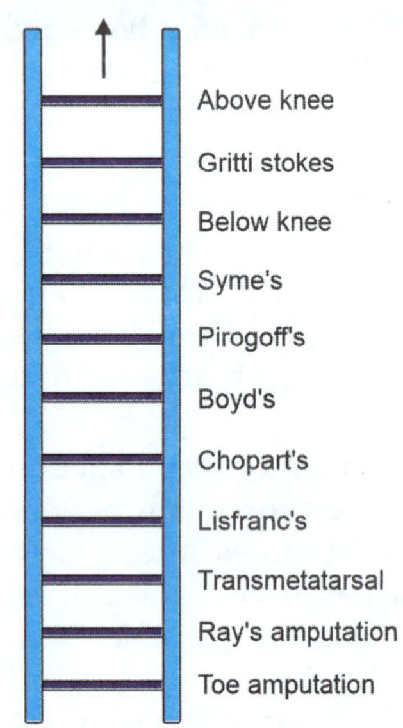

Fig. 26.26: Amit Jain's amputation ladder

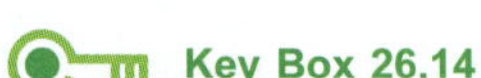

Key Box 26.14

Remember following ladders

- Reconstructive ladder: Wound closure options
- Destructive ladder (Amit Jain's): Amputation options
- WHO analgesic ladder: Pain relief options

Revascularization is done if limb is ischemic and wound is nonhealing. Today, peripheral angioplasties are more commonly done compared to peripheral bypass procedure.

Once the wound has good granulations, then it can be allowed to close by secondary healing, sutured, split skin grafting can be done in case of large wounds or flaps may be required (reconstructive ladder).

6. **Care of the patient as a whole** (Table 26.10): Recovery and healing of diabetic foot ulcer may range from a few weeks to a few months. During this period, there are various other aspects to be looked after, other than infection and insulin. Ensure patient's blood pressure and lipids are under control. If patients are on blood thinning agents like aspirin, then they should be stopped prior to surgery and restarted later.
7. **Revascularisation of the foot:**
   - Ankle brachial pressure index is *misleading* because of calcified vessels (incompressible).
   - Duplex ultrasound assesses both anatomical and functional abnormality. If there is stenosis, the peak systolic velocity ratio will be >2 across the arterial lesion.
   - Angiography is still the gold standard.
   - For short stenotic lesions, balloon angioplasty with or without stent placement is performed.
   - Infrainguinal bypass surgery—popliteal to tibial or pedal artery using the long saphenous vein.
   - Even after successful surgery, the amputation rate is about 35%. The 2-year patency rate is around 70%.

   Patients are given aspirin and lipid lowering agents like Atorvastatin in post-revascularization period.

Table 26.10 Various problems and their solutions

Problems	Solutions
Nutritional factors	Diabetic diet should be given
A bedridden patient may have difficulty in passing urine, situation worsened by pre-existing benign prostatic hypertrophy	Catheterisation (Foley's catheter) under aseptic measures, frequent change of catheter and catheter care
Chest infection such as pulmonary tuberculosis or static pneumonia	Control of tuberculosis, pneumonia, chest physiotherapy
Development of bedsores	Frequent change of position and nursing care
More sensitive to carbohydrate metabolism, protein depletion and changes in water and electrolyte metabolism	Frequent checking of Hb%, total proteins, blood glucose and electrolyte levels, etc.

8. **Vacuum assisted closure (VAC) therapy:** It is also called vacuum therapy, *vacuum sealing*, or topical negative pressure therapy. It is used to drain blood or serous fluid from a wound or operation site.

Technique

- Foam with an open-cell structure is introduced into the wound and a drain is kept and brought out by multiple, lateral holes. The entire area is then covered with a transparent adhesive membrane, which is firmly secured to the normal healthy skin around the wound margin. The drain tube is connected to a vacuum and fluid is drawn from the wound through the foam into a bag (Fig. 26.27).

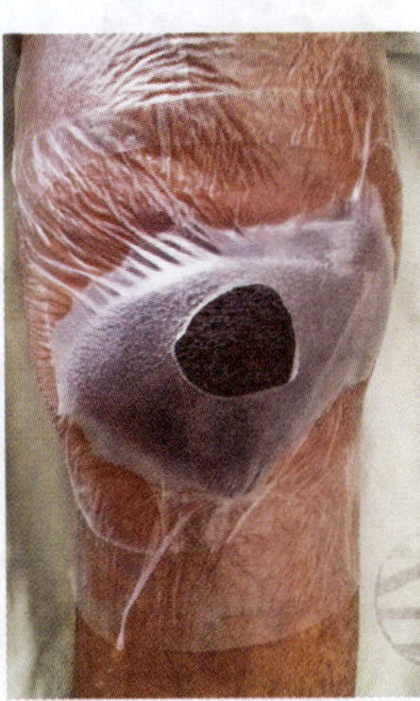

Fig. 26.27: VAC

- The plastic membrane prevents the inflow of air and bacteria. It also allows a partial vacuum to form within the wound, facilitating the removal of fluid.

How does it work?

- **Negative pressure** assists with the removal of interstitial fluid, decreasing localised oedema and increasing blood flow.
- This, in turn, decreases tissue bacterial levels.
- Mechanical deformation of cells occurs, which results in protein and matrix molecule synthesis, which increases the rate of cellular proliferation.
- **Equipment:** Microprocessor-controlled vacuum unit capable of providing controlled levels of continuous or intermittent sub-atmospheric pressure (25–200 mmHg).

Indications

- Venous ulcers, diabetic ulcers, large ulcers following necrotising fasciitis, and any chronic ulcers.
- Patients with open fractures.
- Soft tissue injuries, including sacral pressure ulcers, acute traumatic soft tissue defects, and infected soft tissue defects following rigid stabilisation of lower limb fractures.
- Treatment of burns and wounds in the perineum, hand, or axilla.

Contraindications

- Osteomyelitis—first treat osteomyelitis and then apply VAC
- Internal fistula
- Necrotic tissue in eschar
- Malignancy

9. **Limited access dressing (LAD):** A simple plastic sheet covers the wound and intermittent suction is applied. It is cheaper than VAC (Fig. 26.28).

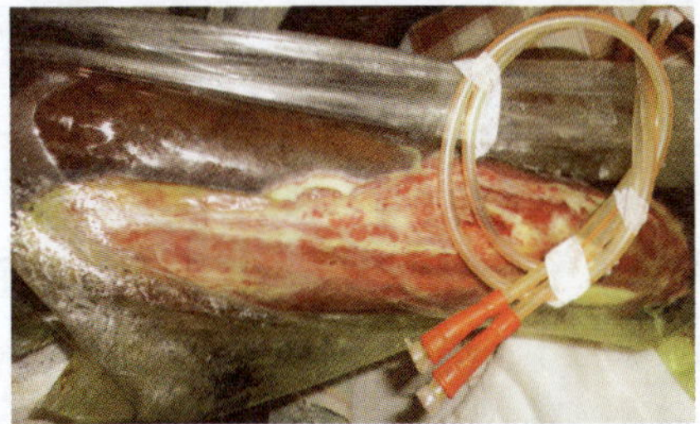

Fig. 26.28: Limited access dressing

Patient Education to Protect the Feet of Patients with Diabetes Mellitus (Key Box 26.15)

- Never walk barefoot. Preferably use ***microcellular rubber sandals,*** which are not only soft, but also allow oxygenation.
- Keep the foot dry after proper cleaning.
- Paring and trimming of toenails should be done carefully. If infection sets in, consult a physician at the earliest.
- **Avoid applying herbal medicines** or lotions to a corn. Consult surgeons for the treatment of corns.
- Proper and regular control of diabetes by diet and frequent measurement of blood sugar.
- Do not consult neighbours[1].
- Reassurance and good rapport with the treating doctors is needed.
- Since these patients have peripheral neuropathy, they will **not be able to appreciate the temperature of water.** Pouring hot water over the foot may cause burns without the patient being aware of it. Hence, a bystander has to check the temperature of water before it is used by the patient. Avoid dipping leg in hotwater.

Key Box 26.15

Public Education in Diabetic Patients

Barefoot walking should be avoided
Avoid herbal/local ointment application
Regular and **r**igorous control of diabetes with diet
Exercises
Foot care—dry, frequent cleaning and corn care
Oxygenation to toes/foot, proper shoes (MCR)
O Do not consult **O**thers
Trimming of nail should be done carefully
Remember as **BAREFOOT**

[1]Remember it is the patient's leg that may have to be amputated and not the neighbour's!

VARIOUS ASPECTS OF DIABETIC ULCER FOOT (Figs 26.29 to 26.39)

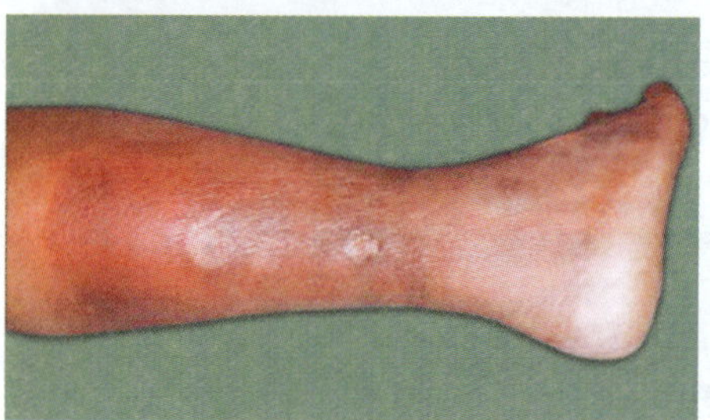

Fig. 26.29: Cellulitis leg

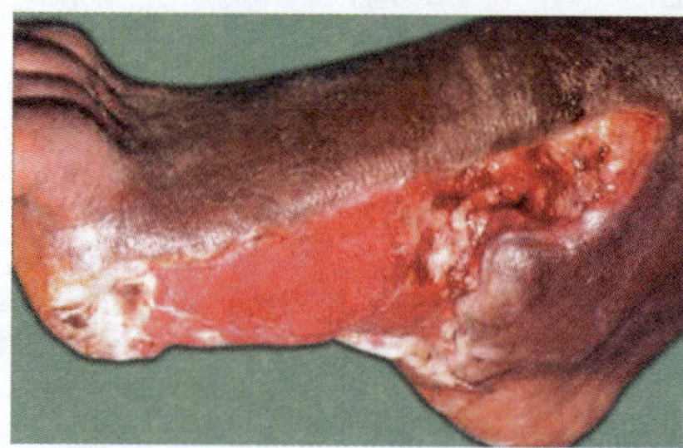

Fig. 26.30: Clawing of toes

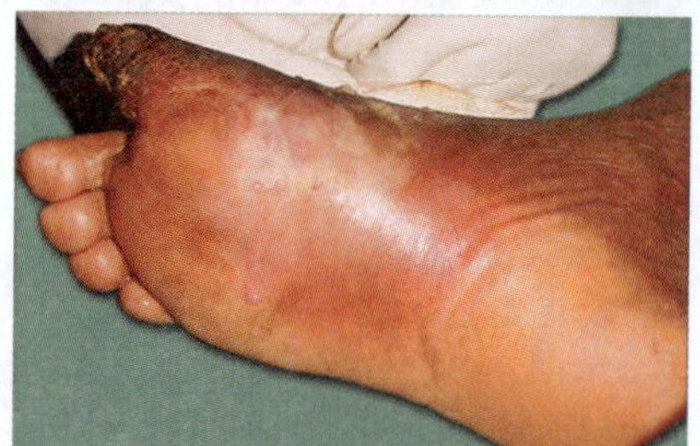

Fig. 26.31: Wet gangrene with abscess foot

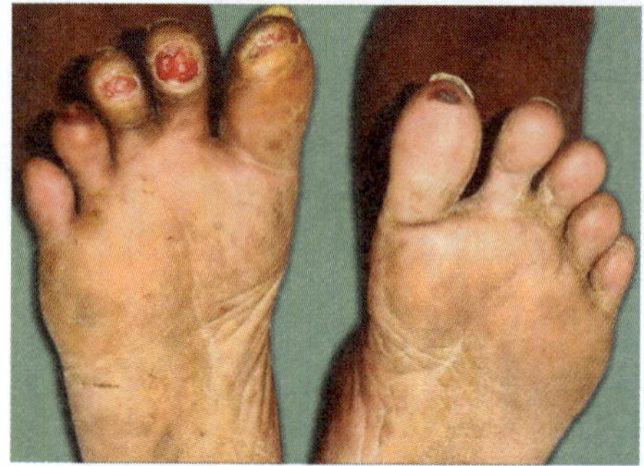

Fig. 26.32: This patient had heat burns following barefoot walking resulting in ulcers

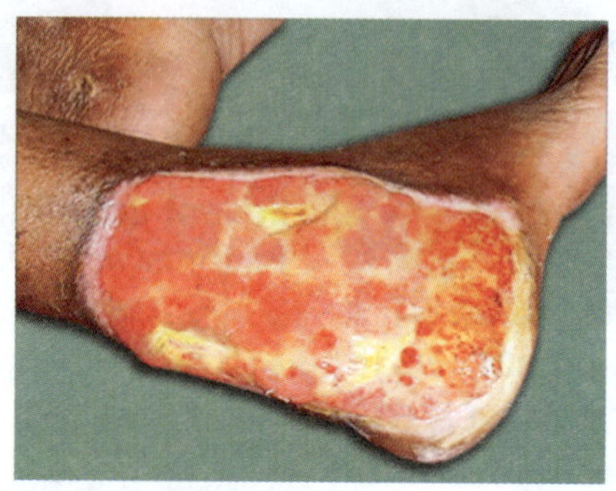

Fig. 26.33: Pale granulation tissue and purulent discharge

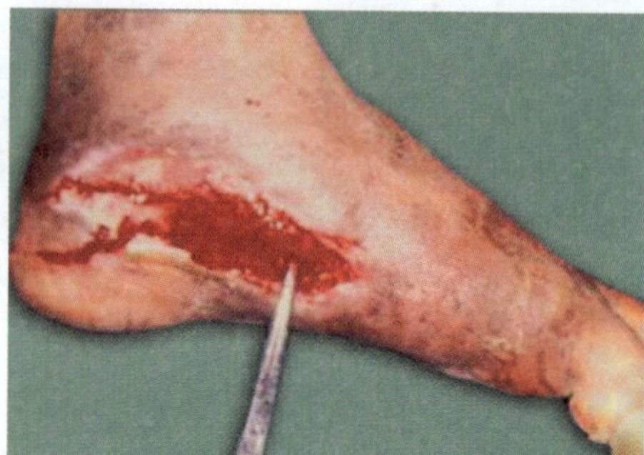

Fig. 26.34: Red granulation tissue-healing after control of diabetes and regular dressings

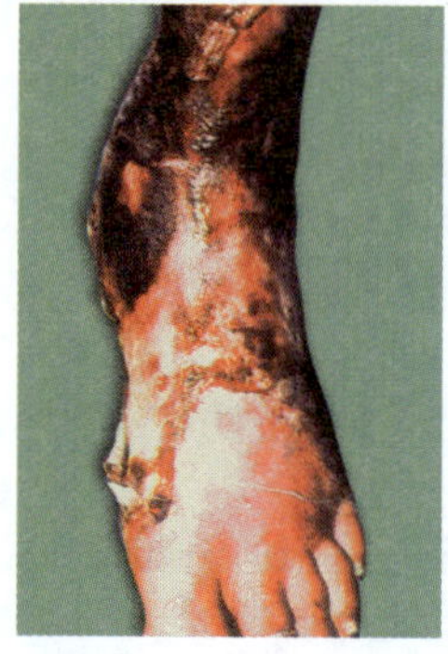

Fig. 26.35: Diabetic ulcer with moist gangrene. Patient had ketoacidosis with septicaemia. In spite of amputation, patient died

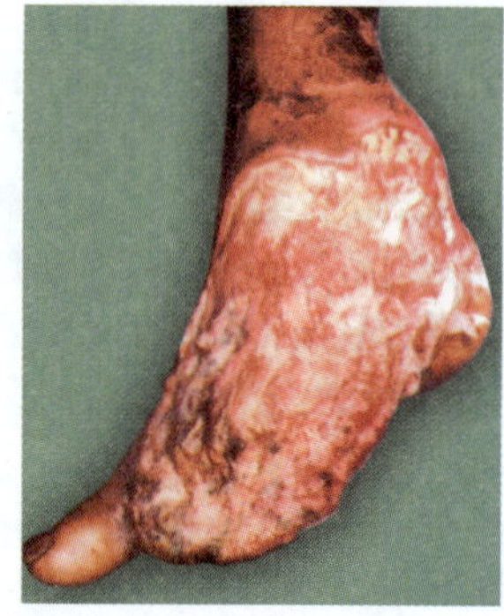

Fig. 26.36: Extensive diabetic ulcer of the foot—needed below knee amputation

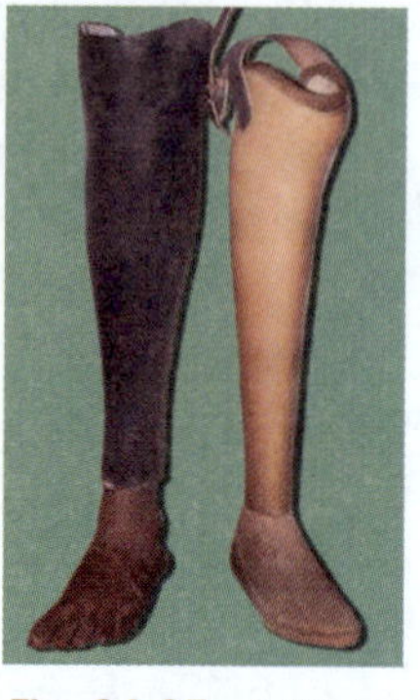

Fig. 26.37: Artificial limb prosthesis

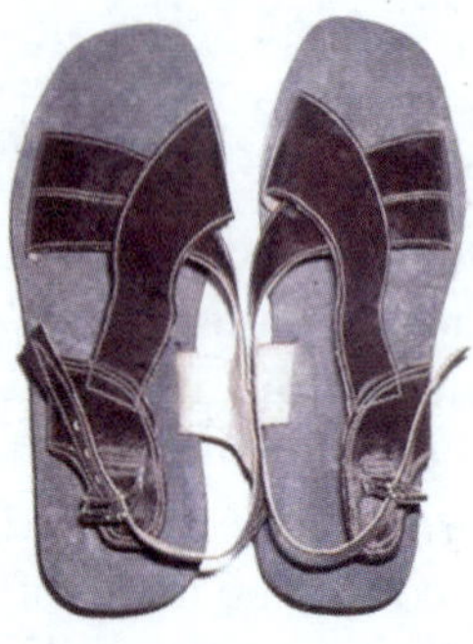

Fig. 26.38: Microcellular rubber (MCR) chappals specially designed for patients with neuropathic foot. They avoid pressure points

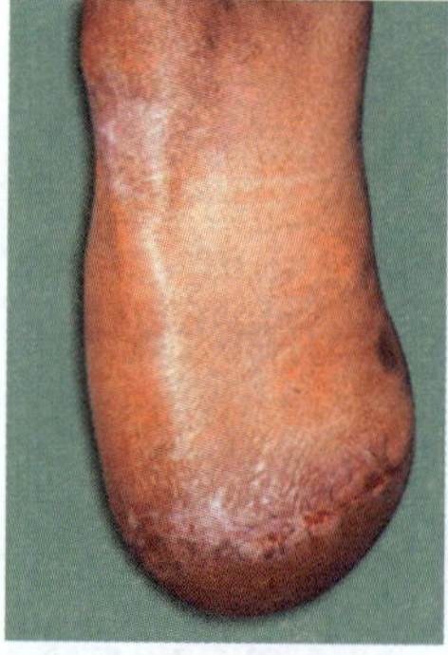

Fig. 26.39: Below knee amputation (see Chapter 70 on amputation under operative surgery for more details)

The best way to avoid complications related to diabetes is by controlling the sugar levels by diet alone or by diet with insulin or oral hypoglycaemic agents.

Screening of foot in diabetes: Diabetic foot is one such disease where prevention is better than treatment and as far as possible one should see that the feet should not be affected. Although physicians are the one to see diabetes patient often, it is responsibility of surgeons also to screen the foot as and when possible. Screening the foot in diabetes can prevent most complications for long period and a diabetic foot storm can be prevented in his life.

Amit Jain's triple assessment for foot: Screening of the foot in diabetic patients should be mandatory by the treating doctor. Amit Jain's screening tool is the simplest and fastest screening tool from India for diabetic foot. It can be performed by any healthcare professional, easy to remember and perform and requires minimal expertise and time for a clinician. It is also known as Amit Jain's linear foot test (LFT) and it has 3 components that address the triad of diabetic foot. It has a look component [check for ulcer/infection over dorsum, plantar and interdigital region], feel component [pulses of foot are palpated] and test component [for sensation].

One can use simple methods to testing sensation like tuning fork, monofilament, pin prick, etc.

The triple assessment should be done annually in every diabetic patient. In case patient comes for follow-up in between, then the look component is enough. This screening tool also has Amit Jain's scoring system and it divides patients into low risk and high risk group

Causes of Death due to Diabetic Foot Ulcer

- Ketoacidosis with septicaemia
- Severe electrolyte abnormalities
- Other causes like silent myocardial infarction, renal failure, etc.

Further Reading (as they are advanced)

1. Amit Jain's Modern Diabetic Foot Surgery Principle and Practice.
2. Amit Jain's Rule of 3 for Diabetic Foot.
3. Amit Jain's Destructive Elevator.
4. Amit Jain's Diabetic Foot Ulcer Scoring.

PRESSURE SORES

Pressure ulcers or bedsores are a serious and **frustrating complication** for paralysed, debilitated, or comatose patients confined to a bed or wheelchair. These ulcers form when soft **tissue is compressed** between a bony prominence (such as the ischium, sacrum, or trochanter) and a supporting structure (such as a bed or wheelchair) (Figs 26.40 and 26.41).

The growing incidence of spinal cord injuries due to automobile accidents and the increased number of debilitated geriatric patients admitted to hospitals have drawn more attention to the prevention and treatment of pressure ulcers. A pressure ulcer is usually the most important factor for delayed rehabilitation in a paraplegic or quadriplegic patient.

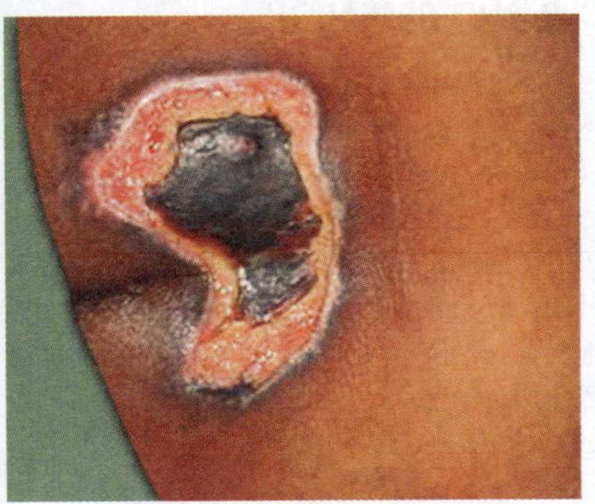

Fig. 26.40: Pressure sore

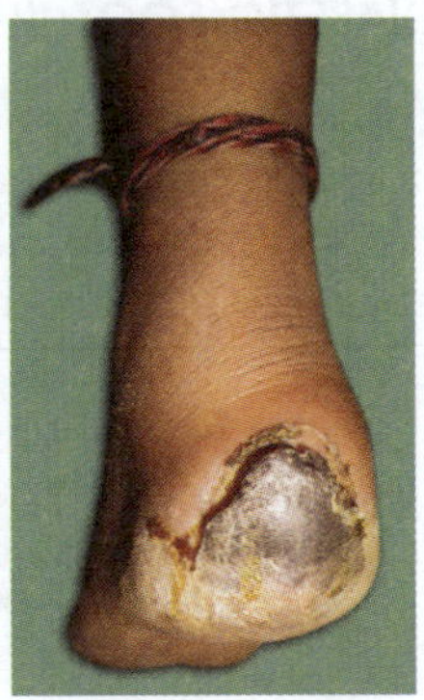

Fig. 26.41: Pressure gangrene—sore over heel

Factors Predisposing to the Formation of a Pressure Sore

The most important factor is **pressure**. Other factors are **paralysis, paresis, shearing forces, malnutrition, anaemia, advanced age, and infection**. A lack of protective sensations in comatose or debilitated patients prevents them from changing posture. The localised pressure continues and a skin ulcer develops. Initially, there is tissue anoxia and cell death. Later, active inflammation and vasodilatation occur, resulting in reactive hyperaemia. If the pressure is removed to allow tissue perfusion and the washing out of toxic byproducts, initial damage may be reversible. If not, permanent damage occurs. This may happen within six hours.

Clinical Features

1. Early Superficial Ulceration

- Erythema, oedema, and punctate haemorrhage
- Moist irregular ulceration with a surrounding erythematous halo

2. Late Superficial Ulceration

- Full thickness skin ulceration
- Spreading necrosis of subcutaneous tissue
- Deep inflammatory response spreads in a cone-shaped fashion to deeper tissues

3. Early Deep Ulceration

- Cicatrization of rolled ulcer edges
- **Eschar** at ulcer base
- Spread of inflammation and bacterial invasion

4. Late Deep Ulceration

- Breakdown of fascial plane
- Chronic inflammation and fibrosis of deep tissue (bursa formation)

There is no such thing as a small pressure ulcer. The visible skin wound is merely the "**tip of the iceberg.**" 70% of the ulcer is below the skin. Pressure is transmitted in a cone-shaped or pyramidal manner from the skin through each layer of tissue to the bony prominence, so that a cone of tissue destruction is created. The point of the cone is at the skin surface, and base is formed by the larger undermined defect overlying the bone.

Preventive Measures

Pressure ulcers may be avoided by meticulous skin care and relief of pressure over the bony prominence (Key Box 26.16).

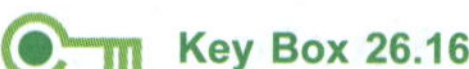
Key Box 26.16

Skin Care

1. Regular, periodical skin inspection, especially over the bony prominences.
2. Any sign of redness, irritation or abrasion—if noted—***all pressure must be taken off*** the area immediately.
3. Keeping the skin clean and dry: Moist areas lead to maceration. Fine talcum powder may be applied to areas where moisture tends to develop. It must be dusted every day after drying the skin.
4. Gentle massage of vulnerable skin with lanolin lotion.
5. ***Care of perineum and genitalia,*** especially in patients with incontinence.
6. Clothing and bedding must be wrinkle-free, made of porous absorbent material to allow air circulation and avoid accumulation of perspiration.
7. ***Pressure relief***—in bedridden patients.
   a. Frequent ***change of posture*** round the clock every 2 hours.
   b. ***Avoid localised pressure*** by proper body alignment.
   c. ***Use of air or fluid-filled floatation*** mattresses also lessens risk of ulcer formation.
   d. Patient and patient's family education.

Treatment

1. **Superficial ulceration:** Debridement and allowing it to heal by secondary intention (takes many weeks)
2. **Deep ulceration** or large superficial ulceration
   - Bedside debridement of obviously necrotic material
   - **'Wet to dry' dressing**
   - Use of **desloughing agents**
   - Systemic **antibiotics**
   - **Nutritional** consideration
   - Correction of spasm and contractures, if present
   - Once it is ready, the defect is closed

   Methods of closure

   a. Primary closure—undermine and approximate the cut edges
   b. SSG—in selected cases only
   c. Skin flaps
      - Transposition flap
      - Rotation flap
      - Advancement flap
   d. **Cultured** muscle interposition for severe and ischial pressure sores.
3. **Education of the patient** and patient attenders to prevent pressure sores.

Miscellaneous

Maggot Therapy

- A **maggot** is the larva of a fly, such as house fly. In practice, any neglected wound on the body, especially over the legs, may get contaminated with maggots. Within 1–2 days, there may be a colony of maggots (Fig. 26.42).

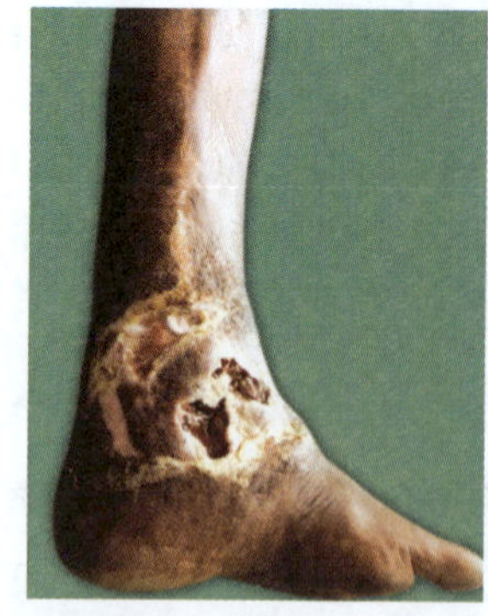
Fig. 26.42: Maggots in diabetic patient who had venous ulcer

- It is a type of biotherapy involving the introduction of live, disinfected maggots into nonhealing wounds.
- The ugly look and feeling of a crawling creature on the body drives the patient to reach the hospital in our country. Maggots may be removed by using turpentine.
- **Mode of action:**
  - Debride wounds by dissolving necrotic, infected tissue.
  - Disinfection of the wound by killing bacteria and healing—doubtful.
  - Maggot therapy may also reduce the need for antibiotics in people with complex, chronic wounds.
  - Maggot therapy has been shown to accelerate the debridement of necrotic wounds.

Indications

- Maggots inhibit and destroy a wide range of pathogenic bacteria including methicillin-resistant *Staphylococcus aureus* (MRSA), group A and B streptococci, and gram-positive aerobic and anaerobic strains. Maggot therapy, therefore, represents a cost-effective method for managing MRSA infection.
- Maggot therapy may also reduce the need for antibiotics in people with complex, chronic wounds.

DIABETIC FOOT ULCER AND RESEARCH

Aldose reductase is the first enzyme in the sorbitol-aldose reductase pathway responsible for the reduction of glucose to sorbitol, as well as the reduction of galactose to galactitol. Too much sorbitol trapped in the retinal cells, lens cells, and the Schwann cells may damage them, leading to retinopathy, cataracts, and peripheral neuropathy, respectively. Aldose reductase inhibitors are currently being investigated as a way to prevent or delay these complications.

Multiple Choice Questions

1. Which of the following statements about tubercular ulcers is false?
A. Undermined edge
B. Edge is thin and bluish in colour
C. Apple jelly granulation tissue
D. Wash leather slough

2. The following are true for squamous cell carcinoma *except*:
A. Keratin pearls are diagnostic
B. Induration at the base is significant
C. Ulcers have everted edges
D. Keratoacanthoma has totally different cytological features than squamous cell carcinoma

3. The following are features of a healing ulcer *except*:
A. Serous discharge
B. Sloping edge
C. Slough is absent
D. Signs of inflammation are present

4. The following are true for induration *except*:
A. Maximum induration is seen in malignant melanoma
B. Brawny induration is seen in chronic abscess
C. Carcinoma tongue may present as an indurated lesion
D. It is overgrowth of fibrous tissue

5. Gummatous ulcer has the following features *except*:
A. Commonly seen in the subcutaneous tissues
B. Floor has wash leather slough
C. Healing results in a hypertrophic scar
D. It has punched out edges

6. Alginate wound dressing has the following advantages *except*:
A. Non-adherent
B. Absorbs exudate
C. It is safe in renal failure cases
D. With silver, it may act against MRSA also

7. The characteristic feature of a venous ulcer in the leg is:
A. Deep and painful
B. Superficial with surrounding pigmentation
C. Penetrating with visible bone
D. Present on the dorsum of the foot

8. The following are true regarding the usage of platelet-derived growth factors in wound dressings *except*:
A. They are used when vascularity is poor
B. They are used in neuropathic ulcers
C. They act through tyrosine kinase receptors
D. They stimulate angiogenesis

9. The following are true for a tropical ulcer *except*:
A. It is caused by Vincent's organisms
B. Minimal inflammation
C. It is also an example of phagedenic ulcer
D. Metronidazole is helpful

10. The following are true about sorbitol *except*:
A. Nerve damage in diabetic foot ulcer is due to sorbitol
B. It results from the reduction of glucose
C. It occurs when the hydroxyl group is changed to aldehyde
D. It may be used as a laxative

11. The following are true for infrainguinal bypass surgery for diabetic ulcer *except*:
A. Long saphenous vein is inferior to PTFE graft
B. Preoperative vein marking is helpful
C. 2-year patency is around 70%
D. Amputation rate after surgery is still high

12. The following are true for cilostazol *except*:
A. It reduces the pain of intermittent claudication
B. It is a phosphodiesterase inhibitor
C. Its action is similar to pentoxyphylline
D. Dose is 50 mg twice daily

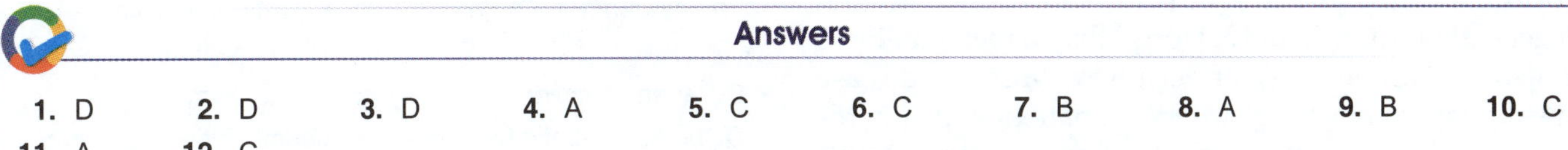

Answers

1. D **2.** D **3.** D **4.** A **5.** C **6.** C **7.** B **8.** A **9.** B **10.** C
11. A **12.** C

CHAPTER

27

Lower Limb Ischaemia and Popliteal Aneurysm

- Causes of lower limb ischaemia
- Collateral circulation
- Symptoms
- Fontaine classification
- Clinical examination
- Differential diagnosis
- Management
- Acute arterial occlusion
- Critical limb ischaemia
- Peripheral aneurysm
- Ainhum
- Frostbite
- Reperfusion injuries
- Fat embolism, air embolism
- ICU gangrene

Competency

SU27.1: Describe the etiopathogenesis, clinical features, investigations and principles of treatment of occlusive arterial disease.

INTRODUCTION

Walking is a fundamental human requirement. Peripheral arterial disease (PAD) is a main cause of disability. Many individuals are conscious about chest pain caused by myocardial ischaemia and arrive at a hospital early. However, patients present relatively late to the hospital with lower limb ischaemia (Figs 27.1 and 27.2). The disease, though benign, is not totally curable, causing financial, social, and psychological burden to the patient and his/her relatives.

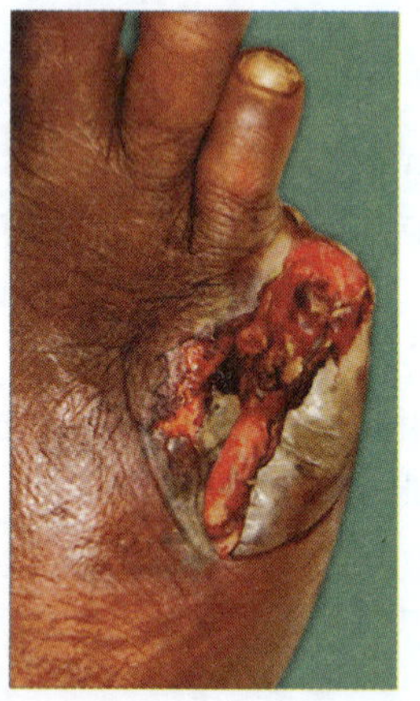

Fig. 27.1: Atherosclerosis with diabetes resulting in wet gangrene—toe has been amputated

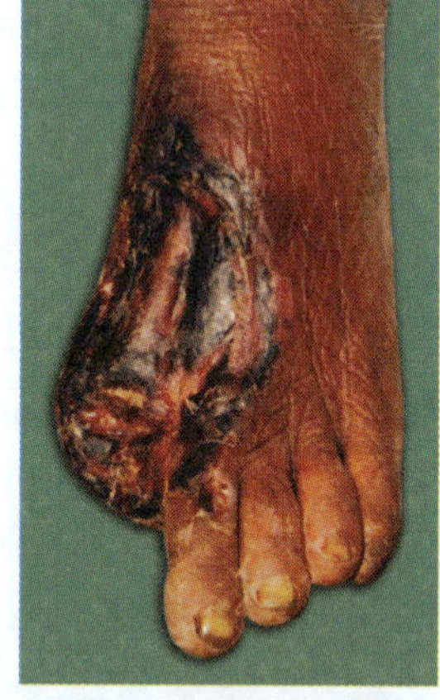

Fig. 27.2: Dry gangrene due to atherosclerotic arterial disease—part is dry, mummified and toe has been amputated

CAUSES OF LOWER LIMB ISCHAEMIA (Table 27.1)

Occlusion refers to obstruction to the lumen of blood vessel. Example being atheromatous plaques or a blood clot, etc. **Stenosis** refers to abnormal narrowing of the vessel. Other rare causes of lower limb ischaemia include popliteal entrapment syndrome and cystic medial degeneration. One should not forget that **diabetes mellitus** is also a common cause of peripheral vascular disease in elderly patients. While treating a patient with atherosclerotic disease, care of diabetes is equally important.

Table 27.1 Causes of lower limb ischaemia

Chronic lower limb ischaemia	Acute lower limb ischaemia
• Atherosclerosis	• Acute thrombosis
• **T**hromboangiitis **O**bliterans (TAO)	• Acute embolism
	• Trauma to the vessels
• Collagen vascular disorders	• Aneurysm
• Diabetes (diabetic foot—neuro-ischaemic foot)	

RISK FACTORS FOR PERIPHERAL ARTERIAL DISEASE (PAD)

- **S**moking: Smoking in any form increases the risk by almost tenfold. It is proportional to 'pack-years' smoked.
- **M**ale (gender): Men are affected 10 years earlier than women.
- **O**ther risk factors: These include hypercholesterolemia (>200 mg/dl), hypertriglyceridaemia, hypercoagulable state (polycythaemia), and hyperhomocysteinaemia.
- **K**nown diabetes: Especially type 2 diabetes mellitus—increases the risk by two to fourfold.
- **E**lderly patients between 60 and 70 years are vulnerable.
- **R**aised blood pressure—hypertension.

You can *remember as* **SMOKER**

HYPERHOMOCYSTEINAEMIA

- It increases the risk of developing PAD by 7%
- Homocysteine levels >15 mmol/L
- Increased levels cause endothelial injury and lead to vascular inflammation
- Defective gene for methylene tetrahydrofolate reductase (MTHFR)
- Prevention is by eating foods containing B_6, B_9, B_{12} and folate, such as potatoes, green vegetables, fish, etc.
- It is also a strong risk for myocardial infarction in young patients.

COLLATERAL CIRCULATION

- Collateral circulation is present in most organs. Hence, even if a major vessel is occluded, the organ may still survive provided collaterals are well-developed.
- In acute ischaemia caused by **thrombus** or **embolism**, there is no time for collaterals to develop. This results in gangrene of the limb in untreated cases (Fig. 27.3).
- Chronic ischaemia caused by TAO or atherosclerosis allows sufficient time for collaterals to develop (Fig. 27.4). Hence, necrosis or gangrene that occurs is minimised and the limb often survives.

SYMPTOMS

1. **Pain** in the limb is the chief symptom of lower limb ischaemia. It is a severe, cramp-like pain due to ischaemia of the muscles that is brought on mainly by exertion, relieved by rest, and **reproducible.** It is called **intermittent claudication** (Key Box 27.1). The most common site of obstruction is the superficial femoral artery which results in classical calf muscle claudication (Key Box 27.2). Blood supply to the great toe comes from the dorsalis pedis artery and a branch from the medial plantar artery, a branch of posterior tibial artery. When these are affected, it results in **instep claudication. The muscle affected is the extensor hallucis longus.**

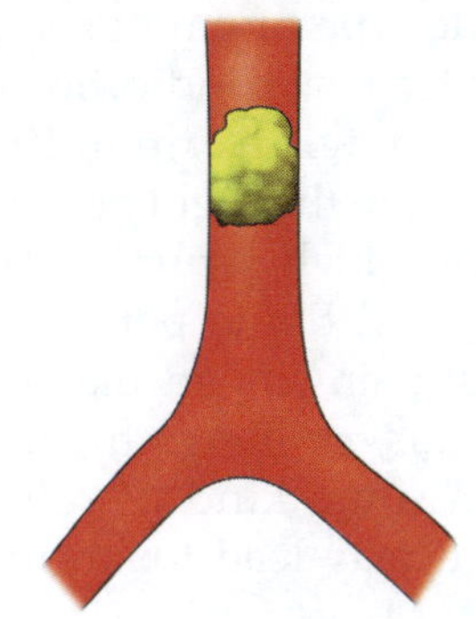

Fig. 27.3: Sudden occlusion. Embolic—no time for collaterals to develop

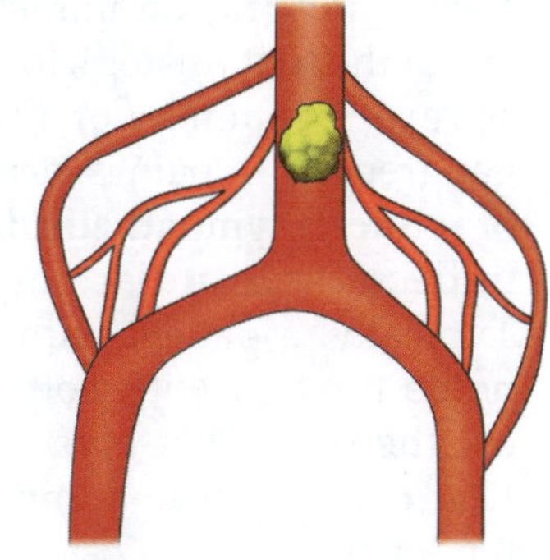

Fig. 27.4: Slow occlusion (atherosclerotic). Collaterals develop

Key Box 27.1

Grades of intermittent Claudication—Boyd's classification

Grade I : The patient walks for a distance, gets the pain, continues to walk and the pain disappears. As a result of ischaemia, anaerobic metabolism takes place, which produces ***substance P, lactic acid***, etc. These produce vasodilatation and the pain disappears.

Grade II: The patient walks for a distance, gets the pain and continues to walk with the pain. He has a limp.

Grade III: The patient walks and gets the pain. He has to take rest. This grade indicates severe muscle ischaemia.

In late stages: Pain at rest is due to ischaemia of nerves* in addition to ischaemia of the muscles.

*Cry of the dying nerves, due to involvement of vasa nervosum

Pain is due to ischaemic neuropathy involving small unmyelinated A, delta and C sensory fibres.

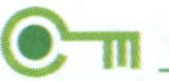

Key Box 27.2

Superficial Femoral Artery Stenosis or Occlusion

- It is the most common cause of intermittent claudication
- Usually calf muscles are affected
- Does not produce life-threatening ischaemia unless profunda femoris is involved.
- Single stenosis less than 3 cm is treated by **P**ercutaneous **T**ransluminal **A**ngiography **(PTA)**

Rest pain:[1] It is an intractable type of pain usually felt in the foot (instep), toes, etc. It is an indication of severe ischaemia of the foot with impending gangrene. Rest pain is increased in the night because of **reduced sympathetic drive,** which in turn results in decreased cardiac output and tissue perfusion. Typically, a patient with rest pain sits on the bed, holds his foot with both hands, or hangs his foot off the bed. This gives him some kind of relief. Rest pain is worse at night. It may lead to suicidal tendency.[1]

- Claudication distance refers to the distance a patient is able to walk before the onset of pain. A patient with severe claudication may not be able to walk even a few yards.
- The site of claudication depends on the level of arterial occlusion (Table 27.2).
- Tables 27.3 and 27.4 list other causes of pain in the leg.

Table 27.2 Site of occlusion and claudication

Level of occlusion	Claudication site
Aortoiliac obstruction	Claudication of both gluteal regions, thighs and calves
Iliofemoral obstruction	Claudication of thigh muscles
Femoropopliteal obstruction	Claudication of calf muscles
Popliteal obstruction	Claudication of the foot muscles, **instep claudication**

Pearls of Wisdom

Intermittent claudication in a young patient may be due to some rare causes such as:

- Popliteal artery entrapment due to abnormal origin of the gastrocnemius muscle
- Cyst in the media of the popliteal artery
- Hyperhomocysteinaemia

2. **Nonhealing ulcer** is the next commonly presenting symptom. It is usually precipitated by minor trauma and occurs in the most distal part of the body, such as the tip of the toes. Ischaemic ulcers are deep and very painful.
3. Some patients present with **gangrenous patches** of skin or subcutaneous tissue (Fig. 27.5). Gangrene affects distal parts such as toes. However, gangrene is minimal because of collaterals.

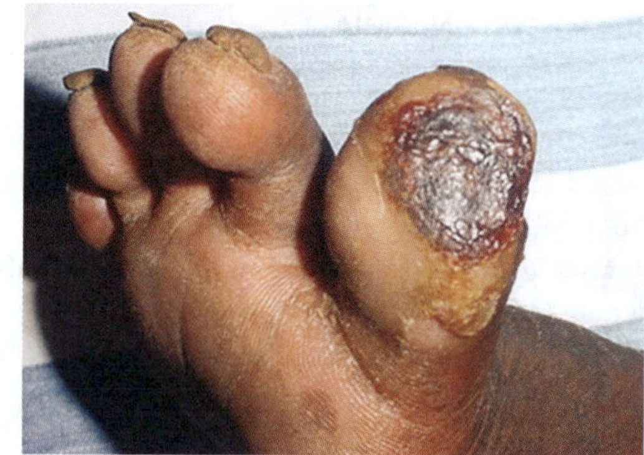

Fig. 27.5: Thromboangiitis obliterans with dry gangrene

Table 27.3 Important causes of pain in the leg

Condition	Aetiology	Nature of pain	Location
• Intermittent (arterial) claudication	Inadequate skeletal muscle perfusion	Burning or cramp like	Calf muscles, thigh or gluteal region. Relieved on rest
• Neurogenic claudication	Lumbosacral nerve root compression	Diffuse radiating deep ache with or without paraesthesia	Pain on first step, decreased on sitting or bending over while walking
• Venous claudication (DVT)	Proximal venous occlusion thrombosis	Bursting	Engorgement during exercise
• Varicosity	Long saphenous varicosity	Diffuse aching/heaviness	Decreases on walking due to calf muscles pump

Table 27.4 Pain in the leg—other causes

	Etiology	Character of pain	Location presentation
• Atheroembolism	Distal embolisation—source may be in the aorta	Aching, severe	Cyanosis, ischaemic changes in toes or distal foot secondary to digital or branch of an artery occlusion
• Lymphatic disease	Idiopathic, iatrogenic or infection. Pain develops secondary to cellulitis or lymphangitis	Localizes	Site of inflammation—redness is a feature

[1]One of our TAO patients with sleepless nights due to rest pain committed suicide by jumping from the 2nd floor of the hospital.

4. History of **bilateral gluteal claudication** with impotence may occur in a young patient due to a saddle thrombus at the bifurcation of the aorta. This is called **Leriche's syndrome**, which presents as a triad of claudication, ***erectile*** dysfunction, and decreased distal pulses. Impotence is due to failure to achieve an erection due to paralysis of the L1 nerve. **Gluteal claudication** is confused for sciatica and many patients are referred to the orthopaedic department. Sciatica causes **neurogenic claudication,** which is present even **at rest** and is aggravated by movements of the spine. Causes of neurogenic claudication include slipped disc, fracture vertebrae, tuberculosis of spine, etc.
5. Coldness, numbness, paraesthesia, and colour changes indicate chronic ischaemia.
6. The majority of patients with peripheral vascular disease are smokers. TAO occurs exclusively in male smokers.[1]

Pearls of Wisdom

Cauda equina claudication or pseudoclaudication is due to compression of cauda equina.

CLASSIFICATION

- Fontaine and Rutherford also categorised chronic lower limb ischaemia into 6 different categories ranging from asymptomatic to major tissue loss (Table 27.5).
- Claudication is classified as either mild, moderate, or severe based on treadmill response and ankle pressure (AP).

Mild: Completes treadmill test. AP is >50 mmHg after exercise.

Moderate: Cannot complete treadmill test. AP after exercise is <50 mmHg.

Severe: Resting AP <40 mmHg (cannot complete treadmill test).

- Normal segmental systolic arterial pressures (mmHg)

Arm	120
Upper thigh	160
Above knee	150
Below knee	140
Ankle	130

Diagnostic criteria of TAO: = Shionoya criteria

- Age at onset <50 years
- Smoking history +
- Distal extremity ischaemia, upper limb involvement, phlebitis migrans
- Typically, infrapopliteal occlusions

SIGNS: CLINICAL EXAMINATION

Inspection

The ***findings are appreciated*** better if a comparison is made with the opposite limb. Evidence of chronic ischaemia of the leg includes:

- ***Attitude of the limb:*** Very often, the patient holds the calf muscles or dorsum of the foot (Fig. 27.6).

Commonly asked question—why does the patient hold his legs and hang them off the bed?

1. Venous stasis and reflex vasodilatation.
2. He compresses the muscles with his hands which may also help in venous return.
3. Warmth of the hands is transferred to the limb. These are explanations given by many experienced senior examiners and teachers. I request student to verify these explanations.
4. Gravity assisted blood flow.

- Flattening of the terminal pulp spaces of toes
- Fissures and cracks between the toes

Table 27.5 Clinical classification of PAOD

Fontaine	Classification	Rutherford	Classification
Stage	Clinical	Grade	Clinical
I	Asymptomatic	0	Asymptomatic
IIa	Mild claudication	1	Mild claudication
IIb	Moderate to severe	2	Moderate to severe
	claudication	3	Severe claudication
III	Ischaemic rest pain	4	Ischaemic rest pain
IV	Ulceration or gangrene	5	Minor tissue loss
		6	Major tissue loss

[1]A 26-year-old female, nonsmoker patient presented to the hospital with ischaemic features of the right upper limb. All causes of upper limb ischaemia were ruled out (Raynaud's, cervical rib, etc.). On careful questioning, she admitted to using Snuff dipping for 10 years (snuff contains nicotine).

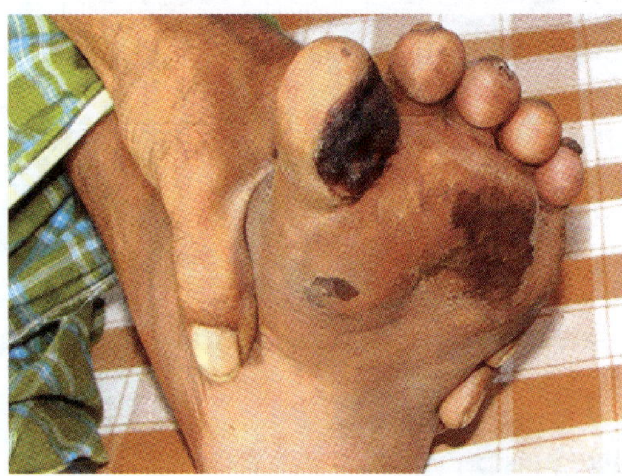

Fig. 27.6: Attitude of TAO patient—foot is tightly held by hand. Observe gangrene, ulcer, skin changes and ridged nails

- Ulceration of toes, interdigital ulcers
- Brittle, flat, and ridged nails, shiny skin
- Loss of hair and subcutaneous fat
- The limb may appear more dark in dark-skinned patients or markedly pale in fair-skinned patients with vasospastic diseases such as TAO.
- Gangrene is usually dry with a clear line of demarcation. It indicates the junction of dead and living tissue. Since the blood supply to the muscle is better, usually the **line of demarcation involves skin and subcutaneous tissue**. The line of demarcation is very well appreciated in senile gangrene, **where it may be skin, muscle, or bone-deep**.
- The limb may show muscle atrophy.
- Multiple toes and finger involvement suggest vasculitis (Fig. 27.7).

Pearls of Wisdom

Why is ischaemic pain more in the night?

Loss of gravity assistance to arterial supply, reduction in cardiac output at rest, reactive dilatation of skin vessels to warmth, and increased attention of the patient to the leg.

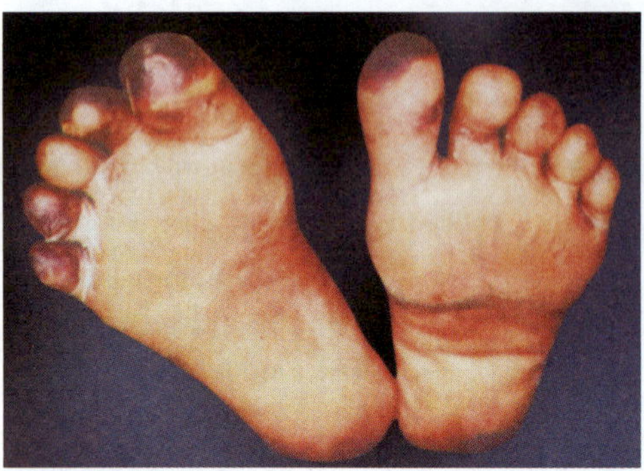

Fig. 27.7: Vasculitis with collagen vascular disorder. It had affected all the ten toes

Palpation

1. **Ulcer:** Examination should be done as described in Chapter 6. Ischaemic ulcers are very tender.
2. **Gangrene:** It is described according to its size, shape, and extent. In dry gangrene, the part is dry and mummified or shrunken. Features of dry gangrene are summarised in Key Box 27.3.

Key Box 27.3

Gangrene

- Loss of temperature
- Loss of pulsation
- Loss of sensation
- Loss of colour
- Loss of function

3. **Limb** above[1]
   - **Ischaemic limb is cold:** Careful palpation from above downwards will reveal the change in temperature from warm to cold. Temperature changes are better appreciated with the dorsum of the hand because it has many cutaneous nerve endings.
   - **Tenderness:** It is tender due to the presence of inflammation.
   - **Sensation:** Ischaemic limb is hypersensitive[2], due to irritation of the nerve endings.
   - **Pitting oedema** may be due to thrombophlebitis or due to nonfunctioning of the limb.
   - Feel pulses in all four limbs and in the head and neck region.
4. **Palpation of pulses**[3] (Table 27.6).
   - After examining the pulses, results are interpreted in **a pulse chart** as shown in Key Box 27.4.
   - In a similar manner, upper limb pulses and head and neck pulses are also recorded in the pulse chart.

Key Box 27.4

Pulse Chart

(For example, classical case of TAO left lower limb)

Lower limb pulses	Right	Left
Dorsalis pedis	++	-
Posterior tibial	++	-
Popliteal	++	+
Femoral	++	++

++ : Normal; + : Weak; – : Absent.

+++ : Indicates prominent pulse such as water hammer pulse as in aortic insufficiency

[1]It is better to palpate the entire limb from the thigh downwards.

[2]Ischaemic limb is like irritable personalities.

[3]A thorough clinical examination of pulses includes not only lower limb vessels but also the head, neck, and upper limb vessels

Table 27.6 Examination of peripheral vessels

Artery	Site where it is felt	Remarks
	Examination of lower limb pulses	
1. **Dorsalis pedis** is the continuation of anterior tibial artery	At the level of ankle joint lateral to extensor hallucis longus. It should not be felt distally where it dips into the plantar space	In 10% of cases, it can be absent
2. **Posterior tibial artery** is a branch of popliteal artery	In between the medial malleolus and medial border of the tendoachilles	For circulation of the foot, any one of these arteries is sufficient
3. **Popliteal artery,** a continuation of femoral artery, extends from the hiatus in adductor magnus to the fibrous arch in soleus. It is about 20 cm long	It is felt in the prone or supine position with knee flexed. It is felt against lower end of femur or against tibial condyles	**The knee is flexed to relax popliteal fascia.** Dorsalis pedis, posterior tibial and popliteal artery are usually not palpable in TAO patients
4. **Femoral artery** is the continuation of external iliac artery	It is felt midway between anterior superior iliac spine and pubic tubercle, just below the inguinal ligament in the upper thigh	Abduction and external rotation of the hip joint may facilitate the palpation in obese patients
	Examination of head and neck vessels	
1. **Subclavian artery** arises from the arch of aorta on the left side and brachiocephalic on the right side	It is felt in the supraclavicular region in the posterior triangle against the first rib	Difficult to feel in obese patients
2. **Common carotid artery** arises from arch of aorta on the left side and from brachiocephalic artery on the right side	It is felt against the carotid tubercle of sixth cervical vertebra (C6) in the carotid triangle (at the upper border of the thyroid cartilage)	Carotid artery bifurcates at the upper border of the lamina of thyroid cartilage (C3 vertebra)
3. **Superficial temporal artery** is the terminal branch of the external carotid artery	It is felt in front of tragus of the ear against the zygoma	This is involved in temporal arteritis, a type of giant cell arteritis

Disappearing pulse: When collateral circulation is very good, peripheral pulses may be normal. However, when the patient is asked to exercise, the pulse may disappear. Exercise produces vasodilatation below the obstruction and arterial inflow cannot keep pace with the increasing vascular space. Hence, the pressure falls and the pulse disappears.

Other Tests of Minor Importance

1. **Buerger's postural test** is relevant in fair-skinned patients. The patient (supine) is asked to raise his legs vertically upwards keeping the knees straight. In cases of chronic ischaemia, marked pallor develops within 2–3 minutes. The angle at which pallor develops is Buerger's angle of circulatory insufficiency. In an ischaemic limb, pallor develops even on elevation of the leg by 15–30°.
2. **Capillary refill test:** Apply pressure over the tip of the terminal pulp space for a few seconds and release the pressure. Rapid return of circulation is observed in normal persons (<2 seconds). The test may also be done in the ischaemic foot by asking the patient to sit up and hang his legs down and observing for colour changes. The time taken for the ischaemic foot to become pink is described as the capillary filling time. This is prolonged in an ischaemic foot.

Pearls of Wisdom

Quincke's sign is pulsation of the capillary nail bed that occurs in cases of aortic regurgitation with a very wide pulse pressure.

Auscultation (Figs 27.8 and 27.9)

1. Systolic bruit over the femoral artery may be heard in atherosclerotic occlusion of the iliofemoral segment due to turbulence created by the blood flow.
2. Auscultation of the heart to rule out mitral stenosis (mid-diastolic murmur, loud S1).

Clinical Notes

An 18-year-old girl was kept in the MBBS examination with ischaemia of the lower limb of 6 days duration. A candidate offered collagen vascular disorder as the first diagnosis and failed.

He had totally missed the cardiac history and findings by not auscultating the heart. It was a case of mitral stenosis with acute embolic gangrene of the lower limb.

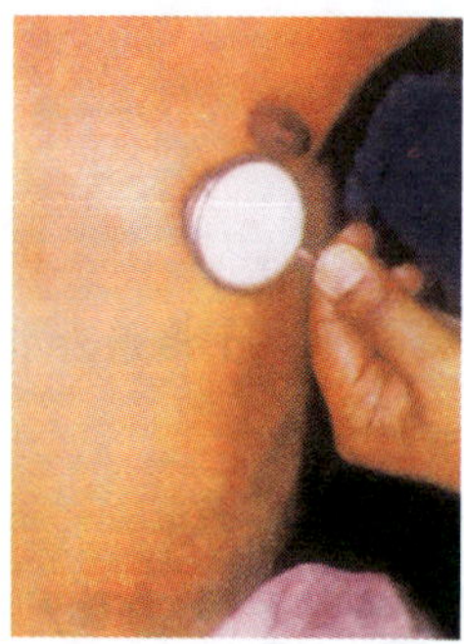

Fig. 27.8: Auscultation of the heart to rule out valvular heart diseases

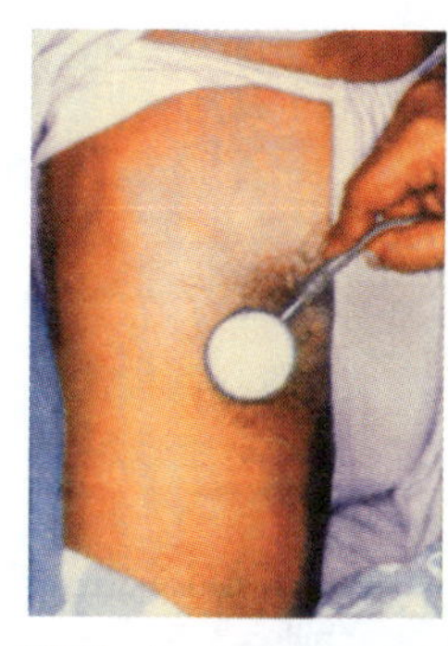

Fig. 27.9: Auscultation over the femoral artery to look for bruit

DIFFERENTIAL DIAGNOSIS

- Even though there are many causes of lower limb ischaemia, thromboangiitis obliterans (TAO) and atherosclerotic vascular disease are the most common causes. Hence, they should be considered before giving other diagnoses.
- TAO is also called Buerger's disease. The details are given in Table 27.7 and Key Boxes 27.5–27.7.
- Atherosclerotic vascular disease is the most common cause of lower limb ischaemia. It may manifest from a simple ulcer to massive gangrene.

Table 27.7 Differential diagnosis[1]

	TAO (Buerger's disease)	Atherosclerosis
1. Age	20–40 years	Around 50 years and above
2. Sex	Exclusively males	Females are also affected
3. Aetiology	1. It is a smoker's disease. Excessive tobacco (nicotine) produces severe vasospasm of the vessels. 2. Excessive smoking produces increased levels of carboxyhaemoglobin which damages these vessels. 3. Low socioeconomic group, recurrent trauma to the foot, poor hygiene are additional factors. 4. Hypercoagulable state 5. Autonomic hyperactivity 6. Autoimmune factors	1. Atherosclerosis is a rich man's disease, who is usually a smoker, diabetic and hypertensive. 2. Strong family history is also present in a few cases. 3. Consumption of high fat diet leading to obesity, lack of regular exercises and hypercholesterolaemia are other factors.
4. **Pathology**	Diffuse inflammatory reaction involving all three coats of vessel **(panarteritis)** causing a thrombus, resulting in occlusion of lumen **(obliterans)**. Polymorphs, giant cells and **micro-abscesses** are found within the thrombus. In severe cases, vein and nerve are bound by fibrous tissue.	Deposition of lipid-rich atheromatous plaque in the intima is the hallmark of atherosclerosis. Plaques tend to be more in **lower abdominal aorta**, coronary arteries, etc. Plaques may undergo **calcification**, ulceration and thrombosis, **dislodge** cholesterol emboli or may weaken the media and produce **aneurysm**.
5. **Vessels involved**	**Small- and medium-sized vessels** such as dorsalis pedis, posterior tibial, popliteal are commonly involved.	Medium-sized and large vessels such as aorta, common iliac, femoral, common carotid arteries are involved.
6. Upper limb involvement	Not uncommon	Rare
7. Nature of vessel wall	Not thickened	Thickened
8. Blood pressure	Normal in the normal limb and low in diseased limb.	Hypertension is commonly present.
9. **Superficial[2] migrating thrombophlebitis**	Seen in about 30% of cases of TAO. Veins of lower limb are involved and are tender and thickened.	Not seen
10. **Raynaud's phenomenon**	Can be present	Not seen
11. Auscultation—femoral artery	Bruit is not heard.	Bruit can be present as in aortoiliac disease.
12. Angiography	**Cork-screw pattern** of vessels	Shows site of block

[1]From MBBS examination point of view, TAO and atherosclerotic vascular disease are to be differentiated.

[2]Migrating thrombophlebitis is also seen in pancreatic malignancy where it is called Trousseau's sign.

Key Box 27.5

Checklist of Features of Chronic Lower Limb Arterial Occlusion

- **C**old and numbness
- **L**imb elevation: Slow venous refilling. Line of demarcation present
- **A**ltered/diminished sensation
- **U**lcerations
- **D**ead toe—gangrene—dried and mummified
- **I**ntractable pain—rest pain
- **C**racks, fissure—interdigital
- **A**rterial pulsations decreased or absent
- **T**hrill/bruit may be present
- **I**ntermittent claudication
- **O**edema—if thrombophlebitis or cellulitis occurs
- **N**arrow calf muscle girth—muscle atrophy

Remember as **CLAUDICATION**

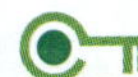

Key Box 27.6

Classification of Buerger's Disease

Type I: Upper extremity

Type II: Crural (leg and foot)

Type III: Femoral type—femoropopliteal

Type IV: Aortoiliac

Type V: Generalised type

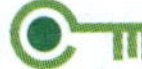

Key Box 27.7

Buerger's Disease—Summary

- Male smoker
- Progressive, nonatherosclerotic, segmental, occlusive, inflammatory condition
- ***Occlusion of small- and medium-sized vessels, superficial thrombophlebitis and Raynaud's phenomenon constitute the 'triad' of TAO.***
- Microabscesses, polymorphs, giant cells (pathology) are found.
- Distal, infrapopliteal, segmental occlusion with skip lesions and corkscrew collaterals in angiogram.
- Stop smoking
- Start analgesics
- Lumbar sympathectomy is of some value

Key words can be *remembered as* **PRISON**

Progressive, **I**nflammatory, **S**egmental, **O**cclusive, **N**onatherosclerotic

MANAGEMENT

Investigations

1. **Complete blood picture:** Anaemia definitely delays wound healing and decreases tissue perfusion. High total count indicates secondary infection.
   - Elevated **platelet count** suggests risk of thrombosis.
   - Fasting blood glucose and **glycosylated haemoglobin.** HbA1c is an important test as it reflects the duration of diabetes.
   - Increased creatinine indicates renal disease.
2. **Lipids:** Fasting total cholesterol, high density lipoprotein, low-density lipoprotein, and triglyceride concentration—hyperlipidaemia should be controlled to prevent progression of peripheral arterial disease and death from coronary artery diseases.
3. **Hypercoagulable status:**
   - Protein C deficiency is identified as a risk factor for arterial thrombosis, especially in patients who will be treated with heparin.
   - Heparin-induced platelet aggregation and heparin-induced thrombocytopaenia.
   - Antiphospholipid antibody (APLA) syndrome (APLS) is also called Hughes syndrome. It is an autoimmune hypercoagulable state resulting in thrombosis of veins (deep vein thrombosis), thrombosis of artery (stroke), and pregnancy-related complications. It is treated by aspirin and heparin.
   - **Homocysteine levels (4 to 15—normal, >15 mmol/L can be dangerous).**
4. **Hand held Doppler ultrasound blood flow detector:** **This is an extension of clinical examination.** This test is based on the Doppler principle. An ultrasound signal is beamed at an artery and the reflected beam is picked up by a receiver. Frequency changes of the beam due to moving blood are converted into audio signals which may be heard by a probe. Thus, a Doppler probe may be used to detect the pulse even when the pulse is clinically not palpable (Figs 27.10–27.13). Using a sphygmomanometer, systolic blood pressure (SBP) of the limb can be measured by positioning the cuff at a suitable level and the pressure index can be calculated. This is called ankle brachial index (ABPI).

$$\textbf{Ankle brachial pressure index} = \frac{\text{Ankle blood pressure}}{\text{Brachial blood pressure}}$$

   - Normal values are >1. However, in patients with peripheral vascular disease of the lower limb, the values are <1 (indicative of vascular obstruction).

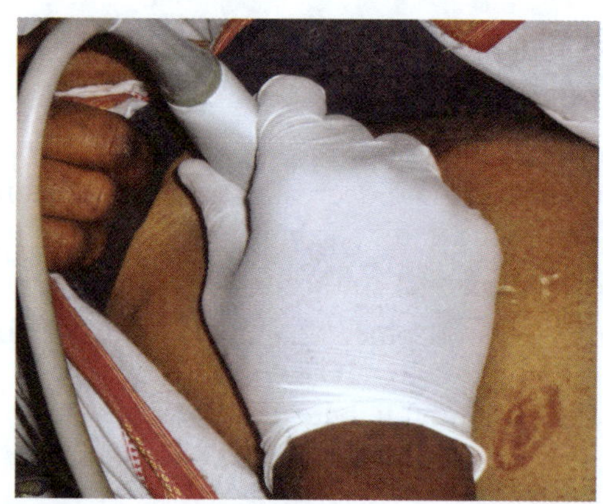

Fig. 27.10: Doppler probe over the femoral artery

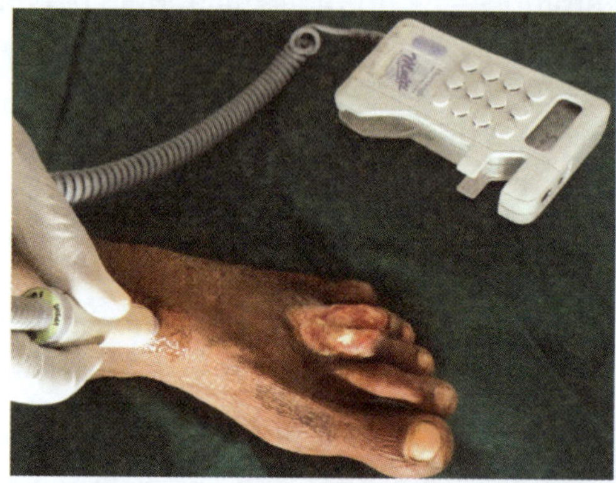

Fig. 27.11: Handheld Doppler checking the dorsalis pedis artery

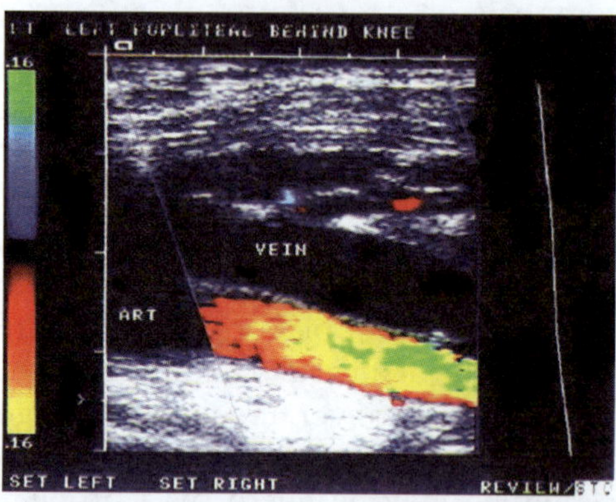

Fig. 27.12: Colour Doppler showing femoral artery and vein

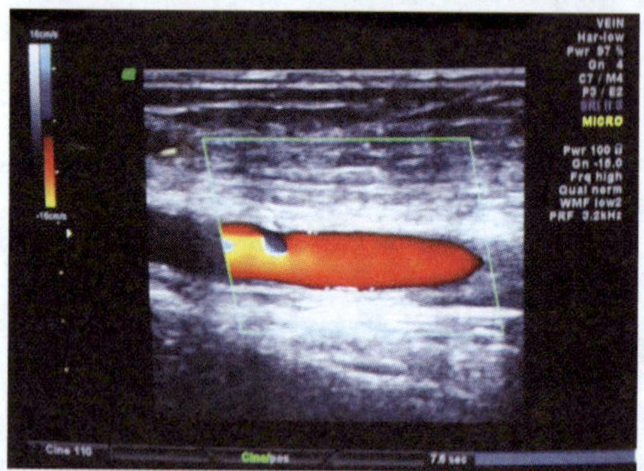

Fig. 27.13: Colour Doppler showing atherosclerotic narrowing

ABPI—Ankle Brachial Pressure Index

Normal ABPI >1

>1.30	Noncompressible
1.00–1.29	Normal
0.91–0.99	Borderline (equivocal)
0.41–0.90	Mild to moderate PAD
0.00–0.40	Severe PAD
Toe-ankle index	
0.6 + 0.2	Normal

- In diabetic patients, ABPI may be increased due to arteriosclerosis. In such patients, toe pressure is measured. If toes are not available (postoperative status), transcutaneous oxygen tension ($TcPO_2$) should be measured instead.
- Normal toe pressure is 20–40 mmHg less than ankle pressure.
- <30 mmHg of toe pressure is associated with ischaemic symptoms.
- Foot ulcers heal only if toe pressure is >30–40 mmHg.
- When ankle pressure is <30 mmHg, gangrene may be imminent.

Uses of Doppler probe

- To detect normal pulses in operation theatres
- To detect clinically nondetectable pulse in peripheral vascular disease
- To measure BP (blood pressure) in ischaemic limbs
- To remeasure BP in the lower limb after exercise to differentiate ischaemic claudication from neurogenic claudication

5. **Duplex scan** (Key Box 27.8)
   - Duplex ultrasound involves using **high frequency sound waves** to look at the speed of blood flow. This is the investigation of choice today. Duplex scan is a combination of Doppler and B mode ultrasound (Fig. 27.14). B mode ultrasound is used

Key Box 27.8

Duplex Imaging Scan

- It yields both anatomic and blood flow information
- No nephrotoxic contrast agent is used
- It gives a **triphasic** wave pattern systolic, diastolic and elastic recoil
- Elastic recoil is absent in calcified arteries
- Thus biphasic and monophasic wave patterns indicate 'PAD'
- Overall sensitivity of 92% and specificity of 99% in occlusive cases
- Limiting factors are extensive ulcers, calcification and oedema of leg

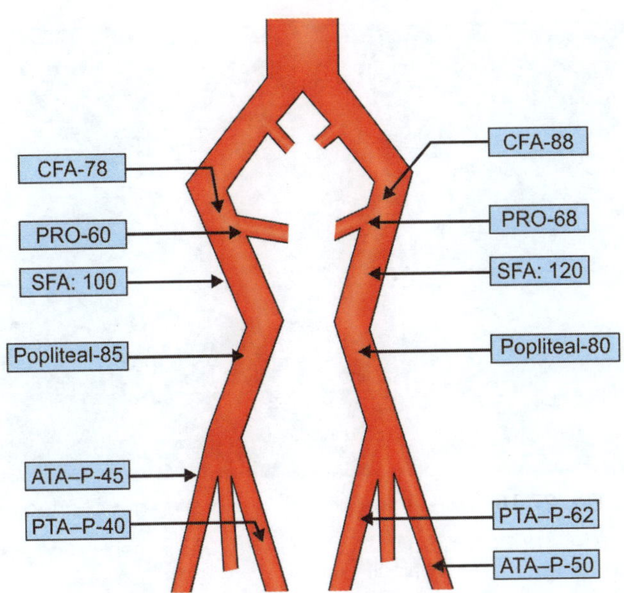

CFA—Common femoral artery; PRO—profunda; SFA—Superficial femoral artery; ATA—anterior tibial artery; PTA—posterior tibial artery

Fig. 27.14: Duplex scan report of a patient with the PAD—the number represents the velocity of blood flow in that artery

to obtain the image of the vessel, and Doppler is used to evaluate the direction and velocity of the blood flow of the vessel. Colour Duplex allows for the assessment of blood flow direction. Red colour indicates that the direction of blood flow is towards the transducer, whereas blue colour indicates that the direction of blood flow is away.

6. **Computed tomography angiography (CTA)**
   - For all patients with chronic limb ischaemia, if revascularisation is planned by surgical/interventional methods, CTA is done. Here, IV contrast–iodine about 300–400 mg/mL is used. An average of about 130 mL of contrast is used. Interpretation of CTA is always based on the axial images. Hydration of the patient should be adequate, and creatinine should be normal, or else renal failure may occur.
   - Advantages of CTA: It gives the vascular anatomy, collaterals, variations (if any), and reformation of the vessels. The most important advantage of CTA over duplex scan is to get the exact information of the level of the block, length of occluded segment/stenosed segment, and distal run off (Figs 27.15 and 27.16).
   - This forms the basis of revascularisation procedures.
   - CTA is the choice of investigation to assess intrathoracic vessels.
   - Because of these advantages and the ease of the procedure, conventional angiogram using Seldinger's technique (details given below) is not done for limb ischaemia.

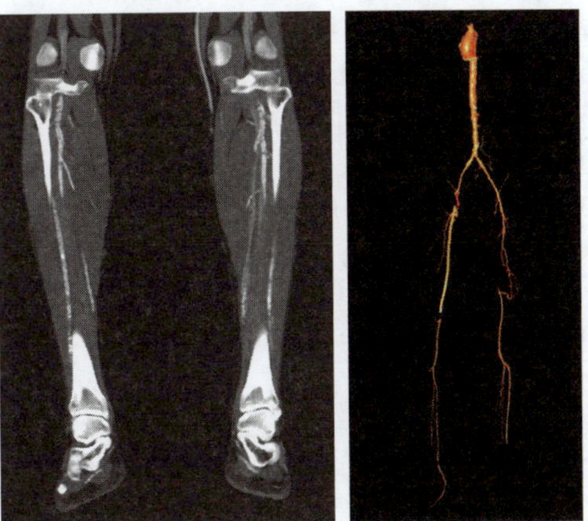

Fig. 27.15: CT angiogram showing narrowing of superficial femoral artery

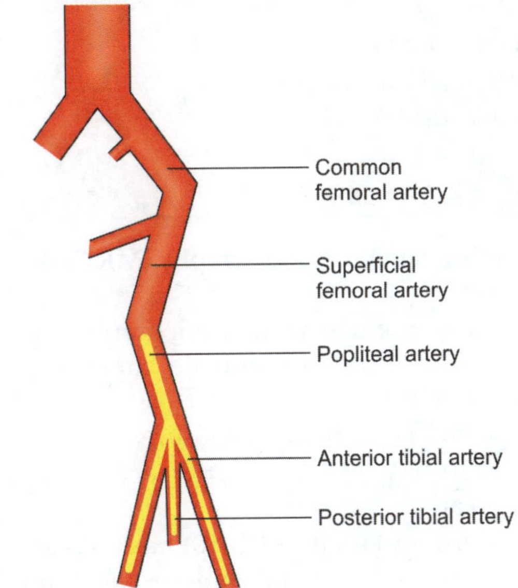

Fig. 27.16: Extensive narrowing of popliteal artery and branches due to atherosclerosis—pictorial representation of a case of CT angiogram

   - Catheter angiography—a catheter is inserted into an artery, and advanced to the area probable blockade, contrast is injected and using DSA, vessels are visualised. This is used more for therapeutic purpose of thrombolysis or dilatation of stenosed segment of the arteries.

7. **Seldinger's technique:** Today it is done to assess cerebral circulation (percutaneous transfemoral method). An incision is made in the upper thigh to expose the femoral artery on the normal side. A Seldinger needle and guidewire are used to introduce the arterial catheter, and a radiopaque dye is introduced after placing the catheter into the aorta. It visualises the entire aortoiliac segment and below. Since the catheter is passed from femoral artery into the aorta, it is also called the retrograde method. **When conventional angiogram is done, subtracting soft tissues,**

bones etc, improves the quality of the images. This is called digital subtraction angiography (DSA). DSA gives excellent pictures of the carotid and large central vessels.

Complications of angiography (Key Box 27.9)

- Contrast allergy, anaphylaxis, which can be avoided by a trial injection.
- Paraplegia due to spasm of spinal arteries.
- Infection
- Renal failure

Key Box 27.9

Complications of Angiography

Thrombus
Rarely paraplegia
Arterial dissection
Unexpected infection/sepsis
Massive bleeding
Anaphylaxis
Remember as **TRAUMA**

8. **Magnetic resonance angiography (MRA)** (Figs 27.17 to 27.20)
   - It is more popular than arteriography because of no arterial puncture and no contrast-induced nephropathy.
   - It also has no radiation exposure.
   - Unlike CTA, MRA is not affected by arterial calcification.
   - Gadolinium-enhanced MRA may visualise the entire arterial tree and pattern, including small pedal vessels.
   - Patients with newly placed metallic implants are advised to avoid undergoing MRA.
   - MRA may overestimate the degree of stenosis because of turbulence, and metal clips may cause artefacts that mimic vessel occlusions.

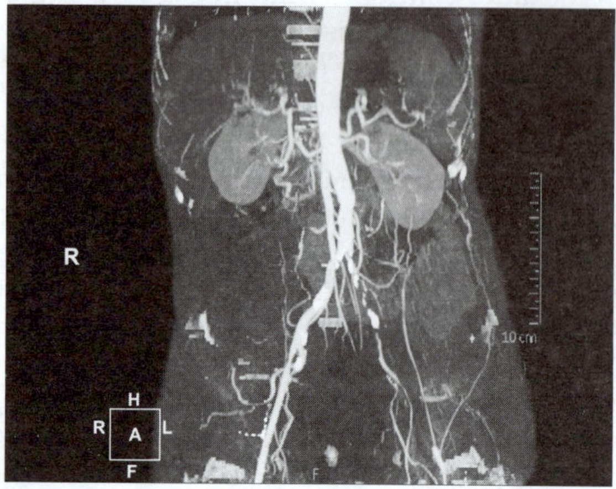

Fig. 27.17: Left common iliac artery occlusion

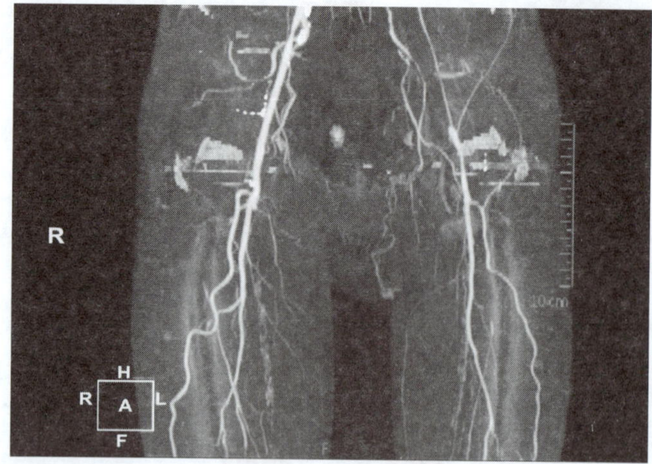

Fig. 27.18: Distal formation at common femoral artery

(Courtesy: Dr Chandrakanth Shetty, Professor, Department of Radiology and Imaging, KMC, Manipal)

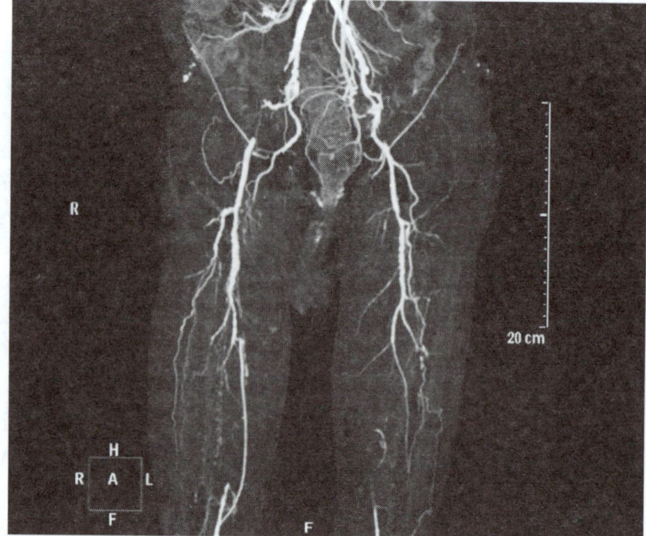

Fig. 27.19: Right common iliac artery occlusion

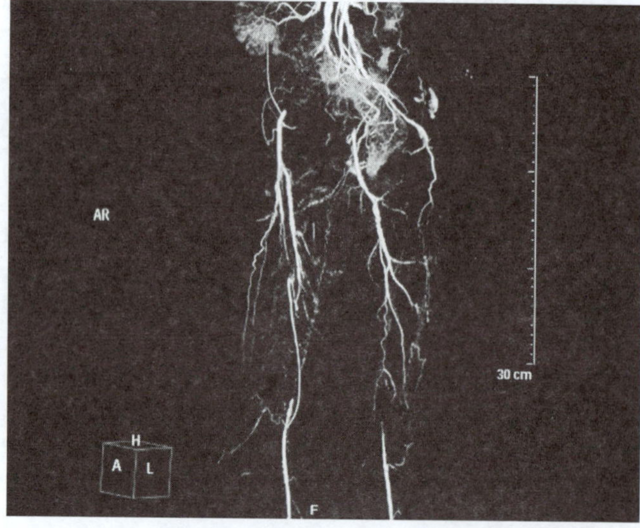

Fig. 27.20: Right common iliac artery occlusion—another view

TREATMENT OF PERIPHERAL ARTERIAL DISEASE (TAO AND ATHEROSCLEROSIS)

- In all patients with peripheral vascular disease, the following general measures must be taken which will help in better perfusion of the lower limb tissues.
- Anaemia must be treated with haematinics and, if necessary, blood transfusion. If ejection fraction is low, drugs are given to improve cardiac output.
- Lifestyle modification of decreasing weight, avoid fat rich food and control of diabetes

Principles (Key Box 27.10)

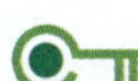 **Key Box 27.10**

Principles of Treatment

- To relieve the pain
- To arrest the progression of the disease
- Medical treatment
- Surgical methods

I. To Relieve the Pain

As already discussed, the pain is very severe and distressing. Some amount of pain relief may be obtained with:

Analgesics: Simple analgesics may not help these patients. Paracetamol 650 mg 1 tablet 2–3 times a day, Tramadol (50 mg) one tablet, 3 times a day. Narcotic analgesics (used judiciously) in cases with rest pain.

Buerger's position, by elevating the head-end of the bed, causes venous congestion and reflex vasodilatation.

Buerger's exercises by elevation and dependency of the limb for a few minutes.

Heel raise by 1–2 cm, to increase claudication distance by decreasing the work load on the calf muscles.

II. To Arrest the Progression of the Disease

- **Stop smoking:** This is more beneficial in TAO patients than in atherosclerotic patients.
- Supervised walking on treadmill of 1 hour or more three times a week as exercise program for 3 months with control of diabetes and cessation of smoking will improve claudication.
- **Diet:** Avoid fatty foods to reduce serum cholesterol. This is more useful in patients with hyperlipidaemia.
- Avoid injuries.

III. Medical Management (Table 27.8)

Cilostazol

- Is the drug of choice in atherosclerotic occlusive disease.
- It is an antiplatelet drug and a vasodilator.
- It helps improve claudication symptoms.
- It helps stabilise atherosclerotic plaques.
- It is a selective inhibitor of phosphodiesterase type 3.

Aspirin/clopidogrel

75 mg/day of clopidogrel or 75 mg of aspirin is advised to all these patients as an antiplatelet. It has been shown to reduce the mortality rate due to cardiac events in these patients.

IV. Surgical Procedures

- In TAO: Lumbar sympathectomy and amputations.
- In atherosclerotic arterial disease (aortoiliac disease and femoropopliteal disease): Percutaneous transluminal angioplasty and bypass grafts.

1. A. **Lumbar sympathectomy** is the indirect surgery done for TAO patients since direct arterial surgery is not possible (Key Box 27.11).
   - **Indications:** Cutaneous ulcer and rest pain.
   - **Structures which may be confused** for the lumbar sympathetic trunk include:
     1. The genitofemoral nerve
     2. Tendon strip of the psoas muscle
     3. The lymphatic chain and fatty tissue
   - By depriving sympathetic nerve supply to the lower limb blood vessels, vasomotor tone is reduced,

Table 27.8 Medical management of peripheral vascular disease—drugs, dosage and their role

• Antiplatelet	Aspirin 75 mg with or without clopidogrel 75 mg	Decreases vascular death by 25%
• Antismoking	Stop smoking	Smoking cessation can decrease 10-year mortality rate from 54% down to 18%
• Anticholesterol	Statins 10 mg/per day—to decrease LDL cholesterol to at least 100 mg/dl. This drug will stabilise the plaques	Slow release niacin is emerging as an important therapy in patients with dyslipidaemia
• Antihypertensives	Decrease blood pressure to <130/85 mmHg	ACE inhibitors, β-blockers
• Antidiabetes	Glycosylated haemoglobin level of <7%	Oral hypoglycaemic agents or insulin
• Antivasospasm (vasodilator)	Cilostazol—50 mg twice a day (doubtful value)	Inhibits platelet aggregation and is a direct arterial vasodilator

Key Box 27.11

Salient Features of Lumbar Sympathectomy

- Transverse loin incision
- Extraperitoneal approach, and it is a preganglionic sympathectomy.
- Lumbar sympathetic trunk is identified in the paravertebral gutter lateral to the psoas muscle as a cord-like structure.
- **2nd lumbar ganglion is large** and has white rami joining it.
- Sympathetic trunk is divided below the first lumbar vertebra and removed up to the 4th lumbar vertebra.
- This is a **preganglionic sympathectomy** because fibres supplying the vessels of the limb have their cell stations in the sacral ganglia which are not disturbed.

which in turn reduces some amount of vasospasm. Thus, rest pain improves and minor ulcerations heal due to cutaneous vasodilatation. However, the duration of the effect of lumbar sympathectomy is not clear.

- Both sides may be done in one sitting. However, during bilateral operation, the 1st lumbar ganglion on one side should be spared since removal of both ganglia may cause sterility due to paralysis of the ejaculatory mechanism.
- ***One should be careful not to damage lumbar veins[1] which join the inferior vena cava.***

B. **Conservative amputations** should be done if the toes are gangrenous.

C. **Below knee amputation**[2] is the last resort. It is indicated in severe rest pain cases in which all other modalities of treatment have failed. The risk of amputation after ten years of the disease is around 10%. **Risk of amputation is more with patients having ABPI of less than 0.5.**

2. **Surgery in atherosclerotic vascular disease:**
   - Avoid or treat risk factors (Key Box 27.12).
   - The decision to revascularise the limb is taken after an angiography. The success of reconstruction depends on a number of factors (Key Box 27.13).
   - **Intermittent claudication alone is not an indication for surgery.** Rest pain and pregangrenous changes in the limb are definite indications for reconstruction with acceptable mortality and morbidity.
   - Surgery can be classified as surgery for aortoiliac disease, ileofemoral disease and femoropopliteal disease.

Key Box 27.12

Major Risk Factors for Atherosclerosis

Lipids: Dyslipidaemia
Inhalation of tobacco: Smoking
Pressure: Hypertension
Insulin deficiency: Diabetes
Disordered metabolism: Hyperhomocystinaemia
Remember as **LIPID**

Key Box 27.13

Prognostic Factors for Limb Revascularisation

- Severity of the disease
- Presence of collaterals
- Presence of diabetes
- Chronic smoking
- Site of occlusion
- Age of the patient
- Angina pectoris
- Fitness for anaesthesia

- **Principle of reconstruction:** Wide exposure to allow safe control of vessels, proximal and distal control inflow (proximal) and outflow (distal) anastomosis in disease free area, careful selection of graft depending upon site of surgery. Dacron and ePTFE perform equally well in aortoiliac bypass, but saphenous vein has superior patency in infrainguinal bypass.

I. AORTOILIAC DISEASE

It is treated by bypass grafts or endarterectomy.

A. Bypass Grafts (Figs 27.21 and 27.22)

- Usually, it is bilateral and is treated with an aorto-bifemoral graft to bypass the stenosis. The graft is made from either teflon or dacron. It is also called a Y-graft or trouser graft. It commonly has a 16 mm trunk and two 8 mm limbs.
- In unilateral cases, a unilateral graft is applied.

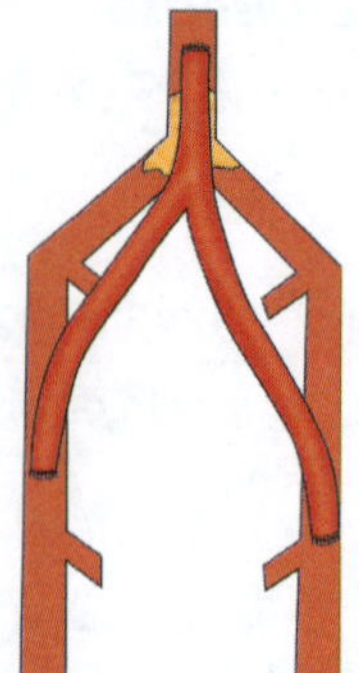
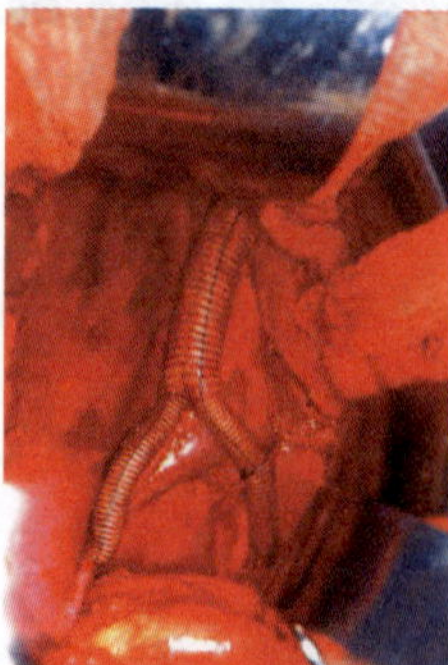

Figs 27.21 and 27.22: Aortobifemoral graft (*Courtesy:* Dr Ganesh Kamath, Professor and Head, Department of Cardiothoracic Surgery, KMC, Manipal)

[1]Lumbar veins, if cut accidentally, retract and cause troublesome bleeding from the inferior vena cava. Pressure packing, waiting for 3–5 minutes and then 'see and ligate' should be the policy.

[2]Students are advised not to tell this as a first treatment modality.

The aorta is approached from a midline incision. The posterior peritoneum is opened to expose the aorta with 2 vertical incisions, and the common femorals are exposed in the groin. Before clamping the vessels, heparin 5000 U is administered intravenously. End-to-side of the graft to aorta above and femoral artery below is done. **Extra-anatomical bypass** refers to any bypass graft, autologous or otherwise, that is placed in a site different to that of the arterial segment that is being bypassed.

For example, axillo-bifemoral bypass in a case of hostile abdomen (previous surgeries, mycotic aneurysms, aortoenteric fistulae), obturator bypass (hostile groin after radiation or previous surgery), femoro-femoral bypass.

B. Aortoiliac Endarterectomy

They are usually not done.

Indications: Short segment, large artery such as aorta and single artery.

Types:

- **Open endarterectomy:** An arteriotomy is done first and the diseased intima, atheromatous plaque, and thrombus are removed. An arteriotomy incision can either be closed directly or with a vein patch graft to close the defect to avoid narrowing.
- **Closed endarterectomy** is indicated in a longer-diseased segment. In this procedure, after an arteriotomy, a wire loop is used to strip out a core of atheroma by introducing it through the lower arteriotomy and removing the atheromatous plaque from the upper end. However, results of bypass graft are better than endarterectomy. The modern tendency is to do bypass graft.

II. ILIOFEMORAL STENOTIC DISEASE

A. Transluminal angioplasty: Any arterial stenosis can be dilated in angioplasty. The technique can be repeated if stenosis recurs. The procedure is done under local anaesthesia and is indicated in poor-risk patients. **Ideally suitable for iliofemoral segment,** not suitable for stenosed vessels below knee. A balloon catheter is inserted into the artery under local anaesthesia and is inflated at high pressure around 30 seconds and deflated. By inflation and dilatation 2–3 times, the stenosed segment can be dilated. Complications include: internal dissection, distal embolisation, thrombosis, and even rupture of the vessel may occur.

B. Ilio-femoral bypass grafts: Generally recommended when the diseased segment is beyond 15 cm in length. Technique is similar to what is mentioned above.

- This can be repaired by a **bypass graft** which is sutured to the normal common iliac artery above and to the normal femoral artery below (Figs 27.23 and 27.24).
- In this procedure, a **balloon catheter** is inserted into the artery and inflated. Its correct position is confirmed by radiopaque markers which are present in the balloon.

A summary of revascularisation surgery is given in Key Box 27.14.

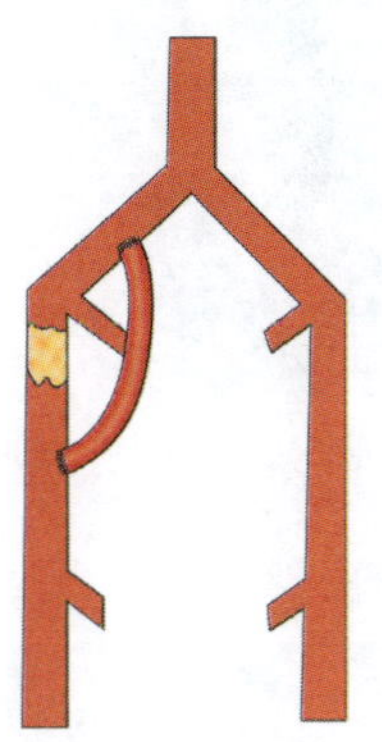

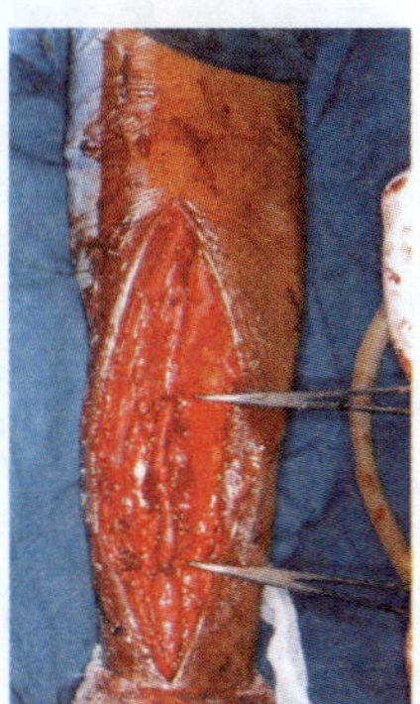

Figs 27.23 and 27.24: Iliofemoral graft by using reversed long saphenous vein

Key Box 27.14

Summary of the Revascularisation Surgery
(Figs 27.25 to 27.31)

Aortoiliac disease	Aortobifemoral or aortofemoral moral graft and endarterectomy
Iliofemoral disease	Iliofemoral bypass graft Balloon angioplasty
Femoropopliteal disease	Bypass graft
Profunda artery stenosis	Profundoplasty

III. FEMOROPOPLITEAL OCCLUSION

- This is the most common site of obstruction in atherosclerotic patients. This is treated with a graft extending from the femoral artery above to the popliteal artery below.
- Reversed autologous long saphenous vein is better than other grafts because it is less thrombogenic. If it is not reversed, the valves have to be disrupted using a valvulotome. If the LSV is not available, try the SSV. When no vein is available, try for synthetic grafts.
- Dacron graft and **polytetrafluoroethylene graft (PTFE)** are commonly used grafts.
- In a few other occasions, small vessel bypass like femoro-tibial artery bypass may also be done if the diameter of the distal vessels is ≥3 mm.
- Success in the immediate post-operative period is around 90%, but the 5-year patency is around 50%.

BALLOON ANGIOPLASTY IN ATHEROSCLEROTIC ARTERIAL DISEASE (Figs 27.25–27.31)

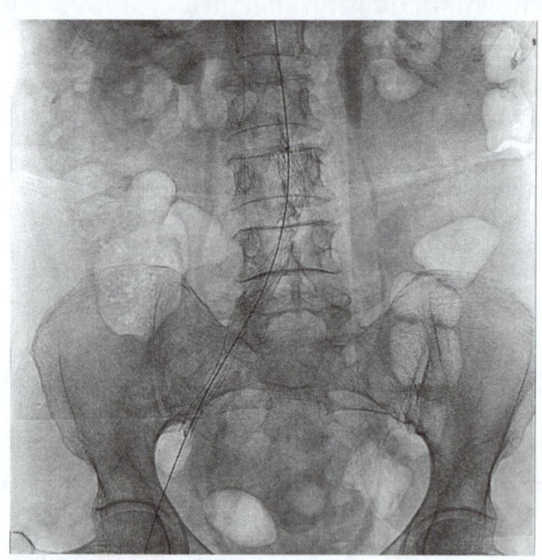

Fig. 27.25: Plain radiograph with guidewire in the aorta

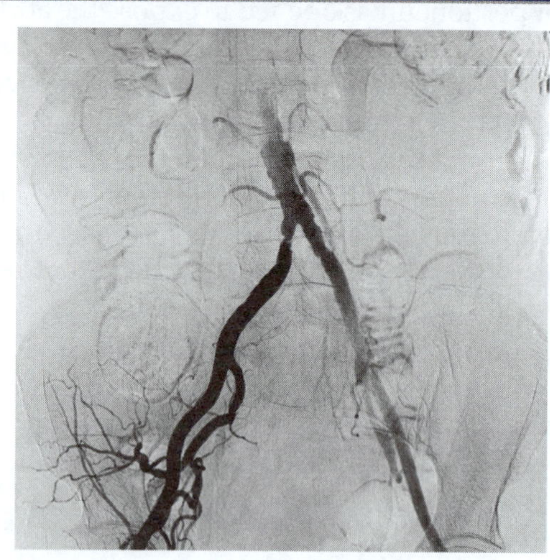

Fig. 27.26: Narrowing of the right common iliac artery

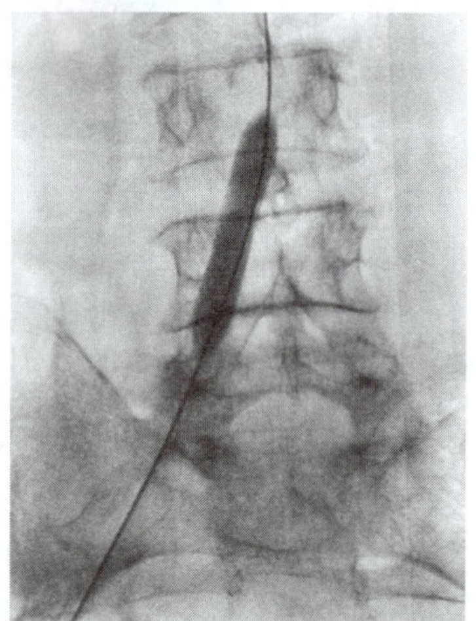

Fig. 27.27: Balloon angioplasty of narrowed right common iliac artery

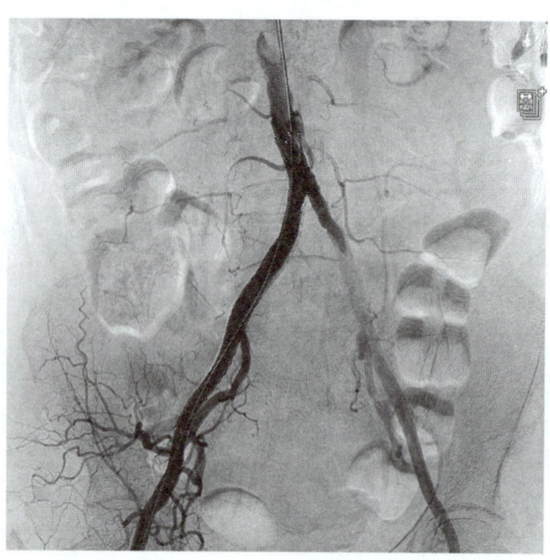

Fig. 27.28: Post-balloon angioplasty

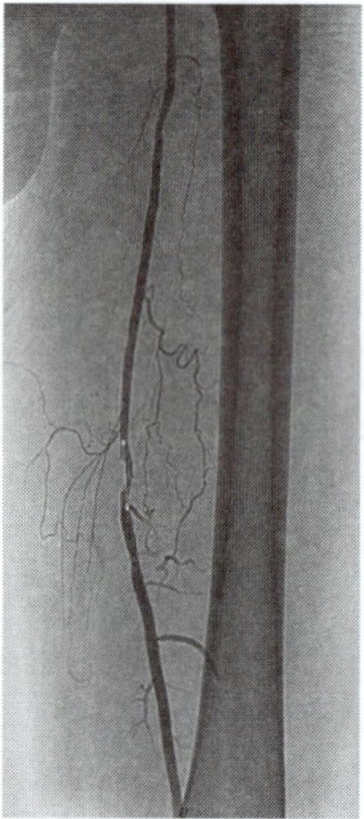

Fig. 27.29: Mid-SFA showing narrowing

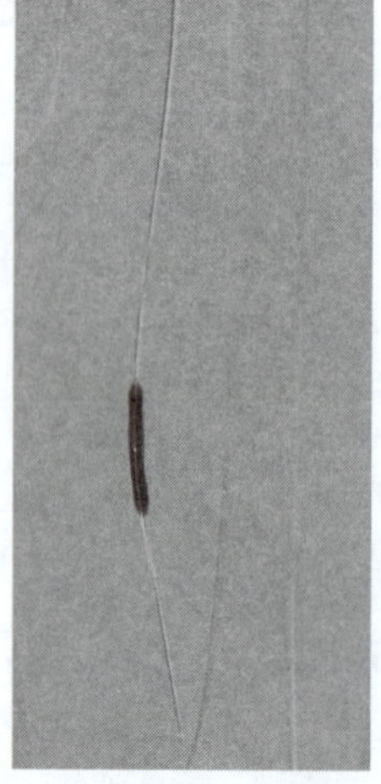

Fig. 27.30: Balloon angioplasty

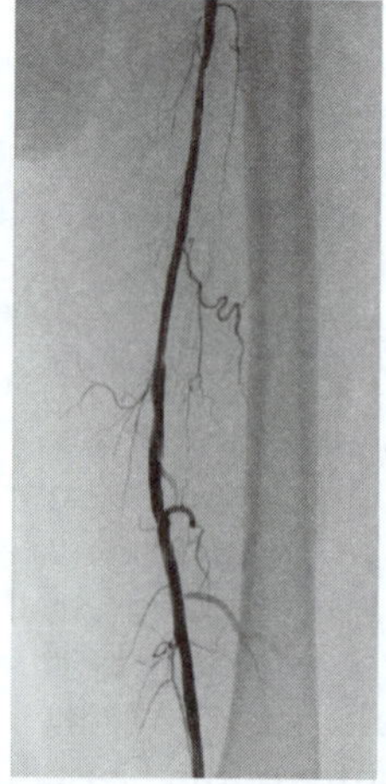

Fig. 27.31: Postangioplasty image showing restoration of lumen of mid-SFA

(*Courtesy:* Prof Chandrakanth Shetty and Dr Praharsha, Resident, Department of Radiodiagnosis and Imaging, KMC, Manipal)

Profunda Artery Stenosis

- Significant occlusion of the profunda is demonstrated by oblique views in an arteriography. If there are no significant vessels available below the stenosis for reconstruction, profundoplasty is considered. It is done using a patch of Dacron or vein to widen the origin of the vessel after endarterectomy.

Complication of Surgery

Early	Late
Hemorrhage	Graft thrombosis
Limb ischemia	Anastomotic pseudoaneurysm
Renal failure	Sexual dysfunction
Intestinal ischemia	Infection
Spinal cord ischemia	Aortoenteric fistula
Urateric injury	

ACUTE ARTERIAL OCCLUSION

- Sudden occlusion of an artery commonly occurs due to an embolus. The source of the embolus is from the heart or from an atheroma. Increased incidence of road traffic accidents, fall, or war injuries are other causes. Trauma to the artery also produces occlusion.
- Emboli from atheromatous plaques are called athero-emboli. In most of these patients collaterals would have developed, hence the limb ischaemia may not be very critical.

EMBOLIC OCCLUSION

- This commonly occurs in the peripheral arteries (e.g. common iliac, femoral, popliteal).
- An embolus is a foreign body to the bloodstream. It gets lodged in a vessel and produces obstruction, clinically manifesting as severe ischaemia or gangrene and resulting in **critical limb ischaemia (CLI)**.
- Atherosclerotic vascular disease, thromboangiitis obliterans, acute embolic ischaemia, and even diabetes, may present as CLI.

Causes/risk factors:

- Smokers, cardiac diseases, obesity, recent cardiac surgery (Table 27.9)

Pathology

- As a result of sudden occlusion, blood supply to the distal part is cut off resulting in rapid development of tissue death and gangrene. Most of such patients also have atherosclerosis. Tissue hypoxia followed by release of superoxide radicals and thromboxanes result in endothelial damage necrosis and gangrene within a few hours (Fig. 27.32).

Clinical Features (Key Box 27.15)

- No previous history suggestive of intermittent claudication.

Table 27.9 Causes of acute lower limb ischaemia

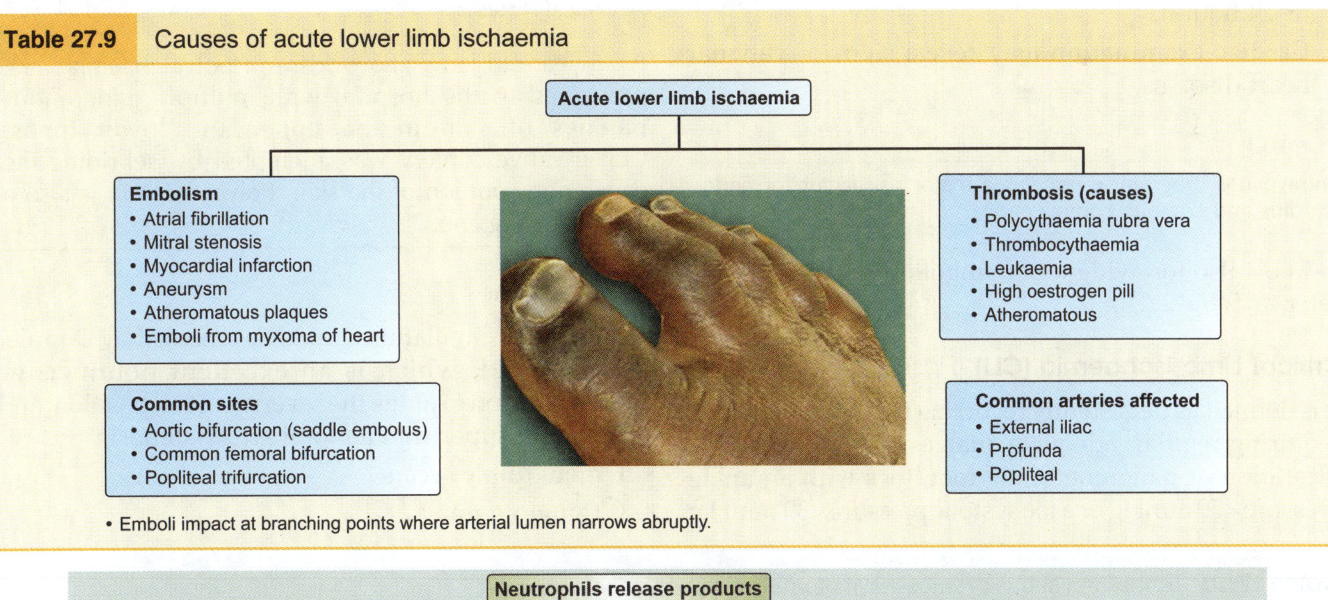

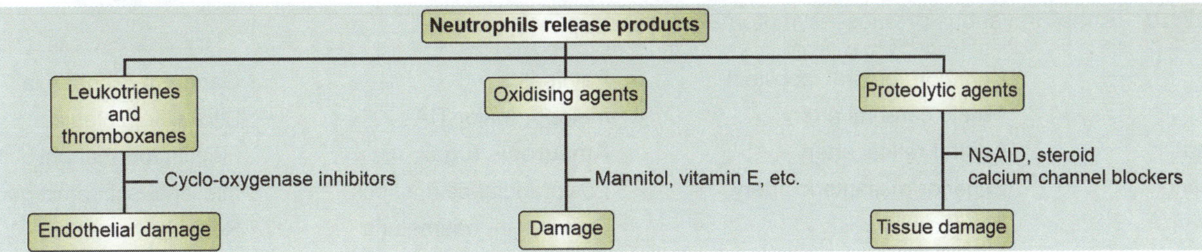

Fig. 27.32: Pathogenesis of tissue damage

Key Box 27.15

Signs of Acute Lower Limb Ischaemia

- Peripheries are cold
- Pallor of the limb
- Poor capillary return
- Positive Buerger's test
- Progressive paralysis
- Pulses are absent

Pulse at ankle by Doppler—undetectable

Observe **7 Ps**

- Sudden dramatic symptoms which are described in the form of **5Ps**—Pain, Pallor, Paresis, Pulselessness, Paraesthesia.
  1. **Pain** is severe, unbearable, and of a burning or bursting type.
  2. The limb is **pale** and cold, and superficial veins are collapsed.
  3. **Paresis:** Depending on the level of occlusion, the function of the limb is lost. Movement of the toes becomes difficult, followed by total paralysis.
  4. **Pulselessness:** Characteristically, peripheral pulses below the level of the embolism are not palpable.
  5. **Paraesthesia:** Altered sensation in the limb.
- If left untreated, necrosis of the muscles followed by gangrene of the limb may occur within a few hours (6–24 hours).
- **Cardiac examination** may reveal signs of valvular heart diseases.

Pearls of Wisdom

Intravenous drug abuse remains a major risk factor for endocarditis and embolic complications.

Look also for evidence of emboli in other arteries—refer to Table 27.10.

Critical Limb Ischaemia (CLI) (Figs 27.33 and 27.34)

It is defined as persistently recurring ischaemic rest pain requiring regular, adequate analgesia for >2 weeks or ulceration or gangrene of the foot/toes with an ankle pressure <50 mmHg or a toe systolic pressure <30 mmHg.

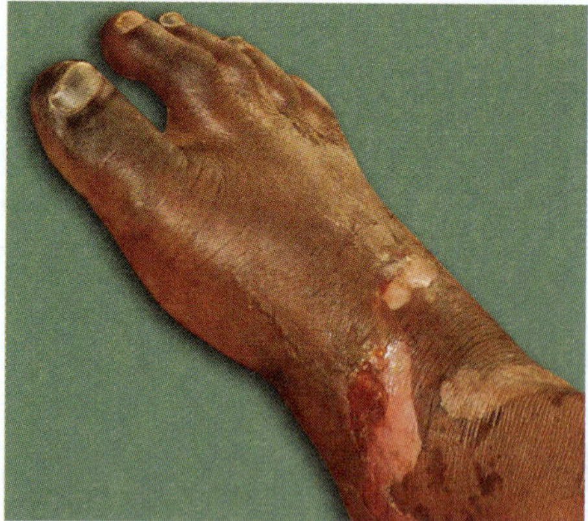

Fig. 27.33: Critical limb ischaemia (CLI)

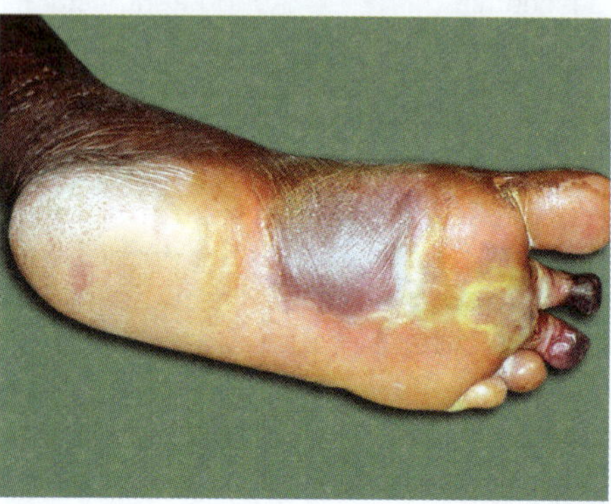

Fig. 27.34: CLI due to diabetes and atherosclerosis

Clinical Notes

A 75-year-old lady, known case of polycythaemia vera, presented to the hospital with multiple gangrenous patches of skin in the upper and lower limbs. Conservative surgery was attempted by debriding the gangrenous portion of the skin. Polycythaemia is also a cause of gangrene.

Investigations

- Peripheral circulation should be assessed by Doppler ultrasound, which is an excellent noninvasive investigation to judge the severity, level, position, and length of superficial femoral artery stenosis.
- Urgent duplex scan
- CT angiogram

Table 27.10 Emboli in various arteries—symptoms, signs and effects

1. Leg	Common femoral, popliteal	Pain/pallor	Gangrene/ischaemia
2. Brain	Middle cerebral artery	Minor or major TIA	Stroke/hemiplegia
3. Retina	Central retinal artery	**Amaurosis fugax**	Fleeting/permanent blindness
4. Intestine	Superior mesenteric artery	Postprandial pain, shock	Intestinal ischaemia/gangrene
5. Kidney	Renal artery	Pain in loin, haematuria	Renal ischaemia
6. Upper limb	Brachial artery	Pain, ulcer upper limb	Gangrene

Treatment

I. **Angioplasty:** Percutaneous transluminal angioplasty (PTA) is **indicated in short stenotic lesions in a large vessel** (e.g. iliac and femoropopliteal lesions).
- First, the balloon catheter is introduced percutaneously over a guidewire across the lesion. Under fluoroscopic control, the balloon is dilated until satisfactory widening of the lumen is achieved.
- It is a relatively safe and simple procedure.
- Immediate intravenous infusion of heparin (10,000 IU) is necessary to reduce extension of the thromboembolism.

II. **Emergency embolectomy** is done under GA or local anaesthesia either by a direct arteriotomy incision and removal of the clot or by using a Fogarty balloon catheter to remove the embolus remotely (Figs 27.35 and 27.36).
- **Embolectomy:** Under local or general anaesthesia, a transverse incision is given over the common femoral artery. A Fogarty catheter is introduced through the incision for about 1–2 cm and the balloon is inflated.
- The catheter is then withdrawn, and the emboli are removed. The procedure is repeated until bleeding occurs. The catheter can be passed by the ankle to remove distal emboli as well. Post-operatively, anticoagulants are continued.

III. **Intra-arterial thrombolysis:**
- It is indicated in acute or acute on chronic ischaemia where in ischaemia is not so severe.
- **Intra-arterial thrombolysis:** A catheter is passed into the 'clot' after performing arteriography and ***t-PA*** (***tissue plasminogen activator***) is infused through the catheter. Repeat angiogram check films are taken to see the results, such as clot lysis, revascularisation, etc.
- It will reopen the occluded lumen within 24 hours.

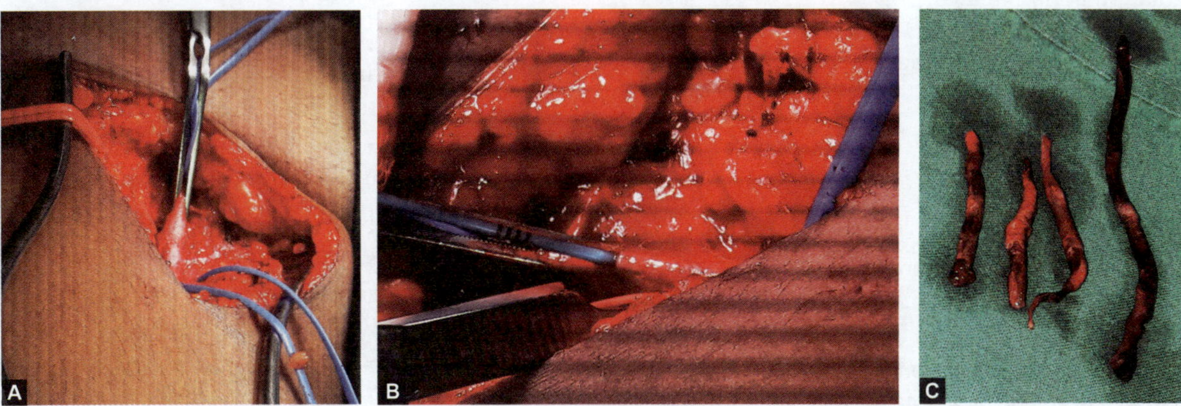

Fig. 27.35A to C: (A) Femoral artery is exposed in the groin, (B) Fogarty balloon catheter is introduced within femoral artery (C) Embolectomy—clots (*Courtesy:* Dr Ganesh Kamath, Head, Department of CVTS, KMC Manipal)

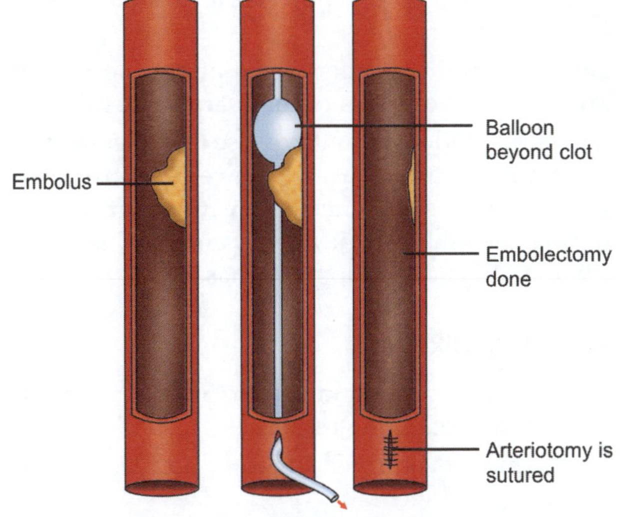

Fig. 27.35D: Fogarty embolectomy

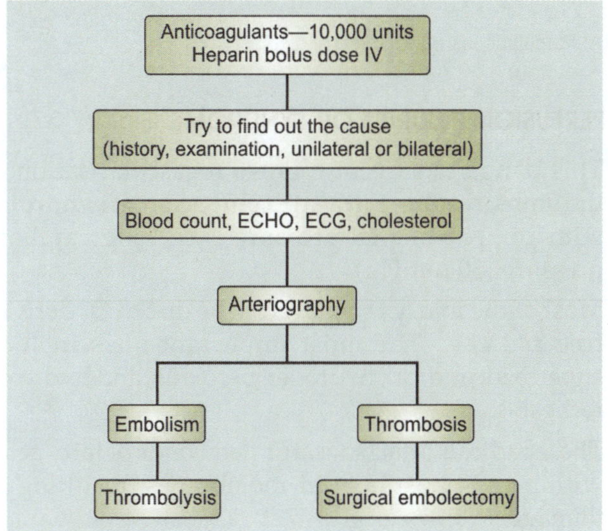

Fig. 27.36: Management of acutely ischaemic limb

- Procedure should be abandoned if the clot does not undergo dissolution.
- Repeat angiogram is necessary to check for patency.

Contraindications for thrombolytic therapy: Key Box 27.16.

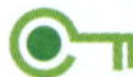
Key Box 27.16

Contraindications to Thrombolytic Therapy

Absolute
- Recent major bleeding
- Recent major surgery
- Recent ophthalmologic procedure
- Recent stroke

Relative
- Active peptic ulcer disease
- Pregnancy
- Uncontrolled hypertension
- Coagulation abnormalities

Recent advances: Trans-Atlantic inter-Society Consensus: TASC guidelines.

Type	RX
A. Single stenosis <10 cm Single occlusion ≤5 cm	PTA
B. Multiple stenoses (or) occlusions each ≤5 cm Single stenosis (or) occlusion ≥15 cm	PTA (or) open surgery
C. Multiple stenoses (or) occlusions totalling >15 cm with or without heavy calcifications	PTA (or) open surgery
D. Chronic occlusion of CFA (or) SFA >20 cm (or) involving the popliteal artery	Open surgery

PTA: Percutaneous transluminal angioplasty

REPERFUSION INJURIES OR SYNDROME (Fig. 27.37)

- This dangerous event follows revascularisation of the limbs, resulting in **acute compartment syndrome** with compartmental pressure exceeding capillary pressure (30 mmHg).
- Most of the injury is believed to be due to O_2 derived free radicals. The most important ones include superoxide radical, hydrogen peroxide, and hydroxyl radical.
- These radicals attach unsaturated bonds of fatty acids within the phospholipid membranes, resulting in damage.
- Oedema and swelling of the muscles take place.

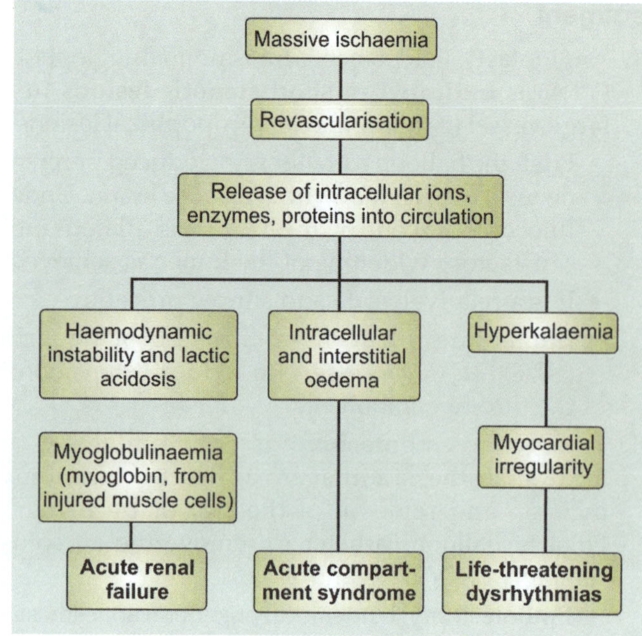

Fig. 27.37: Pathophysiology of reperfusion injuries

Management

- Diagnosis is clinical, as suggested by severe pain in the limb, oedema of the leg, and muscle tenderness.
- Raised intra-compartmental pressure measured by a transducer cannula will help in the diagnosis.
- Creatinine is elevated (renal failure).
- Creatine kinase is elevated (rhabdomyolysis).
- Treated by urgent multiple fasciotomy and decompression, followed by debridement of dead tissues.
- Supportive treatment such as antibiotics and hydration, is given.

PERIPHERAL ANEURYSMS

- These can affect the popliteal artery, femoral artery, iliac artery, etc.
- **70%** of peripheral aneurysms affect the popliteal artery, and **two-thirds of them are bilateral.**
- However, students should realise that aneurysms are uncommon (rare) causes of lower limb ischaemia. Early diagnosis and effective treatment are essential to save the limb. **Aortic aneurysms** are discussed in Chapter 37 under abdominal mass.

POPLITEAL ANEURYSMS

They are the most **common peripheral aneurysms** because of the following reasons:

- Turbulence beyond stenosis at the adductor magnus hiatus.
- Repeated flexion at the knee.

Clinical Features

- They affect elderly patients and are caused by atherosclerosis. Age at presentation is 65 years.
- **One-third** of the cases are associated with aortic aneurysm.
- Striking preponderance in **males**. Male : female ratio is 20–30 : 1.
- Presents as a swelling behind the knee.
- Dull aching pain is common. Severe **bursting pain** indicates **rapid expansion** and impending rupture.
- Pulsatile, tense, cystic, fluctuant swelling behind the knee in the popliteal fossa, in the line of the popliteal artery.
- Its **size diminishes on extending the knee** as the aneurysm is deep to popliteal fascia.
- **Proximal compression test:** On occluding the femoral artery proximally, the swelling may diminish in size.

Pearls of Wisdom

In all cases of popliteal aneurysm, please search for a femoral or aortic aneurysm.

Investigations

- **Duplex ultrasonography** is the investigation of choice, which can measure the diameter and determine the extent of mural thrombus.
- **Angiography** can demonstrate the extent of the involved segment to look for patency and check the quality of runoff vessels.

Complications

1. **Thrombosis** causes severe acute ischaemia of the lower limb (incidence: 40%).
2. **Embolisation** causes ischaemic ulceration of the lower limb.
3. **Rupture** causes pain and haematoma (rare: 2–5%).
4. **Compression** on the popliteal vein causes pain, tenderness, and swelling of the leg.
5. **Compression on the lateral peroneal nerve** causing foot drop, due to paralysis of the peronei and the extensors of the foot.

Treatment

- **Proximal and distal ligation of the artery** followed by reversed saphenous vein bypass graft is the treatment of choice. This results in total obliteration of the sac and revascularisation of the limb.
- **Excision of the sac is better avoided** because of the risk of injury to the popliteal vein and nerves. Lateral popliteal nerve injury causes foot drop, and tibial (medial popliteal) nerve injury causes thinning of the calf region, loss of plantar flexion, and clawing of the toes due to paralysis of the intrinsic muscles of the foot.

MISCELLANEOUS

AINHUM (Fig. 27.38)

It affects those who do not use footwear/walk barefoot. It starts as a fissure at the level of the interphalangeal joint of a toe, usually the fifth. Repeated minor trauma may be present. The tissue becomes a fibrous band resulting in tight constriction and necrosis. If it continues, it may culminate in autoamputation.

- Division of the band or early Z-plasty may be needed to avoid amputation.
- In early cases—thrombolysis with catheter *in situ*.

FROSTBITE

- It occurs due to excessive exposure to cold weather.
- High altitudes with excessive cold precipitate vasospasm and damage the blood vessel wall. It causes sludging of blood and thrombosis.
- Malnutrition and aging are the other precipitating factors. Severe burning pain, discolouration of the foot, and development of blisters suggest that gangrene is imminent.

Treatment

- Slow warming of the parts and protection with cotton wool.
- Analgesics and antibiotics.
- Paravertebral injection into the sympathetic chain may help in a few patients.
- Elevation of the foot to reduce oedema.
- Frank cases of frostbite with gangrene require conservative amputation.

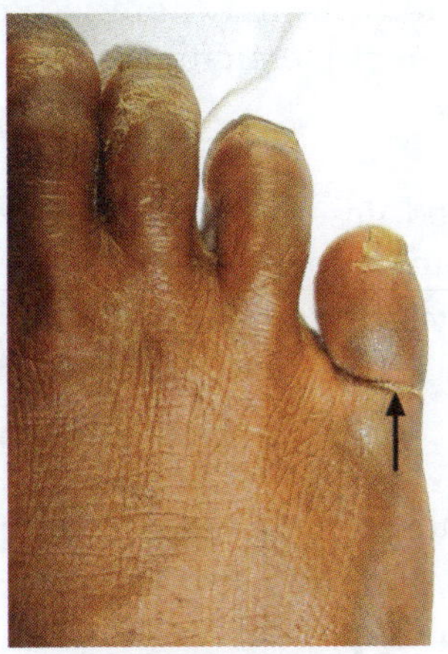

Fig. 27.38: Ainhum

FAT EMBOLISM

Definition

Often a potentially lethal condition which occurs due to blockage of major arteries by the aggregation of chylomicrons.

Causes

- Fracture femur (long bones)
- Orthopaedic surgery, multiple fractures
- Liposuction
- Sickle cell disease
- Pancreatitis
- Diabetes mellitus

Pearls of Wisdom

Triad of fat embolism syndrome—respiratory failure, confusion, and petechial haemorrhages. Early diagnosis and prophylactic administration of oxygen to patients at risk is recommended.

Clinical Features

- **Pulmonary:** Central cyanosis, tachypnoea, right heart failure, and froth in the mouth and nostrils. ***Respiratory distress is the most common presenting feature.***
- **CNS:** Drowsiness, disorientation, restlessness, constricted pupils, pyrexia, and coma.
- **Retinal artery:** Striate haemorrhages, fluffy exudates on fundoscopic examination, and cotton wool spots.
- **Cutaneous:** Petechial rashes in the nondependent parts of the body—chest, axilla and conjunctiva.

Pathogenesis

- 50% of cases occur within 72 hours.
- **Free fatty acids (FFAs),** released at the time of trauma or breakdown of fat in the lung, directly affect pneumocytes resulting in **A**cute **R**espiratory **D**istress **S**yndrome **(ARDS)**.
- Another theory is that there is blockage by the **aggregation of chylomicrons**.

Investigations

- Arterial blood gases—hypoxaemia and respiratory alkalosis from hyperventilation.
- Chest X-ray—bilateral interstitial and alveolar infiltrates in severe cases (**'snowstorm'** pattern).

Treatment

- **Close monitoring** with pulse oximetry.
- **Supportive therapy** with oxygen and mechanical ventilation as required.
- **Surgical**—early internal fixation of the fracture.

AIR EMBOLISM (Key Box 27.17)

Definition

It is a **potentially fatal condition** that occurs due to blockage of the pulmonary artery by a **large volume of air** in the venous circulation.

Causes

- **Neck surgeries** in which a large vein is inadvertently opened and the patient is in head-elevated position (thyroid surgery) or sitting position (posterior fossa surgery).
- Rapid infusion of intravenous fluids where emptying of the bottle and infusion set may go unnoticed and a fresh bottle is connected and infused without eliminating air from the infusion set.

Effects

Formation of an air lock within the pulmonary artery and right heart failure.

Treatment

- Position the patient **head down** (Trendelenburg position) so that air entrainment is stopped.
- Turn the patient to his/her **left side** so that air will float to the ventricular apex, reducing its entry into the pulmonary artery.
- Administer **oxygen and resuscitate as necessary**.

Key Box 27.17

Air Embolism

- Large veins get opened in the neck
- Open heart surgery or if pulmonary vein is punctured
- Fallopian tube insufflation
- Illegal abortion (through paravertebral veins)
- Paradoxical embolism, reaching coronary artery through patent foramen ovale

INTENSIVE CARE UNIT (ICU) GANGRENE (Fig. 27.39)

- It is as a rare clinical entity. It was first described by Jonathan Hutchinson in 1891 as multiple extremity ischaemia and was termed 'symmetrical peripheral gangrene.'
- Possible aetiological factors include sepsis, DIC, and the use of vasopressor agents. The possible responsible drug is noradrenaline.
- Patients in ICU have multiple arterial punctures for securing intra-arterial line for invasive monitoring. These arterial punctures may also be a possible aetiological factor.

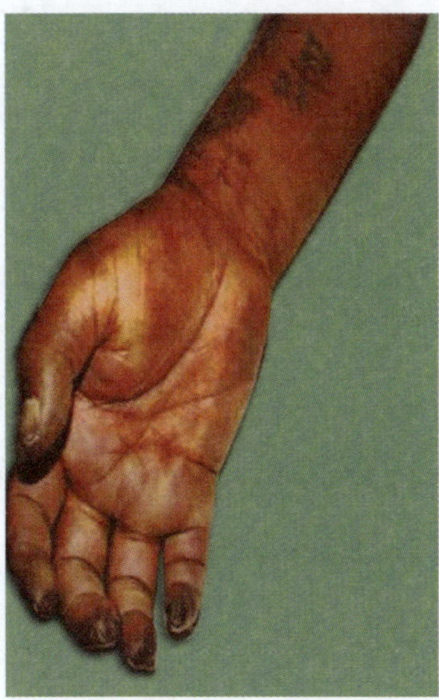

Fig. 27.39: ICU gangrene

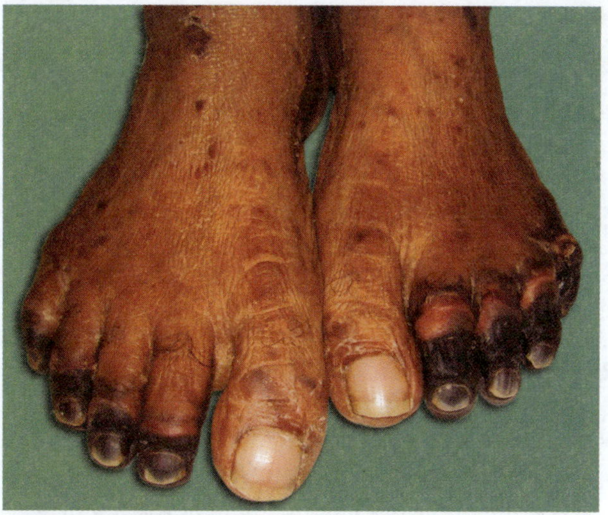

Fig. 27.40: Bilateral symmetrical digital gangrene due to atherosclerosis, diabetes, sepsis and hypotension

- Sepsis in the presence of sluggish blood flow has been described to be responsible for the development of symmetrical peripheral gangrene (Fig. 27.40).
- Vasospastic conditions, small vessel obstruction, and very low cardiac output states (perfusion pressure falling to 35–60 mmHg) may also contribute.
- Medical conditions, such as diabetes mellitus, malignancy, protein C or S or antithrombin III deficiency are other contributing factors.
- The usual manifestation is pallor or cyanosis, coldness, and pain in the extremity. They become erythematous and there is dusky discolouration of skin with bullae or blisters, followed by gangrene.
- Pulses may be intact in the early stages. Large vessels are often spared. Low flow states result in occlusion of the microcirculation of the affected parts.
- The first line of management is immediate discontinuation of vasopressors as soon as discolouration is seen.
- Aggressive treatment of sepsis with intravenous antibiotics and anticoagulation for DIC are the suggested measures.
- Local debridement and secondary skin grafting have been unsuccessful.
- Amputation should be considered only after a clear line of demarcation develops. The condition has a high mortality rate of 40%.

Please note: Aortic aneurysm is discussed in Chapter 62 under cardiothoracic surgery.

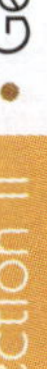

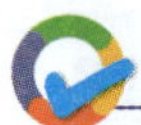

Multiple Choice Questions

1. Which of the following is false regarding thromboangiitis obliterans?
   A. The dorsalis pedis and posterior tibial arteries are often affected
   B. The radial artery may also be affected
   C. The superficial femoral artery is also affected
   D. Bruit is present over the femoral artery

2. The following are true for atherosclerotic arterial disease *except*:
   A. Large-sized arteries are affected
   B. The upper limb is often affected
   C. It may be associated with an aortic aneurysm
   D. A bruit may be present over the artery

3. The following are features of thromboangiitis obliterans *except*:
   A. Raynaud's phenomenon
   B. Migrating thrombophlebitis
   C. Segmental panarteritis
   D. Polymorphs and giant cells are absent on histopathology

4. The following are uses of a Doppler probe *except*:
   A. To feel the nonpalpable pulse
   B. To look for pressure index
   C. To measure blood pressure
   D. To detect triphasic pattern

5. Lumbar sympathectomy has the following advantages *except*:
   A. Rest pain improves to a small extent
   B. Ulcerations heal
   C. Claudication and claudication distance improve
   D. Nutritive value of the blood flow improves

6. A Fogarty catheter is used in:
   A. Chronic arterial occlusion
   B. Acute arterial embolic occlusion
   C. Vasospastic disease
   D. Femoral vein thrombosis

7. The characteristic feature of critical limb ischaemia is:
   A. Intermittent claudication
   B. Ankle pressure <70 mm of Hg
   C. Toe systolic pressure <30 mmHg
   D. Absent pulses

8. The triad of fat embolism includes:
   A. Respiratory failure, confusion, petechial haemorrhages
   B. Respiratory failure, confusion, large purpuric spots
   C. Respiratory failure, alertness, petechial haemorrhages
   D. Cardiac failure, confusion, petechial haemorrhages

9. The following are true for popliteal aneurysm *except*:
   A. It is caused by atherosclerosis
   B. It is the most common type of peripheral aneurysm
   C. It is always unilateral
   D. Foot drop may occur

10. The following are true about lumbar sympathectomy *except*:
   A. It is a postganglionic sympathectomy
   B. The sympathetic trunk is divided below the first sympathetic ganglion
   C. It is a preganglionic sympathectomy
   D. It is usually done by an extraperitoneal approach

11. The following are true for infra-inguinal bypass surgery for diabetic ulcer *except*:
   A. Long saphenous vein is inferior to the PTFE graft
   B. Preoperative vein marking is helpful
   C. 2-year patency is around 70%
   D. Amputation rate after bypass surgery is still high

12. The following are major risk factors for atherosclerosis *except*:
   A. Dyslipidaemia
   B. Tobacco smoking
   C. Hyperhomocystinaemia
   D. Alcohol intake

13. The following are true for profundoplasty *except*:
   A. It is done using a patch of Dacron
   B. It is done using a vein graft
   C. It is done after endarterectomy
   D. It is done in TAO patients

14. The following are true about tissue plasminogen activator *except*:
   A. It was first purified from melanoma cells
   B. It is an endogenous enzyme like urokinase
   C. It is sometimes elevated in carcinoma stomach
   D. Streptokinase also has plasminogen activating action

Answers

1. D **2.** B **3.** D **4.** D **5.** C **6.** B **7.** C **8.** A **9.** C **10.** A
11. A **12.** D **13.** D **14.** C

CHAPTER

28

Upper Limb Ischaemia and Gangrene

- Raynaud's disease
- Thoracic outlet syndrome
- Axillary vein thrombosis
- Vasculitis syndromes
- Gangrene, cancrum oris
- Acrocyanosis
- Drug abuse and gangrene
- Intra-arterial drug and gangrene
- Subclavian steal syndrome

INTRODUCTION

Upper limb ischaemia (ULI) is a well-recognised clinical entity like lower limb ischaemia, though it is less common. There are certain specific conditions (such as cervical rib, Raynaud's disease, etc.) responsible for causing ULI. It is important to note that reconstructive surgery is rarely done in the upper limb, as opposed to the lower limb.

Causes of Upper Limb Ischaemia

1. Raynaud's disease and Raynaud's syndrome—vasospastic.
2. Embolic causes.
3. Thoracic outlet syndrome (Fig. 28.1).
4. Trauma.
5. Buerger's disease—vasospastic.
6. Axillary vein thrombosis.
7. Ergotism: These drugs are used for severe headache due to migraine.
8. Vinyl chloride exposure can give rise to vasospasm (Raynaud's phenomenon).
9. **Vasculitis syndromes:** Takayasu's arteritis, giant cell arteritis, polyarteritis nodosa, systemic sclerosis—scleroderma—**CREST syndrome.**

RAYNAUD'S DISEASE

(Primary Raynaud's Phenomenon)

- It occurs in young women, commonly.
- The upper limb is more involved than the lower limb.

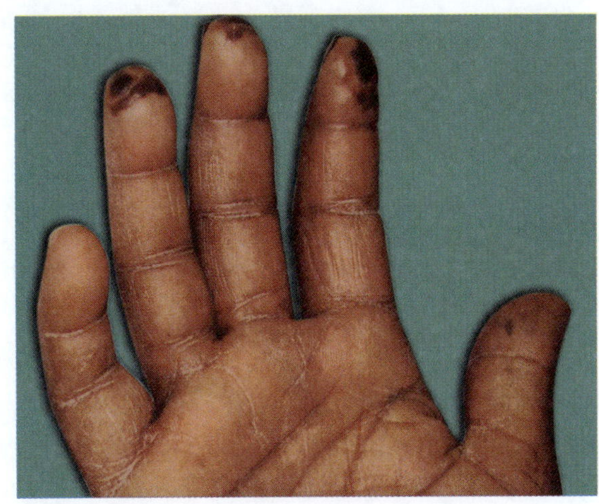

Fig. 28.1: Gangrene of the tip of fingers due to cervical rib

- It is commonly seen in Western countries in white-skinned people. Cold climate is possibly a precipitating factor. It was first described by Raynaud as **bilateral episodic digital ischaemia of the upper limb** on exposure to cold and emotions. **It is also referred to as primary Raynaud's phenomenon.**
- Raynaud's phenomenon is the blanket term used to describe cold-related digital vasospasm (*see* pathophysiology). Raynaud's phenomenon is subdivided into Raynaud's syndrome (associated disorder present) and primary Raynaud's disease (no associated disorder).
- **CREST syndrome: C**alcinosis circumscripta, **R**aynaud's phenomenon, (O) **E**sophageal defects, **S**clerodactyly, **T**elangiectasia.

- Causes of **Secondary Raynaud's phenomenon** are given in Key Box 28.1.

  Currently, both primary and secondary varieties have been grouped together.

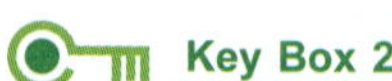
Key Box 28.1

Causes of Secondary Raynaud's Phenomenon

- Atherosclerosis
- Cervical rib
- Systemic lupus
- Carpal tunnel syndrome
- Scleroderma
- Vibrating tools—vibration white finger

Pathophysiology

On exposure to cold[1], some kind of discomfort and colour changes are observed. This is due to abnormal sensitivity of the arterioles to cold. Three stages have been described.

1. **Stage of syncope:** Arterioles undergo constriction as an abnormal response to cold. As a result of this, the part becomes blanched and severe pallor develops.
2. **Stage of asphyxia:** After a brief period of vasoconstriction, capillaries dilate and fill with deoxygenated blood, resulting in a bluish discolouration of the part (cyanosis).
3. **Stage of recovery or stage of rubor:** As the attack passes off, the arterioles relax, circulation improves, and redness occurs. Because of capillary dilatation, there is red engorgement of the part and tingling, burning, or bursting pain in the fingers.

Clinical Features

- Affects young women.
- Typically causes bilateral episodic digital ischaemia on exposure to cold.
- **Thumb is usually spared.**
- **Peripheral pulses are normal.**
- Pallor, cyanosis, and rubor are the colour changes that occur during the attack, which are accompanied by pain.
- In a few patients, because of **recurrent attacks**, gangrenous patches occur on the tip of the fingers (superficial necrosis).

Differential Diagnosis

- Cervical rib
- Vasculitis syndromes
- TAO affecting the upper limb usually affects male smokers. Peripheral pulses are feeble or weak.

Raynaud's Phenomenon—Investigations

- Blood counts, ESR: Increased ESR suggests autoimmune etiology
- ANA: Antinuclear antibody (ANA) test for antinuclear antibodies
- **Nailfold capillaroscopy:** It is to analyse microvascular abnormalities in autoimmune rheumatic diseases. It can detect capillaries, haemorrhages, angiogenesis in cases of scleroderma.
- Thermography: To differentiates primary and secondary Raynaud's phenomenon. In case of primary Raynaud's disease, temperature gradients normalize.
- Wrist–Brachial Index
  a. Normal—0.85–1.0
  b. Abnormal <0.85

Treatment

I. Conservative line of treatment

- Reassurance
- Avoid unnecessary exposure to cold
- Avoid smoking
- Calcium antagonists such as nifedipine 10–20 mg, two times a day may be beneficial.
- If these measures fail, surgery is performed.

II. Cervical sympathectomy (Key Boxes 28.2 and 28.3)

- In this operation, the sympathetic trunk from the lower half of the stellate ganglion to just below the 3rd thoracic ganglion is removed.
- **The upper ½ of the stellate ganglion is preserved** to avoid Horner's syndrome.

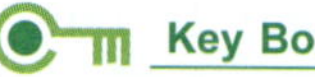
Key Box 28.2

Indications for Cervical Sympathectomy

- Raynaud's disease
- TAO
- Hyperhidrosis
- Cervical rib
- Causalgia

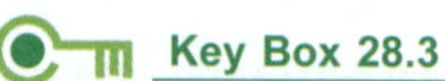
Key Box 28.3

Complications of Cervical Sympathectomy

- Perforation of pleura causing pneumothorax
- Lymph fistula due to injury to thoracic duct
- Horner's syndrome
- Injury to the accessory nerve
- Haemorrhage

[1]Cold refers to temperature—cold climate (winter), cold environment (refrigerator), or cold substance like cold water or ice. Erythromelalgia is a condition wherein heat provokes an attack of burning pain of hands and feet.

- All rami communicantes associated with the 2nd and 3rd ganglia are removed.
- **Nerve of Kuntz,** a grey ramus which springs from the 2nd thoracic ganglion to the 1st thoracic nerve, is also divided.
- It is commonly done through a supraclavicular or axillary route. Thoracoscopic sympathectomy is becoming popular.
- Sympathectomy **raises the threshold** at which spasm occurs (but the effect seems to be temporary). However, the severity of the disease is reduced.

Other Vasospastic Disorders (Key Box 28.4)

These are rare.

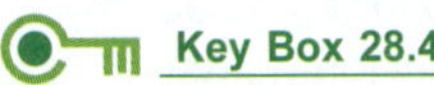
Key Box 28.4

Other Vasospastic Disorders

Acrocyanosis
- Women with cyanosis of hands and feet
- Cutaneous vasoconstriction is the cause

Livedo reticularis
- Spasm of arterioles and dilatation of venules
- Worsening by cold
- May be associated with systemic lupus erythematosus (SLE)

Erythromelalgia
- Burning sensation of hands and feet due to heat

THORACIC OUTLET SYNDROME

SURGICAL ANATOMY OF THE THORACIC OUTLET

- The thoracic outlet is a tight space with bony structures all around (Key Box 28.5), such as the manubrium sternum anteriorly, the spine posteriorly, and first rib laterally.
- At the root of the neck, the brachial plexus and subclavian artery pass through the scalene triangle into the axilla.
- The scalene triangle is the posterior compartment of the costoclavicular space. It is divideyd into anterior and posterior compartments by the scalenus anticus. The anterior compartment contains the subclavian vein.

Key Box 28.5

Introduction to Thoracic Outlet
- Tight space with bones all around
- Brachial plexus and subclavian artery are chief contents
- Scalenus anticus muscle is the muscle for landmark
- Vascular compression is more dangerous
- Neurological symptoms are often undiagnosed

- **Boundaries of scalene triangle** (Fig. 28.2)
  Base: First thoracic rib
  Anteromedially: Scalenus anticus
  Posterolaterally: Scalenus medius

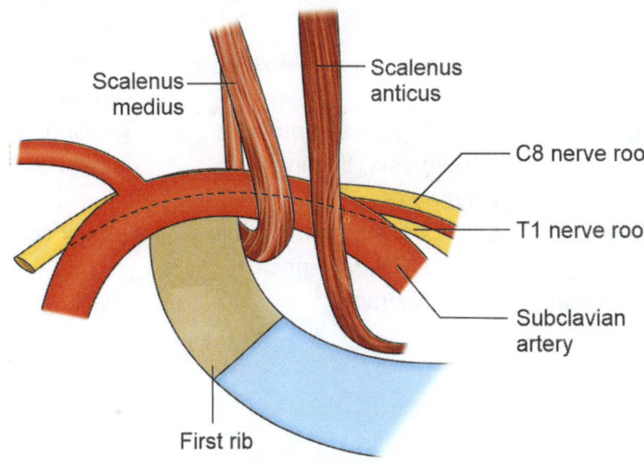

Fig. 28.2: Scalene triangle

- If the base (first thoracic rib) is raised by interposition of the cervical rib or any other cause (Key Box 28.6), it results in compression of the subclavian artery.

The thoracic outlet can be divided into 3 anatomical spaces

A. Scalene triangle is the most common site of brachial plexus compression
   Cervical rib and anomalous 1st rib compress the plexus in this location
B. Costoclavicular space is the space between the 1st rib and clavicle traversed by all 3 structures (subclavian artery, vein, and brachial plexus)
   - It is the most common site of subclavian vein compression
C. Pectoralis minor and ribs of the chest wall, an extension of the thoracic outlet area. It is also called axillary compression syndrome.
   - Types of thoracic outlet syndrome are given in Table 28.1.

Key Box 28.6

Thoracic Outlet Syndrome: Causes
- **T**ransverse process of C7—long
- **H**yperabduction syndrome—compression by pectoralis minor
- **O**perative scars—fibrous bands
- **R**ib—cervical rib
- **A**nomalous first rib—abnormal
- **C**ostoclavicular syndrome—compression between clavicle and first rib
- **I**nsertion of scalenus—anomalous (Scalenus anticus syndrome)
- **C**allus—malaligned fracture clavicle

Remember as **THORACIC**

Table 28.1	Types of thoracic outlet syndrome		
	Neurogenic	**Venous**	**Arterial**
Incidence	95%	30%	1%
Aetiology	Neck trauma, whiplash injury	Repeated overhead shoulder movements, sportsmen	Cervical rib (or) Anomalous 1st rib, rarely congenital band
Pathology	Scalene muscle fibrosis	Subclavian vein stenosis with or without thrombosis	Subclavian artery stenosis, thrombosis (or) Aneurysm
Symptoms	Neurological symptoms paresthesia, tingling Raynaud's	Swelling of whole arm, cyanosis, pain—**Paget-Schroetter syndrome**	Pain, pallor, paraesthesia, digital ischaemia
Diagnosis	Duplex scan, phenomenon EMG, NCS, MRI neck	Duplex scan, venogram	Neck X-ray, duplex scan, arteriogram
Nonsurgical treatment	Physiotherapy	Fibrinolysis, anticoagulants	None (only surgical)
Surgical treatment	–	–	1st rib resection, anterior scalenectomy, embolectomy, thrombectomy, arterial grafting.

PATHOPHYSIOLOGY OF CERVICAL RIB WITH COMPRESSION (Key Box 28.7)

- Due to slow compression, the artery distal to the compression dilates due to a jet-like effect and turbulence of blood flow. This is described as **post-stenotic dilatation** (Venturi effect) (Fig. 28.3).
- In this dilated segment, multiple small thrombi develop, which, when dislodged, result in emboli and distal ischaemia. Vascular symptoms are strictly unilateral.

Cervical Rib

- This is an **extra rib** presents in the neck in about 1–2% of the population.
- It is commonly unilateral but may be bilateral in some cases.
- It is **more frequently** encountered on the **right side.**
- It is the **anterior tubercle** of the transverse process of the 7th cervical vertebra, which attains **excessive development** and results in cervical rib.

Key Box 28.7

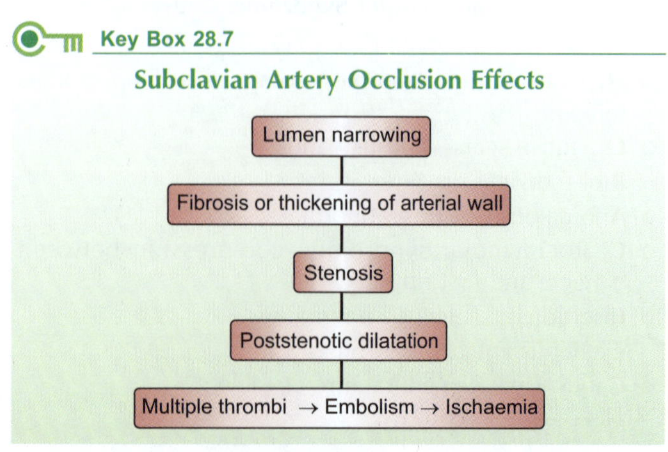

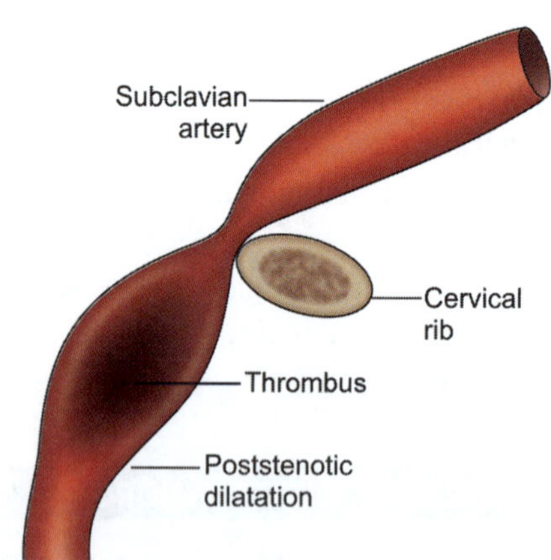

Fig. 28.3: Poststenotic dilatation of subclavian artery caused by cervical rib

Types of Cervical Rib (Fig. 28.4)

Type I	The free end of the cervical rib is **expanded** into a hard, **bony mass** which can be felt in the neck.
Type II	**Complete** cervical rib extends from C7 vertebra posteriorly to the manubrium anteriorly.
Type III	Incomplete cervical rib, which is partly bony, partly fibrous.
Type IV	A complete fibrous band which gives rise to symptoms but cannot be diagnosed by X-ray.

Clinical Features

- Common in **young females**. Even though it is congenital, symptoms appear only at or after puberty. This is because of development of the shoulder girdle muscles and sagging of the shoulder, which narrow the root of the neck. Nerve roots C8 and T1 are stretched by around 25 years of age (completion of growth).

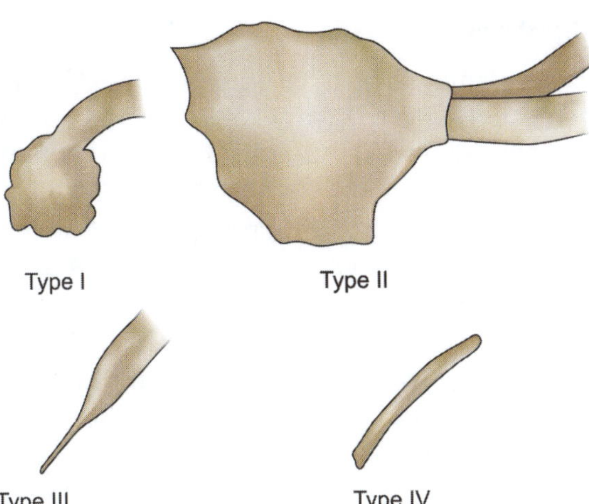

Fig. 28.4: Four types of cervical rib (see text)

- Dull-aching pain in the neck is caused by the expanded bony end of the cervical rib.
- **Features of upper limb ischaemia:** Claudication pain is apparent when the arm with muscle wasting is used. Low temperature, pallor, excessive sweating (vasomotor disturbances), **splinter haemorrhages**, ischaemic ulcers in fingers, and gangrene of the skin of the fingers are the other features. Peripheral pulses may be absent/feeble. Oedema and venous distension are very rare. These are called vascular symptoms of cervical rib.
- **Features of ulnar nerve** weakness (involvement of the lower nerve roots involvement, mainly T1) manifest as tingling and numbness or paraesthesia in the distribution of C8 and T1. The following tests confirm ulnar nerve weakness. It includes sensory disturbances and motor disturbances (performing fine action—writing, buttoning, etc.)
  A. **Card test[1]:** The patient is asked to hold a thin paper or card between the fingers. In cases of ulnar nerve paralysis, due to weakness of the interossei muscles, the patient will not be able to hold the card tightly (Fig. 28.5).

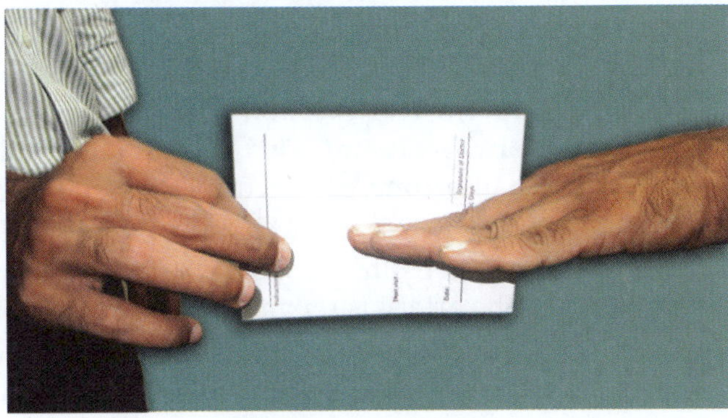

Fig. 28.5: Card test

  B. **Froment's sign:** The patient is asked to hold a book between the hand and the thumb. In cases of ulnar nerve paralysis, since the adductor pollicis is paralysed, there is flexion at the distal interphalangeal joint of the thumb. This is because **flexor pollicis longus**, which is **supplied by the median nerve, contracts** (Fig 28.6).
- **Adson's test:** Feel the radial pulse, ask the patient to take deep inspiration, and turn the neck to the same side. The pulse may disappear or become feeble. This test indicates compression on the subclavian artery (Fig. 28.7).
- **Hyperabduction test (Halsted test):** This test is done to rule out hyperabduction syndrome caused by pectoralis minor. The radial pulse becomes weak on hyperabduction due to angulation of axillary vessels and the brachial plexus, which gets compressed between pectoralis minor and its attachment to the coracoid process.
- **Military attitude test:** When shoulders are set in backward and downward positions, the radial pulse becomes weak. This is due to compression of the subclavian artery between the clavicle and the first rib. **This is seen in costoclavicular syndrome.**

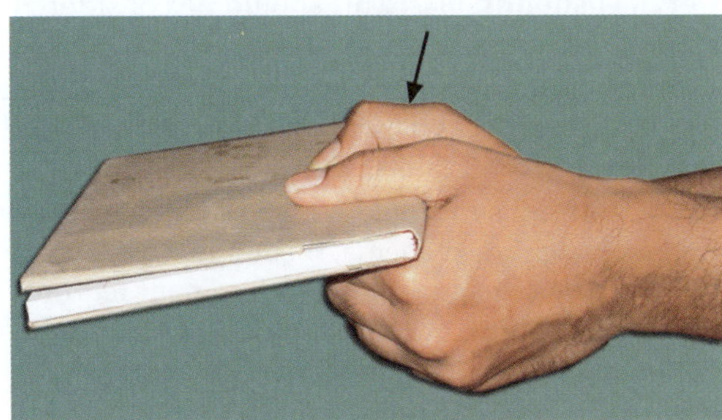

Fig. 28.6: Froment's sign

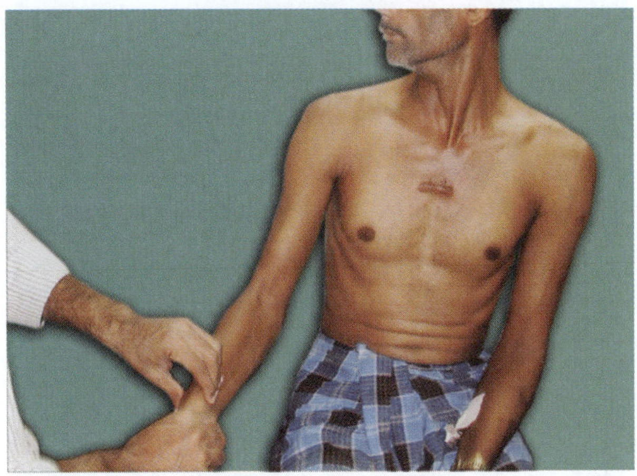

Fig. 28.7: Adson's test

[1]Card test and Froment's sign are not seen in cases of cervical rib.

- **Allen's test:** Ask the patient to clench his fist tightly. Compress the radial and ulnar arteries at the wrist with your thumbs. Wait for 10 seconds and ask the patient to open his hands. Pallor can be seen in the palm. Now release pressure on the radial artery and watch for blood flow. Repeat the test for the ulnar artery. If there is occlusion in either artery, colour changes occur slowly in the fingers (Fig. 28.8).
- **Elevated Arm Stress Test (EAST):** The patient is asked to abduct the shoulders to 90 degrees and to flex the elbow. Then he is asked to pronate/supinate the forearms continuously. Appearance of symptoms suggests thoracic outlet syndrome.
- **A hard mass** may be visible or palpable in the root of the neck (Type I).
- On palpation of the supraclavicular region, a **thrill** may be felt, and on auscultation, a **bruit** may be heard in cases of post-stenotic dilatation.

Differential Diagnosis

A patient who presents with a few neurological symptoms and signs in the upper limb with a cervical rib may be having some other causes for those symptoms. Hence, it is important to exclude other causes.

1. **Cervical spondylosis:** This should be considered as a possibility in patients >40 years.
2. **Cervical disc protrusion and spinal cord tumours** may mimic cervical rib with prominent neurological features.
3. **Carpal tunnel syndrome** may occur due to various causes such as myxoedema, rheumatoid arthritis, and malunited Colles' fracture. Predominant features of median nerve involvement, more so in menopausal women, give a clue to the diagnosis.
4. **Raynaud's phenomenon**
5. **Costovertebral anomalies**
6. **Pancoast tumour**

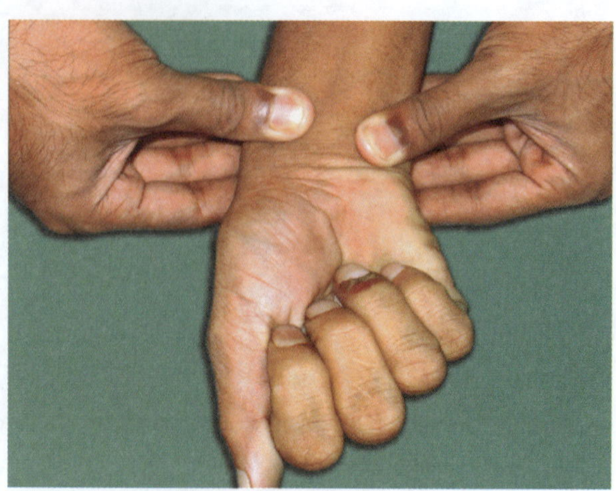

Fig. 28.8: Allen's test

Investigations

1. **X-ray neck** may show a cervical rib (Types I, II, and III). Interestingly, Type IV variety—a fibrous band which cannot be diagnosed by X-ray or by any other investigation—usually gives rise to symptoms (Fig. 28.9).
2. **Cervical disc** protrusion and spinal cord tumours may have prominent neurological features and, thus, may mimic cervical rib. **When in doubt, ask for an MRI.**
3. **Duplex scan** of the affected limb to detect any aneurysm. It may also detect a thrombus.
4. **CT angiography** to define the exact nature of the arterial dilatation and thrombus.

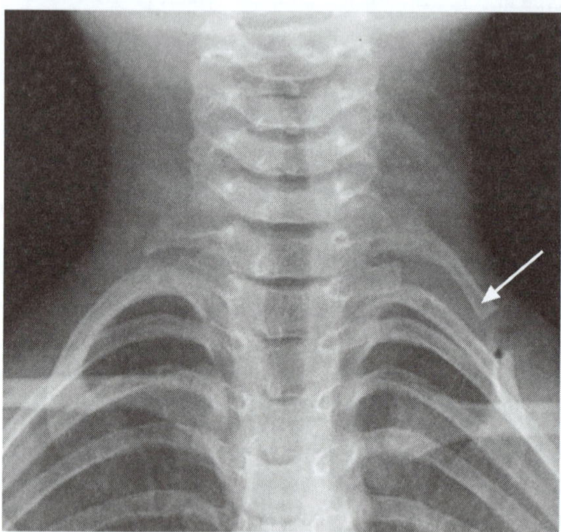

Fig. 28.9: X-ray of the neck showing cervical rib

Treatment

I. Conservative

- Patients with mild neurological symptoms are managed by shoulder girdle exercises or correction of faulty posture.

II. Surgery (Key Box 28.8)

- Presence of **vascular symptoms** and signs are the definite indications for surgery.
- Excision of the cervical rib including the periosteum is called **extraperiosteal excision** of cervical rib (so that it will not regenerate). This is combined with **cervical sympathectomy** if vascular symptoms are predominant.
- If there is a thrombus in the subclavian artery, it is removed and the artery is repaired (Fig. 28.10).
- At exploration, if a cervical rib is not found, the scalenus anterior muscle is divided. This is called scalenotomy. If **hyperabduction syndrome** is diagnosed, **pectoralis minor is divided** at its insertion into the coracoid process (Key Box 28.9).

Key Box 28.8

Cervical Rib Surgery (Figs 28.11 and 28.12)

- Remove cervical rib
- Repair subclavian artery
- Restore circulation
- Reduce vasospasm—sympathectomy
- Recognise other causes

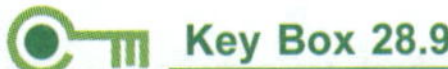

Key Box 28.9

If Cervical Rib is not Found

- Scalenotomy
- Division of pectoralis minor, scalenus anterior
- Extraperiosteal resection of the first rib

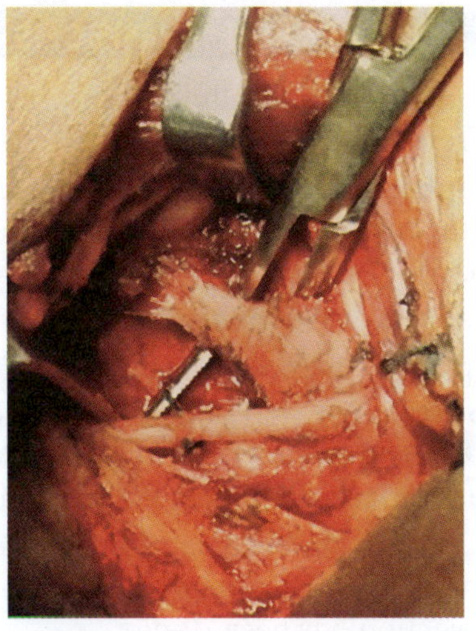

Fig. 28.11: Cervical rib at surgery

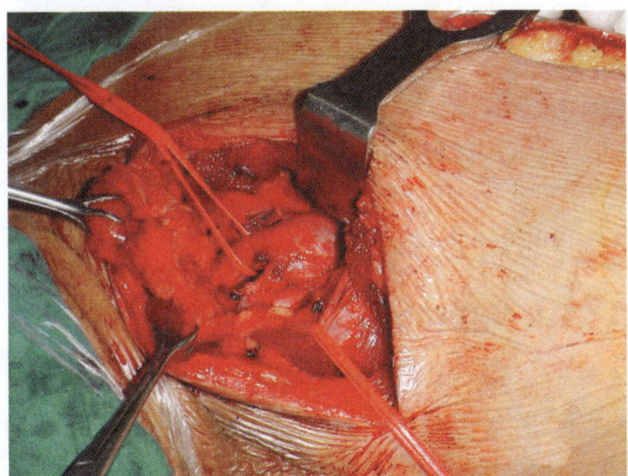

Fig. 28.10: Subclavian artery is exposed to repair the dilatation and remove the thrombus

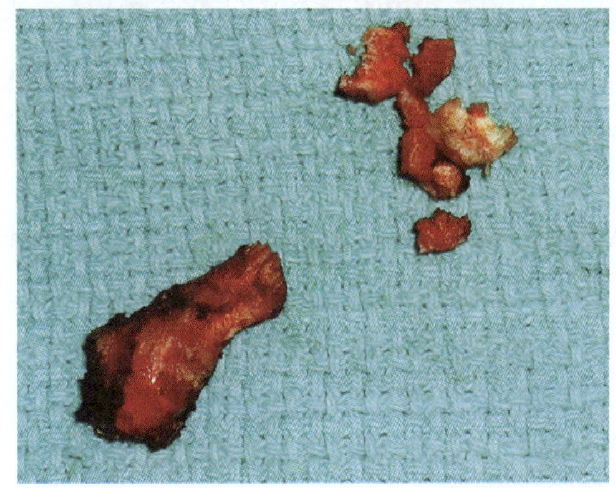

Fig. 28.12: Cervical rib removed

A summary of cervical rib is given in Fig. 28.13.

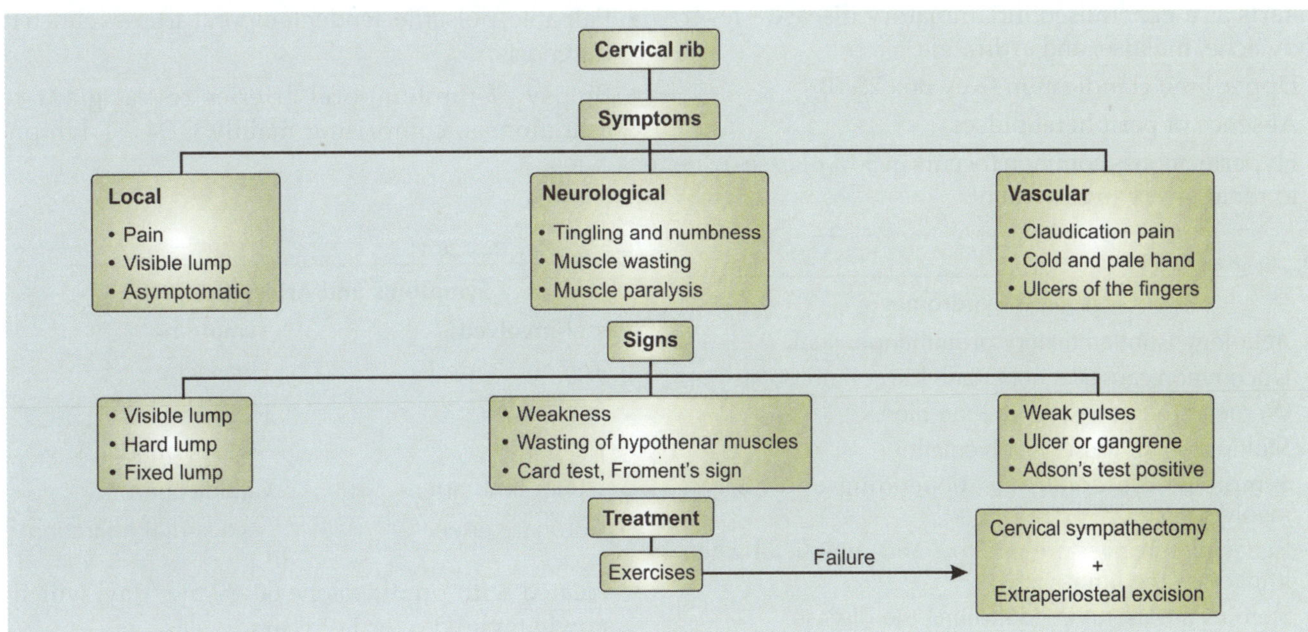

Fig. 28.13: Summary of cervical rib

AXILLARY VEIN THROMBOSIS

- Patients present with swelling of the arm after intense activity from the dominant hand
- **Hypertrophy of the subclavius muscle** may also cause compression of the subclavian-axillary vein (sportsman)
- Peripheral pulses will be normal
- Venography to diagnose thrombus
- **Thrombolysis** or, if necessary, venotomy and removal of the thrombus and 1st rib (if it is the cause of obstruction) are the treatment modalities.
- Axillary vein thrombosis is also a complication of axillary block dissection, especially where extensive nodal dissection has been done.

VASCULITIS SYNDROMES

Competency

SU27.3: Describe clinical features, investigations and principles of management of vasospastic disorders.

TAKAYASU'S ARTERITIS (Pulseless disease, large vessels arteritis)

- It is of unknown aetiology.
- Commonly affects females (85%).
- It is a panarteritis involving the aortic arch and its branches. The subclavian artery is involved in 85% of cases.

Clinical Features

It starts as a generalised inflammatory disease—fever, body ache, malaise, and arthralgia.

- Upper limb claudication (Key Box 28.10)
- Absence of peripheral pulses
- Hypertension is common (occurs in 50% of cases) due to renal artery involvement.

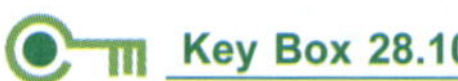

Key Box 28.10

Vasculitis Syndromes

- Aetiology is inflammatory or immunological.
- Uncommon causes of upper and lower limb ischaemia.
- Women are affected more than men.
- Multiple small vessel involvement.
- Symptoms are confusing, depending upon organ involvement.
- Ischaemic changes are minimal and superficial when it involves the limbs.
- Steroids are useful in controlling the disease.
- Immunosuppression should be tried carefully.

- A bruit may be heard over the subclavian artery
- Visual disturbances may occur due to involvement of retinal arteries. Late blindness may occur.

Pathology

It is a **panarteritis**, involving all layers of elastic arteries. Thrombosis and stenosis may occur later.

Investigations

- C-reactive protein is elevated as part of an acute phase response (nonspecific).
- **Duplex-Doppler ultrasound and MR angiography** may diagnose the site of obstruction and blood flow pattern.

Treatment

- Very early cases benefit with steroid therapy, e.g. tablet **prednisolone 30–50 mg/day** (anti-inflammatory effect). Cyclophosphamide may be tried when other measures fail (immunosuppressive effect).
- Vascular reconstruction—difficult.

GIANT CELL ARTERITIS

- It is also called **temporal arteritis**.
- An elderly woman presenting with severe headache is the common presentation.
- Fever and malaise may also be present.
- Involvement of various arteries results in various symptoms (Key Box 28.11).
- Palpable, pulsatile, tender temporal arteries clinch the diagnosis.
- Biopsy of the temporal arteries reveal giant cell granulomas, comprising mainly CD4+ T lymphocytes.

Key Box 28.11

Symptoms and Artery Involved

Vessel involved	Symptoms
Temporal artery	Headache
Facial artery	Jaw pain
Retinal artery	Sudden blindness
Upper limb artery	Claudication
Coronary artery	Myocardial infarction

- Treated with prednisolone 60–80 mg/day, which is slowly tapered over 1–2 years.
- Relapses and remissions are common.

POLYARTERITIS SYNDROME

- This includes microscopic polyarteritis (more common) and polyarteritis nodosa (less common).
- This syndrome also has an inflammatory reaction.
- Ischaemia of the lower limbs and upper limbs may occur due to involvement of small vessels.
- Abdominal pain is due to the involvement of visceral vessels.
- Involvement of renal arteries causes loin pain, haematuria, and hypertension.
- Treatment is similar to the other diseases mentioned above.

SYSTEMIC SCLEROSIS

- It was earlier called 'collagen vascular disorder' because there is obstruction of the small vessels by collagen deposition.
- Now it is included under vasculitis syndromes because of its association with an inflammatory reaction.
- Ischaemic changes occur in the fingers and toes. Necrosis and ulceration are common.
- Oesophageal involvement results in dysphagia.
- Small bowel sclerosis results in disordered motility and malabsorption.
- Sympathectomy and vasodilators may be useful.
- Raynaud's symptoms may be controlled with calcium channel blockers and nitrates.

GANGRENE

Competency

SU27.4: Describe the types of gangrene.

Please note: Principles of amputation are given in operative surgery chapter, page no. 1282.

Definition

Macroscopic death of tissue with superadded putrefaction. It affects the limbs, intestines, appendix, etc. In this chapter, differential diagnoses of gangrene of the limbs are considered.

Pregangrene (Key Box 28.12)

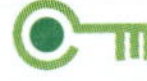

Key Box 28.12

Pregangrene—Symptoms

- Rest pain is the main symptom
- Pallor on elevation
- Congestion on dependent position
- Guttering of veins
- Poor capillary filling
- Thickening or scaling of skin

Rest pain, colour changes at rest and with exercise, oedema, hyperaesthesia, and skin ulcerations are due to inadequate blood supply to the limb. These changes are described as pregangrenous changes in the limb.

Classification of Gangrene

1. **Cardiovascular causes**
   - TAO
   - Atherosclerotic gangrene
   - Acute embolic gangrene
   - Syphilitic gangrene
   - Raynaud's disease
   - Cervical rib
   - Vasculitis syndrome
   - Polycythaemia
2. **Neurological causes:** Hemiplegia, paraplegia, bedsore.
3. **Traumatic gangrene:** Direct—thrombosis; indirect—crush injuries.
4. **Physical causes:** Sunrays, radiation, corrosive acids.
5. **Drugs:** Ergotamine.
6. Diabetic gangrene.
7. **Acute infective gangrene:** Boil, carbuncle, cancrum oris, gas gangrene.

Clinical Features of Gangrene (Key Box 28.13)

- A part which is gangrenous is a dead portion of the body. It has **no arterial pulsations**, venous return, or capillary filling.
- It has no sensation.
- The colour is initially pale and later changes to dusky grey and finally black. The **black colour** is due to the disintegration of haemoglobin and the formation of iron sulphide.
- The gangrenous part has to be treated with surgical excision or debridement, which may amount to disarticulation of the toe or even amputation.
- Gram-positive, gram-negative, and anaerobic organisms multiply in this segment and may produce septicaemia. Thus, this may precipitate multiorgan failure, including renal failure, adult respiratory distress syndrome (ARDS), cardiac failure, etc.

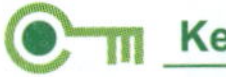

Key Box 28.13

Signs of Gangrene

- Loss of pulsation
- Loss of colour
- Loss of temperature
- Loss of sensation
- Loss of function

Clinical Types (Table 28.2)

Table 28.2 Comparison of dry gangrene and wet gangrene

	Dry gangrene	Wet gangrene
Cause	Slow occlusion of the arteries	Sudden occlusion of the arteries
Involvement of part	Small area is gangrenous due to presence of collaterals	Large area is affected due to absence of collaterals
Local findings	Dry, shrivelled and mummified	Wet, turgid, swollen, oedematous
Line of demarcation	Usually present	Absent
Crepitus	Absent	May be present
Odour	Absent	Foul odour due to sulphurated hydrogen produced by putrefactive bacteria
Infection	Not present	Usually present
Diseases	TAO, atherosclerosis	Emboli, ligatures, crush injuries
Treatment	Conservative amputation	Major amputation is necessary

VARIOUS TYPES OF GANGRENE (Figs 28.14 to 28.19)

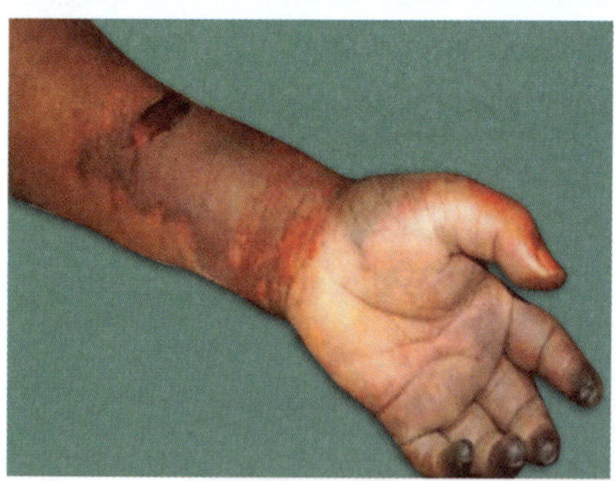

Fig. 28.14: Peripheral gangrene due to sepsis and vasopressors

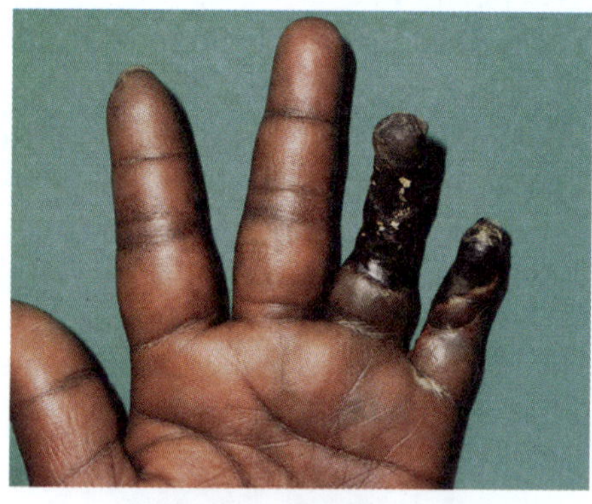

Fig. 28.17: Left medial 2 fingers gangrene due to TAO

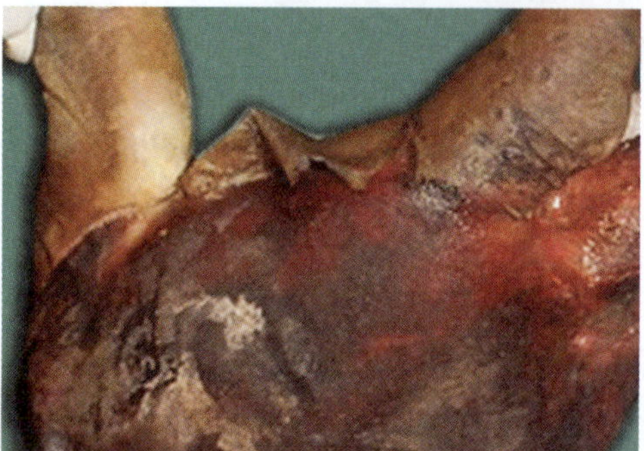

Fig. 28.15: Emboli at the brachial artery resulting in massive gangrene of the hand (wet gangrene)

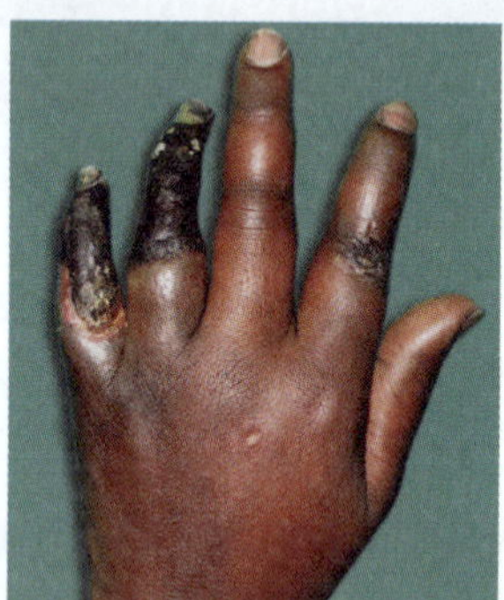

Fig. 28.18: View of the dorsum of the hand

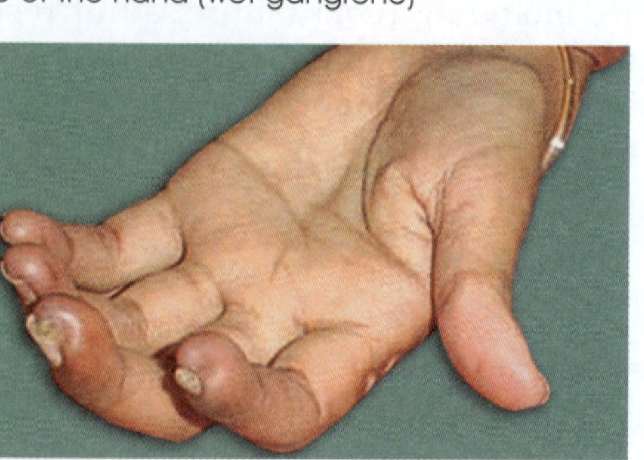

Fig. 28.16: Case of SLE. Observe pulp of fingers

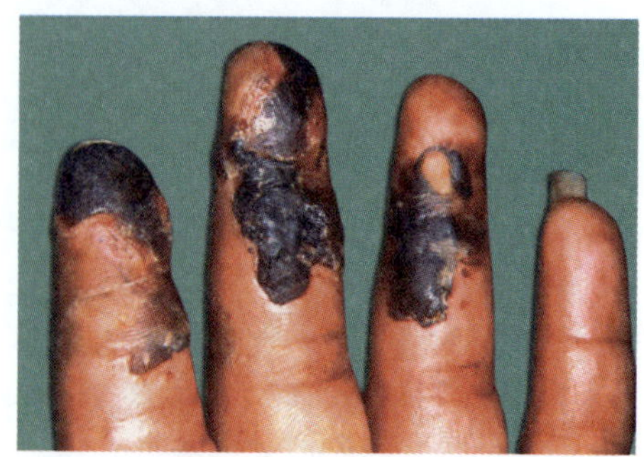

Fig. 28.19: Embolic gangrene of fingers

SPECIAL TYPES OF GANGRENE

CANCRUM ORIS

- It is an extensive ulcerative disease of the cheek mucosa occurring in malnourished children.
- **Precipitating factors** are:
  - Malnourishment
  - Major infectious diseases, such as diphtheria, whooping cough, typhoid, measles, and kala azar.
- As a result of these factors, opportunistic organisms, such as Vincent's organisms (*Borrelia vincentii* and *B. fusiformis*) multiply and cause multiple ulcers, erosions, and later, fibrosis.
- Occasionally, as the disease progresses, the whole thickness of the cheek may be lost.

Treatment of Cancrum Oris

1. Ryle's tube feeding
2. Improve nutrition—IV fluids, parenteral nutrition (in severe cases)
3. Appropriate antibiotics: Penicillin + Metronidazole 400 mg three times a day for 7–10 days.
4. Reconstructive surgery may be necessary later.
5. Chlorhexidine mouthwash

Complications of Cancrum Oris

- Fibrosis causing restriction of jaw movements.
- Septicaemia, toxaemia, and death.

ACROCYANOSIS

- It is also called 'hereditary cold extremities'.
- It presents as persistent cyanotic discolouration of the hands when exposed to cold due to intermittent spasm of small peripheral vessels.
- It commonly affects the hands and, rarely, the feet.
- Generally, it is mild and nonprogressive.

DRUG ABUSE AND GANGRENE

- Abuse of the drugs is an important cause of gangrene in modern days.
- Inadvertent injection of drugs into an artery may lead to thrombosis of the artery, resulting in acute ischaemia—commonly in the brachial artery.
- Emergency treatment in symptomatic cases includes heparinisation and infusion of dextran.
- In severe cases, emergency angiography and intra-arterial thrombolysis is considered.

GANGRENE FOLLOWING INTRA-ARTERIAL DRUG INJECTION

- Inadvertent **intra-arterial injection of thiopentone** into one of the high divisions of the brachial artery, (*congenital anomaly*)—usually the ulnar—will result in severe burning and blanching of the hand (Figs 28.20 and 28.21).
- After the injection, initial signs and symptoms occur very fast (within 15–20 seconds). It consists of intense forearm pain and mottling of the skin over the hand.
- Minutes later, discolouration and nail bed pallor become evident. Approximately 3 to 4 hours later, the symptoms progress to paraesthesias and pronounced hand weakness.
- Rapid development of signs indicative of necrosis (by the eighth day) requires the patient to undergo fasciotomies, multiple debridements, and skin grafts for cosmesis.
- If this complication is noticed, the following steps (measures) have to be taken immediately.

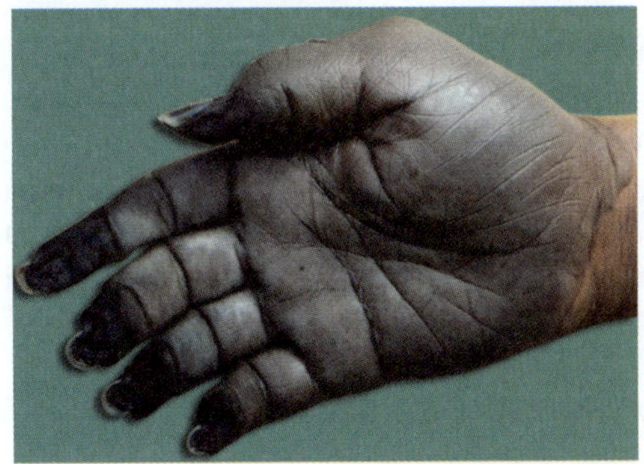

Fig. 28.20: Gangrene following intra-arterial injection

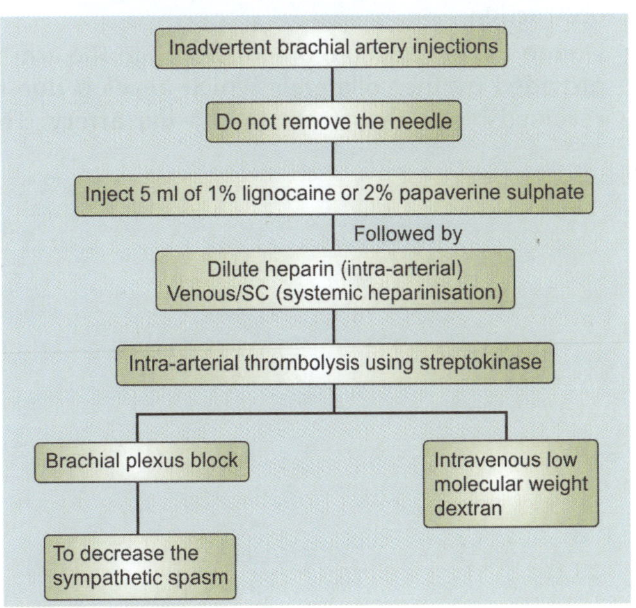

Fig. 28.21: Management of inadvertent brachial artery injections

Treating a Case of Inadvertent Intra-arterial Injection

Step 1: If iatrogenic, maintain the intra-arterial catheter in place—do not remove it.

Step 2: Identify the progression of the disease—colour changes, necrosis, gangrene.

Step 3: Initiate anticoagulation—diluted heparin, intravenous and subcutaneous.

Step 4: Institute symptomatic relief and plan for rehabilitation—analgesics, brachial plexus block (analgesia and vasodilatation) physiotherapy.

Step 5: Elevation of extremity, antibiotics, antiplatelet anticoagulant therapy.

Step 6: Perform specific interventions—angiogram, intra-arterial thrombolysis, vasodilators, prostacyclins, sympathectomy, corticosteroids.

Step 7: Aim is to save the limb—last resort is amputation.

MISCELLANEOUS

Ergot and Gangrene

- Ergot preparations are used over a long period in patients with migraine.
- Ergotamine gangrene occurs in those who eat bread infected with *Claviceps purpurea.* Example: Dwellers on the shores of the Mediterranean Sea and the **Russian Steppes.**

SUBCLAVIAN STEAL SYNDROME (Fig. 28.22)

- It refers to the development of symptoms in either the brain or in the arm due to subclavian artery obstruction.
- Due to the obstruction, blood supply to the arm is provided by the collaterals which develop due to reversed blood flow from the basilar artery. The basilar artery is formed at the base of the skull by the joining of 2 vertebral arteries. The basilar artery supplies blood to cerebellum, brain stem, and occipital lobes. Thus, symptoms may be vertebrobasilar or may occur in the arm (Key Box 28.14).

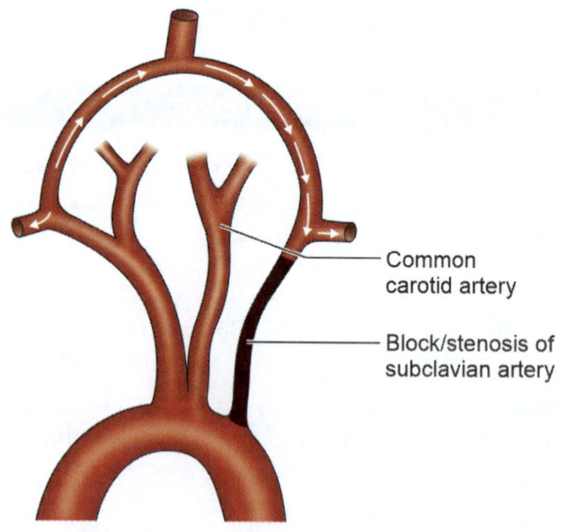

Fig. 28.22: Subclavian steal syndrome

- **Javid test:** Pressure on the common carotid artery produces a weak radial pulse on the ipsilateral side.
- Surgical correction is by endarterectomy, a bypass graft, or transluminal balloon angioplasty is another alternative.

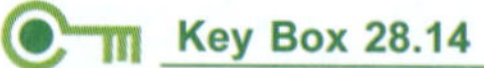

Key Box 28.14

Subclavian Steal Syndrome

- It is more common on the left side
- **Vertebrobasilar symptoms**—dizziness, vertigo, imbalance
- **Arm symptoms**—fatigue, pain with exercise, paraesthesias, coolness and heaviness on the affected side
- Asymmetrical radial pulses or difference of 20 mmHg systolic pressure between the upper limbs.

Multiple Choice Questions

1. **Which of the following is usually not a feature of Raynaud's disease?**
   A. Radial artery pulsations are absent
   B. The upper limb is involved
   C. Cervical sympathectomy is helpful
   D. Pallor, cyanosis, and rubor are the colour changes during the attack

2. **The following are true for cervical sympathectomy *except*:**
   A. It raises the threshold at which spasm occurs
   B. The entire stellate ganglion has to be removed
   C. It is the treatment of choice in hyperhydrosis
   D. Up to the 3rd thoracic ganglion has to be removed

3. **Which muscle is the landmark to the thoracic outlet?**
   A. Scalenus anticus B. Scalenus medius
   C. Scalenus posterior D. Levator scapulae

4. **The following are components of giant cell arteritis *except*:**
   A. Severe headache is a presenting complaint
   B. The temporal artery is usually not involved
   C. A biopsy from the artery reveals giant cell granulomas
   D. CD4+ T lymphocytes are found in histopathology

5. **Hypertension is a common finding in the following conditions *except*:**
   A. Polyarteritis nodosa
   B. Phaeochromocytoma
   C. Polycystic disease of kidney
   D. Hyperthyroidism

6. **Which of the following is the treatment of choice for cervical rib with ischaemia?**
   A. Excision of the rib
   B. Excision of the rib with cervical sympathectomy
   C. Excision of the rib with division of the pectoralis minor
   D. Excision of the rib with division of the scalenus anticus

7. **The following are true for the subclavian artery *except*:**
   A. A cervical rib may compress it
   B. It gives rise to the internal mammary artery
   C. Post-stenotic dilatation occurs once it is compressed by a cervical rib
   D. It continues as the axillary artery at the medial border of the first rib

8. **Compression of the subclavian artery is detected by which clinical test?**
   A. Froment's sign B. Adson's test
   C. Allen's test D. Halsted test

9. **The following are causes of splinter haemorrhages *except*:**
   A. Bacterial endocarditis B. Cervical rib
   C. Scleroderma D. Aortic regurgitation

10. **The following are true about subclavian steal syndrome *except*:**
    A. It is more common on the left side
    B. It presents with vertebrobasilar symptoms
    C. Both radial arteries are normal
    D. Significant arm symptoms are present

11. **The following are the causes of upper limb ischaemia *except*:**
    A. Ergotamine alkaloids
    B. Cervical rib
    C. TAO
    D. Atheroma of the brachial artery

12. **Which is the test to detect the dominant arterial supply for hand circulation?**
    A. Froment's sign B. Adson's test
    C. Allen's test D. Halsted test

13. **Nicoladoni Branham sign refers to:**
    A. Compression causing bradycardia
    B. Compression causing tachycardia
    C. Hypotension
    D. Systolic filling

14. **The most common cause of an acquired AV fistula is:**
    A. Bacterial injection B. Fungal infection
    C. Blunt trauma D. Penetrating trauma

15. **Bilateral pulseless disease in the upper limbs is caused by:**
    A. Aortoarteritis
    B. Coarctation of the aorta
    C. Fibromuscular dysplasia
    D. Buerger's disease

Answers

1. A	2. B	3. A	4. B	5. D	6. B	7. D	8. B	9. D	10. C
11. D	12. C	13. A	14. D	15. A					

CHAPTER

29

Lymphatics, Lymph Vessels and Lymphoma

- Lymphoedema—anatomy and physiology
- Lymphatic circulation
- Primary (congenital) lymphoedema
- Secondary lymphoedema (acquired)
- Lymphangiography
- Hodgkin's lymphoma
- Non-Hodgkin's lymphoma
- Burkitt's lymphoma
- Sézary's syndrome
- Chyluria

INTRODUCTION

Lymphatics and lymph vessels play the role of draining waste fluid from the body. Hence, they are vulnerable to various infections. The lymphatics are connected to a group of lymph nodes and drain into veins. Hence, infections of the lymphatics give rise to enlarged lymph nodes. In this chapter, significant surgical diseases affecting the lymphatics and lymph nodes are discussed.

LYMPHOEDEMA

Competency

SU27.7: Describe pathophysiology, clinical features, investigations and principles of management of lymphedema, lymphangitis and lymphomas.

Definition

Accumulation of lymph in the ***extracellular, extravascular compartment*** and subcutaneous tissues resulting in enlargement of the limb. It is a **protein-rich** interstitial fluid.

Common Sites of Lymphoedema

- Lower limbs are the most common site.
- Upper limbs.
- Scrotum: Elephantiasis of the scrotum is caused by filarial organism (*Wuchereria bancrofti*).

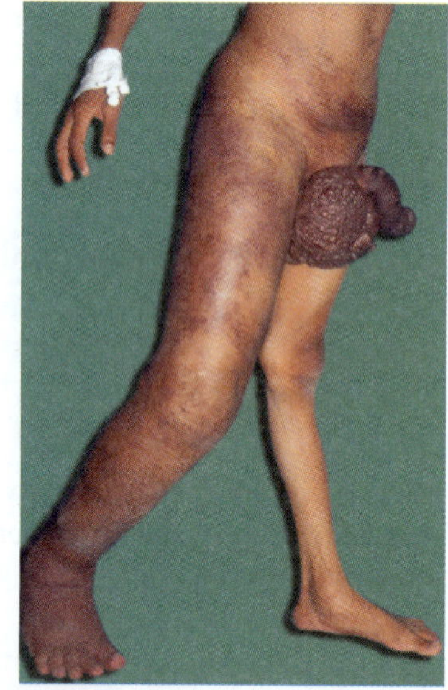

Fig. 29.1: Complication of filariasis—elephant leg, elephantiasis of scrotum and ram's horn penis

- Elephantiasis of the penis caused by filarial organisms produces ***ram's horn penis*** (Fig. 29.1).

Anatomy and Physiology

Surgical Anatomy of the Lymphatic System

- Lumbar trunks: Receive lymphatics from the lower limbs
- Intestinal trunk: Receive lymphatics from the GIT
- These trunks combine to form the cisterna chyli, which later twins into the thoracic duct (45 cm)

- The thoracic duct also drains lymph from left jugular, left subclavian, and left bronchomediastinal trunks.
- The right lymphatic duct (1.25 cm) drains lymph from right jugular, right subclavian, and right broncho-mediastinal trunks and enters into the junction of right IJV and subclavian veins.
- The cisterna chyli is a lymphatic channel that receives lymphatic drainage from the lower limbs and GIT. It is found inferior to the aortic hiatus of the diaphragm, beyond which it continues as the thoracic duct.

Functions of the Lymphatic System

- To return protein-rich fluid to circulation through ***lymphaticovenous junctions*** in the jugular area.
- This fluid includes water, electrolytes, and low molecular weight substances such as polypeptides, growth factors, and cytokines.
- It also includes **macromolecules, such as fibrinogen, albumin,** and globulin.
- **Transport of cholesterol**, long chain fatty acids, triglycerides, and fat-soluble vitamins (A, D, E, K) by intestinal lymph into circulation. They bypass the liver and enter circulation through the cisterna chyli and thoracic duct into the left internal jugular vein (lymph from lower limbs, abdomen, and left arm).
- The right lymphatic duct drains into the right internal jugular vein (lymph from head and right arm).

Components of the Lymphatic System

- Lymphatic channels (Fig. 29.2).
- Lymphoid organs—lymph nodes, spleen, Peyer's patches, thymus, tonsils.
- Circulating cells—lymphocytes and mononuclear immune cells.

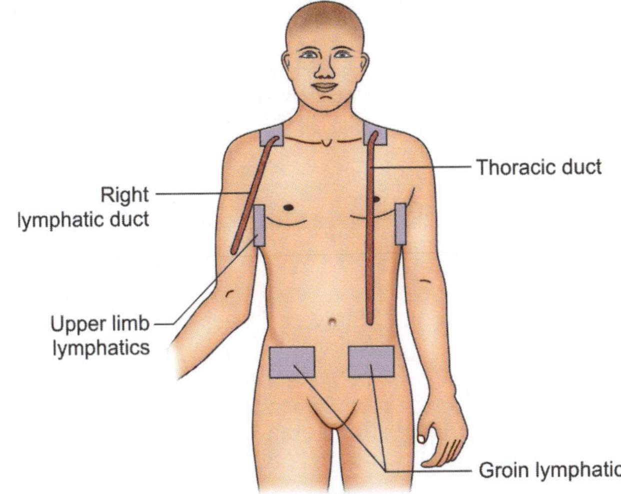

Fig. 29.2: Major lymphatics and lymphatic ducts

Lymphatic Circulation (Fig. 29.3)

- Lymph flow is largely due to **intrinsic lymphatic contractility** by lymphangiomas (segment of lymphatics).
- A transient increase in interstitial pressure secondary to exercise and limb movements also helps to a certain extent.
- Valves prevent reflux in the lymphatics.

Types of Lymphoedema

1. Primary (congenital) lymphoedema
2. Secondary lymphoedema

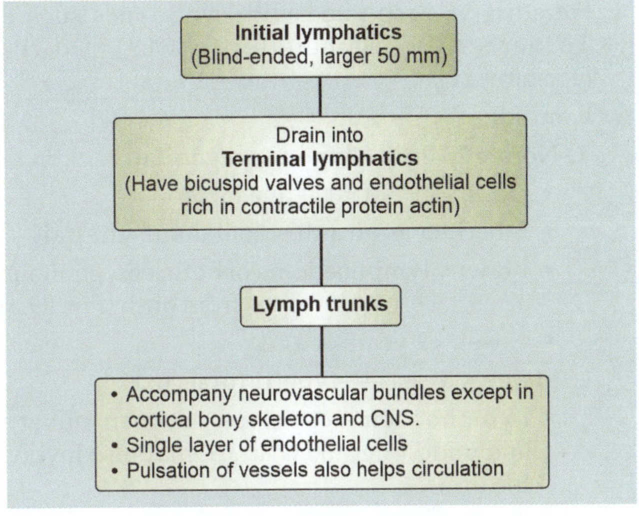

Fig. 29.3: Lymphatic circulation

Risk factors for lymphoedema (Key Box 29.1)

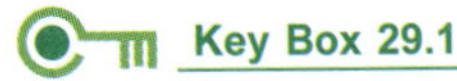

Key Box 29.1

Risk Factors for Lower Limb Lymphoedema

- Inguinal block dissection, e.g. carcinoma penis, melanoma
- Postoperative pelvic radiotherapy
- Varicose vein stripping and vein harvesting
- Obesity

Risk Factors for Upper Limb Lymphoedema

- Axillary block dissection, e.g. carcinoma breast
- Radiation fibrosis, scar formation
- Advanced cancer—breast with axillary lymph nodes
- Obesity
- Chronic infection

PRIMARY (CONGENITAL) LYMPHOEDEMA

INTRODUCTION

- Incidence is 1 in 6000 persons.
- Lymphoedema is confined to the epifascial plane.

- It is due to an inherited abnormality of the lymphatic system.
- A few cases which occur later in life may be due to unnoticed factors—repeated bacterial and fungal infections, trauma to feet, etc.
- **Loss of venoarteriolar reflux (VAR),** which protects the lower limb capillaries from excessive hydrostatic forces in the erect posture, occurs in advanced age. Diseases such as diabetes and chronic venous insufficiency may also contribute.

Causes of Primary Lymphoedema

I. **Hereditary:** Associated with syndromes such as Turner's (XO), Klinefelter's (XXY), Down's (Trisomy 21).

II. **Familial**

1. **Nonne-Milroy—type I (congenital)**
   - Occurs in 1 of 6000 live births
   - Inherited as an autosomal dominant trait
   - Brawny lymphoedema of both legs, genitalia, arms, face, etc. develops from birth (Fig. 29.4).
   - Onset: <2 years of age
2. **Meige's disease—type II (praecox)**
   - Lymphoedema develops between puberty and middle age (50 years). It may also involve the arms.
   - A few are inherited in an autosomal dominant manner.
   - Onset: 2–35 years of age.
3. **Tarda onset after 35 years of age**

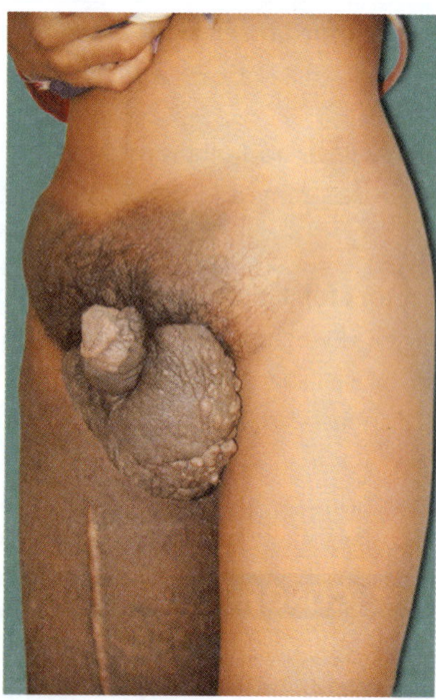

Fig. 29.4: Congenital lymphoedema—observe the right leg. One attempt has been made to decrease lymphoedema by excision

Pathophysiology (Fig. 29.5)

Pearls of Wisdom

Lymphoedema leads to impaired immune surveillance and predisposes to other malignancies (Key Box 29.2).

Types of Primary Lymphoedema

- ***Lymphatic aplasia:*** Number of lymphatic channels and nodes are grossly reduced.
- ***Lymphatic hypoplasia:*** Lymphatic channels are of a small calibre.
- ***Milroy's disease:*** A familial type of lymphoedema congenita.
- Based on the time at which lymphoedema appears, it is classified as either:

  Birth: Lymphoedema congenita.

  Puberty: Lymphoedema praecox.

  Later: Lymphoedema tarda.

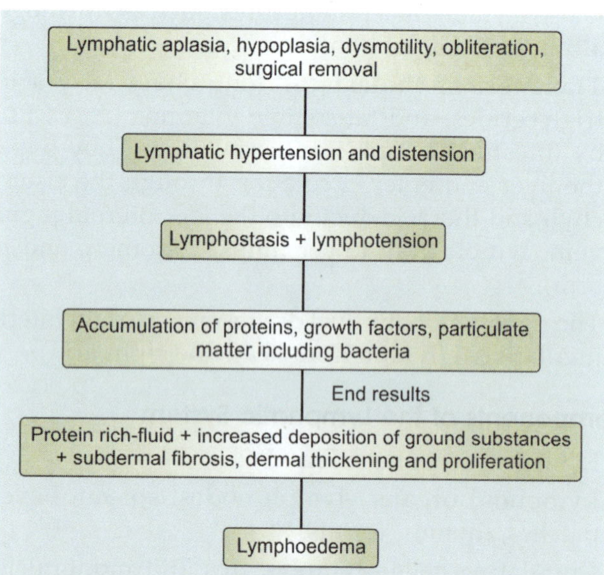

Fig. 29.5: Pathophysiology of lymphoedema

Key Box 29.2

Malignancies Associated with Lymphoedema

Skin cancers

- Squamous cell carcinoma
- Malignant melanoma
- Basal cell carcinoma

Sarcomas

- Lymphangiosarcoma (Stewart-Treves syndrome)
- Kaposi's sarcoma
- Liposarcoma
- Malignant fibrous histiocytoma

Systemic disease

- Lymphoma

SECONDARY LYMPHOEDEMA (ACQUIRED)

1. **Filarial elephantiasis** (Fig. 29.6) is caused by *Wuchereria bancrofti,* transmitted by the mosquito *Culex fatigans.* The disease is caused by adult worms which have an affinity towards lymphatic vessels and nodes. **Microfilariae do not produce any lesions.**
   - Initially, it causes **lymphangitis** which clinically presents with high grade fever, chills and rigors, red streaks in the limb, tenderness, and swelling of the spermatic cord and scrotum (Table 29.1).
   - The lymph nodes are swollen and tender. **Retroperitoneal lymphangitis** produces acute abdominal pain.
   - Due to repeated infections, fibrosis occurs and results in **lymphatic obstruction**. Later, this gives rise to **lymphatic dilatation.** Lower limb lymphatics are dilated and tortuous (lymphangiectasis).
   - Initially, lymphoedema is **pitting** in nature but progressively becomes nonpitting. Lymph (protein) provides good nourishment for fibroblasts.
   - After repeated infections, the skin over the limb becomes *dry and thickened,* and is thrown into folds and even *nodules* that *break open* and result in ulcers. Hence, it is called ***elephant leg***. Malnutrition and infection precipitate lymphoedema. Oedema is also due to reflux of lymph from para-aortic vessels into the smaller lymphatics draining the lower limb. ***The subcutaneous tissue is grossly thickened. The presence of deep fascia prevents involvement of the deep muscles of the lower limb*** (Key Box 29.3).

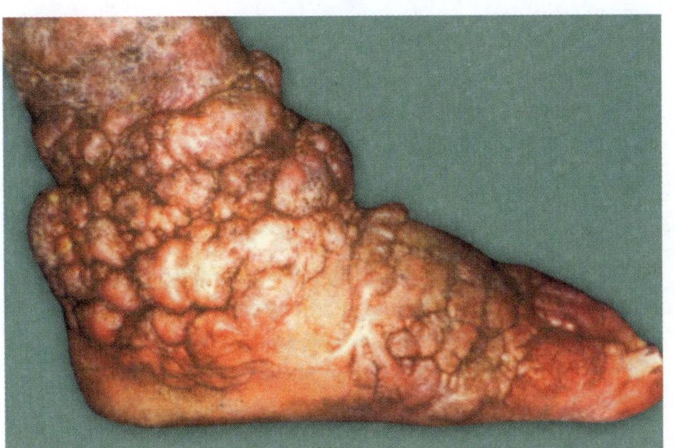

Fig. 29.6: Filarial lymphoedema

Key Box 29.3

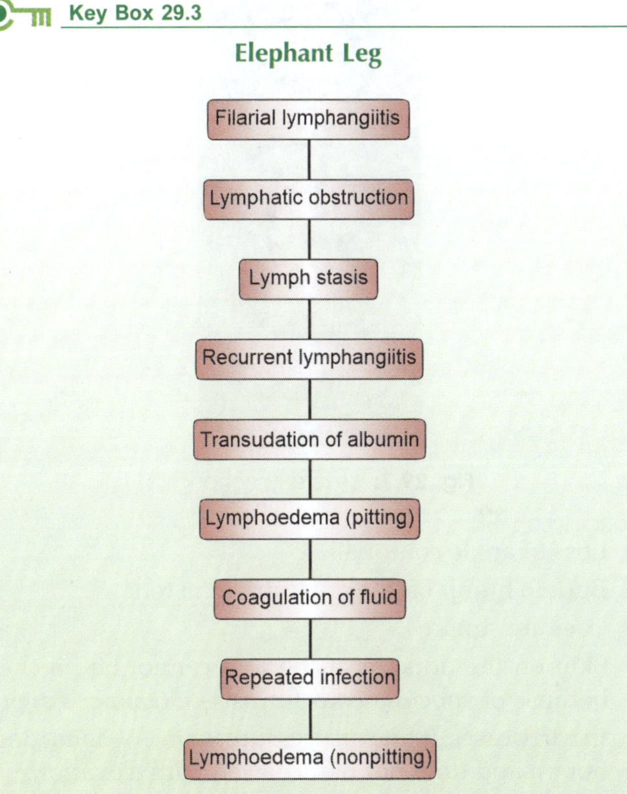

2. After inguinal block dissection for secondaries in the lymph nodes (upper limb lymphoedema following axillary block dissection).
3. Following radiotherapy to lymph nodes.
4. Advanced malignancies.
5. Repeated infections due to barefoot walking (Fig. 29.7).

Symptoms (Table 29.2)

- Swollen limb, dull-aching pain
- Tiredness, pins and needles, cramping pain

Table 29.1 Clinical manifestations of lymphatic filariasis

Site of involvement	Acute	Chronic
Lower limbs	Lymphangiitis, lymphadeniitis	Lymphoedema, chronic lymphadenitis
Scrotum	Lymphangiitis	Lymphoedema, chylocele
Spermatic cord	Acute funiculitis	Chronic thickened cord
Epididymis and testis	Acute epididymo-orchitis	Chronic epididymo-orchitis
Abdomen	Acute retroperitoneal lymphangiitis	Chyluria, lymphadenovarix
Breast	Lymphangiitis	Lymphoedema

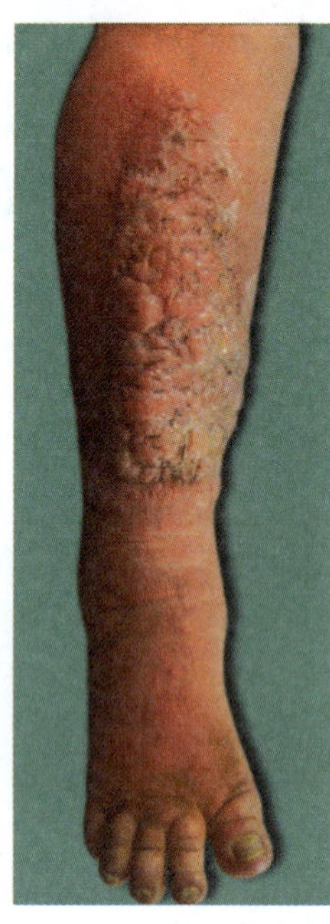

Fig. 29.7: Severe lymphangiitis

- Loss of ankle contour
- Buffalo hump on the dorsum of the foot
- Toes are square
- Skin on the dorsum of the toes cannot be pinched because of subcutaneous fibrosis—*Stemmer's sign*
- In early cases, it pits on pressure. Later, oedema does not pit and does not reduce even with elevation.
- ***Advanced cases:*** Chronic eczema, fungal infections of skin (dermatophytosis) and nails (onychomycosis), fissuring, warts.
- Ulceration is unusual.
- However, once ulcers start, recurrent bacterial infections are common, thus worsening the disease process.

Diagnosed by detecting: Microfilariae on blood smear complement fixation test.

Treatment: Diethylcarbamazine (DEC) 100 mg bid × 14 days.

Grades of Filarial Lymphoedema

Grade I	**Oedema pitting:** Completely relieved on rest and elevation. No skin changes.
Grade II	**Oedema pitting:** Partially relieved on rest and elevation. No skin changes.
Grade III	**Oedema nonpitting:** Skin involvement, subcutaneous thickening present.
Grade IV	**Oedema nonpitting:** Not relieved, warty projections, elephantiasis, lymphorrhoea present.

Differential Diagnosis of Unilateral Elephantiasis of the Leg

1. **Filariasis** is the most common cause of secondary elephantiasis of the leg in endemic areas—coastal Karnataka, coastal Andhra Pradesh, Tamil Nadu, etc. (Table 29.3).

Table 29.2 Clinical features of lymphoedema

Early signs	Change into	Late/advanced cases—signs
1. Loss of ankle contour	1. Fibrosis	1. Chronic eczema
2. Buffalo hump on the dorsum of feet	2. Dermal thickening	2. Fungal infection—dermatophytosis
3. **Stemmer's sign:** Skin on dorsum of 2nd toe cannot be pinched because of subcutaneous fibrosis.	3. Hyperkeratosis	3. Fungal infection of nails—onychomycosis
4. Early pitting on pressure, less on rest, elevation		4. Fissuring, verrucae, papilla
5. Squaring of toes		5. Grossly thickened leg with skin

Table 29.3 Comparison of primary and secondary lymphoedema

Primary lymphoedema	Secondary lymphoedema
It is due to congenital aplasia and hypoplasia	Filariasis is the common cause
Slowly progressive	Rapidly progressive
It is seen in younger age group	Middle age group
Females are more often affected	Males are more commonly affected
Unilateral, begins distally, spreads proximally	Sometimes, it can start proximally—unilateral or bilateral
Capillary haemangioma may be present	Absent
Regional lymph nodes are absent	Lymph nodes are grossly enlarged
Excisional operations are indicated	Excisional operations and other types of surgery

Table 29.4 Causes of secondary lymphoedema (Figs 29.8 to 29.10)

	Cause	Pathology
1. Infections	Filariasis Tuberculosis Chronic lymphadenitis	Recurrent lymphangiitis Lymphadenitis Lymphatic destruction
2. Surgery	Lymph node block dissections (inguinal or axillary)	Excision of lymph nodes as part of treatment
3. Lymph node obstruction	Postradiotherapy large nodes—metastasis lymphoma	Scarred and obliterated lymphatics
4. Tissue damage	Burns scarring	Loss of lymphatics
5. Venous diseases	Chronic venous insufficiency, venous ulcer	Lymphatic destruction
6. Endocrine	Pretibial myxoedema	Obliteration of initial lymphatics by mucin

2. **Congenital AV fistula** may present with unilateral gigantism of the leg. Dilated veins, continuous murmur, gigantism, and a nonhealing ulcer in the leg in a young boy give the clue to the diagnosis.
3. **Elephantiasis neuromatosa** of the leg may cause diffuse enlargement of the leg. The leg is tender on palpation with a soft to firm diffuse swelling.
4. **Extensive lipomatosis** of the leg.

The causes of lymphoedema are summarized in Key Box 29.4 and Table 29.4.

Investigations (Lymphangiography)

By and large, no investigations are done in secondary lymphoedema. In selected cases of primary lymphoedema, investigations may be done but are largely of academic interest.

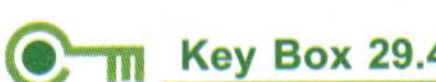 **Key Box 29.4**

Summary of Causes of Lymphoedema

- **A**plasia, hypoplasia (familial and genetic)
- **P**arasitic (filariasis)
- **L**ymph node obstruction—advanced malignancies
- **A**ltered motility—dysmotility (genetic)
- **S**urgical extirpation—block dissection
- **I**nflammatory/infection—recurrent
- **A**fter radiotherapy, after barefoot walking 'silica particles'

Remember as **APLASIA**

LYMPHANGIOGRAPHY

A dye is injected into the lymphatics and the entire draining lymphatics and lymph nodes are visualised.

Indications for Lymphangiography

1. Lymphoedema, if surgery is planned.
2. Lymphoma, to detect pelvic nodes, para-aortic nodes, etc. (but **now CT is preferable**).

Procedure

- Commonly, pedal lymphangiograms are done.
- 5–10 ml of methylene blue (patent blue) is injected into the web spaces intradermally between the toes. This delineates the lymphatics of the dorsum of the foot which are identified. Then, an oily dye such as "ultra fluid lipiodol" is injected (10–15 ml).
- It may take 12–24 hours to delineate the inguinal and para-aortic nodes.
- Isotope lymphangiography refers to injection of albumin labelled with technetium 99m colloid or ^{131}I.

Results

- Metastases appear as irregular filling defects in the lymph nodes.
- It may demonstrate hypoplasia or hyperplasia, as in primary lymphoedema.
- If there is obstruction, the dye may return back (dermal back flow).

Lymphangiographic Classification

Three types are recognised

1. **Congenital hyperplasia (10%):** This is a condition wherein lymphatics are increased in number. These *megalymphatics* are defective, resulting in chylous ascites, chylothorax, and protein-losing enteropathy. Being congenital, it manifests at birth. It is progressive, involves the whole leg, and shows a variable response to compressive therapy.
2. **Distal obliteration (80%)** (Key Box 29.5).
3. **Proximal obliteration (10%)**
   - It is less common.
   - Obstruction is at the region of the aortoiliac or inguinal nodes.
   - Whole leg/thigh is involved (Fig. 29.11).
   - No family history.
   - Rapid progression and poor response.

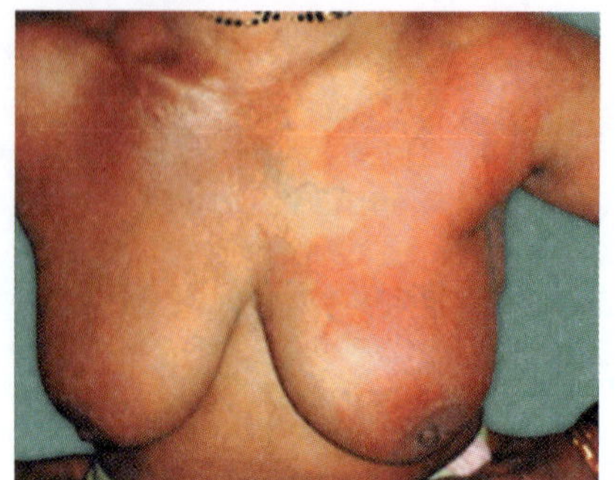

Fig. 29.8: A case of carcinoma of the breast presented with lymphangiitis

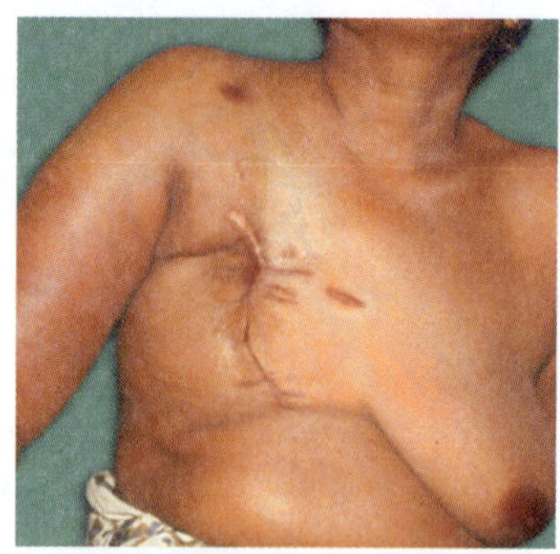

Fig. 29.9: Post-mastectomy lymphoedema of the right upper limb

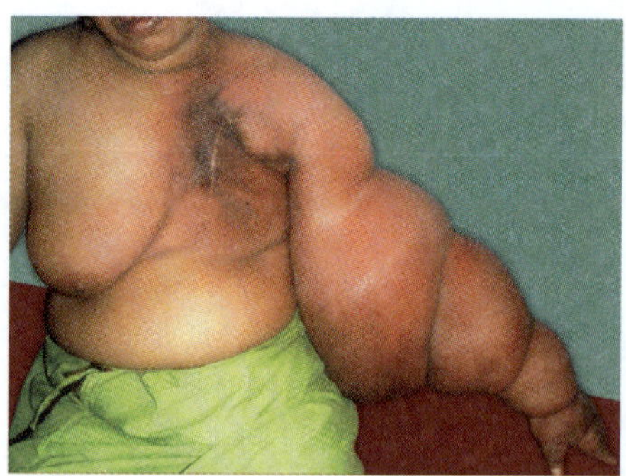

Fig. 29.10: Post-mastectomy lymphoedema—progressive since 6 years (*Courtesy:* Dr Srijayan, Professor, Department of Surgery, Calicut Medical College, Calicut)

Key Box 29.5

Distal Obliteration (80%)

Distal lymphatics are commonly affected
In and around puberty—praecox involved
Sex: Common in females
Treatment is by compression, good response
Ankle, calf region is involved
Lymphatics are decreased or absent (aplasia)
Remember as **DISTAL**

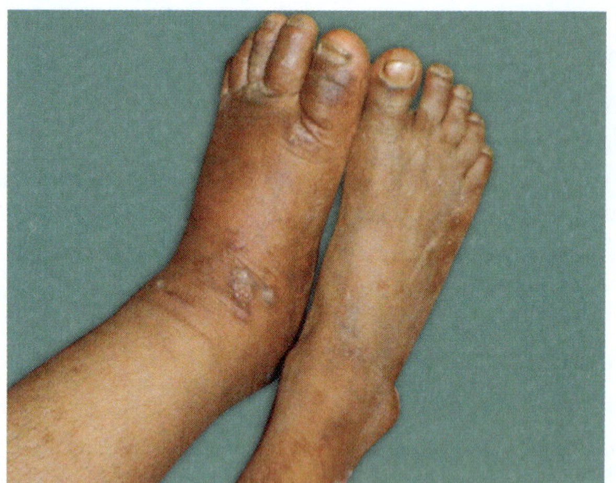

Fig. 29.11: Unilateral limb oedema due to proximal obliteration

Complications of Lymphangiography

1. Lymphangiitis and toxaemia
   - It is not routinely done nowadays because of the availability of ultrasound, CT, and other non-invasive investigations.
2. Rapid infusion should be avoided to prevent the risk of lipid pulmonary embolus.

Lymphoscintigraphy

- It has a sensitivity and specificity of 92% and 100%, respectively.
- It has replaced lymphangiography.
- Radiolabelled (technetium 99m) colloid is injected into the web space between the 2nd and 3rd toes or fingers. The limb is exercised periodically and images are taken.
- If there is an abnormal accumulation of tracer with collaterals, it is a sign of lymphoedema.
- MRI and CT are the latest investigations in addition to lymphangiography for the evaluation of gross swelling of the limb.

Treatment of Lymphoedema (Key Box 29.6)

Pearls of Wisdom

Surgery has a small role in lymphoedema

Key Box 29.6

MLLB

- Graduated pressure highest at ankle (100%) to lowest in the groin (40%) should be applied.
- It requires about 40–60 mmHg to leg and 30–40 mmHg to arm.
- MLLB should be worn at the start of the day and removed at bed time.
- However, limb should be kept elevated at night.
- The aim is to get a graduated pressure in applying. If it is applied wrongly, it may result in increase in lymphoedema.

I. CONSERVATIVE

1. **Control of swelling:** Decongestive lymphoedema therapy (DLT)
   - Bedrest, elevation
   - ***Bandaging:*** Multilayered lymphoedema bandaging (MLLB—Key Box 29.7).
   - Compression garments
   - ***Massage:*** Manual lymphatic drainage (MLD)

Key Box 29.7

Guidelines for Treatment of a Patient with Lymphoedema

- **L** } Lymphoedema bandage is multilayered
- **Y**
- **M**anual lymphatic drainage (MLD) or massage
- **P**rophylactic antifungal treatment to prevent athlete's foot
- **H**ygiene of skin and foot
- **A**dvice on diet—weight reduction
- **T**reatment of infection—early and aggressive
- **I**nstructions about exercises
- **C**ompression garments
- **S**urgery consultation as and when required.

Remember as **LYMPHATICS**

- It aims at draining fluid and protein from ISF space.
- It also stimulates lymphangion contraction.

2. **Care of skin**
   - Wash daily with warm water
   - Moisturiser or liquid paraffin should be applied for dry skin
   - Avoid injuries
   - Hyperkeratosis should be treated by a keratolytic agent such as 5% salicylic acid.
   - Avoid ointments/herbal medicines/soaps, etc., which are allergic.
   - Antifungal treatment
   - Treat infections early and effectively.
3. **Relief of pain**
   - Pain is multifactorial. It may be due to swelling, infection, involvement of nerve/bone, etc.
   - However, it is often psychosomatic and affected by mood and morale.
   - Antianxiety drugs may help.
4. **Control of infections**
   - Usually it is due to streptococci/staphylococci.
   - Oral or injectable penicillin and flucloxacillin or clindamycin are the drugs of choice.
   - Other drugs are co-amoxiclavulinic acid, cephalosporins.
5. **Exercises**
   - 40% of lymph is formed within skeletal muscle.
   - It is directly proportional to central inflow.
   - Slow systemic, isotonic movements such as swimming and massage increase venous and lymphatic return.
   - Foot-end elevation of the bed.
6. **Drugs**
   - **Oxerutins** are the drugs used for venous disease. These are not yet licensed in the UK but are used in India.
   - They reduce capillary permeability, **improve microcirculatory perfusion**, stimulate interstitial macrophage proteolysis, and reduce erythrocyte and platelet aggregation.
   - **Diuretics:** 20 mg of furosemide every day/alternate days. This helps in early cases of lymphoedema.
   - **Antifilarial treatment:** Diethylcarbamazine citrate (DEC) 100 mg 3 times/day for 21 days with every attack of lymphangiitis and once in 6 months.
   - **Warfarin** has been used to reduce lymphoedema due to filariasis. It acts by ***enhancing macrophage activity and extralymphatic absorption of interstitial fluid.***
   - **Antibiotics** are used in cases of cellulitis and lymphangiitis.

II. SURGERY

Aim: To reduce the limb size.

1. **Swiss-roll operation (Thompson's):** A skin flap containing dermis is raised and buried into the deep tissues (close to the vascular bundle). This is a dermal flap prepared by denuding epidermis (Fig. 29.12).
2. **Charles excision operation:** It is indicated in primary lymphoedema. It is performed for extensive swellings and skin changes (Fig. 29.13). Thickened and diseased skin and subcutaneous tissue are excised till the healthy underlying structures are seen, followed by split skin grafting. The skin has *dermal lymphatics which are never involved in filariasis.* Thus, the subcutaneous lymph may flow *via* dermal lymphatics.
3. **Nodovenous shunt:** Dilated, enlarged inguinal lymph node is anastomosed to a vein nearby, e.g. long saphenous vein or femoral vein (Fig. 29.14).

Thus, these are 3 types of surgery commonly done for filarial leg (Fig. 29.15). There are many other surgeries which are of historical interest. However, the results of surgery for filarial leg are disappointing. Many patients develop intractable ulcers and wetting of the limb due to loss of protein. The wound gets secondarily infected resulting in sepsis, recurrent lymphangiitis, etc. As a last resort many patients beg for amputation to get rid of the 'useless limb.' After amputation, the limb can be fitted with a prosthesis.

Lymphoedema and Chronic Venous Insufficiency (CVI)

- Superficial venous thrombophlebitis (SVT) and deep vein thrombosis (DVT) can lead to lymphatic destruction and secondary lymphoedema. Lymphoedema can also predispose to DVT.

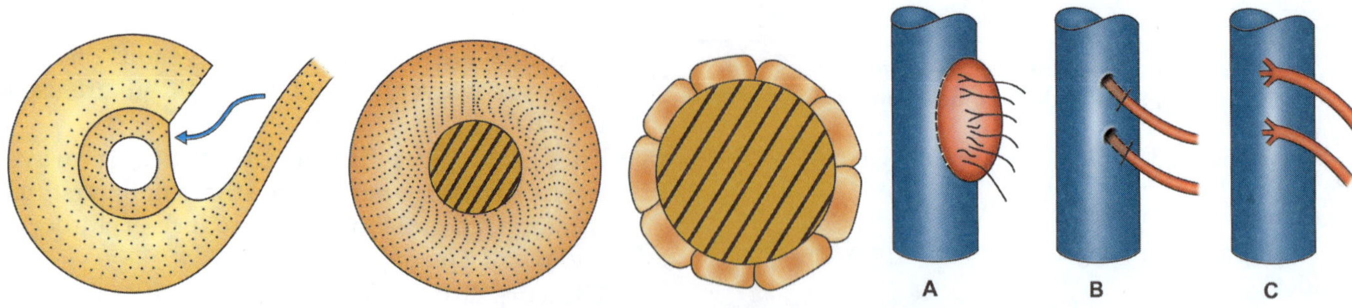

Fig. 29.12: Swiss-roll operation—skin flap is raised

Fig. 29.13: Excision and grafting

Figs 29.14A to C: (A) Node to vein, (B) Lymphatics threaded into a vein and (C) Microvascular anastomosis

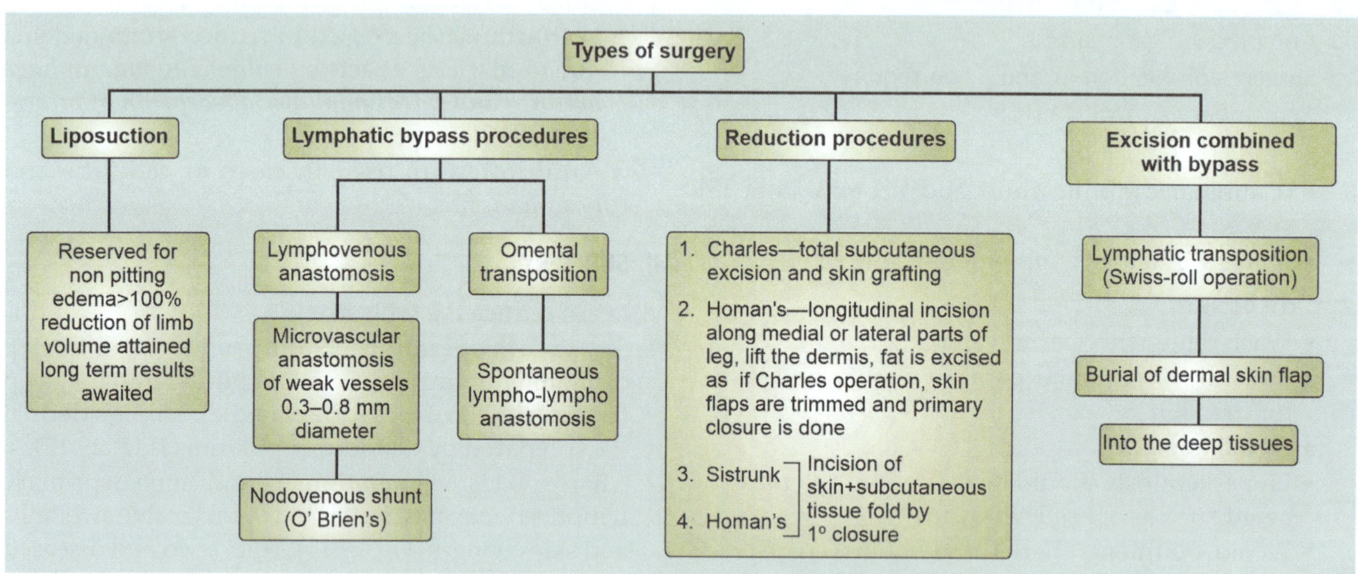

Fig. 29.15: Various surgeries for lymphoedema

- Some degree of superficial reflux may be present in lymphoedema patients that must be managed conservatively rather than by 'blunder surgery.'

HODGKIN'S LYMPHOMA (HL)

Definition

It is a malignant neoplasm of the lymphoreticular system. Thus, it can involve the lymph nodes, spleen, and liver.

Risk Factors for Hodgkin's Lymphoma

- History of ***infectious mononucleosis*** increases the risk of HL two to threefold. ***Epstein-Barr virus (EBV)*** may be a causative agent.
- Immunosuppression caused by the drugs increases the risk of HL. The incidence of HL is significantly higher in the HIV-infected population than in the general population. Patients with systemic lupus erythematosus and rheumatoid arthritis on immune suppression and immunosuppression due to organ transplantation have increased risk of Hodgkin's lymphoma.
- ***Genetic/molecular:*** At least 95% of HL represent monoclonal B cell disorders.

Pathology

- The disease usually starts in one of the lymph nodes as a painless swelling.
- Commonly, it involves the left supraclavicular region. The nodes are ***enlarged and not matted***. It spreads to other nodes in a downstream lymphatic drainage (contiguous spread).
- Cut surface of lymph nodes are smooth and homogeneous.
- **The axial lymphatic system is almost always affected.**
- **Microscopy:** 'Cellular pleomorphism'—lymphocytes, histiocytes, eosinophils, and fibrous tissue with **Reed-Sternberg cells,** giant cells containing mirror-image nuclei.

WHO Classification/REAL (1994)—Revised European American Lymphoma

I. **Lymphocyte predominance, nodular** (both Hodgkin's lymphoma and low grade B cell lymphomas)

II. **Classic Hodgkin's lymphoma (HL)**
- Lymphocyte-rich
- Nodular sclerosis—most common
- Lymphocyte depletion
- Mixed cellularity

However, classical HL and nodular lymphocyte predominant HL—LPHL are now the more practically used classification (Table 29.5).

Clinical Features

- **Age:** Bimodal distribution. First peak in the 3rd decade and second peak after 50 years.
- **Sex:** Increased incidence in males.
- It presents as a generalised lymphadenopathy (more than one group of lymph nodes are significantly enlarged non-contiguous). **Significant lymphadenopathy refers to a lymph node of 2 cm size in the groin,** 1 cm size in nodes in the neck or axilla, firm to hard in consistency, palpable left supraclavicular node of any size.
- The disease starts in the left posterior triangle as a group of lymph nodes with a 'bunch of grapes' appearances. This is seen in about 80% of cases.
- ***The nodes are firm (India rubber consistency) without matting. In advanced cases and in poorly differentiated variety, matting can occur*** (Fig. 29.16).
- By means of ***contiguous and centripetal spread,*** other lymph nodes in the neck, axillary, mediastinal, para-aortic and inguinal lymph nodes get enlarged (Fig. 29.17).
- Abdominal pain can occur due to hepatosplenomegaly. The enlarged liver and spleen are smooth and firm with round borders.
- **Para-aortic nodes** (Key Box 29.8) are felt in the umbilical region, more so on the left side. Its clinical features are:
  - Nodular, firm to hard mass, fixed mass
  - Does not move with respiration
  - Being retroperitoneal, the mass does not fall forward on knee-elbow position
  - Pulsations may be felt over the mass (transmission from aorta)
- Alcohol-induced pain in the involved lymph nodes is a rare symptom.

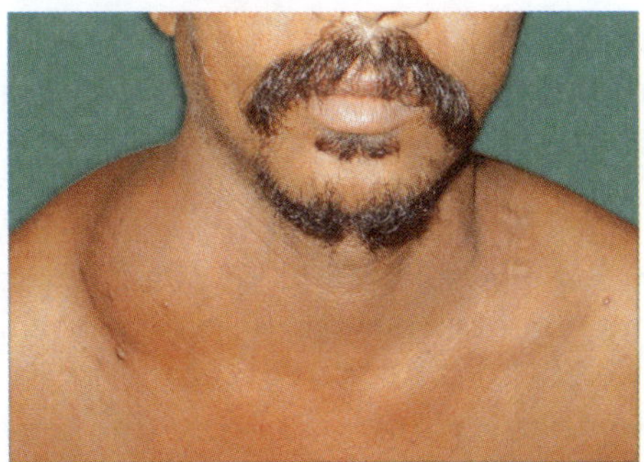

Fig. 29.16: Massive cervical lymph node enlargement. Observe the scar of the lymph node biopsy on the opposite side, reported as normal

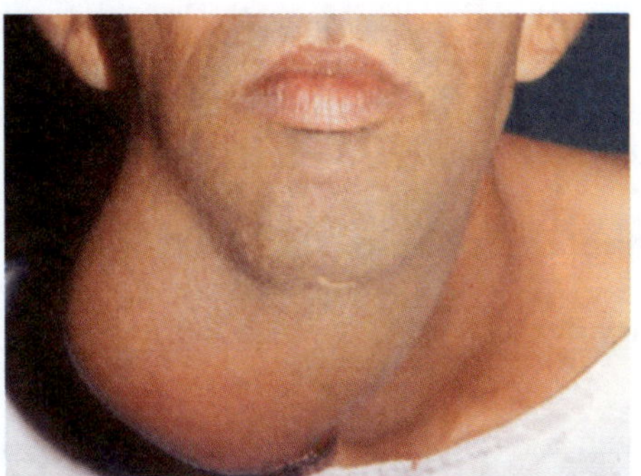

Fig. 29.17: Advanced stage of Hodgkin's lymphoma: Bilateral massive enlargement of nodes

Key Box 29.8

Para-aortic Node Enlargement Common Causes
- Lymphoma
- Testicular tumours
- Malignant melanoma
- Gastrointestinal malignancy

Table 29.5 Hodgkin's lymphoma (HL)

	Classical HL	Nodular lymphocytic predominant HL
1. Cells	Large atypical cells (Reed-Sternberg cell)	LPHL (popcorn cell—L and H cell)
2. Immunohistochemistry	Express CD15 and CD30 (20 and 45 negative)	Express CD20+, CD45+
3. Progress	Slow (No 'B' symptoms, no bulky disease)	Indolent, favourable prognosis
4. Spread	Contiguous pattern of spread	Does not have contiguous pattern of spread
5. Treatment	Extended field	Involved field RT only
6. Prognosis	Good. Depends on staging	Excellent

- There may be ascites.
- **Intermittent fever** (irregular) is sometimes seen. Skin rashes[1] are rare in Hodgkin's lymphoma. Severe pruritus without obvious skin lesions on clinical examination may suggest occult Hodgkin's lymphoma. They may not respond to topical and systemic agents and can be an early clue to the presence of clinically occult HL23.
- **Multiple bony pains** may occur due to secondary deposits, especially in the lumbar vertebrae. The secondary deposits are usually osteoblastic giving rise to ***ivory vertebrae***.
- **Superior vena caval obstruction** indicates enlarged mediastinal nodes. This is tested by asking the patient to raise the hand above the head. Engorgement of the veins indicates obstruction and the test is said to be positive **(*Pemberton's test*).**

Mediastinal Lymphoma (Key Box 29.9)

 Key Box 29.9

Mediastinal Lymphoma

- It is the most common malignancy in the mediastinum.
- Anterior compartment is most commonly involved (posterior—rare).
- Most commonly used treatment is chemotherapy/radiation.
- Most dramatic response to the chemotherapy/radiotherapy with a cure rate of 90% in early Hodgkin's and 60% in advanced stage.
- Even in patients with mediastinal bulky lymphoma, symptoms of cough, chest pain, dyspnoea or SVC obstruction is not common.
- **Mediastinal mass ratio (MMR),** defined as the ratio of maximum transverse diameter of mediastinal mass to the maximum transverse intrathoracic diameter, must be calculated. MMR greater than 0.33 by chest X-ray or 0.35 by CT predicts a worse prognosis.

Pearls of Wisdom

Generalised pruritus occurs in 25% of patients with Hodgkin's lymphoma. It may be the only presenting feature, preceding the diagnosis by months.

Staging (Table 29.6)

Table 29.6 Cotswolds revision of the Ann Arbor staging system

Stage	Description
I	Involvement of a single lymph node region or lymph node structure
II	Involvement of two or more lymph node regions on the same side of the diaphragm
III	Involvement of lymph node regions or structures on both sides of the diaphragm
IV	Involvement of extranodal sites beyond "E" sites

Annotation description

A—No B symptoms

B—Fever, weight loss >10% over 6 months, or night sweats

E—Involvement of a single extranodal site contiguous or proximal to known nodal site

X—Bulky disease as defined by >1/3 widening of mediastinum at T5–T6, or >10 cm maximum dimension of nodal mass

Investigations

1. **Complete blood count (CBC):** Peripheral smear to rule out leukaemia. Anaemia indicates widespread bone narrow metastases.
2. **Elevated creatinine and blood urea nitrogen (BUN)** indicate ureteral obstruction or direct involvement of kidneys (increased uric acid levels indicate aggressive non-Hodgkin's lymphoma).
3. **Alkaline phosphatase, calcium, and albumin levels.** First two are elevated, whereas albumin and haemoglobin levels are lowered.
4. **Uric acid levels:** Increased levels indicate tumour burden or activity. It is associated with B symptoms. Also, when the tumour responds to chemotherapy, **tumour lysis syndrome** develops, and large amount of uric acid is liberated which may result in obstructive nephropathy also.
5. **Chest X-ray** is taken to rule out mediastinal lymph nodes, mediastinal widening, and/or pleural effusion.
6. **Abdominal USG:** To look for para-aortic nodes, splenomegaly, secondaries in the liver or hepatomegaly.
   - However, CT scan of the abdomen is better.
7. **CT scan**
   - The investigation of choice for staging. CT scans of the chest, abdomen, and pelvis are mandatory. CT of the neck is optional.
   - CT to define para-aortic nodes when there is minimal enlargement (≥0.5 cm).
   - To calculate MMR (*see* mediastinal lymphoma).
   - To assess renal function and detect back pressure hydronephrosis.
8. **PET scan:** It is better investigatory modality today.

[1]Mycosis fungoides: It is not a fungal infection but is caused by non-Hodgkin's lymphoma with infiltration of the skin with malignant lymphocytes. Dermatitis and papular rashes are common which progress to tumour formation. It is a variety of cutaneous T cell lymphoma.

9. **Lymph node biopsy:** Incision biopsy is done and a neck node is usually removed. Fine needle aspiration cytology (FNAC) may give the diagnosis but a definite histological pattern cannot be made out by FNAC. A trucut biopsy may also give the diagnosis.
10. **Mediastinoscopy** (Chamberlain procedure) is done if peripheral nodes are not available.

TREATMENT OF HODGKIN'S LYMPHOMA

- Chemotherapy has made a great revolution in the treatment of lymphoma. It is given in almost all stages. Radiotherapy is given in early stage 1cases as involved field therapy protecting the surrounding structures such as abdomen.
- There are several regimens for the treatment of Hodgkin's lymphoma. Students are advised to refer medical oncology books, if necessary. However, a few commonly used regimens are given below. Please note: MOPP regimen is no longer followed because of toxicity.

Regimen 1

ABVD: Adriamycin Bleomycin Vinblastine Doxorubicin. 4 to 6 Cycles has become the standard chemotherapy regimen (details are given below). Doxorubicin 25 mg/m^2 IV, days 1 and 5, Bleomycin 10 mg/m^2 IV, days 1 and 5, Vinblastine 6 mg/m^2 IV, days 1 and 5 and Dacarbazine 375 mg/m^2 IV, days 1 and 5.

Early Complications of ABVD Regimen

- Adriamycin: Acute cardiac toxicity.
- Bleomycin: Pulmonary toxicity.
- Vinca alkaloids: Nausea, vomiting, tumour, neutropaenia, peripheral neuropathy.
- DTIC: Hair loss.

Late Complications of ABVD Regimen

- **Life-threatening cardiovascular disease:** This is due to mediastinal radiation—pericarditis, cardiomyopathy, cardiac failure.
- **Development of second cancer:** *Acute leukaemia:* Incidence is less now as MOPP regimen is rarely used. Lung cancer, breast cancer, melanoma, soft tissue sarcoma, thyroid cancer—may develop after 30 years.
- **Hypothyroidism and hyperthyroidism (Graves' disease).**

Regimen 2

AAVD: Bleomycin is replaced by brentuximab vedotin. AAVD is given every 2 weeks for 6 months. Brentuximab vedotin is an antibody-drug conjugate. Ideally patients who have CD 30 positive respond well to this drug as it delivers chemotherapy only to these cells.

Regimen 3

BEACOPP: Bleomycin, etoposide, doxorubicin, cyclophosphamide, vincristine, procarbazine and prednisone.

STAGEWISE TREATMENT OF HODGKIN'S LYMPHOMA

Stage 1 and stage 2

- Chemotherapy followed by involved site radiotherapy if the disease is favourable. It means the disease is not bulky, disease is in less than 3 different lymph node sites on one side of diaphragm without any B symptoms and ESR is not elevated.
- Otherwise, if these criteria mentioned above are present, treatment remains the same with or without addition of immunotherapy using brentuximab vedotin or nivolumab, etc.
- Consider bone marrow transplant also.

Pearls of Wisdom

Extended mantle field radiotherapy may cause carcinoma of the breast. Pelvic radiotherapy (inverted Y) may cause infertility. Hence, they are not commonly used now.

Stage 3 and stage 4

The treatment remains the same except radiotherapy. Different varieties of chemotherapy are given not only ABVD but other regimens such as **BEACOPP, immunotherapy and stem cell transplant.**

Complications of Disease (Natural History)

1. **Mediastinal disease**—pleural effusion, superior vena caval obstruction
2. HL decreases cell-mediated immunity. It causes depressed CD4+/CD8+ ratio. These patients are vulnerable for **opportunistic infections**—mycobacteria, herpes zoster, cytomegalovirus (Key Box 29.10).

Key Box 29.10

Advanced HL—Independent Prognostic Factors

- **A**lbumin less than 4 g/dl
- **L**ymphocytopaenia <600/mm^3
- **B**lood Hb less than 10.5 g/dl
- **U**nder 44 years of age
- **M**ale sex
- **I**nvolvement of liver, bone (advanced)
- **N**eutrophils (WBC) >15,000 cells/mm^3, leukocytosis

Remember as **ALBUMIN**

What is no Longer followed in Hodgkin's Lymphoma?

1. **Staging laparotomy:** With the availability of CT, ultrasound, and lymphoscintigraphy, all details of intra-abdominal visceral involvement or pathology can be detected.

2. **Splenectomy:** Spleen is required for immunological functions.
3. **Gallium scan:** Detection of lymph nodes is done by scintigraphy, if required.
4. **Bipedal lymphangiogram:** Same reasons as mentioned above.
5. **Intravenous pyelography:** Renal function can be easily assessed by CT scan.
6. **MOPP regimen:** Not favoured—because of toxicity
7. **Pelvic RT (responsible for infertility):** Not favoured.
8. **Classification:** Ryle's classification is no longer used.

NON-HODGKIN'S LYMPHOMA (NHL)

Aetiology

1. **Age and sex**
   - Small lymphocytic lymphoma: Elderly patients
   - Lymphoblastic lymphoma: Male adolescents and young adults
   - Follicular lymphoma: Middle-aged adults
   - Burkitt's lymphoma: Children, young adults
2. **Viruses**
   - RNA viruses: Human immunodeficiency virus (HIV) produces AIDS. These patients may develop high grade B cell lymphoma.
   - DNA viruses: Epstein-Barr viruses (EBV) may produce Burkitt's lymphoma.
3. **Bacteria:** *H. pylori:* Gastric extranodal marginal zone B cell lymphomas of MALT type.
4. **Immunodeficiency states and immune disorders:** AIDS and organ transplantation treated with immunosuppression. Sjögren's syndrome, rheumatoid arthritis, systemic lupus erythematosus.
5. **Genetic syndromes:** Down syndrome and Klinefelter's syndrome.
6. Inflammatory bowel disease in particular Crohn's disease and its treatment.
7. **Radiation exposure,** to atomic bombs and nuclear reactor accidents are at an increased risk of developing NHL after 10–20 years.

Classification of Non-Hodgkin's Lymphoma

I. **Low grade**
   - Small lymphocytic
   - Follicular, predominantly small cleaved cell

II. **Intermediate grade**
   - Follicular, predominantly large cell
   - Diffuse, small cleaved cell
   - Diffuse mixed small and large cell
   - Diffuse large cell

III. **High grade**
   - Large cell immunoblastic
   - Lymphoblastic
   - Burkitt's or non-Burkitt's lymphoma

Pathological Classification

I. **B cell NHL:** Small lymphocytic lymphoma, follicular lymphoma, Burkitt's lymphoma (Key Box 29.11).

II. **T cell NHL:** Cutaneous T cell lymphoma, mycosis fungoides and Sézary syndrome, lymphoblastic lymphoma.

Key Box 29.11

Follicular Lymphomas (FL) or Small Lymphocytic Lymphoma (SLL)

- Called indolent lymphomas
- Can be of many years' duration
- Present as painless lymphadenopathy
- Spontaneous regression in 20% of patients
- Also called waxing and waning adenopathy
- 'B' symptoms are unusual
- Uncommon before the age of 50
- Good prognosis
- Remission duration and survival improvement with **'rituximab'** (anti-CD20 antibody specific for B lymphocytes)

Clinical Features

- **Outer horizontal group of lymph nodes are commonly enlarged.** Refer to Table 29.7.

Investigations

- Complete blood count
- Liver function tests including LDH: Increase LDH represents tumour burden
- Creatinine, calcium
- Ultrasound, CT scan
- Core needle biopsy, lymph node biopsy, bone marrow biopsy
- ***Immunohistochemistry*** is required for subclassification. *Examples:* Small lymphatic lymphoma (CD5+, CD23+), Mantle cell (CD5+, CD23–), etc.

Pearls of Wisdom

If Waldeyer's ring is involved, an upper GI scopy should be considered since the incidence of gastric involvement in such cases is increased.

Table 29.7 Comparison of Hodgkin's and non-Hodgkin's lymphomas

	Hodgkin's lymphoma	Non-Hodgkin's lymphoma
Age	Bimodal age	More than 50 years
Involvement of lymph nodes	Left supraclavicular, axillary, inguinal	External Waldeyer's ring, submental, submandibular, preauricular, postauricular, occipital nodes
Retroperitoneal nodes	Uncommon	Common
Tonsil enlargement	Not enlarged	Tonsils may be enlarged
Epitrochlear node	Not enlarged	Can be enlarged
Hepatomegaly	Uncommon	Common in low grade
Involvement of bone	Uncommon (10%)	In 40% of cases, iliac crest is involved by the time of diagnosis
Alcohol-induced pain	Characteristic	Absent
Fluctuating fever	Present	Absent
Prognosis	Better prognosis	Poor prognosis
Common presentation	Lymphatic organ	Extralymphatic
Mediastinal nodes	Common	Very few patients with DLC (diffuse large B cell lymphoma)

DIFFERENT SITES OF LYMPH NODES IN NHL (Figs 29.18 to 29.23)

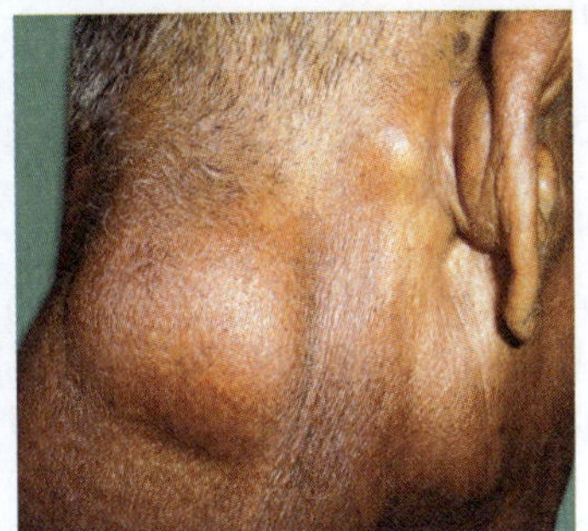

Fig. 29.18: Large occipital lymph node

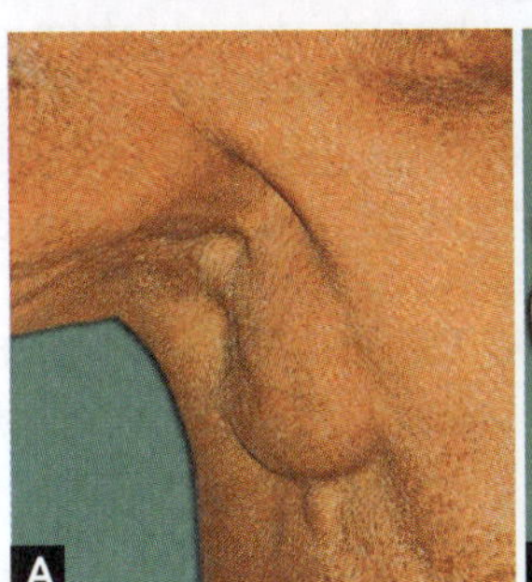

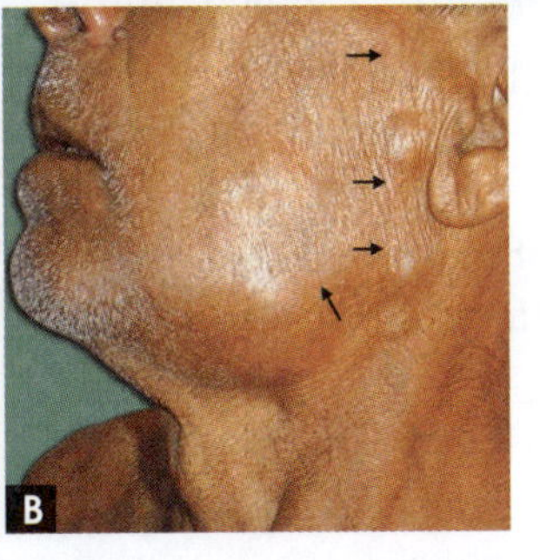

Figs 29.19A and B: Massive axillary lymphadenopathy and enlargement of submandibular, upper deep cervical and preauricular lymph nodes

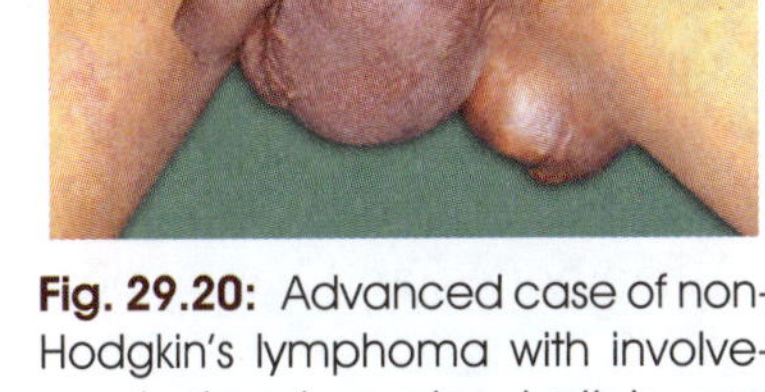

Fig. 29.20: Advanced case of non-Hodgkin's lymphoma with involvement of groin nodes, testicle and skin deposits in the thigh

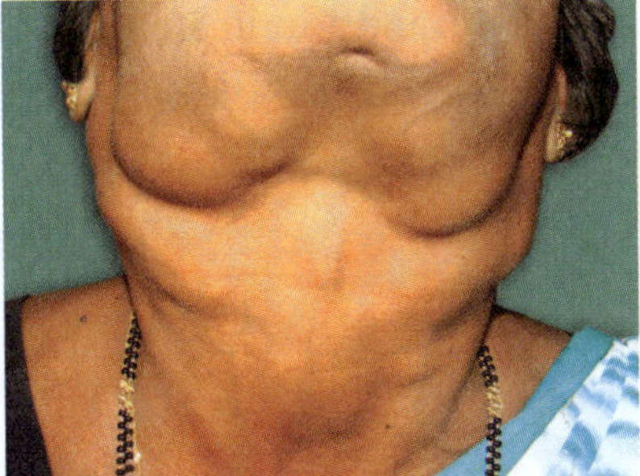

Fig. 29.21: Bilateral lymph nodes in the upper neck

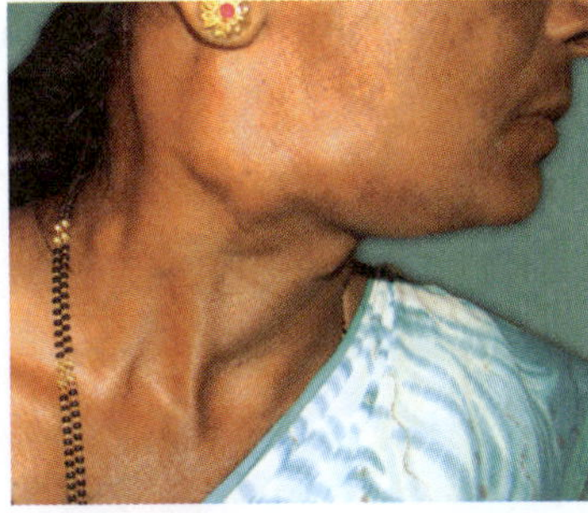

Fig. 29.22: Preauricular, post-auricular and facial lymph nodes

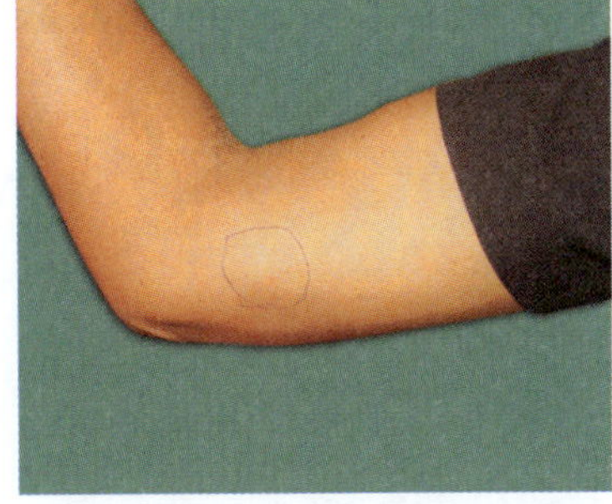

Fig. 29.23: Epitrochlear lymph node enlargement

Management of Non-Hodgkin's Lymphoma

Depends on the Grade of the tumour, Stage of the disease.

- Stages I and II: Low grade—radiotherapy/chemotherapy with CHOP—Cyclophosphamide, Doxorubcin, Oncovin and Prednisone in cases of indolent or low-grade lymphoma. If relapses another regimen is added.
- Stages I and II: Intermediate and high grade—CHOP-chemotherapy.
- Stages III and IV and high-grade Rituximab is added. R-CHOP.
- Those who relapse can be treated with Rituximab monotherapy.

Aggressive large B cell lymphomas with CD20 positive cases are treated with R-CHOP.

Gastric MALT lymphomas may completely regress with therapy against *H. pylori* with appropriate antibiotics and proton pump inhibitors.

Anaplastic large cell lymphoma (ALCL): It is treated with **immunotoxins:** They act as homing devices to deliver the toxins directly to the cancer cells. An example of this is brentuximab vedotin, which contains an antibody to CD30 attached to a cell poison. This has been shown to help treat patients who are unresponsive to chemotherapy

MISCELLANEOUS

BURKITT'S LYMPHOMA (SMALL NONCLEAVED LYMPHOMA)

- It is a type of high grade non-Hodgkin's lymphoma, first described by Burkitt, affecting the jaw bone (maxilla, mandible).
- It is rare everywhere except in a few places where malarial infestation is heavy.
- It is caused by ***Epstein-Barr virus*** (EBV), which multiplies in the presence of heavy malarial infestation.

Types

- **Endemic:** Parts of Africa and other tropical locations. It is associated with EBV. It affects the jaw and orbit and has a good prognosis.
- **Sporadic:** Throughout the world. It is not associated with EBV. It affects the abdomen and GI tract, rather than bones, and has a poor prognosis.

Diagnosis

- Biopsy will reveal typical 'starry sky' appearance with primitive lymphoid cells and large clear histiocytes.

Treatment

- Endemic cases respond well to cyclophosphamide.
- Sporadic cases need to be treated with combination chemotherapy.

SÉZARY'S SYNDROME

It is also a type of cutaneous T cell lymphomas. Here, skin involvement is manifested clinically as a generalised exfoliative erythroderma along with an associated leukaemia of Sézary cells.

These cells are characterised by a cerebriform nucleus. They are indolent tumours so patients have a good survival time.

CHYLURIA

- It is the most common manifestation of ruptured lymph vessels due to filariasis (others being chylocoele, chylous ascites, and chylothrax).
- It occurs when intestinal lymphatics are obstructed by filarial fibrosis and the lymphatics are diverted to renal lymphatics.
- The dilated and tortuous lymphatics, due to high pressure, rupture into the renal pelvis and ureter, leading to chyluria. Passage of a large amount of chyle leads to a loss of protein and fat, resulting in malnutrition. Such patients are also debilitated with loss of immunity.
- Oral ingestion of fat labelled with Sudan red III turns the urine pink in these cases.
- It is treated by diethylcarbamazine, bed rest, foot-end elevation of the bed, and administration of a high protein diet.

Multiple Choice Questions

1. Which of the following is false regarding functions of the lymphatic system?
A. Lymph circulation occurs through lymphatico-venous junctions
B. Lymphatic fluid contains macromolecules
C. The right lymphatic duct drains into the internal jugular vein
D. The lymphatic fluid from the intestines pass through the liver

2. The following are true for lymph trunks *except*:
A. They are lined by a single layer of endothelial cells
B. Pulsations of the vessels help in lymph circulation
C. The thoracic duct drains into the right internal jugular vein
D. They do not accompany neurovascular bundles in the central nervous system

3. The following are risk factors for lower limb lymphoedema *except*:
A. Inguinal block dissection
B. Pelvic radiotherapy
C. Obesity
D. Alcohol abuse

4. Stemmer's sign refers to:
A. Gross thickening of the subcutaneous tissue in a lymphoedematous leg
B. Deep muscle of the leg is not involved
C. Skin on the dorsum of the toes cannot be pinched
D. Buffalo hump on the dorsum of the foot

5. The following are true for filarial elephantiasis of the leg *except*:
A. It is caused by *Wuchereria bancrofti*
B. It is transmitted by *Culex fatigans*
C. Microfilariae do not produce any lesion
D. Significant changes occur deep to the deep fascia

6. The majority of primary lymphoedema is due to:
A. Congenital hyperplasia of lymphatics
B. Distal obliteration of lymphatics
C. Proximal obliteration of lymphatics
D. Central obliteration of lymphatics

7. Oxerutins used in lymphoedema act by the following mechanisms *except*:
A. Decrease capillary permeability
B. Improve microcirculatory perfusion
C. Stimulate interstitial macrophage proteolysis
D. Increase platelet aggregation

8. Which of the following is true regarding lymphoedema?
A. Dermal lymphatics are never involved in filariasis
B. Oxerutins are not used in lymphoedema
C. Lymphoedema pressure bandage requires 0 mmHg pressure in the leg
D. Lymphoedema does not predispose to malignancies

9. Contiguous and centripetal spread occur in:
A. Hodgkin's lymphoma
B. Non-Hodgkin's lymphoma
C. Burkitt's lymphoma
D. Sézary's syndrome

10. The following are true for lymphocytic predominance nodular lymphoma *except*:
A. It has large atypical cells
B. It expresses CD20+
C. It is indolent
D. It has a favourable prognosis

11. The following are true about classical Hodgkin's lymphoma *except*:
A. Spread is contiguous
B. Large atypical cells are seen
C. B symptoms are characteristic
D. CD15 and CD30 are expressed

12. The following are the features of a Reed-Sternberg cell *except*:
A. It is a giant cell
B. It contains mirror-image nuclei
C. It is a large multinucleated cell
D. It is not derived from B lymphocytes

13. The following are true for mediastinal lymphoma *except*:
A. It is the most common malignancy in the mediastinum
B. Its response to chemotherapy is dramatic
C. It is Hodgkin's lymphoma
D. The posterior compartment is commonly involved

14. The following are no longer followed in lymphomas *except*:

A. Pelvic radiotherapy
B. Splenectomy as a staging procedure
C. Rye's classification
D. ABVD regimen is commonly given

15. The following are causes of epitrochlear node enlargement *except*:

A. Hodgkin's lymphoma
B. Non-Hodgkin's lymphoma
C. Secondary syphilis
D. Cat-scratch fever

16. The following are true for Rituximab *except*:

A. It is a monoclonal antibody against protein CD20
B. It is used to treat leukaemia
C. It can also be used to treat follicular lymphomas
D. It has no role in transplant rejections

17. The following are true for Burkitt's lymphoma *except*:

A. It is associated with Epstein-Barr virus
B. It is not associated with heavy malarial infestation
C. It affects the jaw and orbital bones
D. It gives a starry sky appearance on histopathology

Answers

1. D	**2.** C	**3.** D	**4.** C	**5.** D	**6.** B	**7.** D	**8.** A	**9.** A	**10.** A
11. C	**12.** D	**13.** D	**14.** D	**15.** A	**16.** D	**17.** B			

CHAPTER

30

Varicose Veins and Deep Vein Thrombosis

INTRODUCTION

Varicosity is the penalty for verticality against gravity. This is the common statement made in lecture classes. The blood has to flow from the lower limbs into the heart against gravity because of the upright posture of human beings. In many cases, varicose veins are asymptomatic. Raised intra-abdominal pressure may also precipitate varicose veins, which is more common in females due to repeated pregnancy. The complications of varicose veins lead to hospitalisation.

Examples of varicosity: Long saphenous varicosity, short saphenous varicosity, oesophageal varices, fundal varices, haemorrhoids, etc. In this chapter, varicosity of the leg is discussed.

DEFINITION

Dilated, tortuous, and elongated superficial veins of the limb due to reflux are called varicose veins. They are about 3 mm in diameter.

PRIMARY VARICOSE VEINS

- Primary varicose veins occur as a result of ***congenital weakness*** in the vein wall due to defective connective tissue and smooth muscle.
- They may also result from muscular weakness or ***congenital absence of valves.***
- Factors that predispose to varicose veins are given in Key Box 30.1.
- Very often, the valve at the saphenofemoral (SF) junction is incompetent/absent. The valves may also be absent at the junction of superficial veins joining the deep veins.
- **Klippel-Trénaunay syndrome** is a congenital venous abnormality wherein superficial and deep veins do not have any valves. It is also called **valveless syndrome** (Key Box 30.2). It is not a hereditary condition.
- Primary varicosity may also be **genetic**. Some patients inherit abnormalities in the FOXC2 gene. These factors, in addition to prolonged standing (agriculturists, traffic police, hotel workers), contribute to the development of varicose veins.

Key Box 30.1

Factors which Predispose to Varicose Veins

- **Height:** Tall individuals suffer more
- **Weight:** Obesity may weaken vein wall
- **Occupation:** Hotel workers, policemen, shopkeepers, tailors
- **Side:** Left is affected more than the right
- **Age and sex:** Not very clear

Key Box 30.2

Klippel-Trénaunay Syndrome

- Incidence 1 in 1,00,000 population.
- Also called angio-osteohypertrophy syndrome
- Characterised by nevus flammeus (port-wine stain), venous malformations, lymphatic malformations and soft tissue hypertrophy of the affected limb.
- Can also have large arteriovenous malformations.
- Patients can complain of pain heaviness in the limbs, difficulty in walking due to abnormal length of the limb.
- Excision of veins, sclerotherapy, laser treatment for port-wine stain are a few methods to treat the veins.

SECONDARY VARICOSE VEINS

- Women are more prone to varicose veins because of the following reasons:
  - **Pregnancy and pelvic tumours** cause proximal obstruction to the blood flow.
  - **Pills** (oral contraceptive pills) alter the viscosity of blood.
  - **Progesterones dilate the vessel wall.**
- **Congenital arteriovenous (AV) fistula** increases blood flow and increases venous pressure.
- Deep vein thrombosis may occur postoperatively, as a result of road traffic accidents, etc. These may lead to the **destruction of valves,** resulting in varicose veins.

Competency

SU27.5: Describe the applied anatomy of venous system of lower limb.

SURGICAL ANATOMY OF THE VENOUS SYSTEM OF LEG

It may be discussed under the following headings:

1. Superficial venous system—long and short saphenous veins and their tributaries
2. Perforators
3. Deep venous system

SUPERFICIAL VENOUS SYSTEM

Anatomy of the Long Saphenous Vein (LSV)

LSV starts in the foot from the tributaries of the dorsal venous arch which runs in front of metatarsal heads in the subcutaneous tissue in the dorsal aspect of foot. It ascends in front of the medial malleolus, and runs along the medial side of the leg. It then ascends in the thigh and ends at the saphenofemoral (SF) junction by joining the femoral vein, which is 1.5 inches (4 cm) below and lateral to the pubic tubercle. SF junction can be variable, more superiorly located sometimes. Today the junction is marked before surgery during venous ultrasound which helps in placing the incision accordingly. It has 15–20 valves. Absence of valves results in varicose veins (Key Box 30.3 and Fig. 30.1).

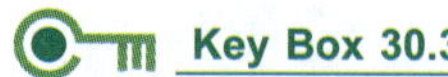

Key Box 30.3

Superficial System—Salient Features

- As the name suggests, they are in the **superficial fascia** and are often visible (saphenous means easily seen).
- **They are low pressure and poorly supported system.**
- They are provided with **numerous valves.**
- The middle coat of these veins consists mostly of **smooth muscle.**
- The **middle coat** is also thicker than that of other veins.
- Normal blood flow is from **superficial to deep system** of veins.

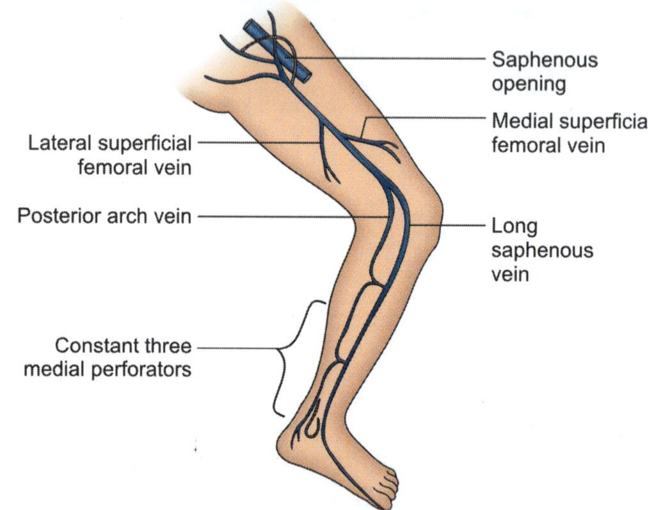

Fig. 30.1: Long saphenous vein, tributaries, communicating veins

Tributaries: These tributaries connect the long saphenous with the short saphenous vein (SSV). They are also known as communicators. They are as follows.

Tributaries Near its Termination

1. Superficial circumflex iliac vein
2. Superficial epigastric vein
3. Superficial external pudendal vein

Tributaries in the Lower Thigh

1. Lateral superficial femoral vein
2. Medial superficial femoral vein
3. Transverse suprapatellar vein
4. Transverse infrapatellar vein

Tributaries in the Leg

1. Anterior vein of the leg—also called anterior (accessory) saphenous vein (ASV).

2. Posterior arch vein—lies parallel to and behind the main trunk of long saphenous vein. It anastomoses with small venous arches connecting the medial perforating veins.

PERFORATORS (Fig. 30.2)

These are the veins which connect long saphenous vein with the deep system of veins. Since they perforate the deep fascia, they are called perforators. There are 5 constant perforators in the lower limb on the medial side.

- **Leg perforators:** They are 3 in number. The lowest perforator is below and behind the medial malleolus, the middle perforator is 10 cm above the tip of the medial malleolus, and the upper perforator is 15 cm above the medial malleolus.
- **Knee perforator:** It is just below the knee.
- **Thigh perforator:** It is a palm-breadth above the knee.

A knowledge of perforators forms the basis of the **multiple tourniquet test**. Most of the perforators contain valves. Weakness of or damage to these valves results in varicosity.

DEEP VENOUS SYSTEM

This comprises the femoral and the popliteal veins, veins or 3 pairs of venae comitantes accompanying the anterior tibial, posterior tibial, and peroneal arteries, and the valveless veins draining the calf muscles (soleal venous sinus).

- **Formation of popliteal vein:** It is formed by these 6 venae comitantes which unite and form popliteal vein in the popliteal fossa. Short saphenous vein (SSV) as the name implies is short and ascends behind the lateral malleolus joins popliteal vein at sapheno-popliteal junction (SP junction). Termination point can be variable often it is inferior. Near the termination it pierces popliteal fascia. Popliteal vein also receives **Giacomini vein** and **gastrocnemius** veins.
- **Formation of femoral vein:** Popliteal vein continues upwards in the sub-sartorial canal as femoral vein and receives long saphenous vein at SF junction. All tributaries mentioned above would have joined the vein and before it pierces it not only receives named 3 tributaries but also receives deep profunda vein. Femoral vein continues as external iliac vein above the inguinal ligament.
- **Soleal plexus of veins:** These are called deep veins of the calf region or also called calf muscle pump. Blind ended soleal sinusoids join them and help in pumping the blood. These veins are also called capacitance vessels. This is because they have the capacity to accumulate large volume (60%) of blood inside. Using this principle, simple elevation of both legs is done in hypovolaemic shock patients as initial step to resuscitate.

Salient Features of the Deep Venous System

- It is a high pressure system, well-supported by powerful muscles.
- They are connected to the superficial veins through perforators.
- The powerful calf muscle contraction returns blood to the heart.
- The deep veins also contain valves (Fig. 30.3).

Venous pathophysiology: Pressure at the capillary side of venule is very low, around 10 to 12 mmHg. Pressure

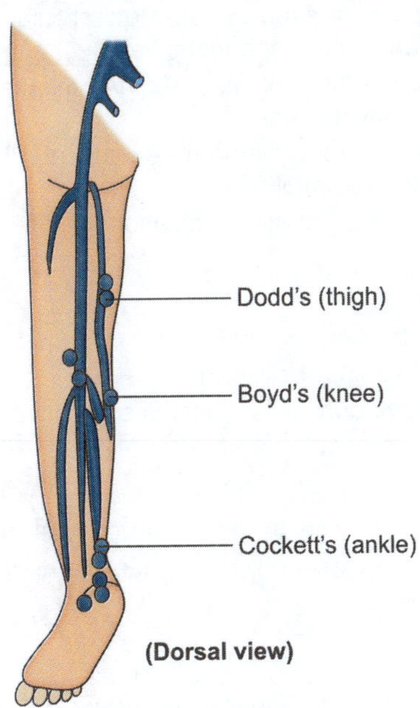

Fig. 30.2: Perforators

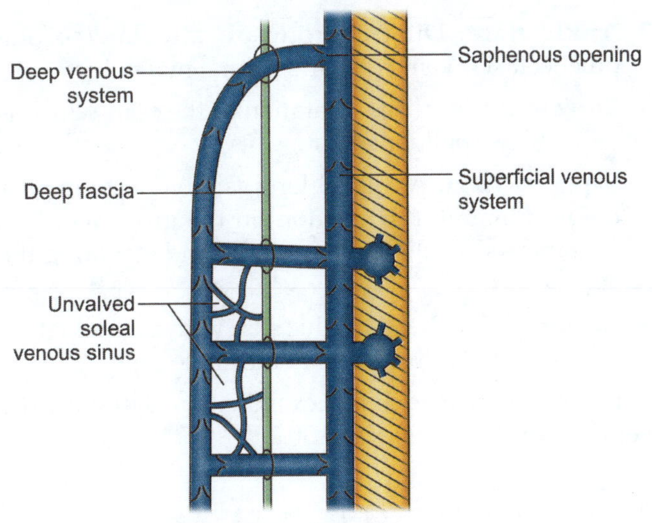

Fig. 30.3: Deep venous system

becomes less and less as the vein is traced upwards. For example: In inferior vena cava it is about 5 mmHg. Blood is returned to the heart from the lower limbs through the following mechanisms:

- **Calf muscle pump:** In standing position blood pressure at the venule is about 100 mmHg. It refers to the alternate contraction and relaxation of the muscles of the leg (the major factor). The pressure within the calf compartment rises to 200–300 mmHg during walking.
- Negative intrathoracic pressure during inspiration resulting in increase in intrathoracic volume.
- **Competent valves** (unidirectional) in the leg (Key Box 30.4): When these valves are absent or weak, perforator incompetence develops, which results in varicose veins.
- ***Vis-a-tergo* of the circulation:** The pressure transmitted from the arterial tree passes the capillary bed to the venous side, which helps return blood to the heart at rest.
- Venae comitantes.

Key Box 30.4

Distribution of Valves

- Inferior vena cava : No valve
- Common iliac vein : No valve
- Long saphenous vein : 10–14 valves
- Short saphenous vein : 1 valve

A Few Terminologies for Dilated Veins

1. **Telangiectasia:** Confluence of dilated intradermal venules of <1 mm diameter.
2. **Reticular veins:** Dilated subdermal veins of 1–3 mm diameter.
3. **Ankle flare:** Dilated group of reticular (corona phlebectasia) veins near the medial malleolus.
4. **Blowout:** A localised dilatation of the vein which is 'dome' like/ballooned out.
5. **Saphena varix:** A dilated long saphenous vein near the termination (SF junction) in the groin which is soft and reducible on lying down and elevating the leg.
6. **Atrophic blanche:** Atrophic skin with pigmentation and reticular veins—seen in the ankle region.

Before we start the clinical examination of the varicose veins study Tables 30.1 and 30.2.

Table 30.1 Classification[1] of chronic lower extremity venous disease

Classification	Definition
C	Clinical signs (grades 0–6): A for asymptomatic or S for symptomatic
E	Etiologic classification (congenital, primary or secondary)
A	Anatomic distribution (superficial, deep or perforator, alone or in combination)
P	Pathophysiologic dysfunction (reflux or obstruction, alone or in combination)

Table 30.2 Clinical (C) (Figs 30.4 to 30.10)

Grade	Characteristics
C0	No visible or palpable signs of venous disease
C1	Telangiectases, reticular veins
C2	Varicose veins
C2r	Recurrent varicose veins
C3	Oedema without skin changes
C4	Skin and subcutaneous changes
C4a	Pigmentation, eczema
C4b	Lipodermatosclerosis or atrophic blanche
C4c	Corona phlebectasia
C5	Healed ulceration
C6	Active ulceration
C6r	Recurrent active ulceration
Etiological classification (E)	
Ep:	Primary
Es:	Secondary: Esi Secondary intravenous, Ese Secondary extravenous
Ec:	Congenital
En:	No cause identified
Anatomical	
As	Superficial: example: As- **Ret:** reticular veins, As-SSV means short saphenous vein.
Ad	Deep veins—example Ad IVC means inferior vena cava Involvement.
Ap	Perforator involvement—example: TPV means thigh perforator involvement.
An	No venous anatomic location identified.
Pathological	
Pr	Reflux
Po	Obstruction
Pr,o	Reflux and obstruction
Pn	No pathophysiology identified

Competency

SU27.6: Describe the pathophysiology, clinical features, investigations and principles of management of DVT and varicose veins.

[1]The 2020 revision of CEAP: Summary of clinical (C) classifications. Ref: Lurie et al, Journal of Vascular Surgery: Venous and Lymphatic Disorders, 2020.

CLINICAL EXAMINATION OF A CASE OF LEG VARICOSITY

Symptoms

- The patient often complains of swelling of the legs. It is due to an increased volume of fluid in skin and subcutaneous tissues, increased interstitial fluid, impaired lymphatic drainage, and increased hydrostatic pressure. Most patients present with dilated veins in the leg. They are minimal at the start of the day and are sufficiently large by the end of the day due to venous engorgement.
- **Dragging pain** in the leg or a dull ache due to heaviness. Night cramps occur due to change in the diameter of veins. Aching pain is relieved at night by taking rest or elevating the limbs. Night cramps also occur due to the prevention of nutrients and oxygen from reaching the muscles due to pooling of deoxygenated blood, which results in lactic acid accumulation. Night cramps are more common in women.
- Sudden pain in the calf region with fever and oedema of the ankle region suggests deep vein thrombosis (DVT). Some patients with DVT may be asymptomatic.
- Patients may present with ulceration, eczema, dermatitis, and bleeding.
- Symptoms of pruritus/itching and skin thickening.

Pearls of Wisdom

Interestingly, pain due to varicose veins is relieved with exercise in contrast to pain due to arterial diseases, which worsen with exercise.

Signs

Inspection (should be done in standing position)

- **Dilated veins** are present in the medial aspect of leg and the knee. Sometimes they are visible in the thigh (Figs 30.4 to 30.10).
- A single dilated varix at the SF junction is called saphena varix. It is due to **saccular dilatation** of the upper end of the long saphenous vein at the saphenous opening (Tables 30.1 and 30.2).
- Veins are **tortuous and dilated**.
- A localised, dilated segment of the vein, if present, is an indication of a **blowout**. It signifies an underlying perforator (Fig. 30.11).

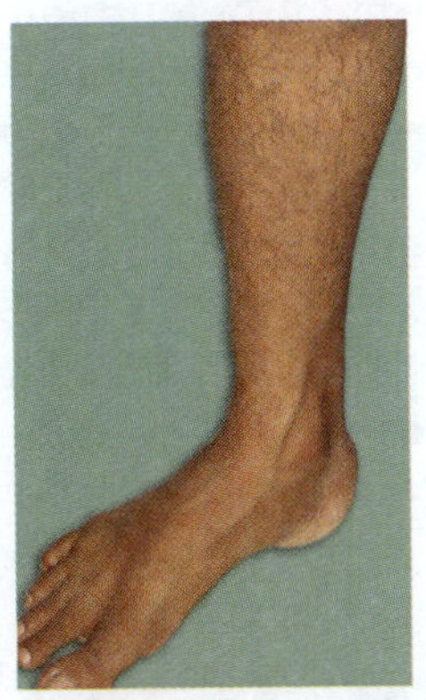

Fig. 30.4: Grade 0

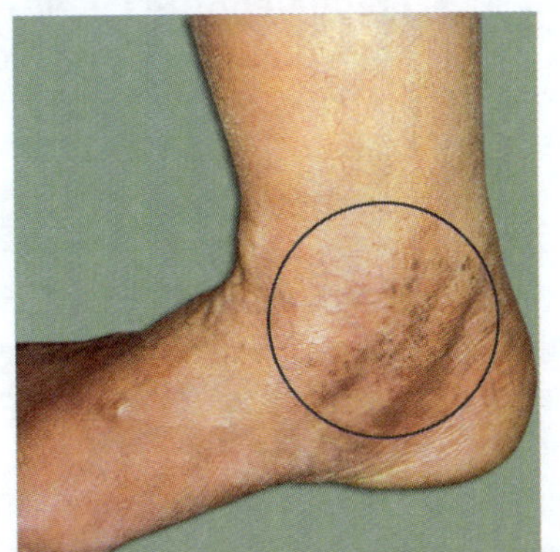

Fig. 30.5: Grade 1

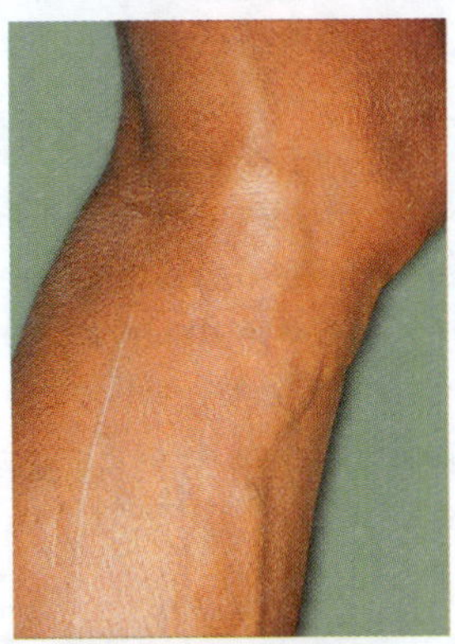

Fig. 30.6: Grade 2

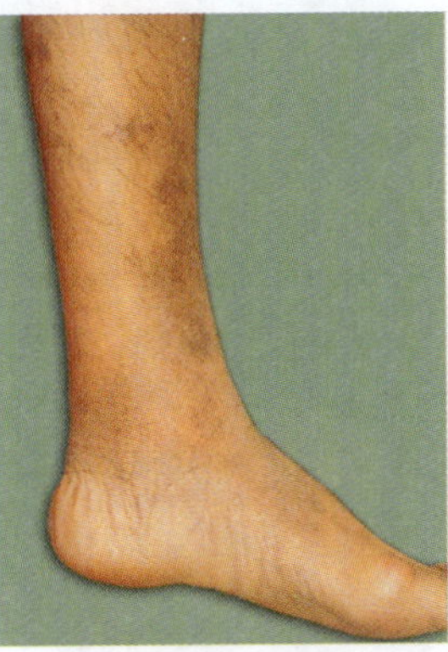

Fig. 30.7: Grade 3

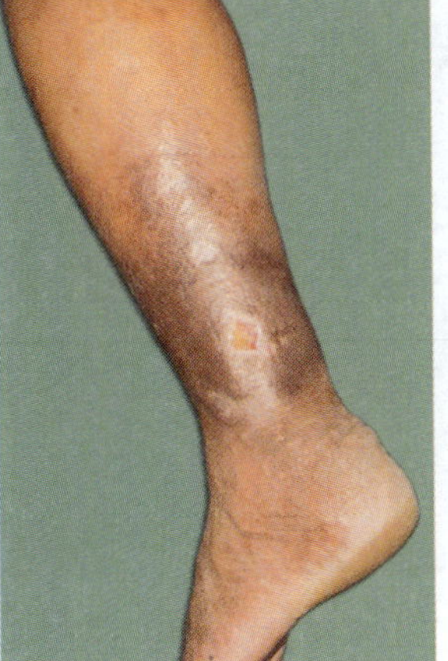

Fig. 30.8: Grade 4

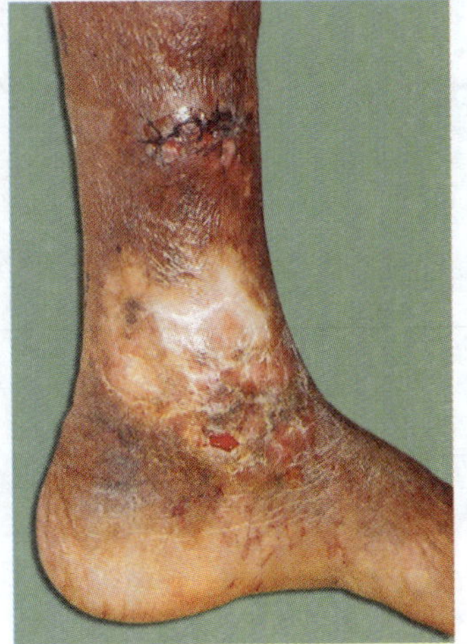

Fig. 30.9: Grade 5

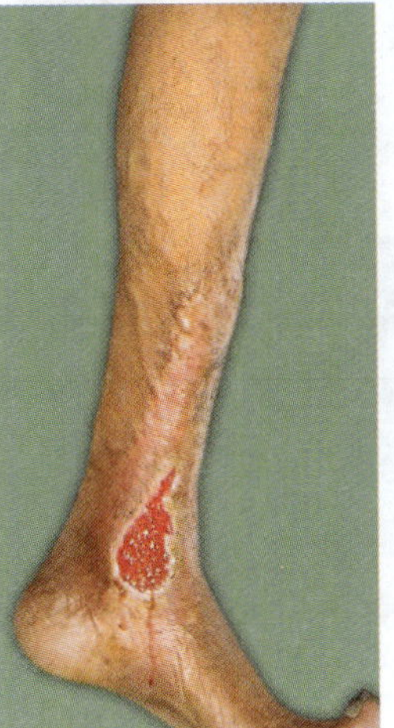

Fig. 30.10: Grade 6

See Table 30.2 for description of various grades of chronic lower extremity venous disease

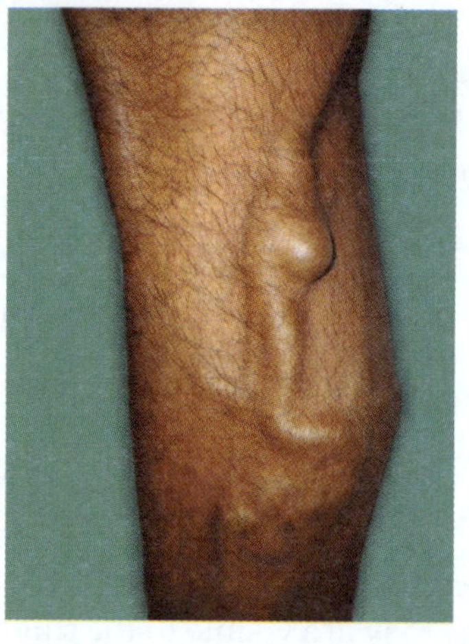

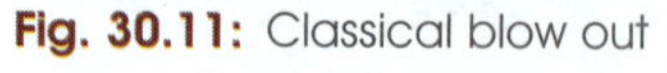

Fig. 30.11: Classical blow out

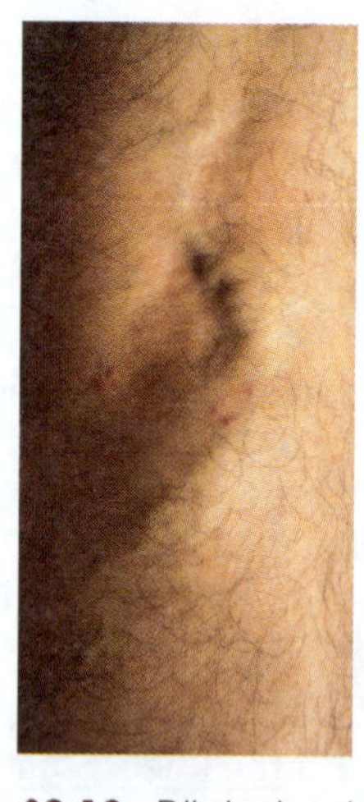

Fig. 30.12: Dilated vein in popliteal region

- **Ankle flare** is a group of reticular veins near the medial malleolus.
- Complications such as ulceration, bleeding, eczema, and dermatitis may be present. Pigmentation is often seen. It is due to subcutaneous microangiopathy, acute cellulitis, fasciitis, and panniculitis.
- Healed scar indicates previous ulceration.
- A dilated vein may be present over the popliteal fossa region as well (Fig. 30.12).

Palpation

- First palpate along the whole length of vein for tenderness. If present, it indicates thrombophlebitis. A thrombosed vein will feel like a firm/hard nodule.
- The following tests are performed (Key Box 30.5).

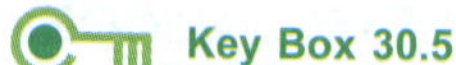

Key Box 30.5

Tests for Varicose Veins

- Cough impulse test: SF incompetence
- Trendelenburg I: SF incompetence
  Trendelenburg II: Perforator incompetence
- Multiple tourniquet test: Site of perforator incompetence
- Schwartz test: Superficial column of blood
- Modified Perthes' test: Deep vein thrombosis
- Fegan's test: To locate the perforators in the deep fascia

1. **Cough impulse test (Morrissey's test):** This test should be done in the standing position. The examiner keeps the finger at the SF junction and asks the patient to cough. Fluid thrill, an impulse felt by the fingers, is indicative of *'saphenofemoral incompetence'*.
2. **Trendelenburg test:** This test is done in 2 parts (Figs 30.13–30.15).
   - *Method:* The patient is asked to lie on the couch in the supine position. The leg is elevated above the level of the heart and the vein is emptied. The SF junction is occluded with the thumb (or a tourniquet) and the patient is asked to stand.
   - **Trendelenburg I:** Release the thumb or tourniquet immediately. ***A rapid gush of blood from above downwards indicates saphenofemoral incompetence.***
   - **Trendelenburg II:** The pressure at the SF junction is maintained without releasing the thumb or tourniquet. The patient is then asked to stand. ***Slow filling of the long saphenous is seen which indicates perforator incompetence*** (retrograde flow of blood).

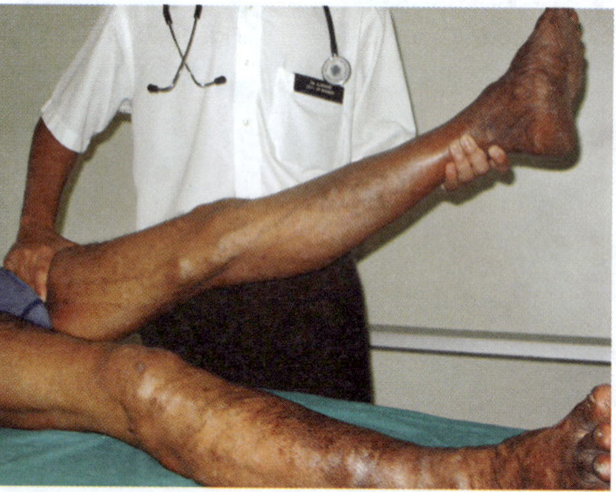

Fig. 30.13: Trendelenburg test part I

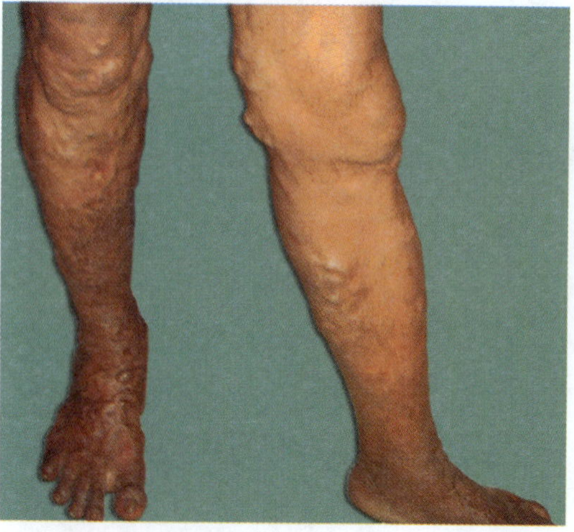

Fig. 30.14: Rapid filling on releasing pressure

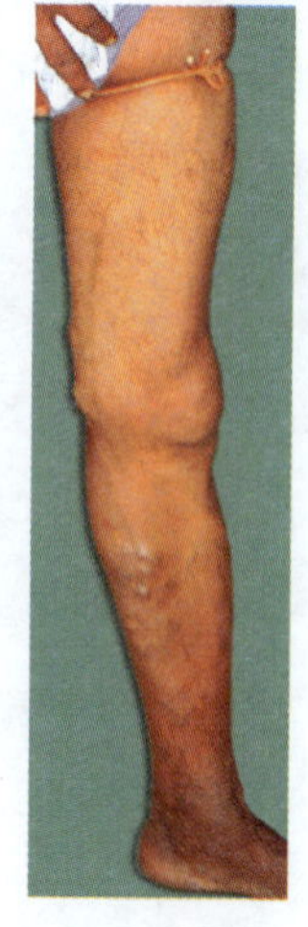

Fig. 30.15: Trendelenburg test part II—slow filling is seen

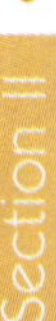

3. **Multiple tourniquet test:** It is done to determine the exact site of the perforators (Fig. 30.16).
   - *Method:* The patient is asked to lie supine on the couch. The vein is emptied by elevation. As the name suggests, 3–4 tourniquets (multiple) may be applied. Applying more tourniquets is not practical. **There are mainly ankle, knee, and thigh perforators.** Hence, four tourniquets may be applied at the following levels:
   - **1st tourniquet:** At the level of the SF junction.
   - **2nd tourniquet:** At the level of middle of the thigh, to occlude the perforator in the Hunter's canal.
   - **3rd tourniquet:** Just below the knee.
   - **4th tourniquet:** Palm breadth (lower third of the leg) above the medial malleolus/ankle.

   Ask the patient to stand and observe the appearance of veins.

   Inference: Appearance of veins between the first and second tourniquets indicates incompetence of thigh perforators, between the second and third indicates incompetence of knee perforators, and below the fourth indicates incompetence of ankle perforators. Most commonly, below-knee and ankle perforators are incompetent.

   On releasing the tourniquets one by one from below upwards, sudden retrograde filling of the veins occurs.
4. **Schwartz test:** It is done with the patient in the standing position. Place the fingers of the left hand over a dilated segment of the vein and tap the vein with the right index finger. A palpable impulse suggests a **superficial column of blood in the vein and incompetent valves between the segment** (Fig. 30.17).

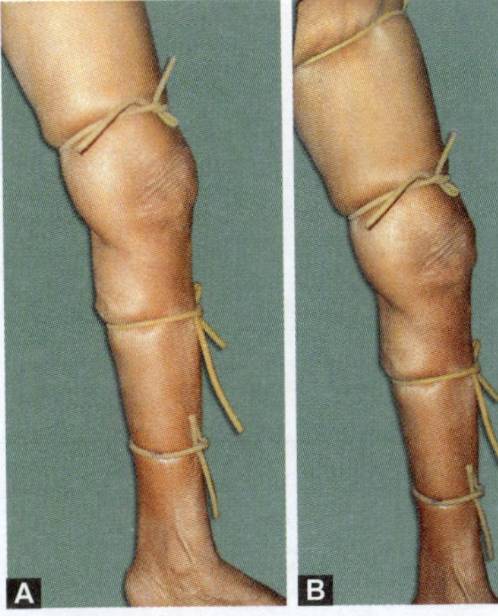

Figs 30.16A and B: Multiple tourniquet test (3 or 4)

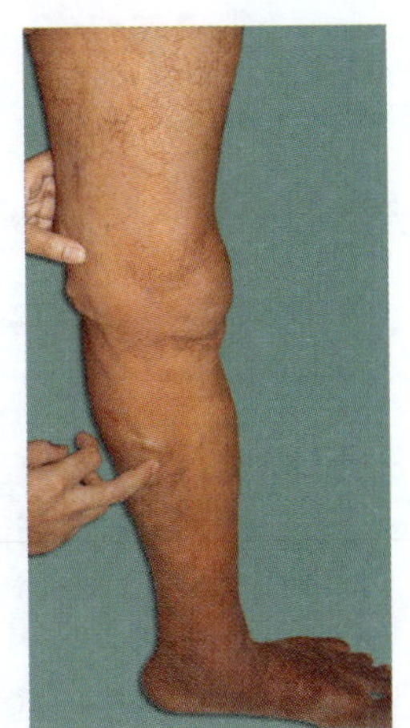

Fig. 30.17: Schwartz test (should be done in the standing position)

5. **Modified Perthes' test[1]:** It is done to rule out deep vein thrombosis. The patient is asked to stand and a tourniquet is applied at SF junction. He is then asked to take a brisk walk-tip toe walking

   Inference: If the patient complains of severe pain in the calf region or if superficial veins become more prominent, it indicates **deep vein thrombosis** and is a contraindication for surgery.

Pearls of Wisdom

Please note: The vein is not emptied in modified Perthes' test.

6. **Fegan's method (test):** It is done to detect the site of perforators. The patient is asked to stand and the varicosity is marked with methylene blue. Patient is then asked to lie down. The leg is elevated to empty the vein and the vein is palpated throughout its course. The defects in the deep fascia have a circular, buttonhole consistency.

Examination of varicose ulcer: It should be done by inspection and palpation.

Evidence of deep vein thrombosis: Homan's test must be done in chronic DVT. Moses' test *(vide infra) not to be done.*

Examination of the abdomen: To rule out pelvic tumours. Look for inferior vena caval obstruction in the form of dilated veins in the lateral abdominal wall.

CLINICAL DISCUSSION

At the end of clinical examination, you should be ready to answer the following questions:

1. **Which system is involved?**
   - Medial veins: LSV—long saphenous vein
   - Lateral veins: SSV—short saphenous vein
2. **Is the SF junction incompetent?**

   Yes—Trendelenburg I is positive, No—Trendelenburg I is negative
3. **Is there perforator incompetence?**

   Yes—Trendelenburg II is positive, No—Trendelenburg II is negative
4. **Which group of perforators is incompetent?**

   According to the results of multiple tourniquet test—usually ankle and below knee.
5. **Is there deep vein thrombosis?**

   Yes—Perthes' test is positive, No—Perthes' test is negative.
6. **Is there any abdominal mass?**

   There may be a pelvic tumour.

[1]In original Perthes' test, the limb is wrapped and elastic bandage is applied.

7. **Are any complications present?**
   Eczema, dermatitis, ulcer, etc.
8. **Is it unilateral or bilateral?**
   Determine by hand-held Doppler—extension of clinical examination.
9. **What is the CEAP classification?**
   Example: C1 Ep A-LSV Pr.
10. **What is the gait of the patient?**
    Equinus deformity in long standing ulcers.

INVESTIGATIONS

1. **Hand-held Doppler** is the first, minimum-level investigation done before treating a patient with venous disease. Patient is asked to stand.
   - When the blood flows, the **wave** emits a signal—the Doppler signal.
   - If there is SF incompetence, forward and backward flow may be detected.
   - **Biphasic signal:** Gently squeeze calf muscles and assess the flow in the SF junction with the Doppler probe.
   - It may also pick up an accessory long saphenous vein in the groin.
   - Can be used to mark the SF junction and SP junction.
   - Patient can be asked to cough and reflux can be confirmed at SF junction.
   - It is not used to identify perforators (Key Box 30.6).
2. **Duplex ultrasound imaging:** In this investigation, high resolution B-mode ultrasound imaging and Doppler ultrasound are used (Figs 30.18 and 30.19).
   - It provides images of the veins and measures the flow in them.
   - The origin of venous ulcers and varicose veins may also be assessed.
   - Retrograde flow in the veins may be demonstrated by compression, release, and the Valsalva manoeuvre.

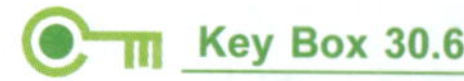
Key Box 30.6

Doppler Ultrasound

- This investigation is carried out with the patient standing/sitting.
- Incompetence of SFJ and saphenopopliteal junction (SPJ) can be assessed by this method—reflux.
- **Gentle squeezing** of calf muscles helps in detecting saphenopopliteal incompetence.
- To identify and locate perforators.
- It also helps to **rule out arterial** diseases.
- It can detect **patency of veins**.
- It can detect deep vein thrombosis.

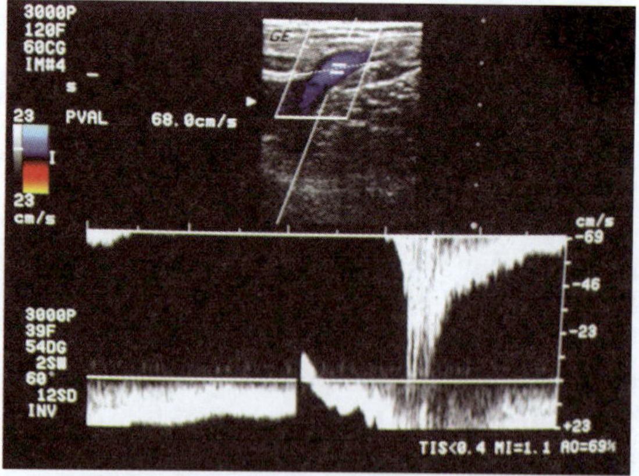

Fig. 30.18: Duplex scanning showing venous reflux

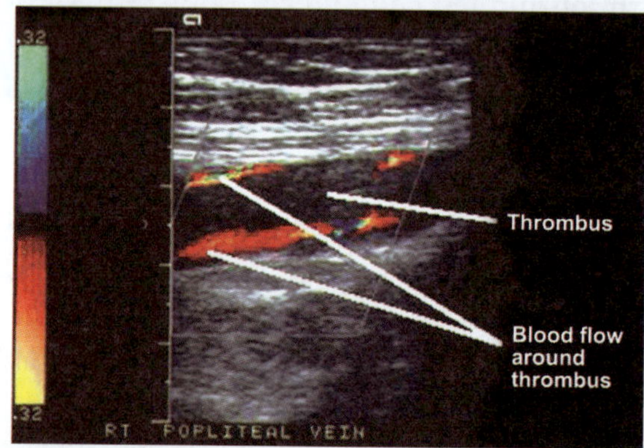

Fig. 30.19: Popliteal vein thrombosis

(*Courtesy:* Dr Rajgopal, Head, Department of Radiology and Imaging, KMC, Manipal)

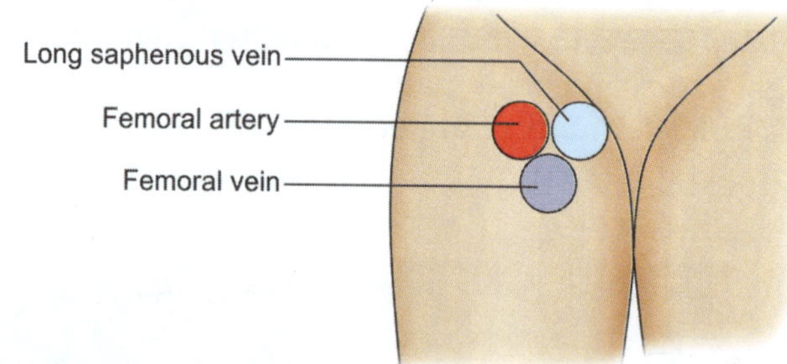

Fig. 30.20: Mickey Mouse sign—as seen in duplex ultrasound

- **Mickey Mouse sign:** The three prominent structures—the common femoral artery and the great saphenous vein above and the common femoral vein below **mimic Mickey Mouse** (Fig. 30.20).
- **Saphenous eye sign:** In the fascial compartments of the thigh, the dilated saphenous vein in cross-section resembles an 'eye' in transverse 'B' mode scan. .

3. **Venography:** Both ascending and descending venographies may be done in a case of deep vein thrombosis. It is an invasive procedure and carries the risk of spreading infection and septicaemia. Duplex ultrasonography has largely replaced this investigation (rarely done now). Varicography refers

to injecting contrast into surface veins (indicated in recurrent varicose veins). It may be followed by sclerosant injections.

4. **Plethysmography:** It is based on the measurement of volume changes in the leg. By placing a light-emitting diode above the medial malleolus and having the patient perform tip-toe movements, venous recovery time may be measured. This is called photoplethysmography (PPT).

With the advent of venous duplex scan, venography and plethysmography are rarely done.

TREATMENT

A. Pharmacotherapy: It helps reduce oedema of the leg, and thereby improves night cramps. Flavanoids affect leucocytes and vascular endothelium, which helps heal cutaneous ulcers. Diosmin and hesperidin are the two commonly used vasoactive drugs. Diosmin prolongs the vasoconstrictor effect of norepinephrine on the vein wall. Thus, venous tone is increased and the venous volume, distensibility, and stasis are reduced. This increases the venous return, which helps patients with CVI.

B. Non-surgical treatment:

1. Elastic compression stockings
2. Injection line of treatment (compression sclerotherapy)
3. Foam sclerotherapy
4. Endovenous laser ablation
5. **R**adio-**F**requency **A**blation (**RFA**)

1. Elastic Compression Stockings (Key Box 30.7)

These are also called graduated compression stockings. It is the fundamental treatment for varicose veins. This may be advised in asymptomatic cases of varicose veins and in cases of venous oedema and secondary varicose veins.

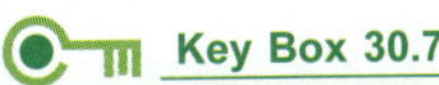

Key Box 30.7

How Graduated Compression Stockings Work?

- Increases the interstitial pressure
- Promotes fluid reabsorption
- Improves ambulatory venous pressure
- Improves skin micro-circulation

- Usually 20–30 mmHg stockings are sufficient.
- It should be worn from the ankle to below the knee.
- It should be worn during working hours (entire day).
- It should be removed while lying down but the legs should be kept elevated.
- ***Above knee stockings should never be prescribed as they are difficult to put on and tend to roll down.***

Advantages

- Require minimal patient involvement
- Provide continuous compression (Table 30.3)
- Provide topical therapy

Disadvantages

- Bulky and uncomfortable
- Ulcers cannot be monitored once applied
- Dermatitis

Indications

- Pregnancy, pelvic tumour
- Perthes' test—positive patient
- AV fistula

Contraindication: Occlusive arterial disease.

Pearls of Wisdom

Extreme care to be taken while applying compression stockings in a patient with arterial occlusive disease. Incidences of gangrene has been reported.

2. Injection Line of Treatment (Compression Sclerotherapy) (Key Box 30.8)

Key Box 30.8

Compression Sclerotherapy

- **E**ndothelial cells in the vein wall are damaged
- **E**ffective sclerosant
- **E**mpty vein
- **E**lastic compression stockings
- **E**xercises *Observe* **5 Es**

Table 30.3 Compression stockings

Class	Pressure	Strength	Indication	CEAP
I	15–20 mmHg	Mild	Minor varicosities, mild oedema	1, 2, 3
II	20–30 mmHg	Moderate	Moderate varicosities, phlebitis, moderate oedema, postoperative ablation	3, 4
III	30–40 mmHg	Firm	Severe varicosities, active ulcer, DVT	4, 5, 6
IV	>40 mmHg	Extra firm	Lymphoedema	N/A

Indications

Below knee varicosity and recurrent varicosity after surgery.

Procedure

Varicose veins are **marked** in the standing position. Doppler can be used to puncture the vein. The veins are punctured with a needle attached to a syringe containing a sclerosant agent and the patient is asked to lie down. **3% sodium tetradecyl sulphate or 1–2 ml of ethanolamine oleate or hypertonic saline** is injected into the column of vein. **Aseptic thrombosis** and fibrosis occur, which shrinks the vein. A tight elastic compression bandage is applied. Success of sclerotherapy depends on the use of an **effective sclerosant**, injection into an **empty vein,** and **compression followed by exercise**.

Pearls of Wisdom

Injection sclerotherapy is useful in varicose veins <3 mm in diameter. Large veins require surgery.

Complications of Compression Sclerotherapy

Allergy, pigmentation, deep vein thrombosis, thrombophlebitis and skin necrosis.

3. Ultrasound-guided Foam Sclerotherapy by Tessari (Key Box 30.9)

- 2 syringes are used here with a 3-way stopcock is used to inject the foam. It was described by Lorenzo Tessari.
- Very useful and better when there are large veins.
- Foam is visible in ultrasound, thus obliteration of veins can be visualised better.
- Foam sclerosant C (polidocanol) is used. It is prepared by mixing air with a sclerosant.

Key Box 30.9

Foam Sclerotherapy

- Used to treat small and medium-sized varicose veins.
- Sclerosant is mixed with air or preferably carbon dioxide plus oxygen.
- Carbon dioxide plus oxygen is soluble in blood and hence safe.
- Foam causes inflammation of vein wall, obliteration of venous lumen and vein occlusion.
- Success rates range from 60 to 90%.
- Complications include cutaneous ulceration, thrombophlebitis, deep vein thrombosis and allergy.
- Foam displaces blood (unlike sclerosant which mixes with blood), requires small quantity to be in touch with vein wall.
- Extravasated foam is much better tolerated.
- It is echogenic.

- It is injected into the superficial veins under ultrasound guidance.
- LSV should be compressed in the upper thigh to prevent entry of foam into the femoral vein.
- The leg should be elevated to prevent entry of foam into the calf veins.

Complications of Foam Sclerotherapy

- Skin ulceration due to extravasation.
- Deep vein thrombosis due to escape into deep veins.
- Headache and stroke due to air entry into the brain.

4. Endovenous Laser Ablation (EVLA) (Fig. 30.21)

It is a minimally invasive, outpatient procedure that uses lasers to ablate varicose veins. It gives excellent cosmetic and functional results and is ideal for veins >12 mm in diameter. It is done after giving tumescent anaesthesia. Tumescent means tissue is swollen and firm. It is done by extensive regional anesthesia of skin and subcutaneous tissue with a high total dose (200 ml of 0.1% lignocaine with adrenaline and bicarbonate) but a low risk of systemic toxicity. Thus it avoids skin burns and other reactions.

Advantages

- Simple outpatient procedure
- Ideal for junctional and truncal incompetence
- Less expensive than radiofrequency ablation

Disadvantages

- Expensive and not ideal for smaller, tortuous, and/or thrombophlebitic veins.

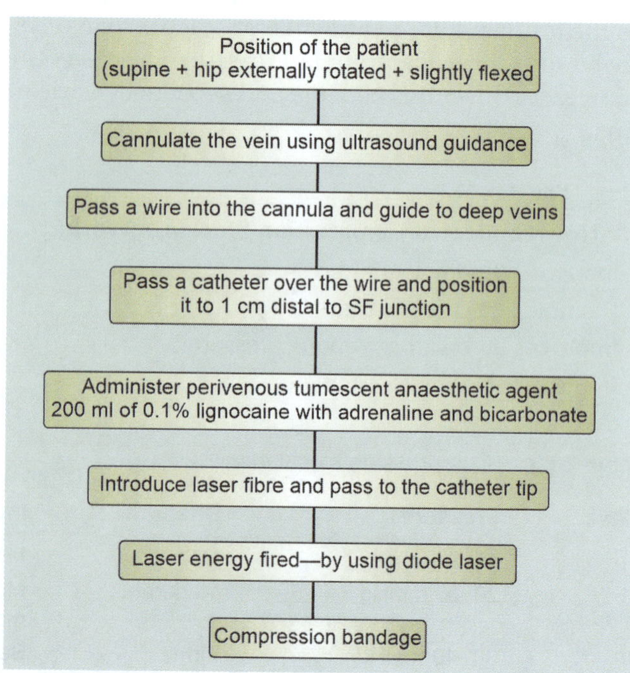

Fig. 30.21: Endovenous laser ablation

5. Radiofrequency Ablation (RFA)

- Ideally suited for long saphenous vein with a diameter <12 mm.
- It is also a minimally invasive ablation technique that uses a bipolar catheter electrode at a temperature of 110–120°C with a power of 2–4 W. It is a high-frequency alternating radiofrequency current that leads to venous spasm, collagen shrinkage and physical contraction.
- The position of the patient, accurate marking of the veins, and tumescent anaesthesia are similar to that of EVLA. The vein is cannulated with a 7F sheath.
- The catheter tip should be placed 2.0 cm inferior to the saphenofemoral or saphenopopliteal junction.
- A vein segment >7 cm long may be ablated in 20 seconds cycles.
- Compression stockings to be used after the RFA.
- Complications include thrombophlebitis, pain, and skin burns.
- It is a safe and effective treatment for varicose veins.

6. Surgery

1. **Trendelenburg's operation** (Figs 30.22–30.27):
   - An inguinal incision is made, the long saphenous vein is identified, and the 3 tributaries are ligated. The long saphenous vein is ligated close to the femoral vein and divided. Up to this step is called Trendelenburg operation (***juxtafemoral flush ligation***).
   - An incision is made on the medial side of the upper leg and the long saphenous vein is isolated. The lower end is ligated and the vein is incised. A long metallic stripper is introduced within the vein and brought out from the long saphenous vein below a knee incision. A metallic head is connected to the stripper and the vein is avulsed. A tight crepe bandage is applied, the inguinal incision is sutured, and the limb is elevated (retrograde avulsion).

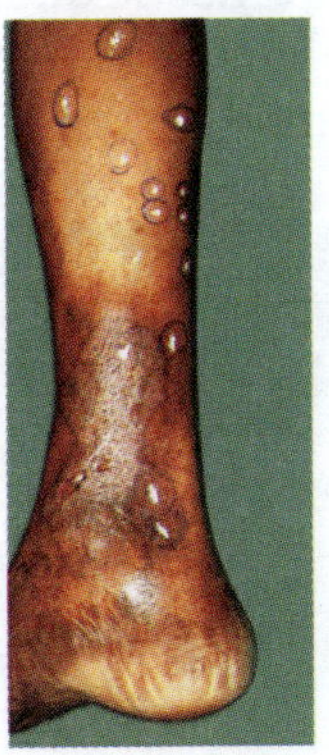

Fig. 30.22: Perforators marked

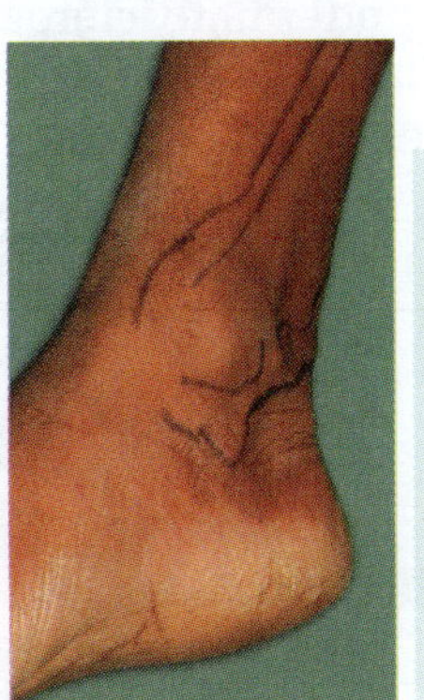

Fig. 30.23: Ankle veins marked

Perforators are marked before surgery to facilitate identification of perforators and communicating veins so that they can be ligated and excised (Fig. 30.22). You can see in this picture the prominent veins are marked (Fig. 30.23).

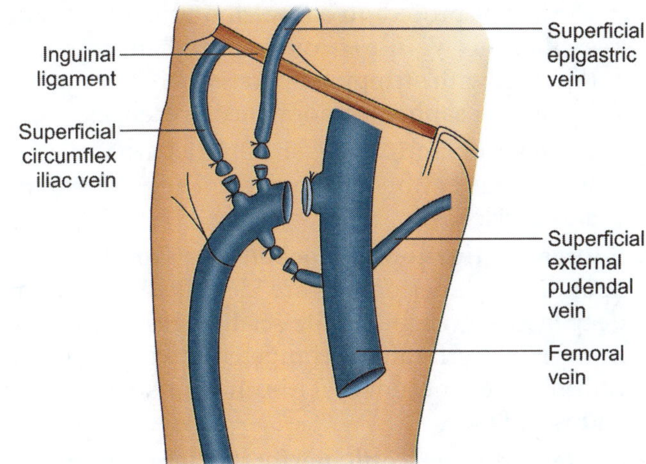

Fig. 30.24: Trendelenburg operation. Long saphenous vein should never be ligated in the groin **unless you demonstrate 'T' junction**—LSV joining femoral vein (Key Box 30.10)

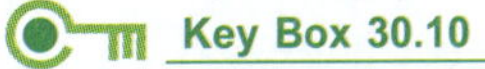

Key Box 30.10

Wisdom in Juxtafemoral Flush Ligation

1. Demonstrate T junction—long saphenous vein joining femoral vein.
2. Demonstrate 3–4 tributaries before ligation.
3. Double saphenous vein can be present as an anomaly.
4. Receives large anterolateral thigh veins and posteromedial thigh veins.
5. Demonstrate femoral vein for a centimetre both above and below the SF junction.

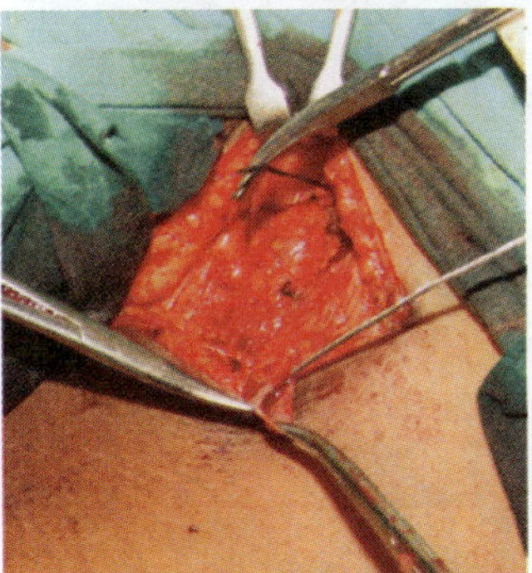

Fig. 30.25: LSV is divided at the groin and stripper is introduced within the lumen

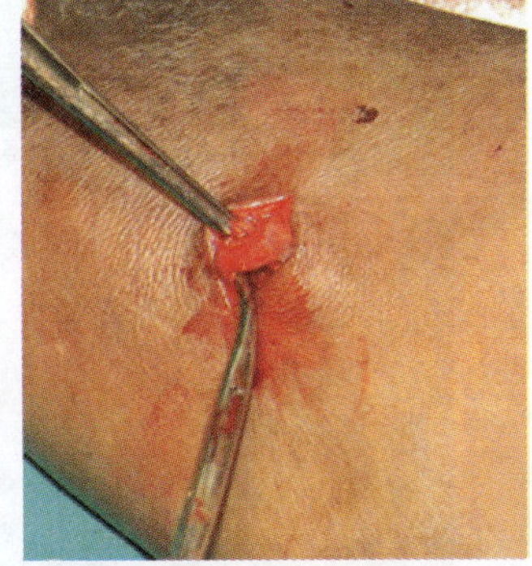

Fig. 30.26: One segment of the vein is isolated followed by ligation at both ends and if it is very tortuous, it is excised

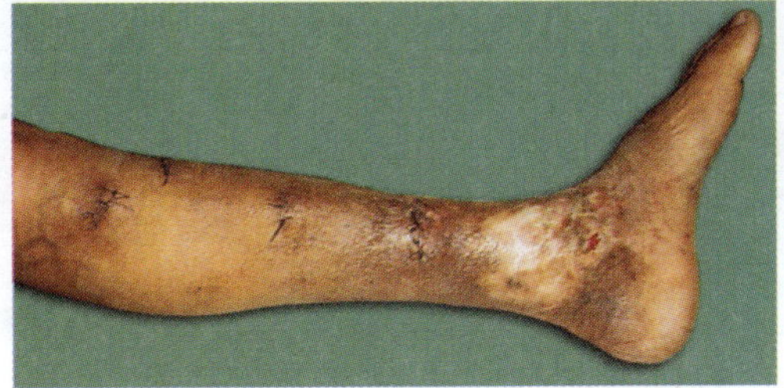

Fig. 30.27: Multiple ligation

- During the procedure, **a few tributaries of the long saphenous vein get avulsed** and thrombosed (ligation with stripping operation). It is indicated in cases of saphenofemoral incompetence.
- Once stripping is done, small incisions are given where perforators are marked. They are ligated and excised.

2. **Subfascial ligation of Cockett and Dodd:** In this operation, the perforators are identified deep to the deep fascia and ligated subfascially. This is indicated in cases of perforator incompetence with saphenofemoral competence. This may also be done endoscopically.
3. **Subfascial endoscopic perforator surgery (SEPS)** (Fig. 30.28)
   - **Small port incisions** are made in the skin over the calf region and deepened through the fascia.
   - **Carbon dioxide** insufflation is done. A balloon expander may also be used to distend the subfascial plane.
   - **2–6 perforators** are identified and ligated.
   - The procedure is simple and quick with least morbidity and is becoming popular.
   - It is indicated for below-knee perforators.
4. Smaller veins have also been treated with phlebectomies.

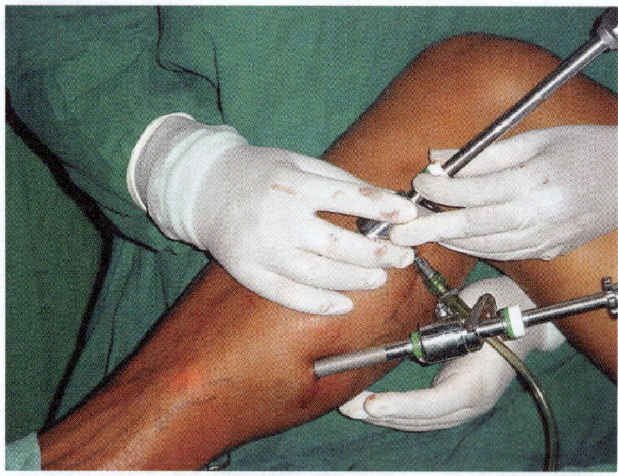

Fig. 30.28: SEPS

Competency

SU27.6: Describe the pathophysiology, clinical features, investigations and principles of management of DVT and varicose veins.

COMPLICATIONS OF VARICOSE VEINS

1. **Eczema and dermatitis** (Figs 30.29 and 30.30)**:** It occurs due to extravasation and breakdown of RBCs in the lower leg. It gives rise to itching, which precipitates varicose ulcer. It is treated by applying zinc oxide cream or silver sulfadiazine cream (stasis dermatitis).
2. **Lipodermatosclerosis** (Figs 30.31 and 30.32) refers to various skin changes in the lower leg associated with varicose veins such as **thickening of subcutaneous tissue, indurated wood-like feel,** pigmentation, etc. It is due to increased venous pressure resulting in capillary leakage with extravasation of blood and fibrin into the surrounding tissues. Blood is broken down and haem is released, which combines with iron to form haemosiderin, which is responsible for pigmentation. Classically, this affects the gaiter area of the leg just above the malleoli.
3. **Haemorrhage:** It occurs due to trauma or eczema. It may be controlled by elevating the leg and applying a crepe bandage. Do not try to catch bleeders with artery forceps.
4. **Thrombophlebitis** (Key Box 30.11)**:** It refers to inflammation of a superficial vein. The vein is tender, hard and cord-like. The skin is inflamed and pyrexia is usually present. It is treated with bedrest, elevation, crepe bandage, antibiotics, and anti-inflammatory drugs.
5. **Venous ulcer** (Figs 30.32–30.35)**:** It is also called **gravitational ulcer**. Its precipitating factors are **venous stasis** and **tissue anoxia.** *Deep vein thrombosis* is also an important cause of venous ulcer wherein valves are either destroyed or incompetent due to damage. **Sustained venous pressure** results in extravasation of cells and activation of capillary endothelium, resulting in the **release of free radicals.** These free radicals cause tissue destruction and ulceration. **Lipodermatosclerosis and tissue anoxia** are the other factors. The following hypotheses may explain the genesis of varicose ulcers.

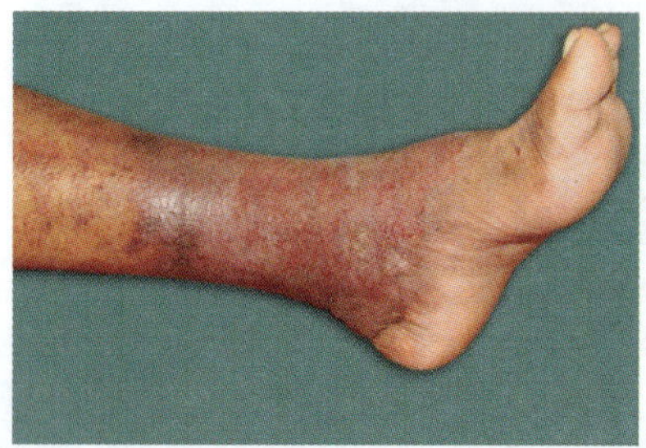

Fig. 30.29: Eczema

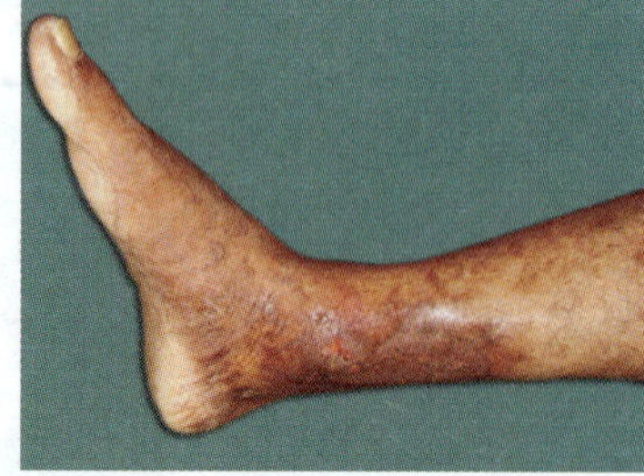

Fig. 30.30: Dermatitis

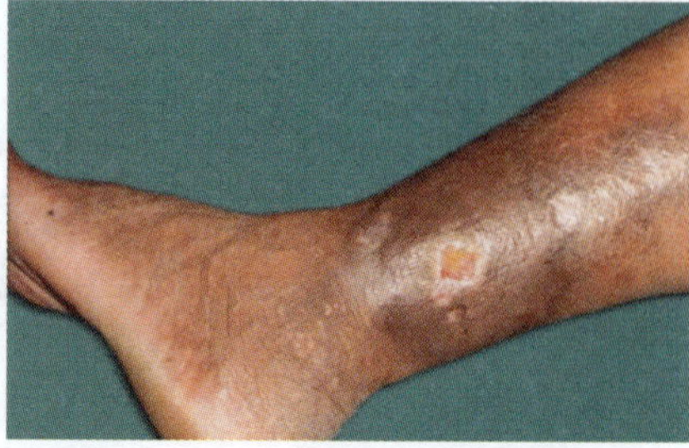

Fig. 30.31: Observe pigmentation, lipodermatosclerosis and ulcer formation

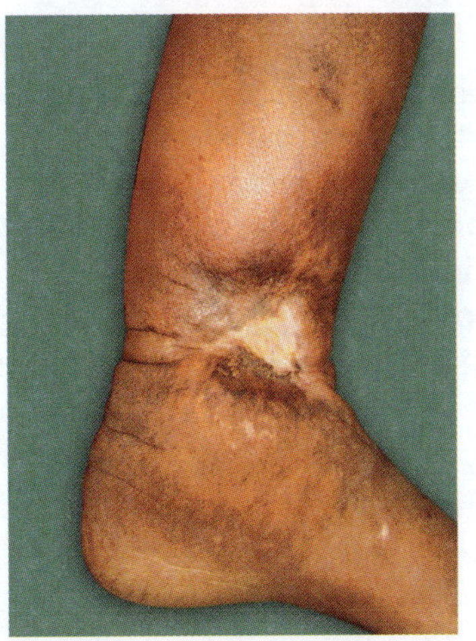

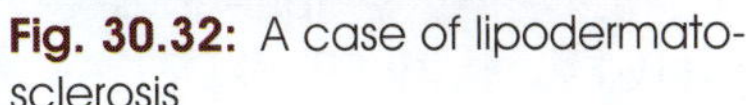

Fig. 30.32: A case of lipodermatosclerosis

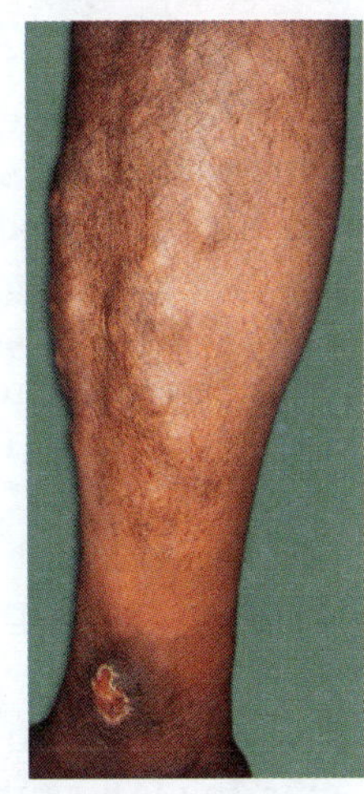

Fig. 30.33: Varicose vein with venous ulcer

(*Courtesy:* Dr Maruthu Pandyan, Government Medical College, Madurai, Tamil Nadu)

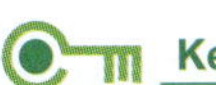

Key Box 30.11

Thrombophlebitis—Causes

- Spontaneous TAO, malignancy
- Trauma
- Blood transfusion
- IV fluids, chemotherapeutic drugs
- Varicose veins

Fibrin cuff hypothesis: The combination of capillary proliferation and inflammation (in the form of macrophages) is a major factor in the development of venous ulcers. As a result of chronic inflammation, a perivascular cuff develops around the capillaries. This perivascular cuff is made up of many connective tissue proteins, including fibrin, collagen IV, and fibronectin. Slowly, a venous ulcer develops.

White cell trapping hypothesis: Venous hypertension causes trapping of leucocytes, which become activated and release proteolytic enzymes that cause damage to the capillary endothelium.

Pearls of Wisdom

Whatever be the exact mechanism of ulceration, ambulatory venous hypertension is the only accepted cause of ulceration (Fig. 30.34).

Features of a venous ulcer (Fig. 30.35)

- Typically situated just above the medial malleolus.
- Oval, small, painless, and superficial with surrounding pigmentation.
- Dilated veins above the ulcer give a clue to the diagnosis (Key Box 30.12).

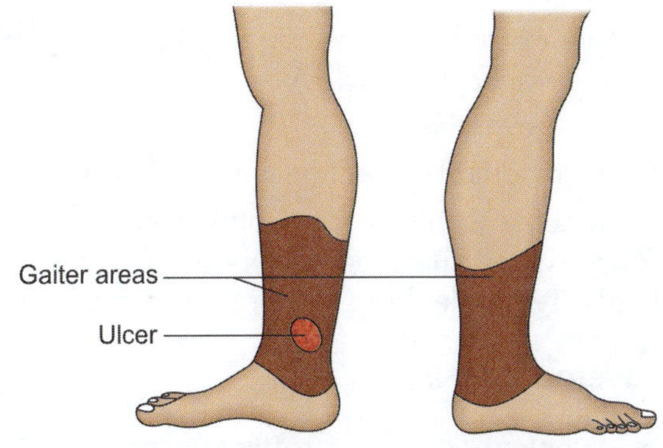

Fig. 30.34: Gaiter areas are those areas where **skin changes** and **venous stasis ulcer occurs** due to **ambulatory venous hypertension** and incompetent perforators. Damage to capillaries results in protein-rich fluid and blood extravasation

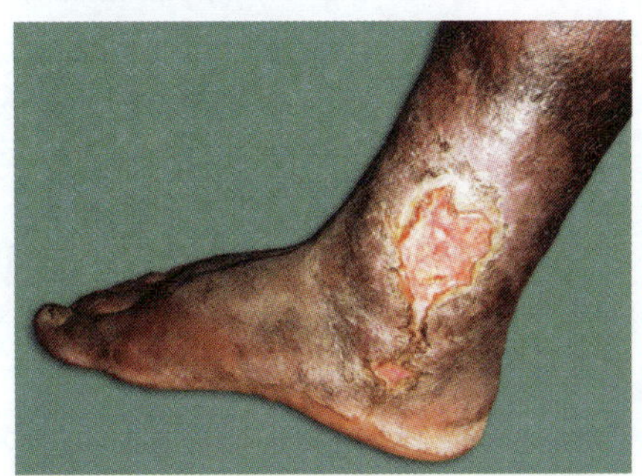

Fig. 30.35: Venous ulcer (*Courtesy:* Dr Maruthu Pandyan, Professor of Surgery, Government Medical College, Madurai, Tamil Nadu)

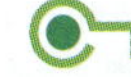

Key Box 30.12

Factors Predisposing to Nonhealing Venous Ulcers

1. Ambulatory venous hypertension.
2. Perivascular fibrin cuff resulting in poor diffusion of oxygen to the tissues.
3. White cell trapping.
4. Reactive oxygen species are increased and they generate free radicals leading to tissue damage.
5. Inhibition of growth factors leading to poor repair.

Treatment of venous ulcers: ***Bisgaard's method*** (Nowadays, it is not recommended)

- Rest with **elevated limb** (Fig. 30.36).
- **Elastic crepe bandage** helps in venous return.

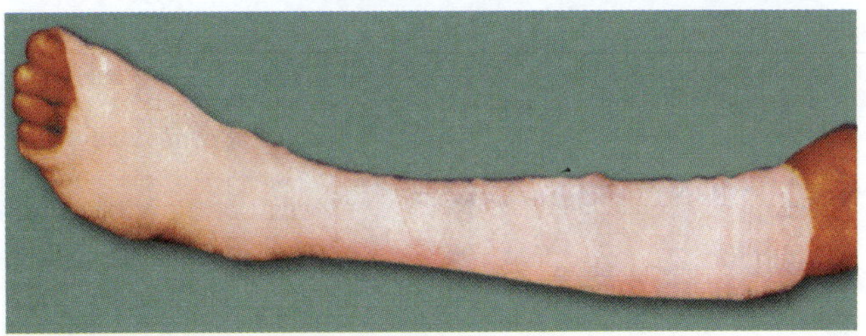

Fig. 30.36: Elastic crepe bandage for varicose ulcer. Elevation of the leg is the most important factor for healing of the ulcer

- **Active exercises** should be taught to the patients (to contract calf muscles).
- **Passive exercises**
- Correct method of walking with the **heel down first**.
- If the ulcer is infected, antibiotics are given and a four-layered dressing is applied. Once the ulcer heals, Trendelenburg's operation is performed.

Four-Layered Dressing

	Content	Uses
Layer 1	Wool bandage	Absorbs exudates. Redistributes pressure around the limb and protects bony prominences.
Layer 2	Crepe bandage (light compression) (15 mmHg)	Holds stockings better and provides padding in place.
Layer 3	Bandage (medium compression)	Applied with graduated compression. 300% extensible and 100%, elastic.
Layer 4	Cohesive bandage	Self-adhesive bandage of added reinforcement. Holds 3 layers in place, thereby retaining the compression.

6. **Calcification** may be seen in the walls of the vein.
7. **Periostitis** of the tibia may occur due to the location of the ulcer on the medial surface of the leg. Due to involvement of the periosteum, there is severe pain.
8. **Equinovarus deformity** occurs due to improper habit of walking on the toes which results in shortening of the tendo-Achilles.
9. **Marjolin's ulcer** is a squamous cell carcinoma arising from a healed varicose ulcer with scarring.

SHORT SAPHENOUS VARICOSITY

The short saphenous vein originates from the lateral part of the dorsal venous arch and ends in the popliteal vein in the popliteal fossa (Fig. 30.37). Incompetence of the saphenopopliteal valve results in short saphenous varicosity. It produces prominent veins on the lateral aspect of the leg with or without ulceration. These are treated by ligation of the short saphenous vein in the popliteal fossa (Table 30.4).

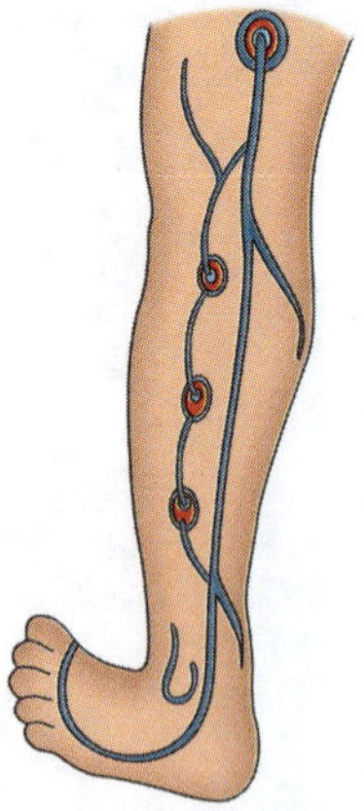

Fig. 30.37: Short saphenous vein and its perforators

Ligation of the Saphenopopliteal Junction

- Preoperative ultrasonographic marking is essential.
- The vein should be ligated deep to the deep fascia.
- Branches—the **Giacomini vein** and **gastrocnemius** veins may be seen. They must be ligated.
- It may be stripped up to the mid-calf to avoid **injury to the sural nerve**.
- It is important to close the deep fascia to avoid an unsightly cosmetic bulge behind the knee.

TEN COMMANDMENTS OF VENOUS ULCER TREATMENT

1. Should lose weight
2. Should perform venous Doppler to rule out deep vein thrombosis or thrombophlebitis
3. Should take rest with the leg elevated above the level of the heart
4. Should receive antibiotics if infection is present
5. Should apply a wound cover with suitable dressings
6. Should apply compression stockings
7. Should consider surgery only once infection is under control
8. Should ligate long or short veins if they are incompetent
9. Should ensure that all perforators are ligated
10. Should look for an accessory long saphenous vein near the termination of the vein—if present, it should be ligated to avoid recurrence

Table 30.4 Comparison between long saphenous and short saphenous veins

Features	Long saphenous vein	Short saphenous vein
1. Origin	Medial part of dorsal venous arch	Lateral part of dorsal venous arch
2. Location	Front of medial malleolus	Behind lateral malleolus
3. Relation with nerve	Saphenous nerve	Sural nerve
4. Number of valves	15–20 valves	1 valve
5. Termination	Saphenofemoral junction	Saphenopopliteal junction

RECURRENT VARICOSE VEINS

- Incidence is about 10–30%.
- Important causes of recurrence include failure to ligate the LSV at the SF junction, failure to ligate tributaries at the SF junction, and a possible accessory long saphenous vein (Fig. 30.38).
- Other factors for failure include neovascularisation and reflux in residual veins.
- Recurrence is less after stripping of veins than after multiple ligation.
- Injection sclerotherapy and EVLA/RFA may be done.
- Re-surgery may be performed. However, wound infection, wound gaping, and lymph leak are more common.

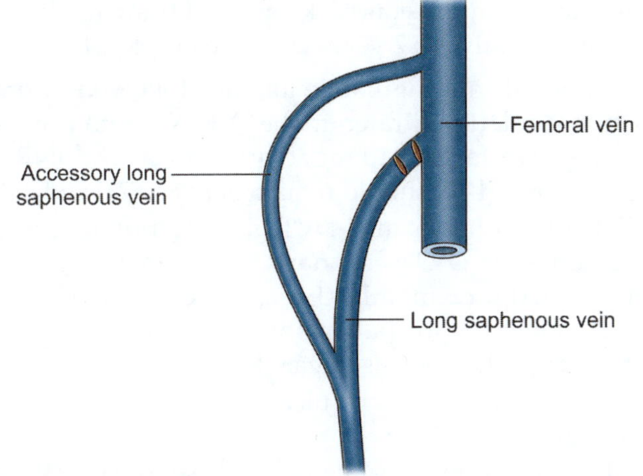

Fig. 30.38: Accessory long saphenous vein

DEEP VEIN THROMBOSIS (DVT)

ACUTE DEEP VEIN THROMBOSIS

It is also called phlebothrombosis. It can be acute or chronic. Acute deep vein thrombosis is very common in western countries, the exact cause of which is unknown. Postoperative immobilisation, pressure on the calf muscles, sluggish blood flow, and prolonged bedrest are some of the precipitating factors for deep vein thrombosis. It commonly affects venous sinuses in the soleal muscles. It is a common starting place. It may also involve pelvic veins. The various factors responsible for deep vein thrombosis can be remembered as THROMBOSIS (Key Boxes 30.13 and 30.14). It should be suspected in the postoperative period when patient complains of pain in the calf region or complains of limb oedema. The maximum incidence occurs on the 2nd and 5th–6th postoperative days.

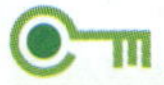
Key Box 30.13

Thrombosis—Virchow's Triad

- Endothelial injury
- Stasis
- Increased coagulability

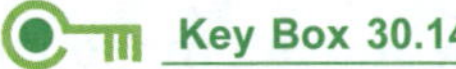
Key Box 30.14

Causes of Deep Vein Thrombosis (Lower Limb DVT)

Trauma—injury to the vessel wall
Hormones—increased coagulability
Road traffic accidents
Operations—cholecystectomy
Malignancy—sluggish blood flow
Blood disorders—polycythaemia
Orthopaedic surgery, obesity, old age
Serious illness—stroke, MI
Immobilisation
Splenectomy

Remember as **THROMBOSIS**

Upper limb DVT is rare. Can occur due to trauma or surgery.

Signs of Acute DVT

1. **Homan's test:** Forcible dorsiflexion of the foot results in severe pain in the calf region.
2. **Moses' test** (ideally should not be done due to risk of embolism): Tenderness over the calf muscle on squeezing the muscle from side to side.
3. **Pitting oedema**
4. Low grade fever with an increased pulse rate is characteristic.
5. **Phlegmasia alba dolens** refers to white leg. It occurs when the thrombus extends from the calf region to the iliofemoral vein.
6. **Phlegmasia coerulea dolens** refers to blue leg with loss of superficial tissues of the toes.
7. Superficial blebs in the skin—can be confused for necrotising fasciitis.

Treatment

Acute DVT

1. Bedrest and limb elevation.
2. **Injection heparin** 10,000 units IV bolus with continuous infusion of 30,000–45,000 units/day. During heparin therapy, **activated partial thromboplastin time (APTT)** should be maintained at twice the normal value. Heparin is given for 7–10 days. **Warfarin**, an oral anticoagulant, is started 2–3 days before heparin is withdrawn because of its slow onset. Treatment with warfarin should continue for 6–12 months. A repeat Duplex scan should be done to look for recanalisation of the veins. The dose of warfarin should be 10 mg twice a day. **Treatment is**

monitored with prothrombin time and international normalized ratio (INR). INR should be 2.0–3.0.

3. **Low molecular weight heparin (LMWH)** is given once or twice a day, in the form of injection. **No blood monitoring is required.** Incidence of bleeding is less with LMWH. **More details are given at the end of this chapter.**
4. **Inferior vena caval filters indicated if thrombus is extensive and recurrent.** They can be inserted percutaneously *via* the femoral vein in patients who have contraindications for **lytic therapy**.
5. Compression stockings.

Pearls of Wisdom

IVC filters are more commonly indicated in patients with recurrent DVT and symptomatic pulmonary embolism.

CHRONIC DEEP VEIN THROMBOSIS

- DVT lasting for >4 weeks is defined as 'Chronic DVT'. Signs and symptoms include pain, oedema, telangiectasia, hyperpigmentation, lipodermatosclerosis, ulceration, and venous claudication.
- The clinical manifestations are secondary to post-thrombotic sequelae (PTS) and occur after an episode of DVT, as thrombosis leads to venous hypertension from venous obstruction and reflux. Classically, the limb is described as having an **inverted beer bottle or champagne bottle appearance** (Fig. 30.39).

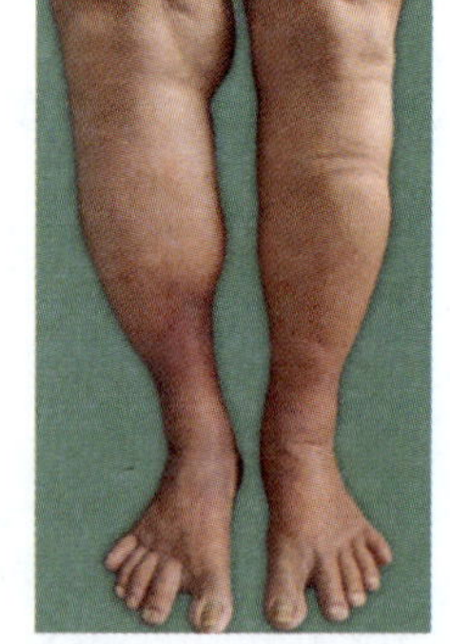

Fig. 30.39: Patient with DVT. (*Courtesy*: Dr Siddesh, senior consultant, Mysore, Karnataka.)

Investigations

1. **Doppler study:** It is ideal for femoral vein thrombosis or if the thrombus extends into the popliteal vein. Normal femoral vein gives a wind storm sound which completely disappears at the end of inspiration. No sound is heard if there is femoral thrombosis (Key Box 30.15).

Key Box 30.15

Duplex Scanning in Deep Vein Thrombosis (B-Mode)

- Vein is larger than normal because of occlusion
- Not completely compressible
- Lacks respiratory variation
- Does not show flow augmentation with calf compression
- May have collateral flow

- Chronic thrombosis is diagnosed by luminal filling defect on gray-scale images, noncompressible vein, narrow vein, absence of color Doppler, and loss of augmentation.

2. **Contrast venography:** It is done by injecting a radio-opaque dye into the dorsal venous arch with an inflatable cuff both above the ankle and above the knee. The clot appears as a filling defect. However, venography is not routinely done because it is expensive and invasive.

Treatment

Chronic DVT

- Graded compression stockings and anticoagulation therapy. Compression stockings (30–40 mmHg) should be worn daily for 2 years from the onset of DVT.
- Parenteral anticoagulation initially, followed by oral anticoagulation titrated to the INR. Vitamin K antagonist (warfarin 5–10 mg/day) is given and INR is monitored (INR should remain between 2.0 and 3.0).
- Patients with proximal DVT (iliofemoral), recurrent episodes, or DVT secondary to malignancy should be treated for 6 months–1 year. Indefinite therapy is recommended for patients with recurrent episodes of venous thrombosis, regardless of the cause.
- Post-phlebitis limb with ulcers may heal with aspirin and pentoxifylline.
- **Chronic thrombosed veins are treated by balloon dilatation—venoplasty, thrombolysis.** Venous stenting is frequently needed of the IVC and iliac veins to maintain flow and venous patency.
- **Surgery** is not done routinely. However, in chronic cases, venous bypass has been attempted with moderate success. **Palma** operation is performed for iliofemoral thrombosis wherein the common femoral vein below the block is anastomosed to the opposite femoral vein using the long saphenous vein from the opposite side. **May-Husni** operation, wherein the popliteal vein is anastomosed to long saphenous vein above.

Complications

1. **Permanent oedema** of the limb. The limb has an **inverted beer bottle** appearance.
2. **Pulmonary embolism** because the thrombus is not attached to the vessel wall.
3. **Secondary varicosity** and **nonhealing ulcer**.

PROPHYLAXIS OF DVT (Key Box 30.16)

- Decrease obesity and advise exercises before surgery.
- **Low dose heparin** 5,000 units subcutaneously, 2 hours before surgery and 24 hours after surgery, then 12 hourly for 5 days in cases of major surgeries

Key Box 30.16

Prophylaxis: Risk Groups

- Low risk : >40 years
  Minor illness
  Operation <30 minutes
- Moderate risk : >40 years
  Debilitating illness
  Major surgery <30 minutes
- High risk : >50 years, medical conditions—MI, stroke, recent thromboembolism, orthopaedic surgeries, major surgery, malignancy, obesity.

like cholecystectomy, abdominoperineal resection, etc. Low molecular weight heparin decreases chances of bleeding.

- **Intermittent pneumatic compression** of the calf throughout the operation maintains blood flow in the lower limbs. Inflation pressure is around 30–50 mmHg.
- Dextran 40 inhibits sludging of red blood cells and platelet aggregation.
- **Aspirin** with dipyridamole has been used (antiplatelet agents).
- **Early mobilisation, walking, and adequate hydration.**

MORE DETAILS OF ANTICOAGULATION AND DVT

Treatment should be initiated at the earliest. The main aims are to reduce the morbidity and risk of pulmonary thromboembolism (PTE) and to decrease post-thrombotic sequelae.

Treatment Modalities

1. **Anti-thrombotic therapy:**

   A. **Heparin:** It is a natural anti-coagulant. It is also unfractionated heparin (UFH). Initial IV/SC heparin therapy is continued for a minimum of 5 days. Heparin acts by binding to antithrombin, which in turn inhibits factors IIa, Xa, XIa, and XIIa. It also binds to tissue factor pathway inhibitor, which inhibits the conversion of X to Xa and IX to XIa. It also catalyses inhibition of thrombin by cofactor II, independent of the antithrombin mechanism.

   Dose of heparin: 80 U/kg IV bolus infusion at 18 U/kg/hour or 10000 units IV 8th hourly. The route is later changed to subcutaneous.

   Complications of heparin:

   - Haemorrhage, which may be reversed by protamine sulphate (up to 50 mg IV over 10 mins)
   - **HIT (heparin-induced thrombocytopaenia)** due to heparin-associated antiplatelet antibodies directed against **platelet factor IV**
   - Osteopenia
   - Rarely—skin necrosis/hypersensitivity
   - Hypoaldosteronism and osteoporosis

   Contraindications to heparin therapy:

   - Eye surgery, neurosurgery
   - Bleeding disorders
   - Uncontrolled, severe hypertension
   - Cirrhosis, renal failure

   B. **Low molecular weight heparin (LMWH):** They are safe and efficacious. They may be administered easily once or twice daily subcutaneously. Enoxaparin and dalteparin are a few drugs. Enoxaparin 0.5 mg/kg is given for prophylactic dosing. The therapeutic dose is 100 U/kg twice daily. They act by selectively inhibiting factor Xa. They do not require laboratory monitoring. Compared to heparin, they have a very low chance of resulting in thrombocytopaenia. Since they have lesser anti-platelet action, there are less chances of haemorrhage.

   C. **Fondaparinux:** It is a synthetic pentasaccharide factor Xa inhibitor. The dose depends on the weight of the patient—5 mg OD (once daily) for 50 kg, 7.5 mg OD for 50–100 kg, 10 mg OD for ≥100 kg given as subcutaneous injections.

   D. **Direct thrombin inhibitors:** Examples include hirudin, agatroban, and bivalirudin. They are indicated in patients with HIT. They are usually given for 7 days till platelet counts normalize and then heparin is re-introduced. Dosing is as follows. Hirudin 4 mg/kg IV bolus f/b infusion T½—30–60 min with APTT at 1.5 to 2.5 times. Agatroban 2 µg/kg/min infusion, T½—40–50 min with APTT at 1.5 to 3 times.

   E. **Warfarin (Wisconsin Alumni Research Foundation coumARIN):** It is given orally, 2–10 mg/day. It interferes with hepatic synthesis of vitamin K-dependent soluble anticoagulation factors. An advantage of warfarin is that it is given orally. Its disadvantage is that it requires more frequent monitoring than heparin. Bleeding may occur, if the INR ratio is high.

   F. **Acitrom (Acenocoumarol)** is another anticoagulant used in the treatment and prevention of abnormal blood clots. It is similar to warfarin but has a longer half-life and less interactions. It does not dissolve formed blood clots but may prevent them from becoming larger and leading to more serious problems like embolism.

2. **Thrombolysis:** It is popularly called catheter-directed thrombolysis. Streptokinase, urokinase, etc. are used. They convert plasminogen to plasmin which in turn degrades fibrin, thereby dissolving the clots.

Advantages of thrombolysis include early recovery of symptoms and signs, early prevention of pulmonary thromboembolism, and prevention of post-phlebitis syndrome. However, clot propagation and re-thrombosis cannot be prevented.

Alteplase: Recombinant tissue plasminogen activator (rtPA). It is given as a 10 mg IV bolus, followed by a 90 mg infusion over 90 minutes.

3. **IVC (inferior vena cava) filters:** Patients with recurrent embolism, pelvic vein thrombosis, or large calf venous thrombosis may be treated with IVC filters. The IVC filter is placed through a small incision in a vein in the groin or neck. A thin, flexible tube (catheter) is inserted inside the vein. The catheter is then gently guided into the IVC. An IVC filter is introduced into the vein in a collapsed state. The filter is left in place, and the catheter is removed. The filter then expands and attaches itself to the walls of the IVC. In a few cases of recurrent thromboembolism, it may be left in place permanently. In some cases, it may be removed after a period of time.
4. **Operative thrombectomy:** It is definitely indicated for pulmonary embolism but is rarely performed for leg veins.

MISCELLANEOUS

PELVIC CONGESTION SYNDROME

A few premenopausal patients complain of dull aching/severe pain in the pelvis. Clinical examination may reveal tenderness in the hypogastrium. A few salient features are given below.

Premenopausal patients
Excessive micturition, excessive bleeding during menstruation
Leg varicosity in atypical sites, such as the thigh
Varicosity of the ovary, vulva, pelvic veins
Increased on standing
Chronic, noncyclical pelvic pain

Remember as **PELVIC**

Management

- Ultrasound, CT, and MRI may be necessary to rule out a pelvic pathology.
- Psychotherapy and nonsteroidal anti-inflammatory drugs are of some help.

PULMONARY THROMBOEMBOLISM

- Mostly thrombus originates in the leg veins—from deep veins and cause pulmonary embolism. Prolonged immobilisation, postoperative patients, major fracture long bones are a few important causes. Patients present with the following features. Recently COVID-19 infections have been associated with many cases of thrombosis.
- Tachypnoea and tachycardia
- Chest pain cough with or without streaks of blood
- Breathlessness
- ECG may show an S1Q3T3 pattern (S wave in lead I, Q and inverted T waves in lead III).

Investigations

- Ventilation perfusion scan (V/Q)
- CT angiography of the thorax

Treatment

- Rest, compression bandage, elevation
- Anti-DVT treatment

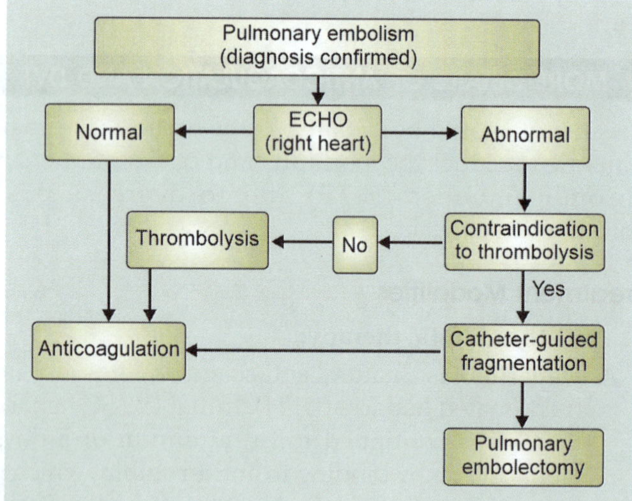

Clinical Notes

Heparin was started on the 5th day for 5 days. He was advised 4 mg of warfarin postoperatively for 6 months, with frequent monitoring of APTT and INR. The dose of warfarin was adjusted after 1 month. He was also advised to wear elastic compression stockings. At the end of 6 months, his DVT was completely cured.

Multiple Choice Questions

1. Which of the following statements is false regarding long saphenous vein anatomy?
A. It starts from the dorsal venous arch
B. It ascends in front of the medial malleolus
C. It has 15–20 valves
D. The posterior arch vein is not a tributary of long saphenous vein

2. The following are true for the short saphenous vein *except*:
A. It has 6 valves
B. It ascends behind the lateral malleolus
C. Its termination is often not constant
D. Incompetency results in an ulcer on the lateral side of the leg

3. The following are features of the deep venous system *except*:
A. High pressure system
B. Has valves
C. Present in the soleal group of muscles
D. Connected to the superficial veins

4. The following are true for perforators *except*:
A. They communicate between the superficial and deep veins
B. They are present in the leg
C. They do not have valves
D. SEPS is the endoscopic surgery performed for perforators

5. Trendelenburg test is performed to determine:
A. Saphenopopliteal incompetence
B. Saphenofemoral incompetence
C. Deep vein thrombosis
D. Site of perforators

6. Perthes' test is done to determine:
A. Saphenopopliteal incompetence
B. Saphenofemoral incompetence
C. Deep vein thrombosis
D. Site of perforators

7. The characteristic feature of a venous ulcer in the leg is:
A. Deep, painful ulcer
B. Superficial ulcer with surrounding pigmentation
C. Penetrating ulcer with visible bone
D. Ulcers on the dorsum of the foot

8. Plethysmography is based on the measurement of which of the following?
A. Volume changes
B. Pressure changes
C. Sound changes
D. Velocity

9. The following are true for Doppler ultrasound *except*:
A. It can detect patency of veins
B. It can detect arterial pulses
C. It acts by the Doppler principle
D. It is used to visualise movement of blood within a vessel

10. The following are true about injection sclerotherapy for treating varicose veins *except*:
A. The vein has to be full during injection
B. Below-knee varicosity may be treated with sclerotherapy
C. Recurrent varicosity may be treated with sclerotherapy
D. It is useful in veins with <3 mm diameter

11. Which of the following is true about radiofrequency ablation?
A. Long saphenous varicosity may be treated
B. Hepatoma >6 cm is often an indication for treatment
C. May be used for Barrett's oesophagus
D. Nerves and cardiac muscles are not stimulated during the treatment

12. The following are true for venous ulcer formation *except*:
A. Ambulatory venous hypertension
B. Free radical release
C. Fibrin, fibronectin, collagen IV
D. Haem deposition

13. The earliest sign of DVT is:
A. Calf tenderness
B. Rise in temperature
C. Swelling of calf muscles
D. Homan's sign

14. The following are seen in DVT *except*:
A. High fever
B. Increased local temperature
C. Pain
D. Tenderness

Answers

1. D	**2.** C	**3.** C	**4.** C	**5.** B	**6.** C	**7.** B	**8.** A	**9.** D	**10.** A
11. B	**12.** D	**13.** A	**14.** A						

CHAPTER

31

Skin Tumours

- Classification of skin tumours
- Premalignant lesions
- Basal cell carcinoma
- Squamous cell carcinoma
- Melanocytic tumours
- Malignant melanoma
- RECIST criteria
- Other malignant skin tumours
- Other skin lesions

INTRODUCTION

The skin, the outermost coat of the human body, functions as a protective cover against various insulting agents, such as ultraviolet radiation, excessive heat, and various chemical agents.

- Hence, it is one of the commonest cancers in elderly patients. However, more than 90% of skin tumours are curable because they are diagnosed early and easily (unlike intra-abdominal malignancies). Many of them are low-grade cancers. Among skin cancers, about 70% are basal cell carcinomas, 20% are squamous cell carcinomas, and 5% are melano-carcinomas.
- Other rare skin cancers are sebaceous carcinomas, dermatofibrosarcomas, etc. In this chapter, only common malignant skin tumours and some common skin lesions, such as corn and wart, are discussed.

CLASSIFICATION OF SKIN TUMOURS

I. Epidermal Tumours

A. Benign

- Papilloma
- Seborrhoeic keratosis
- Verrucous naevus

B. Malignant

- Basal cell carcinoma
- Epithelioma and Marjolin ulcer

II. Melanocytic Tumours

A. Benign

- Junctional naevus
- Compound naevus
- Intradermal naevus
- Hutchinson's freckle
- Hairy and blue naevus

B. Malignant

- Superficial spreading melanoma
- Nodular melanoma
- Lentigo maligna melanoma
- Amelanotic melanoma
- Acral lentiginous melanoma
- Desmoplastic melanoma

III. Sweat Gland Tumours (Malignant)

- Hidradenocarcinoma
- Adenoid cystic carcinoma

IV. Sebaceous Gland Tumours

- Sebaceous adenoma
- Sebaceous carcinoma

V. Other Tumours

- Dermatofibrosarcoma protuberans
- Trichofolliculoma (hair follicle tumour)

PREMALIGNANT LESIONS OF THE SKIN AND RISK FACTORS

1. **Chronic irritation** to the skin may occur due to various carcinogenic chemicals, such as dyes, tar and inorganic arsenic. Coal tar contains polycyclic aromatic hydrocarbons, such as benzopyrenes which are carcinogenic, arsenic, soot, mineral oil.
   - Chimney Sweeps' carcinoma, is a scrotal skin cancer caused by an environmental carcinogen-soot. This was observed and brought to the notice of the British Parliament, and the Chimney Sweepers Act was introduced due to the work of Sir Percivall Pott.
2. **Solar keratosis (actinic keratosis):** Prolonged exposure to sun rays may cause *hyperkeratosis* of the skin (solar keratosis). Skin changes occur due to the accumulated effect of ultraviolet rays over a period of many years. Ultraviolet rays are also present in phototherapy used to treat psoriasis (**PUVA** therapy—**P**soralen **U**ltra **V**iolet-**A**).

   Common sites: Back of hands, face, rim of ears.
   - *Age group:* Middle age, more than 50 years.
   - Clinically, the lesion is an irregular, firm, and irritating patch which is flat or raised, and is better felt than seen.
   - Malignancy should be suspected when the lesion becomes indurated, when a nonhealing ulcer develops, when the central crust sheds, or when regional lymph nodes are palpable.
3. **Chronic scar:** Squamous cell carcinoma that develops in scar tissue is called ***Marjolin ulcer*** (Fig. 31.1). **Burns scar** is the most common cause, followed by a varicose ulcer scar, snakebite scar, chronic osteomyelitis scar, and lupus vulgaris (tuberculosis of face) scar.
   - Marjolin ulcer differs from squamous cell carcinoma by the characteristics in Table 31.1.

Pearls of Wisdom

Once Marjolin ulcer infiltrates the normal skin, it behaves like squamous cell carcinoma.

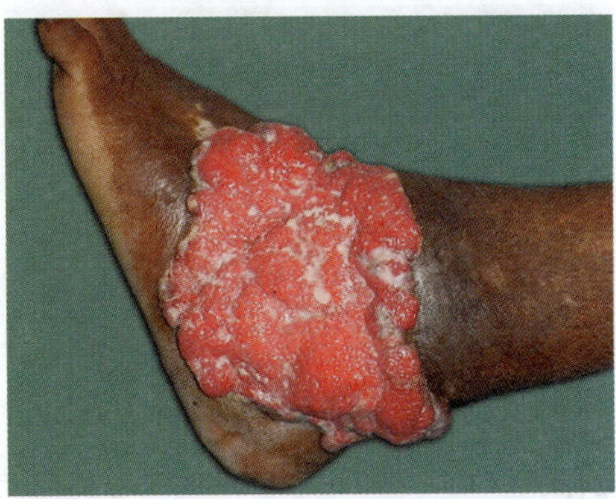

Fig. 31.1: Marjolin ulcer arising in a burns scar

4. **Radiodermatitis:** An increased incidence of skin cancer was initially found in persons who worked in the radiology department. Now, the incidence is less due to the usage of protective gear. Radiation changes in the skin may vary from simple erythema to atrophy or hyperpigmentation. Later, this lesion develops into squamous cell carcinoma.
5. **Bowen's disease** is an intraepidermal carcinoma. Chronic solar damage, inorganic compounds, and human papillomavirus (HPV)-16 are possible aetiological factors. It is rare, and occurs in middle-aged patients. It occurs on the skin of the trunk as scaly, erythematous plaques, which are often multiple. They are brownish patches with raised margins. Microscopically, large clear cells are found (these cells are also found in Paget's disease of the nipple). Topical application of 5-FU and/or imiquimod is an effective treatment (Figs 31.2 and 31.3).
6. **Leukoplakia** (*see* page 350).
7. **Autosomal recessive disorders:** In this group, one or more of the DNA repair enzymes are defective or deficient. As a result, sites exposed to the sun are vulnerable to the development of various skin cancers. **Xeroderma pigmentosum** and **albinism** increase the risk of skin cancer (Fig. 31.4). Muir-Torre syndrome, dystrophic epidermolysis bullosa, Werner syndrome, nevoid basal cell carcinoma, Li-Fraumeni syndrome are the other genetic syndromes with skin cancers.

Table 31.1 Comparison of Marjolin ulcer and squamous cell carcinoma

Marjolin ulcer	Squamous cell carcinoma
Grows very slowly because of scar tissue	Grows slowly
It is painless as scar does not contain nerves	It can be painful if it infiltrates the nerve fibres
Lymphatic metastasis does not occur because lymphatics are destroyed or occluded	Lymphatic metastasis is the chief method of spread
It is less malignant	Comparatively more malignant
Surgery cures the disease, radiotherapy is not very useful	Both surgery and radiotherapy are used

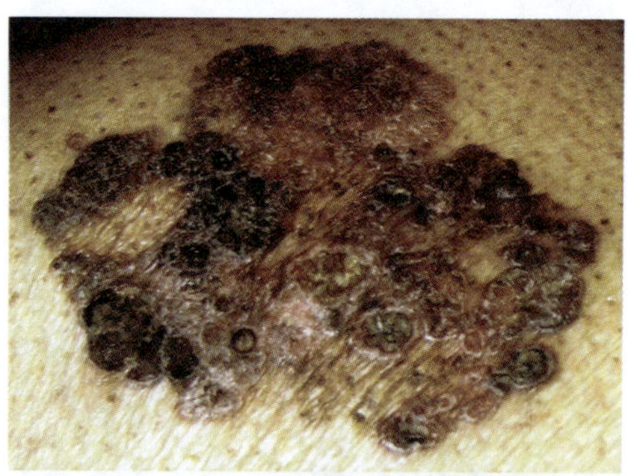

Fig. 31.2: Bowen's disease—premalignant condition

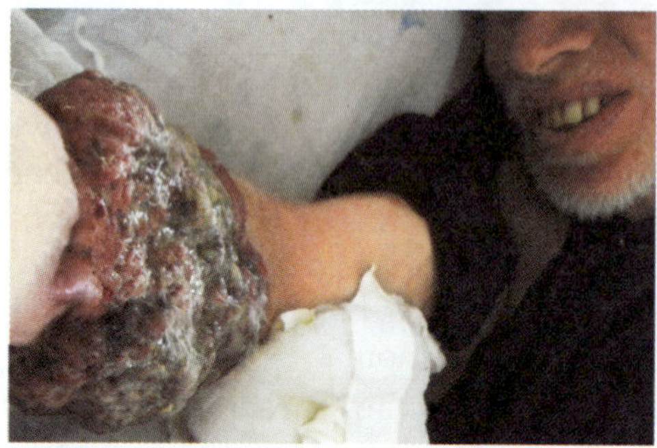

Fig. 31.3: Albinism with squamous cell carcinoma of the right elbow region—patient also has photophobia (*Courtesy*: Dr Satish Deshmukh and Dr Murtaza Akhtar, NKP Salve Medical College and Research Center, Nagpur)

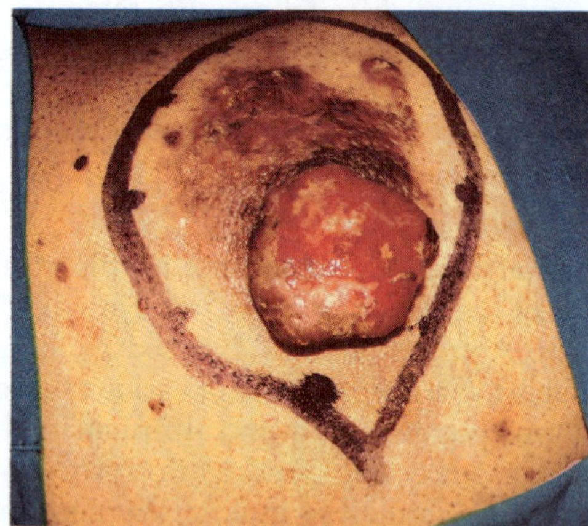

Fig. 31.4: Bowen's disease with ulcerated squamous cell carcinoma

8. Immunosuppression:

- Squamous cell carcinoma develops in 50% of patients within 20 years of organ transplantation due to immunosuppression. Skin cancer is the most common neoplasm after solid organ transplantation.
- Patients with lymphoma, leukaemia, and autoimmune diseases on treatment may also develop skin cancers.
- 30% may be aggressive

> *Pearls of Wisdom*
>
> White race is a definite risk factor for skin cancer. Previous diagnosis of cutaneous carcinoma—increases the risk to 35% at 3 years and 50% at 5 years.

BASAL CELL CARCINOMA (BCC)/RODENT ULCER

It is the ***most common malignant skin tumour.*** It arises from basal cells of the pilosebaceous adnexa and occurs only on the skin. Generally, it is a slow-growing neoplasm which may present as an ulcer of a chronic (many years) duration. ***Metastasis and death from this disease is extremely rare.*** In some cases, it may present as a locally penetrating, ulcerative, and destructive lesion. The majority of lesions are found on the face, above a line from lobule of the ear to the angle of mouth.

Common Sites (Figs 31.5 to 31.8)

- Inner canthus of the eye, outer canthus of the eye, eyelids, bridge of the nose.
- Around the nasolabial fold. These sites are the areas where tears roll down. Hence, BCC is also known as **tear cancer** cell carcinoma (Figs 31.6–31.8).
- **Naevoid basal cell carcinoma syndrome (NBCCS) : Gorlin syndrome** is an inherited medical condition with multiple body systems which are defective, such as the skin, nervous system, endocrine system, eyes, and bones. Inborn kyphoscoliosis and anomalies in the ribs may be present. Other lesions are ovarian fibroma and odontogenic tumours.

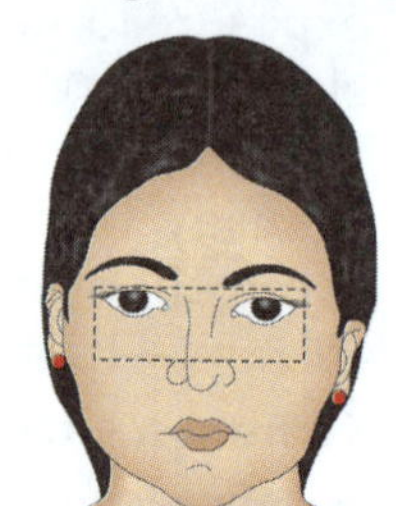

Fig. 31.5: Sites of basal cell carcinoma (BCC)

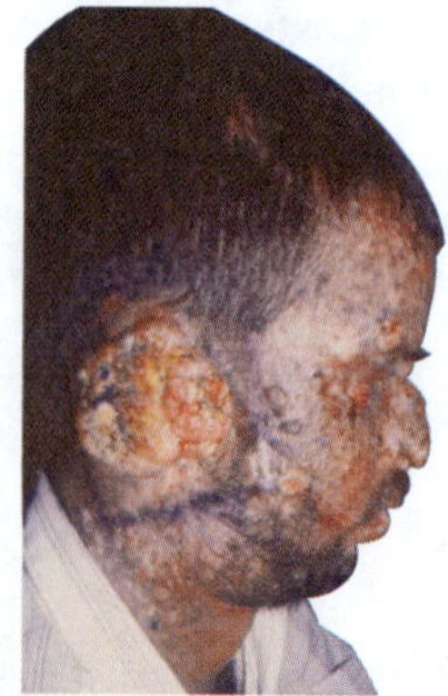

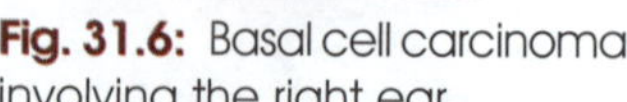

Fig. 31.6: Basal cell carcinoma involving the right ear

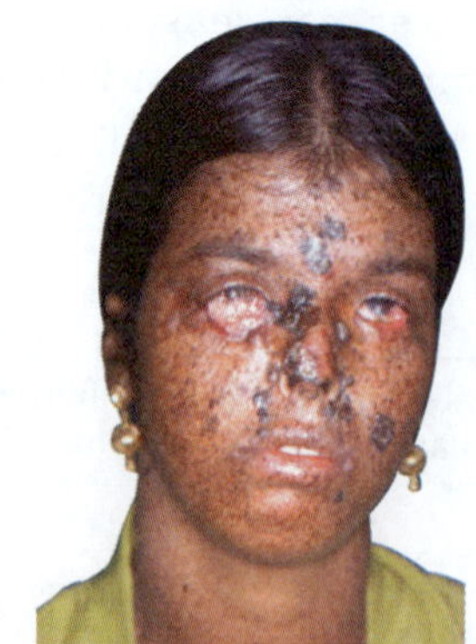

Fig. 31.7: Basal cell carcinoma involving nasolabial fold skin

A brother and sister with **xeroderma pigmentosum** developed 33 and 26 skin malignancies respectively which included basal cell carcinoma, squamous cell carcinoma and malignant melanoma, since the age of 5 till 22 years. Eventually the boy died at 22 years of age (Fig. 31.6). This is the sad part of this distressing and frustrating disease. I have not seen this girl since 20 years now

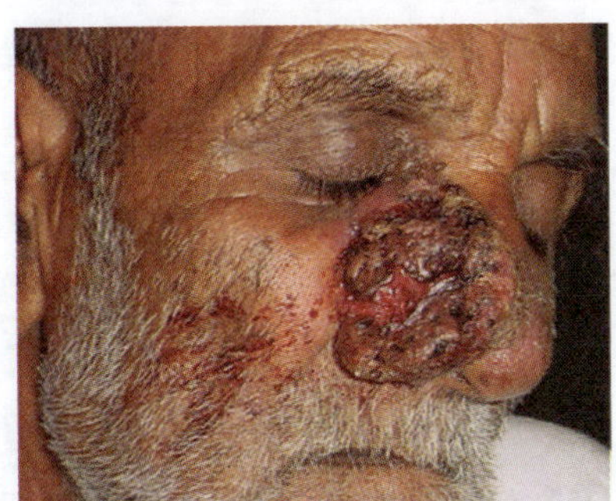

Fig. 31.8: Basal cell carcinoma—typical site

Pearls of Wisdom

Basal cell carcinoma cannot occur in mucosal surfaces that do not have pilosebaceous adnexa (e.g. cervix, lips, tongue).

Precipitating Factors

- **Ultraviolet (UV) rays:** Broad-spectrum short-wavelength **UVB radiation** (290–320 nm) also called as sunburn **rays** are probably responsible for basal cell carcinoma. Basal cell carcinoma is common in Australia[1] and New Zealand because of this reason. Latent peroid between skin damage to development of BCC is about 20 years.
- Fair skin is vulnerable to the development of basal cell carcinoma.
- Arsenic, which was once used in skin ointments, also increases the risk of basal cell carcinoma.

Clinical Features

- The most common clinical presentation is an ulcer that never heals (Fig. 31.9). Sometimes, healing takes place with scabbing, which later breaks down and forms an ulcer again. The ulcer has ***a raised and beaded edge***, may be indurated, and bleeds on touch. The base may be subcutaneous fat or deeper structures, like muscle or bone, depending on the level of invasion.
- When the ***lesion is big***, it is called a ***rodent ulcer*** (Figs 31.10 and 31.11).

Pearls of Wisdom

Scabbing typically occurs only in benign ulcers. Basal cell carcinoma is the only malignant ulcer which shows scabbing.

- It may also present as a ***painless, firm, nodule,*** which is pigmented with fine blood vessels on its surface (Key Box 31.1).
- It may be present in a ***noduloulcerative form*** (Fig. 31.8).
- Rarely, it may be a ***nodulocystic*** variety, which does not show fluctuation.
- **Field fire rodent ulcer** is a rapidly growing rodent ulcer, with destruction and disfigurement of the facial skin. It has an advancing edge with a healed, central scar.
- The more aggressive, infiltrative form is ***morphea-form,*** and the ***more common*** form is the ***nodulo-ulcerative form. Less aggressive:*** Nodular, superficial and micronodular, basosquamous

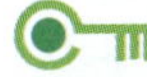

Key Box 31.1

Basal Cell Carcinoma: Types

- Nodular: Nodulocystic or noduloulcerative—70%
- Pigmented
- Superficial: Occur on the trunk
- Cystic
- Infiltrative
- Basosquamous: Rare

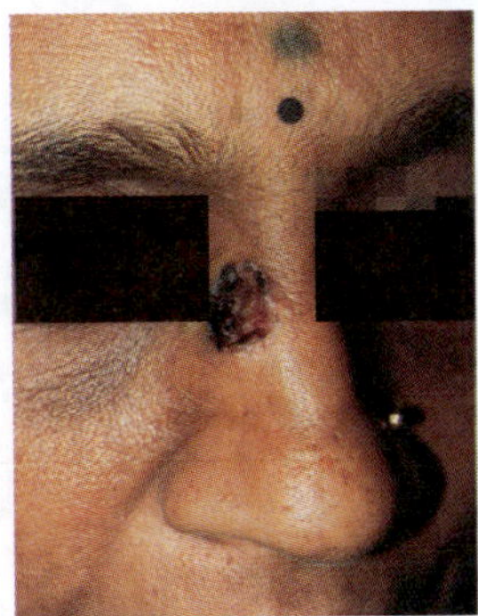

Fig. 31.9: Nonhealing ulcer of 3 years duration—lesion that does not heal and grows slowly—classical history of BCC

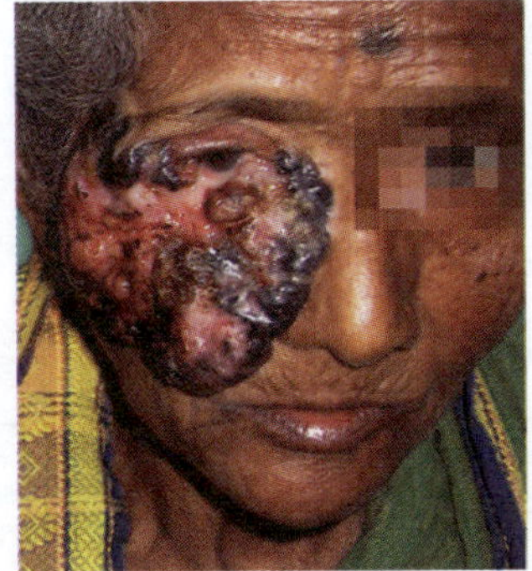

Fig. 31.10: Pigmented large destructive BCC (*Courtesy:* Dr Vidyadhar Kinhal, HOD, Surgery, VIMS, Bellary, Karnataka)

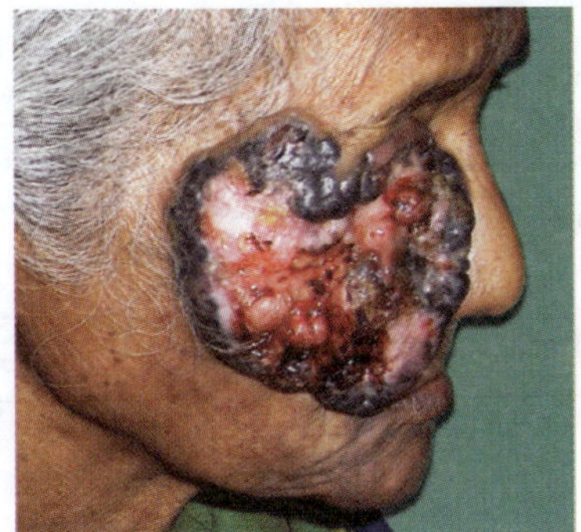

Fig. 31.11: Lateral view of the same patient showing elevated edge, a few areas of scab and slough

[1]This may be the reason why Australian and New Zealand cricket players apply some protective cream to the potentially risky sites while playing the match.

Differential Diagnosis

- **Keratoacanthoma:** It occurs only over the face. The edge may be raised with ulceration, resembling basal cell carcinoma.
- **Sclerosing angioma**
- **Malignant melanoma:** Pigmented basal cell carcinoma may be mistaken for malignant melanoma.
- **Squamous cell carcinoma**

Spread

- It spreads by **local invasion**. Even though it is slow-growing, it slowly penetrates and destroys the deeper underlying tissues, such as bone, cartilage, or even the eyeball (hence, the name rodent ulcer). It **does not spread by lymphatics** because of its large tumour emboli. Blood spread is extremely rare.
- Morpheaform BCC synthesises type IV collagenase and, therefore, spreads rapidly. White scar-like growth pattern is seen in the morpheaform variety.

TNM Staging

TNM STAGING	Skin cancer other than melanoma
T1	Tumour <2 cm in greatest dimension with less than 2 high-risk features
T2	Tumour >2 cm in greatest dimension (or) tumour of any size with 2 or more high-risk features.
T3	Tumour invasion of maxilla, mandible orbit or temporal bone.
T4	Tumour with invasion of skeleton or perineural invasion of skull base
N0	No regional lymph nodes
N1	Metastasis in a single ipsilateral lymph node ≤3 cm
N2	Metastasis in a single ipsilateral lymph node >3 cm but <6 cm; or B/L or contralateral lymph nodes none >6 cm in greatest dimension
N3	Metastasis to lymph node >6 cm in greatest dimension
M0	No metastases
M1	Distant metastases

Investigations

Wedge biopsy from the edge of the ulcer. The edge is selected because of the following reasons:

- The edge is the growing part, so malignant cells are numerous
- The centre has slough or scabs, which may not reveal malignancy
- Comparison with normal skin is possible

Histology (Key Box 31.2, Fig. 31.12)

Types: 1. Basosquamous, 2. Morpheaform, 3. Adenoid, 4. Infiltrative.

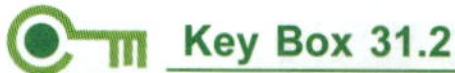

Key Box 31.2

Microscopic Picture

- Central mass of polyhedral cells
- Cells are darkly stained
- With peripheral palisade layer of columnar cells. Cell nests, keratinisation and mitotic figures are absent.

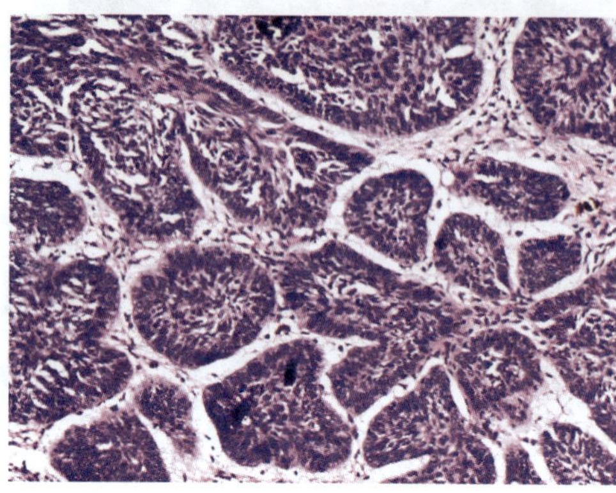

Fig. 31.12: Palisading islands of basaloid cells seen in BCC (*Courtesy:* Dr Laxmi Rao, Head, Department of Pathology, KMC, Manipal)

Treatment

Surgery followed by reconstruction is the main line of treatment.

I. Surgery is indicated when the lesion is very close to the eye, adherent to cartilage or bone, in easily accessible sites, such as the neck or hand and in radiation failure cases. **Wide excision is done in all cases:** This means excision of the growth with at least 3–4 mm of healthy margin all around, including at the base. The resulting defect is closed by:

a. **Primary suturing** of the defect if the lesion is small.

b. **Skin grafting** if defect is big, as in the neck or the dorsum of the hand.

c. **Rotation flaps** in the face for a better cosmetic effect (Figs 31.13–31.20).

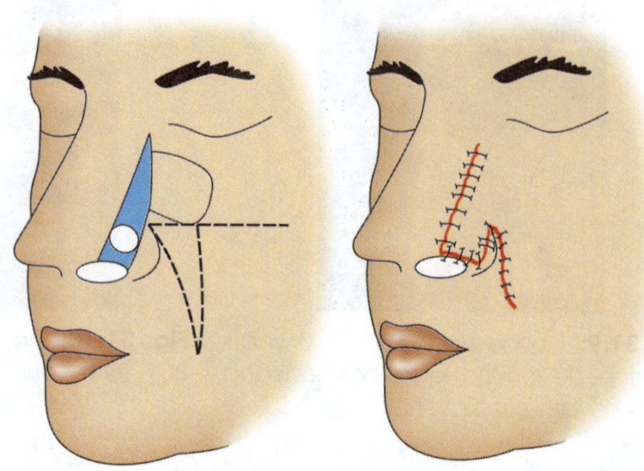

Fig. 31.13: Reconstruction with nasolabial flap following excision

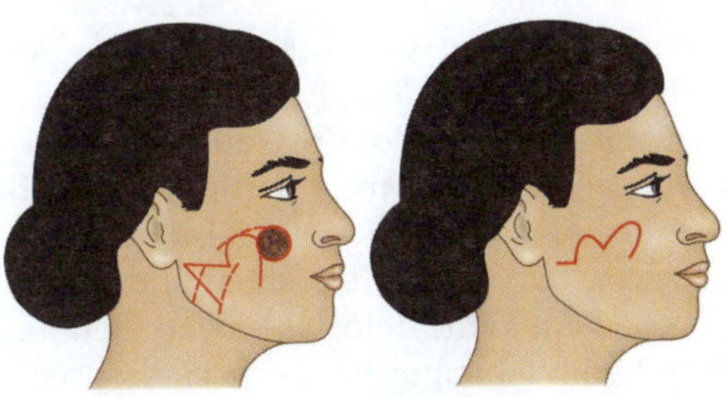

Fig. 31.14: BCC excision and reconstruction by using bilobed flap

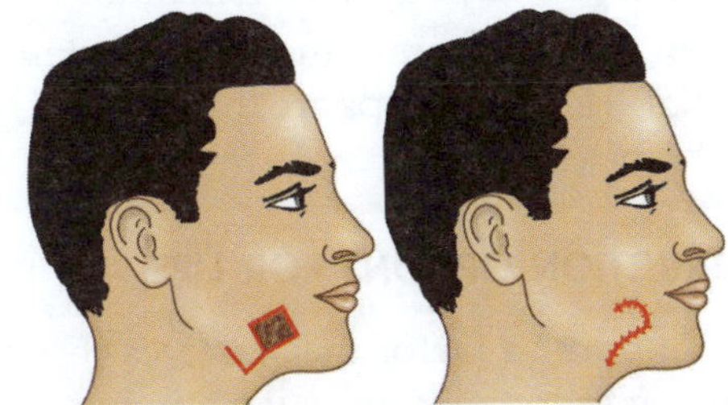

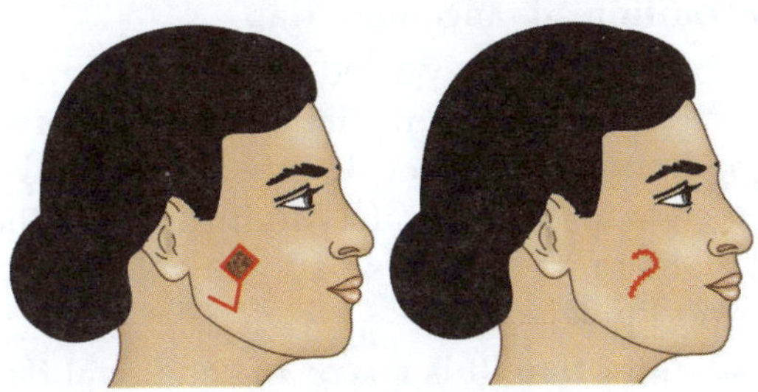

Figs 31.15 and 31.16: BCC reconstruction

Basal cell carcinoma

- **Surgery**
  - Radiorecurrent cases
  - Accessible areas
  - Nearer the eye, nose, cartilage, ear, etc.
- **Radiotherapy**
  - Unfit patients for surgery
  - Large lesions which need complicated surgical procedure
  - **Dosage** 4000—6000 cGy units

Wide excision

Types

- Direct closure (small lesion)
- Split skin grafting (big lesion)
- Flaps (better cosmetic effect)

Fig. 31.17: Treatment of BCC

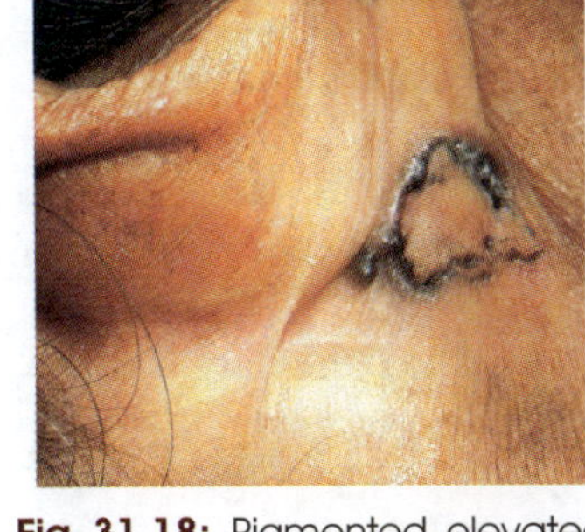

Fig. 31.18: Pigmented, elevated lesion—5 years duration

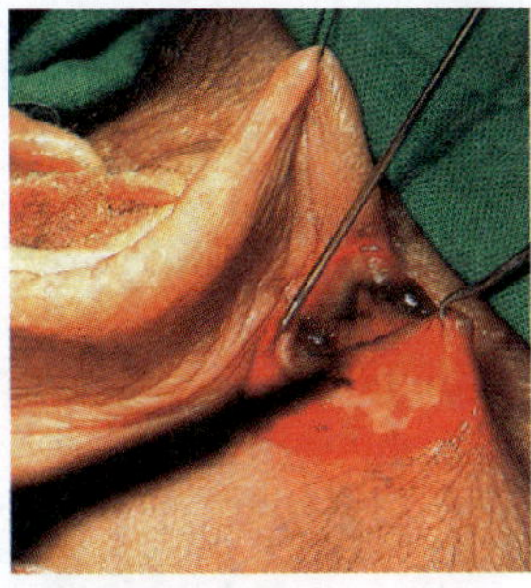

Fig. 31.19: Wide excision in progress

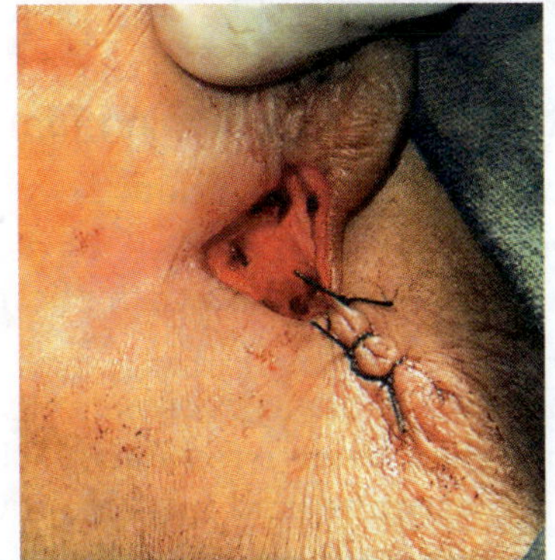

Fig. 31.20: Wide exersion and suturing

Mohs' micrographic surgery: It is a special surgical technique which involves excision of skin cancer under microscopic control. It minimises the chance of recurrence and maximises conservation of the surrounding normal tissue. The technique offers complete evaluation of the lateral and deep margins of the tumour site. This procedure gives better cosmetic results, since only a minimal amount of normal tissue is removed.

Indications for Mohs' procedure are:

- Centrofacially located tumours
- Large tumours, poorly defined tumour margins
- Lesions with perineural/perivascular involvement
- Tumours at the site of prior radiation therapy
- Tumours in the setting of immunosuppression
- High-risk histological subtype of BCC
- Recurrent lesions

II. Radiation is indicated in elderly patients who have an extensive lesion requiring a complicated plastic reconstruction. ***Dosage:*** 4000–6000 cGy units. Radiation chondritis and osteitis are the complications.

III. Other forms of treatment

- Small and superficial: Curettage with electro-desiccation.
- Liquid nitrogen for tumours <1 cm in diameter.
- **CO_2 laser** (Key Box 31.3).

Key Box 31.3

CO_2 Laser in Basal Cell Carcinoma

- Useful in superficial BCC that are confined to epidermis and papillary dermis.
- At least 4 mm surrounding healthy skin should be removed.
- Patients with multiple tumours or in hereditary Gorlin's syndrome—laser is very useful.
- Acts by superficial vaporisation.
- Pathological margins cannot be examined.
- Indication in high risk BCC—large (>2 cm), located near eye, nose, ear.
- Precancerous/low grade BCC.

Flaps and Reconstruction following Tumour Excision

1. **Healing by secondary intention:**

   Simplest method: Suitable only if the defect is <1 cm, superficial, and located in a cosmetically inconspicuous site.

   Disadvantage: Not always cosmetically acceptable; may result in contour irregularity, distortion of surrounding structure, and unstable coverage.
2. **Primary closure:** **In the majority of cases, this is possible.** Simple, but the defect needs to be small. Possible only if excessive tension and distortion can be avoided.
3. **Skin graft:**
   - A skin graft does not look like normal skin, but provides a good skin cover.
   - Cannot be used across a joint. Cosmetically acceptable, but does not give colour and contour match. Preferred if the patient has a high risk of local recurrence, such as in malignant melanoma. Two types of skin garft : Split and full thickness grafts.
   - *Skin grafts will not take on* in following situations: Cortical bone without periosteum, Cartilage without perichondrium, tendon without paratenon and in irradiated tissues.
4. **Commonly used skin flaps:**
   - ***Rotation flap:*** It is a semicircular flap of skin and subcutaneous tissues which rotate about a pivot point into the defect to be closed. A small triangle of skin may be removed to facilitate rotation.
   - ***Advancement flap:*** The defect is closed by stretching the skin. It may be a single, double, or V-Y advancement flap. V-Y flap is an example: Good for defects on the medial cheek and ala of the nose. **V-shaped incision** is made and then advanced to cover the defect, which is later sutured in a 'Y' shape.
   - ***Transposition flap:*** Bilobed and rhomboid flaps are a few examples. A rectangular piece of skin and subcutaneous tissue is rotated. Types of transposition flap are: 1. **Banner flap:** Provides excellent contour and a reasonable colour match. It can only be used for small defects. 2. **Bilobed flap:** Banner flap uses a single lobe. In this flap, however, two lobes are created and then rotated. It is used when the defect is too large enough to be closed with a banner flap, especially useful in the area around the nose. It produces a conspicuous scar and is less desirable than a banner flap. **3. Rhomboid flap:** Geometric modification of the banner flap. It may be used for medium-sized defects.
5. **Complex flaps:** Pectoralis major myocutaneous flaps and radial artery free flaps are the complex flaps used for reconstruction.

RECONSTRUCTION OPTIONS FOR LIPS

The most important factor that dictates reconstruction is the amount of remaining lip vermilion.

A. **Primary closure for small defects**

B. **Vermilion advancement flap**

C. **Abbe flap:** Mainly used for the upper lip. It is harvested based on the labial artery. It provides a good cosmetic effect. It causes minimal loss of function in the lower lip. Modification of the Abbe flap, like reverse Abbe flap, may also be used for lower lip defects.

D. **Estlander flap:** It is a type of rotational flap from upper lip to lower lip. It produces a round commissure and loss of the normal taper of vermilion.

E. **Webster-Bernard flap:** It is a medial advancement of cheek tissue to create a new lower lip. It gives a good result. **Disadvantage:** Results in significant facial scarring.

F. Very large lower lip defects may also be closed with 'double central severe Abbe's flap' or **bilateral Karapandzic flap** (*see* page 364).

SQUAMOUS CELL CARCINOMA (SCC)/EPITHELIOMA

It is the **second most common malignant skin tumour,** after basal cell carcinoma. It arises from the prickle cell layer of the Malpighian layer of the skin. It usually affects elderly males. All the premalignant conditions listed earlier apply to this condition as well. It may also occur *de novo.* Basosquamous carcinoma is the term applied to squamous cell carcinoma arising in a pre-existing basal cell carcinoma. It is interesting to note that a variety of names have been given to squamous cell carcinoma, based on its site (Table 31.2). Also Table 31.3 summarizes the typical sites of SCC, in terms of skin, mucous membrane, and junction involvement.

Table 31.2 Sites of squamous cell carcinoma

Site	Name	Reason/explanation
Skin of the abdomen or back of thigh in Kashmiri patients	**Kangri cancer**	**Kangri** is the name given to the **pot containing hot charcoal** which is applied to the abdominal wall because of excessive cold in Kashmir (India)
Buttocks, heels, elbows	**Kang cancer**	Tibetans sleep on the **oven bed** due to excess cold
Scrotum	**Chimney sweep cancer**	Seen in **chimney sweepers** due to prolonged irritation by chemicals such as tar
Abdominal wall	***Saree* cancer and *Dhothi* cancer**	Due to chronic irritation caused by wearing *dhothi* or *saree* too tight
Lower lip	**Countryman's lip**	Carcinoma lower lip is common in **agriculturists** (outdoor occupation)

Table 31.3 Typical sites of squamous cell carcinoma

Skin	Junction	Mucous membrane
• Dorsum of hand • Limbs • Face • Abdominal wall	• Between skin and mucous membrane • Lip • Penis • Vulva	• Lined by stratified squamous epithelium as in oral cavity and oesophagus • Lined by columnar epithelium, wherein squamous metaplasia occurs, such as gallbladder, bronchus • Lined by transitional cell epithelium with metaplasia as in urinary bladder

Pathological Types

- Ulcerative variety—most common
- Proliferative growth—cauliflower like
- Ulcero-proliferative

Clinical Features (Figs 31.21–31.27)

- Most lesions are preceded by actinic keratosis. Such lesions grow slowly and are locally invasive without metastasis. If not from keratosis, the lesion is aggressive and metastatic.
- Typically, it is an ulcerative or cauliflower-like lesion (Fig. 31.21).
- The edge is everted and the base is indurated and it may be subcutaneous tissue, muscle or bone. The floor contains **cancerous tissue which looks like granulation tissue.** It is pale, friable, and bleeds easily on touch (Figs 31.22–31.23).
- The surrounding area is also indurated.
- Mobility is usually restricted, due to infiltration of the underlying structures. In very early cases, the ulcer can be moved along with skin over the underlying structures.
- Regional lymph nodes, such as inguinal lymph nodes (both vertical and horizontal groups), may get

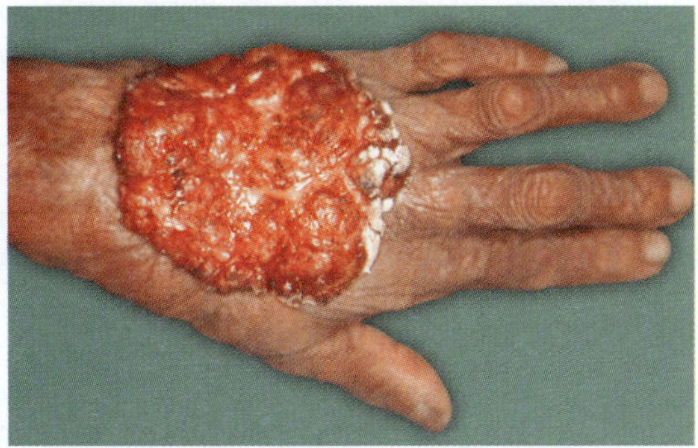

Fig. 31.21: Squamous cell carcinoma affecting dorsum of the hand—ulceroproliferative lesion

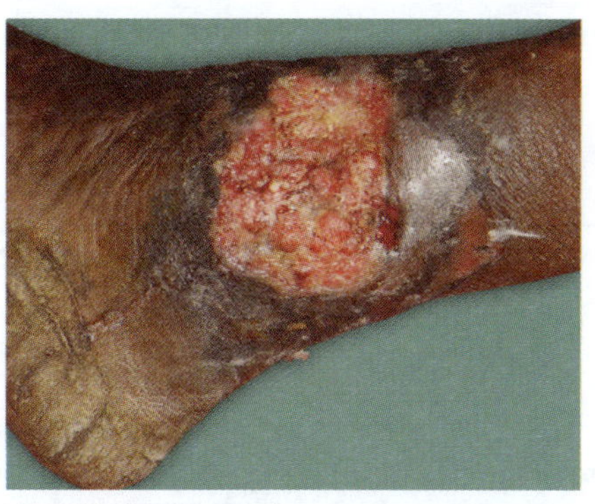

Fig. 31.22: Squamous cell carcinoma—bleeds on touch

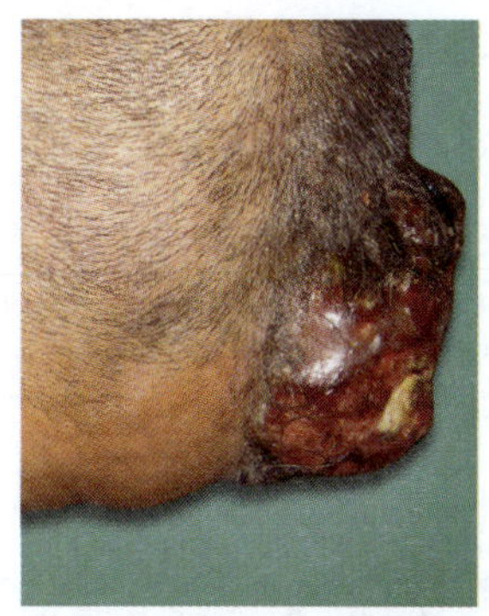

Fig. 31.23: Epithelioma scalp—large ulcerating bleeding lesion

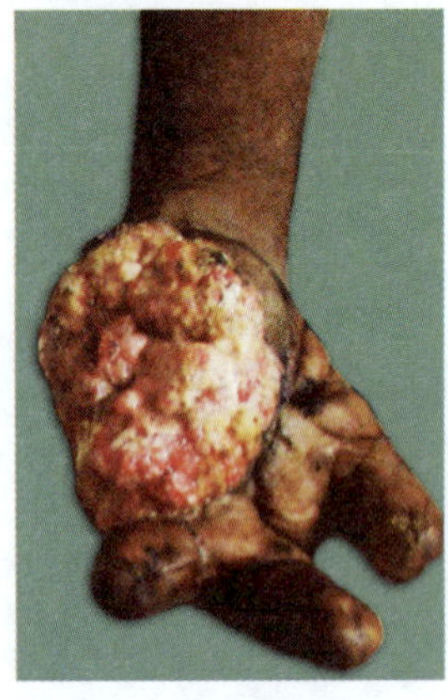

Fig. 31.24: Squamous cell carcinoma arising in leprosy scar

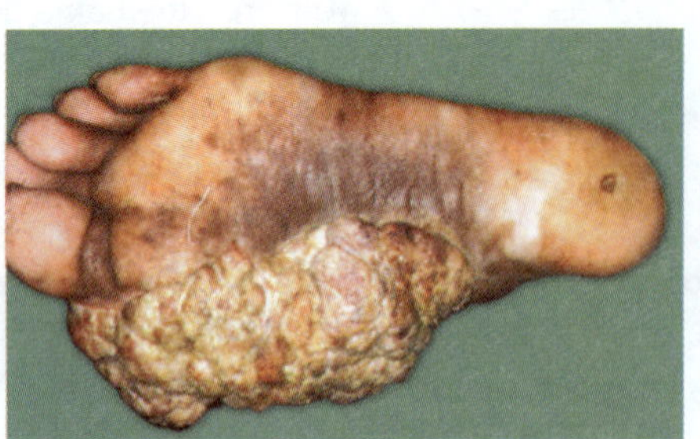

Fig. 31.25: Squamous cell carcinoma of the sole

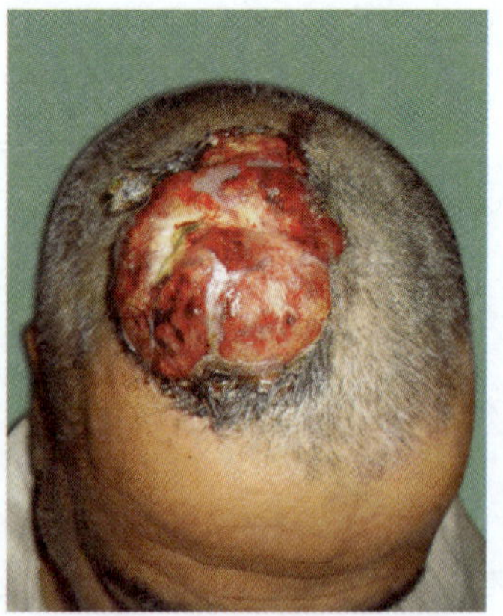

Fig. 31.26: A large epithelioma of the scalp—biopsy proved squamous cell carcinoma

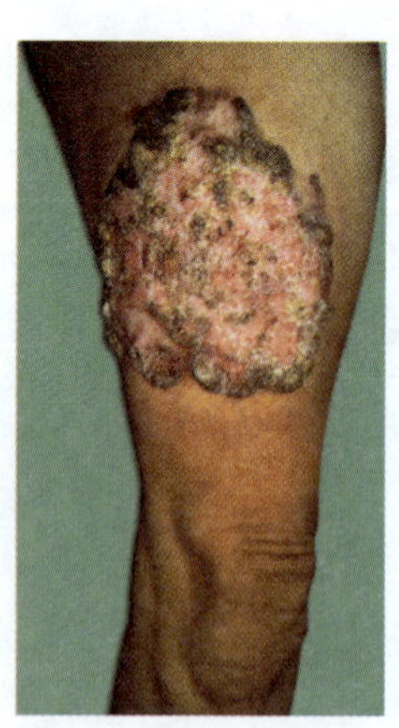

Fig. 31.27: Bowen's disease with squamous cell carcinoma

enlarged when squamous cell carcinoma affects the lower limb or abdominal wall. Hard lymph nodes are suggestive of secondaries.

Spread

1. **Local spread** occurs by infiltration into the surrounding tissues. Depending on the site, various structures may be involved. Some examples are:
   - Tendon involvement in the dorsum of the hand.
   - Muscle involvement in the abdominal wall.
   - Bone involvement (e.g. tibia is involved in carcinoma developing in a varicose ulcer or mandible in carcinoma cheek).
2. **Lymphatic spread** is the chief mode of spread, though it occurs relatively late. Regional nodes are involved first.
   - Nodes which are soft to firm and tender are due to secondary infection.
   - Nodes which are hard, nontender, with or without fixity are due to secondary deposits.
   - In untreated cases, nodes start ulcerating through the skin and result in bleeding and pain.
   - As already stated, nodes are not involved in Marjolin ulcer.
3. **Blood spread** is rare and late.

Differential Diagnoses

Various benign skin lesions may look like squamous cell carcinoma in early cases (Key Box 31.4).

Investigations

- A wedge biopsy from the edge of the ulcer/growth is taken. Main reason being edge is the most proliferative area in malignancies. However, in proliferative lesions, punch biopsy may also be taken.

Pearls of Wisdom

Epithelial pearls are absent in poorly differentiated carcinomas.

Key Box 31.4

Differential Diagnosis

Basal cell carcinoma	:	Typical sites
Keratoacanthoma	:	Benign self-limiting
Papilloma	:	Benign lesion
Pyogenic granuloma	:	Painful, short duration
Tuberculous ulcer	:	Uncommon

- **Microscopic picture:** 80% of these cancers are well-differentiated (Key Box 31.5), characterised by a central, structureless mass of keratin, surrounded by normal looking squamous cells arranged in **concentric manner like onion skin.** This appearance is known as an **epithelial pearl or cell nest** (Fig. 31.28). In 20% of cases, cells are **undifferentiated** with numerous mitoses and without keratinisation.

Key Box 31.5

Broder's Classification

I. Well differentiated	75% keratin pearls
II. Moderately differentiated	50% keratin pearls
III. Poorly differentiated	25% keratin pearls
IV. Anaplastic	<25% keratin pearls

Treatment

I. Treatment of the primary: Epithelioma is treated by wide excision or radiotherapy.

A. Surgery (Figs 31.29 and 31.30): It is indicated when lesion is small and superficial, lesion involving deeper tissues, such as muscles, cartilage, or bone or in radio-recurrent cases. Excision involves removal of the growth along with 1 cm of normal healthy tissue from

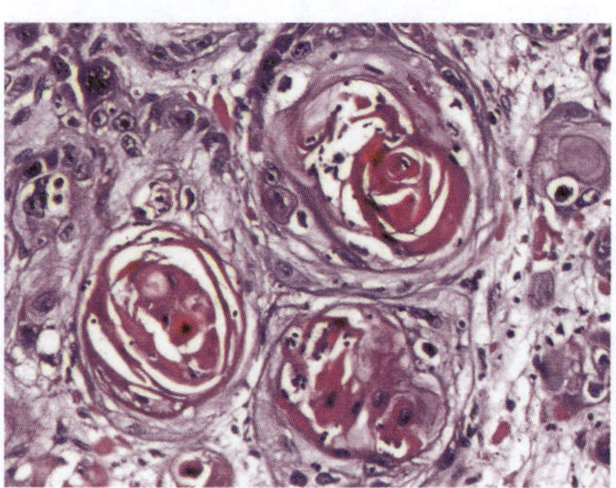

Fig. 31.28: Classical keratin pearls—well-differentiated squamous cell carcinoma (*Courtesy:* Dr. Laxmi Rao, Head, Department of Pathology, KMC, Manipal)

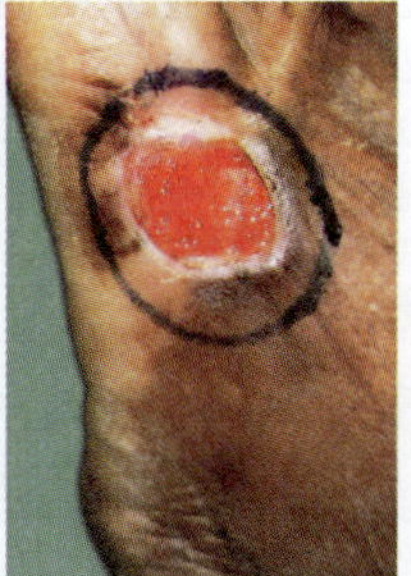

Fig. 31.29: Wide excision of squamous cell carcinoma

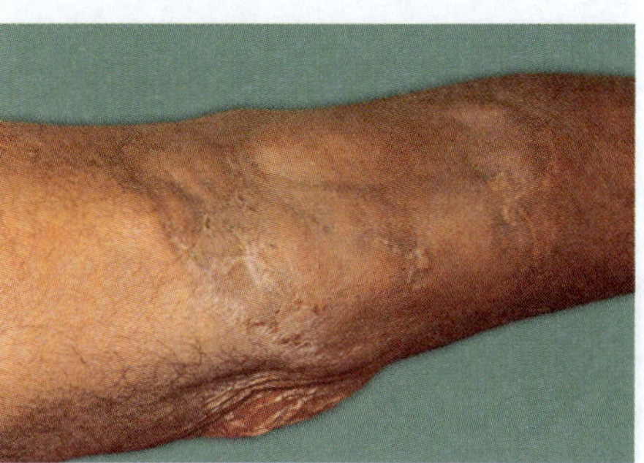

Fig. 31.30: Wide excision followed by skin grafting on 3rd year follow-up

the palpable, indurated edge of the tumour in high-risk cases. In low-risk patients, lesions may be excised with a 4–6 mm margin. After wide excision, the defect may be closed with a split skin graft or with a flap to reconstruct the part, depending on the extent of resection. If the growth is fixed to the tibia, growth can be removed with involved periosteum followed by radiotherapy. One attempt should be aimed at preserving the limb. If it recurs then below knee amputation is performed.

B. Radiotherapy: Is indicted for the following reasons

Primary

1. Patients unable or unwilling to undergo surgical treatment for the primary lesion
2. Clear margins cannot be obtained by surgery
3. Adjuvant treatment
4. Histologically aggressive (e.g. perineural invasion)
5. High grade
6. Bone invasion (Fig. 31.31)
7. Lymph nodes—adjuvant or palliative intent

II. Treatment of the metastasis in the lymph nodes

- In about 20% patients, enlarged regional nodes are due to secondary infection. In all such suspected

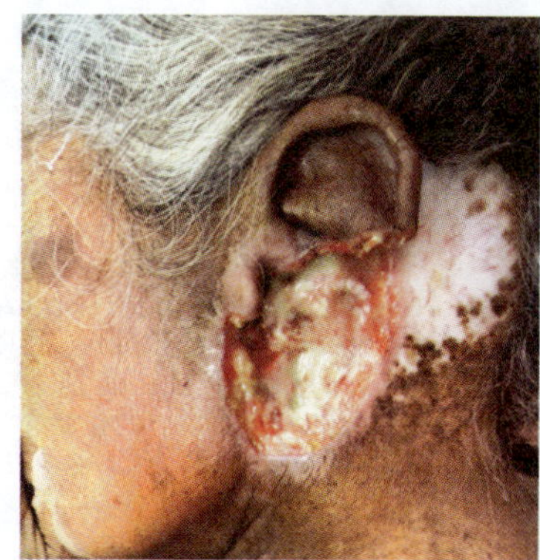

Fig. 31.31: Large penetrating baso-squamous cell carcinoma with destruction of the left ear and infiltrating mastoid process and external ear

cases, ultrasound guided FNAC is done. If found negative, treat the primary. Once the primary is treated and antibiotics are administered, lymph nodes may regress. During follow-up 'wait and watch policy' is observed.
- If the lymph nodes are positive for malignancy, radical block dissection is done. Thus, squamous cell carcinoma of the leg requires inguinal block dissection.

  If lymph nodes are hard and fixed to the femoral vessels, chemo-radiotherapy is given first. combinations of cisplatin with 5-fluorouracil (5-FU), doxorubicin, or bleomycin have been used. Radiotherapy dose is 3000–4000 cGy units over 3–4 weeks, 200 units/day.
- Lymph nodes may regress following chemoradiotherapy and block dissection is done.
- Even in advanced fungating lesions, the response rate to radiotherapy is reasonably good. Dose: 3000 to 4000 cGy units over 3 to 4 weeks 200 units/day.

Structures Removed in Inguinal Block Dissection

(More details in page 270)

- The superficial group of nodes, consisting of a horizontal chain which lies below inguinal ligament and a vertical chain which lies along the upper 5–6 cm of the long saphenous vein (these two groups of nodes form the letter T).
- The deep glands, located along the proximal end of the femoral vein and one lying within the femoral canal.
- Fat, fascia, and lymphatics are cleared from 2 cm above the inguinal ligament up to 2 cm below the saphenofemoral junction. The medial clearance is important up to the femoral canal. Around 8–10 cm of the long saphenous vein near its termination is removed to facilitate lymph node clearance.
- The saphenous vein may be preserved if nodal tissue is removed from the vessel circumferentially; otherwise, it is sacrificed.

- Cloquet's node is sent as a separate specimen for frozen section examination.

Pearls of Wisdom

Fixity to muscle, veins, fascia and bones is not a contraindication for block dissection. Carotid and femoral artery infiltration make it inoperable. Preoperative chemo-radiotherapy should be given all such cases to downstage the disease. Reassessment is done again. If operable, then radical block dissection is done.

Complications of Inguinal Block Dissection and Treatment

- Wound infection → Broad-spectrum antibiotics
- Lymphorrhoea → Adequate drainage
- Haemorrhage → Perfect haemostasis
- Flap necrosis → Edges to be trimmed. At surgery Avoid sharp corner
- Femoral blow-out → Dangerous complication. Sartorius muscle slide to cover femoral vessels at the end of surgery should be done.

Summary of the Treatment of Squamous Cell Carcinoma (Fig. 31.32)

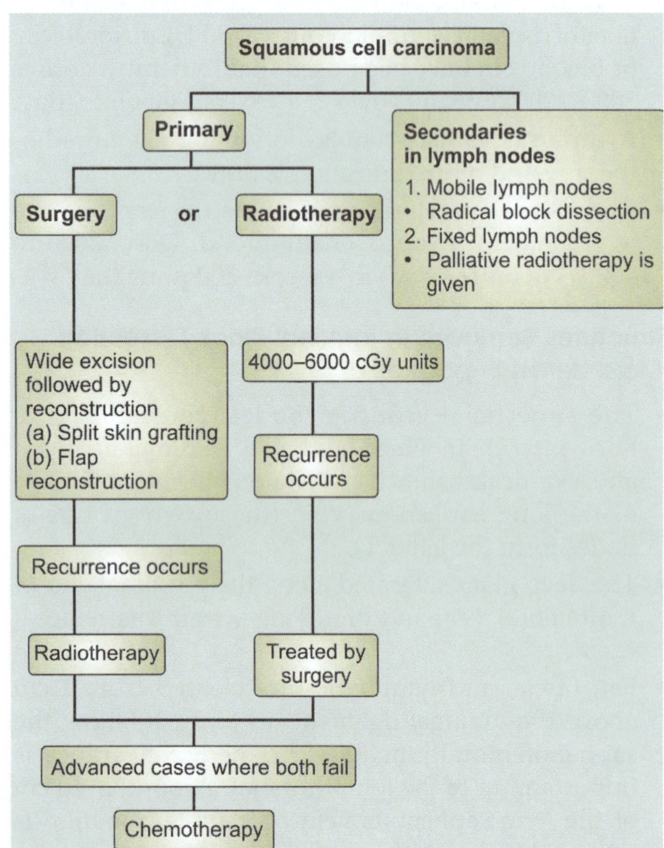

Fig. 31.32: Fixity to major vessels such as carotid and femoral artery is a contraindication. After palliative radiotherapy—reassessment should be done for the feasibility of surgery.

Prognostic Factors (Key Box 31.6)

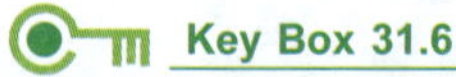

Key Box 31.6

Prognostic Factors of SCC

- *Invasion:* Deeper the lesions or SCC less than 2 mm, metastasis is unlikely. If it is greater than 6 mm—15% SCC may have metastasised
- *Broder's grade higher:* Worse prognosis
- *Site:* Lip and ear—high chances of recurrence
- *Immunosuppression:* Poor prognosis
- *Perineural involvement:* Worse prognosis

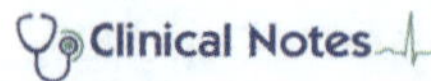

Clinical Notes

This patient with large epithelioma was examined by postgraduate student and he offered the correct diagnosis. However, he did not examine the inguinal region. The groin had 3–4 hard nodes (Figs 31.33 and 31.34). He failed in the examination.

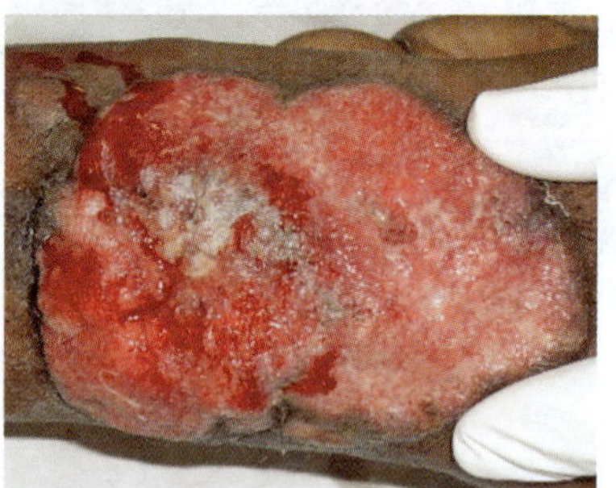

Fig. 31.33: Large epithelioma below knee region

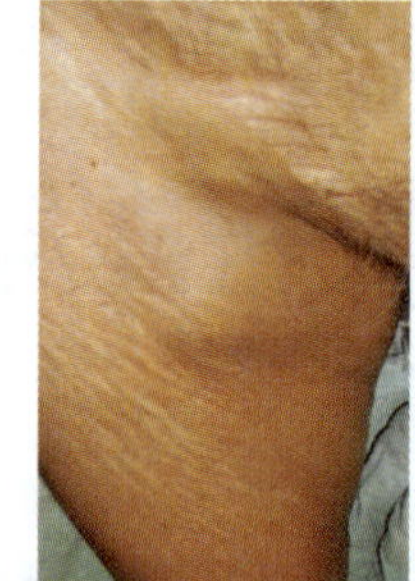

Fig. 31.34: Large lymph nodes in the groin

MELANOCYTIC TUMOURS

Simple Melanocytic Tumours

- As the fetus develops, melanocytes migrate to different parts of body, such as the skin, meninges, mucus membrane, eyes, etc.
- Pigmented naevi are composed of modified melanocytes derived from the neural crest. All naevi have excess melanin pigmentation which makes them tan-brown or black in colour. They are located in the basal layer of the epidermis and are benign. They are of following types:

1. **Junctional naevus:** Located within the epidermis at the dermo-epidermal junction. They are common in children. They appear as tan-brown to black macules. They are smooth, flat, and hairless moles. As they enlarge, they become slightly raised and may evolve into an intradermal or a compound naevus. It has no malignant potential.

   Junctional naevi commonly occurs over the palm, sole, digits, and genitalia.

2. **Compound naevus:** As the mole enlarges, naeval cells also appear in the dermis along the intraepidermal cells. Such moles are described as compound naevi. These are typically found in adolescents and are usually benign.
3. **Intradermal naevus:** It is the most common mole in adult. Because of its deep seated nature, it appears blue (hence, the name blue naevus). It is seen over the scalp and face. It contains hair and does not become malignant.
4. **Spitz naevus:** Commonly occurs over the face and legs. It grows rapidly initially, and then remains static. It appears as a reddish-brown nodule, and is occasionally deeply pigmented.
5. **Spindle cell naevus:** Occurs in women, commonly over the thigh. It has malignant potential.
6. **Congenital pigmented naevus:** It is present at birth, and has a **greater potential for malignant change**. It may involve extensive areas of the skin **(giant)**.

   Giant congenital pigmented naevus (GCPN) or giant hairy naevus (>20 cm size)
   - It is an example of a hamartoma of naevomelanocytes. It involves extensive areas of the skin.
   - Naevus cells are present not only in epidermis, but also in the subdermal fat and muscle.
   - The risk of malignant melanoma is about 10%.
   - Malignant melanoma tends to be axial.
   - Removal is performed for aesthetic and oncological reasons.
7. **Dysplastic naevi** are different from acquired naevi in the following ways:
   - Malignant potential is more (Figs 31.35 and 31.36).
   - Family members may have such lesions.
   - Such syndrome is described as **familial dysplastic naevus syndrome**.

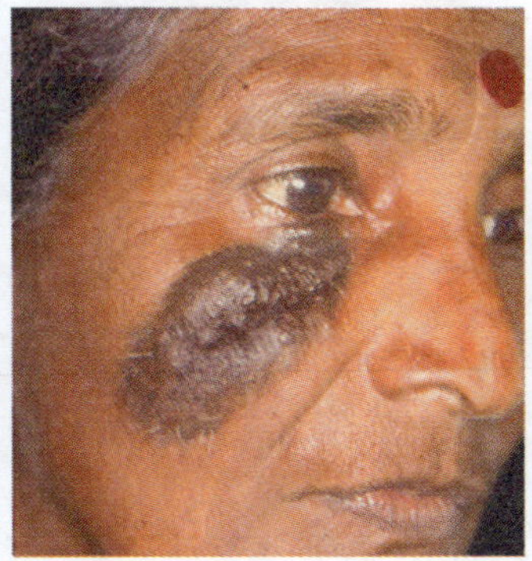

Fig. 31.35: Dysplastic naevi over the face

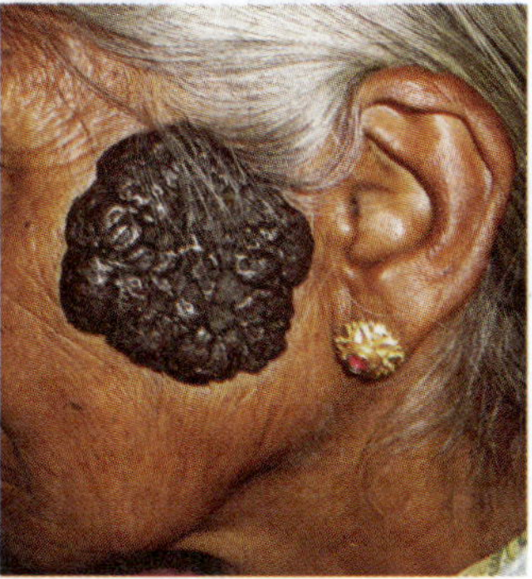

Fig. 31.36: Dysplastic naevus left parotid region

[1]Choroid has no lymphatics. Hence excellent prognosis.

MALIGNANT MELANOMA (MELANOCARCINOMA)

It is a malignant tumour arising from pigment-forming cells (melanoblasts) which are derived from the neural crest. Melanoblasts and melanocytes convert dihydroxyphenylalanine (DOPA) into melanin. This is known as a positive DOPA reaction (Key Box 31.7).

It is a potentially curable tumour in early stages. If it is left untreated or is not treated properly, it disseminates rapidly, showers the body with tumour emboli, and offers a very painful death.

Some interesting 'mosts' about malignant melanoma are listed in Key Box 31.8.

Key Box 31.7

Positive Dopa Reaction

TYROSINE
↓
DOPA
↓
MELANIN

Key Box 31.8

Interesting 'Most' for Malignant Melanoma

- Most benign form of melanoma is lentigomaligna melanoma.
- Most common form of melanoma is superficial spreading melanoma.
- Most malignant type of melanoma is nodular melanoma.
- Most reliable independent prognostic indicator in malignant melanoma is tumour thickness based on Breslow classification.
- Most of them (majority) arise from pre-existing moles.
- Most of the melanoma are pigmented. However, pigmentation is not mandatory for diagnosis of melanoma.

Common Sites of Malignant Melanoma

- Head and neck: 20–30%
- Lower extremity: 20–30%
- Trunk: 20–30%
- Remaining cases occur in the upper extremities, genitalia, and choroid of the eye[1].

Aetiopathogenesis (Fig. 31.37)

Risk factors for malignant melanoma are listed in Key Box 31.9.

1. **Ultraviolet rays:** It is more common in white-skinned people. There is a linear correlation between the

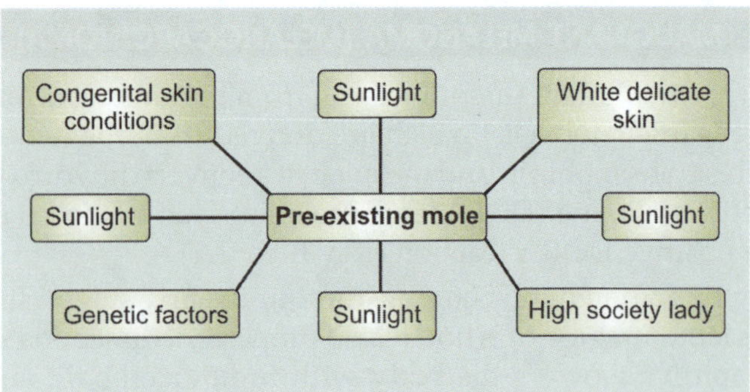

Fig. 31.37: Aetiopathogenesis

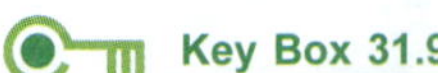

Key Box 31.9

Risk Factors for Developing Malignant Melanoma (MM)

- **P**igmentosa xeroderma
- **I**mmunocompromised—HIV, Hodgkin's disease treated with cyclosporin
- **G**enetic—History of dysplastic naevus
- **M**elanoma excised earlier
- **E**arly childhood burns and eyes blue, red hair
- **N**aevus: GCPN and total number >20 naevi
- **T**endency to freckle

Remember as **PIGMENT**

intensity of exposure to sunlight and malignant melanoma in white-skinned people[1]. White-skinned people who live close to the equator have an increased risk of developing malignant melanoma. The highest incidence is found in Queensland (Australia). For the same reason, malignant melanoma is common in the United Kingdom, North America and Australia. Ultraviolet A (UVA) rays have a long wavelength and deep penetration, causing tanning and wrinkling.

2. **Age and sex:** Malignant melanoma is more common in females. The higher incidence of the disease is found during the reproductive age period. Even though oestrogen and progesterone receptors are found in malignant melanoma in some patients, their true role is not yet established. The leg is the most common site in females. The incidence of melanoma is 1.7 times higher in women than men <39 years of age. After 70 years of age, the incidence of melanoma is 2.2-fold higher in men than women.
3. **Genetic factors:** Tumour suppressor gene mutation 9p21, Deletion or rearrangement of chromosomes 10 and 8p. Familial, atypical, multiple, mole, melanoma syndrome—previously known as familial, dysplastic naevus syndrome . Multiple, large (> 5 cm), atypical dysplastic nevus in areas covered by clothing are characteristic. The disease is also common in individuals of the Celtic race who give a family history of malignant melanoma (3–5%).
4. **Pre-existing mole:** Approximately 2/3rd of melanomas arise in a pre-existing mole, and the remaining 1/3rd arise *de novo*. Malignant change occurs in the junctional or compound naevus. Malignancy should be suspected when certain changes occur in a mole (Key Box 31.10). Patients with atypical mole, large naevus in those with red hair, blue eyes, and Fitzpatrick skin type are predisposed to malignant melanoma.
5. **Immunosuppression:** Increased incidence of malignant melanoma has been found in patients with renal transplantation, leukaemia, and AIDS.
6. **Xeroderma pigmentosum and albinism** patients are susceptible to melanomas.

Key Box 31.10

Glasgow—Check List (Figs 31.38 and 31.39)

1. Change in size
2. Change in shape
3. Change in colour
4. Inflammation
5. Crusting, ulceration, bleeding
6. Sensory change
7. Diameter >6 mm

Ugly duckling sign: Patients with multiple moles, which are having similar characteristics and when malignancy develops in one of the moles, it deviates from the normal. (It will be different).

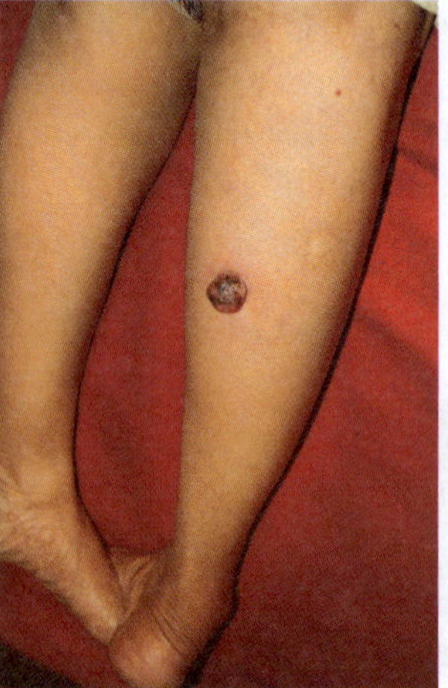

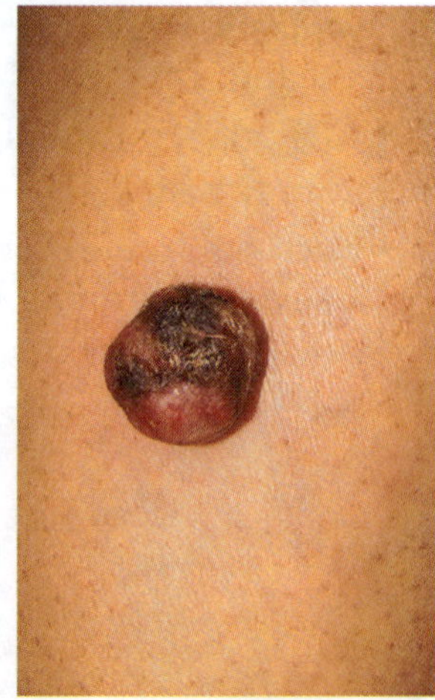

Figs 31.38 and 31.39: Only complaint of this 28-year-old lady was an increase in the size and oozing from the lesion

Pearls of Wisdom

"Bronzed, blue-eyed, blond, body beautiful—high chances of malignant melanoma"

[3]Malignant melanoma is the killer of whites. Bronzed body beautiful concept should be discouraged.

Pathology (Fig. 31.40)

Microscopic picture: Anaplastic, pigment-laden melanocytes confined to the epidermis. The cells which have vacuolated cytoplasm (Paget's cells resembling those seen in Paget's disease of the breast) are found. Cells also invade the dermis. Along with pigment-laden macrophages, dermal infiltration of lymphocytes[1] may be present. Rarely, anaplastic melanocytes do not form pigment **(amelanotic melanoma)**.

All melanomas (except nodular) show **radial growth initially,** in the form of intraepidermal growth. However, **nodular melanoma** has a **vertical growth phase,** which involves the dermis and results in nodule formation. This has poor prognosis.

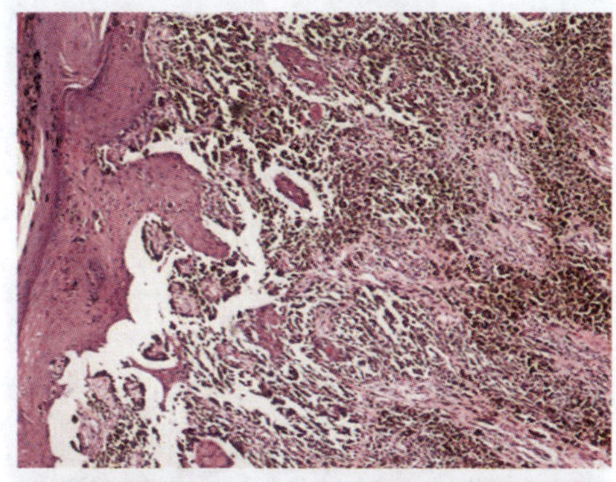

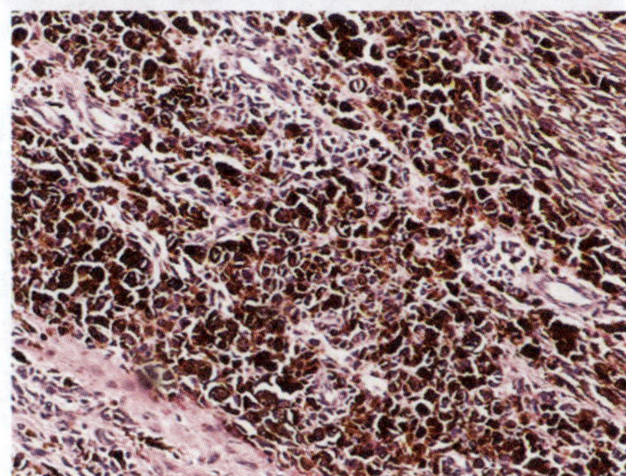

Fig. 31.40: Malignant melanoma with malignant cells showing dark melanin pigment inside. Second picture is a close-up view (*Courtesy:* Dr Laxmi Rao, Head, Department of Pathology, KMC, Manipal)

Pathological Grading of Malignant Melanoma

Breslow described staging depending on the maximum thickness at the centre of the lesion.

Stage I: Thickness <0.75 mm

Stage II: 0.76–1.5 mm

Stage III: 1.51–3.0 mm

Stage IV: >3 mm

- <1 mm is regarded as thin melanoma.

Please note: Clarke's level of invasion (it is no longer followed).

Clinical Types (Table 31.4)

Clinical Features

- Malignant melanoma may present as changes in the pre-existing mole (Key Box 31.11).
- The patient may present as a nonhealing ulcer of the sole of the foot.
- It is a painless ulcer with irregular borders. Ulcer bleeds easily on touch. Lesion is firm in consistency and **induration is absent**. A **halo** may be present around the ulcer.
- **Ugly duckling sign:** A lesion that stands out as different from the patient's own nevi
- Typically, the **ulcer is pigmented** (Fig. 31.41). In 10% of patients, pigment is absent. They are called amelanotic melanoma.
- The lesion moves with the skin and is usually not fixed to underlying structures.

Key Box 31.11

ABCDE of Evaluating a Changing Mole

- **A** Asymmetry: One half does not match the other
- **B** Border irregular: Ragged or blurred
- **C** Colour variation: Tan, black, brown
- **D** Diameter: >6 mm
- **E** Evolving (elevation): Change in a pre-existing lesion

Table 31.4 Clinical types of malignant melanoma (Figs 31.41 to 31.44)

Name	Nature	Behaviour
Lentigo malignant melanoma	Arises from Hutchinson's melanotic freckle Occurs in old people on face and temporal region	Least common (5%) Least malignant
Superficial spreading	Any part, more in the trunk	Most common (70%)
Nodular	Any part, more in the leg, raised papular lesions	Most malignant, invasive (15–30%)
Acral lentiginous	Located on the palm, sole, digits	Presents late, aggressive (4–8%)
Amelanotic	Difficult to diagnose	Rare, nonpigmented (5%)
Desmoplastic (neurotropic)	Often involves nerve fibres	Invasive melanoma

[1]Presence of lymphocytes may be an indication of host response 'Fight' against cancer.

- **Satellite nodules** (within 5 cm of the primary) may be found surrounding the lesion and are due to intradermal lymphatic spread (Fig. 31.42). Such patients will have greatly enlarged, firm, nontender nodes.
- **In-transit lesion**—disease found in the dermis or subcutaneous tissue >5 cm away from the primary melanoma, but before the regional lymph node basin (Figs 31.43–31.47).
- *See* Key Box 31.12 for the acral lentiginous variety.

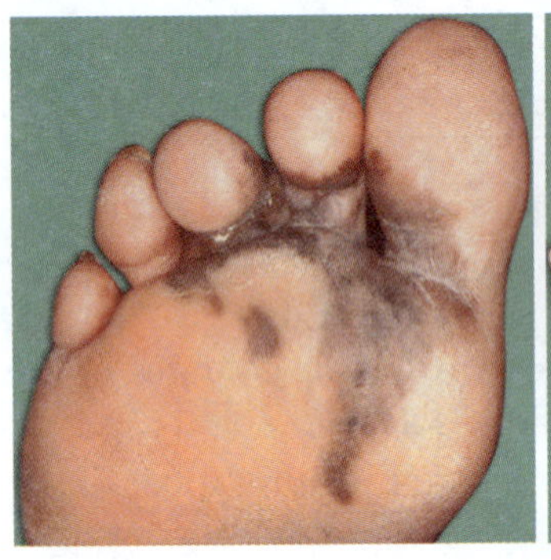
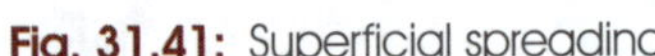

Fig. 31.41: Superficial spreading

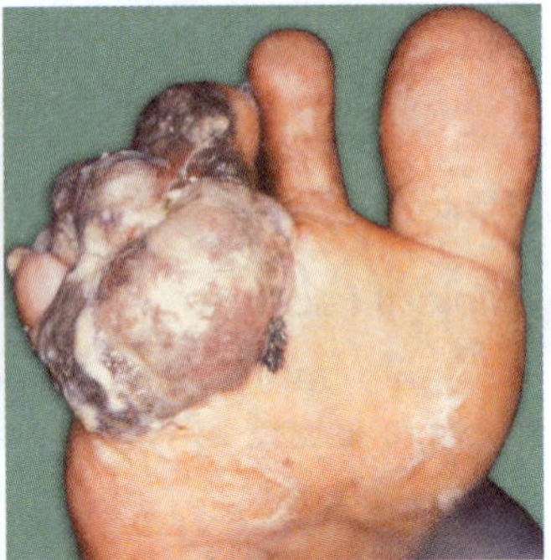

Fig. 31.42: Nodular

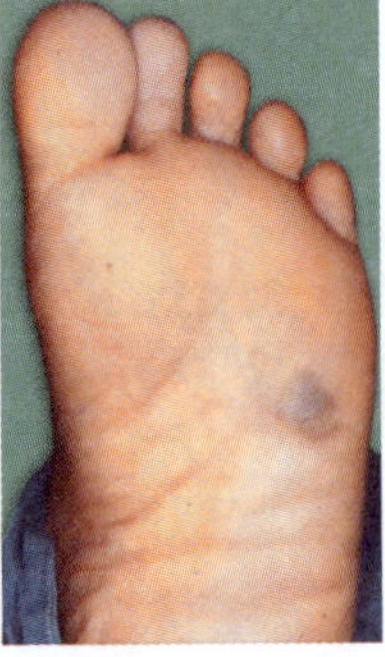

Fig. 31.43: Acral lentiginous variety with early changes—never incise or cauterise such melanomas

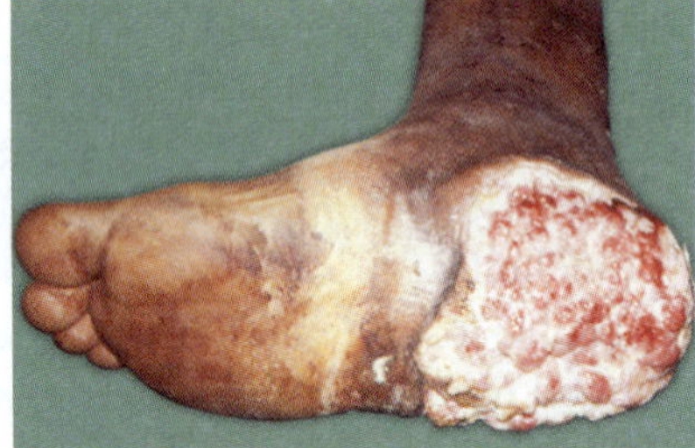

Fig. 31.44: The lesion resembles squamous cell carcinoma. Punch biopsy reported as amelanotic melanoma

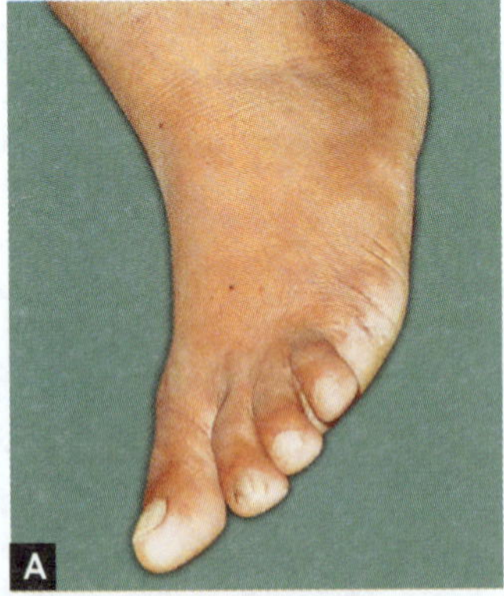

Fig. 31.45A: Observe the foot, little toe has been amputated five years back for malignant melanoma

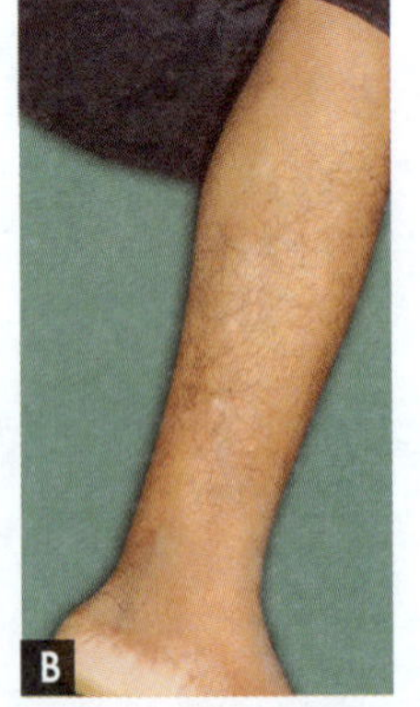

Fig. 31.45B: Same patient as in Fig. 31.45 A presented to the hospital with in-transit deposits

Key Box 31.12

Acral Lentiginous (Fig. 31.48)

- Least common subtype
- Popularly called hand and foot melanoma
- Occurs in palms and soles
- This subtype occurs in dark-skinned people (21–22%)
- In subungual region—blue black discolouration of posterior nail fold (most common on great toe or thumb)
- **Pigmentation in proximal or lateral nail folds (Hutchinson's sign) due to radial spread**

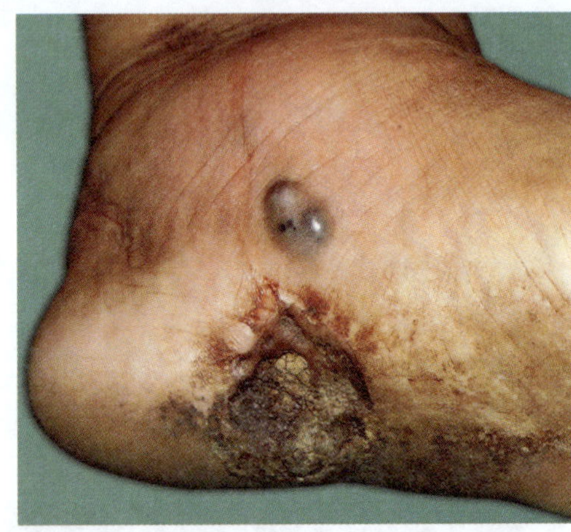

Fig. 31.46: Malignant melanoma operated—recurrence after 8 months with satellite nodule. It is important that the first surgery should be the best surgery. Every attempt should be made to do a three-dimensional excision

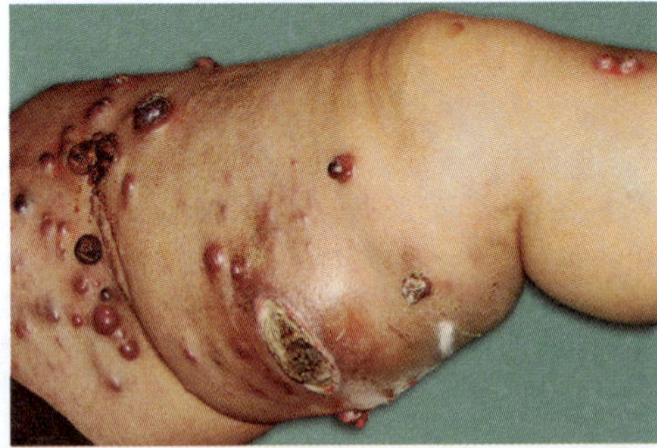

Fig. 31.47: Whole leg is studded with tumour. In-transit deposits from malignant melanoma of the foot

AMELANOTIC MELANOMA (Fig. 31.47)

- Lesion appears pink.
- It has a poorer prognosis than nodular melanoma.

Pearls of Wisdom

In all cases of suspected melanomatous skin lesions, examine the axillae, scalp, soles, genitalia, oral cavity, and interdigital webs also.

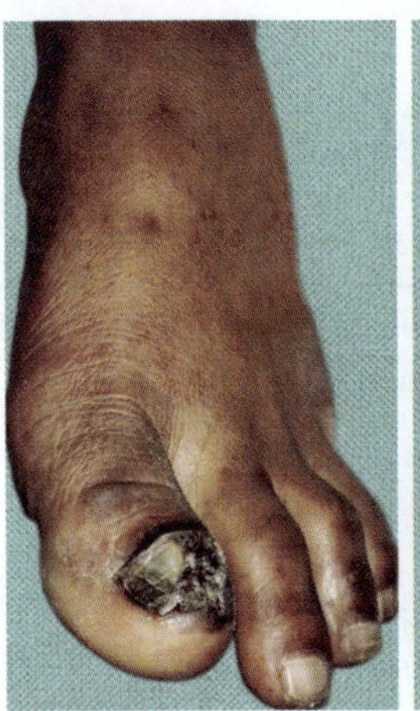
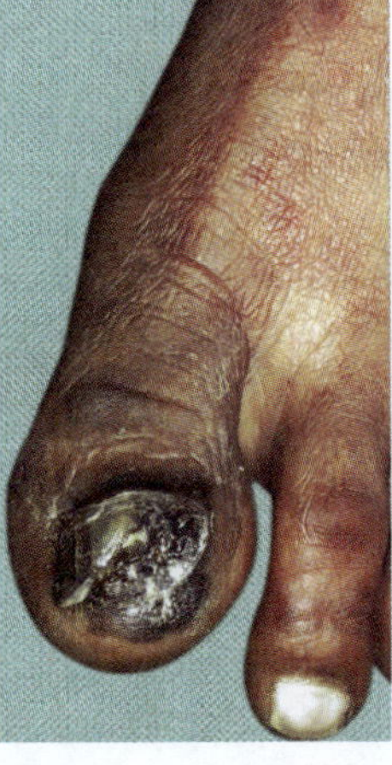

Fig. 31.48: Hutchinson's sign—close-up view

Differential Diagnosis

- Pigmented basal cell carcinoma, histiocytoma (sclerosing angioma)
- Naevus, Kaposi's sarcoma, cavernous haemangioma.

Spread

1. **Local spread** occurs mainly by continuity and contiguity. **Satellite nodules** are due to local and lymphatic spread, situated within 5 cm of the primary lesion. Malignant melanoma rarely infiltrates the deep fascia unless and until a 'blunder biopsy' is done. **Inadequate local excision may result in local recurrence later. Hence, initial surgery should attempt at achieving cure.**
2. **Lymphatic spread** is the principal mode of spread. Regional nodes get involved very early, altering the prognosis. Thus, nodes may get very enlarged even when the lesion looks innocent. Spread occurs by both permeation and embolisation. Permeation produces satellite nodules and in-transit nodules which develop between primary and secondaries. Embolisation occurs rapidly, producing massive regional nodes early (Key Boxes 31.13 and 31.14).

   In-transit metastases appear in the skin as intracutaneous metastases. They are thought to be due to melanoma cells trapped within lymphatic vessels.

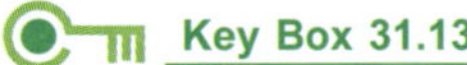

Key Box 31.13

Malignant Melanoma Sole

Inguinal nodes
↓
Iliac nodes
↓
Para-aortic nodes
↓
Mediastinal nodes
↓
Supraclavicular nodes

Key Box 31.14

Lymph Node Metastasis in Malignant Melanoma

- It is the single-most important prognostic index and it presents stage III disease.
- **Number of nodes is more important** than size of nodes.
- **Poor survival in ulcerated** malignant melanoma, even if node-negative.
- **Extranodal extension** has poor prognosis.
- Lymph node metastasis proceeds as an orderly process. Thus, evolved the concept of the **first node to get involved—sentinel node (SN).**
- **Elective lymphadenectomy** is **not indicated in thin melanoma** (1 mm).
- In **thick melanoma**, do a sentinel node biopsy. If positive, proceed to complete lymphadenectomy (block dissection).

3. **Blood spread** occurs relatively early and causes secondaries in the liver, lung, brain, and bones, producing miserable, pathetic situations (Table 31.5).

Clinical Notes

A 55-year-old lady presented to the hospital with enlarged inguinal lymph nodes. Clinical examination revealed nodules in the leg with firm to hard enlarged nodes in the inguinal region. On careful observation, the little toe was missing. On questioning, the patient admitted that the toe had been amputated elsewhere five years back for a painless, blackish lesion (Figs 31.45A, B).

Table 31.5 Spread of malignant melanoma

Spread	Diagnosis	Problems
Metastasis in lung	Cannonball appearance, pleural effusion	Respiratory failure
Metastasis in liver	Massive hepatomegaly, ascites	Abdominal discomfort
Metastasis in brain	Raised intracranial tension	Coma
Metastasis in bone	Bony pains, pathological fractures	Paraplegia, quadriplegia
Metastasis in bowel	Bleeding	Anaemia

Staging

TNM STAGING	Definition of regional lymph node (N)	
N Category	**Number of tumour-involved regional lymph node**	**Presence of in-transit, satellite, and/or microsatellite metastases**
Nx	Regional nodes not assessed (e.g. SLN biopsy not performed, regional nodes previously removed for another reason)	No
N0	No regional metastases detected	No
N1	One tumour-involved node or in-transit, satellite, and/or microsatellite metastases with no tumour-involved nodes	
N1a	One clinically occult (i.e. detected by SLN biopsy)	
N1b	One clinically detected	No
N1c	No regional lymph node disease	Yes
N2	Two or three tumour-involved nodes or in-transit, satellite, and/or microsatellite metastases with one tumour-involved node	
N2a	Two or three clinically occult (i.e. detected by SLN biopsy)	No
N2b	Two or three, at least one of which was clinically detected	No
N2c	One clinically occult or clinically detected	Yes
N3	Four or more tumour-involved nodes or in-transit, satellite, and/or microsatellite metastases with two or more tumour-involved nodes, or any number of matted nodes without or with in-transit, satellite, and/or microsatellite metastases.	
N3a	Four or more clinically occult (i.e. detected by SLN biopsy)	No
N3b	Four or more, at least one of which was clinically detected, or presence of any number of matted nodes	No
N3c	Two or more clinically occult or clinically detected and/or presence of any number of matted nodes	Yes

TNM STAGING	Definition of primary tumour (T)	
T Category	**Thickness**	**Ulceration Status**
TX: Primary tumour thickness cannot be assessed (e.g. diagnosis by curettage)	Not applicable	Not applicable
T0: No evidence of primary tumour (e.g. unknown primary or completely regressed melanoma)	Not applicable	Not applicable
Tis (melanoma *in situ*)	Not applicable	Not applicable
T1	≤1.0 mm	Unknown or unspecified
T1a	<0.8 mm	Without ulceration
T1b	<0.8 mm	With ulceration
	0.8–1.0 mm	With or without ulceration
T2	>1.0–2.0 mm	Unknown or unspecified
T2a	>1.0–2.0 mm	Without ulceration
T2b	>1.0–2.0 mm	With ulceration
T3	>2.0–4.0 mm	Unknown or unspecified
T3a	>2.0–4.0 mm	Without ulceration
T3b	>2.0–4.0 mm	With ulceration
T4	>4.0 mm	Unknown or unspecified
T4a	>4.0 mm	Without ulceration
T4b	>4.0 mm	With ulceration

a = without ulceration, b = with ulceration

CLINICAL STAGING*			
Stage 0	Tis	N0	M0
Stage IA	T1a	N0	M0
Stage IB	T1b	N0	M0
	T2a	N0	M0
Stage IIA	T2b	N0	M0
	T3a	N0	M0
Stage IIB	T3b	N0	M0
	T4a	N0	M0
Stage IIC	T4b	N0	M0
Stage III	Any T, Tis	≥N1	M0
Stage IV	Any T	Any N	M1

*Clinical staging includes microstaging of the primary melanoma and clinical/radiologic evaluation for metastases. By convention, it should be used after complete excision of the primary melanoma with clinical assessment for regional and distant metastases

TNM STAGING **Definition of distant metastasis (M)**

M Category	Anatomic site	M Criteria LDH level
M0	No evidence of distant metastasis	Not applicable
M1	Evidence of distant metastasis	See below
M1a	Distant metastasis to skin, soft tissue including muscle, and/or nonregional lymph node	Not recorded or unspecified
M1a(0)		Not elevated
M1a(1)		Elevated
M1b	Distant metastasis to lung with or without M1a sites of disease	Not recorded or unspecified
M1b(0)		Not elevated
M1b(1)		Elevated
M1c	Distant metastasis to non-CNS visceral sites with or without M1a, M1b	Not recorded or unspecified
M1c(0)		Not elevated
M1c(1)		Elevated
M1d	Distant metastasis to CNS with or without M1a, M1b, or M1c	Not recorded or unspecified
M1d(0)		Not elevated
M1d(1)		Elevated

- Serum lactate dehydrogenase (LDH)
- Suffixes for M category: (0) LDH not elevated, (1) LDH elevated.
- No suffix is used if LDH is not recorded or is unspecified.

*Each stage classified based on LDH level

Important Changes in the New AJCC Staging of Malignant Melanoma

1. Thickness and ulceration in T-category rather than level of invasion.
2. Number of metastatic nodes is more important.
3. LDH (details are given later) is included in 'M' category (metastatic spread).
4. If there is ulceration, 3 stages are upgraded.
5. Satellite nodules and in-transit deposits are grouped into stage III disease.

CUTANEOUS MELANOMA—AMERICAN JOINT COMMITTEE ON CANCER (AJCC 8th Edition)—4 STAGES

- **Stage 0:** *In situ* carcinoma.
- **Stages I and II:** Primary tumours confined to the skin without regional lymph node involvement—depending on the thickness (depth) of the tumour, the presence or absence of ulceration of the overlying epithelium

  Stage IA: <0.8 mm thick, **NO ulceration**

  Stage IB (T1B): <0.8 mm thick **with ulceration** or 0.8–10 mm thickness ± ulceration

  Stage IB: T2a or **Stage II: >10 mm** thick with any features
- **Stage III:** With clinical or pathological evidence of **regional lymph node + OR the presence of in-transit or satellite metastases.**
- **Stage IV:** Disease is defined by the presence of distant metastasis—biopsy proven.

Investigations

1. **Blood tests** such as haemoglobin, total RBC, and WBC counts are done. Lactic dehydrogenase (LDH) has been included under M (Metastasis) category. LDH represents a strong prognostic factor in unresectable, metastatic (stage IV) melanoma. Levels >500–1000 U/L suggest a high tumour burden. LDH which is present in the normal cells gets released when the cells are destroyed by the tumour.
2. **A chest X-ray is taken**—if it shows metastasis, it is stage IV disease. However, a negative chest X-ray does not rule out metastasis.
3. **Biopsy:** A **full-thickness biopsy of the lesion with a narrow (1 to 2 mm) margin of grossly normal skin is made.** The depth of excision should include the full thickness of the dermis and, thus, should extend into the subcutaneous tissue. Accurate measurement **of tumour thickness** is important because it is critical for the prognosis and affects surgical recommendations. Incision biopsy is indicated only in advanced lesions. Once the specimen is removed, the following details have to be studied—Breslow thickness, ulceration, dermal mitotic rate, microsatellitosis, pure desmoplasia, and deep and peripheral margin status. **In subungual melanomas, biopsy may be taken after removal of all or a large part of the nail and one or more punch biopsies** of the base of the nailbed.

Pearls of Wisdom

In cases of melanoma *in situ*, blood tests and imaging are not required.

4. **Imaging:** Ultrasound abdomen is economical and easily available. Presence of iliac or para-aortic lymph nodes and secondaries in the liver can easily be made out. However, in all cases of stage III melanomas (lymph nodes positive), contrast-enhanced CT scan of the chest and abdomen should be done (Fig. 31.49).
5. **PET with fluorodeoxyglucose (FDG):** It is used for staging patients with advanced melanoma, but its role in earlier stages is unclear because it is expensive and associated with substantial radiation exposure.
6. **FNAC of the lymph nodes:** Clinically palpable lymph nodes may be subjected for ultrasound-guided aspiration. In melanoma even a palpable lymph node is enough to decide about block dissection (Figs 31.50 and 31.51).

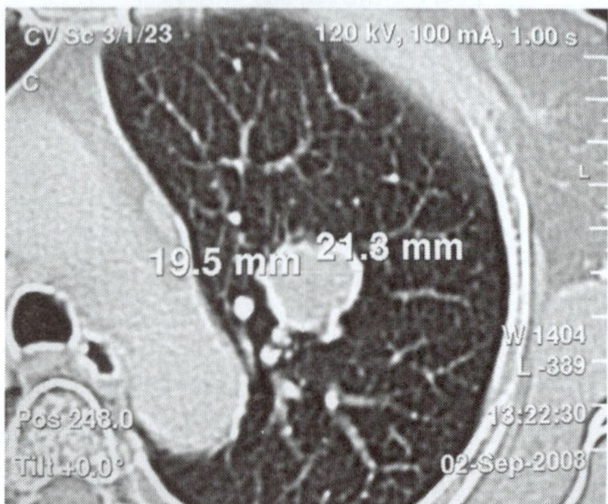

Fig. 31.49: Lung metastasis in CT of the chest. It was not visible in X-ray chest

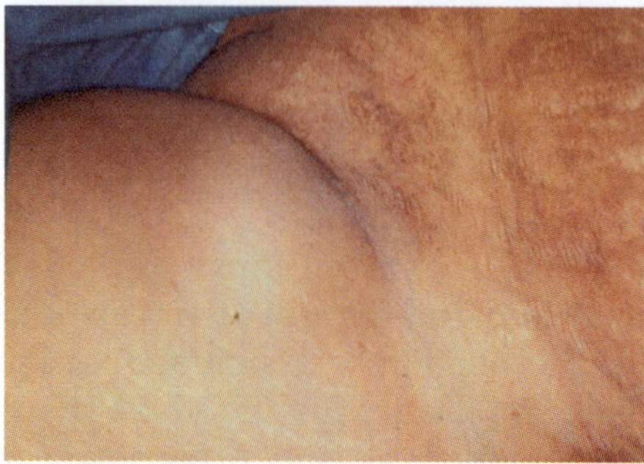

Fig. 31.50: Hugely enlarged inguinal lymph nodes—the nodes can be firm to hard. Sometimes, they are soft due to degeneration

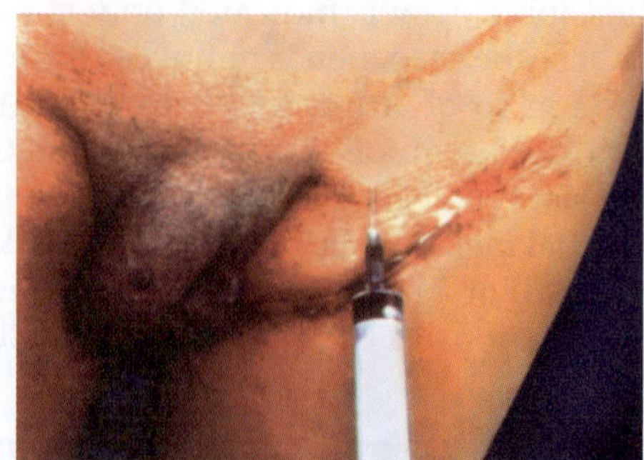

Fig. 31.51: FNAC of the recurrent inguinal node secondaries—bluish black aspirate

7. **Genetic:** Melanocyte protein, also known as pre-melanosome protein (PMEL), is a protein that is encoded by the *PMEL* gene. This may be used as a specific immunohistochemical marker for melanoma.

Treatment

Surgery is the main treatment modality for malignant melanoma. All other modalities are only palliative and supportive. In early stages without lymph node enlargement and the tumour with good histology, it is still a curable cancer. Surgery can be divided as treatment of the primary lesion and of metastatic lymph nodes.

A. Treatment of the Primary

1. **Excision biopsy-wide excision:** A small lesion of 1 mm may be excised even under local anaesthesia with 1 cm of healthy margin around (narrow excision). Defect may be closed by primary suturing. While excising the tumour, it is better not to handle the tumour. It is possible to remove the tumour by strictly adhering to the principle of 'No touch' technique (Figs 31.52 and 31.53). Wide excision is based on principle of 'centrifugal spread of melanoma.' One of the causes of recurrence is inadequate excision (Fig. 31.54).

Tumour thickness (mm)	*Wide excision margin*
<1 mm	1 cm
1–2 mm	2 cm
>2 mm	2 cm

– Desmoplastic melanoma: Has a high rate of recurrence; hence, a wide margin of excision is required.

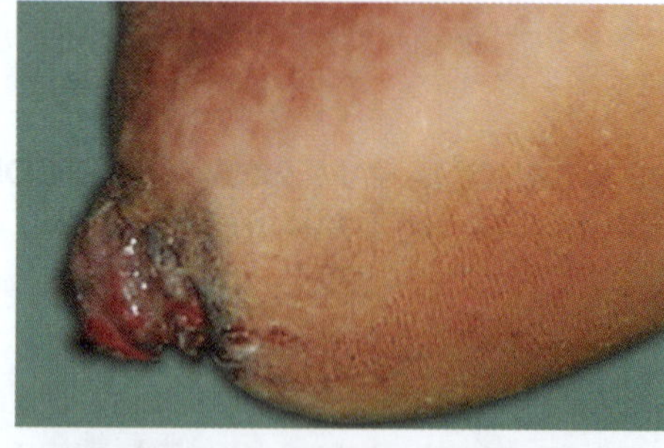

Fig. 31.52: Ulcerated melanoma over the heel—poor prognosis

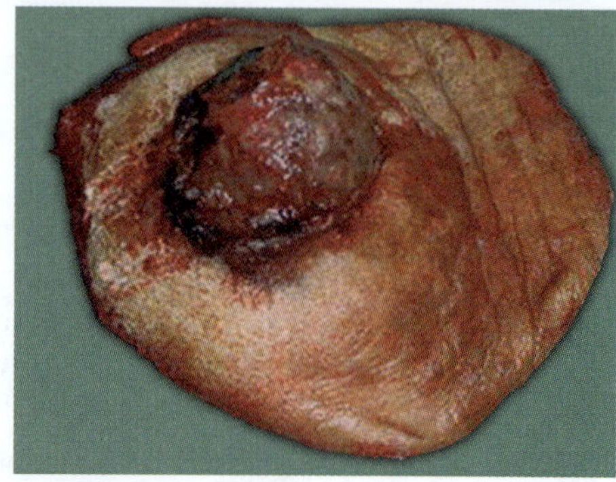

Fig. 31.53: Wide excision (minimum 2 cm) specimen

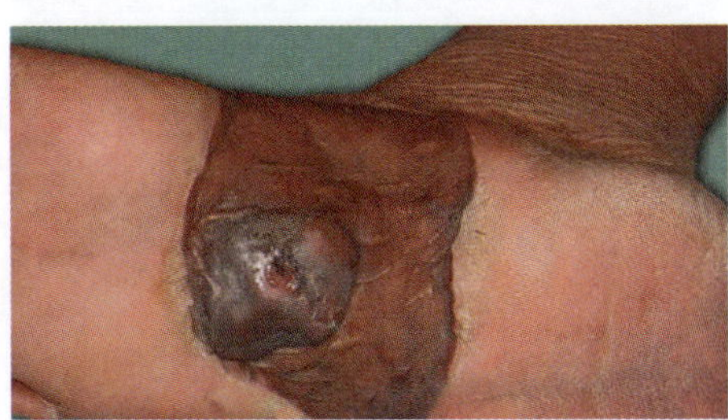

Fig. 31.54: Local recurrence after 2 years probably because of inadequate local excision—you can see the previous skin graft

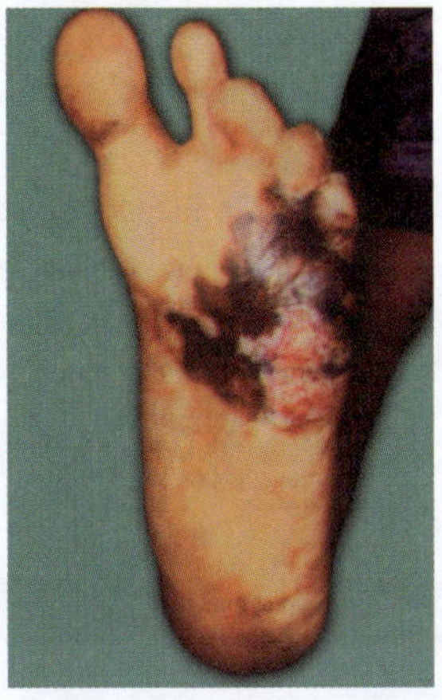

Fig. 31.55: 8 cm ulcerated pigmented lesion in the foot—malignant melanoma foot required amputation

2. **Subungual malignant melanoma** is treated by amputation of the digit.
3. **Amputation (advanced and large lesions)** (Fig. 31.55).
4. **Malignant melanoma of the choroid** has good prognosis. Choroid does not have lymphatic drainage. However, metastasis may occur through the haematogenous route even after many years. It is treated by enucleation of the eye.

B. Treatment of Lymph Nodes

1. If lymph nodes are situated adjacent to the primary lesion, block dissection is done along with the primary lesion in continuity to include 'in-transit' deposits also.
2. If lymph nodes are away, radical block dissection is done. *Example:* For a lower limb malignant melanoma, inguinal nodes along with the iliac nodes are removed (**ilioinguinal block dissection**). If these groups of nodes are positive on frozen section, lymph node clearance should include lymph nodes of obturator vessels (**ilio-obturator block dissection)** (Figs 31.56 and 31.57), or if pelvic CT scan is positive or Cloquet node is positive, the obturator group of lymph nodes is removed. To get the best results if facilities are available sentinel lymph node mapping is done. Depending upon the results of the findings, lymph node dissection is done. Details are given below.

- **Sentinel lymph node mapping:** Isosulfan blue is injected intradermally and the node that gets stained is identified and sent for frozen section (haematoxylin and eosin stains and immunohistochemical technique). **If the node is positive, regional lymphadenectomy is done even if the nodes are clinically not palpable.** At least 20–30% of patients who are in stage I will be identified as stage III after sentinel node biopsy (SNBx). There is a **definite survival advantage in patients** who undergo SNBx and regional lymphadenectomy when the nodes are not palpable.

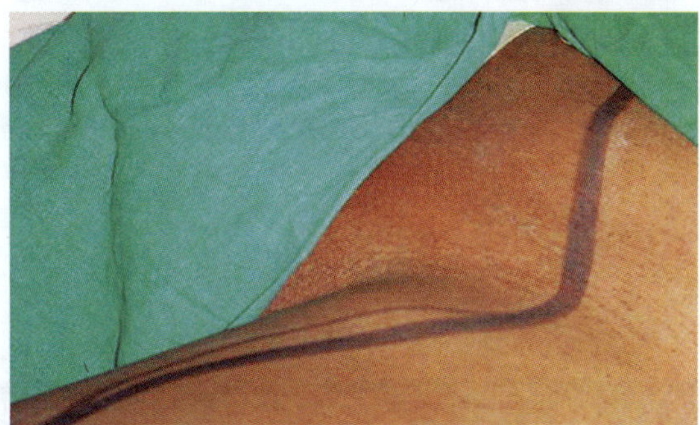

Fig. 31.56: Lazy S incision is given for inguinal block dissection—this incision decreases incidence of flap necrosis

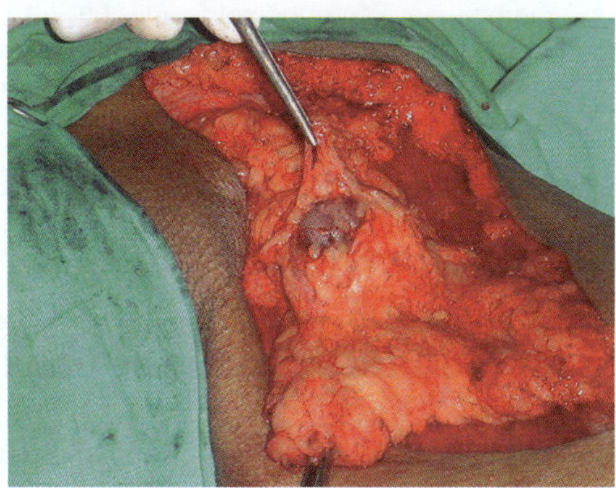

Fig. 31.57: Observe pigmented lymph nodes

Types of lymph node dissections:

- If sentinel node biopsy is negative, prophylactic block dissection is indicated only if the melanoma has poor prognostic histological factors.
- If lymph nodes are positive after FNAC: **TLND**—therapeutic lymph node dissection is done.
- In patients with no clinical lymph nodal metastasis but ELND—elective or prophylactic lymph node dissection is beneficial. In cases of 1–4 mm thick melanoma, melanoma without ulceration, extremity melanoma, patients <6 years of age. In these patients only 25% of patients show occult metastasis.

Summary of skin tumours is given in Table 31.6.

Table 31.6 Summary of skin tumours

	Squamous cell carcinoma	Basal cell carcinoma	Malignant melanoma
Incidence	Common (20–30%)	Most common (60–70%)	Less common (10–20%)
Origin	Prickle cell layer	Basal layer	Melanoblasts
Aetiology	Chronic irritation	Ultraviolet rays, fair skin	Ultraviolet rays, fair skin, pre-existing mole
Site	Trunk, leg, hand, oral cavity	Tear cancer	Head and neck, face, digits, palm and sole
Types	Ulcerative or cauliflower	Nodular or ulcerative	Nodular or ulcerative
Edge	Everted	Rolled out and beaded	Irregular
Induration	Maximum	Moderate	Minimum
Scab	Never occurs	Occurs	Never occurs
Pigmentation	Absent	Absent	Present in 90% of cases
Spread	Mainly by lymphatics. Blood spread is rare and late	Does not spread by lymphatics Blood spread is very, very late Spreads by local spread. Hence the name, rodent ulcer	Mainly by lymphatics, also by blood spread, does not infiltrate like rodent ulcer
Cytokeratin	Expression	No	No

STAGEWISE TREATMENT (MORE DETAILS) AND RECENT ADVANCES

Please note: Recent advances in the treatment of melanoma are very complicated. It not only includes surgery, radiotherapy, and chemotherapy, but also bio-chemotherapy, vaccines, monoclonal antibodies, kit inhibitors, etc. Those of you who would like to get more marks can refer these.

Surgery in the form of wide excision is the most important curative treatment in stage I and stage IIB. Other various forms of treatment are available in Fig. 31.58.

STAGEWISE TREATMENT: CLINICAL TISNOMO, STAGE 0: CLINICALLY LOCALIZED MELANOMA OR MELANOMA *IN SITU*

- Melanoma *in situ* by definition **is not invasive** or metastatic. However, metastatic melanoma to regional nodes has been observed occasionally from melanoma *in situ* with histologic evidence of regression.
- **Examine the nodes clinically.**
- Radiological studies are not necessary.
- **Wide excision alone in the majority of cases.**

PRINCIPLES OF WIDE EXCISION

- Full-thickness excision of skin and subcutaneous tissue to the underlying deep fascia.
- A **5 mm margin** is the standard recommendation, but **melanoma *in situ*** may extend beyond its visible extent. Thus, if cosmetically acceptable, it is reasonable to obtain a margin of as much as **1 cm**, especially if the original biopsy was incomplete.

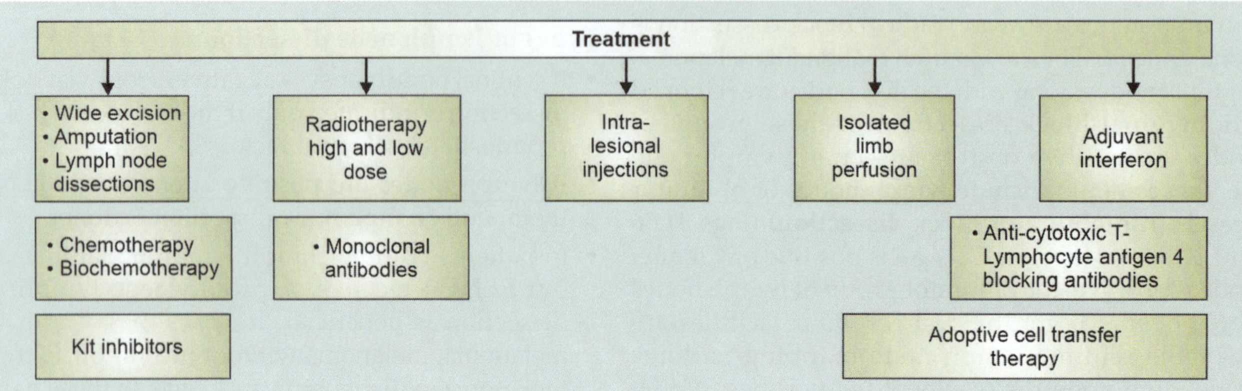

Fig. 31.58: Various treatment available for malignant melanoma

STAGE I: CLINICAL T1A

1. Thin Primary Melanoma

Thin melanomas, such as T1a melanomas, are **those <1 mm thick**, with **<1 mitosis** per mm^2, and **without ulceration**. In the absence of any clinical evidence of metastasis, these are clinical stage IA melanomas. 5-year survival rate of 94%.

Treatment of T1A

- **Wide excision with a 1 cm margin** (including skin and all underlying subcutaneous tissue to the deep muscle fascia).
- The margin should be measured from the **visible edge** of the pigmented lesion or from the biopsy scar, whichever is larger.
- After excision, primary closure is performed. However, if on the face, palms, or feet, skin grafts or rotation flaps are used.

2. Melanomas of the Trunk and Proximal Extremities

- Wide local excisions should involve measuring the appropriate margin (usually 1–2 cm) around the entire scar from the biopsy, or
- From the visible edge of residual melanoma, and extending the **incision to make an ellipse** that is approximately three times as long as it is wide.

Incision/Excision Principles

- Extremities—ideally, the direction of the scar should be longitudinal.
- Over the joints, on the trunk and neck—along skin lines.
- On the upper back—it is usually best for the scar to run transversely.
- The excision should include all skin and subcutaneous tissue up to the deep fascia (but not including the fascia).
- When a major cutaneous nerve runs along the deep fascia to innervate distal cutaneous structures—preserve the nerve.
- Wide excisions can almost always be performed under local anaesthesia.

3. Clinical T2A, T2B Melanomas

- Melanomas 1–2 mm thick, with or without ulceration.
- **History and physical examination**—may suggest metastatic disease.
- In the absence of such findings, very low yield of additional staging studies—hence, **not recommended**.
- No evidence of metastasis—**wide excision with a 1–2 cm margin and SNBx.**

4. Primary Melanomas of the Fingers and Toes

- **Subungual melanomas** of any finger or toe—amputation at the interphalangeal joint of the toe or just proximal to the distal inter-phalangeal joint of the finger (Fig. 31.59).
- **SNBx should** usually be performed for melanomas of the fingers or toes if they are at least T1b lesions.

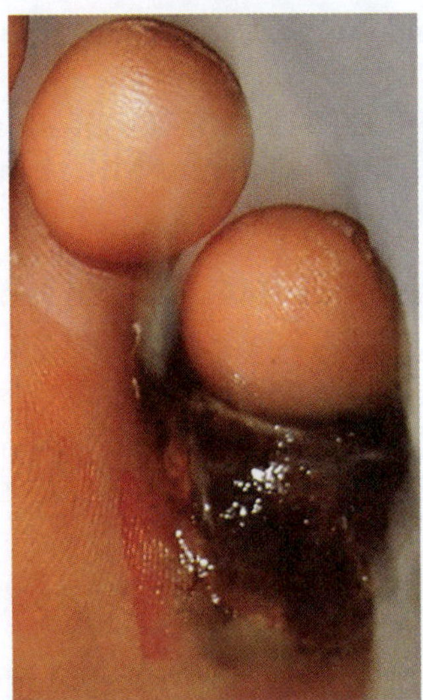

Fig. 31.59: Ulcerated melanoma—Stage IIB

5. Sentinel Node Biopsy

- **If the SNBx is negative**, then the patient is pathologically staged as T2aN0M0 (stage IB) or T2bN0M0 (stage IIA).
- No additional surgical management is required, and no adjuvant systemic therapy is indicated.

STAGE II: MELANOMA (T2B–T4B)

A. Clinical T3A Melanomas (Clinical Stage IIA)

- Melanomas 2–4 mm thick without ulceration represent T3a lesions, and in the absence of metastases, these are clinical stage IIA lesions.
- **Serum LDH level: LDH** is a key enzyme **in** the process of energy production **in cancer** cells. It catalyzes the conversion of pyruvate to lactate **in** hypoxic conditions. **LDH levels are** increased in response to tissue injury or during disease states. **LDH** may be a marker of **tumour burden** for advanced **cancer** patients.
- Wide excision with a 2 cm margin plus **SNBx.**

B. Clinical T3B Melanomas (Clinical Stage IIB)

- Wide excision with a 2 cm margin plus SNBx.
- If the nodes are negative, treat like stage IIB (T3bN0M0).

- No additional surgical therapy required.
- **HDI (high-dose IFNα-2-b) and pegylated-interferon—** postsurgical adjuvant therapy in resected stage IIB–III melanoma.

C. Clinical T3B Melanomas (Clinical Stage IIB)

- **Melanomas 2–4 mm thick with ulceration** represent T3b lesions—clinical stage IIB (Fig. 31.60).
- If symptoms **suggest metastatic disease**, perform imaging.
- **Staging with CT scans of the chest, abdomen, and pelvis (or PET/CT scan) plus MRI scan of the brain—symptomatic cases.**

D. Thick Melanomas (T4A, T4B, >4 mm Thick)

- **Thick melanomas:** A 50% risk of metastasis and mortality over 5–10 years.
- **Ulceration increases this risk:** T4a melanomas are clinical stage IIB, whereas T4b melanomas are clinical stage IIC.
- CT scans of the chest, abdomen, and pelvis plus MRI of the head.
- Wide excision with ≥2 cm margin plus SNBx.
- **In patients with negative sentinel nodes, adjuvant low dose interferon (LDI) should be considered.**
- *If the sentinel node biopsy is positive:* These are melanomas >10-mm thick with or without ulceration. Subsequent management should follow recommendations given later for stage IIIA melanoma (T2a with positive SNBx involving 1–3 nodes) or stage IIIB melanoma (T2b with positive SNBx involving 1–3 nodes).
- **Low-dose interferon alfa (LDI-α):** Interferon-α-2a is approved for clinically lymph node negative melanoma patients with a tumour thickness of ≥1.5 mm.

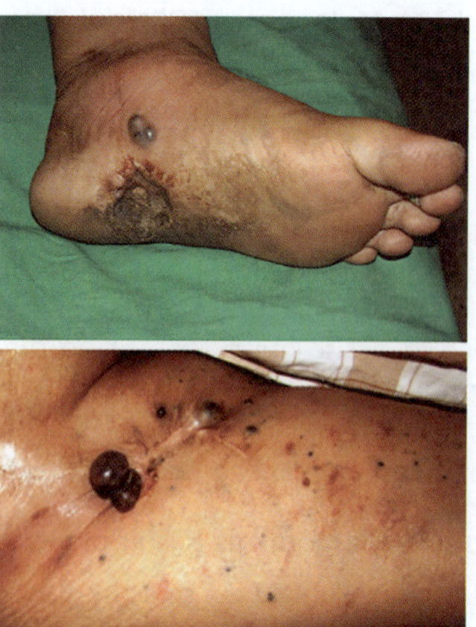

Figs 31.60 and 31.61: Loco regional recurrent melanoma

STAGE III: MELANOMA

Regionally Metastatic Melanoma (Stage III)

Figures 31.61 and 31.62. They should be managed with a curative intent.

- **Primary lesion with lymph node metastasis, satellite lesions, and in-transit metastases**
- Wide excision—maximum of 2 cm margin
- Complete lymph node dissection (CLND)
- Observation or adjuvant immunotherapy with Nivolumab or BRAF mutation gene positive—Tremenitib or IFN-α

Indications for Adjuvant Systemic Therapy (Stages IIb, IIc, and III)

- HDI—for 1 month followed by 1 year of intermediate dosing IFN for 1–2 years. Interferon—at a low dose administered for 1–3 years. Pegylated IFN administered for a target period of 5 years.
- Interferon is administered by IV infusion, 20 million U/m^2, for 5 consecutive days every 7 days for 4 weeks during the "induction" phase.
- For the subsequent 48 weeks, 10 million U/m^2 are administered by subcutaneous injection on alternate days for a total of 3 doses every 7 days in the "maintenance" phase.
- The HDI is used for the treatment of **stage III melanoma patients** (6 µg/kg/week for 8 weeks then 3 µg/kg/week for up to 5 years).
- **Toxicity:** Fatigue, anorexia, hepatotoxicity, flu-like symptoms, injection site reactions and depression.

Management of Palpable Metastatic Melanoma in Regional Nodes: Therapeutic or Completion Lymphadenectomy

- Inguinal block dissection has two components: Block dissection of
  A. Superficial inguinal lymph nodes along the long saphenous vein (vertical) and horizontal group of lymph nodes below inguinal ligament
  B. Deep inguinal node dissection: They are located medial to the femoral vein and under the cribriform fascia. There are approximately 3–5 deep nodes. The superior most node is located under the inguinal ligament and is called Cloquet's node. This node is deep to deep fascia on the medial side of the femoral vein. They are 1–3 in number. One of them may lie in the femoral canal (lymph node of Cloquet). Afferent: From the deep lymphatics of the lower limb and the superficial inguinal LNs. Efferent: To the external iliac LNs. Metastasis to a regional node represents stage III (A, B, or C) disease. It may be curable. Hence complete lymphadenectomy should be done.

- Complete lymph node dissection refers to clearing the anatomically complete dissection of the nodal basin, elective ilio-obturator dissection when inguino-femoral nodes are positive or >3 nodes are positive or when pelvic CT is positive or when Cloquet node is positive. Cloquet node is the transitional node between the inguinal region and the iliac region.
- Lymphatic anatomy of the inguinal canal, the importance of various lymph nodes, and types of dissection are given below (Fig. 31.62).
- **An iliac node dissection** involves skeletonizing the external iliac vessels. It is generally combined with removal of the iliac node-bearing tissue and the **obturator fat pad** (obturator dissection).

Regional Metastases: Definitions

- ***Local recurrence****: Recurrence of melanoma in the scar from the original excision or at the* edge of the skin graft (if used for closure).
- ***Satellite metastases****: Either occur simultaneously with the original diagnosis or arise subsequent to* original excision. Typically, recurrences that are separate from the scar but **within 2–5 cm of it are considered satellite metastases.**
- ***In-transit metastases:*** **Regional recurrences** beyond 5 cm of the scar but proximal to regional nodes.
- ***Regional node metastases*** *are typically in a draining nodal basin near the lesion.*

A. Intratumoral Therapies

- **Intralesional BCG:** Regression of uninjected and injected lesions.

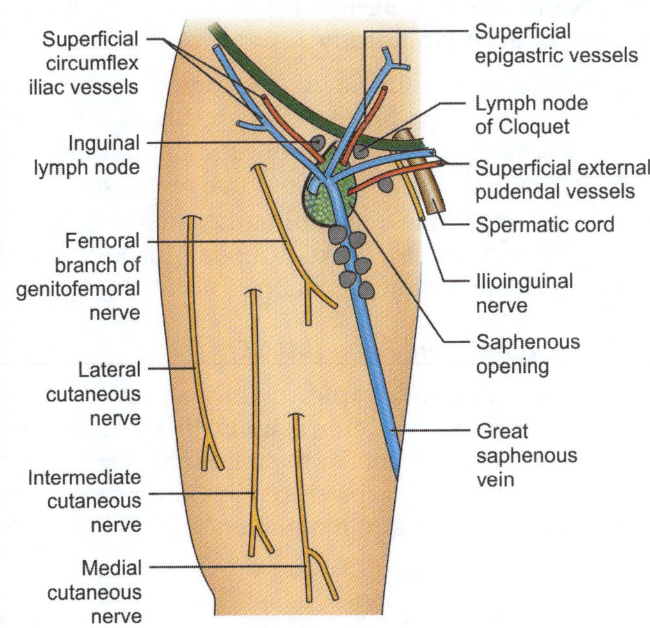

Fig. 31.62: Lymphatic anatomy of the groin region

- Intralesional injection of melanoma metastases with an **oncolytic herpes virus encoding granulocyte macrophage–colony-stimulating factor (GM-CSF).**

B. Solitary In-transit Metastasis or a Localized Cluster of In-transit Metastases

- Excision plus SNBx
- The margin of excision: 5–10 mm

C. Hyperthermic Isolated Limb Perfusion with Melphalan Infusion

- Complete responses in 60–90% of patients
- Risk of limb loss

D. Palliative Treatment of Regional Metastasis

- **Radiation therapy:** After surgical resection.
- **Intralesional therapy with** IFN, IL-2, BCG, or oncolytic replication competent virus injections.
- Highest response rates to intralesional therapy—intratumoral IL-2, intratumoral electrochemotherapy with bleomycin or cisplatin.
- **Dyes like Rose Bengal** or application of diphencyprone.
- **Topical treatment** of superficial metastases with imiquimod.

STAGE IV: MELANOMA

Metastatic disease: M1a: Skin, soft tissue, remote nodes; M1b: Visceral pulmonary and M1c: Visceral nonpulmonary. Stage 4 disease with metastasis and increased LDH is the highest risk category—Stage 1VC.

1. Cytotoxic Chemotherapy and Biochemotherapy

- **Biochemotherapy** consisting of **dacarbazine** 800 mg/m^2 on day 1, cisplatin 20 mg/m^2 on days 1–4; vinblastine 1.2 mg/m^2 on days 1 –4; IL-29 MU/m^2 per day continuous IV administration on days 1–4; **interferon** 5 MU/m^2 subcutaneously on days 1–4, 8, 10, and 12; and **granulocyte colony stimulating factor** 5 μg/kg per day subcutaneously on days 7–16. Biochemotherapy cycles are given every 21 days for 3 cycles (9 weeks total) (Key Box 31.15).

Key Box 31.15

Interferon-α

- It has stimulatory effect on natural killer cells (NK)
- It has anti-angiogenic activity
- It is toxic—weight loss and myelosuppression can occur
- IL-2—can cause capillary leak syndrome—hypotension and renal failure

2. Cytotoxic T-lymphocyte Antigen 4 and PD-1 Blockade in Adjuvant Therapy

Ipilimumab is a fully human immunoglobulin G1 monoclonal antibody that blocks CTLA4, which has demonstrated improvement in OS in the treatment of metastatic melanoma in two randomized clinical trials.

3. Interleukin-2

- IV bolus infusion of 600,000 to 720,000 IU/ kg every 8 hours to tolerance using 2 cycles separated by approximately 10 days (maximum of 15 doses/cycle).
- Significant toxicity (but reversible).

4. Chemotherapy

- Inherent resilience of melanocytes, which have to be naturally resistant to apoptotic death when exposed to UV radiation from the sun.
- Dacarbazine, an imidazole carboxamide, is a classic alkylating agent. It is given intravenously at daily doses of 200 mg/m^2 for 5 days every 3–4 weeks.
- Temozolomide is an orally available prodrug—not superior.
- Combination chemotherapy.
- 20% response for carboplatin-paclitaxel-sorafeniband, and 18% for carboplatin-paclitaxel.

5. Anti-cytotoxic T-Lymphocyte Antigen 4 Blocking Antibodies

- Inactivated tumour vaccines, dendritic cell vaccines or immune-stimulating cytokines like IFN and IL-2 are aimed at turning on T cells against cancer.
- Tumour responses tend to be durable (counted in years) in most cases.
- Thus, there is interest in this mode of therapy for advanced melanoma.

6. Adoptive Cell Transfer Therapy

- **Adoptive cell transfer** (ACT) therapy refers to an immunotherapy approach for the treatment of cancer that involves the infusion to the tumour-bearing host of cells with antitumour activity that may recognize cancer antigens and **result in the destruction of cancer cells**.
- Although it is still experimental, ACT has emerged among the most effective treatments for patients with **metastatic melanoma.**
- 50–70% of patients with metastatic melanoma experience objective cancer regressions as per RECIST criteria when treated with ACT.

RECIST criteria: **Response Evaluation Criteria In Solid Tumours.** Response to the tumour or lymph nodes by chemotherapy/radiotherapy or any other therapies are measured by means of CT scan or X-rays or with callipers. A few other lesions are non-measurable such as pleural effusions, pericardial effusions, etc.[1]

Indications to Radiotherapy

Radiation Therapy for Regional Metastasis

- Melanoma is a radioresponsive tumour and conventional and high dose per fraction schedules are equally effective clinically.
- 8.0 Gy × 4 fractions (32 Gy total) in 21 days delivered once weekly or 2.5 Gy × 20 fractions (50 Gy total) in 26–28 days delivered 5 days a week.

Adjuvant Radiation Therapy in the Management of Primary Melanoma Lesions

- **Lentigo maligna:** Medically inoperable, or if the proposed resection would result in a poor cosmetic outcome.
- **Desmoplastic melanoma:** High chances of recurrence.
- **Neurotropic melanoma:** Propensity to recur at the skull base by tracking along cranial nerves.
- **Palliation of unresectable** primary disease.

GENETIC TESTING AND IMMUNOTHERAPY

- BRAF mutation test may be performed using the mutation-specific PCR tests for the use of **vemurafenib, dabrafenib, or trametinib.**

Melanoma Antigen Gene as in Cancer Immunotherapy

- Immunization against antigenic tumour epitopes is achieved by injecting recombinant tumour antigen protein along with an immunostimulant to induce both humoral and cellular immune responses.
- Patients receiving recombinant MAGE-A3-based vaccine will develop MAGE-A3-specific antibodies and have more clinical benefits.

Melanoma Antigen Gene (MAGE)

- Modern immunotherapies mainly aim to activate immune responses by either stimulating the activities of specific components of the immune system or by counteracting signals produced by cancer cells, such as immune checkpoint modulators and immune cell therapy.

[1]European Journal of Cancer 45 (2009) 228–247.

OTHER MALIGNANT SKIN TUMOURS

Dermatofibrosarcoma Protuberans

- This is a **locally malignant tumour** arising from the dermis.
- Common sites are the trunk and flexor region of limbs. It presents as a nodular (bosselated) ulcerative lesion of many years duration (Figs 31.63 and 31.64).
- **Regional lymph node involvement** is uncommon.
- It is less aggressive and, therefore, curable.
- Treatment is by **local wide excision,** followed by primary closure or skin grafting.

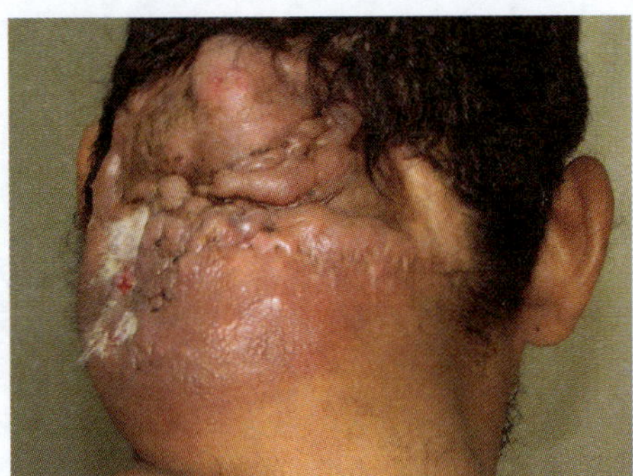

Fig. 31.63: Dermatofibrosarcoma over the nape of the neck

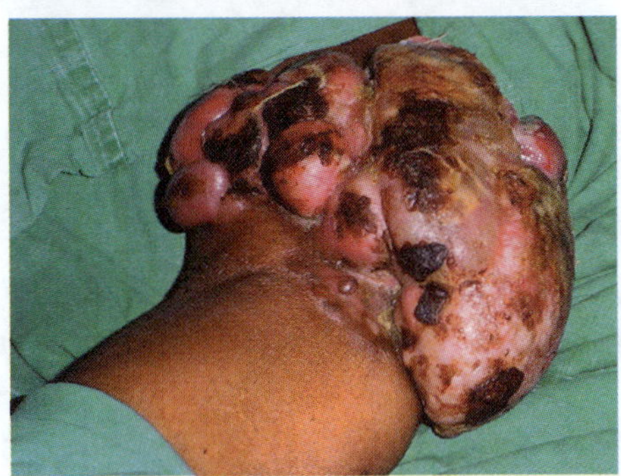

Fig. 31.64: Dermatofibroma protuberans upper limb

Kaposi's Angiosarcoma (Key Boxes 31.16 and 31.17)

- Common among the **Black population**
- It arises from **proliferating capillary vessels** and perivascular connective tissue cells.
- **Multiple, purplish nodules** appear in the limb, which ulcerate and bleed. This is its characteristic feature.
- Regional lymph node involvement may occur.
- Increasing incidence due to AIDS.

Differential Diagnoses

1. Malignant melanoma
2. Soft tissue sarcoma
3. Multiple cutaneous metastases
4. T cell lymphoma

Key Box 31.16

Diseases Associated with Kaposi's Sarcoma

- Diabetes mellitus
- Lymphoma
- Following renal transplantation
- Acute and chronic immunosuppression (HIV)

Key Box 31.17

Types of Kaposi's Sarcoma

- European : Elderly males
- African : Young and children
- Transplant : Due to immunosuppression
- AIDS : Homosexuals

OTHER SKIN LESIONS

They arise from sebaceous glands, sweat glands, hair follicles, etc. Key Box 31.18 describes types of exocrine glands.

- A few examples are syringoma, hidradenoma, tricho-epithelioma, and sebaceous carcinoma.
- They present as a localised swelling and are treated by excision.
- **They have to be kept in mind as a differential diagnosis for malignant skin tumours.** Details of a few skin lesions are given in this chapter.

Keratoacanthoma: Molluscum Sebaceum, Molluscum Pseudocarcinomatosum

- Self-limiting benign neoplasm of viral origin (probably).
- Arises due to overgrowth of the hair follicle.
- Subsequent spontaneous regression is characteristic.
- It is a painless swelling in the skin with a central dark-brown core. After an initial rapid growth of 2–4 weeks, spontaneous regression occurs within 24 hours. After separation of the central core, the lump diminishes in size, leaving a deep indrawn scar.
- Usually single—face is the most common site.
- Like sebaceous cyst, it presents as a hemispherical swelling.
- It is treated by excision.

Key Box 31.18

Types of Exocrine Glands

- ***Holocrine:*** Entire cell dies or disintegrates to liberate secretion, e.g. sebaceous gland.
- ***Apocrine:*** Only the luminal part of the cell disintegrates, cell regeneration takes place from the nucleus and basal portion, e.g. mammary gland.
- ***Merocrine:*** Secretion is discharged without destruction of the cells. Most of the glands belong to this type.

- If associated with sebaceous carcinoma (Fig. 31.65) and visceral malignancy (colon cancer), it constitutes Muir-Torre syndrome.

Turban Tumour (Figs 31.66 and 31.67)

It is the **blanket term** used to describe a tumour occupying the whole scalp, resembling a **turban**.

- It is most often used to describe multiple cylindromata.
- They produce **pink nodular masses.**
- Diagnosis is confirmed by biopsy.
- For differential diagnoses, *see* Key Box 31.19.
- Treatment includes excision and reconstruction by skin grafting or rotational flaps.

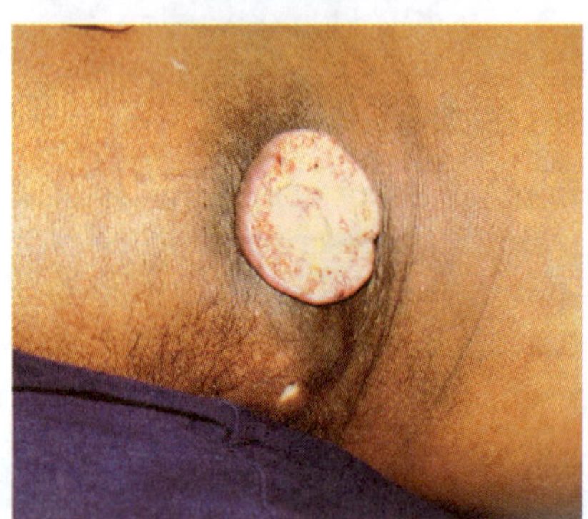

Fig. 31.65: Sebaceous carcinoma

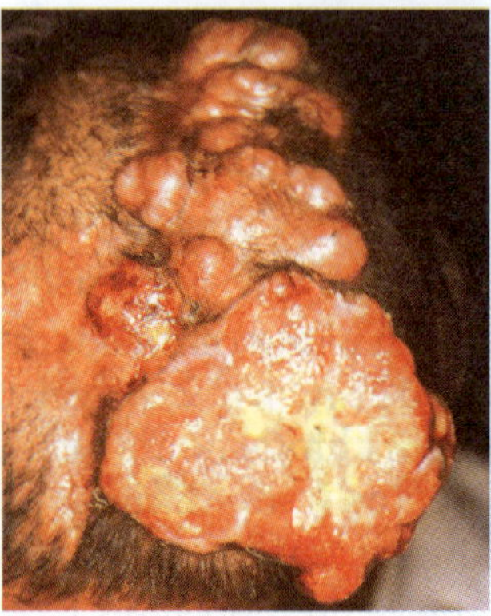

Fig. 31.66: Turban tumour due to squamous cell carcinoma of scalp

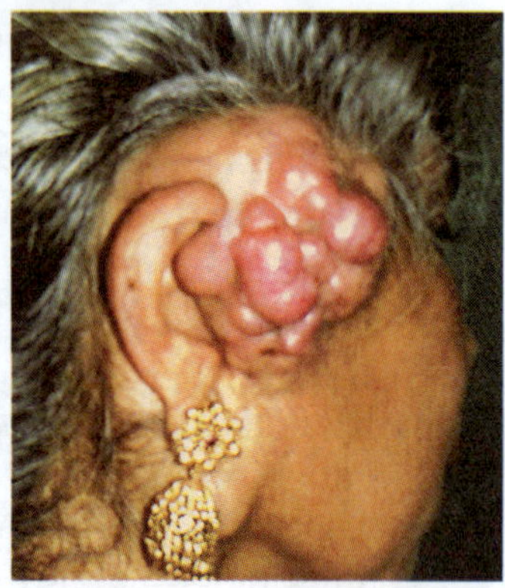

Fig. 31.67: Turban tumour (*Courtesy:* Dr Sreejayan, Professor of Surgery, Calicut Medical College)

Key Box 31.19

Turban Tumour

- Very, very rare

Types

- Multiple cylindromata
- Multiple nodular basal cell carcinoma
- Hidradenomata
- Plexiform neurofibromatosa of scalp

Corn

It is a **popular painful lesion in the plantar surface (sole) of the foot.**

- It affects the plantar surface of toes and the sole of the feet.
- It develops due to intermittent pressure over a limited area.
- Basically, it is a localised area of hyperkeratinisation with a hard central core.
- It is a cone-shaped lesion with a broad surface and is narrow at the deeper plane.
- They are **painful and very tender**.
- Most are **hard corns**.
- **Soft corn** may occur between the toes.

Treatment

- Diabetic patients need to be carefully explained about the consequences of a 'mistreated' corn. Sensations and pulsation have to be checked.
- Symptomatic corns have to be excised. **Excision of a good cone-shaped** tissue is necessary for permanent cure. Otherwise, **recurrence may occur**.

Wart

- A wart is a rough excrescence on the skin
- Papilloma viruses are responsible
- They are pigmented, keratinised, irregular lesions
- Common in young adults
- **Common sites:** Fingers, feet, genitalia, beard area, etc.
- **Venereal warts:** They are also called **papilloma acuminata**. They may occur in the anal region, perineum, and the coronal sulcus of the penis. Some warts may regress spontaneously. **Fulguration** with diathermy is the treatment.

Merkel Cell Carcinoma

- It is derived from neuroendocrine cells that function as touch receptors.
- **It is a highly malignant tumour.**
- Elderly white males are affected.
- Sun-affected areas (such as head and neck regions) are involved, probably due to **ultraviolet rays**.
- Surgery, radiation, and chemotherapy have been tried.
- Histopathological report resembles **metastatic oat cell carcinoma**.

Multiple Choice Questions

1. Which of the following statements about basal cell carcinoma is false?
A. It starts as a nonhealing ulcer of many months duration
B. Outer canthus of the eye is a common site
C. It may spread by lymphatics
D. Haematogenous spread is almost unknown

2. The following are true for basal cell carcinoma *except*:
A. It is the most common malignant tumour
B. It cannot occur in the lips
C. Arsenic used in skin ointments may increase the risk
D. Morpheaform variety grows very slowly

3. The characteristic feature of basal cell carcinoma is:
A. Epithelial pearls
B. Mitotic figures
C. Orphan Annie nuclei
D. Palisading islands

4. The following are used to treat basal cell carcinoma *except*:
A. Wide excision
B. Mohs' micrographic surgery
C. Radiation
D. Radiofrequency ablation

5. The following are true for basal cell carcinoma *except*:
A. Ultraviolet rays may predispose to this condition
B. Mohs' micrographic surgery can minimise the recurrence
C. CO_2 laser may be used to treat deep lesions
D. Gorlin's syndrome is associated with multiple basal cell carcinoma

6. The following skin malignancies may spread by lymphatics *except*:
A. Epithelioma
B. Malignant melanoma
C. Sebaceous carcinoma
D. Basal cell carcinoma

7. The characteristic feature of epithelioma is:
A. Penetrating lesion
B. Elevated, beaded edge
C. Proliferative growth with everted edges
D. Nodular lesion

8. The following are true for epithelioma *except*:
A. The majority are well differentiated
B. Cell nest is characteristic
C. Broder's classification is used
D. Polyhedral cells

9. The following are true for Marjolin's ulcer *except*:
A. It arises from scar tissues
B. It does not spread by lymphatics
C. It is rapidly growing
D. It is painless

10. The following are true about prognostic factors for epithelioma *except*:
A. Metastasis is unlikely if the lesion is >10 mm
B. Broder's high grade means poor prognosis
C. Recurrence is more in the lip
D. Perineural involvement carries poor prognosis

11. Which of the following statements about melanocytes is false?
A. They are derived from the neural crest
B. They convert DOPA into melanin
C. Melanocyte stimulating hormone is released from the intermediate lobe of the pituitary gland
D. Present in the stratum basale layer of the epidermis

12. The following are true for malignant melanoma *except*:
A. Spindle cell naevus has high malignant potential
B. Junctional naevus has very high malignant potential
C. The superficial spreading variety is the most common form
D. Tyrosinase is absent in albinos

13. The following are true for thin melanomas *except*:
A. <1 mm thickness
B. Metastasis in about 10–15 %
C. 20 years survival is almost 95%
D. Local wide excision of 2 cm margin is recommended

14. The following are true for acral lentiginous variety of melanoma *except*:
A. Least common subtype
B. Occurs in the palms and soles
C. Hutchinson's sign may be found
D. Rarely found in Blacks

15. The following are true for superficial spreading malignant melanoma *except*:

A. Most common subtype
B. Trunk is the common site
C. Average age of presentation is the 5th decade
D. It has a long, vertical growth

16. Which of the following treatments is recommended in 2 cm melanoma leg with inguinal nodes?

A. Wide excision with inguinal block dissection
B. Wide excision with ilioinguinal block dissection
C. Wide excision with ilioinguinal obturator dissection
D. Amputation with inguinal block dissection

17. Which of the following drugs is used to decrease cerebral metastasis in malignant melanoma?

A. Adriamycin B. Cisplatin
C. Temozolamide D. IFN-α

18. IFN-α has the following actions *except*:

A. Stimulatory effect on natural killer cells
B. Anti-angiogenic activity
C. Does not cause myelosuppression
D. May cause capillary leak syndrome

19. The following are true for Merkel cell tumour *except*:

A. It is a highly malignant tumour
B. It is derived from neuroendocrine tumours
C. Fingers and digits are the common sites
D. The head and neck are commonly involved

20. The following are true for Kaposi's angiosarcoma *except*:

A. Common in the Black population
B. Paclitaxel is the drug of choice with 75% effectiveness
C. Homosexuals are affected more as a result of AIDS
D. The classic form affects the head and neck more than the legs

21. The following are features of lymph node of Cloquet *except*:

A. It is the transitional node between the inguinal region and the iliac region
B. A superficial groin dissection should include removal of that node
C. If that nodes contain metastatic melanoma, an iliac and obturator dissection is usually indicated.
D. It is an inferior member of the lymph node medial to femoral vein.

Answers

1. C	**2.** D	**3.** D	**4.** D	**5.** C	**6.** D	**7.** C	**8.** D	**9.** C	**10.** A
11. C	**12.** B	**13.** D	**14.** D	**15.** D	**16.** B	**17.** C	**18.** C	**19.** C	**20.** D
21. D									

CHAPTER

32

Burns and Skin Grafting

- Epidemiology
- Classification
- Clinical evaluation
- Burn wound infection
- Inhalation injury
- Contractures
- Electrical burns
- Chemical burns
- Friction burn
- Skin bank
- Skin grafting
- Medico-legal aspects of burns

Burn wounds are one of the most enigmatic and challenging injuries in the medical field. It can vary from small wounds such as sunburn which heal without a trace to larger ones which disproportionately cause initiation of systemic inflammatory response and could lead to immune compromise, multiorgan failure and often death. The ones who survive major burn injuries are frequently left scarred and crippled.

Competency

SU4.1: Elicit document and present history in a case of burns and perform physical examination. Describe pathophysiology of burns.

EPIDEMIOLOGY

A burn is defined as an injury to the skin or other organic tissue primarily caused by heat, radiation, electricity, friction or contact with chemicals.

Heat burns occur when some or all of the different layers of cells in the skin are destroyed by contact with hot liquid (scald), a hot solid (contact burn) or a flame (flame burn). Skin injuries due to ultraviolet radiation, radioactivity, electricity or chemicals, as well as respiratory damage resulting from smoke inhalation, are also considered as burns.

The majority of these injuries occur in low- and middle-income countries, with almost half occurring in the South-East Asia Region.

In India, around 7 million people suffer from burn injuries each year with 1.4 lakh deaths and 2.4 lakh people suffer with disability.

India has one of the highest incidence of burns in the world. Women and children are the victims about 80% of the time (4 out of 5 victims).

Survival following burn injury has significantly improved over the last several years with the introduction of multidisciplinary approach, early aggressive fluid resuscitation, use of effective topical antimicrobial agents, and most importantly the practice of early burn wound excision and wound cover. However, extensive burn injuries remain potentially fatal.

CLASSIFICATION

- Based on causative agent
  1. **Thermal**
     - Moist heat (scalds)
     - Dry heat (flame burn and contact burn)
  2. **Electrical**
  3. **Chemical**
  4. **Cold** (frostbite)
  5. **Ionising radiation**
- Based on depth of burn
  1. First degree—involves only the epidermis
  2. Second degree—involves varying thickness of dermis
  3. Third degree—involves the epidermis, dermis and subcutaneous tissue
  4. Fourth degree—including fascia, muscles or bones

PATHOPHYSIOLOGY OF A BURN WOUND

Jackson's description of the three zones of injury of the burn wound (Fig. 32.1):

- The **zone of coagulation** is at the centre of the wound where no viable cells remain.
- Surrounding it is the **zone of stasis**, characterised as a mix of viable and non-viable cells, capillary vasoconstriction, and ischaemia. This area represents the zone 'at-risk' and may convert to necrosis with hypoperfusion, desiccation, oedema, and infection. With proper wound care management and fluid resuscitation, however, these changes may be reversed.
- The periphery of the burn wound is the **zone of hyperaemia,** with viable cells and vasodilation mediated by local inflammatory mediators. Tissue in this zone usually recovers completely unless complicated by infection or severe hypoperfusion.

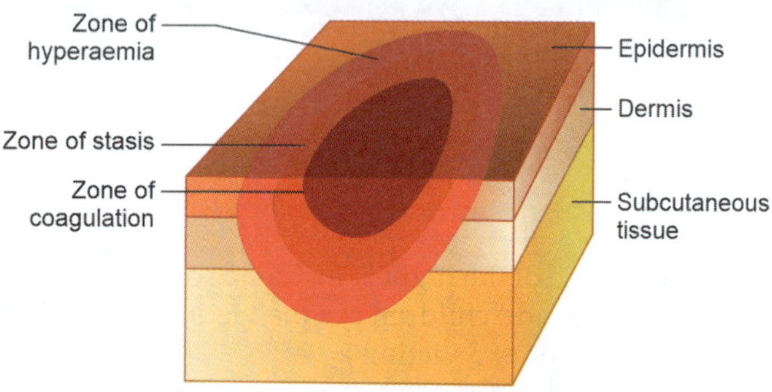

Fig. 32.1: Jackson's zones of burn injury

Burn Shock

Shock is an abnormal physiological situation resulting in insufficient delivery of oxygen and nutrients to tissues and removal of cellular waste products secondary to inadequate intravascular blood volume. Thermal injury results in massive shift of fluid from vascular compartment to the interstitial compartment causing fall in blood pressure and hence shock.

Burn injury releases several inflammatory mediators (histamine, prostaglandins,thromboxane, kinins, etc.) which increase the microvascular permeability and alter cell membrane function which favours fluid shift from blood vessels to interstitial compartment.

Emergency Management

- Burns patients must be considered trauma victims and Advanced Trauma Life Support (ATLS) protocols must be used in their evaluation. Airway, breathing, circulation, disability and examine for major associated injuries such as head injuries, chest injuries, abdominal injuries and fractures must be looked for.
- A—Airway
- B—Breathing
- C—Circulation
- D—Disability
- E—Examine for associated major injuries

First Aid

- Put out the flame!
  - Make the victim roll on the ground
  - Apply a thick wet blanket
  - Using water or fire-extinguishers
- Remove **source of injury,** such as clothing unless stuck to skin.
- Remove items **prolonging injury**
- Remove jewellery, belts, other restrictive items.
- **Cooling** injured areas with running water.
- Gentle **cleansing** of affected area of dirt and soot

Competency

SU4.2: Describe clinical features, diagnose type and extent of burns and plan appropriate treatment.

CLINICAL EVALUATION

Extent of Burns

The extent of body surface area involved is one of the most important indicators of mortality independent of the depth of injury.

Some of the most commonly used methods to clinically estimate the total body surface area (TBSA) burned are:

1. Wallace rule of 9 (Fig. 32.2).
2. Lund and Browder chart (Fig. 32.3).

Wallace rule of 9 is the simplest and most commonly used formula. It delineates the body surface area into anatomical regions as multiples of 9 and genitalia as 1%. Lund and Browder chart is a more accurate formula as the difference in body proportions of children and adults are taken into consideration.

Depth of Burns

The depth of burn is the main factor influencing the ability of the wound to heal itself, as the greater depth of injury will result in fewer surviving dermal and epidermal elements to initiate healing and regeneration. Thus it is important in deciding on wound management and whether or not to intervene surgically.

Depth of burn wound is classified as follows.

1. First degree—superficial burn involving only epidermis

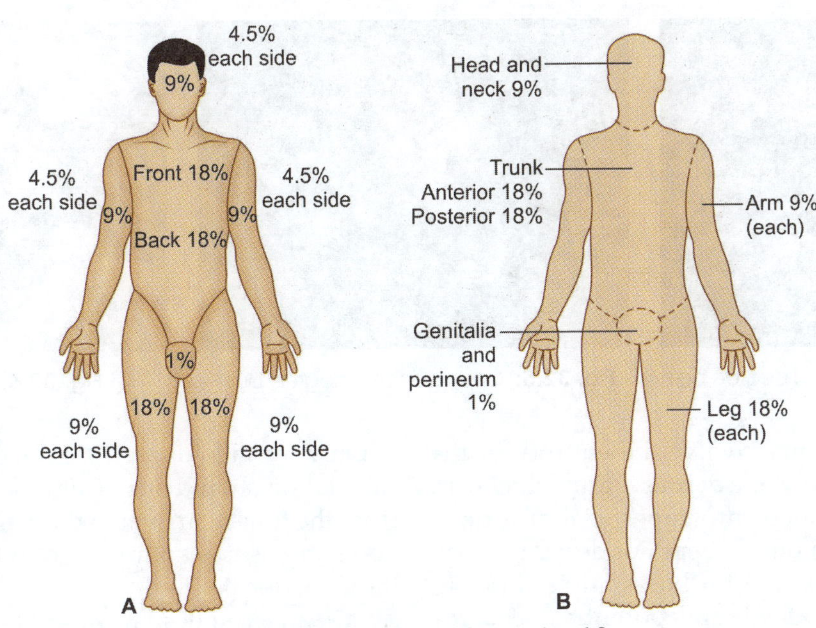

Figs 32.2A and B: Wallace rule of 9

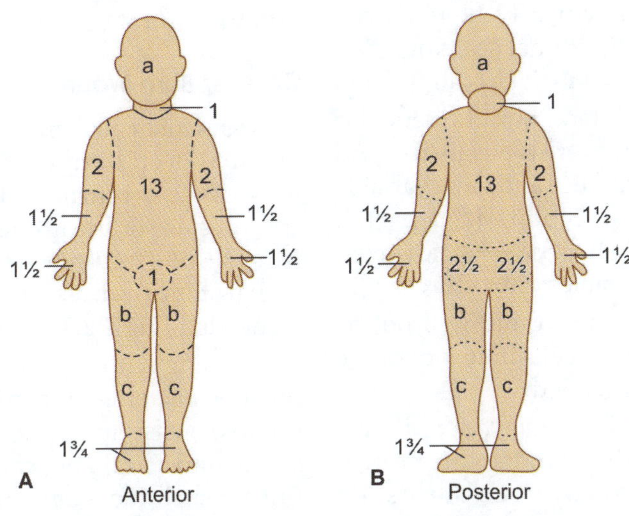

Relative percentage of body surface area (% BSA) affected by growth

Body part	Age 0 yr	1 yr	5 yr	10 yr	15 yr
a = ½ of head	9½	8½	6½	5½	4½
b = ½ of 1 thigh	2¾	3¼	4	4¼	2½
c = ½ of 1 lower leg	2½	2½	2¾	3	3¼

Figs 32.3A and B: Lund and Browder chart

2. Second degree
   - Superficial dermal
   - Deep dermal
3. Third degree–full thickness of skin including subcutaneous tissue
4. Fourth degree—involving muscles and bones

Depth of injury depends on:
- The temperature of the causative agent
- Duration of contact

Superficial or first degree burns involve only the epidermis. It forms erythema, oedema and burning sensation. Heals in about 5–7 days.

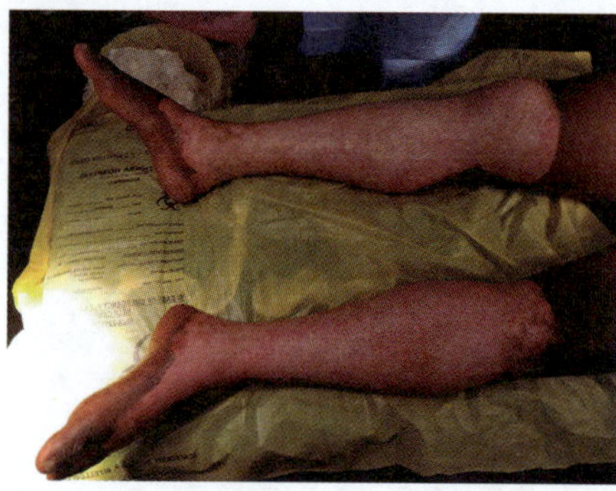
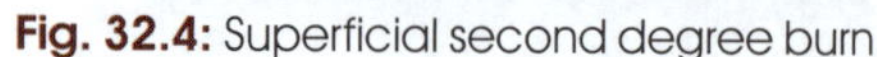

Fig. 32.4: Superficial second degree burn

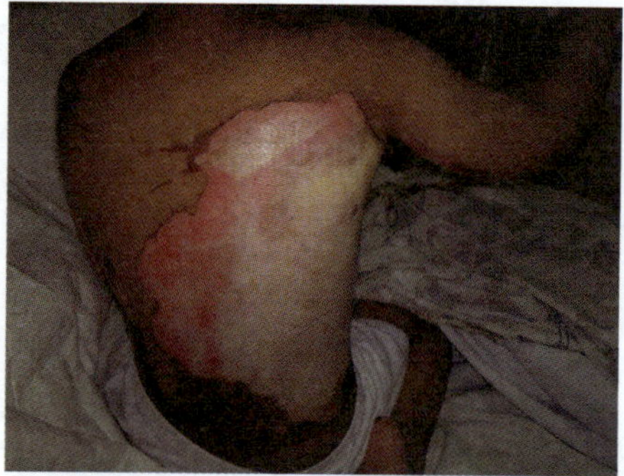

Fig. 32.5: Deep second degree burn

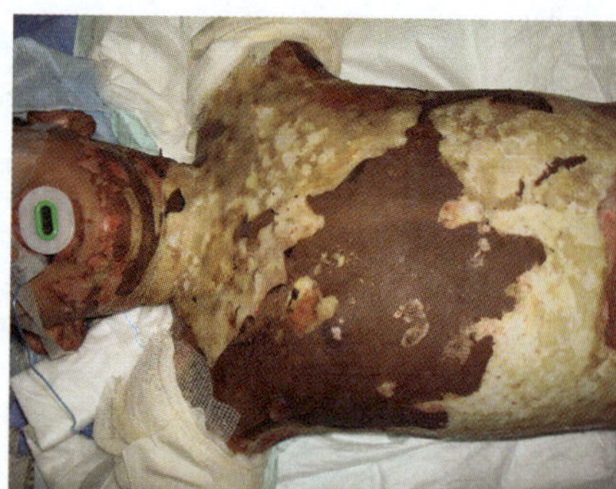

Fig. 32.6: Third degree burn

Partial thickness burns involve the entirety of the epidermis and a portion of the dermis. Partial thickness burns are further divided into superficial and deep partial thickness based on the depth of dermal injury. Superficial and deep partial thickness burns differ in appearance, ability to heal, and potential need for excision and skin grafting. Superficial partial thickness burns are typically pink, moist, and painful to touch (Fig. 32.4). These burns will typically heal within 2 weeks and generally result in minimal scarring.

Deep partial thickness burns (Fig. 32.5) involve the entirety of the epidermis and extend into the reticular portion of the dermis. These burns are typically dry and mottled pink and white in appearance and have variable sensation. If protected from infection, deep partial thickness burns will heal within 3 to 8 weeks, however, typically with scarring and possible contractures.

Therefore, if it appears that the wound will not be completely re-epithelialized in 3 weeks time, operative excision and grafting is recommended.

Full thickness burns (Fig. 32.6) involve the epidermis and the entirety of the dermis. These wounds are brown-black, leathery, and they are usually insensate and do not blanch. Full thickness burns are best treated by excision and grafting.

Resuscitation

- Secure a good IV access.
- For major burns, central venous line is preferred.
- Fluid resuscitation: Various formulas are used for calculating fluid requirement in burns. They include Muir and Barclay, Evans, Brooks, etc. Commonly used is Parkland's formula.
- According to Parkland's formula, total fluid for first 24 hr is 4 ml × body weight (kg) × % of total body surface area burned (TBSA)
  - Half of the calculated fluid given in first 8 hours
  - Next half given in next 16 hours
  - Important to maintain good urine output 0.5–1 ml/kg/hr

Only crystalloids are used during first 24 hours. Fluid calculation should start from the time of burn and not from the time of arrival to the hospital. Colloids are not necessary as it is not retained in the circulation during initial period.

Adequacy of fluid resuscitation is assessed based on monitoring of pulse, blood pressure and signs of dehydration. Better method is monitoring hourly urine output/central venous pressure (CVP).

Care of Burn Wound

Assessment of area and depth of burn. Look for circumferential deep burn on the extremities or chest which may cause a tourniquet effect resulting in vascular compromise or breathing difficulty as the case may be. In case of circumferential deep burn, emergency escharotomy (release of dried necrotic burn tissue) may be needed (Fig. 32.7).

Dressing with topical agents: An ideal topical agent must be bactericidal having broad spectrum coverage, nontoxic, easy to apply, should penetrate deep to the eschar and should not cause any metabolic disturbance. But no such ideal agent is available. Commonly used agents are:

- Silver sulfadiazine
- Silver nitrate gel/solution
- Fucidic acid, etc.

Over the topical agent, cotton pads and bandaging is applied.

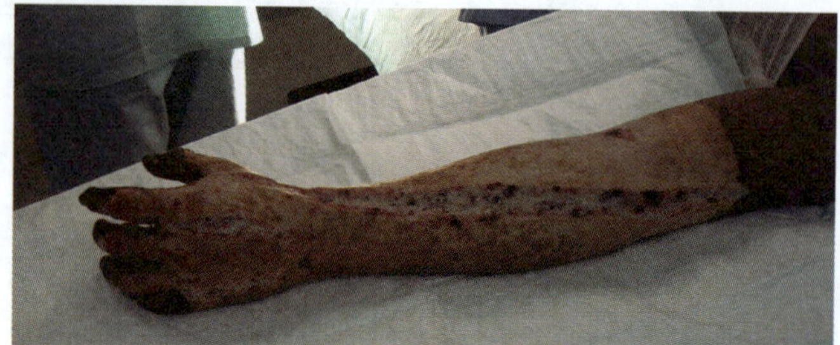

Fig. 32.7: Escharotomy for circumferential burn

Biologic dressings gives temporary covering for the wound alleviating pain and protection from infection, e.g.
- Collagen
- Amniotic membrane.

Surgery

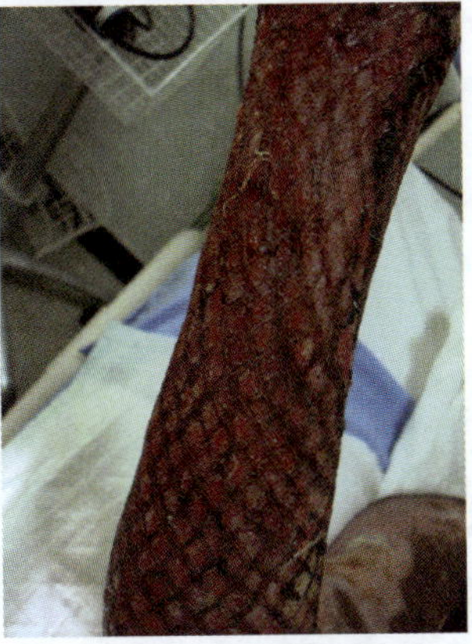

Fig. 32.8: Meshed SSG

Early burn wound excision and cover with autograft or allograft is preferred to reduce the morbidity and mortality. At a time, 15–20% of burn wound can be excised. Adequate blood should be arranged for surgery. Debridement can be full thickness excision or tangential excision depending on the depth of burn. When the burn wound is large, meshed skin grafts (Fig. 32.8) are used to cover wider area. In the absence, adequate autografts skin substitutes like cultured epithelial autografts (CEA), synthetic skin substitutes (e.g. Integra, Biobrane) or skin allografts may be used.

Other supportive measures:
- Good analgesia, e.g. morphine, paracetamol, NSAIDs
- Anti-histamines for decreasing histamine induced adverse reactions
- Gastroprotection: Against Curlings ulcer's (e.g. PPIs such as pantoprazole)

Nutritional Support

Forms an important feature of effective burn patient management. Hypermetabolism occurs following the injury and the diet should accommodate for the higher carbohydrate and protein requirements. This increased metabolic rate begins immediately following injury which can go up to 150 to 200% of normal and persists until complete wound coverage is achieved. The hypermetabolism may extend for months thereafter. Oral feeding should be encouraged and started early. Those who does not tolerate oral feeds, nasogastric tube feeding may be given.

Curreri formula for calculating calorific requirement:

Adults: 25 kcal × weight (kg) + 40 kcal × % TBSA

Protein requirement:

2 g × kg body weight per day

Supplements such as vitamin A, vitamin C, zinc, omega-3 fatty acids, glutamine, iron, etc. are also given routinely.

Burn Wound Infection

Early burn wound is sterile due to the thermal effect. Contamination of the wound occurs either from the environment or by opportunistic pathogens from the patient's own body. Infection remains a significant risk following burn injury. Burn patients are also immunocompromised for a number of reasons.

1. Loss of protective skin barrier
2. Cellular and humoral portions of the immune response are compromised.
3. Hypoproteinemia → Decreased production of antibodies
4. Impaired chemotaxis and phagocytosis

Infection can be bacterial, fungal or viral. Most often the infection is by bacteria and that too aerobic organisms. Common gram-positive infections are by *Staphylococcus* species, streptococci and enterococci. Majority of gram-negative infections are due to *Pseudomonas* species. Others include *Acinetobacter*, *E. coli*, *Klebsiella*, etc. which are often multidrug resistant.

Prophylactic antibiotics are not advisable for minor burns with early presentation. For major burns, all attempts should be made to remove the necrotic tissue under cover of broad spectrum antibiotic after attaining haemodynamic stability. Tissues are taken for bacterial culture at the time of initial debridement.

Following the initial 72 to 96 hours, periodic cultures are important in making a diagnosis of infection. Temperature spikes warrant culturing of wound, urine, blood, and central lines. Selection of antibiotics should be based on culture results.

Inhalation Injury

Inhalational burns are devastating and increase mortality of burn victims by 20% independent of other factors.

Scenarios
- Burns sustained in closed space
- Explosions
- Facial burns
- Prolonged exposure to flames

Suggestive clinical features
- Facial burns with singed facial and nose hair
- Inflamed and oedematous mucosa
- Sooty dark sputum in the mouth or nostrils
- Hoarseness or Stridor
- Laboured breathing

They may have inflamed airway, damaged lung tissue. May require intubation or tracheostomy.

Management

- Oxygenate—high flow O_2
- Establish and maintain patent airway. Intubate or perform tracheostomy early, if necessary.
- Obtain ABGs and blood CO levels, if possible.

Patients are predisposed to ARDS and pneumonia and may require aggressive treatment in the form of:

1. Chest physiotherapy
2. Pulmonary toilet
3. Bronchodilators
4. Intubation and mechanical ventilation
5. Sputum or bronchial lavage-based antibiotic therapy.

Complications of Burns

Early

- Shock, renal failure, wound infection
- Septicaemia
- ARDS, pneumonia
- Multiorgan failure

Late

- Scarring
- Contractures

CONTRACTURES

Definition

Wound contracture is a process that may occur during normal wound healing. When there is excess of wound contraction—an abnormal healing process—leads to physical deformity characterised by skin contraction and functional limitations (Fig. 32.9).

Goals of management:

1. Maximize function
2. Minimize disfigurement
3. Restore appearance

Timing of surgeries for contracture:

A. Exact timing of surgery is tailored to each patient's circumstances.

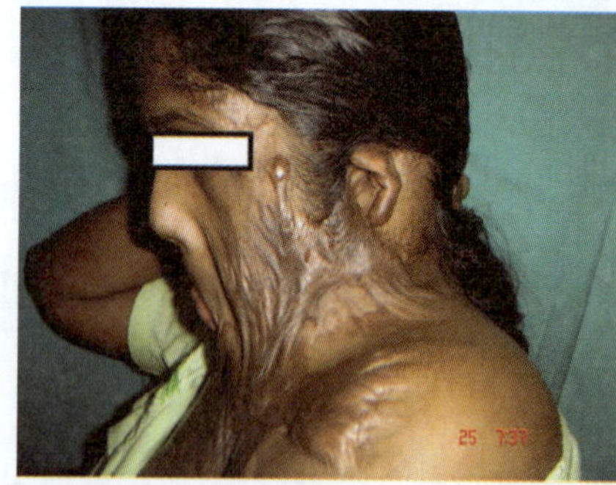

Fig. 32.9: Post-burn contracture

B. At least 3 months post-wound cover so as to attain adequate tissue equilibrium.

Contracture **prevention** and **non-operative** scar treatments:

1. Early and aggressive mobilization therapy with active and passive range of motion (ROM) exercises
2. Splints across joints
3. External pressure garments
4. Silicone gels and gel sheets
5. Intralesional triamcinolone injections
6. Laser resurfacing

Surgical interventions to minimize scar and contracture.

Reconstructive options after excision or release of contractures are:

1. Direct closure: If there is minimal tension across the wound
2. Serial excision
3. Skin grafts: Partial thickness grafts and full thickness grafts
4. Local flaps and tissue adjustments, such as Z-plasty
5. Tissue expansion
6. Distant flaps and free tissue transfer.

ELECTRICAL BURNS (Fig. 32.10)

Passage of electricity through the tissue generates heat depending on the tissue resistance. Low tension injuries are usually localised. High tension injuries can be devastating due to the damage caused in depth than on the surface.

Electrical burn can be:

- Direct contact burn
- Arc burn (current passes from a source to an object)
- Flash burn (similar to thermal burn)

Patients with electrical burn can develop cardiac, renal and neurological complications.

In the extremities can cause compartment syndrome which will require early fasciotomy (Fig. 32.11).

Electrical burns may have associated injuries like fractures following fall secondary to electric shock.

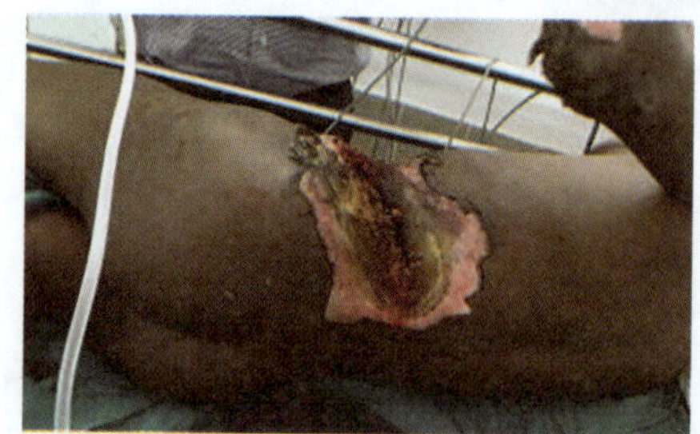

Fig. 32.10: Electrical burn

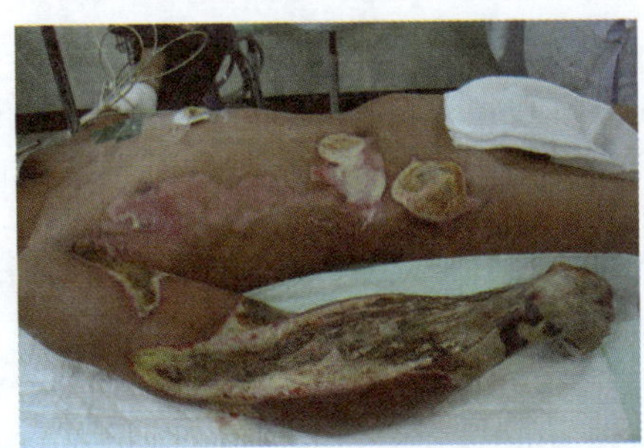

Fig. 32.11: Fasciotomy for electrical burn

Ressuscitation formulas may not be adequate as the extent of injury in the depth cannot be accurately assessed clinically. In the absence of myoglobinuria/ hemoglobinuria, a urine output of 30–50 ml/hour should be maintained with Ringer lactate solution. Higher urine output of 1–2 ml/kg body weight is necessary when associated with myoglobinuria.

After haemodynamic stability, all the devitalised tissues are debrided which may need multiple stages and reconstruction with skin grafts or flaps.

CHEMICAL BURNS (Fig. 32.12)

Chemicals cause irritation and destruction of tissues by different chemical reactions when in direct contact. Severity of chemical burn is determined by:

- Concentration of the chemical
- Duration of contact with the tissues
- Quantity of the chemical
- Mechanism of action

They act as oxidants, reducing agents, corrosives, protoplasmic poisons, vesicants or desiccants.

Common chemical burns are caused by acids or alkali. The latter cause more damage due to liquefaction necrosis, whereas acids act by coagulation necrosis.

Principles of management of chemical burns involve removal of all offending agents from the patients body. The involved part is thoroughly washed under running tap water for ½ to 1 hour. When burn occurs with chemical powder, it should be dusted off first before irrigation. Use of neutralizing agents is controversial.

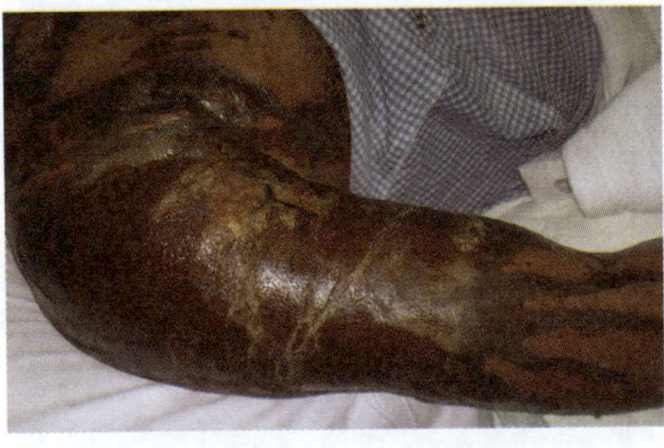

Fig. 32.12: Chemical burn

Special mention is necessary for hydrofluoric acid. It continues to destroy the tissues in the depth until comes in contact with bone. It can cause severe calcium deficiency which may be lethal. Local application of calcium gluconate gel, or subcutaneous/ intra-arterial calcium gluconate injections may be used as antidote.

Friction Burn

Results due to rubbing of the skin against a rough surface (Fig. 32.13). Most common cause is road traffic accidents. Other causes include sports injuries and fall from height. Superficial injuries can be treated conservatively. Deeper wounds may need tangential excision or full thickness excision and skin grafting.

Skin Bank

Skin harvested from cadavers can be stored at 4–8°C for prolonged periods in skin banks (tissue bank). Banked skin allografts are widely used nowadays for the management of major burns. Like other organ donation, skin also can be donated to save burn victims or patients with major skin loss. Being a temporary procedure, skin allotransplant does not need tissue matching. It has reduced the mortality and morbidity in burn patients considerably.

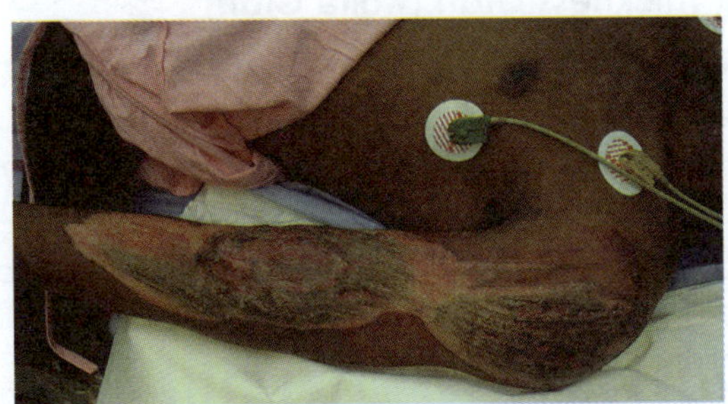

Fig. 32.13: Friction burn

FREE SKIN GRAFTING

Skin grafting is the commonest method of achieving wound cover.

TYPES

1. Split Skin Graft (SSG-Thiersch Graft)

- Also called partial thickness graft.
- Consists of epidermis and a variable portion of dermis (Figs 32.14 and 32.15).
- Split skin graft is usually harvested using Humby's knife (Fig. 32.16). Drum dermatome or a power dermatome may also be used.
- Preferred donor area is thigh.

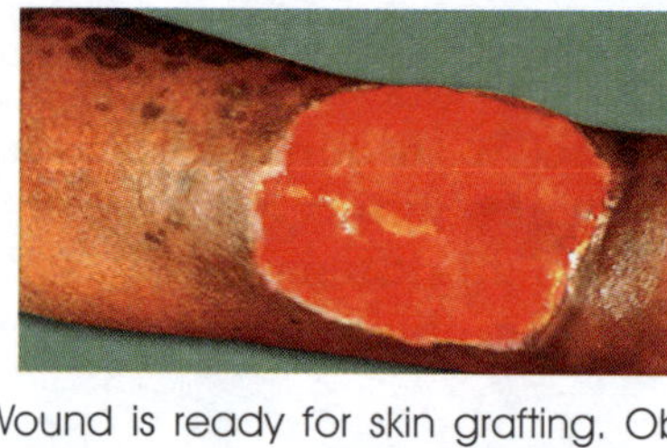

Fig. 32.14: Wound is ready for skin grafting. Observe the red granulation tissue

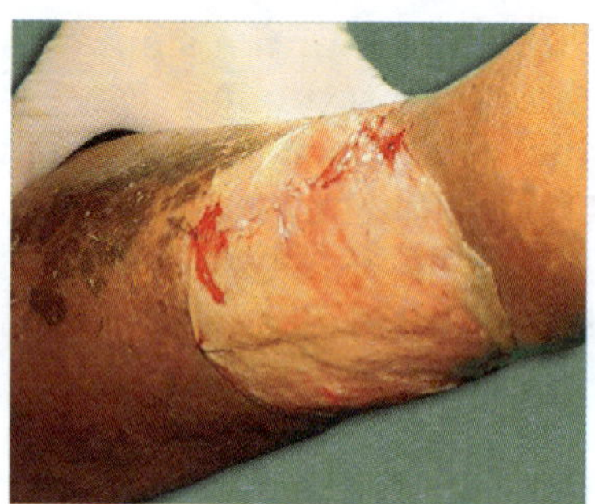

Fig. 32.15: Skin graft is applied over the recipient area

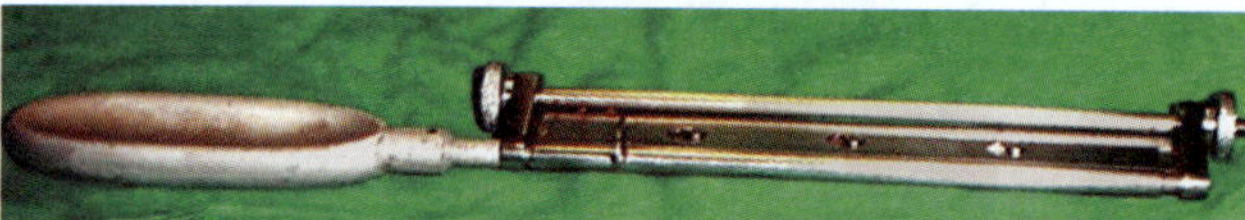

Fig. 32.16: Skin graft is taken from thigh using Humby's knife

2. Full Thickness Graft (Wolfe Graft)

- Consists of epidermis and full thickness of dermis.
- Harvested using ordinary scalpel.
- Needs excellent vascularity of the recipient wound for graft survival.
- Used for small uncontaminated wounds produced after excision of skin lesions or after release of skin contractures (lower eyelids, fingers).
- Donor area needs primary suturing or split skin graft for healing and hence limits the size of the graft.
- Unlike split skin grafts, full thickness grafts do not contract and retain their colour. Hence, they are cosmetically superior.

INDICATIONS OF SKIN GRAFT (Key Box 32.1)

1. Skin loss

- Post-traumatic (e.g. avulsion and degloving injury)
- Post-surgical (e.g. excision of tumours, excision of burn wound)
- As a result of pathological process (e.g. venous ulcer, diabetic ulcer)

2. Mucosa loss

- After excision of lesions of oral cavity, tongue.
- For resurfacing reconstructed vagina in cases of vaginal agenesis.

Key Box 32.1

Ideal Requirements for Free Skin Graft

- Wound should be free from infections such as streptococci and pseudomonas
- Vascular wounds, e.g. wounds with healthy granulation
- Wound should be thoroughly debrided
- Haemostasis must be achieved before placing the graft
- Close and immobile contact between graft and the wound
- Recipient area should be immobilised with POP slab

CONTRAINDICATIONS FOR SKIN GRAFT

- Infection by *beta-haemolytic streptococci.* They produce fibrinolysin which dissolves fibrin.
- Presence of an infected wound with copious discharge in the vicinity.
- Avascular wounds: With exposed bare bone without periosteum, exposed tendon without paratenon and exposed cartilage without perichondrium.

HEALING OF THE DONOR AREA

Donor area of split skin graft heals by epithelialisation from the adnexal remnants of dermis, pilosebaceous follicles and or sweat gland apparatus. Complete healing of donor area occurs by 8–10 days.

THE PROCESS OF GRAFT 'TAKE'

The processes which result in reattachment and revascularisation of the graft to the bed are collectively referred to as "take" of graft.

- The graft initially adheres to its new bed by fibrin. Revascularisation starts by 48 hours and is completed by 4–5 days. This is achieved by the outgrowth of capillary buds from the recipient area to unite with those on the deep surface of graft. For the first 2 days after grafting, the skin graft derives its nutrition from the wound by the process of serum imbibition/ plasmatic circulation.

FLAPS

Flap is a block of tissue transferred from donor to recipient area along with its vascularity.

COMMON INDICATIONS FOR FLAP SURGERY

- To cover defects/wounds where free skin graft cannot be used, e.g. exposed bare bones, bare tendons, bare cartilage.
- Wounds with exposed joints, exposed major vessels and nerves.

- Implant exposure following orthopaedic procedures.
- In wounds with soft tissue loss, where future reconstructive surgery is contemplated.
- Defects which need better contour to improve cosmesis.
- Breast reconstruction following mastectomy.

CLASSIFICATION OF FLAPS

These are broadly classified into pedicled flaps and free flaps.

I. Pedicled Flaps

Pedicle or the base remains attached to the donor site during its transfer to the recipient area (Figs 32.17 to 32.19). Pedicled flaps may be of following types:

1. Local flaps, e.g. rotation, transposition, limberg and bilobed.
2. Pectoralis major myocutaneous (PMMC) flap, deltopectoral (DP) flap for head and neck defects, transverse abdominis myocutaneous (TRAM) flap for breast reconstruction.
   - Regional flap, e.g. PMMC, DP for head and neck defects,
   - TRAM for breast reconstruction.

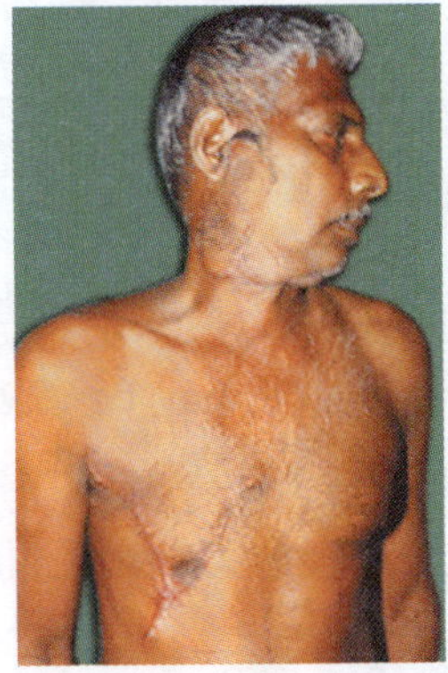

Fig. 32.17: PMMC flap following radical parotidec tomy

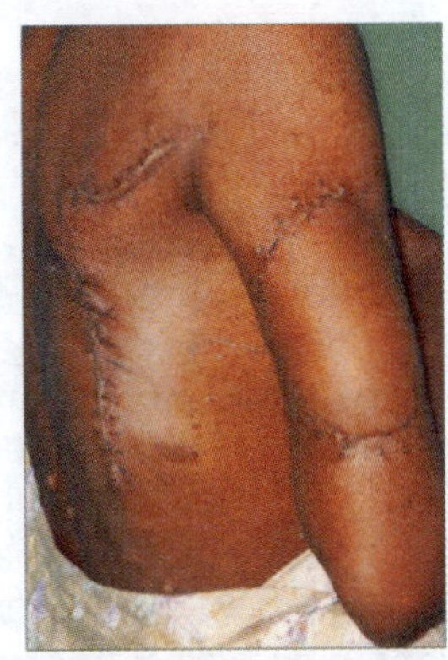

Fig. 32.18: Latissimus dorsi flap used to cover the defect in the arm following radical excision of a sarcoma

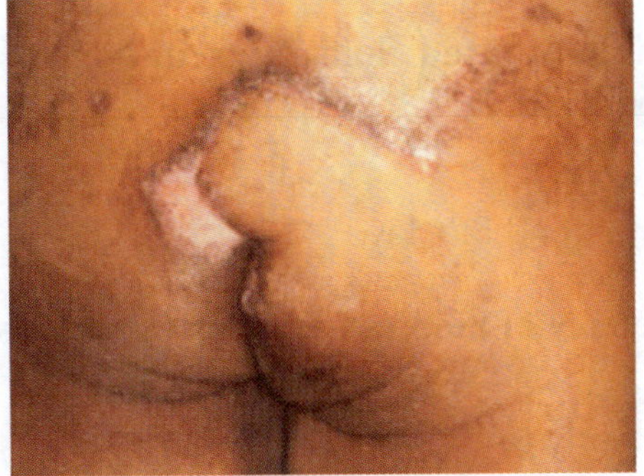

Fig. 32.19: Bedsore covered with local advancement flap

3. Distant flaps, e.g. groin flap, subaxillary flap for hand defects.

   A few examples of the pedicled flap
   - Skin flap
   - Fasciocutaneous flap
   - Muscle flap
   - Myocutaneous flap
   - Adipofascial flap
   - Osteocutaneous flap

II. Free Flaps

These are completely detached from the donor area before being transferred to the recipient area. The vascularity of the flap at the recipient site is immediately restored by anastomosing the vessels of the flap with the vessels at the recipient area using microvascular techniques.

SOME OF THE COMMONLY PERFORMED FLAPS

- **Forehead flap:** Entire forehead skin can be raised based on anterior branch of superficial temporal artery. It bears an unsightly scar of the donor site. Median (Indian) forehead flap based on supratrochlear vessels is a very useful flap in reconstructing defects over nose.
- **Deltopectoral (DP) flap:** It is supplied by upper 4 perforating branches of internal mammary artery and is used to reconstruct defects of neck and lower face. After about 4 weeks, the flap is divided and the base is returned to the chest wall.
- **Pectoralis major myocutaneous (PMMC) flap:** Pectoral branch of thoracoacromial artery is the pedicle of this flap. It is the ideal pedicled flap for reconstruction of head and neck defects following ablative surgeries for various head and neck cancers. Hence, it is described as a workhorse among the flaps. Osteomyocutaneous PMMC flap by including 5th or 6th rib can be used for mandibular reconstruction.
- **Latissimus dorsi flap (LDF):** As a myocutaneous flap, based on thoracodorsal vessels can be used for reconstruction of the lower half of face, neck, breast, chest wall, axilla, and upper arm.

FREE (MICROVASCULAR) FLAPS

Using operating microscope and microvascular techniques, it is possible to do a free tissue transfer of tissues such as skin, muscle, bone, intestine, omentum, etc. The procedure involves anastomosis of vessels of the flap to vessels at the donor site, e.g. latissimus dorsi muscle myocutaneous flap, radical artery forearm flap, gracilis flap and free fibula flap.

MISCELLANEOUS

Skin Substitutes

- This is one of the important requirements wherein large surface area of burns and skin is lost.
- An ideal substitute must be affordable, permanent, provide normal pigmentation, resist scar formation and grow with developing children.
- A few examples of skin substitutes are:
  - Dermal substitutes: They allow for creation of a 'neodermis'. They are formed from patient's own mesenchymal cells. Once 'neo-dermis' is formed, split thickness skin graft is applied. Thus, the burns site is closed quickly with less scarring.
  - Cultured epithelial autograft is another example of dermal substitute. They are cultured from patient's own full thickness biopsy. It will require 3 weeks to grow.
  - Another cultured skin is a biologic dressing from cultured neonatal keratinocytes and fibroblasts. They are all very expensive.

Hydrotherapy in Burns

It refers to usage of external water (may be very cold) to run over the burned part for a few minutes.

Methods used are:

1. Immersion hydrotherapy: It is performed in tubs called hydrotanks or burns tanks. Tanks should be disinfected after usage. Water used is sterile.
2. Shower hydrotherapy: Depending upon severity of burns, the shower can be either in supine or sitting position.
   Showering immediately rinses away dead skin and bacteria.

How does it work?

- Cleans the surface of wound and remove debris
- Removes pus
- Prevents loss of fluid through skin
- Minimises scar formation
- Provides moist environment for wound healing
- Minimises risk of infection

Duration

- It may vary from 10 to 20 minutes

Sedation

- Sedation or general anaesthesia is required as it can be very painful.

Competency

SU4.3: Discuss the medicolegal aspects in burn injuries.

1. **Antemortem or postmortem burns:** Firstly, it has to be determined whether the burns are antemortem or post-mortem in origin.
   Features of antemortem burns are:
   Presence of soot (carbonaceous particle) in airways
   Line of redness surrounding the burn injury
   Blister with serous fluid rich in protein and chloride
2. **Manner of sustaining burns:** It can be accidental, suicidal or homicidal
   Accidental burns: It is the commonest variety encountered. It may happen during cooking, careless burning of various forms of waste, fire cracker accidents or any other industrial/domestic accidents.
   Suicidal: Self-inflicted burns. It may be related in dowry (Section 304 (B) IPC). It may also be a form of protest against government (self-immolation)
   Homicidal: It may be done sometimes related to dowry or any other crime related to women. Sometimes a person may be killed by others using fire or any other inflammable substance.
   Scalds: May be accidental commonly. It may be also seen in child abuse cases where it is done deliberately on the child by the adult.
   Electrical burns: It is mainly accidental. Sometimes it may be suicidal which is however rare.
   Lightening burns: It is accidental in nature.

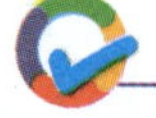

Multiple Choice Questions

1. What fluid is used for IV fluid resuscitation in burns according to Parkland's formula?

A. Crystalloids
B. Colloids
C. Both crystalloids and colloids
D. None of the above

2. Scald burns are caused by:

A. Chemicals B. Dry heat
C. Hot water D. Hot metal

3. Commonly used fluid resuscitation formula for burns is:

A. Evans B. Brooke's
C. Muir and Barclay D. Parkland's

4. Adequacy of fluid resuscitation in burns is assessed by:

A. Hourly urine output B. Volume of IV fluids
C. 24-hour urine volume D. Colour of urine

5. Which of the following is an example of biologic dressing?
A. Human amnion B. Paraffin gauze
C. Burn mesh D. Acticoat

6. Which formula is used for calculating energy requirement in burns?
A. Curreri formula B. Brooke's formula
C. Rule of 9 D. None of the above

7. Advantages of meshed skin grafts are:
A. Wider area of coverage
B. Lets out blood and serum from beneath the graft
C. Better graft take
D. All of the above

8. Fasciotomy is indicated in:
A. Scald burns B. Flame burns
C. Chemical burns D. Electrical burns

9. Antidote for hydrofluoric acid is:
A. Calcium chloride B. Calcium gluconate
C. Sodium chloride D. Sodium gluconate

10. Human skin allografts are usually obtained from:
A. Cadavers B. Live donors
C. Infected persons D. Newborn babies

11. Following factors contribute to burns shock *except:*
A Increased capillary permeability
B. Increased plasma oncotic pressure
C. Increased capillary hydrostatic pressure
D. Depressed myocardial function

12. Bacterial translocation can occur in the following conditions *except:*
A Burns
B. Subacute bacterial endocarditis
C. Intestinal obstruction
D. Myocardial infarction

13. Acute tubular necrosis can occur in burns due to the following factors *except:*
A. Hypovolaemia B. Toxins
C. Myoglobin D. Aldosterone

14. Following metabolic responses to burns occur *except:*
A. Gluconeogenesis is increased
B. Lipolysis is increased
C. Catecholamines are increased
D. Proteolysis is decreased

15. Tangential excision refers to:
A. Excision and leaving the wound open immediately after admission
B. Excision within 6 hours and primary closure
C. Excision after 2–3 days and skin grafting
D. Excision after 10 days

16. Following are true for split skin graft *except:*
A. It is partial thickness graft
B. It is called Thiersch graft
C. Humby's knife is used often
D. Cosmetically it is superior to full thickness graft

17. Following are true for full thickness graft *except:*
A. It is called Wolfe graft
B. It consists of epidermis and dermis
C. Cosmetically it is superior to partial thickness graft
D. Problem with this graft is that it contracts often

18. Following heals by serum imbibition process:
A. Split skin graft B. Musculocutaneous flaps
C. Fracture of bones D. Mesh healing

19. Following are true for pectoralis major myocutaneous flap *except:*
A. It is the flap for head and neck reconstruction
B. Based on pectoral branch of thoracoacromial artery
C. It is an example of pedicle flap
D. It is a free flap

20. Following is true for hydrotherapy in burns *except:*
A. It can be done by immersion
B. Shower can also be used
C. It is painless
D. It rinses away dead skin and bacteria

Answers

1. A	**2.** C	**3.** D	**4.** A	**5.** A	**6.** A	**7.** D	**8.** D	**9.** B	**10.** A
11. B	**12.** D	**13.** D	**14.** D	**15.** C	**16.** D	**17.** D	**18.** A	**19.** D	**20.** C

CHAPTER

33

Tumours and Soft Tissue Sarcoma

- Benign tumours
- Papilloma
- Fibroma
- Lipoma
- Neural tumours
- Neuroma
- Neurofibroma
- Neurilemmoma
- Chordoma
- Malignant tumours
- Paraneoplastic syndromes
- Soft tissue sarcomas
- Aetiology/Epidemiology of STS
- Role of chemotherapy
- Differential diagnosis of soft tissue sarcoma
- Liposarcoma
- Malignant fibrous histiocytoma
- Synovial sarcoma
- Angiosarcoma
- Rhabdomyosarcoma
- Kaposi's sarcoma
- Dermatofibrosarcoma protuberans

INTRODUCTION

A tumour is a new growth consisting of cells of independent growth arranged atypically and serves no function. Broadly classified into:

- Benign
- Malignant

BENIGN TUMOURS

PAPILLOMA

This is a benign tumour arising from skin or mucous membrane. It is characterised by finger-like projections with a central core of connective tissue, blood vessels, lymphatics and lining epithelium (Fig. 33.1). It can be called hamartoma or a skin tag. It is an example of overgrowth of fibrous tissue (Key Box 33.1). It can be pedunculated with narrow base or broad base.

Key Box 33.1

Overgrowth of Fibrous Tissue

- Keloid : Page 106
- Desmoid tumour : Page 975
- Hypertrophic scar : Page 106

Pearls of Wisdom

Acrochordons (skin tags) are fleshy, pedunculated masses located on the axillae, trunk and eyelids.

Types

1. Skin Papilloma

a. *Squamous papilloma* occurs in the skin, cheek, tongue, etc. (Figs 33.2 and 33.3)
   - **Soft papillomas** are squamous papillomas. They are seen in elderly patients on the eyelid as small, soft, brownish swellings.
   - **Squamous papilloma** can also be ***congenital,*** sometimes multiple in number and can be sessile or pedunculated.

b. *Basal cell papilloma* (seborrhoeic keratosis) is seen on the trunk of elderly patients as brownish elevated patch of skin and gives a semitransparent, oily appearance.

2. Arising from Mucous Membrane of Visceral Organs

a. *Transitional cell papilloma* in the urinary bladder as a cause of haematuria.

b. *Columnar cell papilloma* in the rectum as a cause of mucous diarrhoea.

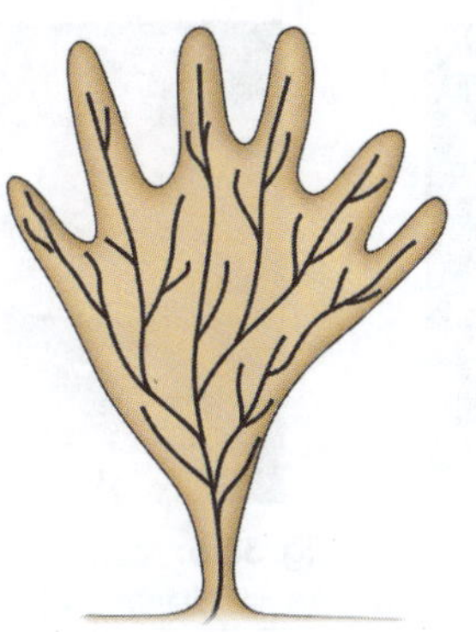

Fig. 33.1: Structure of papilloma

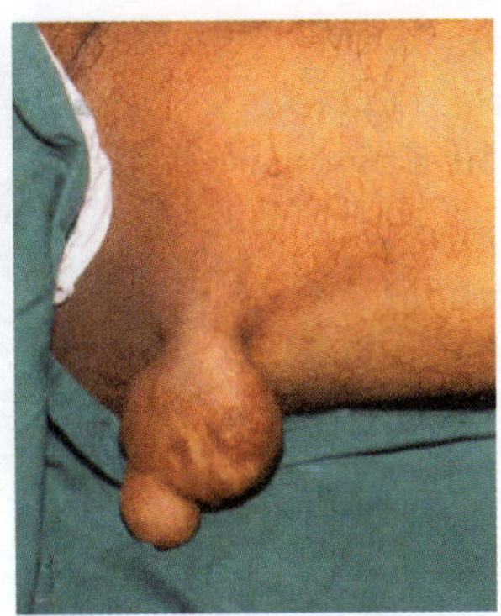

Fig. 33.2: Pedunculated papilloma thigh—broad base

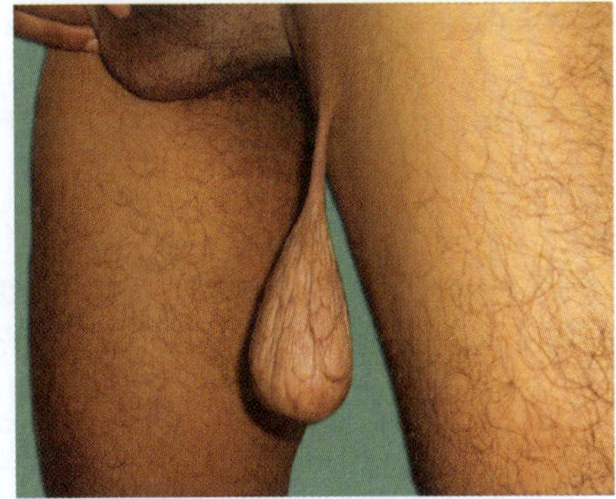

Fig. 33.3: Papilloma thigh with a narrow base—easy to remove it. Ulceration can be a problem here

c. ***Cuboidal cell papilloma*** in the *gallbladder.*
d. ***Squamous papilloma*** in the larynx can cause *respiratory obstruction.*
e. ***Papilloma of breast*** **(duct papilloma) causes bleeding per nipple.**

Treatment

Excision, only if papilloma causes discomfort, or if it is symptomatic.

Complications

1. Skin papilloma can get secondarily infected resulting in pain and swelling.
2. Ulceration and bleeding (trauma).
3. Papilloma in the breast, rectum, tongue and gallbladder can undergo malignant change.

FIBROMA[1]

Fibroma is a benign tumour, consisting of connective tissue fibres only. Clinically, it presents as a firm, subcutaneous swelling. However, ***a true fibroma is rare.*** They are combined with neural elements, muscle tissue or fatty tissue.

Types

1. Soft fibromas: Less fibrous tissue
2. Hard fibromas: More fibrous tissue
   - Neurofibroma: Fibroma mixed with nerve fibres
   - Fibrolipoma: Fibroma mixed with fat
   - Myofibroma: Fibroma mixed with muscle fibres
   - Angiofibroma: Fibroma mixed with blood vessels

Treatment

They are treated by excision because of the possibility of developing into a sarcoma.

LIPOMA: UNIVERSAL TUMOUR

Lipoma is a benign tumour arising from fat cells of adult type. It is also called 'universal tumour' because it can occur anywhere in the body where there is fat (Key Box 33.2).

Key Box 33.2

Diagnostic Features of Lipoma

- Subcutaneous—commonest type
- Soft to firm lobular swelling
- 'Slip' sign positive—a pathognomonic sign
- Semifluctuant swelling
- 'Smart' dimple sign on movement of the skin

Types

1. Single Encapsulated Lipoma

- This is a single, soft, slow-growing, painless and semifluctuant swelling (Fig. 33.4).
- The swelling is soft, may feel cystic with fluctuation. This is also called pseudofluctuation because fat at body temperature behaves like fluid.

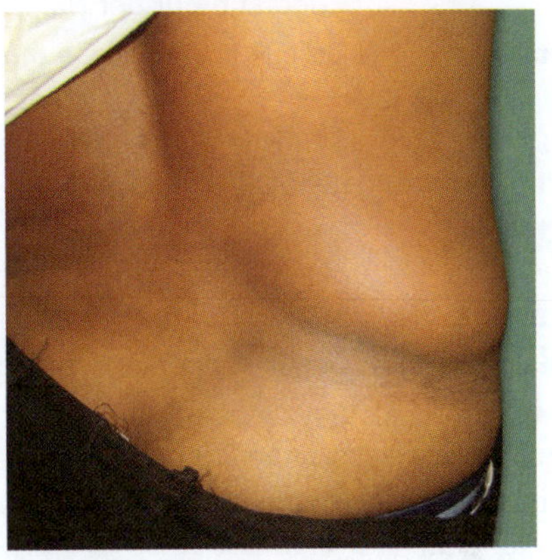

Fig. 33.4: Lipoma in the flank—**commonest site of lipoma**

[1]Students should not give the diagnosis of fibroma because in majority of cases, it is neurofibroma or fibrolipoma.

- Surface is **lobular.** Lobulations are better appreciated with firm palpation of the swelling. Due to the pressure, lobules bulge out between the fibrous tissue strands.
- ***The edge slips under the palpating finger which is a pathognomonic sign of lipoma.***
- Commonly present as a subcutaneous swelling. It is ***freely mobile.*** The flank is the commonest site. Shoulder region, neck, back, upper limbs are the other common sites. (For various locations, refer to Table 33.1, Figs 33.5 and 33.6.) Some lipomas from the chest wall can be of large size.
- ***Dimpling sign:*** **Fibrous bands connect a lipoma to the skin.** When the skin **moved,** a dimple appears **on the skin.**

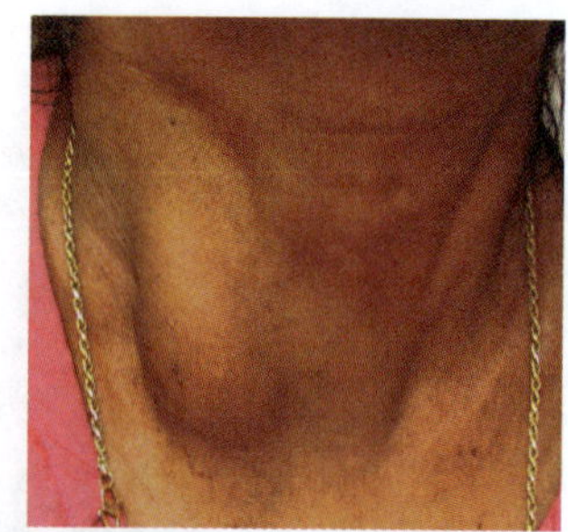

Fig. 33.5: Mediastinal lipoma. The swelling was deep to pretracheal fascia and partly substernal. It was soft and lobular—confused for compressible swelling. Candidate offered haemangioma as diagnosis. [*Courtesy:* Dr Salim, Head, Department of Surgery, Trivandrum Medical College, Kerala (PG exam case 2009)]

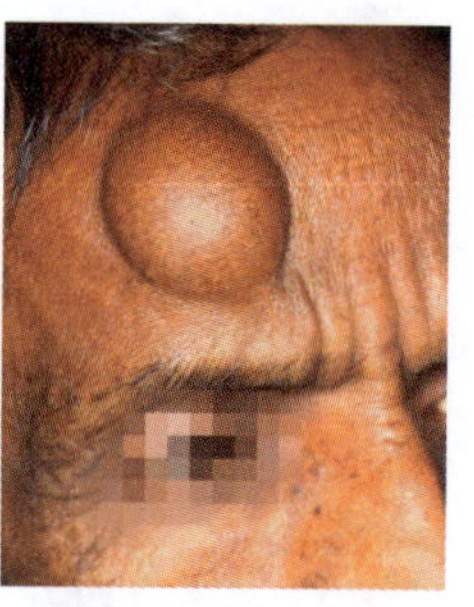

Fig. 33.6: Lipoma forehead. An undergraduate gave the diagnosis as dermoid cyst. You see the location. It is not the classical site of dermoid cyst and the 'slip sign' was positive. Even though face is not a common site, lipoma can occur in this location. Another differential diagnosis for this swelling is sebaceous cyst

2. *Multiple Lipomatosis* (Fig. 33.7)

- Such lipomas are multiple and very often tender because of *nerve elements* mixed with them. Hence, they are called *multiple neurolipomatosis. Dercum's disease* is one example of this variety *(Adiposis dolorosa)* wherein tender, lipomatous swellings are present in the body, mainly the trunk.

3. *Uncapsulated Lipoma (Diffuse)*

- Diffuse variety is a rare type of lipoma. It is called pseudolipoma. It is an overgrowth of fat without a capsule.

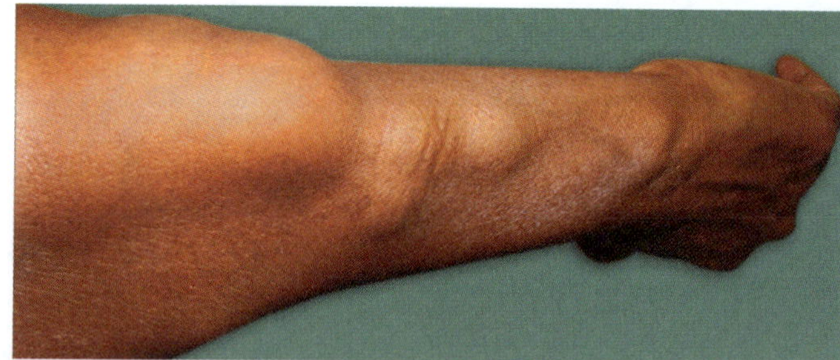

Fig. 33.7: Multiple lipomas—being subcutaneous in location, they become **prominent on contraction of muscles**

Table 33.1 Various types of lipoma

Location	Presentation	Differential diagnosis	Significance
1. **Subcutaneous** Shoulder Flank	Mobile Lobular **Edge slips under palpating fingers**	Neurofibroma	**The most common variety**
2. **Subfascial** Limbs, palm, sole	Difficult to appreciate the edge and lobulation	Implantation dermoid, TB tenosynovitis	Subfascial lipoma of the scalp—erodes bone
3. **Subsynovial, intra-articular**	Swelling in relation to knee joint, elbow joint (Figs 33.10 and 33.11)	Bursa Baker's cyst	Intra-articular lipomas are rare
4. **Intermuscular** Thigh Shoulder region	Swelling of the thigh. On contraction of the muscles, it becomes more firm due to transmitted pressure	Fibrosarcoma Haematoma	Chances of developing liposarcoma are more
5. **Parosteal**	Under the periosteum of bone, feels hard	Bony tumour	Very, very rare
6. **Submucous** Intestines, larynx	Asymptomatic or stridor or pain abdomen	Intestinal tumour Laryngeal tumour	Intussusception
7. **Subserosal** Retroperitoneum	Retroperitoneal swelling	Hydronephrosis Retroperitoneal cyst	Liposarcoma
8. **Extradural**	Very rare	–	–
9. **Intraglandular**	Breast, pancreas	Cystic lesions	Very rare

Histological Types of Lipoma

1. **Fibrolipoma:** Since fibrous tissue is mixed with fat, lipoma feels hard.
2. **Neurolipoma:** *Painful* lipoma, because of presence of nerve elements.
3. **Naevolipoma:** Lipoma is usually relatively avascular but this variety is vascular.

Treatment

- An **incision** is given over the swelling. **Dissection** is carried out all around, separating it from underlying tissues and it is excised (Fig. 33.8).
- **Small lipoma** can be removed by incising the skin followed by squeezing the lipoma out (no dissection method).

Complications

1. **Liposarcoma:** The current view is that lipomas are benign and do not turn into malignancy. However, atypical retroperitoneal lipomas and lipoma in the thigh can turn into liposarcoma after many years of growth. Malignancy should be suspected when:
   - The swelling grows rapidly (Fig. 33.9).
   - It becomes painful due to infiltration of nerves.
   - The swelling becomes vascular and red coloured with dilated veins over the surface.
   - Surface is warm due to increased vascularity.
   - Skin fungation or fixation occurs later
   - Mobility gets restricted because of infiltration into deeper planes such as muscle.
   - Liposarcoma spreads via blood. It rarely spreads via lymphatics. Metastasis in the lung can rarely occur from liposarcoma producing multiple chest secondaries.
   - Liposarcoma is treated by wide excision followed by reconstruction either by split skin graft or by flaps. In the thigh, sometimes radical surgery may amount to compartmental excision. Chemotherapy and radiotherapy can also be used but the benefit is doubtful.
2. **Calcification**

Clinical Notes

A 32-year-old man presented with gross swelling of the right leg. He had seen two surgeons earlier who had told him that he had deep vein thrombosis but no treatment was offered. Examination revealed an obvious mass which was palpable in anteromedial and posterior compartment. MRI revealed an intermuscular mass. At exploration, an intermuscular lipoma weighing 700 g was excised (Figs 33.10 and 33.11).

3. **Myxomatous degeneration:** Occurs only in retroperitoneal lipoma.
4. **Intussusception**—due to submucosal lipoma of terminal ileum is an abdominal emergency.
5. **Saponification** (*see* Key Box 33.3 and Figs 33.10 and 33.11).

Key Box 33.3

Some 'Rare' Facts in Lipoma

- It is rare in children
- Rarely gives rise to transillumination (if size is big)
- Rarely gets infected (because it is relatively avascular)
- Diffuse variety is rare
- Neurolipomas are rare
- Rarely they turn into malignancy

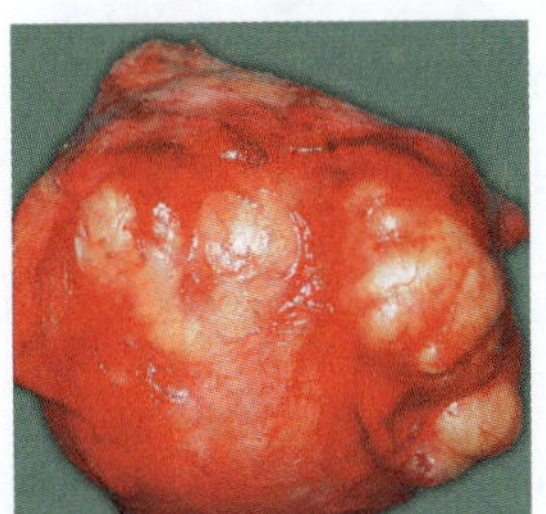

Fig. 33.8: Excised specimen of lipoma—see the lobularity

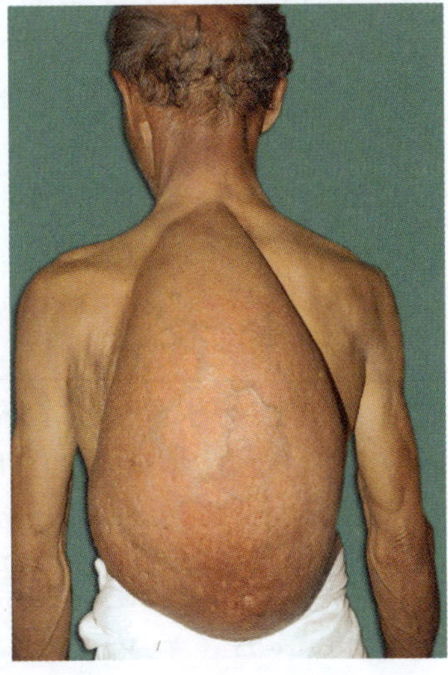

Since 3 months, it is rapidly growing, observe dilated veins and shiny skin. There is local rise of temperature. These features are suggestive of sarcoma.

Fig. 33.9: Pedunculated lipoma of the back of 15 years duration with features suggestive of sarcomatous change

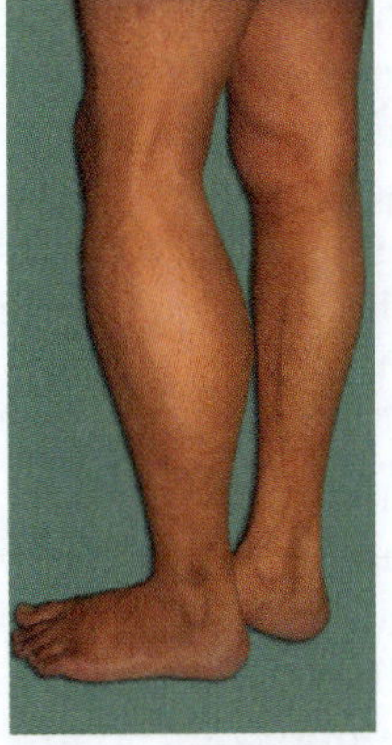

Fig. 33.10: Compare both the legs. Local gigantism can also be caused by extensive lipomatosis involving the leg. This was treated initially as filariasis

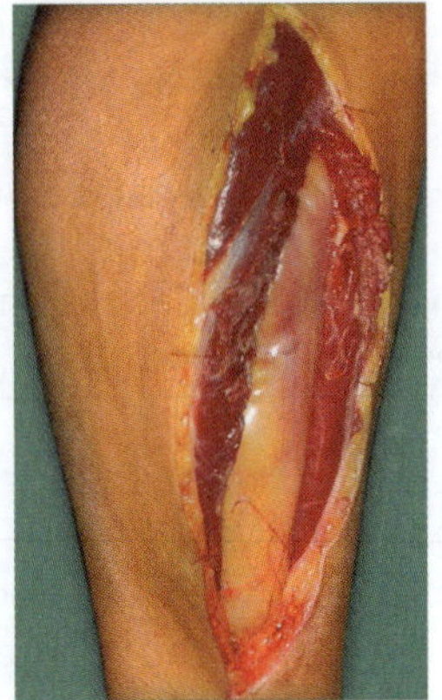

Fig. 33.11: Soleus muscle is cut, lipoma is seen coming out of the deeper plane. Luckily no major neurovascular bundle was involved. The patient had a smooth recovery

NEURAL TUMOURS

NEUROMA

They are uncommon benign tumours which arise from sympathetic nervous system or spinal cord. They can be classified into true neuromas and false neuromas.

True Neuroma

1. **Ganglioneuroma:** It consists of ganglion cells and nerve fibres of sympathetic chain. They are slow-growing tumours. When present in the neck as a *parapharyngeal mass,* it can cause dysphagia. These tumours can occur in the neck, retroperitoneum or mediastinum. Excision of the tumour is the treatment (*see* clinical notes).
2. **Neuroblastoma:** It consists of poorly differentiated cells. It occurs in young children. It is interesting to know that this tumour can undergo spontaneous regression.
3. **Myelinic neuroma:** It is very rare. It arises in relationship with spinal cord made up of myelinic fibres.
   - Does not contain any ganglion cells.

   All these three tumours are called *true neuromas.*

False Neuroma

These tumours arise from the connective tissue of the sheath of nerve endings.

They occur following nerve injuries, lacerations or after amputation. They are of two types:

Clinical Notes

An 18-year-old engineering student who had backache was examined by an orthopaedician and referred to general surgery. CT scan of the abdomen revealed mass in the paraspinal region in the retroperitoneum. Laparotomy and excision of the mass was done. It was a ganglioneuroma. Paraspinal region is one of the common sites of ganglioneuroma.

1. *End-neuroma* occurs after amputation due to proliferation of nerve fibres from the distal cut end of the nerve. This produces a bulbous swelling. If it is caught in the suture line or due to pressure of the prosthesis, it produces severe neuralgic pain. To avoid this, when an amputation is being done, the nerve is pulled downwards and cut as high as possible so that it retracts upwards (Fig. 33.12).
2. *Lateral neuromas* occur due to partial injury to the nerve on the lateral aspect (Fig. 33.13).

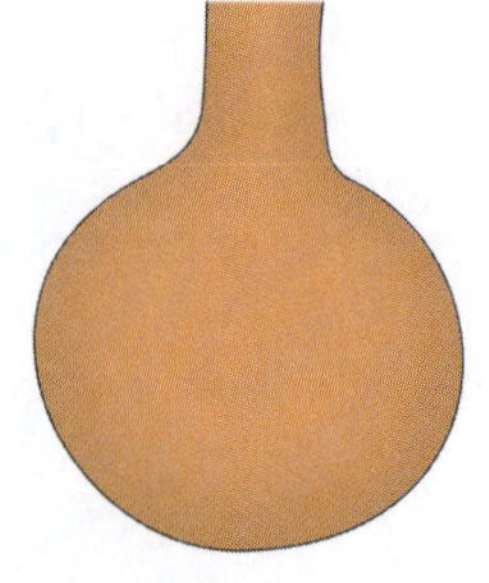

Fig. 33.12: End-neuroma

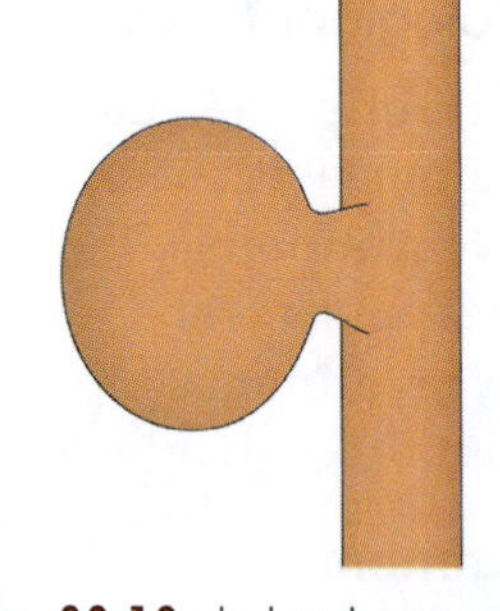

Fig. 33.13: Lateral neuroma

Treatment

Excision of the neuroma.

NEUROFIBROMA

It is a benign tumour arising from the connective tissue of the nerve sheath. Typically, it produces a *fusiform swelling* in the direction of the nerve fibres. The tumour contains both neural (ectodermal) and fibrous (mesodermal) elements.

Clinical Types

1. Single Subcutaneous Neurofibroma (Local)

Commonly affects the peripheral nerves such as ulnar nerve, median nerve or cutaneous nerves. Occurs in adults.

Clinical features

- **Presents as a painful, subcutaneous nodule.**
- Tingling and numbness, paraesthesia in the distribution of the nerve, specially when the nodule is compressed.
- Round to oval swelling in the direction of nerve fibre.
- Smooth surface, with round border. The swelling moves at right angles to the direction of nerve fibres. Vertical mobility is absent.
- Consistency is firm. Sometimes, it is hard.
- Being a subcutaneous swelling, the skin can be lifted up.

Treatment

- It is treated by excision.
- In most of the cases, excision is easy as the tumour is well encapsulated.

2. Generalised Neurofibromatosis: von Recklinghausen's (vR) Disease (Type I) (Figs 33.14 to 33.16)

- This is an autosomal dominant disorder transmitted by both sexes. The whole body is studded with cutaneous nodules of varying sizes. They are soft and nontender.
- Coffee brown pigmentation is characteristic of this condition (*café au lait* spots, Fig. 33.17). *Café au lait*

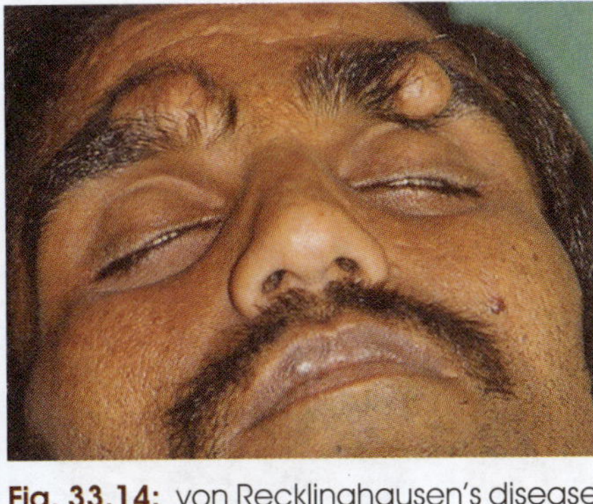

Fig. 33.14: von Recklinghausen's disease with plexiform neurofibromatosis. (*Courtesy:* Dr Prashanth Shetty, Professor, Department of Surgery, KMC, Manipal)

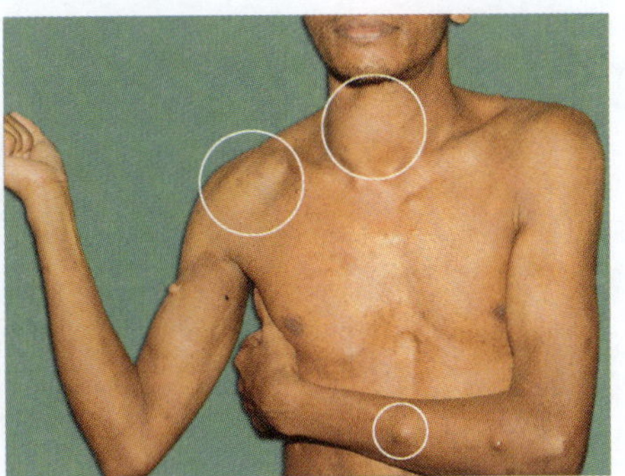

Fig. 33.15: Case of vR disease with multiple nodules, pigmentation and schwannoma of vagus nerve. (*Courtesy:* Dr Siddarth Bhandary, Professor, Department of Surgery, KMC, Manipal)

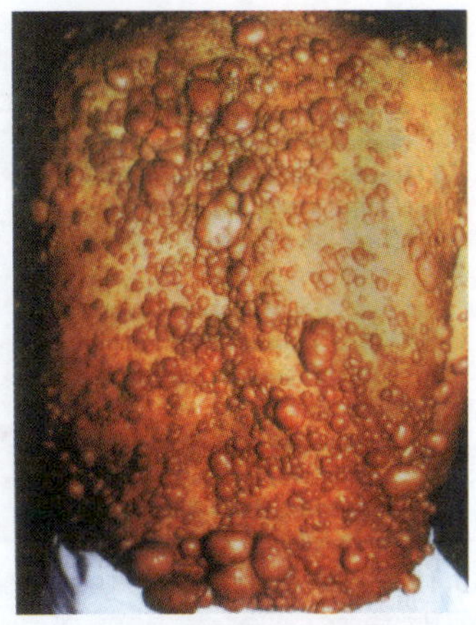

Fig. 33.16: von Recklinghausen's disease—tumours are multiple, congenital, familial

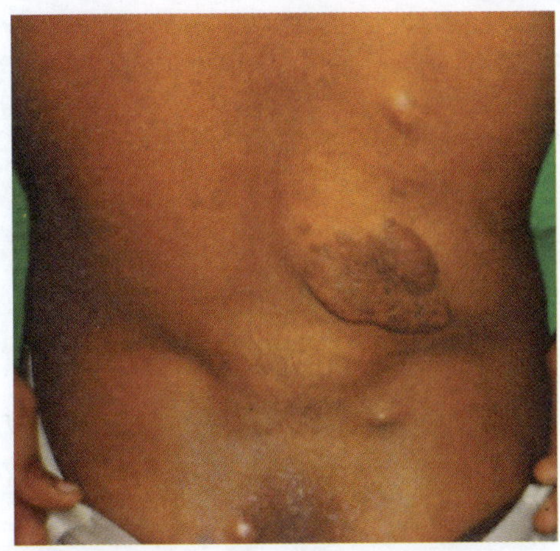

Fig. 33.17: The café au lait spots. More than five such spots will appear by early life. (*Courtesy:* Dr Prashanth Shetty, Professor, Department of Surgergy, KMC, Manipal)

spots can be associated with involvement of cranial nerves—VIIIth nerve (auditory nerve) *acoustic neuroma—**a cerebellopontine angle tumour. Popularly called vestibular schwannoma.***

- Fibroepithelial skin tags are often present.
- Type I is caused by ***gene mu tation on chromosome 17.***
- The presence of skin pigmentation is an indication of the common neuroectodermal origin of nerve sheath cells and melanocytes.
- Skeletal deformities such as kyphoscoliosis or osteoporosis are common.
- It may be associated with phaeochromocytoma (high blood pressure).
- Sarcomatous changes do occur.

Pearls of Wisdom

Record the blood pressure in all cases of von Recklinghausen's disease because it may be associated with phaeochromocytoma.

Bilateral vestibular schwannoma or acoustic neuromas are pathognomonic of neurofibromatosis type 2, a syndrome resulting from chromosome 22 mutation. It is also associated with increased incidence of meningiomas and gliomas.

3. Plexiform Neurofibromatosis (Trigeminal) (Fig. 33.18)

- In this condition, the branches of 5th cranial nerve are commonly affected. It can also involve the peripheries.
- The affected part is grossly thickened due to **fibromyxomatous degeneration.**
- When it involves the branches of trigeminal nerve, following problems can occur:
  - **Tingling paraesthesia** in the distribution of Vth nerve, especially ophthalmic division.
  - When it attains a huge size, it can **obstruct the vision**. As it grows bigger in size, it hangs in front of the neck, as a grossly thickened pendulous fold of skin.
- **Treatment:** Very difficult. Excision can be attempted with plastic surgery repair.

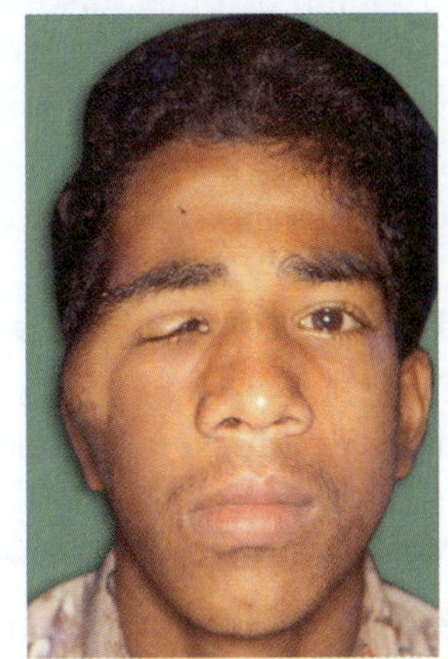

Fig. 33.18: Plexiform neurofibromatosis. (*Courtesy:* Dr Rohit Jain, Assistant Professor, Department of Surgery, KMC, Manipal)

4. Elephantiasis Neuromatosa

- This condition affects the limbs. It represents an advanced stage of plexiform variety. Gross thickening of subcutaneous tissue gives the ap-

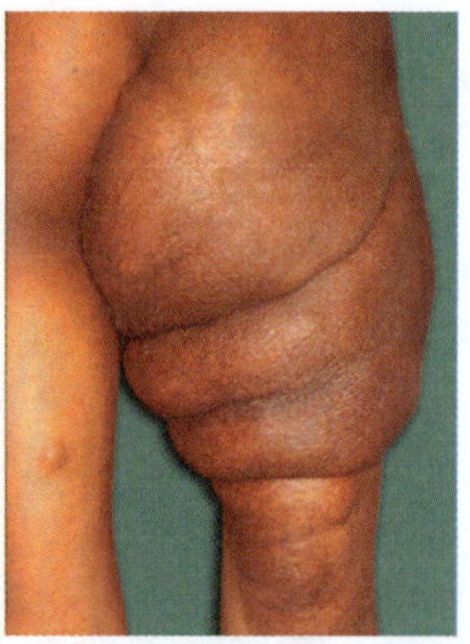

Fig. 33.19: Elephantiasis neuromatosa. (*Courtesy:* Dr Balakrishna Shetty, Professor, Department of Surgery, KS Hegde Medical Academy, Mangalore)

pearance of elephant's leg. The skin is dry and coarse (Fig. 33.19).

Complications of Neural Tumours (Key Box 33.4)

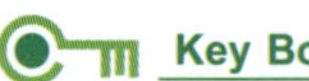

Key Box 33.4

Complications of Neural Tumours

- Atrophy of muscles
- Dumb-bell tumours from dorsal spinal nerve root can cause backache or paralysis
- Acoustic neuroma—deafness
- Cystic degeneration
- Sarcomatous change

5. Pachydermatocoele

This refers to the plexiform lesions mainly found in the neck as a thickened, coiled single mass.

NEURILEMMOMA (Schwannoma)

- This is a benign tumour arising from ***Schwann cells.***
- Commonest site is the ***acoustic nerve.*** However, vagus nerve is the most common peripheral site (Fig. 33.20).
- They can be single or multiple and present with a fusiform swelling in relationship with the nerves.

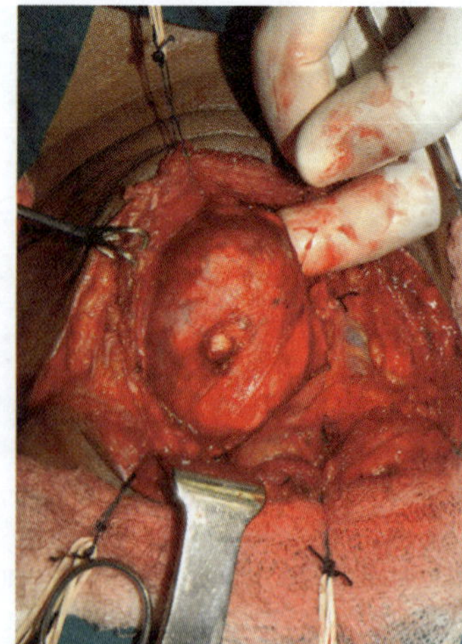

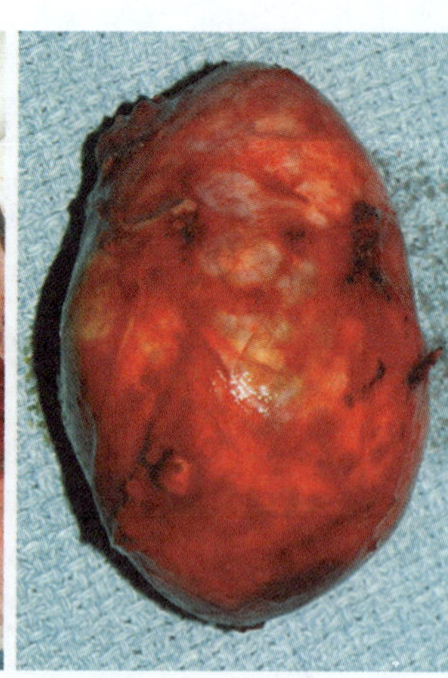

Fig. 33.20: Vagal schwannoma at surgery—you can see the displaced carotid artery and internal jugular vein. Second picture showing the specimen. (*Courtesy:* Prof Balakrishnan, Department of ENT, Kasturba Hospital, Manipal. Initially it was diagnosed as solitary nodule of the thyroid gland but it was not moving with deglutition)

- They can also arise from a peripheral nerve. ***Sensory branches*** are affected more frequently (Table 33.2).
- They can also be seen in mediastinum and retroperitoneum.
- They are ***soft, lobulated, well encapsulated tumours.***
- They are ***benign*** and ***do not turn into malignancy.***

Treatment

Excision of the tumour can be done without sacrificing the nerves because the tumour is well encapsulated and displaces the nerve.

HAMARTOMA

- It is a tumour-like developmental malformation of the tissues of a particular part of the body wherein it is arranged haphazardly.
- Hamartoma is a Greek word which means **fault** or **misfire**. It is not a clinical diagnosis.

Table 33.2 Comparison between neurofibroma and schwannoma

Neurofibroma	Schwannoma
• More common	• Less common
• Ectodermal and mesodermal origin	• Ectodermal origin
• Subcutaneous (forearm) nerves are the commonest site	• Acoustic nerve is the commonest site
• Multiple lesions are common	• Very rare
• Feels firm or hard	• Soft
• Tender	• Nontender
• Can turn into sarcoma	• **Rarely turns into sarcoma**
• Often nerve fibres are entangled with tumour. Hence, excision involves sacrificing nerve also	• Well encapsulated. Hence, **enucleation is possible** without sacrificing nerve

Table 33.3 Pathology of tumours

Terminology	Explanation	Examples
1. Well differentiated	Cells that resemble very closely their normal counterparts	Well-differentiated squamous cell carcinoma
2. Undifferentiated (anaplasia)	Loss of structural and functional differentiation	Poorly-differentiated carcinoma (anaplasia)
3. Dysplasia	Loss in the uniformity, loss in the architectural orientation	Barrett's columnar cell lined oesophagus
4. Carcinoma *in situ*	Dysplastic changes involving **entire thickness** of the epithelium	Cheek, tongue, breast, etc.
5. Apoptosis	Programmed cell death	Seen in malignant tumours

A Few Examples of Hamartoma

Haemangioma, neurofibroma, glomus tumour, benign naevus, lymphangioma.

Characteristic Features

- Being a developmental anomaly, they are seen at birth or in early childhood.
- In adults, there is a long history of swelling.
- **Being a malformation (not a tumour), it does not have a capsule.**
- They can be single or multiple.
- Some may **regress** as in **strawberry angioma**.
- They are benign lesions.

Treatment

- **Excision** is not only curative but also gives a correct diagnosis.
- Care should be taken when it contains vascular tissue such as haemangioma or neural tissue as in cases of neurofibroma.
- Facial nerve and its branches may be damaged while excising hamartomatous lesions over the face.

CHORDOMA

- Rare tumour
- Remnant of notochord (origin)
- Sacrococcygeal region (common site)
- Resection is difficult, chances of neurological deficit and bleeding are high.
- Radioresistant

MALIGNANT TUMOURS

TYPES OF MALIGNANT TUMOURS

- They are of two types: Carcinoma and sarcoma. Carcinoma arises from epithelium—ectodermal, endodermal or mesodermal in origin.
- Sarcomas arise from soft tissues or bone and are derived from mesoblast or mesenchymal tissues.
- It may be observed that mesoderm can give rise to carcinoma and mesenchymal sarcoma also.

Pathology (Table 33.3)

Spread

1. **Local spread:** Generally, local spread occurs into adjacent structures. A few examples are given:
   - Carcinoma cheek—fixity to mandible

     Significance: May necessitate removal of mandible along with wide excision (Fig. 33.21A).
   - Squamous cell carcinoma—fixed to tibia may necessitate an amputation.
2. **Lymphatic spread:** It is one of the most important features of **carcinoma** (Key Box 33.5). As you complete reading this book, you will come across many cases and many examples of lymphatic spread of malignant tumours. A few sarcomas also spread by lymphatics (*see* page 301). Different types of lymphatic spread are given below:
   - ***Embolisation***: More aggressive tumour means more aggressive spread—by embolisation wherein nodes can be enlarged in a far away station, e.g. malignant melanoma (Fig. 33.21B).

Key Box 33.5

Carcinoma

Origin
- Ectodermal—skin cancer
- Endodermal—gut cancer
- Mesodermal—renal carcinoma

Types
- Squamous cell carcinoma
- Basal cell carcinoma
- Glandular

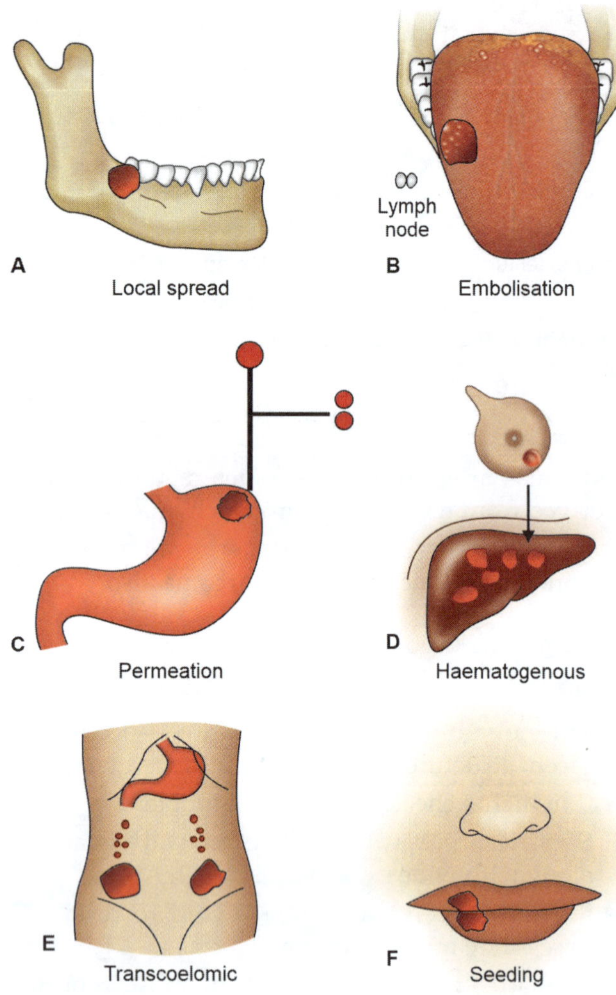

Fig. 33.21: Spread of malignant tumour (see text)

- ***Permeation*:** Refers to tumour cells travelling along the lymphatic vessel, e.g. carcinoma tongue with sub-mandibular node enlargement (Fig. 33.21C).
- ***Retrograde lymphatic spread*:** When main lymphatic pathway is blocked retrograde spread can occur and a node in an unusual location may get enlarged, e.g. **Irish node (left axillary node enlargement in carcinoma stomach).**

3. **Haematogenous spread:** This is most important method of spread of **sarcomas**. Also, a few malignancies such as renal cell carcinoma, follicular carcinoma thyroid, carcinoma prostate, carcinoma breast (Fig. 33.21D) and malignant melanoma commonly spread by blood. Bone metastasis and lung metastasis result from blood spread. Bone metastasis can vary from mild form with only bone pain to severe form with quadriplegia/pathological fracture.
4. **Transcoelomic spread:** Spread through peritoneal cavity by dislodgment of malignant cells, e.g. Ca stomach with Krukenberg's tumour—bilateral bulky ovarian metastasis, commonly seen in premenopausal patients (Fig. 33.21E).
5. **Seeding** (Fig. 33.21F): A few examples are given below:
   - Cancer of lower lip spreading to upper lip, also called kiss cancer. Other example: Cancer of vulva.
   - Incision and 'port' site metastasis (port refers to laparoscopic port).

Comparison of benign and malignant tumours is given in Table 33.4.

Table 33.4 Comparison of benign tumours and malignant tumours

Feature	Benign	Malignant
Growth	Very slow	Rapid
Duration	Long	Short
Pain	Usually not a feature	Pain can be present due to local infiltration
Mobility	Present	Restricted
Fixity	No	Can be present
Consistency	Firm/soft	Hard, irregular
Spread	No	Spreads
Capsule	Capsulated	Uncapsulated
Recurrence after surgery	Does not occur	Can occur if wide excision is **not** done

PARANEOPLASTIC SYNDROMES (PNS)

These are interesting syndromes and are listed in Table 33.5.

Certain cancers produce some specific clinical syndromes (symptom complexes other than cachexia) which cannot be explained by their local or distant spread or by the hormones produced by the tissue of origin of these tumours. These are called paraneoplastic syndromes (Key Box 33.6).

Just to give an example, hypercalcaemia due to skeletal metastasis from carcinoma breast is not considered as PNS, but if it occurs without skeletal metastasis, it is considered as PNS.

Key Box 33.6

Important Featurs of PNS

- Incidence: 10–15% of patients with cancer
- It may be the earliest manifestation (primary can be occult)
- Bronchogenic cancer and breast cancer are most commonly associated with PNS.
- Hypercalcaemia and Cushing's syndromes are the most common clinical syndromes associated with PNS.
- PNS can be a major clinical problem and can be treated.

AETIOLOGY OF CARCINOMA IN GENERAL

1. **Tobacco** is the most important factor in the development of **lung cancer, upper respiratory tract cancer, gastrointestinal tract and genitourinary tract cancer.** Carcinoma pancreas is found more commonly in smokers. Passive smokers also have increased incidence of development of cancers.
2. **Alcohol:** Smoking with alcohol increases the permeability of the upper digestive tract mucosa and respiratory mucosa to the carcinogens. Thus, they increase the incidence of cancer. Hepatocellular cancer is commonly found in alcoholic cirrhotic liver.
3. **Ionising radiation:** Atomic bomb blasts in Japan have definitely resulted in increased number of cases of breast cancer in premenopausal women and leukaemia in children.
4. **Ultraviolet radiation:** **Causes all types of skin cancers.**
5. **Genetic causes** (Key Box 33.7)

Key Box 33.7

Genetic/Defective DNA Repair

1. **Xeroderma pigmentosa**	:	Skin cancer
2. **Bloom's syndrome**	:	Acute leukaemia, various cancers
3. **Fanconi's anaemia**	:	Acute leukaemia, squamous cell carcinoma, hepatoma
4. **Ataxia-telangiectasia**	:	Acute leukaemia, lymphoma, breast cancer

Table 33.5 Paraneoplastic syndromes

Clinical syndrome	Underlying major cancer	Mechanism
1. Endocrinopathies		
• Cushing's syndrome	Small cell Ca lung, Ca pancreas	ACTH or ACTH-like substance
• Hyponatraemia	Small cell Ca lung	ASH or atrial natriuretic peptide
• Hypoglycaemia	Hepatoma	Insulin or insulin-like substance
• Hypercalcaemia	Squamous cell Ca lung Ca breast, Ca kidney	PTH-like substance
• Carcinoid syndrome	Bronchial carcinoid, Ca pancreas, Ca stomach	Serotonin, bradykinin
• Polycythaemia	Renal cell carcinoma, cerebellar haemangioma	Erythropoietin
2. Muscle syndrome		
Myasthenia gravis	Thymoma	Immunologic
3. Bone and soft tissues		
Hypertrophic osteoarthropathy and clubbing of fingers	Adenocarcinoma lung	Unknown
4. Vascular		
• Venous thrombosis	Carcinoma pancreas	Hypercoagulability
• Disseminated intravascular coagulation	Ca pancreas, lung, prostate	Tumour products

Ca: Carcinoma

6. **Hereditary causes**
   - **MEN** syndrome: Medullary carcinoma thyroid (**M**ultiple **E**ndocrine **N**eoplasia)
   - **FPC**: Colonic cancer (multiple) (**F**amilial **P**olyposis **C**oli)
   - Li-Fraumeni syndrome: Familial breast cancer.
   - Retinoblastoma.
7. **Dietary factors**
   - **Red meat:** Carcinoma colon, carcinoma breast.
   - **Fat:** Carcinoma breast, carcinoma colon.
   - **Smoked, charred fish:** Carcinoma oesophagus, carcinoma stomach.
8. **Chemicals**
   - Benzanthracenes: Skin cancer when painted on the skin
   - Benzopyrenes: Lung cancer
   - β-naphthylamine: Bladder cancer
   - Nitrosamines and amides: Cancer stomach
   - Aflatoxin B: Hepatocellular carcinoma
   - Asbestos: Lung cancer
9. **Viral factors**
   - Human T cell leukaemia virus type 1 (HTLV-1): T cell leukaemia/lymphoma (RNA virus)
   - Human papillomavirus (HPV) Cancer cervix, cancer urogenital region
   - Epstein-Barr virus: Burkitt's lymphoma.

SOFT TISSUE SARCOMAS (STS)

These are malignant tumours arising from soft tissues. Thus, they can occur in any part of the body. Examples are given in Table 33.6.

Table 33.6 Soft tissue sarcoma

Tissue of origin	Name
• Mesenchymal tissue	Malignant fibrous histiocytoma (MFH)
• Adipose tissue	Liposarcoma
• Smooth muscle	Leiomyosarcoma (GIST)
• Striated muscle	Rhabdomyosarcoma
• Synovial tissue	Synovial sarcoma
• Neural tissue	Malignant schwannoma
• Uncertain	Epithelioid sarcoma
• Blood vessels	Angiosarcoma
• Lymph vessels	Lymphangiosarcoma

INTRODUCTION

- Sarcomas are relatively uncommon tumours accounting for approximately 1% of all adult cancers. These are heterogeneous group of tumours of mesenchymal cell origin, occurring more commonly in young patients with not a favourable outcome. The overall survival is approximately 40–50% at 5 years.
- These are malignant tumours which are **fatal if untreated** or mistreated. Most of them occur in young patients as painless lumps. CT scan, MRI and incision biopsy (details later) are key investigations. Early diagnosis and curative resection have a major role in the management of soft tissue sarcomas. In addition to TNM staging, pathological grading of the tumour has been included **GTNM staging**.

AETIOLOGY/EPIDEMIOLOGY OF STS (Key Box 33.8)

1. **Genetic factors: Genetic mutations/gene rearrangements** have been implicated in the pathogenesis of STS. Two genes that are most relevant to soft tissue tumours are retinoblastoma **(Rb) tumour suppressor gene and p53 tumour suppressor gene.** Various familial syndromes are associated with STS such as Li-Fraumeni syndrome, Gardner's syndrome and von Recklinghausen's disease. Several oncogenes have been identified.
2. **Exposure to radiation:** 8–50-fold increase in the incidence of STS is reported in patients who are treated for cancer of the breast, cervix and ovary by radiation.
3. **Neurofibromatosis type I:** Specially mentioned here because it is the only benign tumour progressing to STS. 100% lifetime risk of malignant peripheral nerve sheath tumour, in patients with familial neurofibromatosis, caused by mutations in the *NF1* gene.
4. **Exposure to chemicals:** Thorium oxide, vinyl chloride, arsenic have been implicated in hepatic angiosarcomas.
5. **Trauma:** Chronic tissue trauma is blamed as a triggering factor for development of STS. Others believe that trauma draws attention of the patient to the STS.
6. **Immunosuppression:** Kaposi's sarcoma occurs in HIV/AIDS patients.

Key Box 33.8

Aetiology of STS—Summary

Genetic factors
Exposure to radiation
Neurofibromatosis (NF-1)
Exposure to chemicals
Trauma
Immunodeficiency
Chronic lymphoedema
Remember as **GENETIC**

7. **Chronic lymphoedema** can give rise to lymphangiosarcoma. Postmastectomy lymphangiosarcoma is called Stewart-Treves syndrome.

TNM STAGING **Soft tissue sarcomas of (A) trunk and extremity and (B) retroperitoneum**

Definition of Primary Tumour (T) AJCC, 8th Edition

TX Primary tumour cannot be assessed
T0 No evidence of primary tumour
T1 Tumour 5 cm or less in greatest dimension
T2 Tumour more than 5 cm and 10 cm in greatest dimension
T3 Tumour more than 10 cm and 15 cm in greatest dimension
T4 Tumour more than 15 cm in greatest dimension

Definition of Regional Lymph Node (N)

N0 No regional lymph node metastasis or unknown lymph node status
N1 Regional lymph node metastasis

Definition of Distant Metastasis (M)

M0 No distant metastasis
M1 Distant metastasis

Definition of Grade (G): FNCLCC = Fédération Nationale des Centres de Lutte Contre Le Cancer;

GX Grade cannot be assessed
G1 Total differentiation, mitotic count and necrosis score of 2 or 3
G2 Total differentiation, mitotic count and necrosis score of 4 or 5
G3 Total differentiation, mitotic count and necrosis score of 6, 7 or 8.

FNCLCC: Fédération Nationale des Centres de Lutte Contre Le Cancer

Table 33.7 AJCC prognostic stage groups for soft tissue sarcoma in the trunk and extremity and retroperitoneum

Stage	Primary tumour (T)	Regional lymph node (N)	Distant metastasis (M)	Histologic grade (G)
IA	T1	N0	M0	G1, GX
IB	T2, T3, T4	N0	M0	G1, GX
II	T1	N0	M0	G2, G3
IIIA	T2	N0	M0	G2, G3
IIIB	T3, T4	N0	M0	G2, G3
	Any T	N1	M0	Any G
IV	Any T	Any N	M1	Any G

Clinical Features

Sarcomas are rapidly growing vascular growth (Table 33.8).

- Typically patients present with painless lump/swelling in the thigh or forearm.
- When the tumour is increasing in size, size more than 5 cm, deep fascia and painful—suspect STS.

INVESTIGATIONS/DIAGNOSTIC IMAGING

- Few blood tests, cardiac evaluation is done and ECOG performance score is calculated (page 681).
- **Chest radiography:** Presence of cannonball metastasis alters the staging, treatment policy and prognosis.

Pearls of Wisdom

If STS is more than 5 cm (T2), computed tomography (CT) of the chest should be considered.

Table 33.8 Comparison of carcinoma and sarcoma

	Carcinoma	Sarcoma
1. Cell of origin	Ectodermal or endodermal (epithelial)	Mesodermal (mesenchymal)
2. Age group	Elderly, 40–60 years	Young, 10–30 years
3. Rate of growth	Slow	Fast
4. Presentation	**Nonhealing ulcer,** cauliflower-like growth with everted edges and induration. Fixity is a late feature	**Fleshy mass, red and vascular, dilated veins** over the surface, local rise of temperature. Ulceration is a late feature
5. Spread	**Lymphatic spread** is very common, both by emboli and permeation. Blood spread does occur as in renal cell carcinoma, thyroid carcinoma, breast carcinoma, etc.	**Blood spread** occurs very early and results in cannonball secondaries in lung. Rhabdomyosarcoma, synovial sarcoma, epithelioid sarcoma. Malignant fibrous histiocytoma, angiosarcoma spread by lymphatics
6. Microscopy	**Cell nests or epithelial pearls** are seen in well-differentiated cancers	Malignant cells resemble their cell of origin. Thus, **spindle-shaped cells** are found in **fibrosarcoma**
7. Treatment	**Surgery** is the main treatment of ectodermal cancers, surgery or radiotherapy for ectodermal lesions. Chemotherapy is not very useful	**Surgery** is the main modality of treatment. Radiotherapy and chemotherapy are also beneficial when the tumour is more than 5 cm

Imaging

- **CT scan** is useful in evaluating retroperitoneal sarcomas. It can define structures, infiltration into neighbouring structures, hydronephrosis, etc. CT can guide a ***core biopsy also***. It is also used to image chest and pelvis to stage the disease.
- **MRI** is the investigation of choice when STS occurs in **extremities to delineate muscle groups,** bones, vascular structures, etc. (Figs 33.22 and 33.23).

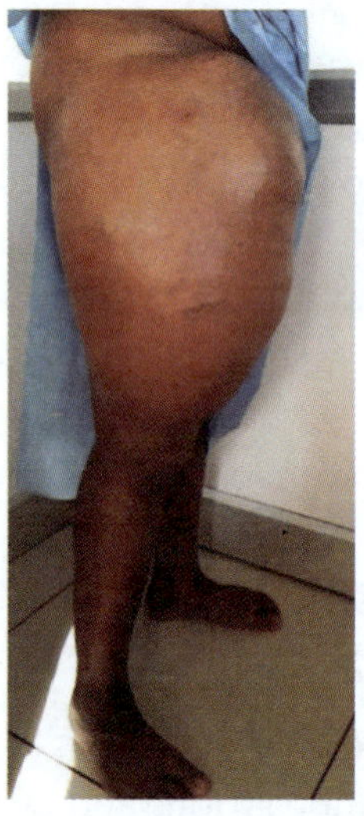

Fig. 33.22: Giant lipoma thigh

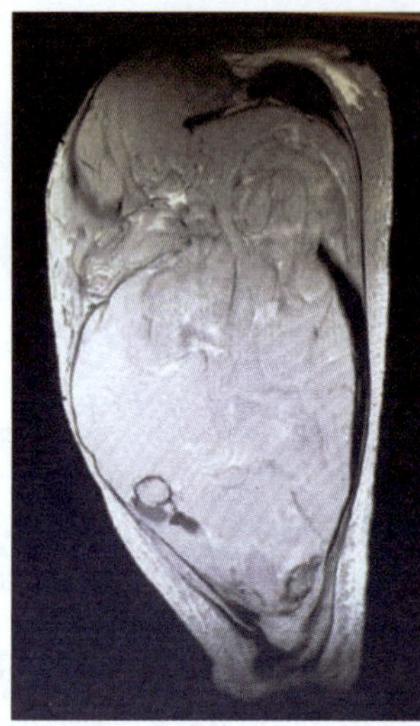

Fig. 33.23: MRI-giant lipoma

- FNAC
  - Useful to detect metastatic disease
  - To detect local recurrence
  - Ideal for superficial lesions
  - **Disadvantage:** Cannot assess tumour grading. Tissue is not sufficient for diagnostic tests.
- **Core needle biopsy:** It is the investigation of choice to confirm or rule out the diagnosis. It can give not only the diagnosis but also the histological type and grade also. Several scores are added to TNM staging such as tumor differentiation score, mitotic score and tumor necrosis score.
  - Safe and accurate
  - Tissue is sufficient for grading, electron microscopy and flow cytometry.
  - With CT guidance, core biopsy can be taken from deeper structures also.
- **Incisional biopsy**
  - When core biopsy tissue is not adequate, incisional biopsy is indicated (Key Box 33.9). Strict guideline to be followed to avoid risk of tumour seeding.
- PET-CT scan is indicated in high grade tumors, metastatic disease or before an amputation.

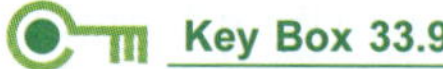

Key Box 33.9

Guidelines while Doing an Incisional Biopsy

- Incision should be oriented longitudinally in STS of extremities to facilitate removal of biopsy site track, scar and tumour *en bloc*. Do not put transverse incision.
- Flaps should not be raised
- Perfect haemostasis should be achieved
- Prevent dissemination, avoid crushing of the tissues
- Avoid drain

TREATMENT (see next page)

- The aim is to achieve local control and to treat metastasis including subclinical metastasis, thus trying for a cure.
- Adult sarcomas are best treated by wide excision with negative margin (R–O) resection. However, near the major and minor arteries, margin need not be wide but it may be microscopically positive margin.
- **Surgery is the first line of treatment** varying from a wide local excision to amputation or disarticulation (5%), when it occurs in the extremities. **Low-grade tumours** can be treated on **1 cm wide excision** of surrounding normal tissue and **high-grade tumours by 2 cm margin** (Key Box 33.10).
- Small tumours less than 5 cm have not been associated with recurrence. Hence, radiotherapy may not be required **but if grade is high, RT is required** (Key Box 33.11).

Key Box 33.10

Surgery for Soft Tissue Sarcoma

- **Surgery is the primary and most effective therapy**
- Local wide excision with 2 cm of surrounding normal tissue should be removed. **1 cm for low-grade and 2 cm for high-grade tumour.**
- **Not to dissect along pseudocapsule** which is composed of tumour cells.
- If necessary, **excision should include nerves** and vessels followed by nerve grafts and arterial reconstruction—when they are directly infiltrated. Otherwise preserve them.
- **STS rarely involve bones** and skin. Hence, wide resections of these structures are infrequently necessary.
- It should also include **previous scars.**
- If amputation can be avoided by giving preoperative radiotherapy, it is preferred first. It is then followed by wide excision/compartmental excision and postoperative radiotherapy. Dose of pre- and postoperative radiotherapy is 50–60 Gy given in 25 fractions. Brachytherapy is also given.
- **Margin negative resection should be the aim.**

Key Box 33.11

Radiotherapy

- *It is not the first modality of treatment in STS.*
- Radiotherapy is given after margin negative resection.
- Surgery + RT has resulted in local control rates up to or more than 90%.
- External beam radiation therapy (electrons, protons or neutrons) is given with a margin of 5 to 7 cm or even more depending on size of tumour. Dose is 50 Gy given in 25 fractions—as preoperative dose.
- Dose is 60 to 70 Gy for postoperative treatment.
- In brachytherapy, multiple catheters are placed in tumour resection bed. Catheters are loaded with seeds containing iridium 192.
- Dose of brachytherapy is 42–45 Gy to tumour bed over 4–6 days.
- Short period of treatment time and less systemic toxicity are advantages of brachytherapy.

- Tumours do respond to radiotherapy and chemotherapy.

Enneking classification of surgical procedures: Once the specimen is subjected for pathology request should be made to look specifically into the margin status. This is very important. Details are given below. Four types of margin have been recognised. If it is *intralesional,* means tumour remains—margin runs through tumour. If it is *marginal,* means surgical plane passes through pseudocapsule. Pseudocapsule is a reactive zone, hence high chances of local recurrence because tumour satellites may be present. When the margin is *wide,* means say 2 cm in all dimensions, recurrence rate is low, because surgical plane is in the normal plane. *Radical,* means tumour is removed including affected compartments and there is a minimal risk of local recurrence.

ROLE OF CHEMOTHERAPY

- High-grade tumours have high potential of metastasis. Hence, combination chemotherapy is to be considered before or after surgery.
- The most favoured combination chemotherapy drugs include Mesna, Adriamycin, Ifosfamide and Dacarbazine (MAID).
- The success rate is around 10–20%. Round cell sarcomas respond better to chemotherapy than spindle cell sarcoma.

Not all sarcomas are chemosensitive. A few details are given below.

Relative chemosensitivity

i. Ewing's sarcoma
ii. Embryonal and alveolar rhabdomyosarcoma

Chemosensitive

i. Synovial sarcoma
ii. Myxoid/round cell liposarcoma

Moderately chemosensitive

i. Pleomorphic liposarcoma
ii. Epithelioid sarcoma
iii. Pleomorphic rhabdomyosarcoma
iv. Leiomyosarcoma
v. Malignant peripheral nerve sheath tumour
vi. Angiosarcoma

Chemo-insensitive

i. Dedifferentiated liposarcoma
ii. Alveolar soft part sarcoma

Sarcomas that Metastasise to Lymph Nodes*

- **R**habdomyosarcoma
- **A**ngiosarcoma
- **C**lear cell carcinoma
- **E**pithelioid sarcoma
- **S**ynovial sarcoma

Remember as* **RACES

Isolated limb perfusion (like melanoma) with high dose chemotherapy (melphalan) and tumour necrosis factor alpha (TNF-α) with hyperthermia to the links can be used by cannulating artery and vein with tourniquet.

PROGNOSIS

- Almost 80% of STS metastasise to lungs within 2–3 years of the diagnosis.
- Prognosis depends on metastatic STS, grade of the tumour, size of the tumour, margins after resection and anatomical location.
- If pulmonary metastasis is resectable, 30% survival may be expected at 3 years.

DIFFERENTIAL DIAGNOSIS OF SOFT TISSUE SARCOMA

LIPOSARCOMA

- It is a malignant fatty tumour (*see* page 749).
- **Common sites:** Proximal extremity (Figs 33.24 to 33.26 MRI of liposarcoma of thigh), trunk or retroperitoneum (Fig. 33.27).
- They are generally large at the time of diagnosis, e.g. retroperitoneum. It results in gross swelling, which is firm to hard (more than 50% will be of >20 cm size) (Key Box 33.12).

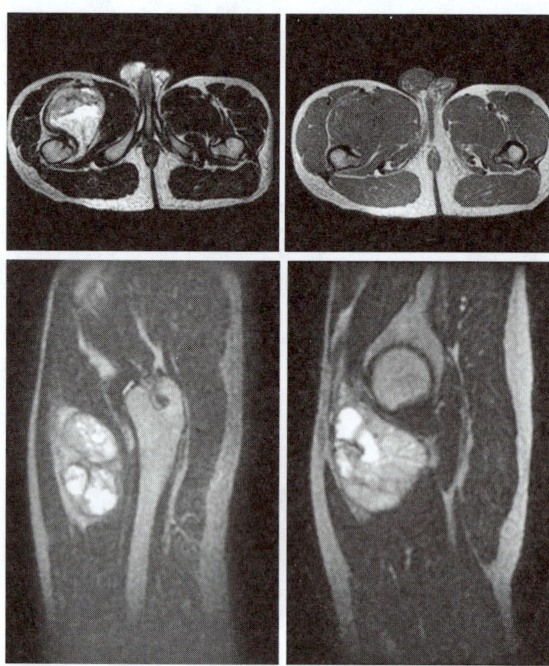

Figs 33.24 to 33.26: T1- and T2-weighted (W) axial MRI. Isointense to hyperintense mass lesion noted in the anterior compartment of right thigh. Sagittal T2-W MRI shows supero-inferior extent of the lesion

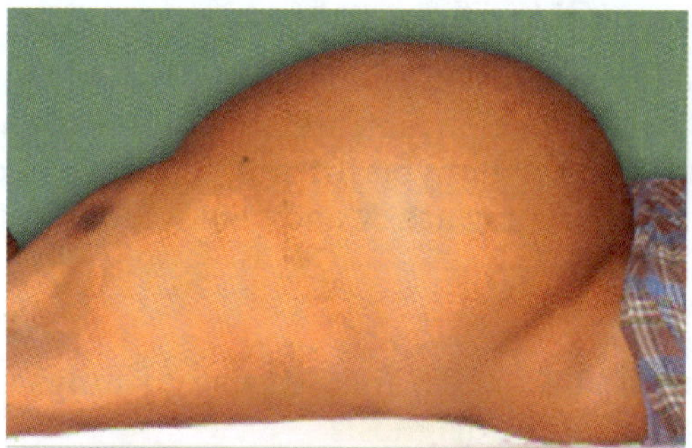

Fig. 33.27: Retroperitoneal liposarcoma

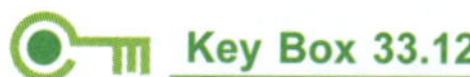

Key Box 33.12

Retroperitoneal Sarcoma (RPS)

- Most common RPS is liposarcoma or leiomyosarcoma.
- They constitute 15% of adult soft tissue sarcomas.
- May present as large masses of more than 20 cm at the time of presentation.
- Local recurrence and intra-abdominal spread is more common.
- Progressive abdominal distension, pedal oedema, young age and firm to hard retroperitoneal mass clinches the diagnosis.
- CT scan of chest and abdomen followed by FNAC/true-cut biopsy for histology/grade of the tumour.
- Margin negative—**complete surgical resection** is the treatment of choice.
- Chemotherapy **has not been effective** against RPS.

- The compression on blood vessels may result in oedema of the limbs when it occurs in retroperitoneum.
- Well-differentiated myxoid liposarcomas **are notoriously known to recur** many times before spreading to lungs. **Hence, prognosis is good** (Fig. 33.34).
- Dedifferentiated liposarcoma can be distinguished from other poorly differentiated STS subtypes on the basis of MDM2 and CDK-4 immunohistochemistry.
- Pleomorphic and lipoblastic liposarcomas tend to be of higher grade and often present with metastasis.
- MRI (Fig. 33.24) followed by wide excision/surgery is the primary treatment.
- They do respond to radiotherapy.

MALIGNANT FIBROUS HISTIOCYTOMA (MFH)

- It is a malignant tumour of mesenchymal tissue (fibrous tissue). This is the recent nomenclature of sarcoma. Fibrosarcoma or pleomorphic rhabdomyosarcomas are included under this. **Most of the so-called fibrosarcomas are presently included under MFH**.
- These are **high-grade tumours** that lack differentiation.
- It can also arise from bone.
- **The MFH: Superficial type rarely metastasises and carries good prognosis.**
- Locations: Retroperitoneum, trunks and limbs (intermuscular septae of adductors, scapulohumeral and pectoral muscles).

Clinical Features and Treatment

- Common in elderly patients (50 years) but can occur at any age.
- Slow-growing, firm to hard mass with restricted mobility.
- As the tumour is locally invasive, it infiltrates the muscles and adjacent structures. Thus, it can cause muscle weakness or pain, etc.
- **Spread:** Local spread is common. Distant metastasis by blood is late (lungs). Lymph node metastasis is rare.
- Like other sarcomas, dilated veins, local rise of temperature, restricted mobility and hardness will clinch the diagnosis.
- **MRI is the investigation of choice to know the extent of the disease**.
- Margin negative surgery should be the aim.

Figures 33.28 to 33.41 depict types of common sarcomas, wide excision and histological features.

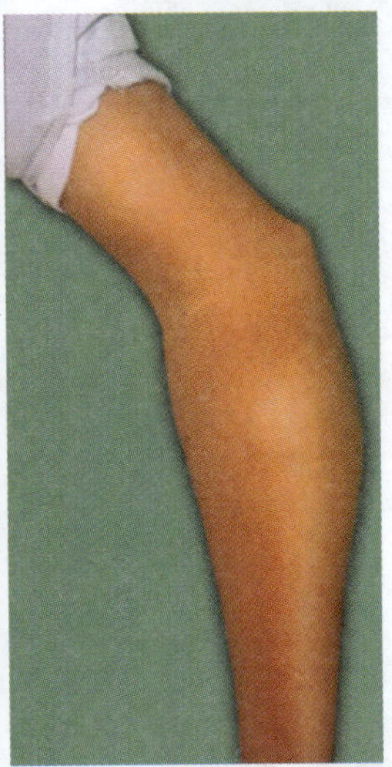

Fig. 33.28: Early stage of liposarcoma—this swelling had local rise of temperature and restricted mobility

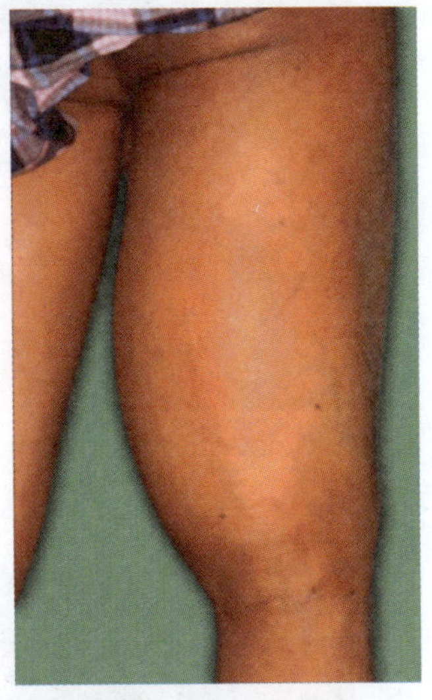

Fig. 33.29: Advanced case of liposarcoma—the swelling was hard and fixed. Dilated veins over the surface and location were characteristic

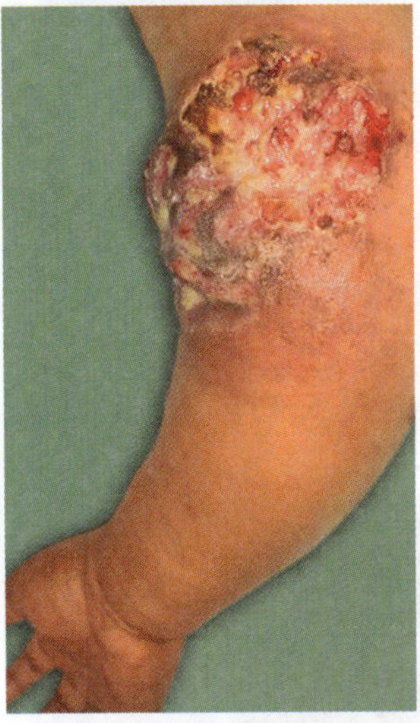

Fig. 33.30: Swelling in the elbow region for two years duration presented to the hospital with bleeding and fungation. Advanced case of epithelioid sarcoma

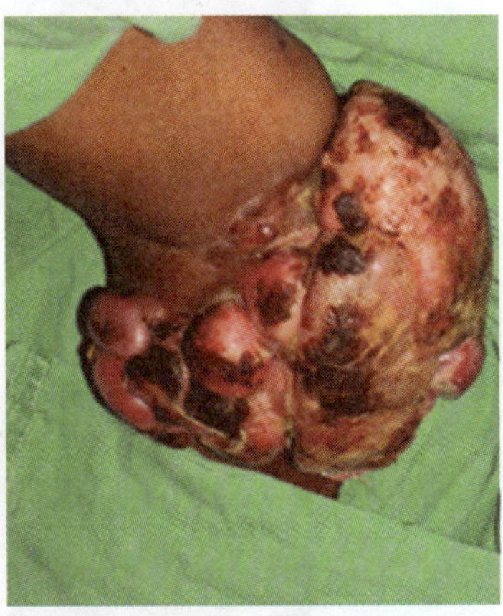

Fig. 33.31: Ulcerated lesion in the elbow region of two years duration presented to the hospital with bleeding. A case of dermatofibrosarcoma protuberans

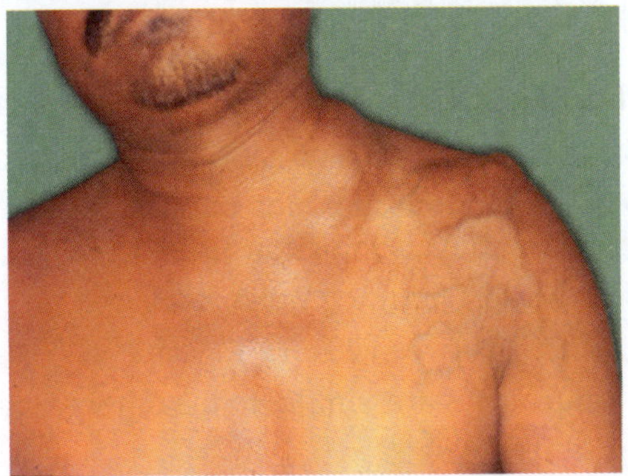

Fig. 33.32: Synovial sarcoma left shoulder region. *See* the secondary varicosity due to pressure effects. Nonextremity sarcomas have poor prognosis

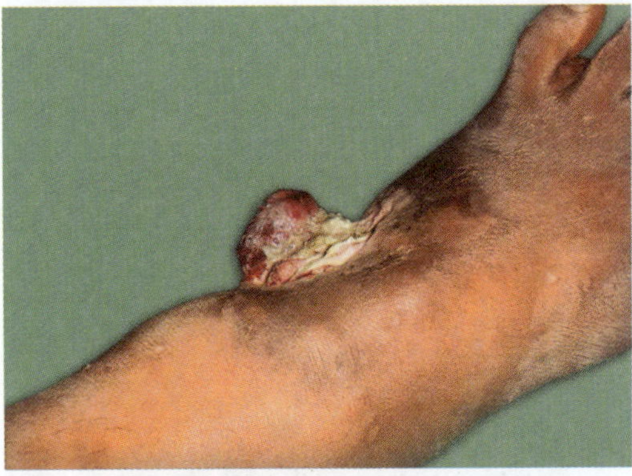

Fig. 33.33: Bleeding vascular lesion in the ankle region—angiosarcoma. (*Courtesy:* Dr Mallikarjuna Desai, Head, Department of Surgery, SDMC, Dharwar, Karnataka)

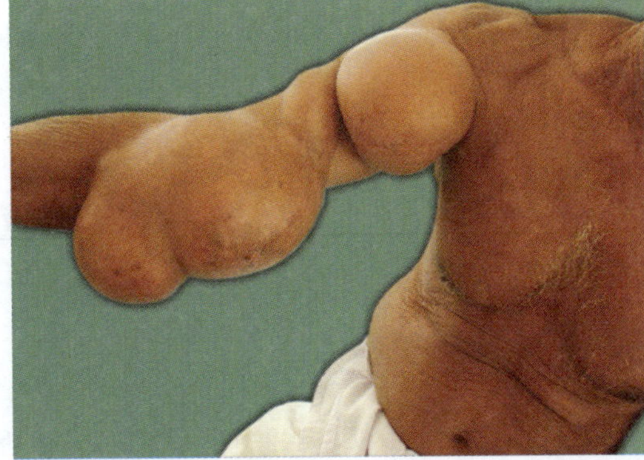

Fig. 33.34: Six times recurrent myxoid liposarcoma since 8 years. It has good prognosis. (*Courtesy:* Dr Shashi, Head, Department of Surgery, Calicut Medical College, Calicut, India)

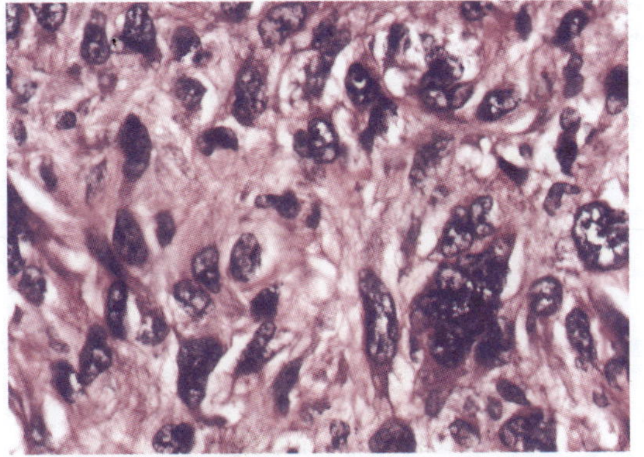

Fig. 33.35: Spindle cell sarcoma. (*Courtesy:* Dr Laxmi Rao, Head, Department of Pathology, KMC, Manipal)

SURGICAL PROCEDURES DONE FOR SOFT TISSUE SARCOMA (Figs 33.36 to 33.41)

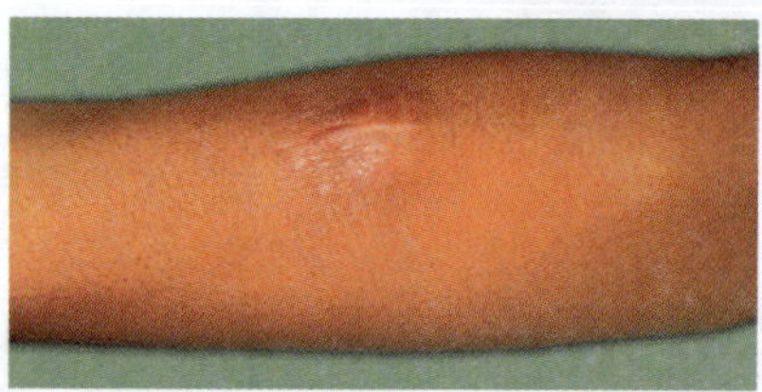

Fig. 33.36: A 24-year-old lady underwent excision of a swelling diagnosed as lipoma in a peripheral hospital which was reported as sarcoma

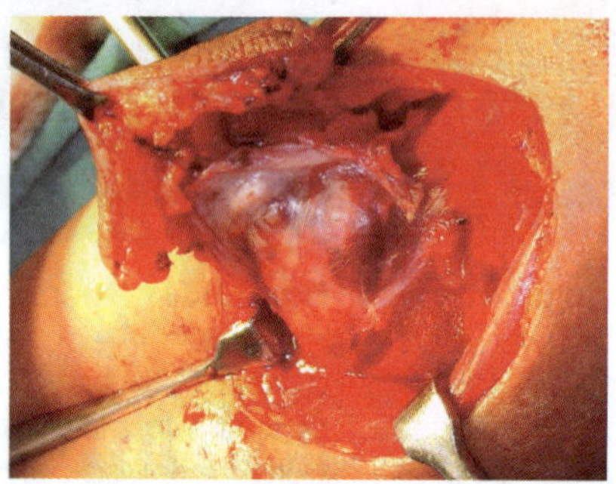

Fig. 33.37: The swelling was explored—as you can see it was infiltrating the muscles—the first surgeon had not excised the swelling completely

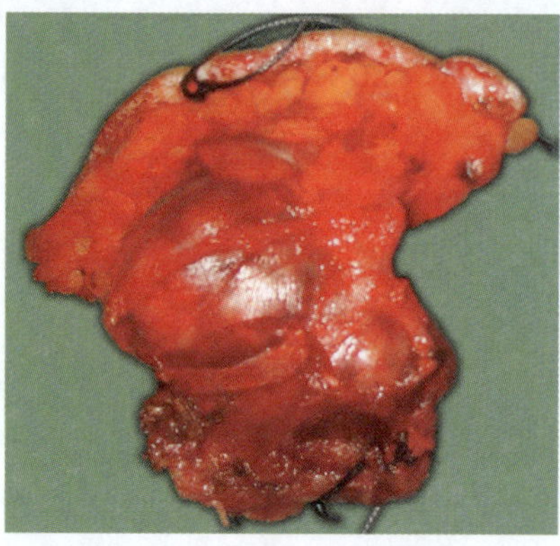

Fig. 33.38: Excised specimen showing skin, tumour and deeper muscle fibres. STS was 3 cm in diameter. Histopathology reported as synovial cell sarcoma. Margins were negative. (*Courtesy:* Dr Ankur Sharma, Assistant Professor, Department of Surgery, KMC, Manipal)

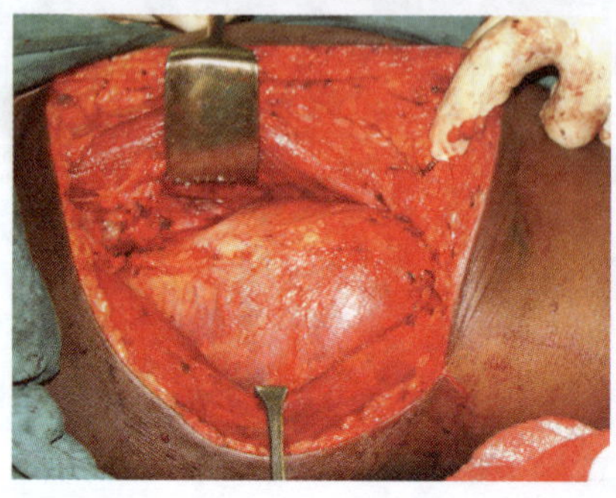

Fig. 33.39: A large (8 cm) liposarcoma of the thigh being explored with a longitudinal incision of the thigh. He had undergone an incision biopsy earlier. The biopsy site is removed along with the skin

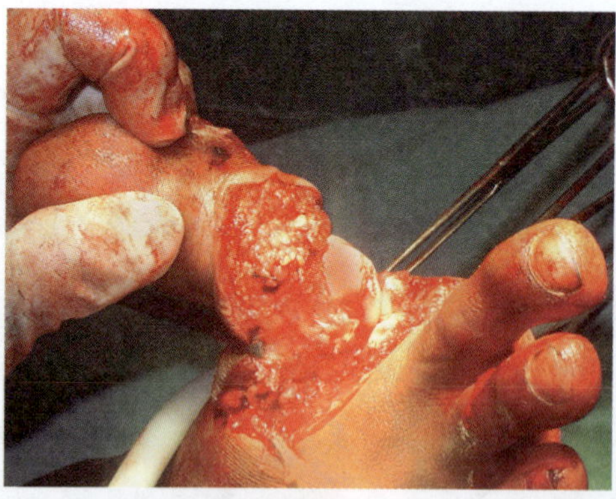

Fig. 33.40: Synovial sarcoma of the toe—disarticulation being done—highly malignant sarcoma

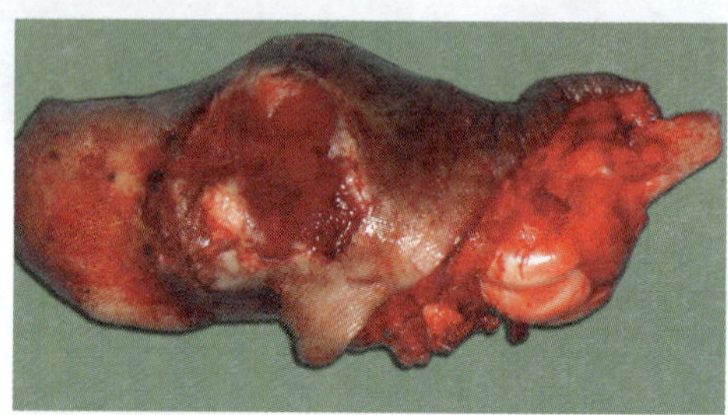

Fig. 33.41: Specimen of the growth along with the toe: Wide excision. No nodes were palpable in the leg

SYNOVIAL SARCOMA (Fig. 33.32)

- Any rapidly growing tumour in the region of joint or near the tendons in young patients (20–40 years), synovial sarcoma is to be considered.
- Common site: Shoulder, wrist, knee, etc.
- Age: Young between 20 and 40 years.
- Clinical features are similar to the other sarcomas—hard, painful mass.
- In addition to the local and blood spread, **it also spreads by lymphatic route**.
- Plain X-ray: It may show characteristic calcification.
- It is aggressive, with high rates of recurrence.
- **In the G-TNM staging system, they are Grade 3.**

ANGIOSARCOMA (Fig. 33.33)

- 1 to 2% of soft tissue sarcomas.
- Affects elderly patients.
- They are high grade and aggressive tumours.
- They arise from skin and subcutaneous tissue rather than deeper tissues.
- Most of them occur in the **head and neck, breast and liver**.
- Surgery (excision) followed by radiotherapy/ combination chemotherapy may have to be given.

RHABDOMYOSARCOMA

- It is the **most common soft tissue sarcoma** seen in children, even though they are rare (under the age of 15).
- It arises from **striated muscle**—painless enlarging mass.
- Resection/chemotherapy/radiotherapy (combination) is tried depending on location.
- **Sites:** Head and neck (30%), genitourinary system (25%), extremities (20%).
- All three varieties: Embryonal, alveolar and pleomorphic are considered as Grade 3 in GTNM staging. Hence, prognosis is not good.
- Complete tumour resection should be the aim. Chemotherapy and RT are also used.
- Rhabdomyosarcomas have a **high propensity for lymph node metastasis**.

KAPOSI'S SARCOMA

- Vulnerable section of people includes Jews, immunocompromised patients such as transplant recipients and AIDS.
- Typical sites: Legs. Other sites include chest, arm, neck in epidemic form (Africa).
- It presents as **multiple pigmented sarcoma nodules** in the leg.
- It is interesting to note that **Kaposi's sarcoma is "not seen" in transfusion related 'AIDS '**.
- It manifests with purplish to red subcutaneous nodules in the leg followed by ulceration and bleeding.
- Combination chemotherapy with doxorubicin, etoposide and interferon have been used to control the disease.

DERMATOFIBROSARCOMA PROTUBERANS (Fig. 33.31)

- Clinically presents as nodular **exophytic 'mass' lesion**—protuberans.
- Locally aggressive tumour which does not metastasise.
- Wide excision should be the aim with negative margin to prevent local recurrence.
- Mohs' micrographic surgery such as basal cell carcinoma has been advocated to get negative margin and thus to get a low recurrence rates.
- Has good prognosis, if treated early.

Malignant Peripheral Nerve Sheath Tumours (MPNST)

- They are malignant form of benign schwannomas.
- They are aggressive tumours and local recurrence rate is about 20%.
- Although arising from nerve sheath they are painless at presentation and usually present in the 20–50 years age group.
- MPNST may occur spontaneously or as part of NF-1
- Treatment is similar to other STS subtypes with an aim towards margin negative resection.

USEFUL TIPS IN A CASE OF SOFT TISSUE SARCOMA (Key Box 33.13)

In undergraduate clinical examination, students are advised to offer soft tissue sarcoma as the diagnosis. When asked the possible type, they only give a possible histological type based on various clinical features mentioned above. **Ask the following questions to yourself** to get ready for the clinical examinations.

1. **Is it soft tissue sarcoma?** Tumour arising from soft tissue, dilated veins, reddish skin, increase in local temperature, firm to hard, rapidly growing swelling, with late involvement of skin (carcinoma starts in the skin) (Key Box 33.13).
2. **What is the age of the patient?**
   - In children – Rhabdomyosarcoma
Undifferentiated sarcoma

Key Box 33.13

Interesting 'Most' to Remember in Soft Tissue Sarcoma

- Most of the soft tissue sarcomas **arise *de novo***.
- Most originate in an **extremity** (60%).
- Most common soft tissue sarcoma in adults is **MFH (28%).**
- Most extremity sarcomas (35%) occur in the lower limbs.
- Most occur in men (4 times more common in men compared to women).
- Most common soft tissue sarcoma in **children** is **rhabdomyosarcoma**.
- Most of the soft tissue sarcomas metastasise by blood.
- Most of the **extremity** soft tissue sarcoma **metastasise to lungs**.
- Most of the **retroperitoneal soft tissue** sarcoma metastasise to liver.
- Most important prognostic factor for soft tissue sarcoma is **size and grade of the primary tumour**.
- Most accurate imaging modality for soft tissue sarcoma is **MRI**.
- Most effective modality of **treatment is surgery**.
- Most effective **chemotherapeutic drugs** are doxorubicin, dacarbazine and ifosfamide.

- In 20–40 years – Liposarcoma
  Synovial sarcoma
  Kaposi's sarcoma
- In elderly patients – Angiosarcoma
  Chondrosarcoma (bone)
  Fibrosarcoma (Fig. 33.21)

3. Which site has it occurred?
- *Head and neck* – Angiosarcoma
  Rhabdomyosarcoma
  Osteogenic sarcoma (jaw)
- *Distal extremity (limbs)* – Synovial sarcoma (Fig. 33.23)
  Epithelioid sarcoma (Fig. 33.34)
  Clear cell sarcoma
- *Retroperitoneum and mesentery* – Liposarcoma (Fig. 33.27)
  MFH, leiomyosarcoma

4. Has it spread to lymph nodes?
- Rhabdomyosarcoma
- Synovial sarcoma
- Epithelioid sarcoma

5. Has it spread to lungs or liver?
- Chest X-ray
- Ultrasound

6. Can I preserve the limb? How?
- Wide excision
- Compartmental excision
- Preoperative radiotherapy combined with surgery and postoperative radiotherapy.

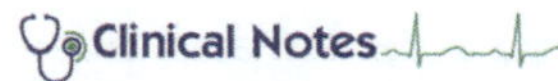

A 34-year-old nondiabetic male patient had a nonhealing ulcer right great toe of 6 months duration. History of minor trauma was present. Examination revealed ulceration, thickening and induration with 'mass' lesion. It was MBBS examination case. The student offered osteomyelitis, foreign body granuloma and tuberculous synovitis as diagnosis. He qualified but he was asked to examine the groin. The patient had 3 hard nodes in the groin. The final diagnosis—synovial cell sarcoma with metastasis in the groin nodes—the student had not examined the groin!

Multiple Choice Questions

1. When do you suspect lipoma turns into liposarcoma?
A. When lipoma gets infected
B. When lipoma causes lymphangitis
C. When it becomes fixed
D. When it undergoes myxomatous degeneration

2. Intussusception is caused by:
A. Submucosal lipoma
B. Subserosal lipoma
C. Retroperitoneal lipoma
D. Intraperitoneal lipoma

3. Myxomatous degeneration occurs only in which lipoma?
A. Retroperitoneal B. Subfacial
C. Submucosal D. Subcutaneous

4. Following are true for von Recklinghausen's disease *except:*
A. It is an autosomal dominant disorder
B. Skin pigmentation is a feature
C. Café au lait spots are characteristic
D. Does not turn into sarcoma

5. Following are true for schwannoma *except:*
A. Commonest site is acoustic nerve
B. Sensory branches are affected more often
C. Well-encapsulated tumour
D. Highly premalignant tumour

6. Following are radiosensitive tumours *except:*
A. Oral cancer B. Seminoma testis
C. Carcinoma breast D. Malignant chordoma

7. Which one of the following does not have a capsule?
A. Hamartoma B. Schwannoma
C. Fibroadenoma D. Branchial cyst

8. Which one of the following is commonly associated with paraneoplastic syndrome?
A. Carcinoma stomach B. Carcinoma colon
C. Carcinoma pancreas D. Carcinoma lung

9. Which one of the following conditions is more commonly associated with paraneoplastic syndrome?
A. Hypernatraemia B. Hyponatraemia
C. Hypercalcaemia D. Hypocalcaemia

10. Polycythaemia is a paraneoplastic syndrome seen in which condition?

A. Hepatoma
B. Wilms' tumour
C. Apudoma
D. Renal cell carcinoma

11. Post-mastectomy lymphoedema is called:

A. Stewart-Treves syndrome
B. Bloom's syndrome
C. Fanconi's syndrome
D. Sturge-Weber syndrome

12. Precautions to be taken while doing an open biopsy in soft tissue sarcoma include following *except:*

A. Incision should be longitudinal
B. Perfect haemostasis should be achieved
C. Drain should be kept
D. Flaps should not be raised

13. Sarcomas metastasise to lymph nodes include following *except:*

A. Rhabdomyosarcoma B. Angiosarcoma
C. Synovial sarcoma D. Liposarcoma

14. Following are true for the treatment of soft tissue sarcomas *except:*

A. Surgery is the best line of treatment
B. Radiotherapy is given after surgery
C. Chemotherapy is also given
D. Radiotherapy is the first line of treatment

15. Following are true for the treatment of retroperitoneal sarcoma *except:*

A. Surgery is the best line of treatment
B. Radiotherapy is extremely helpful
C. Chemotherapy is not very useful
D. Most of them are liposarcoma

16. Following are high grade soft tissue sarcomas *except:*

A. Angiosarcoma
B. Synovial sarcoma
C. Malignant fibrous histiocytoma
D. Liposarcoma

17. Following are true for glomus tumour *except:*

A. It can turn into malignant
B. It is an angioneuromyoma
C. It is radio-resistant
D. It is concerned with heat regulation

Answers

1. C **2.** A **3.** A **4.** D **5.** D **6.** D **7.** A **8.** D **9.** C **10.** D
11. A **12.** C **13.** D **14.** D **15.** B **16.** D **17.** A

CHAPTER

34

Cystic Swellings, Neck Swellings and Metastasis Lymph Node Neck

- Cystic swellings
- Transilluminant swellings
- Differential diagnosis of midline swellings
- Swellings in the submandibular triangle
- Swellings in the carotid triangle
- Swellings in the posterior triangle
- AV fistula
- Lymph node secondaries in the neck
- Different types of neck dissections
- Secondaries in the neck—occult primary
- Pancoast's tumour

CYSTIC SWELLINGS

A cyst is a swelling containing fluid. **True cysts** are lined by endothelium or epithelium. They contain clear serous fluid, mucoid material, pus, blood, lymph or toothpaste like material.

The **false cysts** do not have lining epithelium. They can be ***degenerative cysts*** as in the case of tumours which undergo tumour necrosis or tumour degeneration, or merely a ***collection*** of fluid which is walled off by coils of bowel as in tuberculous encysted ascites or an ***exudation cyst*** as in pseudopancreatic cyst.

Classification of Cyst

I. Congenital Cyst

- Sequestration dermoid cyst
- Branchial cyst
- Thyroglossal cyst
- Lymphangioma
- Cysts of embryonic remnants: Cyst of urachus, vitellointestinal duct cyst.

II. Acquired Cyst

- *Retention cyst:* Sebaceous cyst, galactocele, spermatocele, Bartholin's gland cyst
- *Distension cyst:* Thyroid cyst, ovarian cyst
- *Exudation cyst:* Hydrocele
- *Degenerative cyst:* Tumour necrosis
- *Traumatic cyst:* Haematoma, implantation dermoid cyst
- *Cystic tumours:* Cystadenoma of pancreas, cystadenoma of the ovary

III. Parasitic Cyst

- Cysticercosis
- Hydatid cyst

Clinical Examination of Cysts in General

Students are requested to follow the standard practice of examination of the swelling in the form of inspection, palpation, percussion and auscultation in the clinical examination. Some important tests for cystic swellings are given in the next page.

1. Location: Most of the congenital cystic swellings have a typical location wherein diagnosis can be made with fair accuracy. A few examples are as follows:
   - **Branchial cyst** occurs at the junction of upper one-third and lower two-thirds of the sternocleidomastoid muscle, whereas opening of branchial fistula occurs at junction of upper two-thirds and lower one-third of sternocleidomastoid muscle.
   - **Dermoid cyst:** Midline, outer or inner canthus of the eye.
   - **Meningocele:** Swelling in the newborn at lumbosacral region.
   - **Ganglion:** On the dorsum of the hand and foot
2. Shape: Majority of the cystic swellings are round or oval.
   - ***Subhyoid bursitis:*** Transverse oval cystic swelling in the midline of the neck.
   - ***Thyroglossal cyst:*** Vertically placed oval swelling in the midline of the neck.
   - ***Sebaceous cyst:*** Hemispherical swelling.

3. **Surface:** Almost all the cystic swellings in the skin and subcutaneous tissue have smooth surface.
4. **Consistency:** Fluctuation is positive in all cystic swellings (Fig. 34.1 and Key Box 34.1). However, depending on the contents, the fluctuation may be different, which an experienced surgeon can diagnose.

Key Box 34.1

Rules of Elicitation of Fluctuation

- **Mobile swelling has to be fixed.**
- **Both hands should be used.**
- With the index finger and thumb of one hand, the swelling is pressed—these are 'active' fingers and the impulse is received by the thumb and index finger of the other hand (passive fingers).
- Fluctuation should be elicited in **both directions,** as fleshy muscle in the thigh can be fluctuant across but not in the longitudinal direction.
- When swelling is smaller than 2 cm in size, **Paget's test is done**. Cystic swellings feel soft in the centre and firm at the periphery. Solid swellings feel firm at the centre than periphery.

- ***Soft cystic:*** Thyroglossal cyst, meningocele, lymph cyst.
- ***Tensely cystic:*** Ganglion, tensely cystic swellings in the neck may feel firm or solid, e.g. tense thyroid cyst. Cyst in the breast may feel firm or hard.
- ***Yielding*** in cases of lipoma, as fat at body temperature behaves like fluid (pseudofluctuation).
- ***Soft with firm thickened periphery:*** Cold abscess
- ***Half-filled like a rubber hot water bottle:*** Branchial cyst.
- ***Putty or toothpaste:*** Sebaceous cyst (true fluctuation is not found).
- ***Cross-fluctuation*** for swellings having two components connected to each other, e.g. plunging ranula.

5. **Transillumination test:** Cystic swellings which contain clear fluid show positive transillumination (Fig. 34.2).

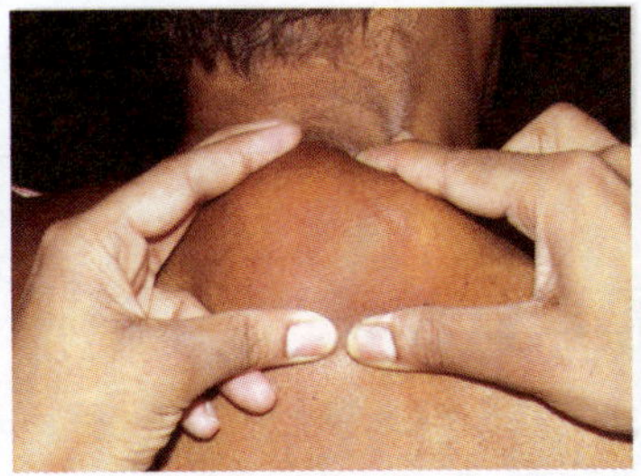

Fig. 34.1: Fluctuation should be elicited using both hands and in both directions

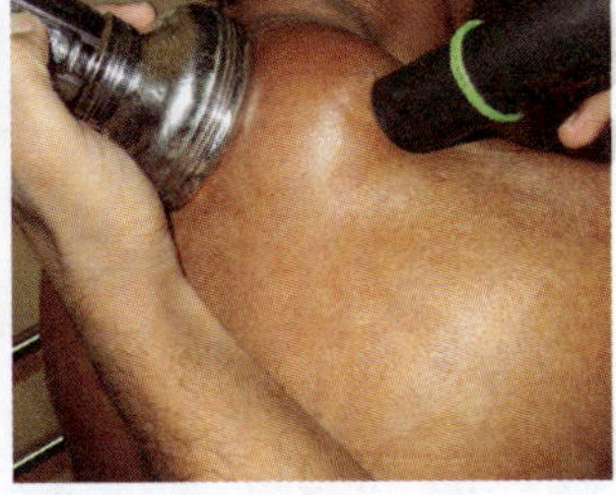

Fig. 34.2: Transillumination test: It should be done in a dark room

6. **Mobility:** Almost all the cystic swellings in the skin, subcutaneous tissue or in the deeper plane are benign and as a rule, they should have free mobility. However, this is not true due to various anatomical factors.
   - ***Branchial cyst:*** Restricted mobility is due to its adherence to the sternomastoid muscle.
   - ***Thyroglossal cyst:*** Transverse mobility is absent because the cyst is tethered by remnant of the thyroglossal duct.
   - ***Sebaceous cyst:*** Limited mobility due to the adherence to the skin.
7. **Sign of compressibility:** The swellings which have communication with a cavity or with tissue spaces give the positive sign of compressibility. Thus, a steady pressure is applied over the swellings. The swelling may disappear completely or may partially disappear. However, when pressure is released the swelling fills up slowly. Hence, it is also called the 'sign of refilling' (Key Box 34.2).

Key Box 34.2

Compressible Swellings

- Haemangioma
- Lymphangioma
- Meningocele

8. **Plane of the swelling**
   - Almost all significant cystic swellings in the neck are deep to deep fascia. Thus, contracting sternomastoid for laterally placed swellings and bending the chin against resistance for centrally placed swellings must be done to define the plane of swelling.
   - Subcutaneous swellings become more prominent when the underlying muscles are contracted as in limbs.
   - Swelling due to semimembranous bursitis, almost disappears on flexion of knee and becomes more prominent on extension of the knee.
   - Sebaceous cysts are attached to the skin at the site of punctum.
9. **Pulsations**
   a. ***Expansile:*** Aneurysms are characterised by expansile pulsations. When two fingers are placed over the swelling on the sides, the fingers are not only elevated but are also separated. Popliteal aneurysms typically give this sign (Key Box 34.3).
   b. ***Transmitted:*** When the swelling is situated over a vessel, the fingers are raised but not separated, e.g. pseudopancreatic cysts. When the swelling pushes the vessel anteriorly, transmitted pulsation can be obtained, e.g. cervical rib pushing the subclavian artery.

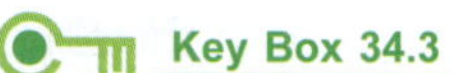

Key Box 34.3

Aneurysm Tests

- Expansile pulsations: Finger separation sign
- Proximal compression test: Decreased size
- Distal compression test: Size may increase
- Thrill and bruit are present and distal pulses may be weak

c. *Pulsation* can also be present in vascular tumours, such as osteogenic sarcoma or secondaries from carcinoma thyroid, etc.

Effects of Aneurysm (Key Box 34.4 and Figs 34.3 and 34.4)

Some Useful TIPS

1. **Thrombosis:** It is one of the common effects of aneurysm particularly aortic and popliteal, resulting in ischaemia in the distal territory.
2. **Ischaemia:** Distal parts may become gangrenous and/or can have ischaemic ulcers or claudication.
3. **Pressure effects**
   a. ***Effect on bone:*** Erosion of the vertebral body as in aortic aneurysm. This does not happen in TB spine.
   b. ***Effect on nerves:*** Popliteal aneurysm can give rise to foot drop due to pressure on lateral popliteal nerve.

Key Box 34.4

Effects of Aneurysm: TIPS

- Thrombosis, Ischaemia
- Pressure, Skin changes

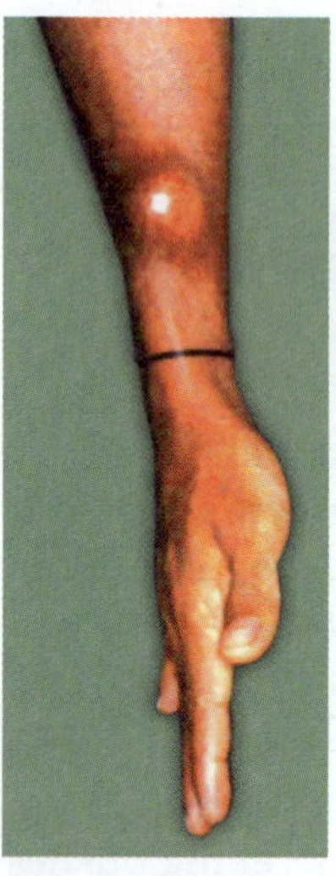

Fig. 34.3: Radial artery aneurysm

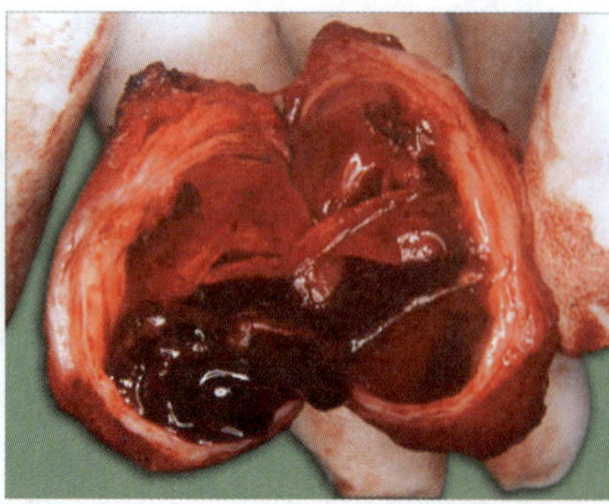

Fig. 34.4: Radial artery aneurysm with clot—excised specimen. (*Courtesy:* Prof L Ramachandra, Professor of Surgery, KMC, Manipal)

   c. ***Effect on the veins:*** Results in congestion and oedema of the leg.
   d. ***On the oesophagus:*** Dysphagia as in aortic aneurysm.
4. **Skin changes** may be in the form of oedema and redness.

Complications of Cysts in General

1. **Infection**, e.g. **sebaceous cyst**
2. **Calcification**, e.g. haematoma, multinodular goitre with cyst, hydatid cyst
3. **Pressure effects:** Ovarian cyst pressing on the iliac veins.
4. **Haemorrhage** within thyroid cyst.
5. **Torsion:** Ovarian dermoid.
6. **Transformation** into malignancy.
7. **Ovarian cachexia:** Large ovarian tumour with pedal oedema, anorexia, loss of weight, lordosis.

DERMOID CYST

This is a cyst lined by squamous epithelium containing desquamated cells. The contents are thick and sometimes toothpaste-like which is a mixture of sweat, sebum and desquamated epithelial cells and sometimes even hair.

Clinical Types of Dermoid Cyst (Key Box 34.5)

I. Congenital/Sequestration Dermoid

- They occur along the line of embryonic fusion, due to dermal cells being buried in deeper plane.
- The cells which are sequestrated in the subcutaneous plane proliferate and liquefy to form a cyst.
- As it grows, it indents the mesoderm (future bone) which explains the bony defects caused by dermoid cyst in the skull or facial bones.
- Even though they are congenital, they manifest as a swelling during childhood or later in life. Often they can be mistaken for lipoma and sebaceous cysts (Fig. 34.5).
- They can occur anywhere in the midline of the body or the face (Key Box 34.5).

Key Box 34.5

Origin of Dermoid Cyst

- The face is developed from 5 processes—2 maxillary, 2 mandibular and 1 frontonasal.
- Dermoid cyst occurs in the line of embryonic fusion of these processes.

1. External and internal angular dermoid cyst: At the fusion lines of frontonasal and maxillary processes (Fig. 34.6).
2. Median nasal dermoid cyst: At the root of the nose at the fusion lines of frontal process (Fig. 34.7).
3. In the suprasternal space of *Burns*
4. Sublingual dermoid cyst (Fig. 34.8)
5. Pre-auricular dermoid cyst—in front of the auricle
6. Post-auricular dermoid cyst behind the auricle (Fig. 34.9).

Pearls of Wisdom

Pinna is formed by the fusion of 6 cutaneous tubercles. Both preauricular and postauricular dermoid cysts occur because of failure of fusion of one of the tubercles with the others as they form pinna.

Complications of Dermoid Cyst

1. Infection
2. Suppuration: Abscess
3. Ovarian dermoid: Torsion

Clinical Features

- Though congenital, the cyst manifests in childhood or during adolescence. A few cases also manifest in 30–40 years age group.
- Typically, the patient presents with a painless, slow-growing swelling.
- Soft, cystic and fluctuant; transillumination is negative.
- Rarely, it may be putty-like in consistency.
- **The underlying *bony* defect gives the clue to the diagnosis.**
- Classical location of the cyst (along the line of fusion) is a feature of sequestration dermoid cyst.

II. Implantation Dermoid Cyst (Fig. 34.10)

- This is common in women, tailors, agriculturists who sustain repeated minor sharp injuries.
- Following a **sharp injury,** a few epidermal cells get implanted into the subcutaneous plane. There, they develop into an implantation dermoid cyst. Hence, it is typically found in the fingers, palm and sole of the foot. As the cyst develops in the areas where the skin is thick and keratinised, it feels firm to hard in consistency.

III. Teratomatous Dermoid Cyst (Figs 34.11 and 34.12)

- Teratoma is a tumour arising from ***totipotential cells.*** Thus, it contains ectodermal, endodermal and mesodermal elements—hair, teeth, cartilage, bone, etc.
- Common sites are ovary, testis, retroperitoneum and mediastinum.

Clinical Notes

A 24-year-old female patient was admitted with acute lower abdominal pain of 2 days' duration. There was guarding and rigidity of the abdominal wall with rebound tenderness. Per vaginal examination was normal. At exploration, there was a twisted ovarian teratoma on the left side with gangrene. It was excised. The opposite ovary, on careful examination revealed a small teratomatous dermoid cyst which could be enucleated. The significance of this case report lies in the fact that both ovaries should be examined in cases of ovarian dermoid cysts.

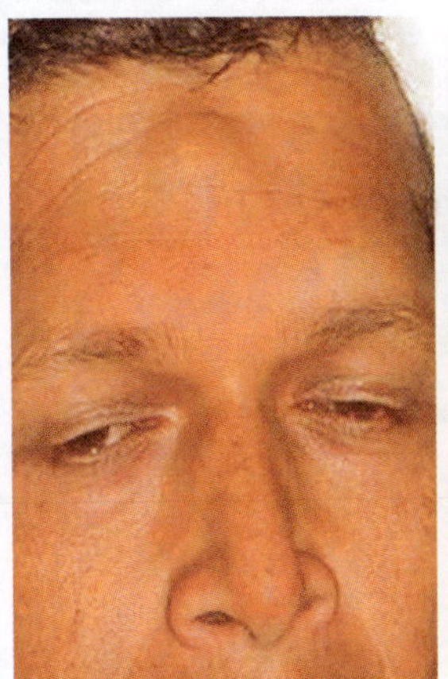

Fig. 34.5: Median frontal dermoid cyst, lipoma, sebaceous cyst are other differential diagnosis

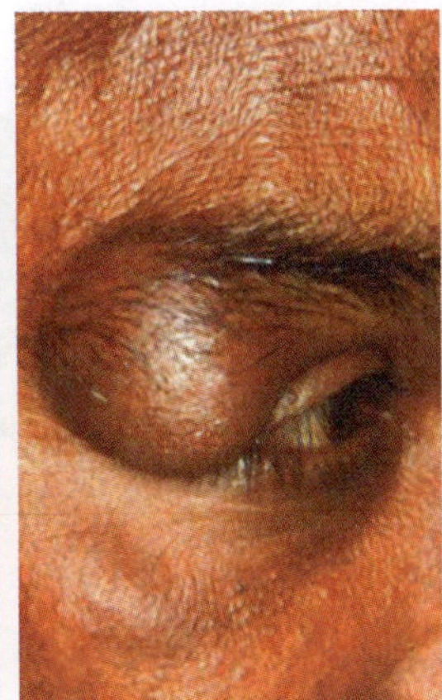

Fig. 34.6: External angular dermoid cyst. Look for bony depression—it is pathognomonic of this swelling

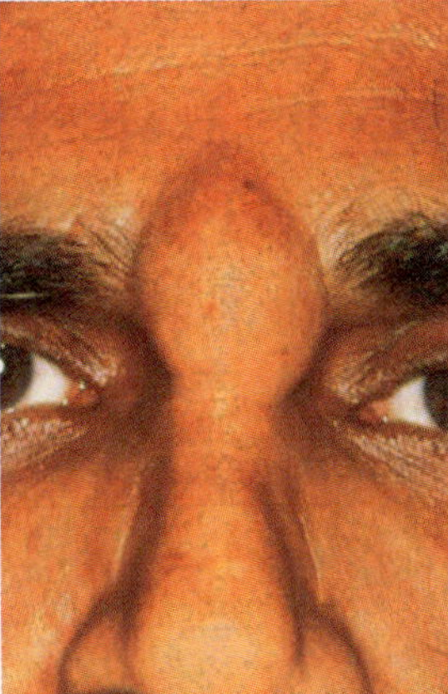

Fig. 34.7: Median frontal dermoid cyst at the root of the nose.Test for cough impulse

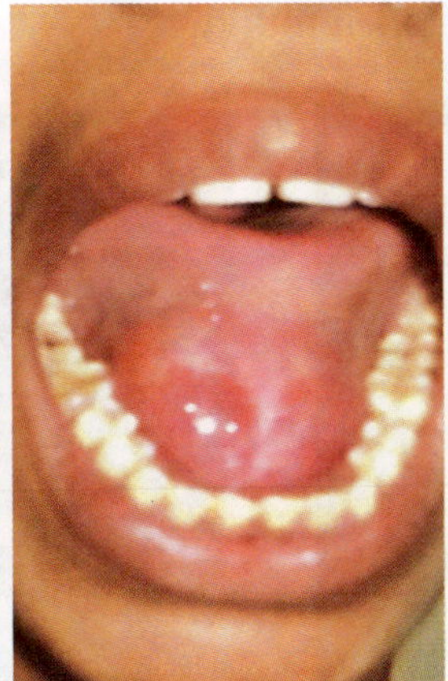

Fig. 34.8: Sublingual dermoid. (*Courtesy:* Dr Sreejayan, Professor of Surgery, Calicut Medical College)

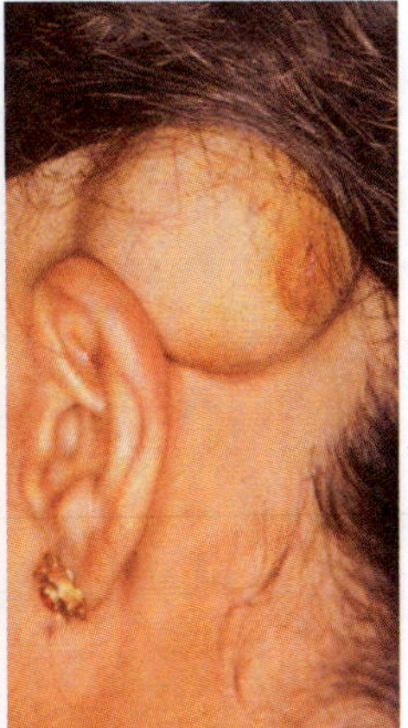

Fig. 34.9: Post-auricular dermoid cyst. Location and soft consistency are characteristic

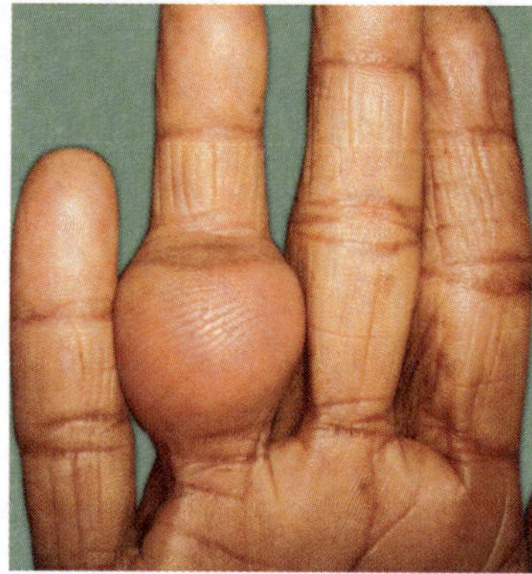

Fig. 34.10: Implantation dermoid cyst. TB synovitis and chronic abscess are the other differential diagnosis

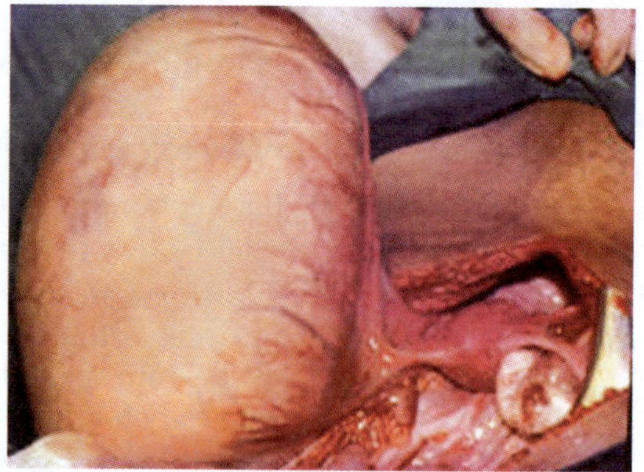

Fig. 34.11: Ovarian teratomatous dermoid cyst. Usually they are bilateral. Large ones with pedicles are vulnerable for torsion. (*Courtesy:* Dr Rajesh Bhakta, Associate Professor, Dept. of OBG, KMC, Manipal)

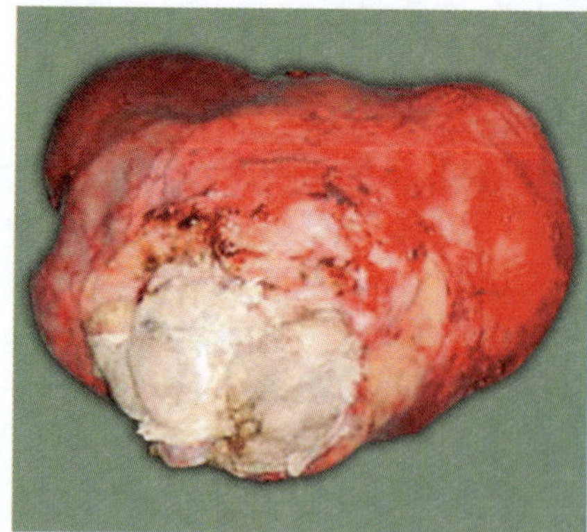

Fig. 34.12: Cut open specimen of epidermoid cyst showing cheesy material

IV. Tubuloembryonic Dermoid Cyst

- They arise from ectodermal tubes. A few examples are thyroglossal cyst, post-anal dermoid cyst.
- Ependymal cyst of the brain.

Treatment of Dermoid Cyst

Excision of the cyst.

EPIDERMAL CYST (WEN)

- This is popularly called **sebaceous cyst**. It is a misnomer. This occurs due to obstruction to one of the sebaceous ducts, resulting in accumulation of sebaceous material. Hence, this is an example of **retention cyst**.
- **Sites:** Scalp, face, back, scrotum, etc. ***It does not occur in palm and sole,*** where sebaceous glands are absent. In the back, scalp and scrotum (Figs 34.13 to 34.16), multiple cysts are often found.

Clinical Features

- They are slow-growing and appear in early adulthood or middle age.
- **Hemispherical** or spherical swelling located in the dermis. A dark spot in the centre (punctum) filled with keratin is a diagnostic feature of this cyst. The punctum indicates blockage of the duct (Fig. 34.17).
- In 20–30% of cases, instead of opening into the skin, sebaceous duct opens into the hair follicle. Hence, punctum is not seen.
- It has a smooth surface, round borders, soft and putty consistency and is nontender.
- The cyst can be moulded into different shapes which is described as ***sign of moulding.***
- **Sign of indentation** refers to pitting on pressure over the swelling (Table 34.1).
- The swelling is mobile over the deep structures, and the skin is free all around except an area of adherence at the site of punctum.

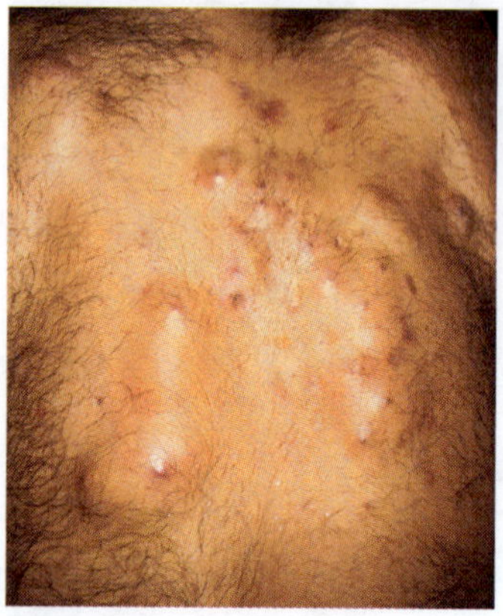

Fig. 34.13: Multiple sebaceous cysts on the back. Troublesome situation

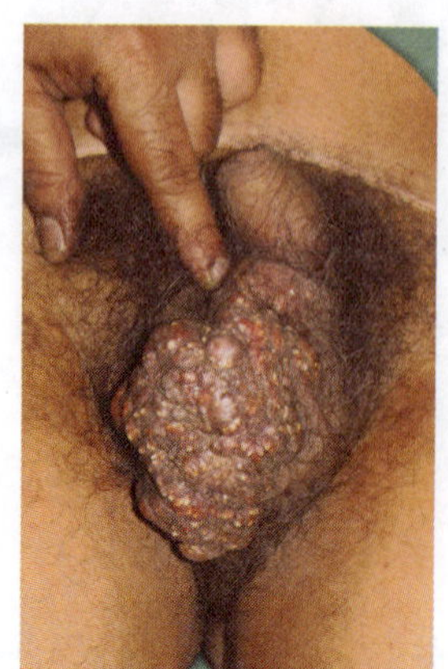

Fig. 34.14: Multiple sebaceous cysts on the scrotum calcified. Requires excision

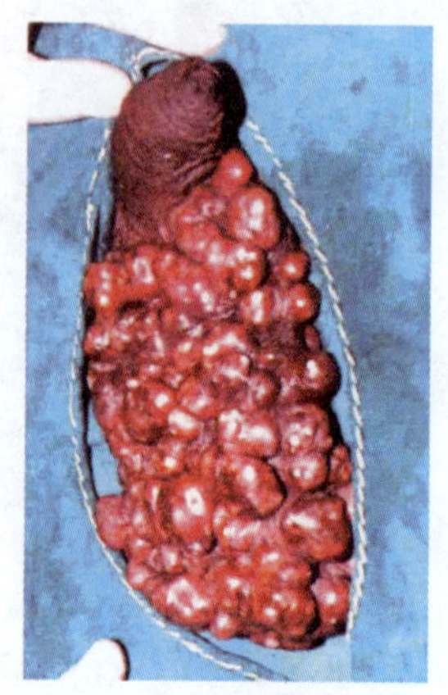

Fig. 34.15: Strawberry scrotum. (*Courtesy:* Dr Umesh Bhat, Surgeon, Kundapur, Karnataka, India)

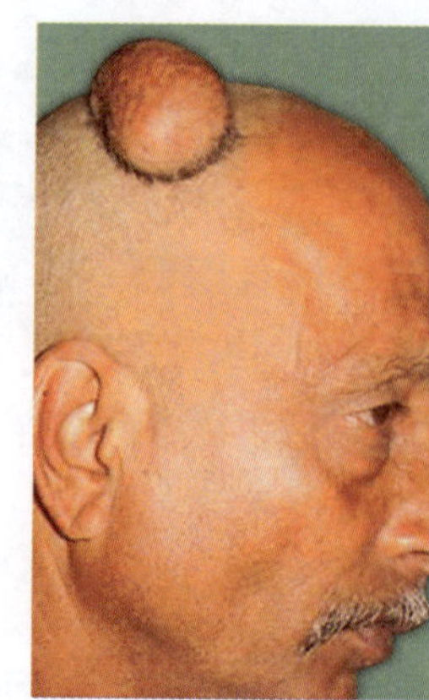

Fig. 34.16: Sebaceous cyst on the scalp. Loss of hair is a feature. When punctum is absent, the differential diagnosis is lipoma

Table 34.1 Comparison of congenital dermoid cyst and sebaceous cyst

	Congenital dermoid cyst	Epidermal cyst
• Aetiology	Congenital—sequestration of the dermal cells in the subcutaneous plane	Acquired—retention cyst due to accumulation of sebaceous contents
• Location	Midline of the body, along the line of fusion	Face, scalp, scrotum, back
• Sign of indentation, moulding	Uncommon	Very common
• Punctum	Absent	Present in 50% of cases—diagnostic
• Skin fixation	Absent	Skin is fixed at the site of punctum
• Bony defect	Present in majority of cases	Absent
• Intracranial communication	Rare, can be diagnosed by cough impulse test	Absent
• Treatment	Excision	Excision or avulsion

- In the scalp, loss of hair is a feature over the swelling because of constant slow expansion of the cyst.

Treatment

- Incision and **avulsion of cyst with the wall**. Very often, during dissection, the cyst wall ruptures. Care should be taken to excise the entire cyst wall. If not, recurrence can occur.
- When it is small it can be excised along with the skin.

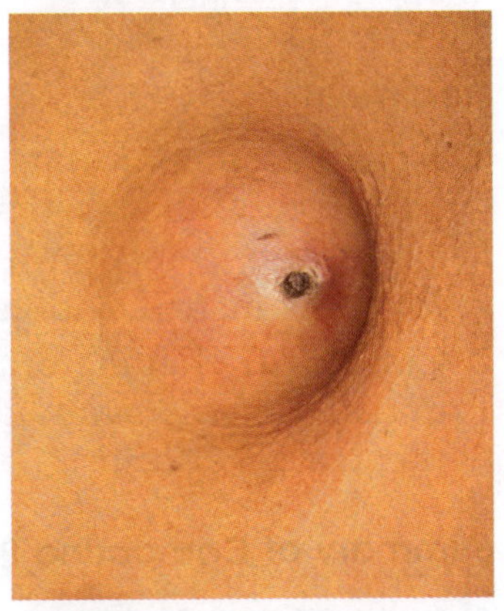

Fig. 34.17: Sebaceous punctum is diagnostic of sebaceous cyst

Complications

1. **Infection** can occur due to injury or scratch resulting in an abscess. The cyst will be tender, red and warm to touch. It should be treated like an abscess by incision and drainage. After one to two months, the cyst can be excised.
2. **Sebaceous horn** results due to slow drying of the contents which are squeezed out, specially if a patient does not wash the part. Thus, it is not common to find a large sebaceous horn nowadays because of better ways of living and sanitation (Fig. 34.18).
3. **Calcification**
4. **Cock's peculiar tumour**[1] refers to infected, ulcerated cyst of scalp with pouting granulation tissue and everted edge resembling epithelioma (Key Box 34.6).
5. **Rarely, basal cell carcinoma** can arise in a long-standing sebaceous cyst.

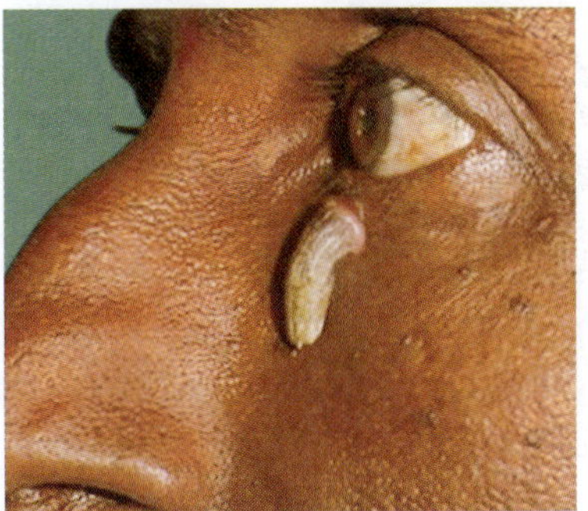

Fig. 34.18: Sebaceous horn

Key Box 34.6

Interesting—Sebaceous Cyst

- Syndrome: Gardner's syndrome
- Tumour: Cock's peculiar tumour
- Parasitic worm: Demodex folliculorum
- Strawberry scrotum: Multiple sebaceous cysts of scrotum

Pearls of Wisdom

Meibomian cysts: They are epidermal cysts found on the free edge of eyelid. Chronic meibomian cyst is called chalazion.

GANGLION

It is a tense, cystic swelling and which occurs due to myxomatous degeneration of the synovial sheath lining the joint or tendon sheath. It is common around joints because of abundant fibrous tissue. It contains gelatinous fluid.

Common Sites

- The dorsum of the hand is the common site, at the **scapholunate** articulation.
- In the foot, dorsal or lateral aspect.
- Small ganglion in relation to flexor aspect of fingers.

[1]Pott's puffy tumour refers to osteomyelitis of the frontal bone with oedema of scalp secondary to frontal sinusitis. This and Cock's peculiar tumour are favourite *viva voce* questions.

Clinical Features

- Majority of patients are between 20 and 50 years.
- A round to oval swelling in the dorsum of the hand, with smooth surface and round borders. Skin over the swelling is normal.
- The swelling is tensely cystic and fluctuant. Transillumination is negative. It is mobile in the transverse direction.
- When the tendons are put into contraction, the mobility of the swelling gets restricted.
- Ganglion is not connected with the joint space. Sometimes, it gives an impression of becoming small due to slipping away between bones.

Treatment

1. Asymptomatic ganglion is ***better left alone***.
2. ***Aspiration*** of the ganglion and injection of sclerosants may reduce the size of ganglion.
3. Sometimes, rupture of the cyst due to trauma may result in permanent cure.
4. ***Surgical excision*** can be done. However, recurrence rate is high.

Differential Diagnosis (DD)

1. Implantation dermoid cyst, when it occurs in the feet or hand.
2. Exostosis of the bone, has to be considered, if *swelling is very hard.*
3. Bursa (*vide infra*)

COMPOUND PALMAR GANGLION

Aetiology

- ***Tuberculous tenosynovitis*** of the tendon sheaths affecting the flexor tendons. This is a common cause in India (Key Box 34.7).
- ***Rheumatoid arthritis*** with involvement of multiple joints causing thickening of synovial membrane—common cause in Western countries.

Pathology

As a result of tuberculous tenosynovitis, typical caseous material collects within the flexor tendon sheaths. The tendons get matted, a swelling develops in the palm and another swelling develops in lower aspect of forearm. The thickening of synovial membrane, fibrin particles in the **fluid and melon seeds** are characteristic of this condition.

Clinical Features

- Majority of patients are below 40 years of age.
- Concavity of the palm is obliterated.
- Soft, cystic, fluctuant, transillumination—negative swelling situated above and below the flexor retinaculum.
- **Cross-fluctuation test** between these two swellings is positive, which is diagnostic of compound palmar ganglion.
- Restricted mobility of the fingers due to matting of the tendons.
- **Wasting of the small muscles** of the hand.
- **Paraesthesia** due to compression on median nerve.

Investigations

1. The ESR may be increased, if it is due to tuberculosis.
2. Aspiration of the swelling and fluid can be sent for acid-fast bacilli.
3. Synovial biopsy.

Treatment

1. **Antituberculous treatment (ATT)** in case of tubercular pathology. If the response rate is not satisfactory—exploration, decompression, synovectomy and release of matted tendons is the treatment.
2. **Control of rheumatoid arthritis**, with complete excision of the synovial sheath, in cases due to rheumatoid arthritis.

Summary of Compound Palmar Ganglion

- Tuberculosis and rheumatoid arthritis—common causes.
- Synovial thickening will clinch the diagnosis.
- Cross-fluctuation test is an important clinical finding.
- Antituberculous treatment, if it is due to tuberculosis.
- Decompression or synovectomy may be required in both conditions mentioned above.

GLOMUS TUMOUR (Key Box 34.7)

- This is also called glomangioma or angioneuromyoma.
- Glomus is a specialised organ.

Key Box 34.7

Glomus Tumour

- Rare and benign tumour
- The **most painful** tumour
- The **smallest benign tumour,** does not turn malignant.
- **Nail bed** is the commonest site.
- Histologically, it is an **angioneuromyoma.**
- It is **radioresistant.**
- **Excision** gives permanent cure.
- Function of glomus is concerned with **heat regulation.**

Structure of Glomus (Glomus Body)

Abundant arteriovenous anastomosis surrounded by large clear cells (glomus cells) and medullated and non-medullated nerve fibres in between the cells is characteristic of glomus.

Clinical Features of Glomus Tumour

(Figs 34.19 and 34.20)

1. Typical site: Under the nail beds of hands and feet.
2. It is purple red in colour, usually single, the size does not exceed 1 cm in diameter.
3. Glomus tumour is usually seen in the 5th decade.
4. Excruciating pain either at rest or on movement of the finger or on pressure is pathognomonic feature of this tumour. Pain is due to compression of the nerve fibres by dilated glomus vessels.
5. The tumour is compressible.

Treatment

Surgical excision results in *permanent cure.*

Differential Diagnosis

1. Subungual melanoma: Painless and pigmented

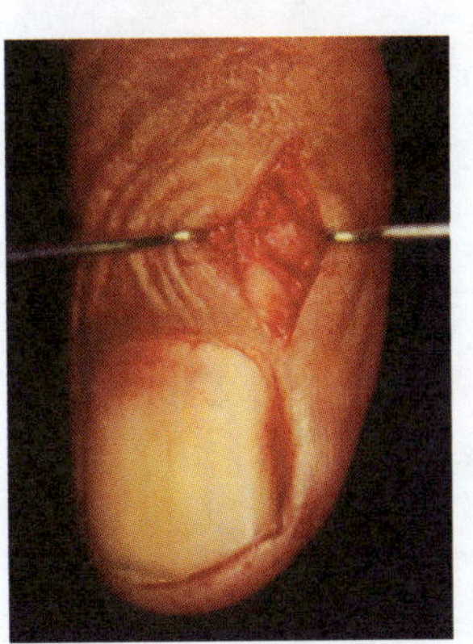

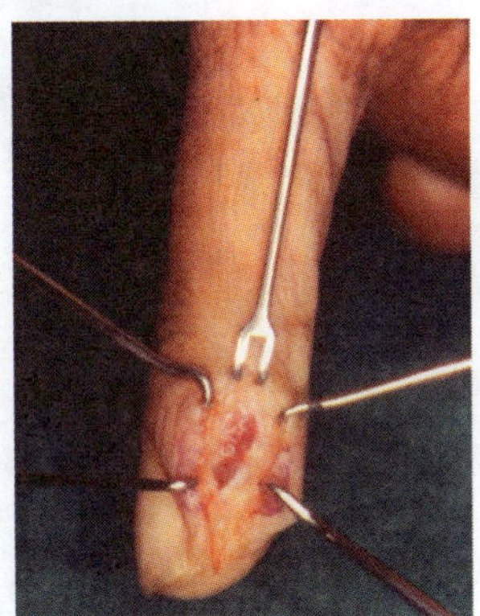

Figs 34.19 and 34.20: Glomus tumour: The most painful condition in the finger. (*Courtesy:* Prof Bhaskarananda Kumar and Dr Anil Bhat, Department of Orthopaedics, KMC, Manipal)

2. Granuloma pyogenicum: Mild pain, bleeds on touch and evidence of infection is present.
3. Chronic infection with granuloma.

BURSA

- Bursa means a sac or a sac-like cavity containing fluid lined by endothelium. It is meant to reduce the friction between tendons of the muscle and the bone.
- Bursitis refers to inflammation of a bursa resulting in accumulation of excessive fluid inside the bursa. This results in a swelling in the anatomical sites of normal bursa.
- The causes of chronic bursitis include constant pressure, constant irritation or minor injuries.
- Some examples of bursitis are given in Table 34.2.

Clinical Features

- A cystic swelling in a known anatomical site of a bursa is a chronic bursitis unless proved otherwise.
- Bursitis produces a soft, cystic, circumscribed or oval swelling with fluctuation.
- As majority of bursitis contain inflammatory fluid, they do not show transillumination.
- In a few cases, signs of inflammation may be present.

Complications

1. Secondary infection may result in an abscess.
2. Frequent friction may result in ulceration.
3. Cosmetic deformity.

Treatment

- Excision is indicated only in the presence of symptoms such as pain or complications mentioned above.
- Chances of recurrence are high.

Table 34.2 Bursae and bursitis

Anatomical site	Popular nomenclature
1. Prepatellar bursa	Housemaid's knee
2. In front of patella tendon (infrapatellar)	Clergyman's knee
3. Olecranon bursa	Student's elbow
4. Under the insertion of tendons of sartorius, gracilis and semitendinosus muscle	Bursa anserina (extension of the bursa along the sides of tendon—resembles goose's foot)
5. Between the tendon of the semimembranosus and the medial condyle of tibia	Semimembranosus bursitis

SEMIMEMBRANOSUS BURSA (Figs 34.21 to 34.23)

This is the commonest swelling in the popliteal space. It presents as a tensely cystic swelling when the knee is extended and it becomes flaccid on flexion of the knee. It is not compressible as it does not communicate with the joint.

The differential diagnosis for semimembranosus bursitis is **Morrant-Baker's cyst**, which is a herniation of the synovial membrane. The differences between these two swellings are given in Table 34.3.

ADVENTITIOUS BURSAE

- This refers to a cyst which develops in an anatomical area where no bursa is present. These also occur due to constant pressure or friction. They are summarised below.
  1. **Tailor's ankle:** Above the lateral malleolus
  2. **Porter's shoulder:** Between clavicle and skin
  3. **Weaver's bottom:** Between gluteus maximus and ischial tuberosity
  4. **Bunion:** Between prominent head of the first metatarsal and skin due to hallux valgus.
- The complications and treatment of adventitious bursae are similar to chronic bursitis (Fig. 34.22).

TRANSILLUMINANT SWELLINGS IN THE BODY

These are the cystic swellings containing clear fluid characterised by **fluctuation and transillumination**.

1. Lymphangioma
2. Ranula
3. Meningocele
4. Epididymal cyst
5. Vaginal hydrocele

LYMPHANGIOMA (Figs 34.24 to 34.26)

- Failure of one of the lymphatics to join the major lymph sac of the body results in a lymphangioma. Hence, it occurs in places where lymphatics are abundant.

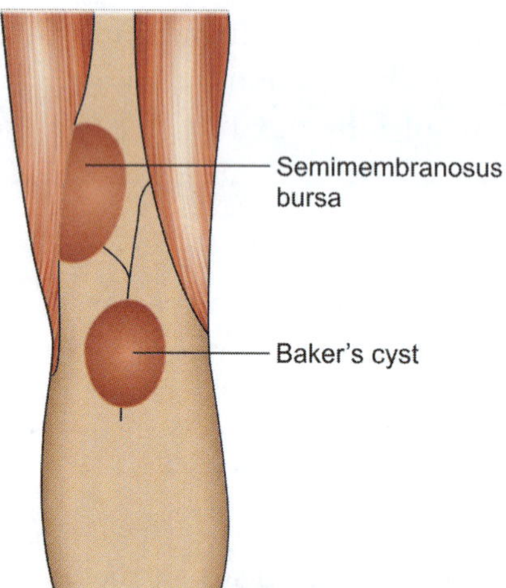

Fig. 34.21: Popliteal fossa swelling

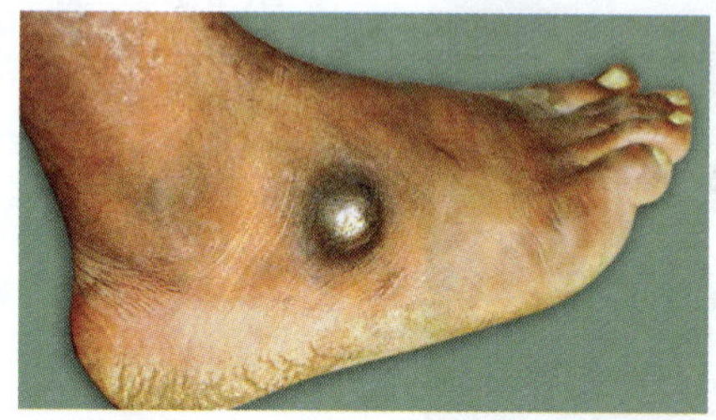

Fig. 34.22: Constant pressure on the lateral aspect of foot resulting in bursa due to the habit of 'squatting position'. Second picture is showing the bursa with pigmentation all around

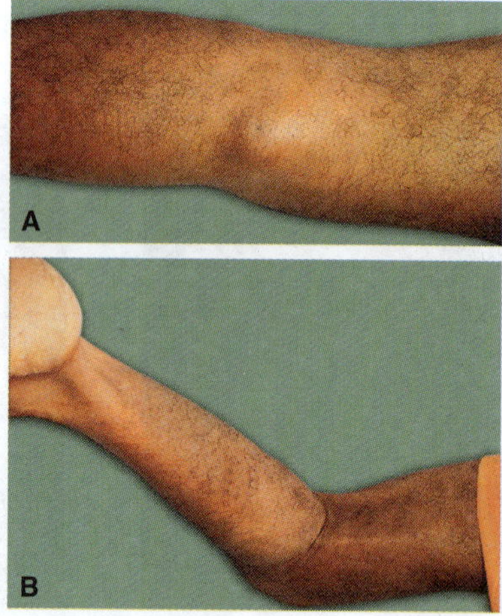

Figs 34.23A and B: (A) Semimembranosus cyst and (B) cyst disappears on flexing

Table 34.3 Comparison of semimembranosus bursa and Baker's cyst (Fig. 34.21)

	Semimembranosus bursa	Baker's cyst
1. Aetiology	Friction or pressure	Rheumatoid or osteoarthrosis of knee joint
2. Age	Young patients	Middle aged
3. Location in the popliteal fossa	Higher up and more medial	Below and midline
4. On flexion of the knee	Disappears	Increases
5. On extension of the knee	Appears and is tense (Figs 34.23A and B)	Diminishes
6. Patellar tap	Absent	Present
7. Compressibility	Absent	Present partially
8. Knee movements	Normal	Restricted

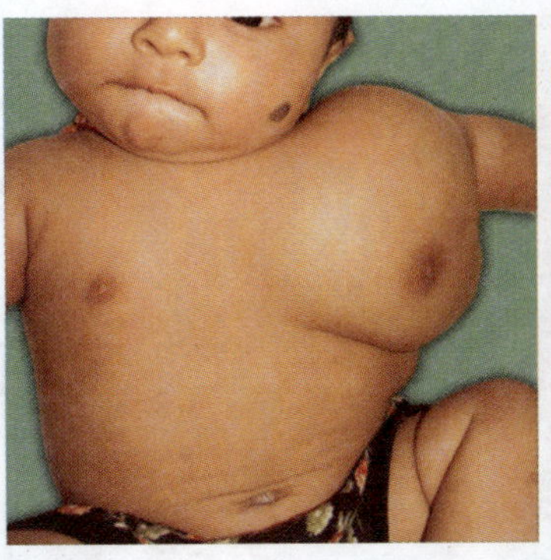

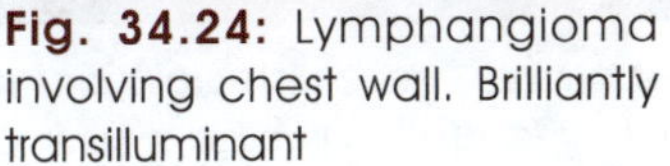

Fig. 34.24: Lymphangioma involving chest wall. Brilliantly transilluminant

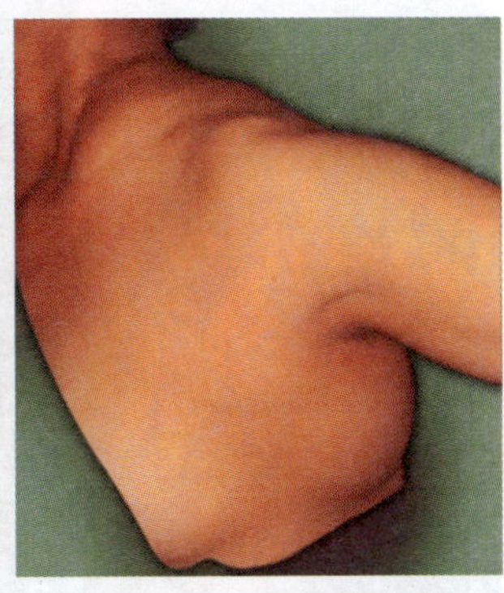

Fig. 34.25: Lymphangioma involving neck and axilla. Cross-fluctuation was positive

- They are dilated lymphatics that project onto the skin surface.
- Common sites: Posterior triangle of the neck, axilla, mediastinum, groin, etc. (Key Box 34.8).

Key Box 34.8

Lymphangioma	Sites
❍ Jugular lymph sac	Neck
❍ Posterior lymph sac	Groin
❍ Cisterna chyli	Retroperitoneum

- In the neck, it is called cystic hygroma of the neck. As the sac has no communication with lymphatics by the time swelling appears, the lymph is absorbed and is replaced by thin watery fluid (mucus) secreted by endothelium. Hence, it is also called hydrocele of the neck.
- When it is largely confined to subcutaneous plane, it is called **cystic hygroma**.

Types of Lymphangioma

1. **Lymphangioma circumscriptum:** If it is less than 5 cm across.
2. **Lymphangioma diffusum:** If they are more widespread.
3. **Lymphoedema *ab igne*:** If they form a reticulate pattern of ridges.

Clinical Features

- Usually, cystic hygroma presents during infancy or early childhood. Occasionally, present since birth and rarely before birth. They can also present as small vesicles.
- When the child cries or strains the swelling increases in size and becomes prominent due to increased intrathoracic pressure which is transmitted through root of the neck.
- Typical locations—lateral aspect of neck (posterior triangle), groin, buttocks.
- Soft, cystic, fluctuant, partially compressible swelling. Lymphangioma is a multilocular swelling consisting of aggregation of multiple cysts. These cysts may intercommunicate and may occasionally insinuate between muscle planes. Hence, it gives the sign of compressibility! However, **complete reducibility is not a feature**.
- The swelling is **brilliantly transilluminant** because it contains clear fluid (watery lymph) (Key Box 34.9).

Key Box 34.9

Transillumination Test

- ❍ Should be done in a dark room
- ❍ Avoid surface transillumination
- ❍ Transillumination may be negative because of infection, sclerotherapy and haemorrhage

Treatment

Surgical excision is the treatment of choice. **All the loculi or cysts should be removed.** Careful search has to be made for the extension of lymphangioma through the **muscle planes** so as to avoid **recurrence** (Figs 34.26 and 34.27). Sclerotherapy was being used earlier for lymphangioma. Since, tissue planes are distorted by sclerosants, dissection becomes difficult. **Thus, injection type of treatment is not favoured at present**.

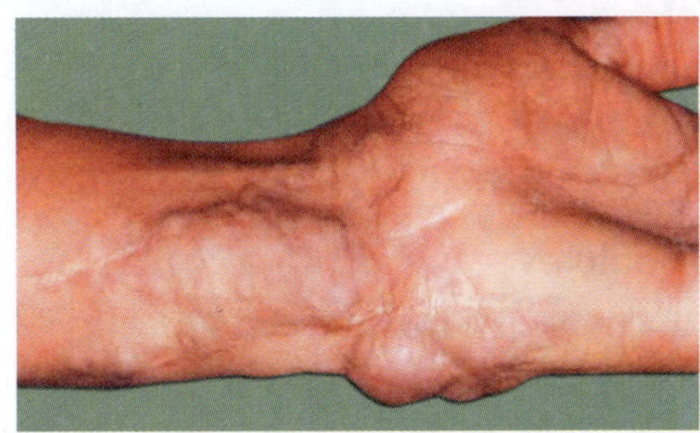

Fig. 34.26: Lymphangioma twice excised—residual lesion. It can be left alone if it is asymptomatic

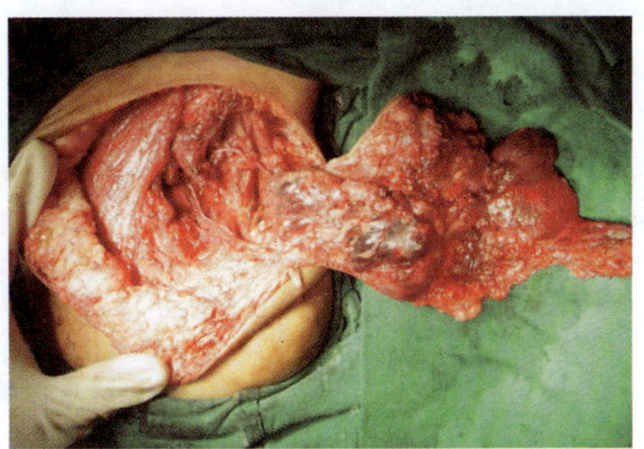

Fig. 34.27: Lymphangioma. Multiple pockets at surgery. All those extensions have to be removed to prevent local recurrence

Differential Diagnosis

1. **Haemangioma:** Posterior triangle of the neck is one of the common sites for haemangioma. Haemangioma is soft, cystic and fluctuant but transillumination is negative and the sign of compressibility is positive.
2. **Lipoma:** This is a soft lobular swelling with fluctuation because fat behaves like fluid at body temperature. However, the edge slips under the palpating fingers. Both transillumination and compressibility tests are negative with lipoma.
3. **Cold abscess** (details follow in a later page).

Complications

1. In neonates and infants, lymphangioma can cause difficulty in breathing due to its large size.
2. Occasionally, secondary infection can occur.
3. Lymphangioma in the mediastinum can give rise to dyspnoea, dysphagia due to compression on the trachea/oesophagus.

RANULA

Ranula is a cystic swelling arising from sublingual salivary gland and from accessory salivary glands which are present in the floor of the mouth called **glands of Blandin and Nuhn**.

The word ranula is derived from the resemblance of the swelling to the **belly of frog—*Rana hexadactyla***.

Aetiology

1. Ranula occurs due to obstruction to the ducts secreting mucus. Hence, it is an example for ***retention cyst.***
2. Some surgeons consider it as an ***extravasation cyst.***

Clinical Features

- Seen in young children and adults.
- The swelling is typically located in the floor of the mouth or **under surface of the tongue,** to one side of the midline.
- Soft, cystic, fluctuant swelling, which gives **brilliant transillumination.**
- It is covered by thin mucosa containing clear, serous fluid. Hence, it is **bluish in colour** (Fig. 34.28).
- Surface is smooth, borders are diffuse, nontender swelling.
- ***Plunging ranula:*** It is an intraoral ranula with cervical extension, where it passes on the side of mylohyoid muscle and produces a swelling in the submandibular region. Thus, one swelling in the floor of the mouth and the other in the neck gives rise to plunging ranula. The diagnosis is confirmed by cross-fluctuation test (Key Box 34.10).

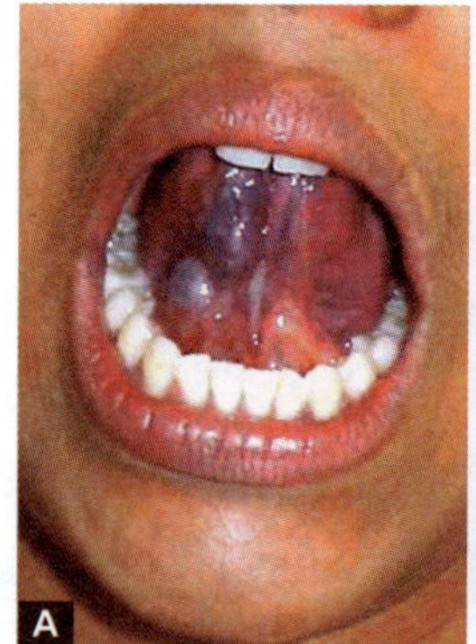

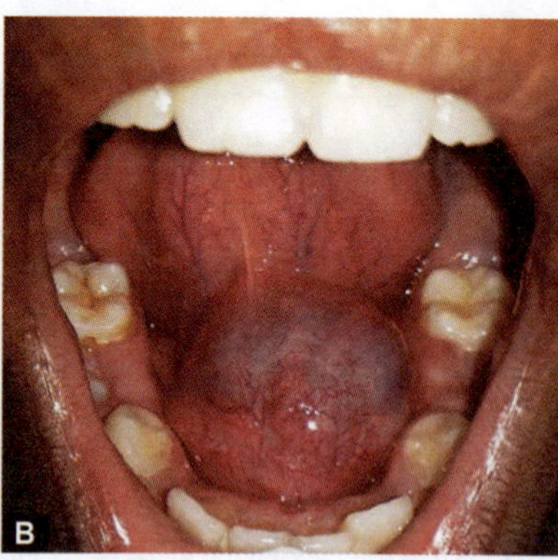

Figs 34.28A and B: Ranula—observe the bluish colour and swelling in the floor of the mouth (*Courtesy:* Dr Adarsh Kudwa, MCODS Manipal)

Key Box 34.10

Cross-fluctuation Test

- Indicated when a cyst has two interconnected components
- When gentle pressure is applied on one component, impulse is felt on the other component
- Demonstrated by bidigital palpation
- Plunging ranula, compound palmar ganglion, iliopsoas abscess, hydrocoele *en bisac*—cross-fluctuation can be felt

Treatment

1. **Complete excision** of the ranula is the treatment of choice in plunging ranula. Since the cyst wall is very thin, it should be carefully dissected and removed.
2. **Marsupialisation** is indicated in simple ranula. The ranula is incised and the wall of the cyst is sutured to the mucosa of the floor of the mouth, so as to leave an opening to the exterior (marsupials, e.g. kangaroo).
   - After 5–10 days, the cyst gets collapsed, fibrosis occurs and the entire cavity gets obliterated.
   - **Marsupialisation avoids surgical dissection** and chances of injury to the submandibular duct.
   - **Plunging ranula can be excised by intraoral approach.** Once the intraoral dissection is completed, the cervical extension can be mobilised by the same incision dissecting close to the cyst wall. However, rupture and chances of leaving behind a portion of the cyst wall are high.

Differential Diagnosis

- Sublingual dermoid cyst is a thick-walled cyst, whitish in colour and **not transilluminant**.
- Mucus cyst.

Complications

1. Rupture of the cyst decreases the size but it can reappear at a later date.
2. When the swelling is big, the tongue is pushed upwards and may cause difficulty in speech or swallowing.

MENINGOCELE

Meningocele is a herniation of the meninges through a weak point in the spine (neural arch) where the bony fusion has not taken place effectively (Fig. 34.29 and Key Box 34.11). The swelling is covered by pia mater and arachnoid mater without a dural covering. The swelling contains cerebrospinal fluid (CSF). **Meningocele is an example of spina bifida cystica.**

Clinical Features

- The swelling is present **since birth**.
- Soft, cystic, **fluctuant with brilliant transillumination** are the typical features of the swelling.
- Sign of **compressibility** is present due to displacement of CSF.
- When the child cries or coughs, an **expansile impulse** is present.
- On palpating the edge of the swelling, a bony defect is usually found.

Treatment (Key Box 34.12)

- CT scan is done to look for hydrocephalus. If it is present, a ventriculoperitoneal shunt is done which will reduce the meningocele.

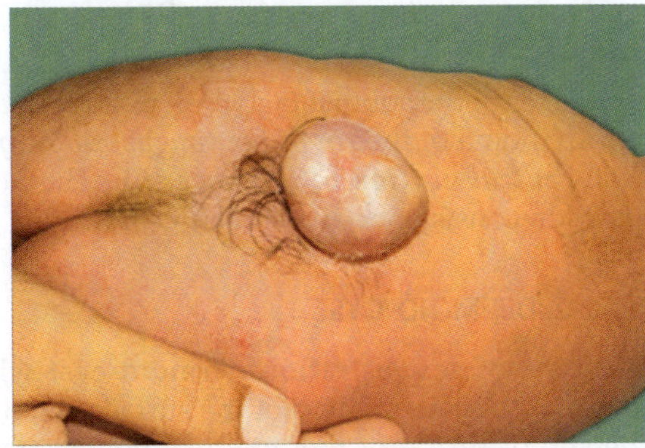

Fig. 34.29: Meningocele

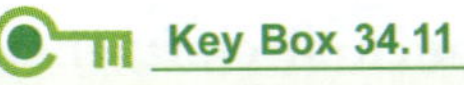 **Key Box 34.11**

Meningocele: Sites

- Lumbosacral: The commonest
- Occipitocervical: Second common
- Root of the nose: Rare

Key Box 34.12

Excision of Meningocele

- Surgery: As early as possible after birth
- Early closure prevents infection
- Transverse elliptical incision
- Excision of the sac
- Closure of the defect by plication
- Approximation of the muscles

- Excision of the meningocele should be done as early as possible to prevent the rupture and secondary infection.

Complications

- Skin covering the swelling is very thin and so is prone to ulceration. Due to ulceration, secondary infection and meningoencephalitis can occur.
- Haemorrhage.

SPINA BIFIDA OCCULTA

- In this condition, the neural arch is defective posteriorly. There is no visible swelling.
- It can be suspected when there is a tuft of hair, lipoma, naevus, pigmented patch of skin overlying the lumbosacral region.
- Child is normal at birth. Neurological symptoms such as weakness, sciatica-like pain may start appearing at puberty (neurogenic talipes equinus—club foot).
- During this time, because of growth, there may be traction on the spinal cord by a ligament called *membrane reuniens.*
- X-ray can demonstrate the bifid spine.
- Surgical excision of the membrane gives permanent cure to the patient, if there are symptoms.

Types of Spina Bifida Cystica

1. **Meningocele**
2. **Meningomyelocele**

} *See* Table 34.4 for comparison.

- Protrusion of meninges, with ***nerve root of* spinal cord or disordered spinal cord** results in meningomyelocele.
- Neurological deficit such as **foot drop, talipes, trophic ulcer** of the foot (S_1 root) may be present.
- Surgical excision may be followed by residual neurological deficit.

3. **Syringomeningomyelocele**

- In this condition, in addition to the meninges, the central canal of spinal cord is also herniated out.

Table 34.4 Comparison of meningocele and meningomyelocele

	Meningocele	Meningomyelocele
Contents	Membranes	Membranes with nerve roots
Consistency	Soft and cystic	Soft to firm
Transillumination	Brilliant	Partially transilluminant
Longitudinal furrow	Absent	Present due to adherence of the nerve roots to the skin
Neurological deficit	Absent	Trophic ulcers, bladder and bowel incontinence, locomotor problems are present
Prognosis after repair	Good	Residual neurological deficit is present

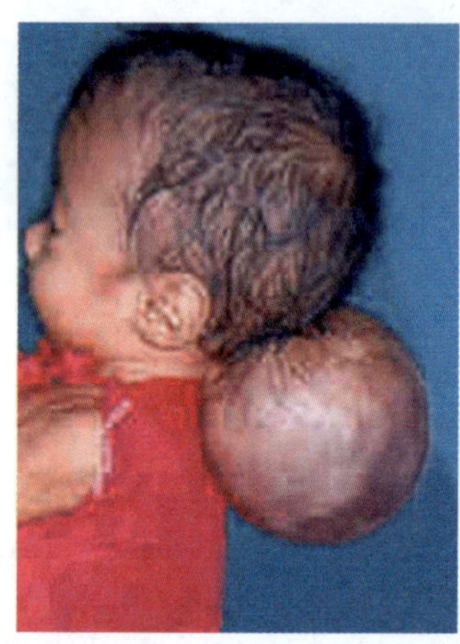

Fig. 34.30: Encephalocele. (*Courtesy:* Prof Vijaykumar, Paediatric Surgeon, KMC, Manipal)

- Most of the children are stillborn.
- Very difficult to treat, if the child survives.

Encephalocele (Fig. 34.30): It is also known as cranium bifidum. It is a neural tube defect characterised by sac-like protrusion of brain and meninges through an opening in the skull.

DIFFERENTIAL DIAGNOSIS OF MIDLINE SWELLINGS IN THE NECK

MIDLINE SWELLINGS (From Above Downwards)

1. Ludwig's angina
2. Enlarged submental lymph nodes
3. Sublingual dermoid cyst
4. Subhyoid bursitis
5. Thyroglossal cyst
6. Enlarged isthmus of thyroid gland
7. Pretracheal and prelaryngeal lymph nodes
8. Retrosternal goitre
9. Thymic swelling
10. Swelling in the suprasternal space of Burns: Lipoma/cold abscess/aneurysm.

LUDWIG'S ANGINA

- This is an inflammatory oedema of the floor of the mouth. It spreads to the submandibular region and submental region.
- Tense, tender, brawny, oedematous swelling in the submental region with putrid halitosis is characteristic of this condition.

ENLARGED SUBMENTAL LYMPH NODES

The three important causes of enlargement:

1. **Tuberculosis: Matted submental nodes,** firm in consistency, with enlarged upper deep cervical lymph nodes, with or without evening rise of temperature, are suggestive of tuberculosis.
2. **Non-Hodgkin's lymphoma** can present with submental nodes along with other lymph nodes in the horizontal group of nodes such as submandibular, upper deep cervical, pre-auricular, post-auricular and occipital lymph nodes (external Waldeyer's ring). Nodes are ***firm or rubbery,*** **discrete without matting.**
3. **Secondaries** in the submental lymph nodes can arise from carcinoma of the ***tip of the tongue, floor of the mouth, central portion of the lower lip.*** The nodes are **hard** in consistency and sometimes, **fixed.**

SUBLINGUAL DERMOID CYST

- It is a type of **sequestration dermoid cyst** which occurs due to sequestration of the surface ectoderm at the site of fusion of the two mandibular arches. Hence, such a cyst occurs in the midline, in the floor of the mouth (Key Box 34.13).
- When they arise from **2nd branchial cleft,** they are found lateral to the midline. Hence, **lateral variety**.
- The cyst is lined by squamous epithelium and contains hair follicles, sebaceous glands and sweat glands. **It does not contain hair**.

Key Box 34.13

Sublingual Dermoid Cyst

- Origin: At the site of fusion of 2nd branchial arches
- Site: **Midline**—common; **Lateral**—uncommon
- **Supraomohyoid** variety is common
- **Bidigital palpation** for demonstration of fluctuation
- Soft, cystic, fluctuant, transillumination negative swelling

Differential diagnosis

- Ranula: Transillumination is positive
- Thyroglossal cyst: Moves with deglutition

Clinical Features

1. Young children or patients between the age of 10 and 20 years present with painless swelling in the **floor of mouth**.
2. Swelling is **soft** and **cystic**. **Fluctuation** test is positive. **Bidigital palpation** gives a better idea about fluctuation with one finger over the swelling in the oral cavity and the other finger in the submental region.
3. **Transillumination test is negative** as it contains thick, cheesy, sebaceous material.

Differential Diagnosis

1. **Ranula:** When a sublingual dermoid cyst is in the midline in the floor of the mouth and above the mylohyoid muscle, ranula is considered as differential diagnosis. However, **ranula is bluish in colour, brilliantly transilluminant.**
2. **Thyroglossal cyst** should be considered as differential diagnosis when the sublingual dermoid cyst is below the mylohyoid muscle. Thyroglossal cyst **moves up with deglutition,** whereas **a sublingual dermoid cyst does not.**

Treatment

Through intraoral approach, excision can be done for both types of sublingual dermoid cyst.

SUBHYOID BURSITIS

- Accumulation of inflammatory fluid in the subhyoid bursa results in a swelling and is described as subhyoid bursitis.
- The bursa is located below the hyoid bone and in front of thyrohyoid membrane.

Clinical Features

- The swelling is in front of the neck, in the midline below the hyoid bone (Fig. 34.31).
- The *swelling is oval in the transverse direction.*
- It moves up with deglutition.
- Soft, cystic, fluctuant and transillumination negative swelling *(turbid fluid).*
- The swelling *may be tender* as it contains inflammatory fluid.

Treatment

Complete excision

Complication

It can develop into an abscess.

Differential Diagnosis

1. Thyroglossal cyst is a vertically placed oval swelling, whereas **subhyoid bursitis** is transversely placed oval swelling (Fig. 34.32).
   - Thyroglossal cyst moves on protrusion of the tongue outside (subhyoid bursitis does not).
2. Pretracheal lymph node swelling.
3. Ectopic thyroid enlargement.

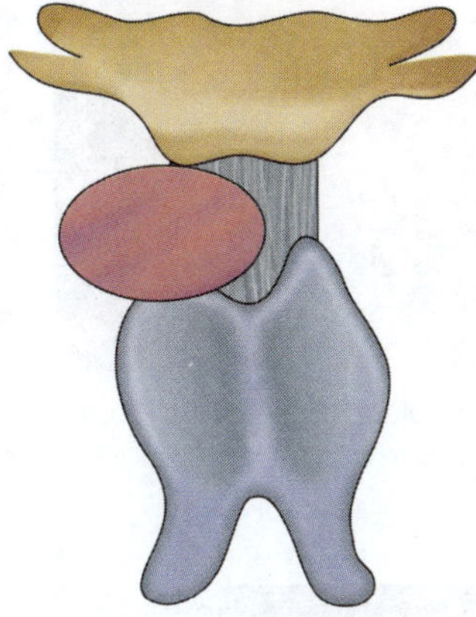

Fig. 34.31: Subhyoid bursitis: Transversely placed oval swelling

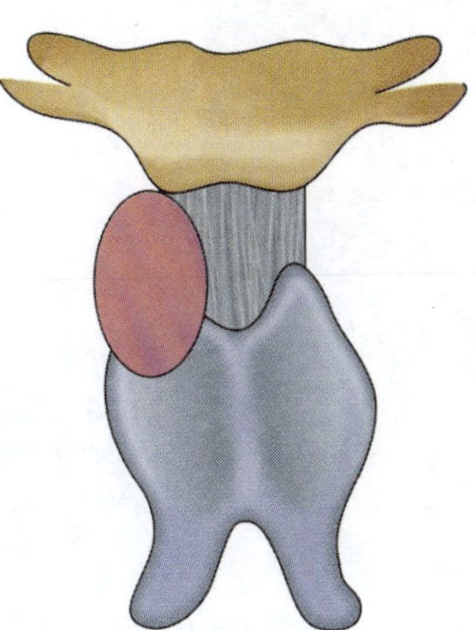

Fig. 34.32: Thyroglossal cyst: Vertically placed oval swelling

MIDLINE SWELLINGS IN THE NECK (Figs 34.33 to 34.40)

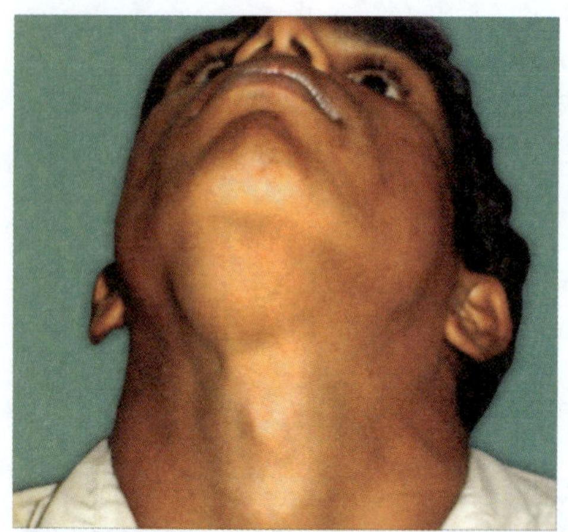

Fig. 34.33: Submental lymphadenitis: Caused by tuberculosis—not a common site

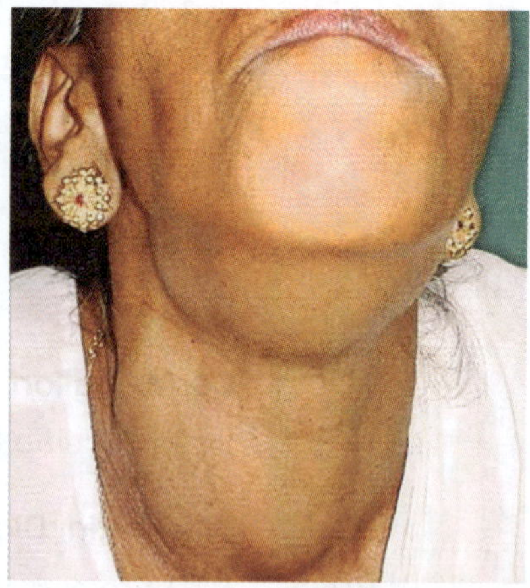

Fig. 34.34: Submental swelling of 30 years duration. (*Courtesy:* Prof. KK Rajan, Calicut Medical College)

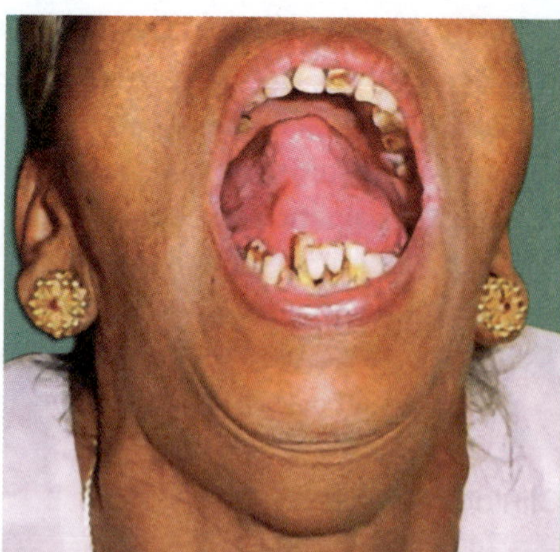

Fig. 34.35: Intraoral examination of patient (Fig. 16.36) reveals swelling also in the floor of mouth—sublingual dermoid cyst

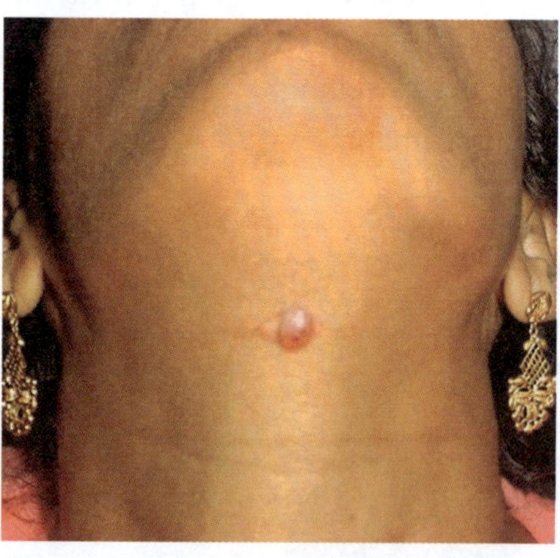

Fig. 34.36: Incompletely treated thyroglossal cyst. Recurred, about to rupture and form thyroglossal fistula

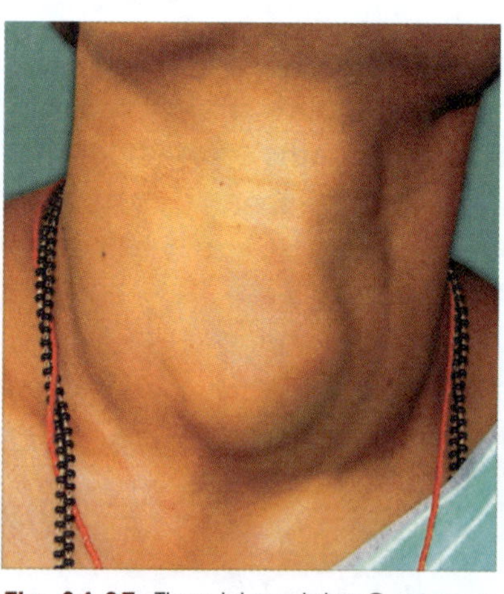

Fig. 34.37: Thyroid nodule: Common swelling—moves with deglutition

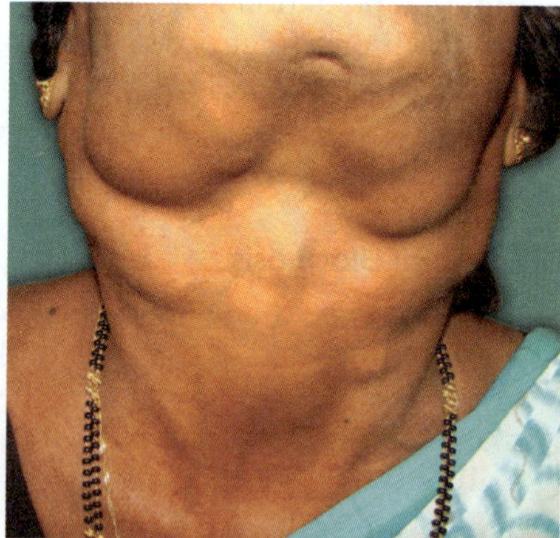

Fig. 34.38: Pretracheal lymph nodes and upper neck nodes: Case of non-Hodgkin's lymphoma

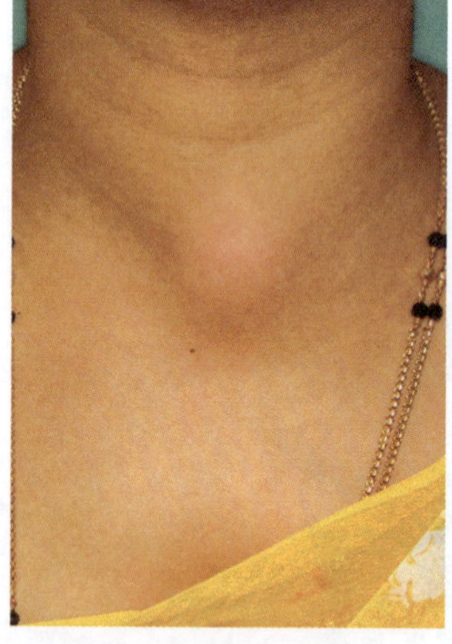

2008: MS Examination short case, KMC, Manipal. (*Courtesy:* Professor BH Ananda Rao, Department of Surgery)

Fig. 34.39: Cold abscess in the suprasternal space of Burns: One of the common sites of cold abscess

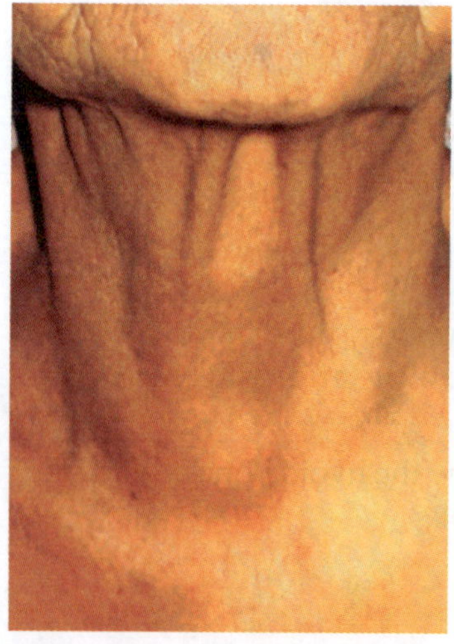

2008: MS Examination short case, Govt. Medical College, Goa. (*Courtesy:* Prof. Dilip Amonkar, Head, Department of Surgery)

Fig. 34.40: Aneurysm of innominate artery. Atherosclerosis is the cause. Before incising a cold abscess in this location, make sure that it is not an aneurysm

THYROGLOSSAL CYST

- This is an example for **tubuloembryonic dermoid cyst.**
- It arises from *thyroglossal tract/duct* which extends from **foramen caecum at the base of the tongue to the isthmus of the thyroid gland.** Hence, the thyroglossal cyst can develop anywhere along this duct. Four anomalies are shown in Fig. 34.41.
- It is lined by **pseudostratified, ciliated, columnar** or squamous epithelium which produces desquamated epithelial cells or mucus at times.

Sites of Thyroglossal Cyst (Fig. 34.42)

1. Subhyoid: **The most common type**
2. At the level of thyroid cartilage: 2nd common site
3. Suprahyoid: Double chin appearance
4. At the foramen caecum: Rare
5. At the level of cricoid cartilage: Rare
6. In the floor of the mouth

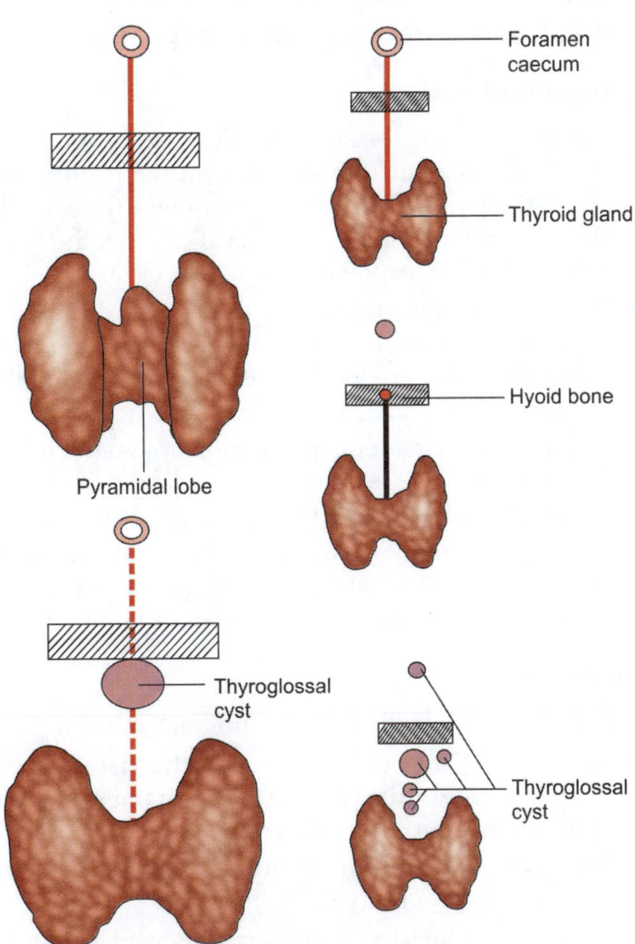

Fig. 34.41: Anomalies/fate of thyroglossal tract

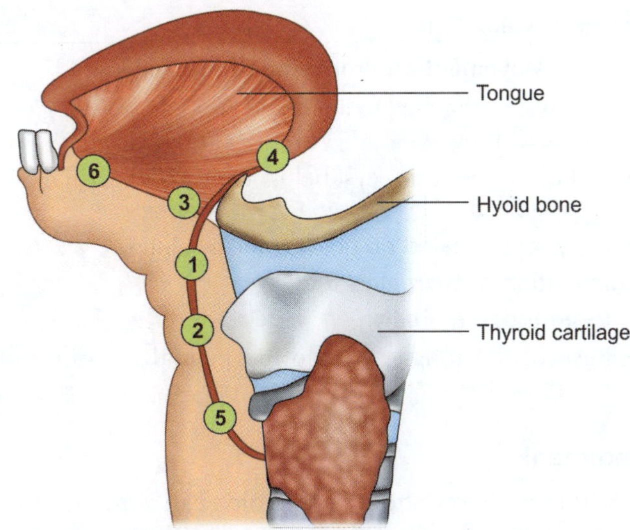

Fig. 34.42: Sites of thyroglossal cyst (see the text)

Clinical Features

- Even though congenital, thyroglossal cyst appears around the age of 15–30 years.
- They are more common in females who present with painless, midline swelling. However, in the region of thyroid cartilage, the swelling is slightly deviated to the left side.
- The cyst is soft, cystic, fluctuant, transillumination-— negative swelling (very rarely, it can give rise to transillumination). It can be firm, if the tension within the cyst is high.
- **Mobility:** Thyroglossal cysts exhibit 3 types of mobility which are characteristic of this condition:
  - The cyst moves with deglutition.
  - **Moves with protrusion of the tongue** (Fig. 34.43 and Key Box 34.14): Hold the thyroglossal cyst with the finger and thumb and ask the patient to protrude the tongue outside. **The movement of the cyst upwards is described as a tug because of its attachment with the hyoid bone.**
  - The swelling moves sideways but not vertically as it is tethered by the thyroglossal duct.

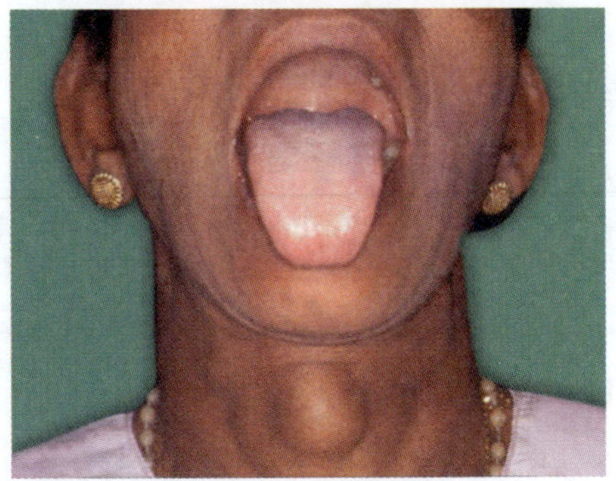

Fig. 34.43: Thyroglossal cyst: It moves upwards with protrusion of the tongue

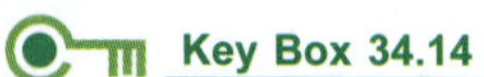

Key Box 34.14

Movement on Protrusion of the Tongue

- The cyst is attached to the hyoid bone. Hence, it gives a classical tug
- Not always present, cyst below the thyroid cartilage—tug is absent
- Better appreciated on holding the swelling

Examination of thyroglossal cyst

- Cyst proper, mobility
- Base of the tongue to rule out lingual thyroid and lymph nodes

Treatment

- Before excision of cyst, a thyroid scan is mandatory since it may be the only functioning thyroid tissue.
- **Sistrunk operation: Excision of the cyst** along with the entire thyroglossal tract which may **include part of the hyoid bone,** is the recommended treatment. The intimate relationship of hyoid bone can be explained by its development from 2nd and 3rd branchial arches.

Complications

1. **Recurrent infection:** The wall of the thyroglossal cyst sometimes contains **lymphoid tissue** which can get infected, resulting in an **abscess**. If it ruptures or is incised, it results in **thyroglossal fistula** (Key Box 34.15).
2. Rarely, a **papillary carcinoma** can occur in the **thyroglossal cyst**.
3. Fistula.

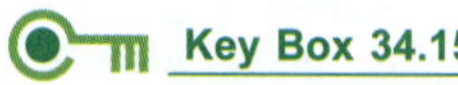

Key Box 34.15

Recurrent Abscess: Rupture Fistula or Sinus

- Thyroglossal fistula
- Osteomyelitis
- Stitch abscess
- Pilonidal sinus
- Median mental sinus
- Cold abscess
- Umbilical sinus

Pearls of Wisdom

Do not forget to feel base of the tongue for lingual thyroid/ ectopic thyroid. Whenever a patient has one congenital anomaly, examine thoroughly for 'more' associated anomalies.

THYROGLOSSAL FISTULA

Thyroglossal fistula is **never congenital**. It is always acquired due to the following reasons (Fig. 34.44 and Key Box 34.16):

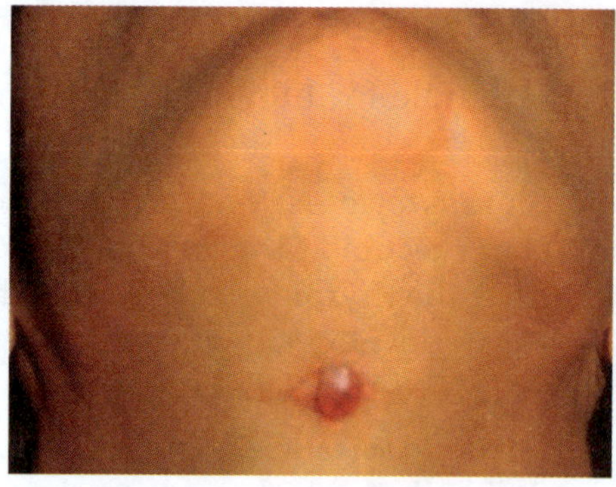

Fig. 34.44: Thyroglossal fistula

Key Box 34.16

Thyroglossal Fistula

- Always acquired
- Fistulous opening is in the midline
- Semilunar sign or hood sign
- It gets pulled up with protrusion of the tongue

1. Infected thyroglossal cyst rupturing into the skin.
2. Inadequately drained infected thyroglossal cyst.
3. Incompletely excised thyroglossal cyst.
   - **The track is lined by columnar epithelium.**

Clinical Features

- Previous history of swelling in front of the neck, which is now **painful, red and ruptured resulting** in discharging pus. Once the pus is drained, the opening closes. However, after an interval of time, the 'pain and discharge' reappear.
- When there is **no infection, the fistula** discharges only mucus and the surrounding skin is normal. Infected fistulae are tender, discharging pus and the skin is red hot.
- Majority of the patients presenting are young in the age group of 10–20 years.
- **A fistulous opening in the centre of neck** which is covered by a hood of skin can occur due to increased growth of the neck, when compared to that of fistula. This is described as **semilunar sign or hood sign.**

Treatment

- Infection is controlled with antibiotics.
- Surgical excision should include the **fistula with removal of the entire tract up to the foramen caecum.** Otherwise, recurrence will occur.
- The **central portion of the hyoid bone is removed** due to close proximity of the fistula.
- An elliptical incision is preferred as it gives a neat scar.

- This operation is called **Sistrunk's** operation. Key Box 34.17 for details about Sistrunk's operation.

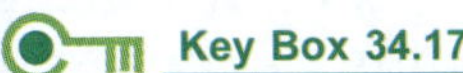

Key Box 34.17

Sistrunk's Operation

- Fistula with **entire thyroglossal tract** is excised.
- **Central portion of the hyoid bone** and lingual muscle are removed.
- Removal is facilitated by **pressing the posterior 1/3rd of the tongue**.
- **Do not perforate** thyrohyoid membrane.
- **Incomplete removal results in recurrence.**

ANOMALIES OF THYROGLOSSAL DUCT

- Thyroglossal duct extends from foramen caecum to thyroid cartilage.
- Various anomalies have been given in Key Box 34.18.
- However, thyroglossal cyst is common. Lingual thyroid and ectopic thyroid tissue are uncommon swellings.
- They have to be kept in mind as a differential diagnosis of the swellings in the midline of the neck.

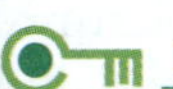

Key Box 34.18

Thyroglossal Duct Anomalies

- Lingual thyroid
- Levator glandulae thyroidae
- Ectopic thyroid tissue
- Thyroglossal cyst

SWELLING ARISING FROM ISTHMUS OF THE THYROID GLAND

Almost all the diseases of the thyroid gland result in enlargement of the isthmus. However, a solitary nodule and cysts can occur in relation to isthmus. The swelling moves with deglutition. However, it does not move on protrusion of the tongue.

PRETRACHEAL AND PRELARYNGEAL LYMPH NODES

These lymph nodes produce nodular swelling in the midline. One or two discrete nodes are palpable. They can enlarge due to the following conditions:

1. **Acute laryngitis:** The nodes are tender, soft.
2. **Papillary carcinoma of thyroid:** The nodes are firm without matting, with or without evidence of thyroid nodule.
3. **Carcinoma of the larynx:** The nodes are hard in consistency.
4. **In India, tuberculosis** should be considered as a possible diagnosis when other diseases are ruled out.

SWELLINGS IN THE SUPRASTERNAL SPACE OF BURNS

1. **Lipoma:** Soft and lobular, edge slips under the palpating finger.
2. **Sequestration dermoid cyst** is a midline, soft, cystic, fluctuant swelling.
3. **Gumma** produces a firm swelling with evidence of syphilis elsewhere in the body.
4. **Thymic swellings, an aneurysm** of innominate or subclavian artery, are the other causes (Fig. 34.45).

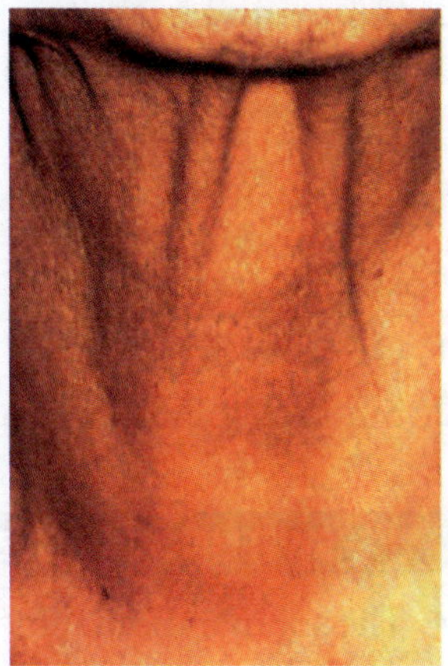

Fig. 34.45: Aneurysm

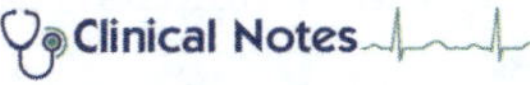

Clinical Notes

A lady of 65 years presented with swelling in the suprasternal space (Fig. 34.82). Candidate gave the diagnosis of lymph node swelling—probably cold abscess. He failed. It had expansile pulsations. It was a case of aneurysm of innominate artery. M.S. exam case 2008, JNMC, Belgaum. (*Courtesy:* Professor Ashok Godhi, Head, Dept. of Surgery)

DIFFERENTIAL DIAGNOSIS OF LATERAL SWELLINGS IN THE NECK

Before we discuss the swellings in the lateral side of the neck, it is essential to know the various triangles in the neck. These are discussed below.

Triangles of the Neck

Each side of the neck is a quadrilateral space subdivided by sternocleidomastoid into anterior triangle and posterior triangle. They are further subdivided as given below (Fig. 34.46).

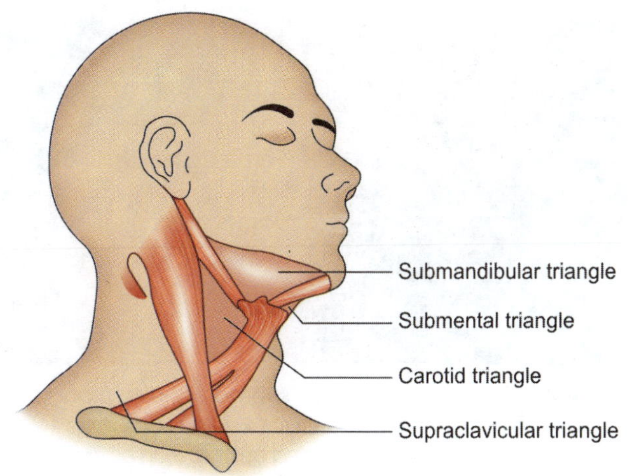

Fig. 34.46: Triangles of the neck

Anterior Triangle

1. Submental triangle
2. Digastric (submandibular) triangle
3. Carotid triangle
4. Muscular triangle

Posterior Triangle

1. Occipital triangle
2. Supraclavicular triangle

SWELLINGS IN SUBMANDIBULAR TRIANGLE

- The submandibular triangle is a part of anterior triangle.
- This is bounded **inferiorly** by anterior and posterior belly of digastric muscles with their tendon, **superiorly** by the attachment of deep fascia to the whole length of mandible.
- This triangle is covered by deep fascia.
- The floor is formed by mylohyoid muscle which arises from mylohyoid line of the mandible, thus closing the space.
- **Swellings in the submandibular triangle are** (Fig. 34.47)**:**
  1. Enlarged submandibular lymph nodes—common
  2. Submandibular salivary gland enlargement—common
  3. Plunging ranula—not uncommon
  4. Ludwig's angina—not uncommon
  5. Lateral sublingual dermoid cyst—rare
  6. Tumours of the mandible—rare

ENLARGED SUBMANDIBULAR LYMPH NODES

They form a nodular swelling which is deep to deep fascia. They are palpable only in the neck (not intraorally). The nodes can get enlarged due to the following conditions:

1. **Acute lymphadenitis:** Very often, poor oral **hygiene** or a **caries tooth** produces painful, tender, soft enlargement of these lymph nodes. Extraction of the tooth or with improvement of oral hygiene, lymph nodes regress.
2. **Chronic tuberculous lymphadenitis** can affect these nodes along with upper deep cervical nodes. The nodes are firm and matted.
3. **Secondaries** in the submandibular lymph nodes arise from carcinoma of the cheek, tongue, palate. The nodes are **hard** with or without **fixity**.
4. **Non-Hodgkin's lymphoma** can involve submandibular lymph nodes along with horizontal group of nodes in the neck. The nodes are **firm** or **rubbery** in consistency.

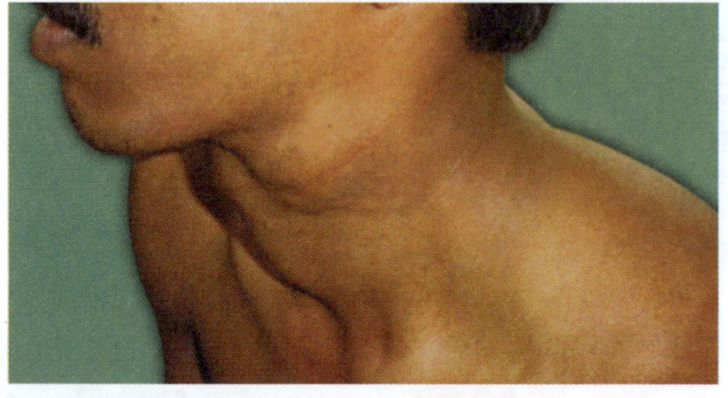

Fig. 34.47: This swelling in the submandibular triangle was bidigitally not palpable. However, it exhibited a doubtful sign of movement with deglutition. It turned out to be an ectopic thyroid swelling. (*Courtesy:* Prof Sampath Kumar, Dept. of Surgery, KMC, Manipal)

SUBMANDIBULAR SALIVARY GLAND ENLARGEMENT

(Key Box 34.19)

The various causes of submandibular salivary gland enlargement have been discussed under the salivary gland chapter. The common causes are chronic sialadenitis with or without a stone, tumours of the salivary gland or enlargement due to autoimmune diseases. They form irregular or nodular swelling. The diagnosis is confirmed by bidigital palpation of the gland. **Enlarged submandibular gland is bidigitally palpable because the deep lobe is deep to mylohyoid muscle.**

Key Box 34.19

Submandibular Salivary Gland Enlargement

- Calculus
- Chronic sialoadenitis
- Cancer
- Chronic diseases: Autoimmune

DIFFERENTIAL DIAGNOSIS OF SWELLINGS IN THE CAROTID TRIANGLE

The carotid triangle has the following boundaries (Fig. 34.48): Laterally by sternomastoid muscle, superomedially by digastric muscle and stylohyoid muscle and inferomedially by omohyoid muscle.

Some important swellings in this triangle are as follows:

1. Branchial cyst
2. Lymph node swelling (cold abscess)
3. Aneurysm of carotid artery
4. Enlargement of the thyroid gland

5. Carotid body tumour—rare
6. Laryngocele—rare
7. Sternomastoid tumour—rare
8. Neurofibroma of the vagus

Omohyoid muscle
Carotid triangle

Fig. 34.48: Carotid triangle

BRANCHIAL CYST

Aetiology

- Branchial cyst arises from ***vestigeal remnants of 2nd branchial arch.***
- The cyst is lined by squamous epithelium and contains desquamated epithelial cells which slowly forms a toothpaste-like material.

Clinical Features

- Even though congenital, majority of patients are young between the age group 15 and 25 years.
- The swelling is typically located in the **anterior triangle of the neck partly under cover of the upper 1/3rd of anterior border of sternomastoid**. This can be explained because of the development of *sternomastoid muscle from the myotome in the ridge of second branchial arch* (Fig. 34.49).
- The swelling has smooth surface and round borders. It is **soft, cystic, fluctuant and transillumination negative.**[1] The consistency is that of a rubber bag half filled with water. The swelling is very often firm due to thick inspissated content. In such situations, it is very difficult to elicit fluctuation. The mobility of the swelling is also restricted because of its adherence to the sternomastoid muscle.
- **Sternomastoid contraction test:** The **swelling becomes less prominent.**
- If contents are aspirated, it contains **cholesterol crystals** (Key Box 34.20).
- No other lesion is found in the neck (lymph nodes).

Key Box 34.20

Swellings Containing Cholesterol Crystals

- Branchial cyst
- Dental cyst
- Dentigerous cyst
- Hydrocele

Treatment

- **Excision** of the cyst along with *its entire epithelial lining* with a curved incision centred over the swelling. One must ensure that epithelial lining should be removed completely or else recurrence will occur.
- Sometimes cyst may grow backwards in between 'fork' of common carotid artery as far as pharyngeal constrictors.

Complication

Since the wall is rich in lymphatic tissue, it can undergo secondary infection with pain and swelling. Hence, the swelling has to be excised (Fig. 34.50).

Differential Diagnosis (Fig. 34.51)

There is no differential diagnosis in a classical case of branchial cyst. However, a few swellings have to be considered as differential diagnosis.

1. **Cold abscess** occurs in young patients due to tuberculosis of jugulodigastric nodes. Presence of multiple lymph nodes in the neck with or without fever gives clue to the diagnosis.

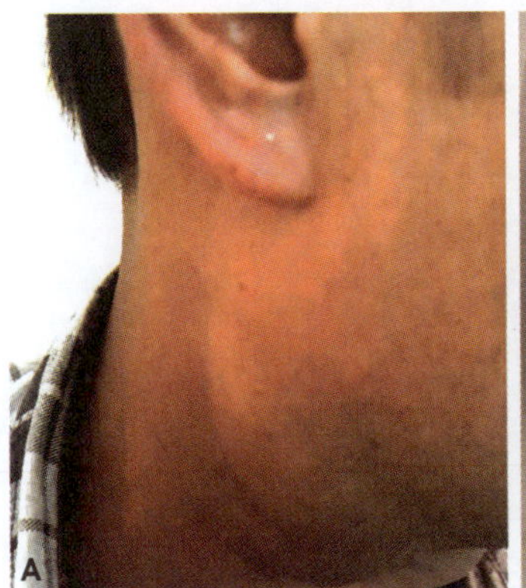

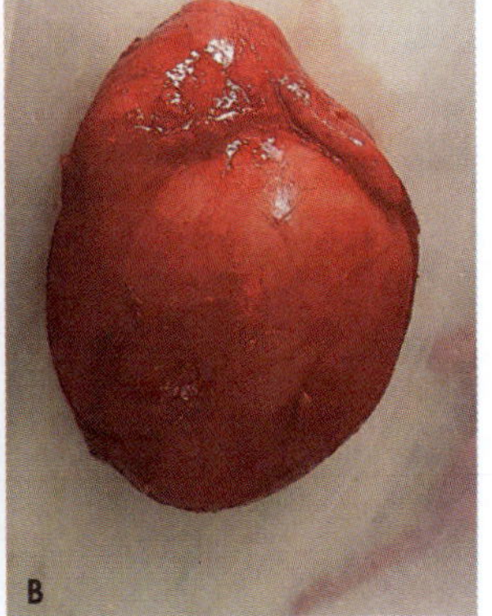

Figs 34.49A and B: (A) Branchial cyst, (B) excised specimen. (*Courtesy:* Dr Dayananda Nooli, Senior Consultant Surgeon, Chikodi, Belgaum)

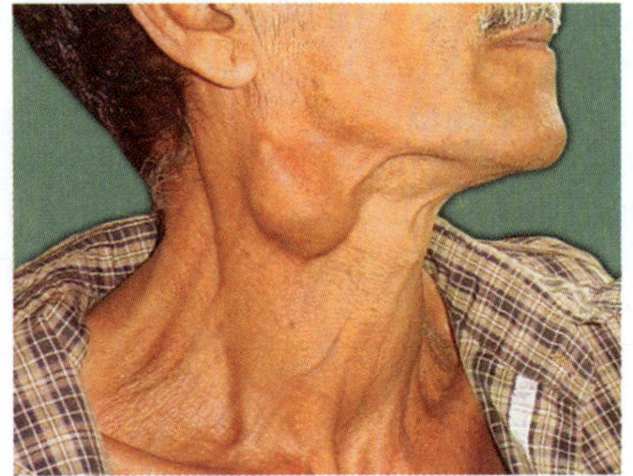

Fig. 34.50: Swelling mimicked branchial cyst. However, it was a subcutaneous swelling with lobularity—it turned out to be lipoma. (*Courtesy:* Dr P Rajan, Calicut Medical College, Calicut, Kerala)

[1]Branchial and thyroglossal cysts rarely give rise to transillumination, if contents are clear and unless the cyst is small, it is difficult to elicit fluctuation. These cysts can be firm or hard swellings also.

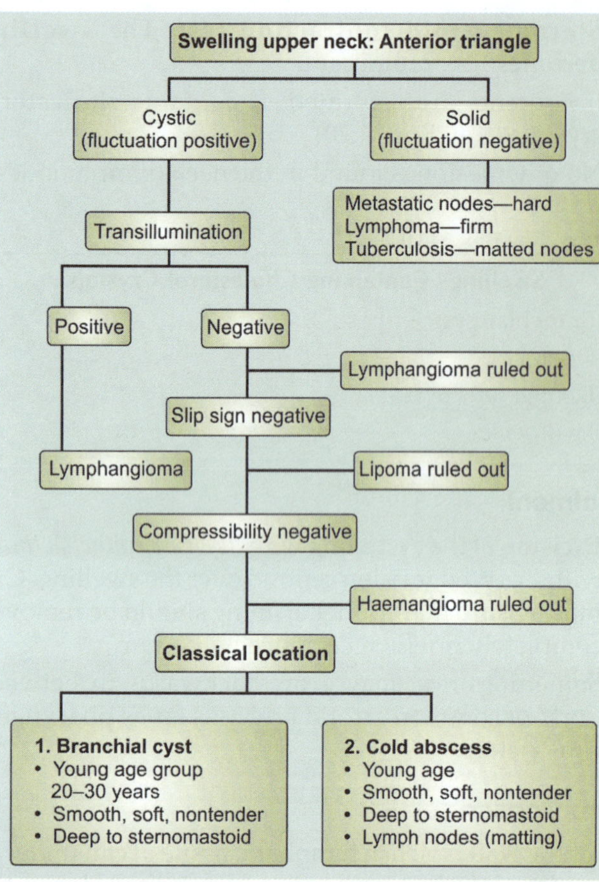

Fig. 34.51: Branchial cyst—one example of diagnosing a case using clinical methods. It is important that each clinical method **elicited carefully**, gives a clue to the diagnosis

2. **Lymphangioma** is a brilliantly transilluminant, partially compressible swelling. However, anterior triangle is not a common site for lymphangioma.
3. **Lipoma** can also occur in the neck, though it is an uncommon site (Fig. 34.50).

BRANCHIAL FISTULA (Key Box 34.21)

- This is always congenital and occurs due to persistent **2nd branchial cleft.**[1]
- External opening is situated at the junction of middle 1/3rd and lower 1/3rd of sternomastoid (Fig. 34.52).
- The tract from the skin passes through the *fork of common carotid artery* deep to the accessory and hypoglossal nerve and opens in the **anterior aspect of posterior pillars of tonsils** (Fig. 34.52). The tract is lined by ciliated squamous epithelium and discharges a mucopurulent discharge. Sometimes, the upper end is blind resulting in a sinus.

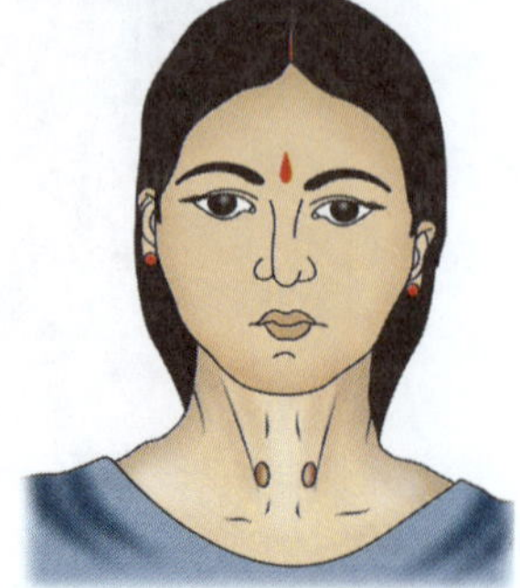

Fig. 34.52: Sites of branchial fistula—commonly bilateral

- The patient may complain of a **dimple, discharging mucus** and the dimple becomes more obvious when the patient is asked to swallow.
- Usually seen in growing adults (30% of cases).
- Can be unilateral or bilateral, equally common in males and females.
- It is also called **lateral fistula of the neck.** (Thyroglossal fistula is called median fistula of the neck.)

[1]Persistent first branchial cleft results in external auditory meatus.

Key Box 34.21

Branchial Fistula Passes Superficial to following Structures

- Internal carotid artery
- Internal jugular vein
- Hypoglossal nerve
- Glossopharyngeal nerve — Derivatives of 3rd arch
- Stylopharyngeous muscle — Derivatives of 3rd arch

Pierces superior constrictor muscle and opens on posterior pillar of the fauces behind tonsil.

Treatment

Fistulogram can be done by injecting methylene blue into the external opening and defining the tract (Fig. 34.53). This is followed by exploration of the tract. At surgery, it should be carefully dissected up to the internal opening and then excised. May have to be done by two different incisions: Upper incision at upper border of thyroid cartilage and lower incision encircling fistula and dissecting upwards.

Complication

Recurrent infection of the fistula.

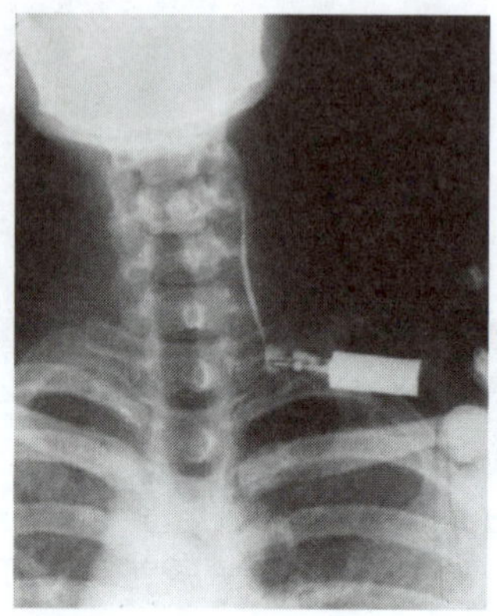

Fig. 34.53: Contrast study demonstrating fistulous tract

COLD ABSCESS DUE TO TUBERCULOSIS

- In India, this is the commonest cystic swelling in the carotid triangle. The cold abscess occurs as a result of caseation necrosis of the lymph nodes. This forms a soft, cystic, fluctuant swelling with negative transillumination. Presence of other lymph nodes in the neck or sinuses in the neck gives the clue to the diagnosis.
- Loss of appetite, weakness and fever with chills may be other features.

ANEURYSM OF THE COMMON CAROTID ARTERY

- ***Atherosclerosis*** is the most common cause of aneurysm. This weakens the vessel walls uniformly and produces fusiform dilatation of the blood vessel. ***Hypertension*** is another factor which adds to the aneurysm.
- ***Abdominal aorta*** is the commonest site for aneurysms followed by ***popliteal artery.***

Types

A. ***Fusiform:*** Atherosclerosis, hypertension (Fig. 34.54A).
B. ***Saccular:*** Due to injury (Fig. 34.54B).
C. ***False:*** In this condition, there is a sac lined by cellular tissue which communicates with the artery through an opening in its wall (Fig. 34.54C).

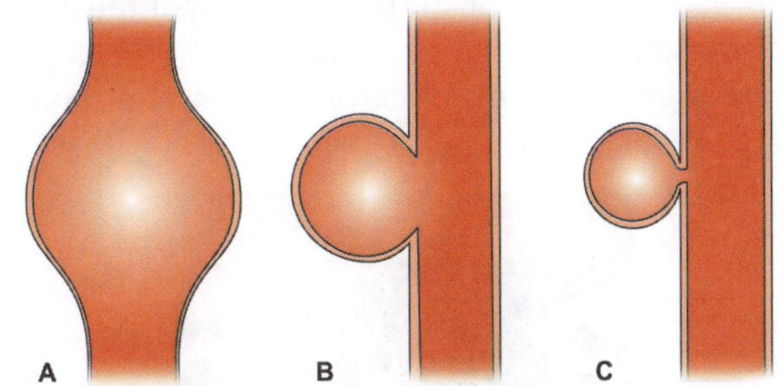

Fig. 34.54A to C: (A) Fusiform, (B) saccular, (C) false aneurysm

Causes (Key Box 34.22)

Key Box 34.22

Aneurysm: Causes

- **Congenital:** Berry aneurysm in the circle of Willis
- **Traumatic**
- **Degenerative:** Atherosclerosis
- **Rare causes:**
  Syphilis: Endarteritis obliterans
  Mycotic: Infective emboli
  Subacute bacterial endocarditis
  Marfan's syndrome
  Polyarteritis

Clinical Features of Aneurysm

1. Elderly patients are commonly affected.
2. Evidence of atherosclerosis in the form of thick-walled vessel is present.
3. Tensely cystic (feels firm), fluctuant, transillumination negative swelling with ***expansile pulsation*** (when the fingers are kept over the aneurysm, *they are not only elevated but they are also separated*).
4. Compressibility is positive.
5. On exerting pressure proximally the swelling diminishes in size—classically it happens in a case of popliteal aneurysms on compression of the femoral artery.
6. Bruit/thrill is characteristic of this condition.

Pearls of Wisdom

Classical signs of an aneurysm described above may be absent, if thrombus is present within it.

Treatment of Aneurysm

- Angiography to confirm the diagnosis followed by repair of aneurysm with graft—PTFE graft (polytetrafluoroethylene graft, Fig. 34.55).

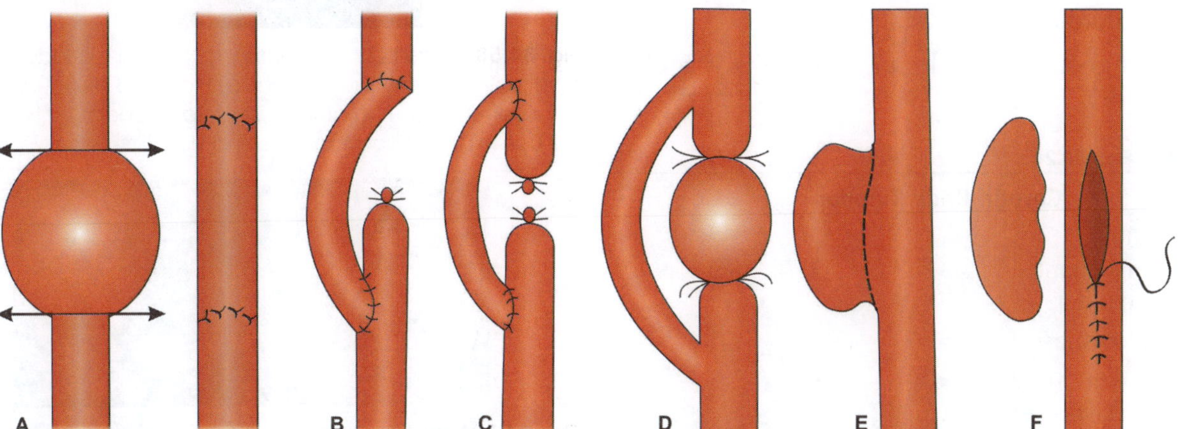

Figs 34.55A to F: Different methods of operation for aneurysm. (A) Excision and end-to-end graft, (B) excision and end-to-side graft, (C) excision and side-to-side graft, (D) excision and bypass grafting, (E and F) matas aneurysmorrhaphy

CAROTID BODY TUMOUR (CHEMODECTOMA)

Introduction

- This is a benign tumour arising from chemoreceptors in the carotid body (Key Box 34.23). They are situated in the tunica adventitia at the bifurcation of common carotid artery (Fig. 34.56).
- Hence, such a tumour is called chemodectoma.
- Function of the carotid body is regulation of pH.

Key Box 34.23

Chemoreceptors: Sites

- The carotid body
- The aortic body
- Brain stem
- Pulmonary receptors
- Myocardial receptors

(All of the above:) Hormonally not active cells

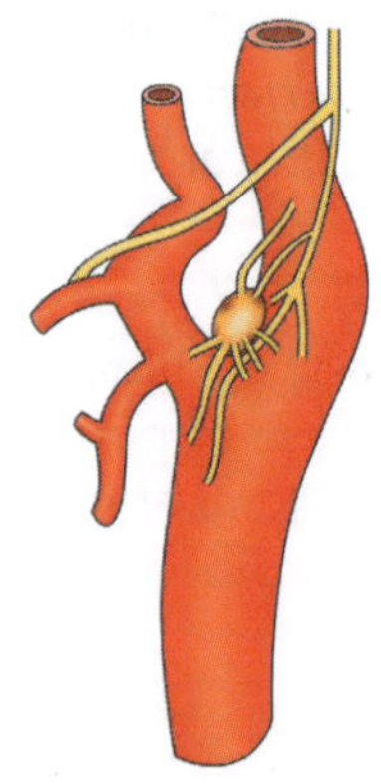

Fig. 34.56: Location of carotid body

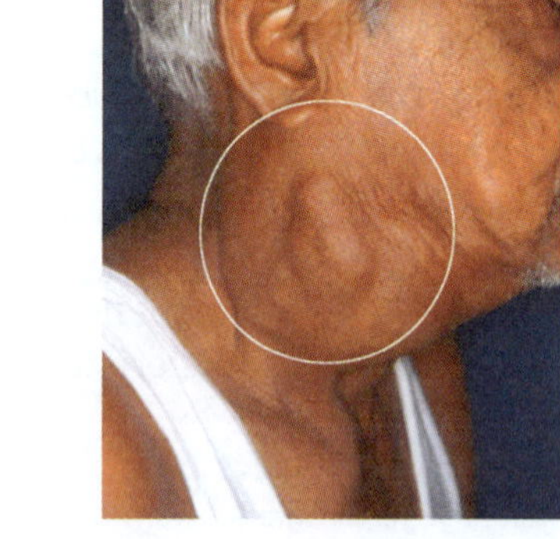

Fig. 34.57: Carotid body tumour—classical site

- It may be associated with phaeochromocytoma.
- **Chronic hypoxia can lead to carotid body hyperplasia. Hence, there is a higher incidence of chemodectoma in people living at higher altitudes.**

Clinical Features (Key Box 34.24)

- Middle-aged or elderly patients are affected (5th decade).

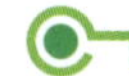

Key Box 34.24

Carotid Body Tumour

- Rare tumour
- Rarely malignant
- Rarely bilateral
- Rarely grows fast
- Rarely patient presents early
- Rarely metastasises
- Experience of a general surgeon with this tumour is very, very rare

- The patient gives long history of painless, slow-growing swelling for many years.
- **Typical location:** In the upper part of the anterior triangle of the neck, at the level of the hyoid bone, beneath the anterior edge of the sternomastoid muscle (Fig. 34.57).
- Surface is smooth or lobulated, borders are round, and is an oval, vertically placed swelling. Consistency is firm to hard. Hence, called **classical potato tumour.**
- **Horner's syndrome and unilateral vocal cord paralysis** can occur due to involvement of the nerves.
- Pressure on the tumour gives rise to syncopal attack due to decrease in the pulse rate **(carotid body syndrome).**
- Moves in the transverse direction.
- Carotid artery is stretched over the swelling and so, transmitted pulsations are felt (Fig. 34.58).
- Intraoral examination shows prolapse of ipsilateral tonsil, unless it grows in parapharyngeal space.

Shamblin classification

Class I: Localized—minimal vascular attachment.

Class II: Partially surrounds carotids.

Class III: Encase carotids—resection difficult and may need temporary interruption of cerebral circulation.

Diagnosis

- Carotid angiography (Fig. 34.59A) should be done, if there are neurological symptoms, such as syncopal attack. It may demonstrate separation of the carotid bifurcation.
- **Lyre sign:** Splaying of carotid artery can be seen (Fig. 34.59B).

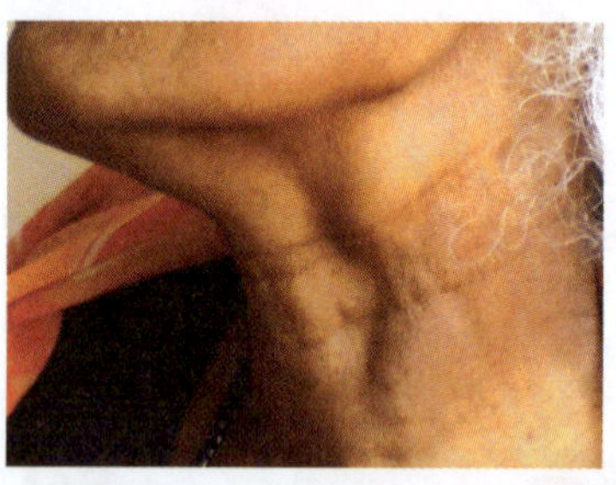

Fig. 34.58: Carotid body tumour in a 45-year-old lady—duration 5 years. (*Courtesy:* Dr MR Srivatsa, Prof. and Head, Prof. Bagali Babasaheb, Prof. Bharathi, Dr Srikar Pai, Department of Surgery, MS Ramaiah Medical College and Hospital, Bangalore)

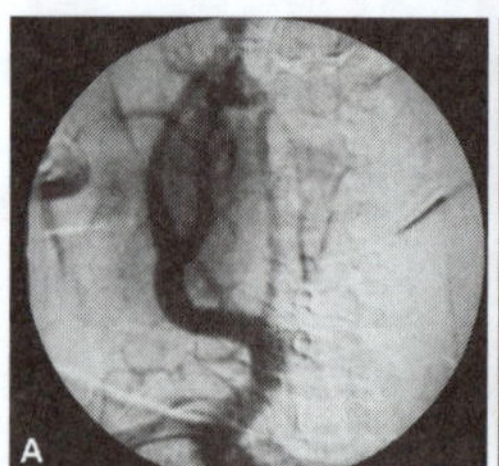

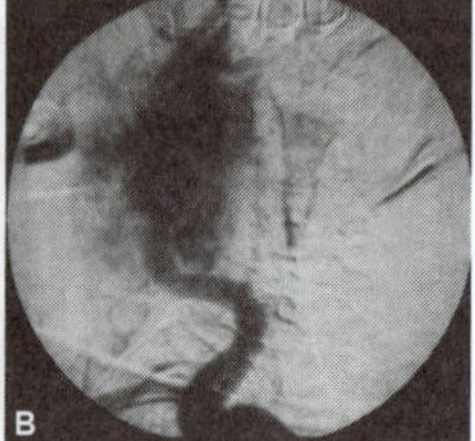

Figs 34.59A and B: Carotid angiography—observe separation of internal and external carotid artery by the tumour (A) and vascular blush (B)

- Incision biopsy is dangerous.
- Colour Doppler should be the first investigation.

Treatment

- Excision of the tumour with reconstruction
- No role for radiotherapy.

Pearls of Wisdom

It is important to preserve cerebral circulation during surgery. Vascular surgeon's help is necessary.

Complications

Very rarely, it can turn into a malignant carotid body tumour with lymph nodal metastasis.

Precautions

- Do not biopsy from within mouth—carotid body tumour can displace tonsil medially.
- Should not do FNAC.
- Should not do open biopsy.
- When you feel some pulsations over a lymph node in the carotid triangle—remember carotid body tumour.

STERNOMASTOID TUMOUR

- This is not a tumour, it is a **misnomer**.
- Injury to the sternomastoid during birth causes rupture of a few fibres and ***haematoma.*** Later, healing occurs with fibrosis, resulting in a swelling in the middle of sternomastoid muscle.
- The other possible theory is that this is a congenital anomaly—**short sternomastoid muscle**.

Clinical Features

- This is seen in infants or children. Firm to hard, 1–2 cm swelling in the middle of the sternomastoid muscle.
- Tender and mobile sideways. Medial and lateral borders are distinct but superior and inferior borders are continuous with the muscle.
- Many cases are associated with torticollis.

Treatment

- Gentle manipulation of child's head
- Physiotherapy to stretch the shortened sternomastoid muscle.
- Division of lower attachment of sternomastoid from clavicle and sternum with or without removal of lump is the surgical treatment.

LARYNGOCELE (Key Box 34.25)

- It occurs due to herniation of the laryngeal mucosa (Fig. 34.60, external laryngocele)

Key Box 34.25

Laryngocele

- Very rare
- Increased laryngeal pressure
- Expansile impulse on cough
- Treatment: Ligation of its neck and division of the whole sac.

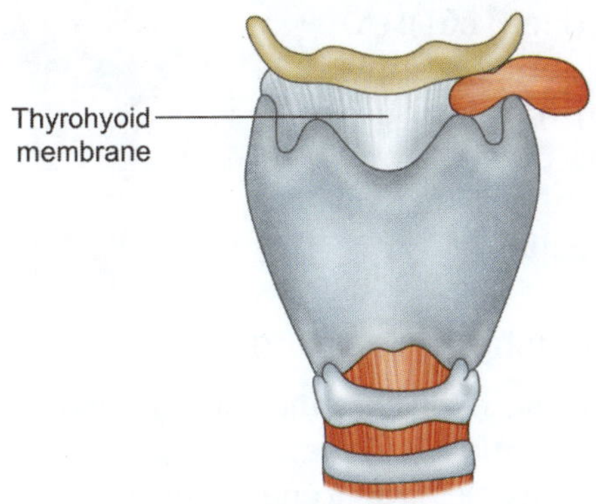

Fig. 34.60: Laryngocele

- When it enlarges within the larynx, it may displace vocal cord, produce hoarseness and is called **internal laryngocele.**

Causes

- Glass blowers, musicians, wind instruments and trumpet players are commonly affected.
- Chronic cough may be one of the predisposing factors.

Clinical Features

- Smooth, oval, boggy swelling which moves upwards on swallowing, in relation to thyrohyoid membrane (subhyoid position).
- Swelling becomes prominent when the patient is asked to cough or blow ***(Valsalva manoeuvre).***
- Expansile cough impulse is present.
- Tympanitic note on percussion (resonant)

Treatment

- Excision of the sac—in external laryngocele
- Marsupialisation—in internal laryngocele.

Differential Diagnosis

Other cystic swellings, such as branchial cyst and lymphangioma, should be ruled out.

Complications

Secondary infection results in laryngopyocele. The opening in the thyrohyoid membrane may be blocked by mucopus in such cases.

PHARYNGEAL POUCH

- Herniation or protrusion of mucosa of the pharyngeal wall through Killian's dehiscence.
- **Killian's dehiscence** is a potential area of weakness in between the two parts of the inferior constrictor muscle (Fig. 34.61): **(A)** Upper oblique fibres (thyropharyngeus) and **(B)** Lower horizontal fibres (cricopharyngeus).

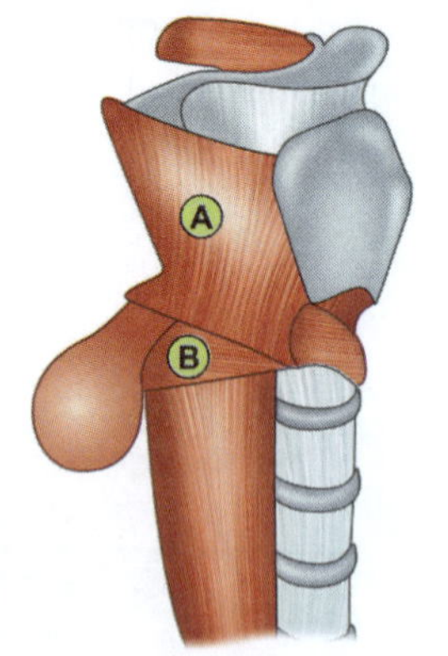

Fig. 34.61: Pharyngeal pouch

Aetiopathogenesis

Due to increase in the intrapharyngeal pressure, mucous membrane bulges in between parts of inferior constrictor muscles due to neuromuscular imbalance. Hence, it is a pulsion diverticulum.

Course of the Diverticulum

Pulsion diverticulum deviates to one side mostly to the left because of the rigid vertebral column in the midline, posteriorly.

Diagnosis

- Initially foreign body sensation is present in the throat. Later, gurgling sound, regurgitation of food on turning to one side, sense of suffocation, cough or dysphagia are present.
- Aspiration may cause dyspnoea later.

Pearls of Wisdom

Pharyngeal pouch is a swelling behind sternocleidomastoid below the level of thyroid cartilage—soft swelling which can be emptied.

Treatment

- Barium swallow followed by excision of the pouch
- Cricopharyngeal myotomy may also be done.

SCHWANNOMA OF THE VAGUS NERVE (Fig. 34.62)

- This condition produces swelling in the carotid triangle in the region of thyroid swelling.
- It is a vertically placed oval swelling
- It is firm to hard in consistency
- On pressure over the swelling, dry cough and in some cases bradycardia may occur.

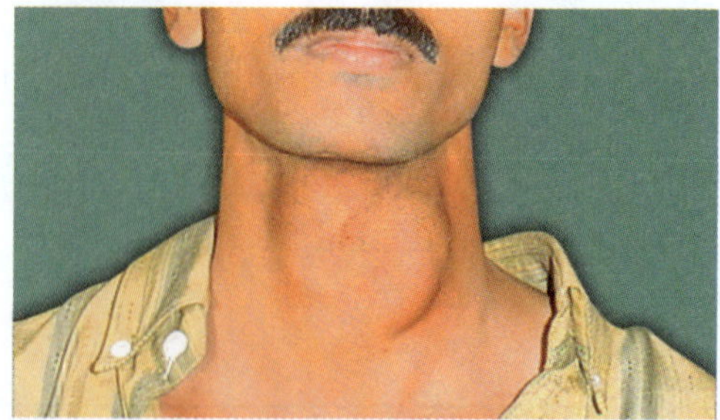
Fig. 34.62: Schwannoma of the vagus nerve. (*Courtesy:* Prof. P Rajan, Calicut Medical College, Kerala. This swelling was not moving with deglutition—candidate offered thyroid nodule as diagnosis—MS exam case 2007)

DIFFERENTIAL DIAGNOSIS OF SWELLINGS IN THE POSTERIOR TRIANGLE

The posterior triangle (Key Box 34.26) is an interesting area as far as swellings are concerned. It is the commonest area of metastasis in lymph nodes from occult primary. Lymphangiomas, haemangiomas, cold abscess, lymphomas commonly occur here. Interesting cases of cervical rib, Pancoast's tumour, aneurysms also occur here.

Key Box 34.26

Boundaries of Posterior Triangle

- Anteriorly : Sternomastoid (posterior border)
- Laterally : Trapezius (anterior border)
- Above : Mastoid process
- Below : Clavicle

Most of the swellings have been discussed under appropriate chapters. Haemangioma, metastasis in the cervical lymph nodes and Pancoast's tumour have been discussed below.

CLASSIFICATION (Table 34.5)

Common swellings in the posterior triangle are given below.

HAEMANGIOMA

Definition

This is a swelling due to congenital malformation of blood vessels. It is an example of ***hamartoma***.

Classification

A. Depending on the Origin

- Capillary
- Cavernous
- Arterial

Table 34.5 Swellings in the posterior triangle

Solid swellings	Cystic swellings	Pulsatile swellings
1. Metastasis in the lymph nodes	Lymphangioma	Subclavian artery aneurysm
2. Tuberculosis	Haemangioma	Vertebral artery aneurysm
3. Lymphoma	Cold abscess	
4. Lipoma		
5. Cervical rib		
6. Pancoast's tumour		

B. Depending on Behaviour of the Lesion

	Terms in common use
I. Involuting haemangioma	
• Superficial	Strawberry naevus Capillary haemangioma
• Deep	Cavernous
• Combined (superficial + deep)	Strawberry naevus Capillary haemangioma Cavernous haemangioma
II. Noninvoluting	
• Port-wine stain	Port-wine stain Capillary haemangioma Naevus flammeus
• Cavernous haemangioma	
• Arteriovenous fistula	

CAPILLARY HAEMANGIOMA (Key Box 34.27)

It consists of dilated capillaries and proliferation of endothelial cells. Hence, it commonly occurs in the skin (Figs 34.63 and 34.64). It can be of the following types:

1. **Salmon patch** is a bluish patch over the forehead, in the midline, present at birth and disappears by 1 year of age. Hence, no treatment is required.
2. **Port-wine stain** is an extensive intradermal haemangioma. This is bluish purple in colour, commonly affects the face or other parts of the skin, is present at birth, usually progresses and does not regress (Key Box 34.28).

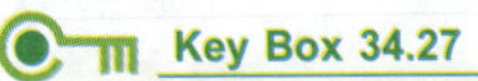

Key Box 34.27

Capillary Haemangioma

- Skin and soft tissue involvement
- Salmon patch: Midline forehead
- Port-wine stain: Head and neck
- Strawberry angioma: Compressible
- Wait and watch policy is the best

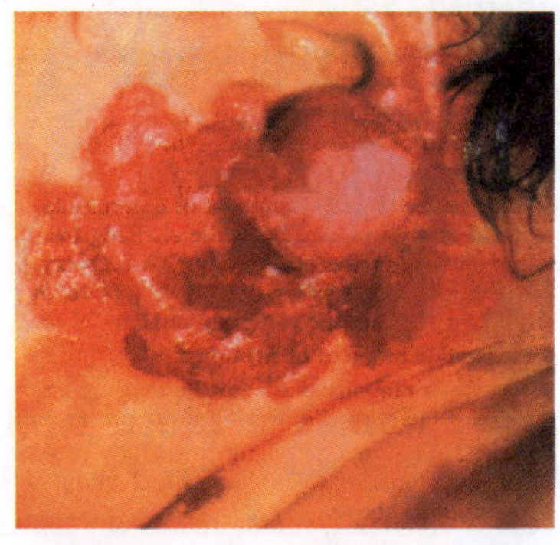

Fig. 34.63: Capillary haemangioma. (*Courtesy:* Prof. Pramod Kumar, Head, Department of Plastic Surgery, KMC, Manipal)

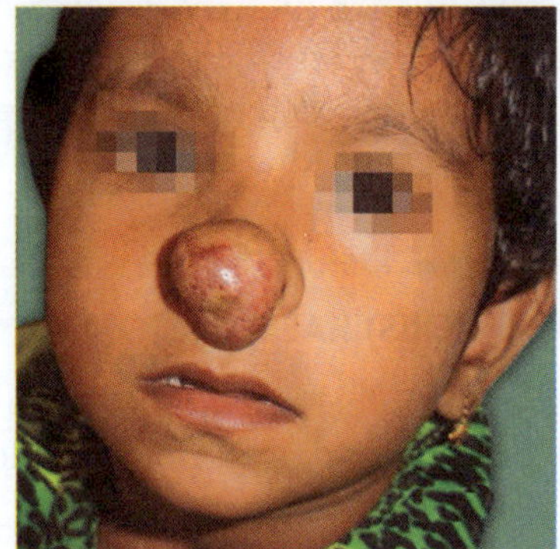

Fig. 34.64: Capillary haemangioma of the nose

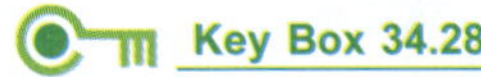

Key Box 34.28

Port-wine Stain

- **P**ort-wine colour even though to start with it is red in colour.
- **O**ccurs usually in the face, can also occur on the shoulder and trunk.
- **R**egression does not occur.
- **T**reatment: Pulsed dye laser, photocoagulation, dermabrasion.
- **W**orrying because it becomes more keratotic and nodular as age advances.
- **I**njection of sclerosants may be needed.
- **N**oninvoluting haemangioma is its another name.
- **E**xtensive intradermal capillary dilatation

Remember as **PORT-WINE**

- It is a non-involuting capillary haemangioma (dilatation due to defective maturation of cutaneous innervations during embryogenesis).
- Area supplied by sensory branches of the fifth cranial nerve is involved.
- Starts with light red colour and progresses to deep colour.
- Pulsed dye laser using light with specific wavelength of 585 or 595 nanometres is **one of the best treatments** available. This process is called **'photothermolysis'.**
- It may be associated with **Sturge-Weber syndrome** (page 335).

Pearls of Wisdom

Flat, patchy lesion on the face in the area of fifth cranial nerve that does not fade is port-wine stain.

3. **Strawberry angiomas** produce swelling which protrude from the skin surface. The child is normal at birth. After a month, a ***bright red swelling*** appears over the head and neck region, which exhibits ***sign of compressibility***. The lesion consists of immature vascular tissue. Even though the lesion grows initially, by 5–7 years of age, ***swelling regresses and colour fades.*** Hence, no specific treatment is necessary. The treatment is indicated only when the swelling persists. 70% resolve by 7 years of age.

VENOUS (CAVERNOUS) HAEMANGIOMA

This occurs in place where venous space is abundant, e.g. lip, cheek, tongue, and posterior triangle of the neck (Key Box 34.29 and Fig. 34.65).

 **Key Box 34.29**

Cavernous Haemangioma

- Compressible swelling
- Bluish warm, nontender swelling
- Associated with arteriovenous communication
- Associated with lipoma: Naevolipoma

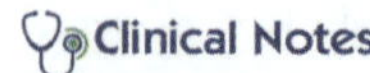

Clinical Notes

Gluteal region is one of the sites of haemangioma, AV fistula, aneurysm and neurilemmoma. A patient presented with this swelling which was firm with a few cystic areas. It was excised in toto. Remember to check whether it is a low pressure (venous) or a high pressure arterial lesion before excising a haemangioma. Massive bleeding can occur, if it is a high pressure lesion.

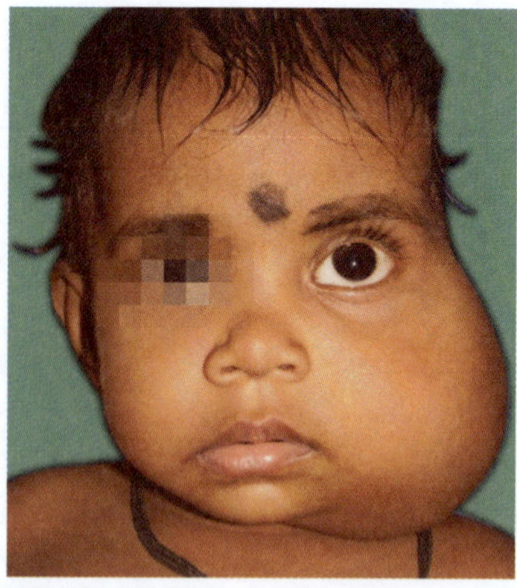

Fig. 34.65: Cavernous haemangioma of the cheek

Clinical Features

- History of a swelling in the neck of long duration. History of bleeding is present when it occurs in the oral cavity.
- The swelling is warm and ***bluish in colour*** but not pulsatile.
- Soft, fluctuant, transillumination is negative.
- **Compressibility** is present. This sign is also called 'sign of emptying' or 'sign of refilling'. When the swelling is compressed between the fingers, blood diffuses under the vascular spaces and when pressure is released, it slowly fills up. Compressibility is a diagnostic sign of haemangioma (Fig. 34.66).

Differential Diagnosis

1. **Lymphangioma is brilliantly transilluminant.** If a lymphangioma is infected or has been treated with preliminary injections, it may not show transillumination.
2. **Lipoma** is not compressible.
3. **Cold abscess**
4. **Branchial cyst** when it is in anterior triangle.

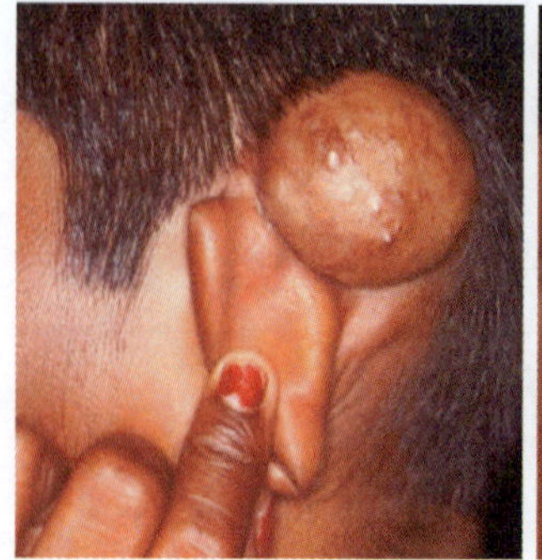

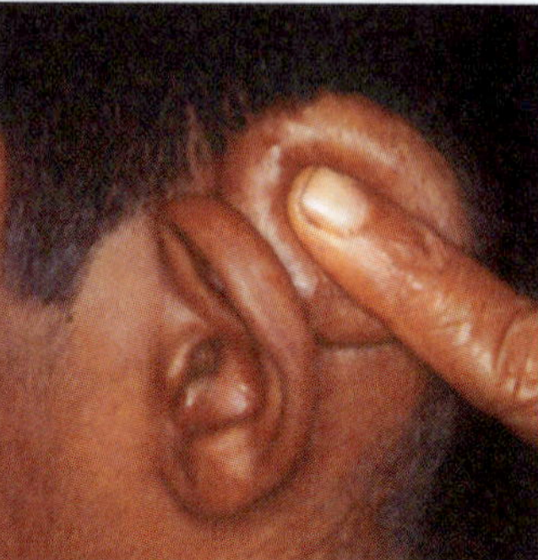

Fig. 34.66: Sign of compressibility was positive in this case. It was initially diagnosed as post-auricular dermoid

Note: Importance of complete clinical examination

Treatment of Cavernous Haemangioma

Principles

1. **Injection** is the first line of treatment of cavernous haemangioma. It makes the swelling **fibrotic, less vascular and small**. Thus, excision can be done at a later date (Key Boxes 34.30 and 34.31).
2. **Excision** of haemangioma in the oral cavity is more difficult than in the neck.
3. It is better to have a control of external carotid artery in the neck, while excising haemangioma in the oral cavity. If necessary, external carotid artery should be ligated in order to control the bleeding.
4. Adequate blood to be arranged.
5. **Previous embolisation** into the feeding artery decreases the size of the haemangioma (therapeutic embolisation).
6. ***Large haemangiomas in the oral cavity*** should be excised only after ***preliminary sclerotherapy*** and taking all the precautions mentioned above.

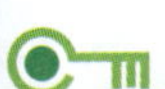 **Key Box 34.30**

Injection Line of Treatment

- Boiling water, hypertonic saline or sodium tetradecyl sulphate (STD solution) can be used
- In multiple spaces, in multiple sittings
- Obliteration occurs due to aseptic thrombosis and fibrosis
- Lesion becomes flat

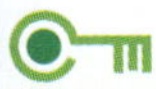 **Key Box 34.31**

Swellings: Treated with Sclerosants

- Haemangioma
- Haemorrhoids
- Prolapse rectum
- Oesophageal varices
- Varicose veins

Syndromes Associated with Haemangioma (Table 34.6)

Table 34.6 Syndromes associated with haemangioma and their findings

Syndromes associated with haemangioma	Findings
1. Klippel-Trénaunay-Weber syndrome	1. Naevus flammeus, osteohypertrophy of extremities, AV fistula and varicose veins
2. Osler-Rendu-Weber syndrome	2. Haemangioma of lip associated with haemangioma of GIT
3. Sturge-Weber syndrome	3. Haemangioma of brain, mental retardation, Jacksonian epilepsy, glaucoma

Complications of Haemangioma (Key Box 34.32)

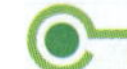 **Key Box 34.32**

Complications of Haemangioma

- Ulceration and bleeding: Commonly occurs with capillary haemangioma
- Infection: Septicaemia usually precipitated by a small ulcer
- High output cardiac failure

CONGENITAL ARTERIOVENOUS (AV) FISTULA (Arterial Haemangioma)

- An abnormal communication between artery and vein, results in AV fistula (Key Box 34.33).
- AV fistula can be congenital or acquired (Figs 34.67 and 34.68).
- Such AV fistula has got structural and functional effects (Figs 34.69A and B).

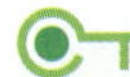 **Key Box 34.33**

Arteriovenous Fistula: Types

- Congenital
- Traumatic
- Iatrogenic: Created in cases of renal failure

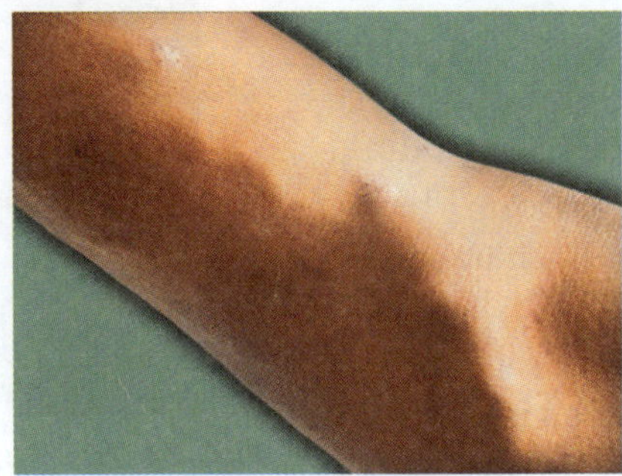

Fig. 34.67: Most common type of AV fistula you see today is in the nephrology ward—created to facilitate haemodialysis

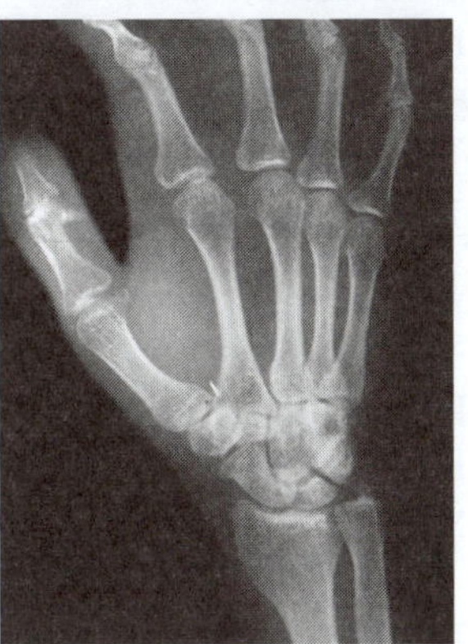

Fig. 34.68: X-ray of the hand— traumatic AV fistula

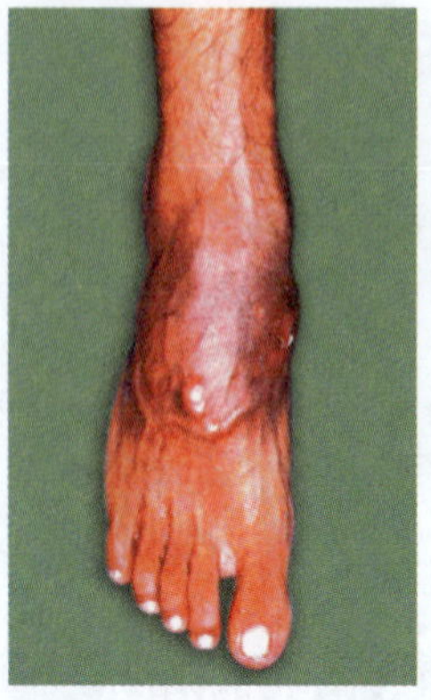

Fig. 34.69A: Traumatic AV fistula. See the arterialisation of the vein

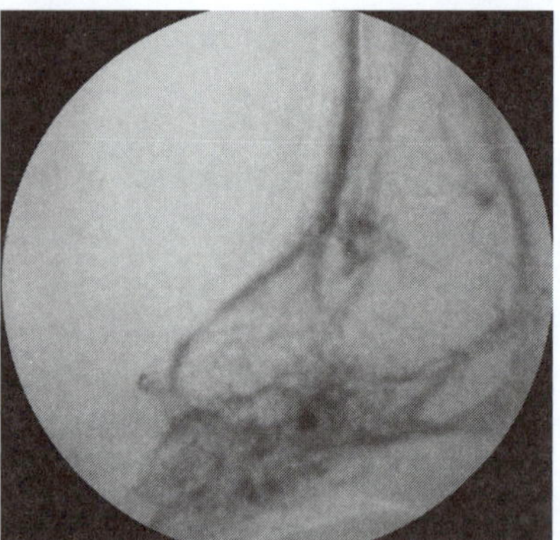

Fig. 34.69B: DSA picture

Structural Effect

Since high pressure blood from an artery flows into the vein, the veins get dilated, tortuous and elongated. This arterialisation of the vein results in secondary varicose veins.

Physiological Effect

Increased pulse rate, increased cardiac output, increased pulse pressure result due to increased venous pressure and arteriovenous shunt.

Functional Effect

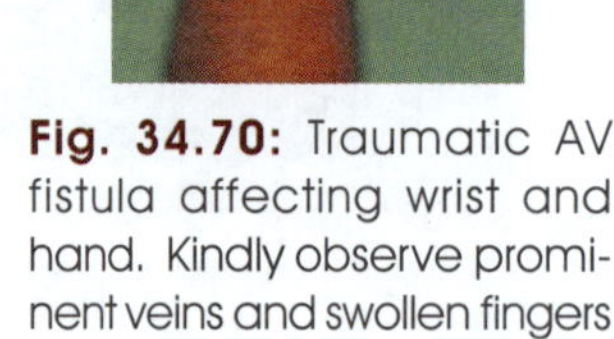

Fig. 34.70: Traumatic AV fistula affecting wrist and hand. Kindly observe prominent veins and swollen fingers

- Soft, cystic, fluctuant, transillumination negative, **pulsatile swelling.**
- A continuous bruit/ murmur is characteristic (Fig. 34.70).
- **Nicoladoni's sign or Branham's sign**
  - On compressing the feeding artery, the venous return to the heart diminishes, resulting in fall in pulse rate and pulse pressure.
  - On compressing feeding artery, pulsation or **continuous murmur** may also disappear and swelling will diminish in size.
- If the AV fistula is big, a **high output cardiac failure** can occur.
- The affected part is swollen (because of high pressure) than—**local gigantism** (Figs 34.71 and 34.72). Thus, overgrowth of the limb or toe can occur.
- Distal to the AV fistula, there are **ischaemic ulcers**, due to comparative reduction in the blood supply.

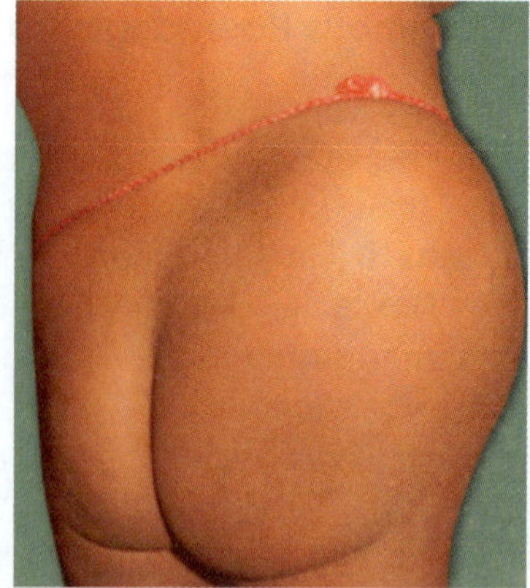

Fig. 34.71: Local gigantism due to haemangioma involving gluteal region

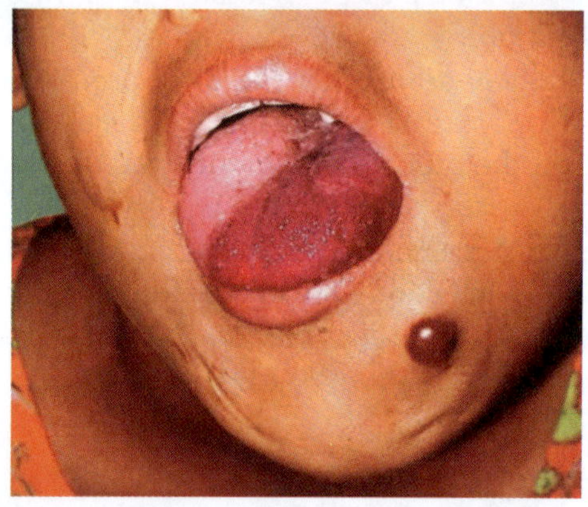

Fig. 34.72: Haemangioma tongue causing macroglossia. She also had haemangioma of the cheek and skin

Clinical Notes

This lady visited many general practitioners for a swelling near the coccyx region (adjacent to natal cleft). The diagnosis which was made in this case was subcutaneous neurofibroma, pilonidal sinus abscess, boil and haemangioma. Careful examinations revealed pulsations. History dates back to 20 years duration. It was a case of congenital AV fistula. Wide excision was done. She has been asymptomatic for 2 years now.

Clinical Notes

A 30-year-old patient who had an injury to the dorsum of hand, had pain and swelling in dorsum of hand for 60 days duration. Many had missed the diagnosis. However, swelling had local rise of temperature, pulsations and reducibility (Fig. 34.70).

Investigations

Angiography with **DSA** (digital subtraction angiography) pictures are essential before treating these patients (Fig. 34.69B).

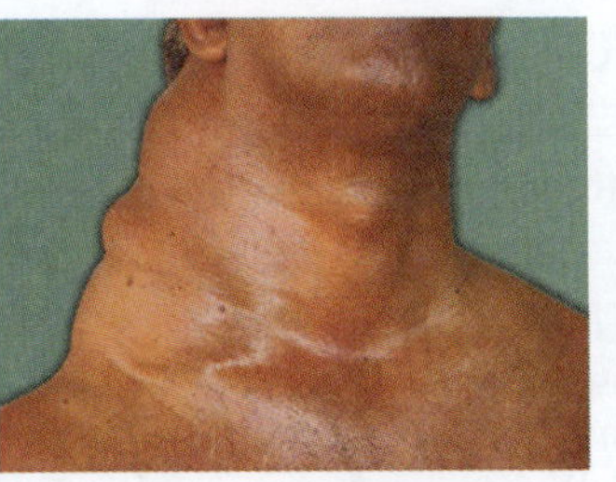

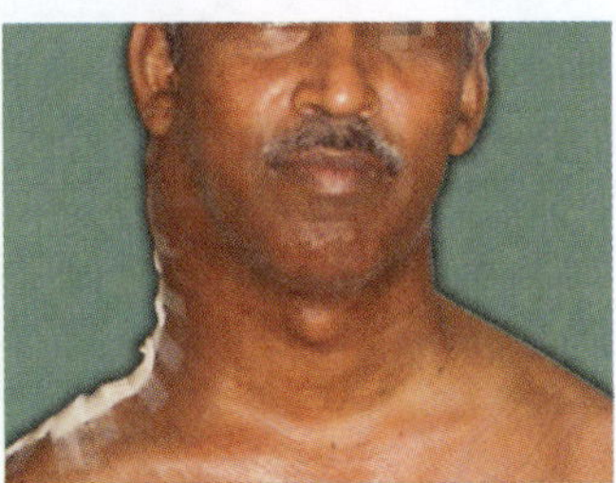

Figs 34.73 and 34.74: Congenital AV fistula of 25 years duration. After therapeautic embolisation, it has regressed by over 70%. Patient is waiting for another course of embolisation. (*Courtesy:* Dr Umesh Bhat, Surgeon, Kundapur and Dr Subhaschandra, Interventional Cardiologist, Manipal Hospital, Bangalore)

Treatment

- Therapeutic embolisation is the treatment of choice for arteriovenous fistula, in congenital cases (Figs 34.73 and 34.74).
- Acquired lesion needs to be observed or treated by quadruple ligation, if needed.

CIRSOID ANEURYSM

- Not an aneurysm
- It is an AV fistula occurring in older people affecting the temporal region.
- The arteries and the veins are dilated and tortuous and are compared to pulsating bag of worms.

COLD ABSCESS IN THE POSTERIOR TRIANGLE (Fig. 34.75)

Causes

1. **Posterior cervical lymph nodes** primarily involved—route of infection from **adenoids** or other lymph nodes in the anterior triangle.
2. Lower posterior lymph nodes or Scalene node—route of infection from **lungs.**
3. **From tuberculous cervical spine: Caries spine**
   - Clinically, it presents as pain in the back, cold abscess and neurological presentation.
   - **Rust's sign:** Child with caries spine will support the head by holding the chin.
   - Cold abscess from caries spine can rupture anteriorly or posteriorly.

   A. **Anterior rupture:** It ruptures deep to prevertebral layer of deep cervical fascia. From here, it can take the following routes:
      - *Upper cervical region:* Presents as deep seated abscess in the posterior wall of the pharynx in the **midline**.
      - *Lower cervical region:* Pus will press on oesophagus and trachea forwards.
      - *Laterally* pus passes deep to prevertebral **fascia behind carotid sheath** in the **posterior triangle** (Fig. 34.76).

   B. **Posterior rupture:** Pus may enter spinal canal and then can travel along anterior primary division of the cervical spinal nerves.

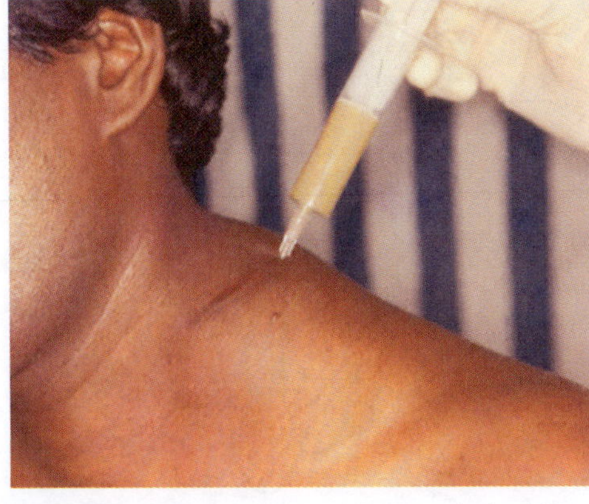

Fig. 34.75: Cold abscess in the posterior triangle

Diagnosis

- **Cervical spine X-ray** to rule out spinal tuberculosis.
- **Chest X-ray** to rule out pulmonary tuberculosis.
- **Nondependent aspiration of the cold abscess** followed by AFB staining.

Treatment

- Antituberculous treatment
- Nondependent aspiration, if cold abscess is present.
- Please refer orthopaedic books for specific treatment of TB spine.

Differential Diagnosis

- Haemangioma—compressible
- Lymphangioma—transilluminant
- Schwannoma (Fig. 34.76)

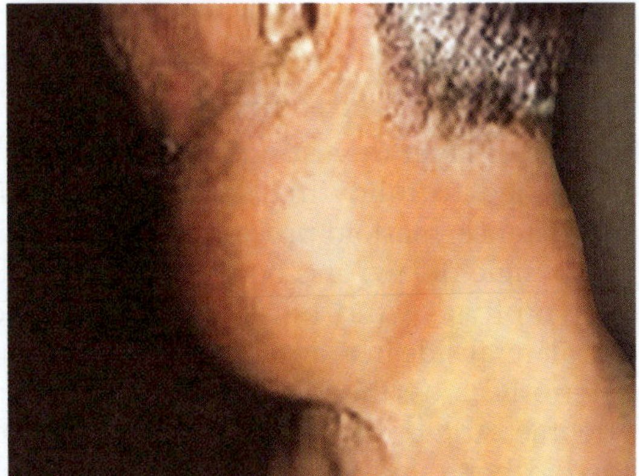

Fig. 34.76: Schwannoma in the posterior triangle. Soft tissue sarcoma is another diagnosis. (Undergraduate clinics at JNMC, Belgaum, Karnataka). (*Courtesy:* Dr Aditya Patil, Prof. Ashok Godhi, Head, Department of Surgery)

LYMPH NODES SECONDARIES (METASTASIS) IN THE HEAD AND NECK

Introduction

Very often, the patients present to the surgeon with lymph node swelling in the neck with or without any complaints. If there is an obvious lesion in the oral cavity, the diagnosis is easy. On the other hand, difficulty arises in locating the primary malignancy, which is hidden or occult. It is important to know the anatomical location of the lymph nodes in the neck and drainage area, so that drainage areas can be investigated.

Before understanding the various lymph nodes, drainage area and block dissection, it is advisable to know surgical anatomy of the neck and lymphatic drainage.

SURGICAL ANATOMY OF NECK

Neck is that region of the body that lies between the lower border of the mandible and the suprasternal notch and the upper border of the clavicle. Its boundaries include mandible, zygomatic process of temporal bone, external auditory canal, mastoid process, superior nuchal line, external occipital protuberance, manubrium sterni, clavicle, acromioclavicular joint and spinous process of 7th cervical vertebra.

Fascial Layers of Neck

- Two fascial layers in the neck: Superficial cervical fascia and deep cervical fascia.
- Superficial cervical fascia corresponds to subcutaneous tissue.
- Deep cervical fascia (fascia colli) is the important layer for functional and selective neck dissection. It is this layer that divides neck into various compartments.

Deep Cervical Fascia

It has superficial and deep components.

A. **Superficial layer (investing or anterior fascia):** It is attached to following structures—occipital protuberance, mastoid process, capsule of parotid gland, angle of jaw, and body of the mandible to the symphysis. And here, it proceeds around contralateral side in a similar manner. It then goes posteriorly across the spinal process of the cervical vertebrae. Anteriorly, it passes from the mandible to hyoid bone. Inferiorly, it attaches to sternum, upper edge of clavicle, acromion, and spine of scapula. At the inferior border, in the midline, superficial layer splits in two different layers just superior to the manubrium of sternum. The space between these two layers is known as the **suprasternal space of Burns**.

   From posterior to anterior, the superficial layer splits to enclose the trapezius, the portion of the omohyoid muscle that crosses the posterior triangle of the neck, and the sternocleidomastoid muscle. In a similar way, it envelops the strap muscles, before ending in the midline. The superficial veins of the neck lie on or within this superficial layer of the deep cervical fascia.

B. **Deep layer (prevertebral fascia):** The deep or prevertebral layer, like the superficial layer, attaches posteriorly to the spinous process of the cervical vertebrae. Above, it reaches the skull base at the jugular foramen and carotid canal, then passes across the basilar process to the opposite side. It covers the muscles of the back that enter into the neck immediately deep to the trapezius muscle. At the upper limit of the posterior triangle, the spinal accessory nerve crosses the posterior triangle at this level, along with some lymph nodes. At the lower end, both fascial layers further separate, the deep layer covers the scalene muscles, whereas superficial layer remains attached to the trapezius muscle and the clavicle.

Lymphatic Drainage of Neck

- The cervical lymphatics are divided into superficial and deep. The superficial lymphatics perforate the cervical fascia and drain into the deep lymphatics. The deep vessels and nodes are most commonly found along blood vessels, nerves and muscles. For example: Along the internal jugular vein classically described as jugular chain of lymph nodes. Look for this finding in ultrasound examination of neck.
- Lymph nodes have been given numbers according to their levels and drainage sites which are given below (Fig. 34.77).

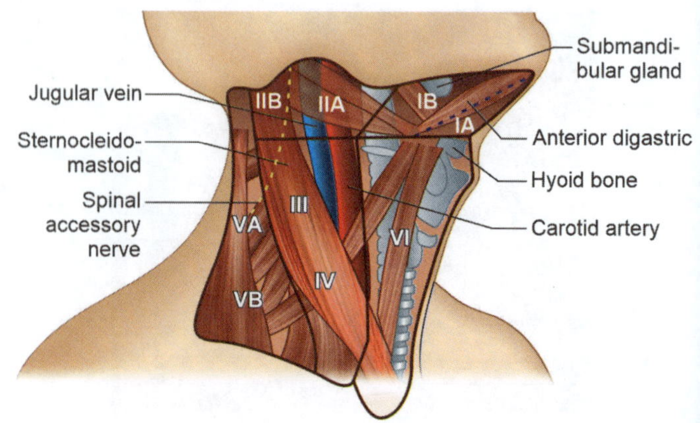

Fig. 34.77: Lymph nodes stations

Memorial Sloan-Kettering Cancer Centre: Lateral Lymph Node Classification

Level I : Lymph nodes in the **submental triangle and submandibular triangle.**

Level II : Upper jugular nodes. Deep to the sternocleidomastoid muscle, anterior to posterior border of sternocleidomastoid, posterior to posterior aspect of the posterior belly of diagastric, superior to level of hyoid.

Level II is further divided into (IIa) which is inferior and in front of the line of spinal accessory nerve, (IIb) is above and posterior to line of spinal accessory nerve.

Level III : **Middle jugular nodes** from hyoid superiorly to cricothyroid membrane inferiorly.

Level IV : **Lower jugular nodes** from cricothyroid membrane superiorly to clavicle inferiorly.

Level V : **Posterior cervical region** from anterior border of trapezius posteriorly to posterior border of sternocleidomastoid anteriorly and clavicle inferiorly.

a. Above the line of spinal accessory nerve.

b. Below the level of spinal accessory nerve.

Level VI : **Anterior compartment nodes** from hyoid bone superiorly to suprasternal notch inferiorly and laterally by medial border of carotid sheath.

Level VII : **Upper mediastinal nodes** inferior to suprasternal notch (no longer used).

Drainage Area

- **Level Ia lymph nodes:** Floor of mouth, anterior oral tongue, anterior mandibular alveolar ridge, lower lip.
- **Level Ib lymph nodes:** Oral cavity, anterior nasal cavity, soft tissue of midface, submandibular gland.
- **Level IIa and IIb nodes:** Oral cavity, nasal cavity, nasopharynx, oropharynx, hypopharynx, larynx, parotid gland.
- **Level III lymph nodes:** Oral cavity, nasopharynx, oropharynx, hypopharynx, larynx.
- **Level IV lymph nodes:** Hypopharynx, thyroid, cervical oesophagus, larynx.
- **Level V lymph nodes:** Scalp, parotid gland, nasopharynx, thyroid gland, etc.
- **Level VI lymph nodes:** Thyroid gland, glottic and subglottic larynx, apex of pyriform sinus, cervical oesophagus (Figs 34.78 and 34.79).

Rational for Subzones (Fig. 34.80)

Level II subzones

- Oropharynx and nasopharynx—IIb
  – XI should be mobilised
- Oral cavity, larynx and hypopharynx—may not be necessary to dissect IIb, if level IIa is not involved.

Level IV subzones

- Level IVa nodes—increased risk in level VI
- Level IVb nodes—increased risk in level V

Level V subzones

- Oropharynx, nasopharynx, and cutaneous—Va
- Thyroid—Vb.

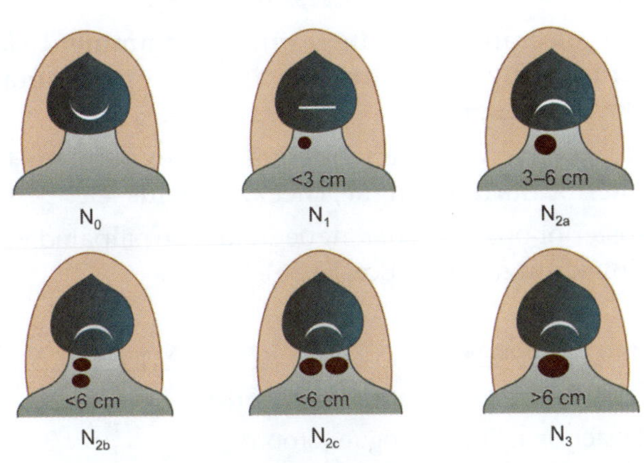

Fig. 34.78

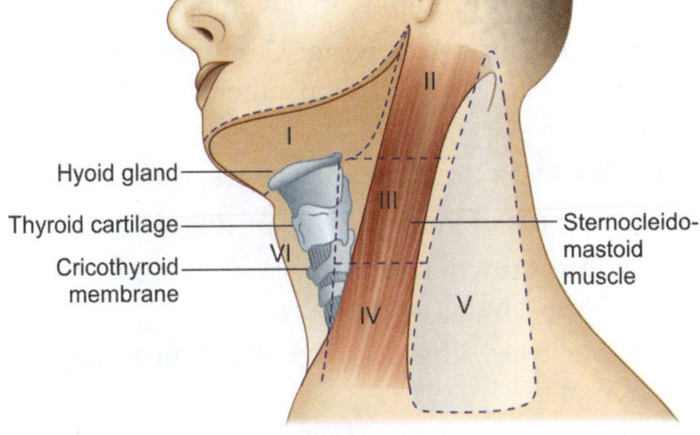

Fig. 34.79

Figs 34.78 and 34.79: Levels of various lymph nodes, nodal-N position and relation to various triangles

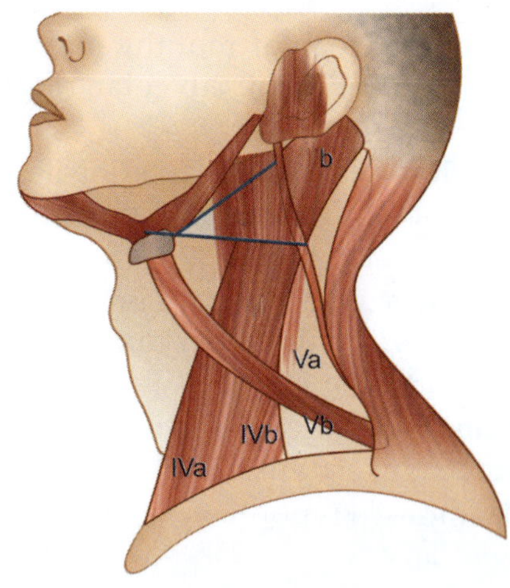

Level	Lymph Node Group
Ia	Submental nodes
Ib	Submandibular nodes
IIa	Upper jugular, anterior to IX
IIb	Upper jugular, posterior to IX (submuscular recess)
III	Middle jugular nodes
IVa	Lower jugular nodes (behind clavicular head of sternocleidomastoid muscle)
IVb	Lower jugular nodes (behind sternal head of sternocleidomastoid muscle)
Va	Posterior triangle nodes (spinal accessory group)
Vb	Posterior triangle nodes (transverse cervical artery group, supraclavicular group)
VI	Anterior (central) compartment lymph nodes (paratracheal, perithyroidal, Delphian)

Fig. 34.80: Subzones of neck lymph node metastasis—level 4b are supraclavicular lymph nodes

Reason why lymphatic spread occurs widely is given in Key Box 34.34

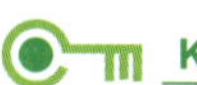 Key Box 34.34

Factors which Accelerate Local and Regional Spread of Malignant Tumour

- Angiogenesis
- Lymphangiogenesis
- Lack of basement membrane on lymphatic vessels
- Extracapsular breakout

Clinical Presentation of Metastatic Deposits in the Lymph Nodes

1. Majority of patients are elderly males (>50 years), present with painless swelling in the neck of a few months duration.
2. The symptoms with which a patient presents to the hospital gives the clue to the site of origin of the primary. A few examples are given below:
   - **Difficulty in swallowing:** Carcinoma posterior 1/3rd of tongue, oropharyngeal carcinoma or carcinoma oesophagus.
   - **Difficulty in breathing:** Laryngeal cancer
   - **Hoarseness of voice:** Larynx or thyroid
   - **Obvious growth in oral cavity:** Carcinoma cheek, alveolus, tongue, etc.
   - Haemoptysis, difficulty in breathing: Bronchogenic carcinoma
   - **Epistaxis, ear pain or deafness:** Nasopharyngeal carcinoma

   Refer to Key Box 34.35 also

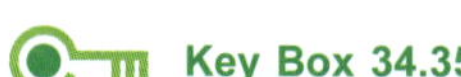 Key Box 34.35

Nasopharyngeal Carcinoma[1]: Trotter's Triad

- Conductive deafness
- Homolateral immobility of soft palate
- Pain in the side of the head due to involvement of 5th cranial nerve.

[1]More details about nasopharyngeal carcinoma are given in page 366 in the chapter on oral cavity.

Clinical Signs

- Lymph nodal metastasis appears as a **hard, nodular** or irregular mass in the anatomical location of the lymph nodes (Figs 34.81 to 34.89).
- Early cases may have some mobility. However, in majority of cases, **nodes get fixed** and they attain a huge size. Very often, what appears as one lymph node, is a complex mass of multiple lymph nodes.
- On sternomastoid contraction test or chin test, these nodal swellings become less prominent.
- Skin ulceration is a late feature. **A prominent skin fold** is due to infiltration into the platysma—**platysma sign**.
- The primary malignancy may be evident in the anterior third of tongue, cheek, alveolus, etc.
- Posterior one-third of tongue should be palpated with gloved finger (Key Box 34.36).

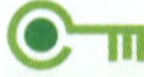 Key Box 34.36

Occult Primary Sites

- Posterior 1/3rd of tongue, oropharynx
- Nasopharynx, sinuses
- Upper oesophagus, bronchus, thyroid

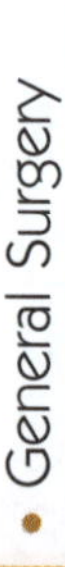

- Secondaries in the lymph nodes can cause pressure effects or may cause paralysis of nerves. Upper anterior deep cervical lymph nodes can cause **hypoglossal nerve paralysis** (Key Box 34.37) where in the tongue points towards the side of lesion. **When there is no evidence of the primary lesion clinically, the situation is described as occult primary** with secondaries in the neck.
- Pain in the distribution of trigeminal nerve (face) suggests nasopharyngeal malignancy infiltrating skull base (foramen lacerum).

Key Box 34.37

Clinical Examination in a Case of Lymph Nodes in the Neck

- Lymph nodes: All groups
- Drainage areas

Pressure effect on

- Hypoglossal nerve
- Accessory nerve
- Cervical sympathetic chain

TYPES OF SECONDARIES IN THE NECK

1. **Secondaries in the neck with known primary**
   - In this case, secondaries in the neck are present and the site of primary tumour is clinically identified either in oral cavity, pharynx, thyroid, etc.
   - Primary may be treated by surgery or radiotherapy as the case may be.
   - Secondaries may need radical neck dissection.
2. **Secondaries in the neck with clinically unidentified primary**
   - Here the hard neck nodes are present but primary is not identified clinically. However, it is detected after investigations. *Example*: Oropharyngeal carcinoma.
   - FNAC is done to confirm the diagnosis.
   - Various investigations like panendoscopy, blind biopsies, CT may be done to establish the primary.
3. **Secondaries in the neck with an occult primary:** It is biopsy proven cancer of neck nodes which even after complete clinical and radiological workup reveals or yields no demonstrable primary lesion.

How do you Suspect Metastasis in the Neck?

Any elderly patient presenting to the hospital with firm to hard lymph node in the neck of short duration with or without fixity. He has no signs and symptoms of inflammation such as fever or pain to begin with.

Having suspected a metastatic deposit, remember the following facts:

- **80%** of them are **metastatic** deposits.
- Majority of malignant neoplasms are **epithelial** in origin.
- Nodes in the **upper half** (level I and II) can be due to **primary in the oral cavity, tongue, oropharynx, larynx.**
- Nodes in the **lower half** (level III and IV) **can be due to primary in the thyroid, tongue.**
- **Nodes in the supraclavicular region** (level V): Carcinoma in the GIT, genitourinary tract, lungs and nasopharynx.
- **Nodes in the pretracheal, suprasternal region** (level VI): Papillary carcinoma thyroid

Rule of 80 in Neck Masses

- 80% of neck masses are neoplastic
- 80% of neoplastic masses occur in males
- 80% of neck masses are malignant
- 80% of malignant neck masses are metastatic
- 80% of metastatic neck masses are from primary sites above clavicle

NECK DISSECTIONS

Introduction

- **Crile** in 1906, first described a standardised dissection of cervical nodes by applying **anatomical and oncological principles** including removal of surrounding fibrofatty tissue from various compartments of the neck.
- Radical neck dissection (RND) causes significant functional and cosmetic morbidity.
- Today adjuvant chemoradiotherapy is an important modality of treatment.
- Thus with better understanding of tumour biology, natural history of disease and availability of adjuvant radiotherapy, radical neck dissection is not **frequently done but its modifications are done.**

Classification of Concepts

1. RND is the standard basic procedure for cervical lymphadenectomy against which all other modifications are compared.
2. Modifications of the RND which include preservation of any non-lymphatic structures are referred to as modified radical neck dissection (MRND).
3. Any neck dissection that preserves one or more groups or levels of lymph nodes is referred to as a selective neck dissection (SND).
4. An extended neck dissection refers to the removal of additional lymph node groups or non-lymphatic structures relative to the RND.

METASTASIS IN CERVICAL LYMPH NODES—VARIOUS LEVELS (Figs 34.81 to 34.89)

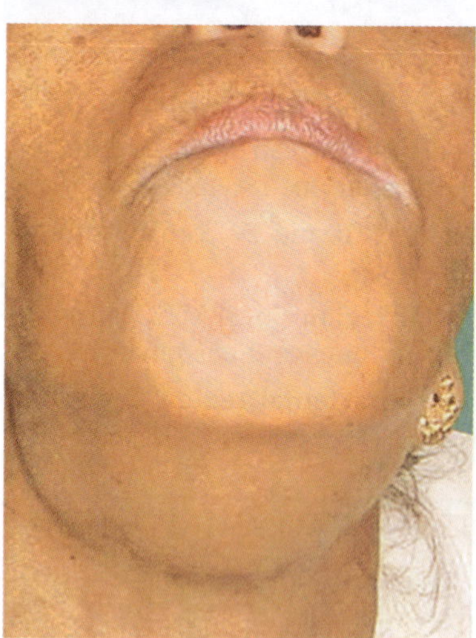

Fig. 34.81: Level I and II nodes. Carcinoma floor of the mouth

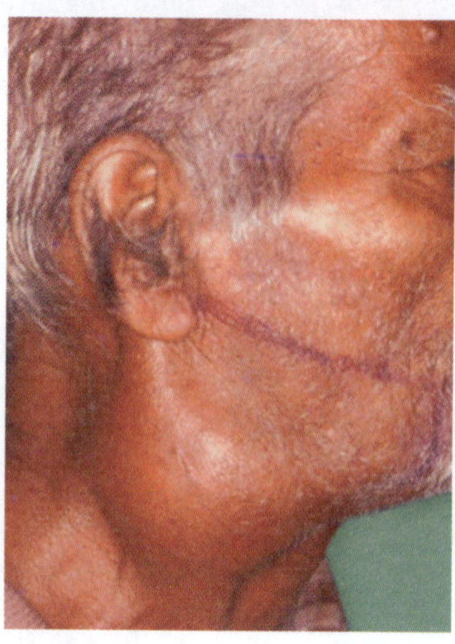

Fig. 34.82: Level II and III nodes: Carcinoma alveolus

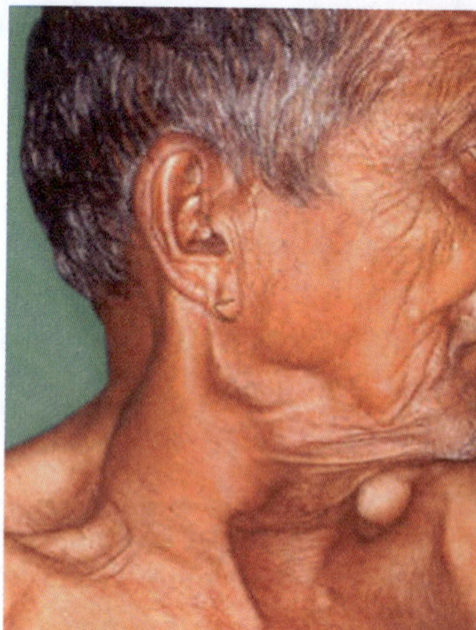

Fig. 34.83: Level III, IV and V nodes: Carcinoma posterior 1/3rd of tongue

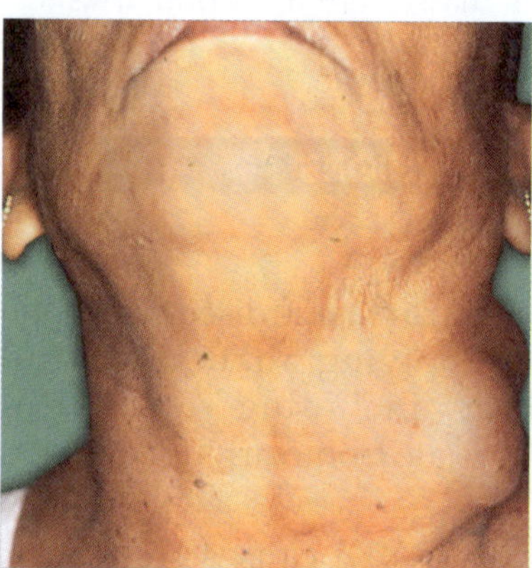

Fig. 34.84: Level V nodes: Post-cricoid carcinoma

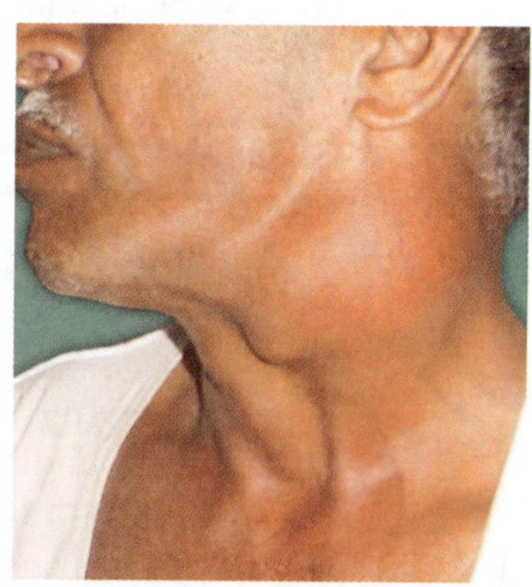

Fig. 34.85: Predominantly level II, III and V nodes: From nasopharyngeal carcinoma

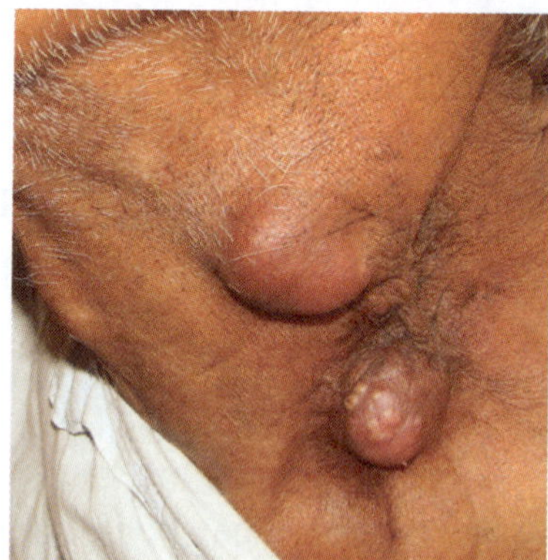

Fig. 34.86: Predominantly level II, III and V nodes: From nasopharyngeal carcinoma

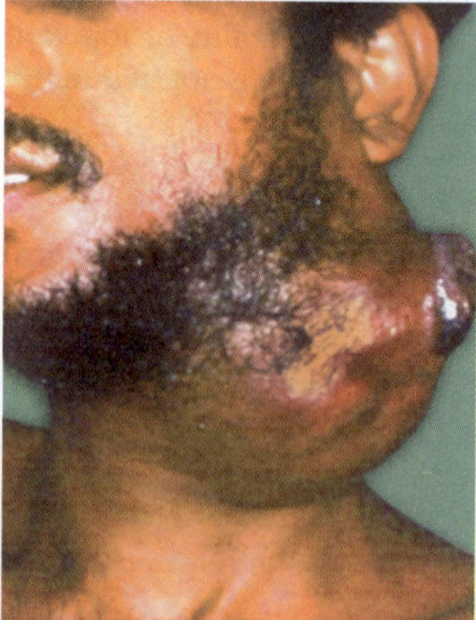

Fig. 34.87: Level I, II, III and V nodes: Primary could not be identified—a case of occult primary

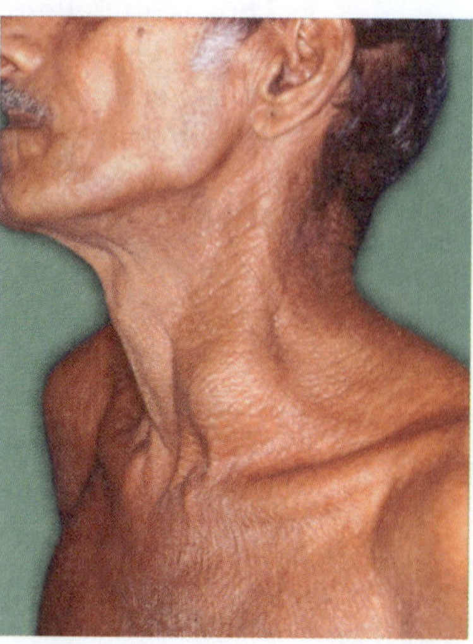

Fig. 34.88: Scalene node: In between the two heads of sternomastoid—a case of bronchogenic carcinoma

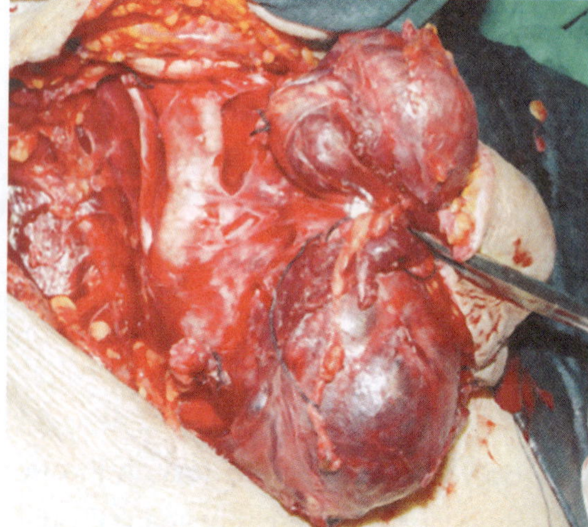

Fig. 34.89: Hugely enlarged lymph nodes which are bluish in colour, pushing the carotid arteries anteriorly—papillary carcinoma thyroid

Classification

1. Radical neck dissection (RND)
2. Modified radical neck dissection (MRND)
   Type I (XI preserved)
   Type II (XI, IJV preserved)
   Type III (XI, IJV, and SCM preserved) *"Functional neck dissection"*
3. Selective neck dissection (SND)
   - Supraomohyoid type
   - Lateral type
   - Posterolateral type
   - Anterior compartment type
4. Extended radical neck dissection
   - Rule of 80 in neck masses

Indications

- Carcinoma tongue, carcinoma floor of mouth
- Malignant melanoma
- Metastatic lymph nodes from pharynx and upper oesophagus.

Contraindications

- Fixed nodes, evidence of distant metastasis
- Untreatable primary cancer

Types (Details of the Neck Dissections)

I. *Classical Radical Neck Dissection* *(Crile's Operation)* (Figs 34.90 to 34.97)

Removal of levels I to V nodes + IJV, sternocleidomastoid + spinal accessory and submandibular salivary gland + Tail of parotid.

Incision

1. *MacFee:* **Two incisions are given** (Fig. 34.90)
   - Upper incision extends from mastoid process to hyoid bone up to the point of chin across intermediate tendon of digastric muscle.
   - Lower incision is given 2 cm above clavicle—from anterior border of trapezius to midline.
   - Gives a very good exposure and vascularity of flaps are good. No corners and hence, no necrosis.
2. *Crile's incision*
   - Upper incision is similar to MacFee. The other incision is oblique along the length of sternocleidomastoid inclining more in the posterior triangle (Fig. 34.91).
   - When sternocleidomastoid has to be removed as a part of neck dissection or to clear the **lymph nodes which** are badly **stuck to jugular vein or to accommodate PMMC flap, Crile's incision is better** (Fig. 34.92).
   - Here all the cervical lymph nodes from level I to level VI are removed **along with nonlymphatic structures** such as sternocleidomastoid muscle, internal jugular vein, accessory nerve (XI), submandibular salivary gland and cervical sympathetic plexus. A few examples wherein radical neck dissection is done are **carcinoma tongue, oropharyngeal** carcinoma, etc.

II. *Modified Radical Neck Dissection (MRND)* (Fig. 34.93)

Type I

- *Preserve one structure:* Spinal accessory nerve
- Classically done for squamous cell carcinoma of upper aerodigestive tract with clinically positive neck dissection.

Type II MRND

Preserve two structures: Spinal accessory and IJV.

Type III MRND or Bocca's functional neck dissection (Fig. 34.94)

- *Preserve three structures:* Spinal accessory, sternocleidomastoid and internal jugular vein.
- Done for metastatic well-differentiated carcinoma thyroid.
  In this, all the lymph nodes from level I to level V are removed but **nonlymphatic structures are preserved**.
- Dissection is from lower border of mandible to clavicle and from anterior border of trapezius to midline.

III. *Selective Neck Dissection*

- Here any of the lymphatic compartments is preserved (which should have been removed as part of classic RND). A few examples are given below.
  a. **Supraomohyoid dissection** (Fig. 34.92): Removal of nodes in levels I, II and III is done for carcinoma oropharynx, carcinoma cheek. Usually done for carcinoma floor, lateral tongue, etc.
  b. **Lateral neck dissection:** Levels II, III, IV are removed as in carcinoma larynx and cervical oesophagus.
  c. **Posterolateral neck dissection:** Levels II to V are removed as in cutaneous malignancy of

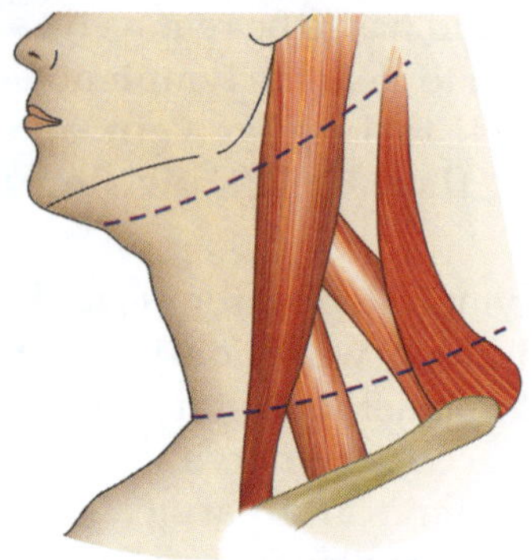

- Double transverse incision
- 3-point intersection is avoided
- Subsequent blow outs of carotid artery can be avoided

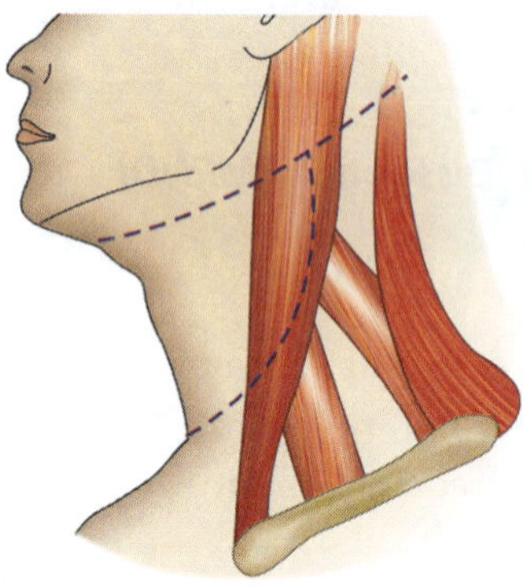

- Furcate incision—otherwise called Y incision
- 3-point intersection occurs which may give rise to necrosis

Figs 34.90 and 34.91: Incisions for block dissection: MacFee and Crile

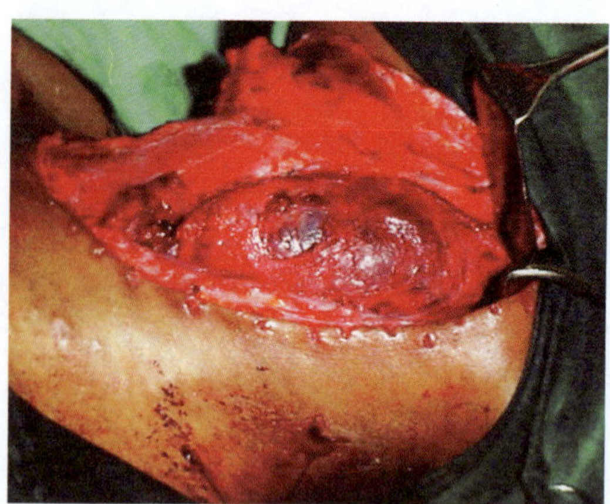

Fig. 34.94: Functional neck dissection—blue nodes of papillary carcinoma thyroid are unmistakable

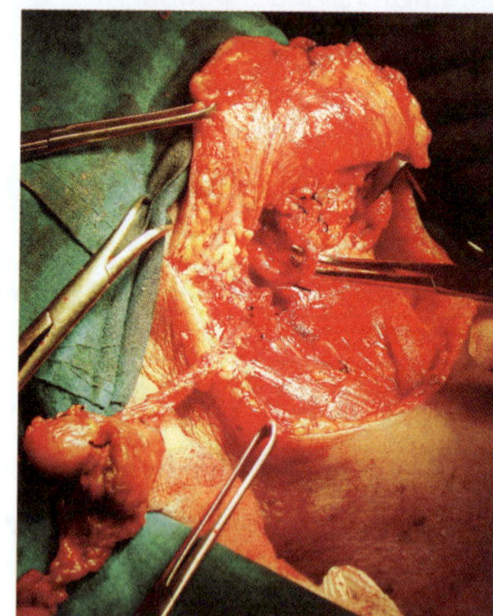

Fig. 34.95: Supraomohyoid neck dissection

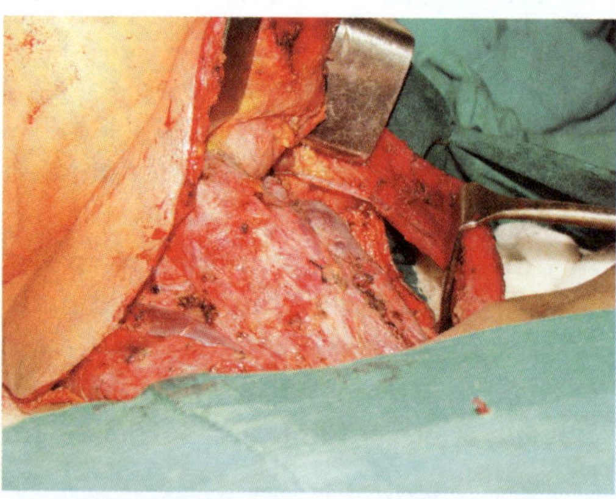

Fig. 34.92: Sternomastoid retracted

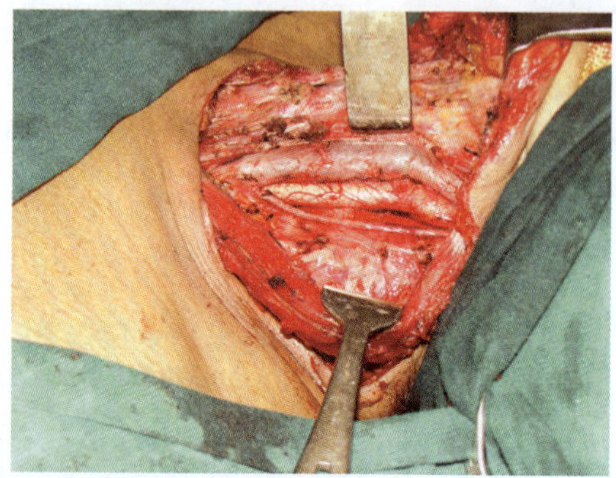

Fig. 34.93: Radical neck dissection

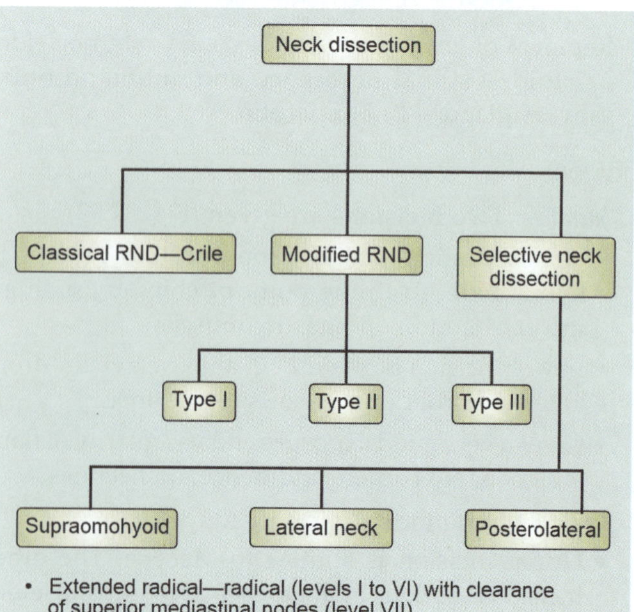

Fig. 34.96: Types of radical neck dissection

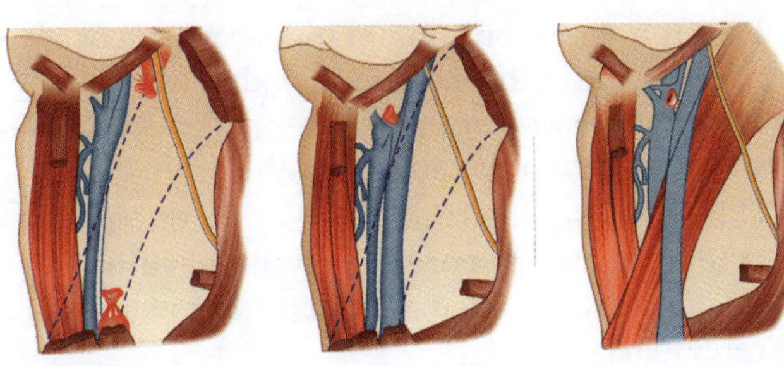

Fig. 34.97: Three types of neck dissections: Radical, modified radical and selective

posterior scalp and neck. Can also be done for thyroid malignancies.

d. **Anterior neck dissection**

- En bloc removal of lymph structures in level VI
- Perithyroidal nodes
- Pretracheal nodes
- Precricoid nodes (Delphian)
- Paratracheal nodes along recurrent nerves

Limits of the dissection are the hyoid bone, suprasternal notch and carotid sheaths.

- Indications
  - Selected cases of thyroid carcinoma
  - Parathyroid carcinoma
  - Subglottic carcinoma
  - Laryngeal carcinoma with subglottic extension
  - Ca of the cervical oesophagus

IV. *Commando's Operation*

RND, hemimandibulectomy with radical glossectomy. It is a very radical and aggressive surgery done for carcinoma tongue.

Investigations

1. **Complete blood picture**
2. **Chest X-ray** can provide the following information:
   - Secondaries in the lungs with cannonball appearance as in cases of malignant melanoma of head and neck.
   - Bronchogenic carcinoma can be suspected by an irregular dense shadow in the peripheral lung fields.
   - Large mediastinal node mass may be seen, with or without tracheal shift.
3. **Biopsy** from clinically obvious lesion (tongue, cheek, lips, etc.).
4. **Triple endoscopy includes**
   - Direct and indirect laryngoscopy
   - Oesophagoscopy
   - Bronchoscopy and biopsy of the suspicious area.
5. **X-ray base of the skull** may show destruction of the bone by the tumour.
6. **CT scan** of the sinuses, or nasopharyngeal area, or skull base to detect a primary growth, its extension, etc.
7. **FNAC** of the lymph nodes can give a diagnosis in more than 90% of the cases, **avoid incision biopsy as it will result in tumour recurrence and wound necrosis.**
8. If primary tumour cannot be detected on endoscopy, a **blind biopsy** is taken from **posterior wall of the fossa of Rosenmüller** and of the **pyriform fossa** on the same side.
9. When aspiration cytology is negative, an excision biopsy is advised as a last resort.

INVESTIGATION AND MANAGEMENT OF THE UNKNOWN PRIMARY WITH METASTASIS IN THE NECK

This is the challenging problem to clinicians to detect primary and to treat the disease. When all investigations fail to come to detect primary, and is called metastasis of unknown origin.

Certain Facts

1. Even though primary is not found initially, rate of emergence of primary tumour is about 3% per year.
2. About 10% of patients are cured of the disease but primary is unknown.
3. About 20–30% of patients who have received complete treatment die sometime later but primary is still unknown.
4. Majority of occult primary nodes are located in level 2 and level 3.
5. Cystic malignant nodes in level 2 can be due to oropharynx as occult primary and **it will be squamous cell carcinoma due to human papillomavirus.**
6. Supraclavicular lymph nodes enlargement is due to a few occult sites, such as bronchogenic carcinoma.
7. Clinical presentation of lymph nodes in the neck can be solid or cystic lesions, or solitary or multiple swellings. The swellings are usually located in level 2, followed by level 3.
8. The clinical N stage at presentation is usually N2a, N2b and N2c. The presence of cystic malignant metastases in level 2 is usually due to human papillomavirus (HPV)-related squamous carcinoma, usually with subclinical primaries in the oropharynx.

Management Principles

1. All patients presenting with confirmed cervical lymph node, metastatic squamous cell carcinoma and no apparent primary site should undergo: **Positron emission tomography–computed tomography whole-body scan.**

2. **Bilateral tonsillectomy:** Few consider this is not necessary because if the lesion is very small-less than 0.5 cm, it will anyhow respond to radiation. So why do tonsillectomy?
3. CECT is done from skull base to diaphragm.
4. **MRI:** If we suspect primary source in the tongue, tonsil, etc. because of level 2/3 lymph node, MRI is done. Extension of tumours in intratemporal fossa can be better appreciated by MRI scan.
5. **Panendoscopy:** This is done to visualise the following sites which cannot be examined clinically
   - Tongue base — Hard palate
   - Tonsils — Soft palate
   - Posterior pharyngeal wall — Vallecula
   - Paranasal sinuses — Post-cricoid fossa
   - Nasopharynx — Pyriform fossa
   - Oral cavity — Glottis, subglottis
6. Performance status should be assessed for major surgery, chemotherapy (ECOG page 681) or radiotherapy.
7. Concomitant chemotherapy with radiation should be considered in patients with an unknown primary. Concomitant chemotherapy with radiation should be offered to suitable patients in the postoperative setting, where indicated.
8. Neoadjuvant chemotherapy can be used in gross 'unresectable' disease.
9. Patients should be followed up at least two months in the first two years and three to six months in the subsequent years.
10. Patients should be followed up to a minimum of five years with a prolonged follow-up for selected patients.
11. Positron emission tomography–computed tomography scan at three to four months after treatment is a useful follow-up strategy for patients treated by chemoradiation therapy.
12. Ultrasound-guided fine needle aspiration (FNA) cytology and/or core biopsy under ultrasound guidance. Most often, the report is squamous cell carcinoma.

Treatment

Surgery is the main principle of treatment for N1 neck nodes.

- If extracapsular spread is present, surgery should be combined with radiotherapy.
- In advance diseases, surgery should be done after chemoradiotherapy.
- Cisplatin is the drug of choice.
- The neck dissection is modified radical neck dissection (MRND) including levels I–V.
- Summary of the treatment is given in Fig. 34.98.

Follow-up

- About 30–40% of treated patients with occult primary with metastatic nodes die with no evidence of the primary later.
- In about 30% of patients, the primary will manifest within 1–2 years time.
- About 10% of patients are **cured** but primary is not detected.

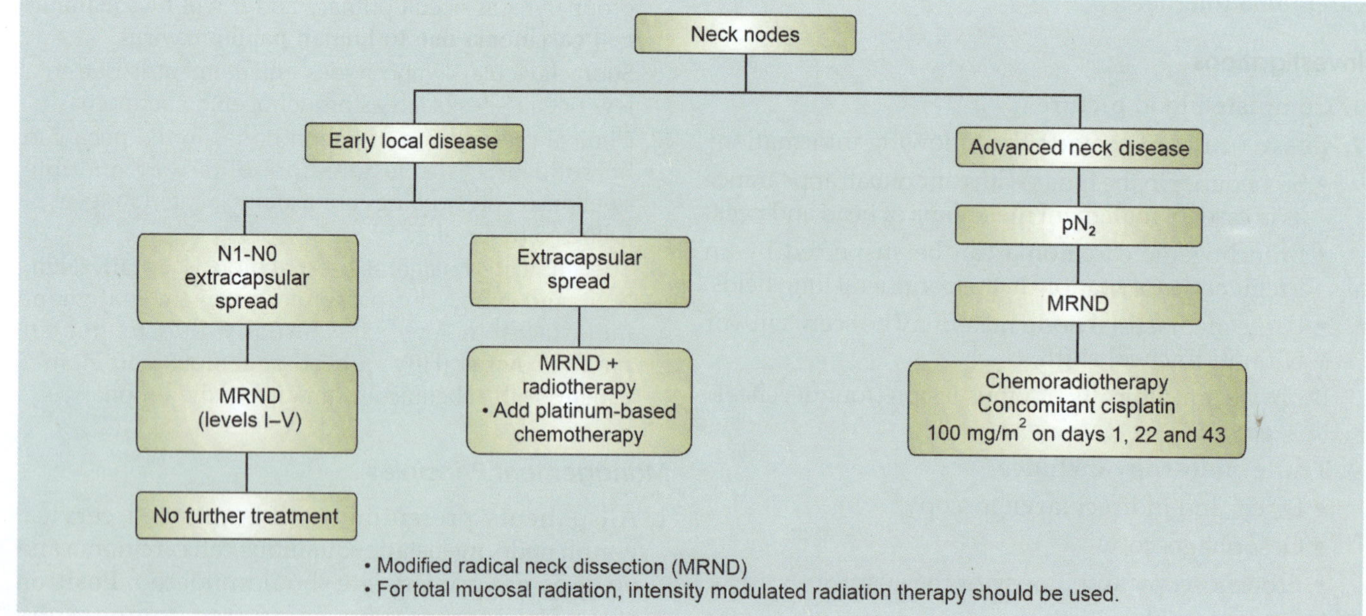

Fig. 34.98: Flowchart showing management of neck nodes

PANCOAST'S TUMOUR

- **Pancoast's tumour** or superior sulcus tumour is a bronchogenic carcinoma arising from the apex of lung.
- Typically, the patient is an elderly male around 70 years, **chronic smoker** who presents with cough, weight loss, dyspnoea and chest pain.
- As the tumour grows, it compresses the **lower roots of brachial plexus C8 and T1** and results in tingling, pain and paraesthesia in the distribution of ulnar nerve.
- The tumour is felt in the lower part of the posterior triangle. It is **hard in consistency, fixed, irregular** and sometimes tender. The lower border of the mass cannot be appreciated.

The Pancoast's syndrome refers to the following components

1. Pancoast's tumour
2. Erosion of the first rib
3. Paralysis of C8 and T1 nerve roots
4. **Horner's syndrome** due to paralysis of cervical sympathetic chain. The preganglionic sympathetic fibres of the head and neck are given from the 1st and sometimes the 2nd thoracic segments of the spinal cord. These nerve fibres synapse with the cells in the three cervical sympathetic ganglia. They give rise to postganglionic fibres to the head and neck region.

Thus, anywhere along this pathway, disruption, damage or infiltration of the nerve roots results in Horner's syndrome. The causes of Horner's syndrome are depicted in Key Box 34.38.

Components of Horner's Syndrome

- Miosis: Small pupil
- Anhidrosis: Absence of sweating.
- Pseudoptosis: Drooping of upper eyelid (Fig. 34.99).
- Enophthalmos: Regression of the eyeball
- Nasal vasodilatation: Nasal congestion

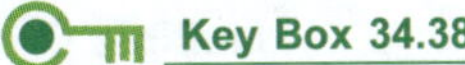

Key Box 34.38

Horner's Syndrome

Common causes

- Posterior inferior cerebellar artery (PICA) thrombosis
- Cervical sympathectomy
- Pancoast's tumour

Uncommon causes

- Syringomyelia
- Injury to lower roots of brachial plexus
- Tumour in the neck
- Aneurysm of carotid artery

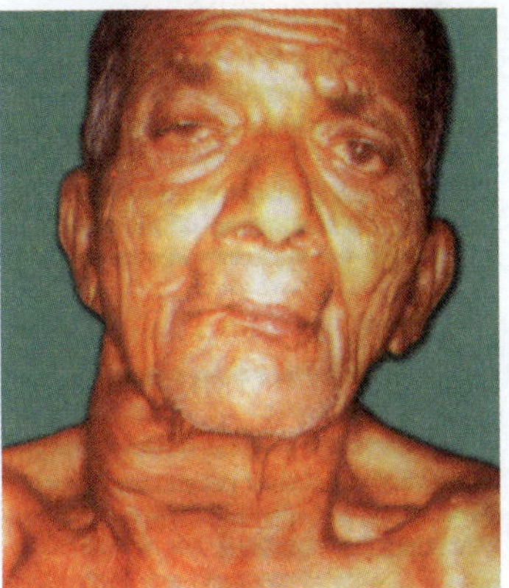

Fig. 34.99: Pseudoptosis due to Pancoast tumour

Investigations

- **Chest X-ray:** May demonstrate a dense mass or collapse of the lobe, etc.
- **CT scan** may demonstrate infiltration of the tumour into ribs or vertebra.
- **Sputum for malignant cells**
- **Flexible bronchoscopy:** Tissue biopsy or sputum sample can be collected.
- **FNAC of the tumour** gives the diagnosis in majority of cases.

Treatment

Palliative radiotherapy. The response rate is poor.

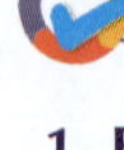

Multiple Choice Questions

1. **Following are true for ranula *except:***
   A. It is a swelling in the floor of the mouth
   B. It is a retention cyst
   C. It is transilluminant
   D. Plunging ranula produces one more swelling in the submental region

2. **Which one of the following does not give rise to cross-fluctuation?**
   A. Iliopsoas abscess
   B. Compound palmar ganglion
   C. Sebaceous cyst
   D. Hydrocele *en bisac*

3. **Following are true for thyroglossal fistula *except:***
   A. Always congenital
   B. It is lined by columnar epithelium
   C. Semilunar sign is seen in adults
   D. Surgery done for this is called Sistrunk's operation

4. **Following are derived/arises from 2nd branchial arch *except:***
   A. Sternocleidomastoid muscle
   B. Branchial cyst
   C. Facial muscles
   D. Anterior belly of the digastric

5. **Which one of the following swellings does not contain cholesterol crystals?**
   A. Branchial cyst
   B. Sebaceous cyst
   C. Dental cyst
   D. Hydrocele

6. **Most important stimulus for carotid body tumour is:**
   A. Hypoxia
   B. Hyperbaric oxygen
   C. Hypothermia
   D. Hypercarbia

7. **Tuberculous cervical spine can give rise to cold abscess in following locations *except:***
   A. Posterior wall of the pharynx in the midline
   B. Behind the carotid sheath
   C. Front of the carotid sheath
   D. Along the anterior primary division of the cervical spinal nerves

8. **Pancoast's tumour has following features *except:***
   A. It is a superior sulcus tumour
   B. It can give rise to Horner's syndrome
   C. It can erode first rib
   D. It is usually resectable

9. **Components of Horner's syndrome are following *except:***
   A. Miosis
   B. Anhydrosis
   C. Pseudoptosis
   D. Exophthalmos

10. **Following organs drain to posterior triangle lymph nodes:**
    A. Adenoids
    B. Thyroid
    C. Retropharynx
    D. Tonsil

11. **Content of sebaceous cyst includes:**
    A. Desquamated epithelial debris
    B. Keratin
    C. Sebum
    D. Pus

Answers

1. D **2.** C **3.** A **4.** D **5.** B **6.** A **7.** C **8.** D **9.** D **10.** D
11. B

CHAPTER

35

Oral Cavity, Odontomes, Lip and Palate

- Oral cancer
- Premalignant conditions
- General principles in the treatment
- Carcinoma of buccal mucosa
- Carcinoma of tongue
- Ulcers of tongue
- Carcinoma of lip
- Carcinoma maxillary antrum
- Nasopharynx—cancer
- Benign lesions in the oral cavity
- Odontomes
- Epulis
- Median mental sinus
- Vincent's angina
- Cleft lip and cleft palate
- Ectopic salivary gland tumour
- Mucous cysts

INTRODUCTION

Oral cavity extends from vermilion junction of lips to junction of hard and soft palate above and the line of circumvalate papillae below or it is bounded by the lips anteriorly, the cheek on each side, tonsils posteriorly, superiorly by the palate and inferiorly by the floor of the mouth. It is lined by squamous epithelium. Oral cavity is a common site of malignancy because it is insulted by various agents such as alcohol, smoking, tobacco chewing. **Oral cancer is the commonest malignant neoplasm** in the **head and neck**. Risk factors are given in Key Box 35.1.

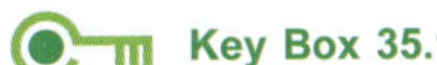

Key Box 35.1

Risk Factors Associated with Cancer of Head and Neck

- **Tobacco quid**[1]—'Pan Masala'
- **O**ropharyngeal Ca—**Plummer-Vinson syndrome**
- **B**arr-Epstein virus
- **Alcohol**, areca nut
- **Cigarette** smoking and reverse smoking[2]
- **Chronic** irritation—dentures
- **O**ral hygiene poor and poor nutrition

Remember as **TOBACCO**

More than 70 to 100 carcinogens have been recognised in the tobacco smoke such as nitrosamines, polycyclic aromatic hydrocarbons, benzene, ammonia, arsenic, butanone, etc.

Competency

SU20.1: Describe etiopathogenesis of oral cancer symptoms and signs of oropharyngeal cancer.

Abuse of tobacco and alcohol are the most common preventable risk factors for development of head and neck cancers. Those who smoke 2 packs/day and drink 4 units of alcohol/day have an odds ratio of 35 for development of carcinoma. Tobacco quid is very dangerous and highly carcinogenic.

An interaction occurs between **redox-active metals in saliva** and **low reactive free radicals in cigarette smoke.** Net result is that saliva loses its **antioxidant** capacity and instead becomes a potent pro-oxidant milieu.

Field cancerisation is a concept based on prolonged exposure of oral and pharyngeal mucosa to carcinogens. 15 to 20% of the survivors of one cancer of head and neck develop another primary head and neck cancer. Oral cavity has many subsites which have been given in Key Box 35.2. Importance of subsites (Fig. 35.1) is related to different methods of management which has been discussed later.

[1]**Betel nut** chewed in combination with lime and cured tobacco is called **'quid'**. It is commonly placed in gingivolabial sulcus. **It is highly carcinogenic.** This type of carcinoma is very common in India called Indian oral cancer.

[2]**Reverse smoking:** Smoking a cheroot with burning end inside mouth. The risk of hard palate carcinoma is 47 times more in these patients.

Key Box 35.2

Oral Cavity Subsites

- Lip
- Lower alveolus
- Oral tongue
- Upper alveolus
- Buccal mucosa
- Retromolar trigone
- Floor of mouth
- Hard palate

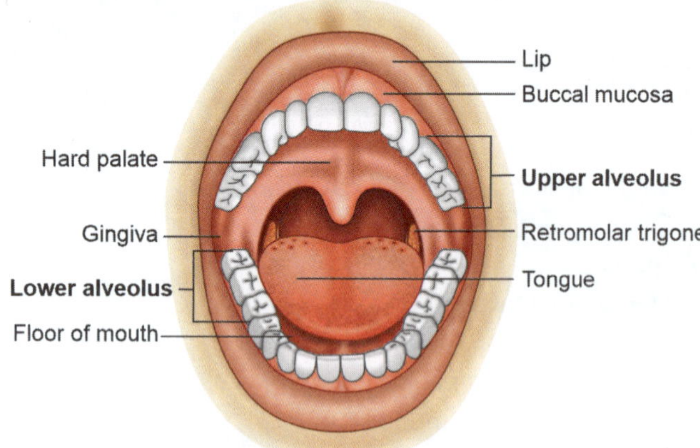

Fig. 35.1: Oral cavity subsites

ORAL CANCER

Incidence of Oral Cancer

- Tongue : 50%
- Cheek : 20–25%
- Floor : 10–15%
- Gums : 10%

Definitions

- **Hyperkeratosis** refers to increase in keratin layers. It occurs due to **constant irritation**. Once the cause is removed, it is **reversible**. It is a microscopic diagnosis.

  For example, smokers' hyperkeratosis of the palate and lips. Once the aetiological agent is withdrawn, the lesion returns back to normal.
- **Leukoplakia** appears clinically as a white patch in the mouth and cannot be scraped off. It is irreversible and not attributable to any known disease. It is important to biopsy leukoplakic portion to rule out malignancy.

Pearls of Wisdom

Sump area or 'Coffin corner' at the posterior tongue/floor of the mouth is a common site for cancer—may be missed on cursory inspection.

PREMALIGNANT CONDITIONS FOR ORAL CANCER

1. Leukoplakia

The causes for leukoplakia are as follows:

- **Smoking** results in hyperkeratosis. Nicotine in the form of cigarettes, chewed tobacco, powdered snuff produces premalignant changes in the oral cavity.
- **Spices**
- **Spirits** have synergistic action with smoking
- **Sharp** tooth, **sepsis**, poor oral hygiene
- **Sunlight** actinic rays
- **Syphilis** causes endarteritis obliterans and results in chronic superficial glossitis of the tongue which is a precancerous condition (rare these days).

Betel nut, and slaked lime with betel leaf and tobacco (pan) is eaten and usually kept inside the cheek for many hours. Over the years, it brings about chronic irritation of mucosa of the cheek and causes leukoplakia. Tobacco contains multiple carcinogens including aromatic hydrocarbons.

Stages in the development of leukoplakia

I. **Keratosis** appears as a milky blush on the surface.
II. **Acanthosis** refers to elongation of rete pegs. This appears as a smooth, white, dry patch—**smooth paint.**
III. **Dyskeratosis** means the formation of keratin cell layer in the deeper aspect of epidermis, before they reach the surface—**like wrinkled paint.**
IV. **Carcinoma *in situ***—*warty.*
V. *Invasive carcinoma.*

Pearls of Wisdom

Speckled leukoplakia appears as multiple, small white patches on an erythematous base. ***It has the highest rate of malignant transformation*** (Figs 35.2 and 35.3).

Treatment of Leukoplakia

- About 10% of leukoplakia patients develop oral cancer. Hence, superficial excision of the lesion followed by skin grafting should be done.
- Even though leukoplakia is irreversible, **isotretinoin** (13-*cis*-retinoic acid) can reverse some cases of leukoplakia and possibly reduce the development of squamous cell carcinoma.

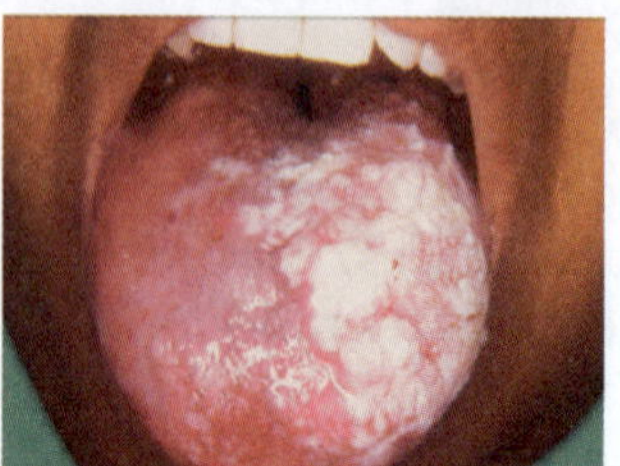

Fig. 35.2: Leukoplakia of the tongue—biopsy was positive for malignancy. He was treated with radiotherapy

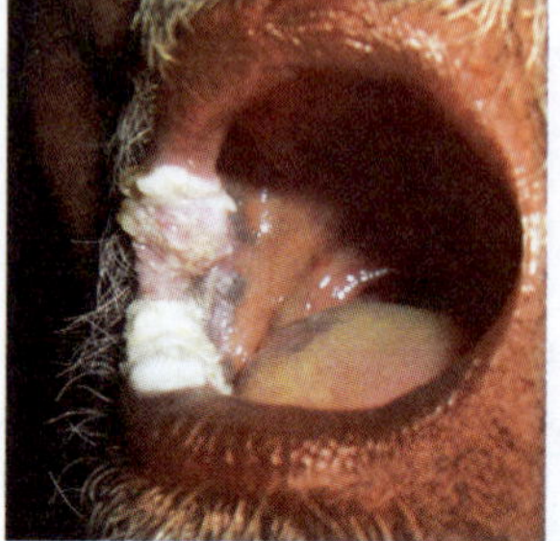

Fig. 35.3: Carcinoma arising from leukoplakia

(*Courtesy:* Dr Keerthilatha Pai, Dean and Professor, Department of Oral Medicine, College of Dental Sciences, Manipal)

2. **Erythroplakia** is a red, velvety lesion with an incidence of malignancy around 15% (17 times more malignant than leukoplakia). It is irregular in outline and may be nodular.
3. **Chronic hyperplastic candidiasis** (Key Box 35.3).

Key Box 35.3

Chronic Hyperplastic Candidiasis (Fig. 35.4)

Commissures of the mouth commonly affected
Albicans Candida invasion
No response to drugs, then surgery/laser treatment
Dense plaques of leukoplakia
Immunodeficiency can precipitate this condition
Dangerous because of malignant potential
Antifungal treatment—Topical application may help
Remember as **CANDIDA**

4. **Submucous fibrosis**
   - This is supposedly due to use of pan masala, arecanut with or without alcohol.
   - Initially it produces ulceration of mucosa of the cheek. These ulcers heal resulting in a dense submucous fibrosis, which appear clinically firm to hard. It can affect the tongue also. It is a progressive disease entirely confined to Asian population.
   - Chances of malignancy are around 10–15%.
   - Mouth opening may be restricted.
   - It is treated by excision with reconstruction.

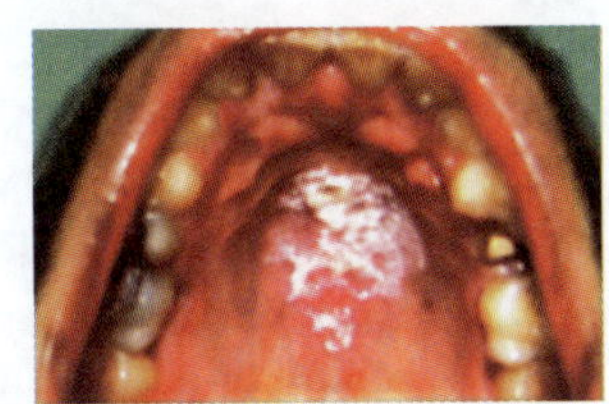

Fig. 35.4: Chronic hyperplastic candidiasis affecting palate

5. **Sideropenic dysphagia** (Plummer-Vinson and Paterson-Kelly syndrome). Iron deficiency occurs in the absence of anaemia in these patients. Common in Scandinavian women. Iron supplements reduce epithelial atrophy.
6. Papilloma of the tongue or cheek
7. Discoid lupus erythematosus
8. **Dyskeratosis congenita**
9. **Syphilitic glossitis:** Tertiary syphilis produces chronic superficial glossitis which can lead to carcinoma of the tongue. However, it is rare these days.
10. Human papillomavirus is an epitheliotropic virus. Its oncoproteins suppress tumour suppressor gene. It can give rise to tonsillar carcinoma and oropharyngeal carcinoma.
11. **Miscellaneous:** Saw dust—sinonasal adenocarcinoma.
    - UV rays—lip cancer
    - Reverse cigarette smoking—palatal cancer.

Upper Aerodigestive Tract Cancers

- Most of them are **squamous cell carcinomas.**
- **Tobacco and alcohol** are the most common aetiological factors.
- Most common premalignant lesion is **leukoplakia.**
- **Multiple anatomic sites** can be involved simultaneously (synchronous).
- **Second primary cancers** develop in 10–15% of cases **(metachronous).**
- Clinical presentation can be **peculiar/misleading** depending on anatomic site.
- **Generous biopsy** and MRI (if necessary) are the investigations of choice.
- Surgery, **radiotherapy and chemotherapy** are used singly or in combination in appropriate cases.

Pearls of Wisdom

Distant metastasis is more common with nasopharyngeal carcinoma than with any other head and neck cancer.

COMMON SYMPTOMS AND SITES (Table 35.1)

Table 35.1 Common symptoms and common sites of oral cancer (Ca: Carcinoma)

Symptom	Site of cancer (Ca)
Pain around the eyes	Nasopharynx
Pain in the ear (otalgia)	Base of tongue, hypopharynx
Hoarseness	Glottis
Trismus	Extension of cancer into pterygoid muscles
Dysphagia	Base of tongue, hypopharynx, oesophagus
Loss of hearing	Auditory canal or nasopharynx

Competency

SU20.2: Enumerate the appropriate investigations and discuss the principles of treatment.

GENERAL PRINCIPLES IN THE MANAGEMENT

Investigations

1. **Wedge biopsy from the edge of the ulcer** is taken because of the following reasons:
   - Tumour cells are concentrated more in the growing edge.

- Centre of the ulcer has slough.
- **Histopathological report** shows squamous cell carcinoma and in majority of the cases it is well-differentiated with keratin pearls.

2. **Orthopantomography:** X-ray of mandible to rule out mandibular involvement (Fig. 35.5A and 35. 5B).
3. **Chest X-ray** to detect inhalation pneumonia.

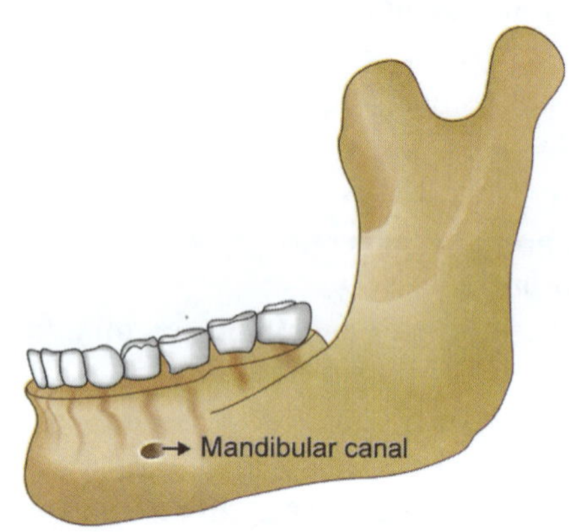

Fig. 35.5A: Mandibular canal in a normal person is well away from occlusive surface

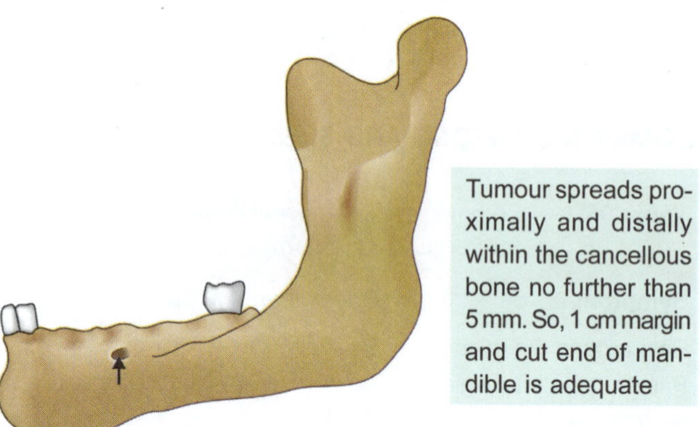

Fig. 35.5B: Mandibular canal in an edentulous patient is close to occlusive surface explaining easy spread in carcinoma buccal mucosa

4. **Ultrasound guided FNAC** of the lymph node.
5. **Magnetic resonance imaging (MRI)**
   - Large advanced lesion can be better assessed by MRI. Soft tissue infiltration can be assessed correctly, thus dictating the extent of resection especially in patients with restricted mouth opening.
   - **It is the investigation of choice to look for involvement of skull base, brachial nerve plexus, bone marrow, spinal nerve roots and lymph nodes.**
   - MRI has no radiation hazards.
6. **CECT** is done when growth is infiltrating mandible.

AJCC—American Joint Committee Cancer staging is followed uniformly while managing these patients.

TNM STAGING — Oral cancer—American Joint Committee Cancer (AJCC)

Primary Tumour (T)

- T0: No evidence of primary tumour
- Tis: Carcinoma *in situ*
- T1: ≤2 cm with DOI (depth of invasion) ≤5 mm
- T2: >2 cm and ≤4 cm with DOI ≤10 mm
- T3: >4 cm with DOI ≤10 mm
- T4: Any cancer invading adjacent structures such as cartilage, cortical bone, deep (extrinsic) muscles of the tongue, skin or soft tissue of the neck.
  T4a: Moderately advanced local disease.
  T4b: Very advanced local disease (skull base, pterygoid plate, internal carotid artery, masticator space)

Regional Lymph Nodes (N)

- Nx: Nodes cannot be assessed
- N0: No lymph node metastasis
- N1: Single positive ipsilateral node less than or equal to 3 cm in greatest dimension
- N2a: Single positive ipsilateral node more than 3 cm but less than or equal to 6 cm
- N2b: Multiple ipsilateral nodes but all less than 6 cm
- N2c: Bilateral or contralateral lymph nodes but all less than 6 cm
- N3: Lymph node more than 6 cm

Distant Metastasis (M)

- M0: No distant metastasis
- M1: Distant metastasis present

Stage Grouping

Stage I	T1, N0, M0
Stage II	T2, N0, M0
Stage III	T3, N0, M0, TI–3, N1, M0
Stage IV	T4, N0, M0 , T, N2–3, M0
	T0, N0, M1

Aim of the Treatment

1. **Cure of the patient:** Cure of the cancer, if possible, with wide excision of the tumour which includes removal of the tumour with 1–2 cm of the normal tissues, with or without bone.
2. **Palliation:** If cure is not possible, palliation should be attempted by surgery or radiotherapy.
3. **Preservation of function** such as swallowing, speech and vision, should also be taken into consideration.
4. **Cosmetic function:** Following wide excision, the cosmetic function must be maintained by reconstruction with myocutaneous/osteomyocutaneous flap.
5. To achieve **minimal mortality and morbidity**.

6. **Metastatic lymph nodes** are treated by neck dissection or curative radiotherapy (RT). Even when nodes are not palpable, follow guidelines given in Key Box 35.4.
7. When nodes are positive—refer to Key Box 35.5.

Key Box 35.4

Clinically 'Node Negative' Neck from Oral Cancer

- Carcinoma lateral tongue, floor of mouth and mandibular alveolus commonly cause occult metastasis.
- Occult metastasis is seen in up to 30% of patients.
- Hence, selective neck dissection of levels I, II and III is indicated in continuity with tumour excision in these cases.

Key Box 35.5

Clinically Node Positive Neck

N1	: Selective supraomohyoid neck dissection
{N2a and N2b}	: Modified radical or radical neck dissection followed by postoperative radiotherapy
N2c	: Bilateral radical neck dissection—preserve at least one internal jugular vein (IJV) + postoperative radiotherapy
N3	: Preoperative radiotherapy, if feasible radical neck dissection later

8. Treatment of advanced tumours—T3 and T4 lesions: These are managed by combination of surgery with postoperative RT. **Usually, surgery is the principal therapeutic modality of treatment followed by postoperative radiotherapy**. The treatment depends upon general condition of the patient, risks of anaesthesia, adequate intensive care management, etc. Chemotherapy also has been tried before or after surgery. However, response rate has improved but it has not affected the survival.

- These are guidelines only, individualise the treatment.

Flowchart showing treatment of primary tumour and metastasis is shown in Figs 35.6 and 35.7.

Role of Chemotherapy in Head and Neck Cancers

- The most important benefit of chemotherapy has been in the treatment of laryngeal and nasopharyngeal carcinomas.
- **Cisplatin** is clearly the most effective drug. Other drugs such as carboplatin, 5-fluorouracil (5-FU), bleomycin, gemcitabine, etc. are also used.
- **Induction chemotherapy:** In advanced cases, chemotherapy is given before surgery or RT. In more than 80% of cases, tumour regression can occur.
- **Concurrent chemoradiotherapy** (CCRT): It improves both local and regional controls, specially in those patients with high risk cancers, e.g. locally advanced cancers of the oral cavity, larynx, oropharynx. Drug

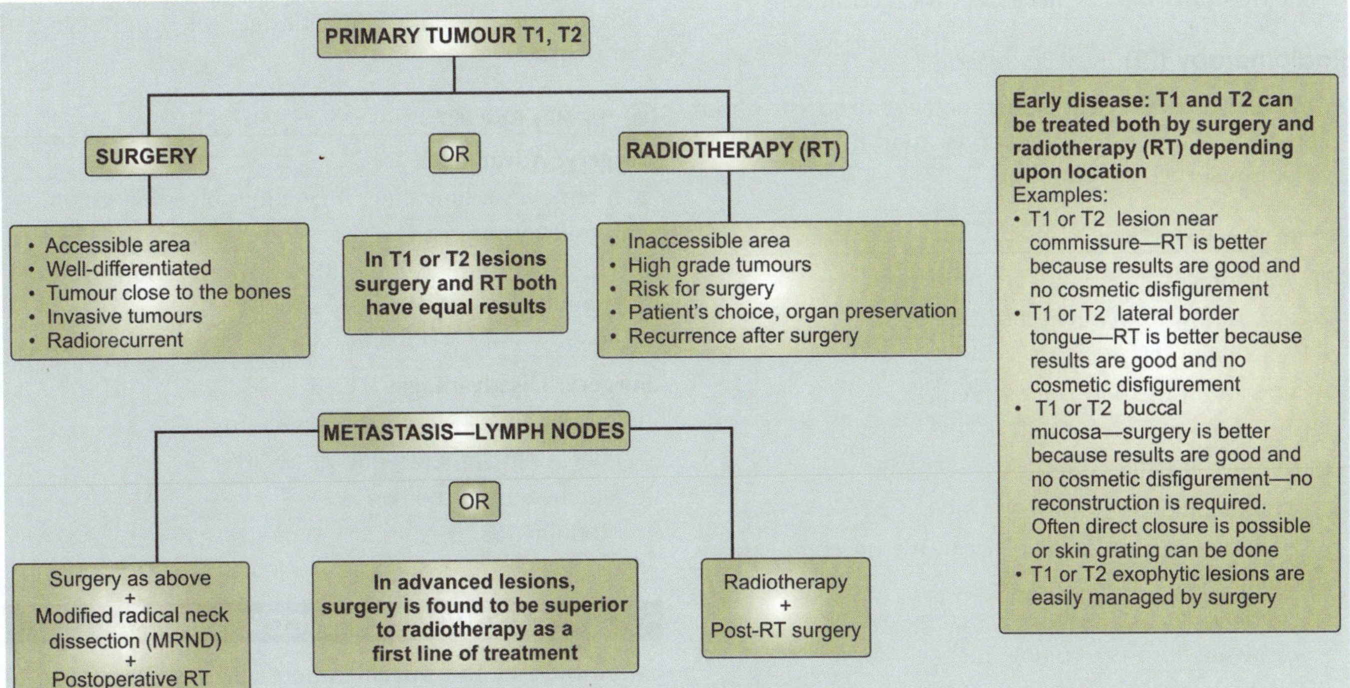

Fig. 35.6: Treatment of primary tumour and metastasis

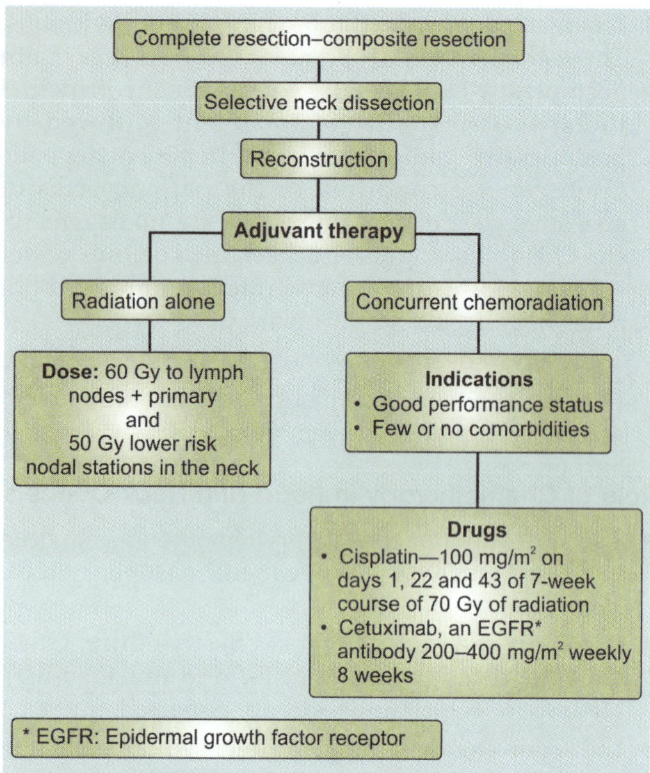

Fig. 35.7: Management of locally advanced nonmetastatic disease (III to IVB)

used in CCRT can be high dose cisplatin—100 mg/m^2 IV for 3 cycles every 21 days concomitantly with RT (for other dosage, kindly *refer* to oncology manual). Side effects include severe mucositis, xerostomia. Gastrostomy may be necessary for feeding.

Radiotherapy (RT) (Key Box 35.6)

- Irradiation of the oral cancers achieves a cure in about 80–90% of patients. It preserves anatomical part and also preserves the function.

Key Box 35.6

RT: Advantages

- Easy, safe with minimal mortality
- Preservation of an organ
- Function of the part is preserved
- Cure rate is around 80–90%
- First line in early cases

RT: Disadvantages

- Long stay in the hospital (can also be taken as an outpatient)
- Tumour cure cannot be assessed by pathology
- Soft tissue fibrosis resulting in ankylostomia
- Adverse effects on skin, loss of hair, mucositis of oral cavity, xerostomia, etc.

- **The dose of RT:** 6500–7500 cGy units are required to eradicate squamous cell carcinoma of head and neck. It is usually given in the daily dose of 180–200 cGy units.
- Radiotherapy is given in T1 and T2 lesions as the first line of treatment and postoperatively in T3 and T4 lesions after surgery.

Role of Surgery (Key Box 35.7)

- Surgery is done in all stages of oral cancers. It may be in the form of wide excision or **wide excision with removal of the bone (composite resection).** In advanced stages it may be palliative surgery such as excision of a fungating, ulcerating, bleeding mass. Surgery is also done for the lymph nodes in the form of radical neck dissection (RND), or modified RND.
- **The pectoralis major myocutaneous flap** (PMMC flap)**:** It is the most widely used flap for the reconstruction of oral cancers.

Indications for Surgery

- Early disease, bulky disease
- Tumour involving mandibular alveolus
- Tumour invading bone
- Advanced disease
- Fungating and bleeding lesion
- Radiorecurrence
- Multiple tumours
- Extensive premalignant changes of oropharyngeal mucosa.

Key Box 35.7

Surgery: Advantages

- It removes a fungating, ulcerating, bleeding lesion
- It relieves the pain
- The specimen is available for histopathological examination for cancer clearance
- 80–90% cure is possible

Surgery: Disadvantages

- Loss of an organ—total glossectomy
- Functional and cosmetic disability
- Significant morbidity
- Mortality: 8–10%

CARCINOMA OF BUCCAL MUCOSA

Carcinoma of the buccal mucosa is very common in India due to the habit of keeping **tobacco quid** in the cheek pouch (gingivoalveolar sulcus).

Pathological Types

1. A **nonhealing** ulcer, with slough in the centre of the lesion.
2. An **exophytic growth**, or a proliferative growth—verrucous carcinoma.
3. An **infiltrative lesion** slowly involves the adjacent structures such as tongue, mandible, floor of the mouth and skin. Skin infiltration results in orocutaneous fistula.

Competency

SU20.1: Describe etiopathogenesis of oral cancer symptoms and signs of oropharyngeal cancer.

Clinical Features

Clinical examination should be thorough—not just visible oral mucosa but also inside and outside of the lip, examine gums by pulling away the lips, retromolar trigone, etc.

- A **nonhealing ulcer** or cauliflower-like growth. Verrucous carcinoma is an exophytic growth.
- **Edges are everted** (Fig. 35.8) with induration at the base as well as at the edge. **Induration** clinically presents as a hard feeling. Pathologically, it is due to fibrosis, caused by malignancy (carcinomatous fibrosis). It is a diagnostic feature of squamous cell carcinoma. Possibly, it is a host reaction indicating good immunity. Due to fibrosis, some lymphatics get obliterated. This delays spread of the disease, thereby improving the prognosis.
- Proliferative lesions are often verrucous carcinoma (Key Box 35.8).

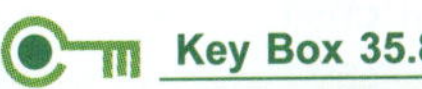

Key Box 35.8

Peculiarities of Verrucous Carcinoma

- Very slow-growing
- Growth is exophytic (than infiltrative)
- Rarely spreads by lymphatics
- It is a well-differentiated carcinoma
- Surgery is the treatment of choice

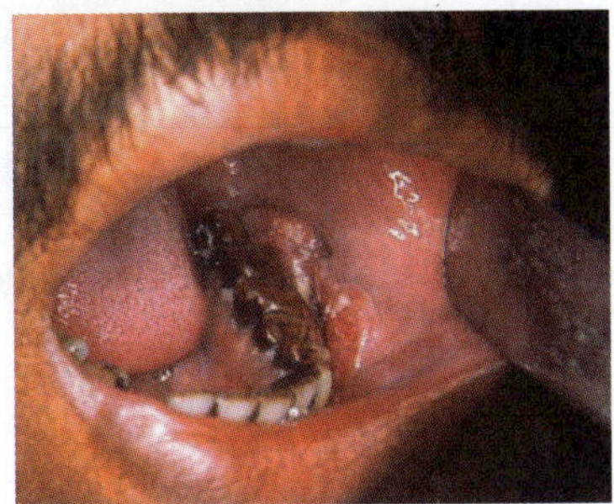

Fig. 35.8: Carcinoma alveolar margin. Look at teeth stains—everted edge

- Ulcer **bleeds on touch**. Due to secondary infection most of the oral cancers are tender to touch (Fig. 35.9).
- **Fixity** to the underlying structures such as mandible may be present.
- **Surrounding area** may also show **induration**.
- Evidence of **leukoplakia** may be present in the oral cavity.
- **Trismus** is due to involvement of pterygoid muscles and masseter. This occurs when carcinoma buccal mucosa **extends into the retromolar trigone**. Trismus can also be due to soft tissue fibrosis caused by radiation. **Once perineural lymphatics are involved, spread can occur in infratemporal fossa resulting in trismus** (Key Box 35.9).
- Retromolar trigone is triangular space behind the third molar tooth with base above. It is over the mucous membrane over the ascending ramus of the mandible.
- **Halitosis** is very characteristic.
- Assessment of fixity to mandible: Severe pain over the jaw indicates periostitis.

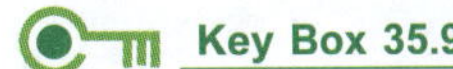

Key Box 35.9

Trismus

Difficulty in opening the mouth is called trismus. Normal mouth opening ranges from 35 to 45 mm.

Grades

- Grade I: Mouth opening is between 2.5 and 4 cm
- Grade II: Between 1 and 2.5 cm
- Grade III: Less than 1 cm

Common causes of trismus

1. Temporomandibular joint involvement—such as ankylosis, dislocation, synovitis, etc.
2. Mandible fractures
3. Pterygoid muscle infiltration by growth in the retromolar region
4. Acute inflammatory lesions in the oral cavity
5. Tetanus and tetany
6. Radiation fibrosis of soft tissues/muscles of mastication

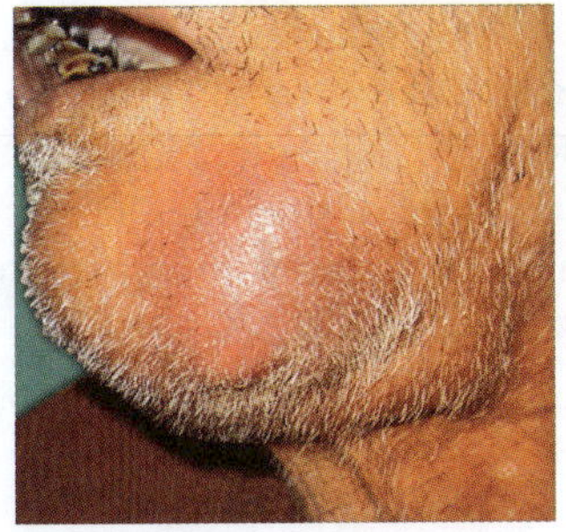

Fig. 35.9: Carcinoma buccal mucosa infiltrating skin—'warning' of fistula

- **Bidigital palpation of mandible** is done by examining with index finger on the outer aspect of the mandible and the thumb on the under surface of the mandible. This test should be done on the opposite side first. Only then, the thickening of the mandible can be appreciated.
- **Gingival cancers** (Fig. 35.10)
  - Early cases present as mucosal change in leukoplakia
  - Loosening of tooth may be a presenting feature.
  - Can present as bleeding and pain
  - Bone involvement occurs early
  - Spread to adjacent structures occurs early.

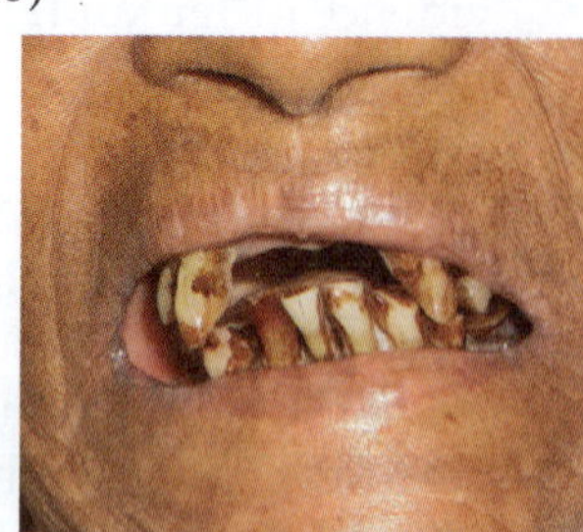

Fig. 35.10: Carcinoma buccal mucosa infiltrating mandible—severe trismus. Also observe tobacco stains

Spread

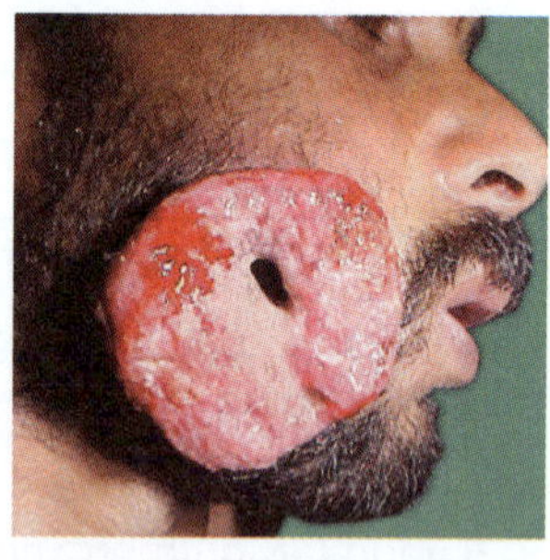

Fig. 35.11: Carcinoma cheek with orocutaneous fistula

1. **Local spread:** Once it involves the entire thickness of the cheek it results in orocutaneous fistula (Figs 35.8 and 35.11). Involvement of mandible results in sinus (Key Box 35.10).
2. **Lymphatic spread:** Submandibular nodes and upper deep cervical nodes get enlarged (levels I and II). In 50% of cases, lymph node enlargement is due to infection and remaining 50%, it is due to metastasis. Metastatic deposits are hard in consistency, indurated and with or without fixity. Significant oedema of face can occur due to lymphatic spread.
3. **Blood spread:** It is very rare and it occurs late.
4. **Perineural spread** along inferior alveolar nerves may occur up to the skull base. In such cases frozen section may be required.

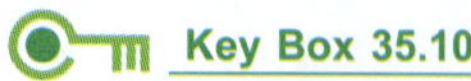

Key Box 35.10

Carcinoma Buccal Mucosa and Mandible

- Direct infiltration by the tumour
- Through mandibular canal
- Through periodontal membrane
- Orthopantomogram or spiral CT can be used for imaging
- Loss of central part of mandible results in pouting of lower lip and continuous drooling of saliva. It is called **Andy Gump deformity**[1]

[1]**Andy Gump** was one of the characters in a popular comic strip, 'The Gumps' created by Sidney Smith in 1917. The character's face seems to end at the upper lip due to 'absence of mandible' and is chinless. A statue of this comic character is on display at Lake Geneva Museum

Pearls of Wisdom

The mandibular canal is close to occlusive surface, in edentulous elderly patients due to decrease in the vertical height of horizontal ramus, thus facilitating easy spread **(Figs 35.11A and B)** of oral cancer to mandible.

Treatment of Carcinoma Buccal Mucosa

It can be classified into early disease and advanced disease.

Early Disease

Two modalities are given in Key Box 35.11.

I. Surgery

1. A small **superficial ulcer** (T1, T2) is treated by wide excision followed by split skin graft (SSG).
2. An **infiltrative lesion** is treated with wide excision followed by a flap reconstruction. Usually, PMMC, flap (pectoralis major myocutaneous flap) is used.
   PMMC flap: This is the most widely used flap now for head and neck reconstruction. The flap is raised along with muscle and an island of skin based on pectoral branch of thoracoacromial artery. It is tunnelled under the skin of chest wall and neck and brought to the area of the defect. It has been described as the **'workhorse'** for head and neck reconstruction.
   - **Radial artery based flap** is the **workhorse of microvascular reconstruction.**

Key Box 35.11

Early Carcinoma Buccal Mucosa

- T1, T2 lesions—surgery/RT
- T1 lesion near commissure—RT
- T2—exophytic and superficial—RT
- T2—deep—surgery is better
- Early disease—no nodes—surgery is better—no other treatment is necessary
- Early disease—positive lymph nodes—same modality to be used for primary and secondary

II. Radiotherapy

As mentioned earlier, early lesions can be managed with radiotherapy (RT). The advantage of RT is that it cannot only cure the disease but also preserve the organ and its function.

Indications for radiotherapy

(1) Patient not willing for surgery, (2) patient not fit for surgery, (3) T1 and T2 lesions and (4) lesion near the commissure.

Types

1. **External radiotherapy:** Large total dose of 6000–8000 cGy units are given at the rate of 200 cGy units/day.
2. **Interstitial radiotherapy** is indicated in infiltrative small lesions. Caesium 137 or iridium wires are placed within the tumour. Advantage of this method is minimal tissue reaction.

Advanced Carcinoma Buccal Mucosa

(Figs 35.12 and 35.13)

Surgery: T3 and T4 lesions require surgery as the main modality of the treatment followed by postoperative radiotherapy. Most of the lesions require full thickness resection leaving behind large defects. Such defects can be repaired using myocutaneous flap.

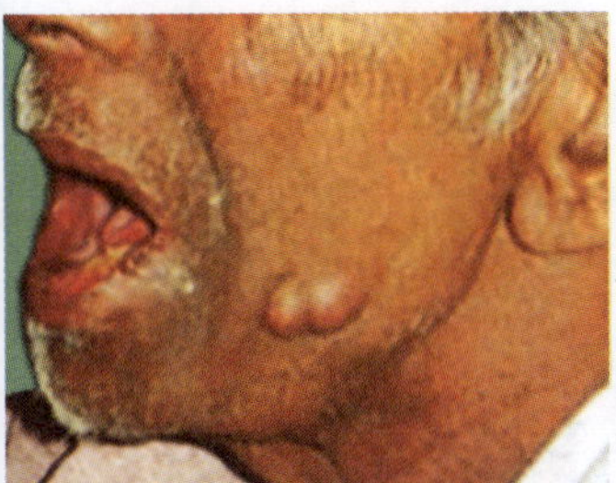

Fig. 35.12: Carcinoma cheek with infiltration into the skin and mandible—locally advanced. Good case for **composite resection**

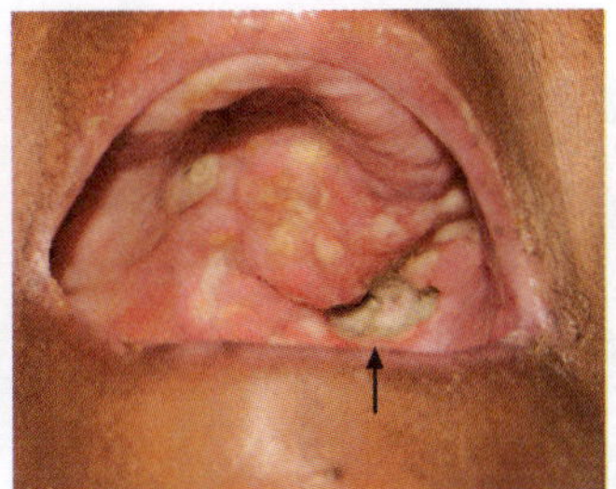

Fig. 35.13: Carcinoma alveolus—excavating ulcer with slough, infiltrating retromolar trigone. RT followed by surgery is the ideal choice of treatment

Pearls of Wisdom

When the primary lesion is removed *en bloc* with mandible and cervical lymph nodes, it is called composite resection.

Examples of Surgeries

1. **Carcinoma buccal mucosa fixed to the mandible:** Wide excision of the growth along with segmental resection of the man-dible or hemimandi-bulectomy is done depending upon the infiltration of the tumour. Very often, whole thickness of the cheek is lost which is reconstructed by using PMMC flap.

Types of Mandibulectomy

A. **Segmental mandibulectomy** (Fig. 35.14)

Indications

- Clinical and radiological involvement of bone
- To obtain wide margins
- To facilitate reconstruction when one has to use 'bulky' PMMC flap
- Excision of full thickness of cheek.

B. **Marginal mandibulectomy:** It can be done for carcinoma floor of the mouth or tongue. This involves removal of either inner or outer table of the mandible or excising the superior rim of the mandible. **However, in large lesions, it is better not to do marginal mandibulectomy.**

C. **Hemimandibulectomy:** Very advanced lesion may necessitate removal of mandible.

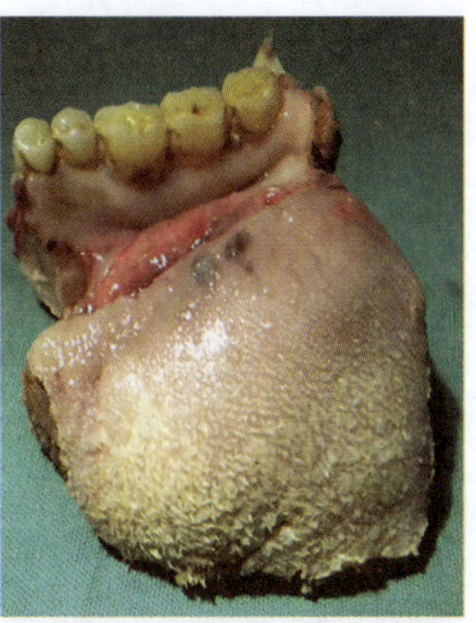

Fig. 35.14: Segmental mandibulectomy. (*Courtesy:* Dr Somshekhar, Head, Department of Surgical Oncologist, Manipal Hospital, Bangalore

Various methods of reconstruction of mandible following excision

• Soft tissue	: PMMC flap
• Soft tissue with bone	: 2.4 mm reconstruction alloplastic material plate and PMMC flap
• Nonvascularised bone grafts	: Titanium tray and cancellous chips from iliac crest
• Vascularised bone grafts	: Fibula, iliac crest

2. **Orocutaneous fistula** is treated by wide excision which refers to removal of the entire thickness of the cheek along with the growth.

   Reconstruction is done by using PMMC flap. Radiotherapy should not be given as it results in persistence of fistula.
3. **Carcinoma of the buccal mucosa with lymph nodes:** Along with the primary, submandibular nodes and upper deep cervical nodes (levels I, II and III) are removed, along with submandibular salivary gland. This is called supraomohyoid block dissection. If surgery has been used to treat the primary, the lymph nodes also should be treated by surgery in the form of neck dissection.
4. **Carcinoma of buccal mucosa with fixed lymph nodes: Both primary lesion and lymph nodes should be treated by radiotherapy** and reassessment done after 3–4 weeks. If residual glands persist or if the glands become mobile, neck dissection can be done at a later date. Fixity to internal jugular vein and sternocleidomastoid muscle are not contra-indications for radical block dissection. Those structures can be removed. However, when the lymph nodes are fixed to the carotid artery, radiotherapy is preferred.

STEPS OF PECTORALIS MAJOR MYOCUTANEOUS FLAP (PMMC FLAP) (Figs 35.15 to 35.21)

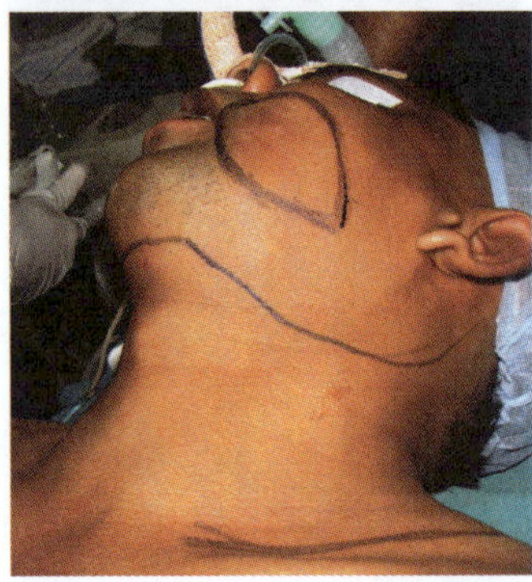

Fig. 35.15: Amount of tissue to be removed (wide excision) is marked. Horizontal incision is given in the neck for block dissection

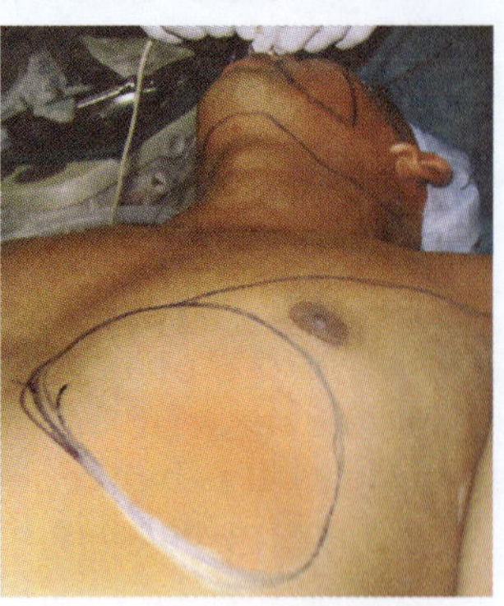

Fig. 35.16: Skin paddle outlined prior to elevation

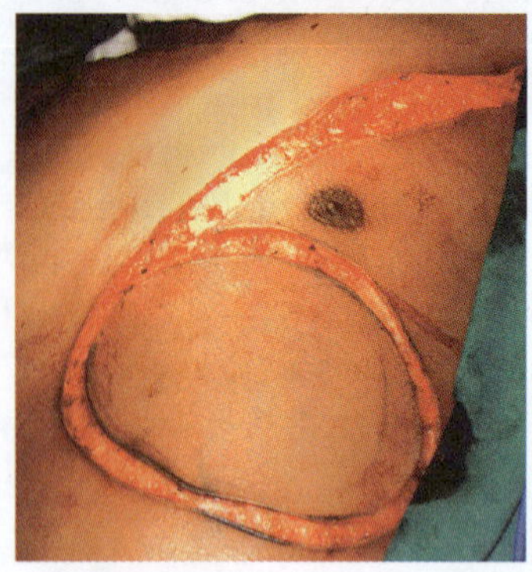

Fig. 35.17: Skin paddle mobilised

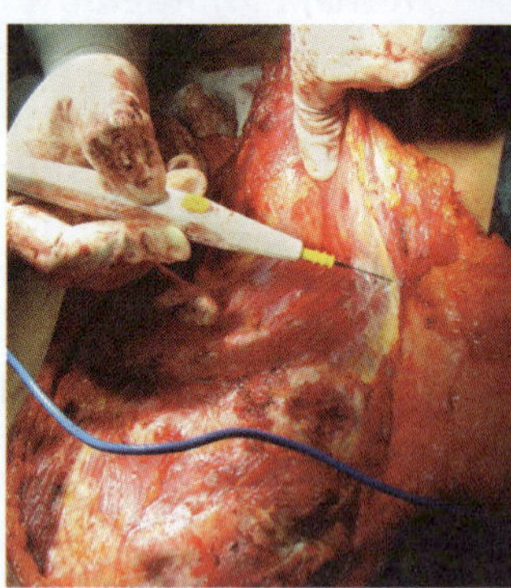

Fig. 35.18: Flap being turned out (bipedaled) to provide inner and outer lining for the tissue loss

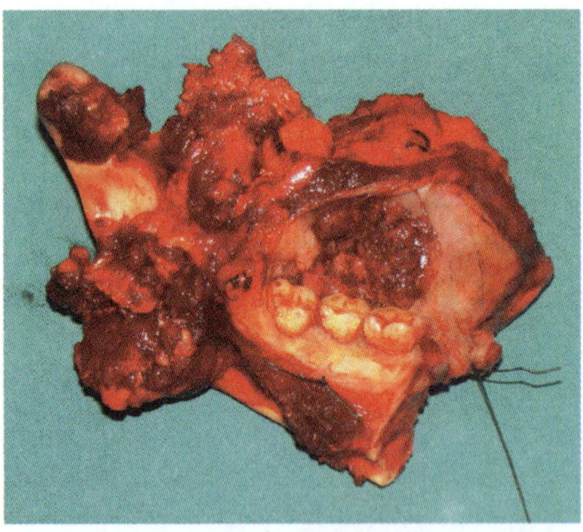

Fig. 35.19: Composite resection: Inner aspect

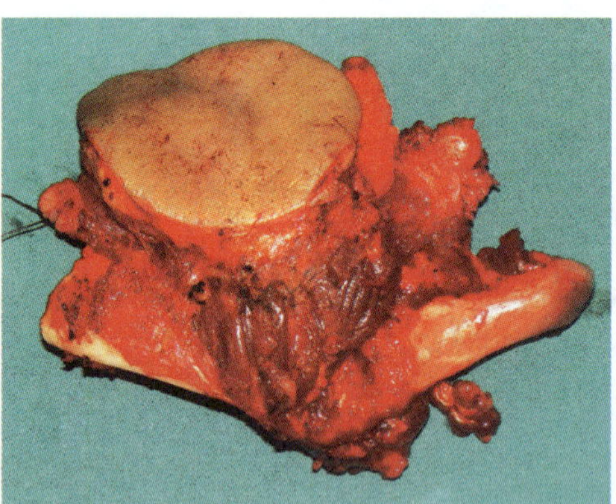

Fig. 35.20: Composite resection: Outer aspect

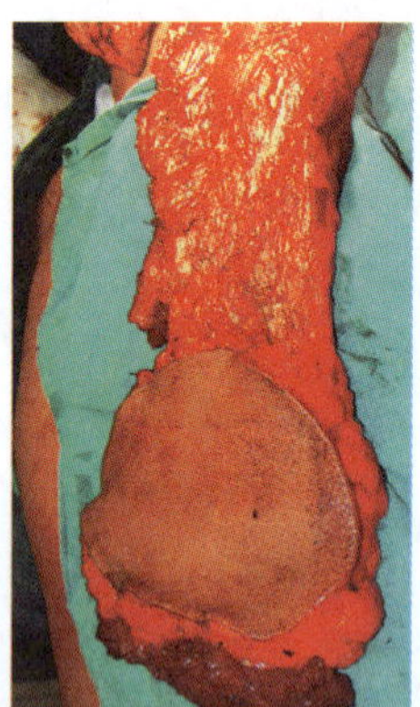

Fig. 35.21: Completely mobilised PMMC flap ready for reconstruction. Main vessels in the paddle are **pectoral branches of acromiothoracic artery.** Mandible reconstruction is not mandatory

(*Courtesy*: Dr Satadru Ray, former Professor and Head, Department of Surgical Oncology, KMC, Manipal)

Prophylactic Neck Dissection

- It is advocated in T3 and T4 lesions irrespective of nodal status. This amounts to minimal supraomohyoid neck dissection with removal of levels I, II and III lymph nodes. It has shown survival benefits.
- It is also indicated in carcinoma mandibular alveolus or buccal mucosa extending into the floor of the mouth.

Complications of Carcinoma Buccal Mucosa

1. Orocutaneous fistula
2. Trismus: It can be due to direct infiltration of pterygoid muscles or masseter or soft tissue fibrosis following RT.
3. Recurrent respiratory tract infection
4. Cancer cachexia

CARCINOMA OF TONGUE

Pathological Types

1. Nonhealing ulcer, commonly on lateral border of tongue in 60% of cases, with slough (Fig. 35.22)
2. A proliferative growth, with everted edge
3. Frozen tongue or indurated variety (Fig. 35.23)

   In this variety, there is maximum induration and sometimes it is more than the size of tumour. The tongue is converted into a hard woody "mass".
4. ***Fissure variety:*** The tongue is indurated with deep fissure.

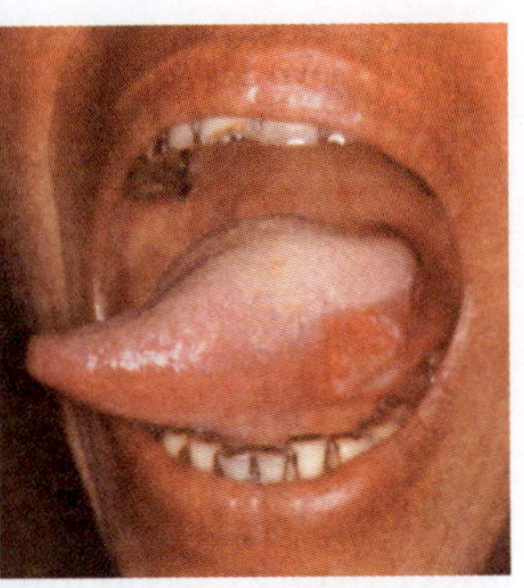

Fig. 35.22: Carcinoma tongue lateral border—the most common site

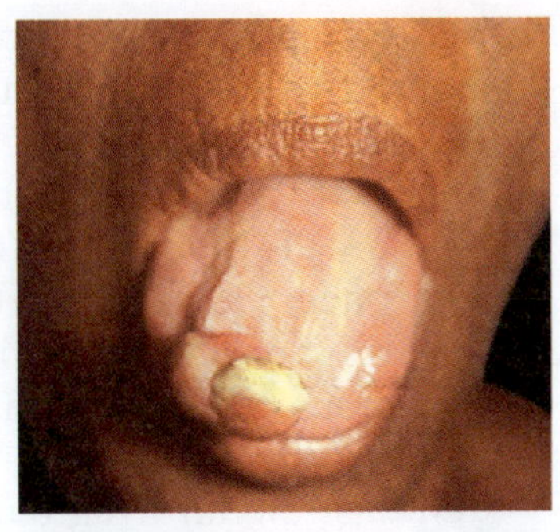

Fig. 35.23: Frozen tongue—ankyloglossia and dysphagia are present

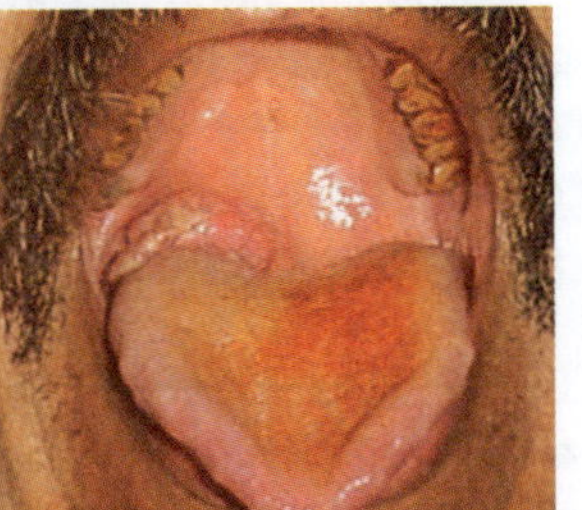

Fig. 35.24: Carcinoma posterior 1/3rd easily missed

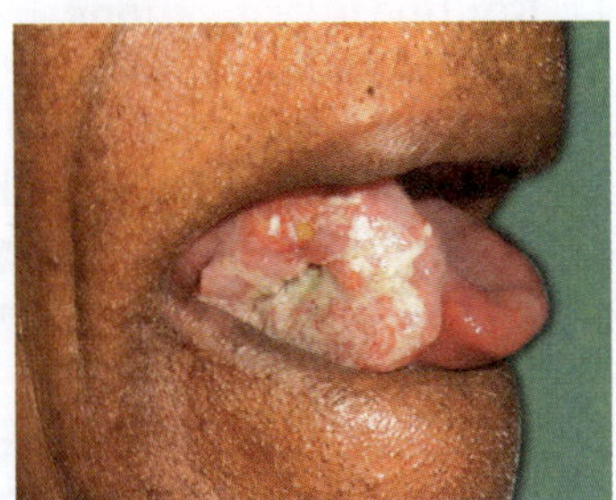

Fig. 35.25: Carcinoma tongue—excavating ulcer

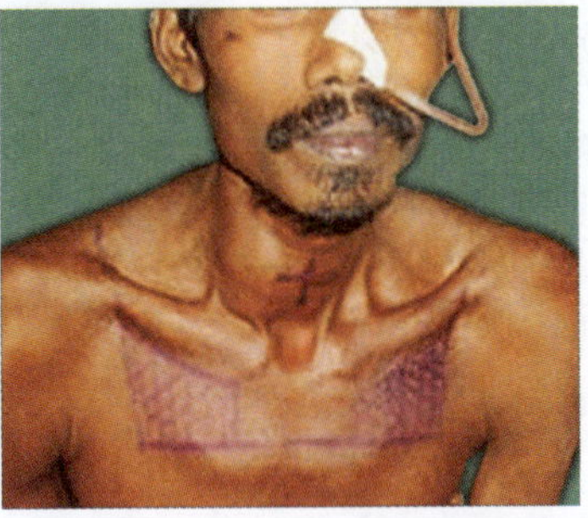

Fig. 35.26: Carcinoma tongue with absolute dysphagia, fixed lymph nodes in the neck and involvement of mediastinal lymph nodes-receiving radiotherapy—on Ryle's tube feeding

Clinical Presentation

- A bleeding ulcer non-healing and progressive
- Pain in the tongue is due to involvement of lingual nerve. In such cases, pain from the tongue can be referred to the ear and lower temporal region.[1]
- **Ankyloglossia** is restricted mobility of the tongue. It is due to infiltration of the floor of the mouth or mandible, or due to an advanced lesion (Figs 35.24 to 35.26).
- **Disarticulation**—difficulty in talking is due to inability of the tongue to move freely.
- **Dysphagia** is a common presentation from carcinoma of posterior 1/3rd (in 20% of cases). An elderly gentleman sitting in the outpatient department spitting blood-stained saliva is suggestive of carcinoma posterior 1/3rd of the tongue.
- **Foetor oris** is due to infected necrotic growth.
- **Bilateral massive enlargement** of lower deep cervical nodes in an elderly patient is suggestive of carcinoma of posterior 1/3rd. The patient may not be aware of growth at all.

Pearls of Wisdom

Tongue cancers tend to be more rapid in their onset than other cancers in the oral cavity. Compared with other cancers within the oral cavity, tongue cancers have greater potential of lymph node metastasis.

Clinical Examination

- Inspection and palpation of the growth or the ulcer should be described in the same manner as that of carcinoma cheek. Typically, the ulcer bleeds on touch with central slough. The edge, base and surrounding area are indurated. Carcinoma of the tongue and carcinoma of the penis are two places in the body wherein induration can be much more extensive than the primary growth or an ulcer. In some cases, induration may be the only finding. Everted edge is commonly seen (Figs 35.22 to 35.26).
- Digital palpation of posterior 1/3rd of tongue should be done with a glove.
- **Test for mobility of the tongue.**
  - **Forward** protrusion—**genioglossus**. This is the muscle commonly involved.
  - **Backward** movement—**styloglossus**
  - **Elevation—palatoglossus**
  - **Depression—hyoglossus**

  All these muscles are supplied by hypoglossal nerve except palatoglossus which is supplied by glossopharyngeal nerve.
- **Bidigital palpation** of the mandible should be done which may show thickening.

Lymphatic Spread (Fig. 35.27)

1. **Apical vessels** drain the tip of the tongue into submental lymph nodes, bilaterally.
2. **Lateral vessels** drain into submandibular lymph nodes, from here to the lower deep cervical lymph nodes and jugulo-omohyoid nodes—level III.
3. **Central vessels** drain into submandibular nodes.
4. **Basal vessels** drain the posterior 1/3rd of the tongue. There is criss-crossing of the lymphatics on both sides. Hence, they drain into bilateral lower deep cervical lymph nodes.

[1]Auriculotemporal nerve and lingual nerve are posterior branches of mandibular division of trigeminal nerve.

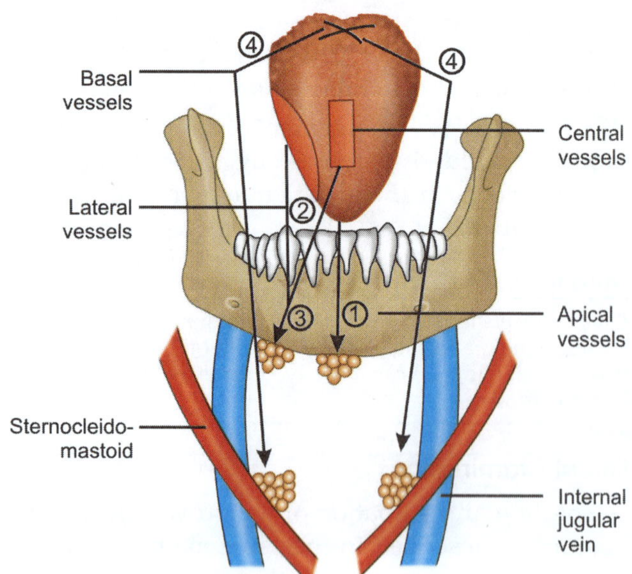

Fig. 35.27: Lymphatic drainage of the tongue—see text for numbers

- In 50% of cases, the lymph node enlargement is due to secondary infection. Such nodes are tender and firm and respond to antibiotics. In remaining cases, they are hard and fixed and hence, significant. However, in all such cases of lymph node enlargement, ultrasound guided FNAC is done.

Pearls of Wisdom

Posterior 1/3rd of tongue has very less cornification but has abundant lymphatics which explains massive nodes **(Key Box 35.12).**

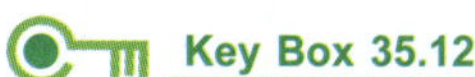

Key Box 35.12

Carcinoma Posterior 1/3rd

- It presents with **dysphagia** or with a change in voice.
- **Easily missed** in a clinical examination
- **Biopsy** should be done under **general anaesthesia** to avoid aspiration and to assess the spread posteriorly.
- Palpation will give the diagnosis—induration
- It is one of the **occult primaries** for lymph node secondaries in the neck.
- Criss-crossing of the lymphatics explain **bilateral lymph** nodes in the neck.
- **Blood spread** is more common.
- Prognosis is **bad** because well-differentiated carcinoma in this location is rare.

Investigations

1. **Wedge biopsy from edge of the ulcer** can be taken under local anaesthesia. In cases of **proliferative growth, punch biopsy is recommended.** In cases of growth arising from posterior 1/3rd of the tongue, biopsy can be taken under general anaesthesia. It also provides an opportunity to examine in detail the posterior spread of the disease into tonsils, pharynx, etc. Biopsy is done to confirm the diagnosis, to know the grade of the tumor (Broder's classification page 256) and depth of invasion. More the keratin pearls means it is well-differentiated squamous cell carcinoma.
2. **Orthopantomogram:** X-ray of the mandible can demonstrate an irregular defect due to **invasion, erosion** or **pathological fracture.**
3. **Chest X-ray** is taken to rule out **aspiration** or **inhalation pneumonia.**
4. **Routine investigations** such as complete blood picture, fasting and postprandial sugar estimation to rule out diabetes and electrocardiography to assess cardiovascular function should be done. These patients will undergo often combined modalities specially in advanced stages. ECOG criteria should be calculated.
5. Tongue lesions respond well to surgery and to decide partial or hemiglossectomy MRI is the ideal investigation.

Treatment

Carcinoma of the tongue is managed similar to a cancer in the oral cavity. However, to preserve the function of the tongue, widespread disease in the posterior one-third tumours, general health of patient (elderly with bad bronchopneumonia) may decide the treatment in favour of radiotherapy. However, results of surgery or radiotherapy for early carcinoma of tongue are equivalent.

Various Types of Surgery

1. **Carcinoma *in situ*:** This type is uncommon in our country. Wide excision with 1 cm margin and a depth of 1 cm is sufficient. Reconstruction of the tongue is not necessary.
2. **Partial glossectomy** is indicated when the lesion is less than 2 cm (T1) and confined to the lateral border of the tongue. The principle is to do wide excision. The wide excision should include at least 2 cm of tissue away from the palpable indurated edge of the tumour (Figs 35.28 to 35.30).
   - Alternatively, radiotherapy can be given.

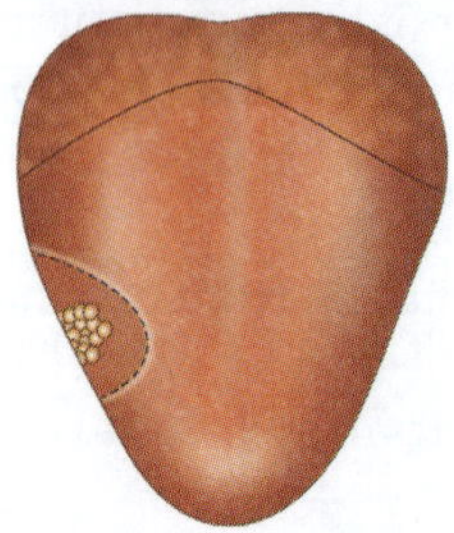

Fig. 35.28: Partial glossectomy

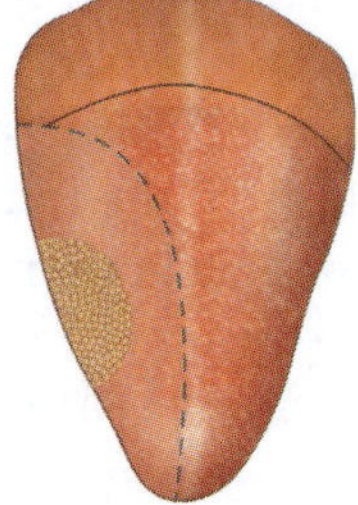

Fig. 35.29: Hemiglossectomy

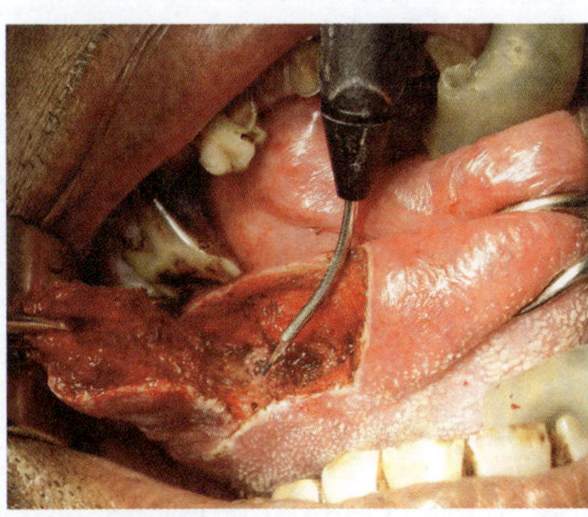

Fig. 35.30: Partial glossectomy done with the help of laser—excellent tool for haemostasis. (*Courtesy:* Dr Balakrishnan, Professor, Department of ENT and Head and Neck, KMC, Manipal)

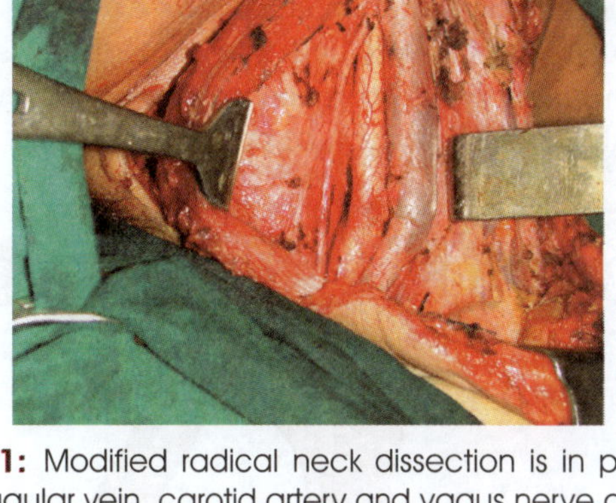

Fig. 35.31: Modified radical neck dissection is in progress—internal jugular vein, carotid artery and vagus nerve are seen

3. **Hemiglossectomy** refers to removal of around 50% of the tongue. This is indicated in a radio-residual tumour, radio-recurrent tumour or where radiotherapy facilities are not available (Fig. 35.29). Reconstruction of the tongue can be done by nasolabial flap and division of pedicle at a later date. Radial forearm free flap can also be used.
4. **Total glossectomy:** Indications are similar to those mentioned above. However, very extensive growth involving the entire tongue is given radiotherapy initially, to reduce the size of the tumour. Surgery can then be undertaken. Total glossectomy carries significant mortality and morbidity.
5. **Commando's operation:** This is indicated when carcinoma of tongue is fixed to the mandible with infiltration of the floor of the mouth. Hemiglossectomy with hemimandibulectomy, removal of the floor of the mouth and radical neck dissection is described as Commando's operation (Key Box 35.13).
   - However, in a few selected cases, removal of the **hemimandible is not necessary**. Growth which is close to the margin of the mandible without infiltration (confirmed by X-ray) needs to be treated by **marginal mandibulectomy**. Carcinoma of the tongue with involvement of only a small portion of mandible can be managed by **segmental excision**. Advantage of this method is that it is not only cosmetic but also **preserves the function of the tongue by preserving genioglossus**. Hence, the tongue may not fall backwards after surgery.

Key Box 35.13

Structures Removed in Radical Block Dissection of the Neck

- The fat, fascia, lymphatics from midline to the anterior border of trapezius, from mandible to clavicle below.
- The lymph nodes—submental, submandibular, upper and lower deep cervical nodes, posterior group of nodes (levels I–V).
- Submandibular salivary gland, sternocleidomastoid and one side internal jugular vein (IJV) are sacrificed.
- Spinal accessory nerve is removed.
- Lower pole of parotid is removed to facilitate lymph node clearance.

Treatment of Lymph Nodes (Fig. 35.31)

- Lymph node metastasis in the neck from squamous cell carcinoma can be managed both by surgery as well as radiotherapy. Radiotherapy can be given in all stages of secondaries in the neck. However, its main indication is a large primary tumour with neck nodes. In such situations both the primary and secondary can be managed with radiotherapy alone which carries minimal morbidity and mortality.
- If the general condition of the patient is good and the lymph nodes are hard and mobile, hemiglossectomy with excision of the floor of the mouth with radical dissection of the neck is done (Commando's operation).
- **If radical neck dissection has to be done on both sides, the IJV should be preserved at least on one side to prevent cerebral oedema. In such cases, radiotherapy is a very good alternative.**

Please note: Details about radical neck dissection is given in Chapter 34, page 341.

Causes of Death in Carcinoma Tongue

1. Recurrent aspirational pneumonia
2. Gross local recurrence, fungation, ulceration, cachexia.

3. **Uncontrolled haemorrhage from growth:** In such cases, ligation of external carotid artery above superior thyroid branch should be done (Fig. 35.32). If ligature is applied below the origin of superior thyroid artery, it results in eddy currents and thrombus at bifurcation of common carotid artery.

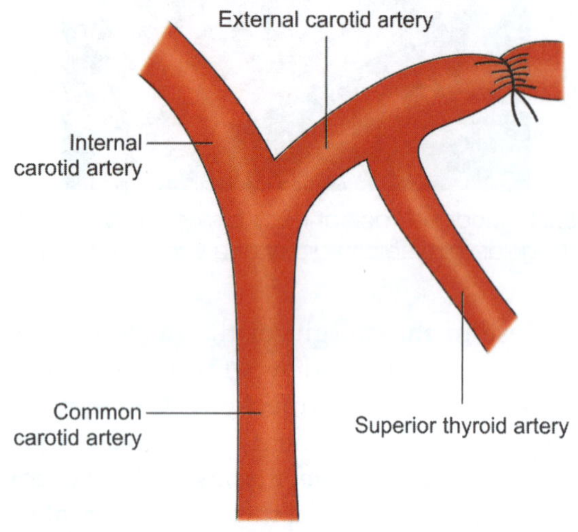

Fig. 35.32: Ligation of external carotid artery

CARCINOMA OF LIP

- Incidence of carcinoma of the lip is about 10 to 12%. It is common in the western, elderly, white people, specially those exposed to sunlight. The actinic rays produces actinic cheilitis—inflammation of the lip, especially lower lip, which over a period of years can turn into malignancy.
- Sinc e this is common in agriculturists, who are constantly exposed to sunlight, it is called **Countryman's lip** (Key Box 35.14).
- Carcinoma lip includes growth arising from vermilion surfaces and mucosa.
- **Leukoplakia** is also responsible for squamous cell carcinoma. Smoking, spirits and spices are the common precipitating factors.

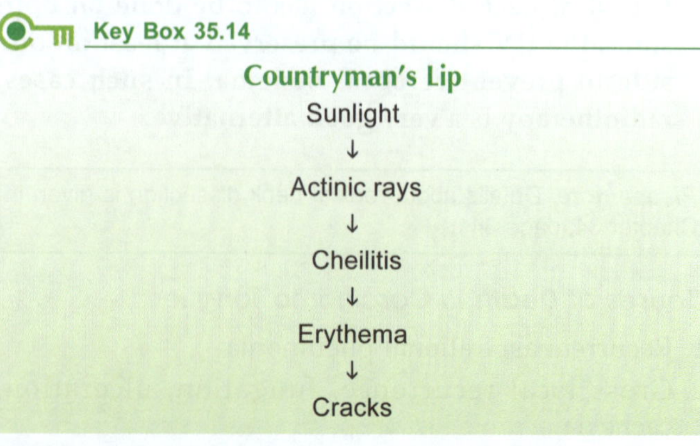
Key Box 35.14

Countryman's Lip

Sunlight
↓
Actinic rays
↓
Cheilitis
↓
Erythema
↓
Cracks

- **Genetic factors** also may play a role. Blacks are less susceptible. On the other hand, **increased incidence** of carcinoma lip has been found in **Caucasians.**
- **Khaini chewers** are more susceptible for carcinoma of the lip (*khaini* is a mixture of tobacco and lime).
- It can also present as verrucous carcinoma of lip.

Clinical Features (Figs 35.33 and 35.34)

- Elderly males are affected in 90% of cases.
- **Nonhealing** ulcer or growth is a common presentation.
- **Edge is everted and indurated.** Induration of the edge and the base is characteristic.
- Floor is covered with slough. Bleeding spots may be visible.
- **Mobility:** Ulcer or the growth moves with the lip, if is fixed to the subcutaneous structures of the lip.
- The entire upper lip and lateral portions of the lower lip drain into **upper deep cervical nodes.** Central portion of the lower lip drains to submental nodes and submandibular nodes. Like elsewhere in the oral cavity, in 50% of the cases, nodes are enlarged due to secondary infections. In remaining 50% of the cases, they are enlarged due to metastasis. Such nodes are hard, with or without fixity. Blood spread is uncommon.

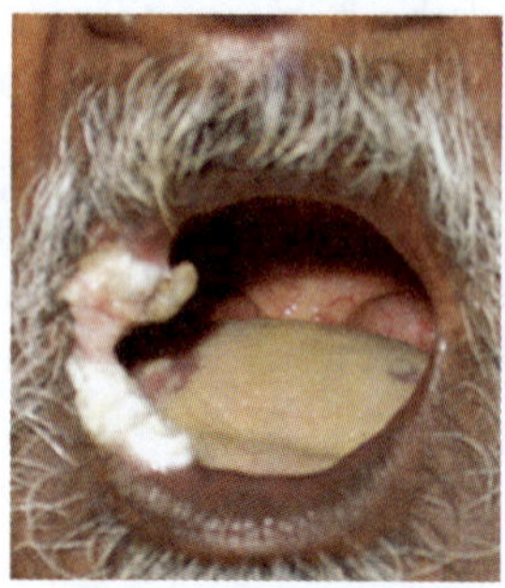

Fig. 35.33: Carcinoma lip—everted edge and exophytic growth—also observe coating of the tongue

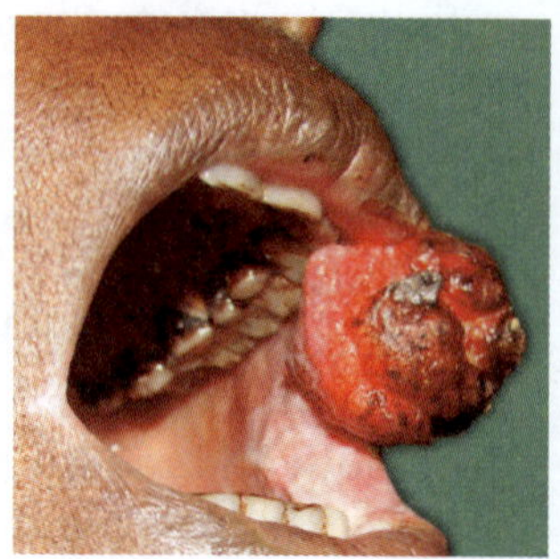

Fig. 35.34: A bleeding exophytic lesion. Better managed by surgery than radiotherapy

Differential Diagnosis (Key Box 35.15)

In a classical case of carcinoma of the lip with everted edges and induration, there is no differential diagnosis. However, following are a few conditions to be remembered:

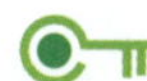
Key Box 35.15

Differential Diagnosis of Carcinoma Lip

- Keratoacanthoma
- Ectopic salivary gland tumour
- Pyogenic granuloma
- Leukoplakia

1. **Keratoacanthoma**
   - It is a cutaneous tumour arising from hair follicles on the lips. It is common in White, Western males between 50 and 70 years of age.
   - Sunlight (actinic rays), chemical carcinogen, viral factors may be responsible for this lesion.
   - The central portion of the nodule may ulcerate. The lesion may progress for 6 weeks and may resolve spontaneously within 4–6 months.
2. **Ectopic salivary gland tumour**
   - The lip is one of the common sites of malignant salivary gland tumours. This presents with submucous nodules that grow slowly and ulcerate and may mimic squamous cell carcinoma (Fig. 35.35).
   - They are also indurated lesions.
   - However, the characteristic everted edge may not be seen.
   - These are adenocarcinomas which are treated by surgery.
3. **Pyogenic granuloma**
   - Recurrent infections or trauma produces a polypoidal mass with significant bleeding.
   - It is rich in granulation tissue and resembles a polyp.
   - It is devoid of epithelium.
   - Histologically, it is a capillary haemangioma.
   - Absence of induration gives the diagnosis.
4. **Leukoplakia**

   A slow developing leukoplakia presents as whitish nodule or an ulcer. However, biopsy confirms the diagnosis.

Treatment

Surgery and radiotherapy are the two modalities available for the treatment of carcinoma of the lip.

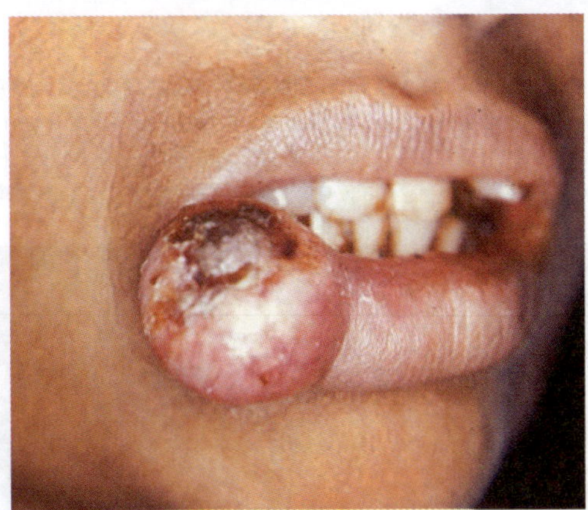

Fig. 35.35: This lesion was diagnosed as carcinoma lip. However, it did not have everted edges. It was indurated. Biopsy reported as ectopic salivary gland tumour. On careful questioning, patient says it started as a swelling not as an ulcer

I. Surgery

- T1 and T2 lesions can be excised followed by direct suturing without much functional problems. This is described as "V" excision which includes removal of growth with 1 cm healthy margin. Care should be taken to excise full thickness of the lip.
- When removal of more than 1/3rd of the lip is required, flap reconstruction may be necessary. The primary goal in lip reconstruction surgery is oral competence.

  Examples

  1. **Abbe flap:** Based on upper labial artery—a pedicled flap is rotated down and sutured to the defect at the lower lip (Fig. 35.38).
  2. **Estlander's flap:** Wedge-shaped flap is used to reconstruct carcinoma of lower lip, when it involves the angle (Fig. 35.37).
- **Larger tumours:** T3 and T4 lesions are irradiated first. If the tumour persists after radiotherapy, excision of the entire lip may be necessary followed by PMMC flap reconstruction.
- Significant lymph nodes can be removed along with the primary tumour—**supraomohyoid block dissection**.

II. Radiotherapy

- It is indicated in all stages of carcinoma of the lip. Radiotherapy produces tumour necrosis resulting in a slow-healing rate. Treatment lasts for several weeks and it delays the wound healing. Elderly patients who are not fit for surgery and carcinoma lip with fixed nodes are treated by irradiation.
- Commissure involvement is treated with RT than surgery.
- Dose: 4000–6000 centigray (cGy) units.

Reconstruction of the Lips

- There are various methods available to reconstruct the lip
- Up to 1/3rd of the lip can be sacrificed with direct closure
- Details are given on page 364 and summary (Table 35.2).

Please note: Students are advised to refer plastic surgery books for more details. Knowledge of some of these flaps will help you in getting more marks in the examinations.

Table 35.2 Reconstruction following resection of oral malignancy. Ca—carcinoma

Anatomic site of cancer	Surgery	Reconstruction
1. Ca lip (<2 cm)	**V** or **W** excision	Direct closure
2. Ca lip (large lesion)	Wide excision	**Bernard rotational flap:** Advancement flap
3. Advanced Ca lip	Total excision of lip (chin also)	Total lip reconstruction by using forearm flap
4. Small lesions lateral tongue	Partial glossectomy	Primary closure or secondary healing
5. Large defect tongue (>2 cm)	Partial glossectomy	Reconstruction by radial forearm flap
6. Advanced lesions tongue	Total glossectomy	Reconstruction by using rectus abdominus flap
7. Floor of mouth T1 or T2	Wide excision	Radial artery forearm flap
8. Floor of mouth T3 or T4	Wide excision with removal of anterior mandible	Fibula flap or iliac crest graft—deep circumflex iliac artery (**DCIA**) is used
9. Buccal mucosa	Wide excision with removal of underlying buccinator muscle also	Direct closure or radial artery forearm flap
10. Lower alveolus	Wide excision with segmental resection of mandible	Primary reconstruction with fibula flap for enentulous mandible and DCIA for dentate mandible

LIP RECONSTRUCTION PICTURES (Figs 35.36 to 35.41)

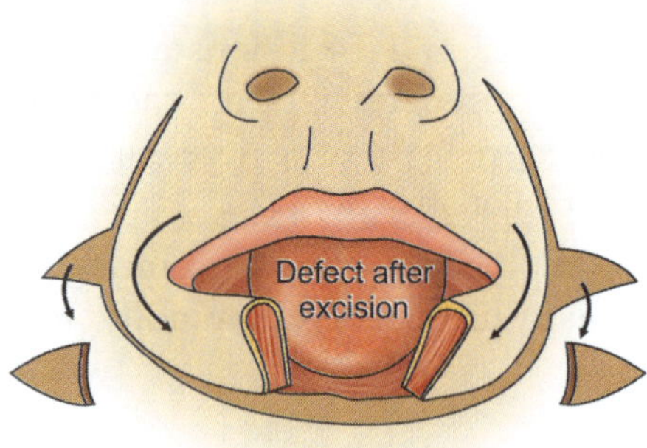

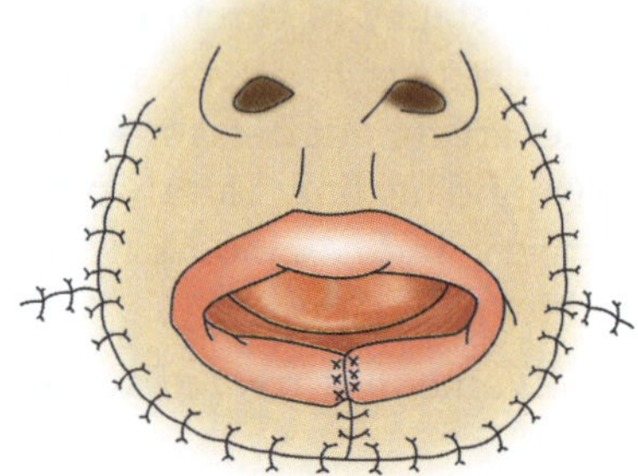

Fig. 35.36: Karapandzic flap—used for defect up to 2/3rd of lip size. Good functional result, good colour and texture match

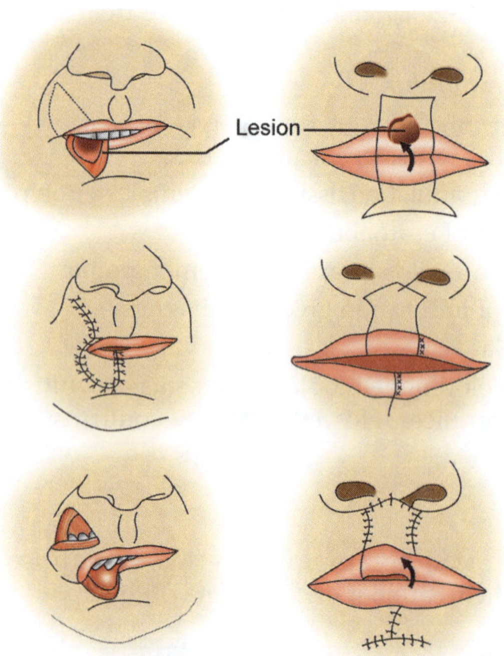

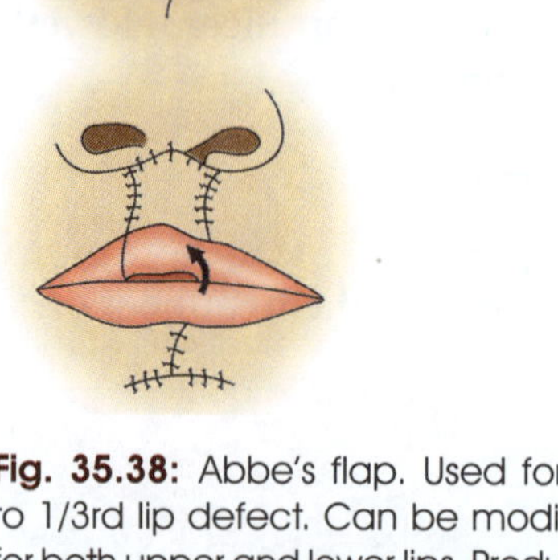

Fig. 35.37: Estlander flap. Used for lateral lip defects up to 1/3rd size. Good functional result

Fig. 35.38: Abbe's flap. Used for up to 1/3rd lip defect. Can be modified for both upper and lower lips. Produces good functional and cosmetic result

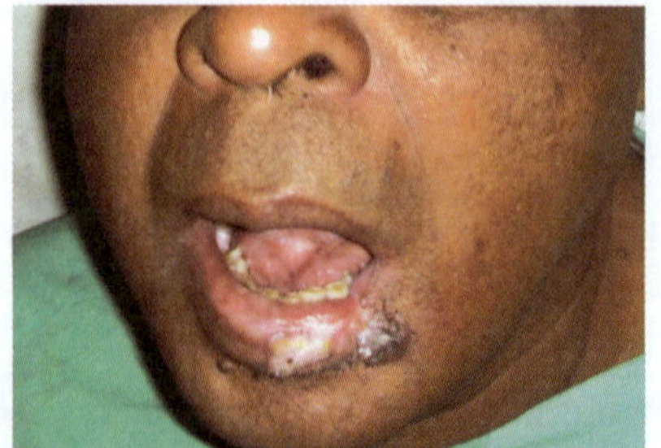

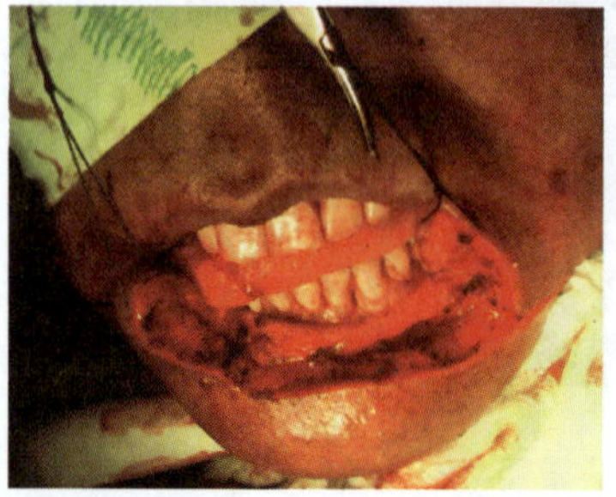

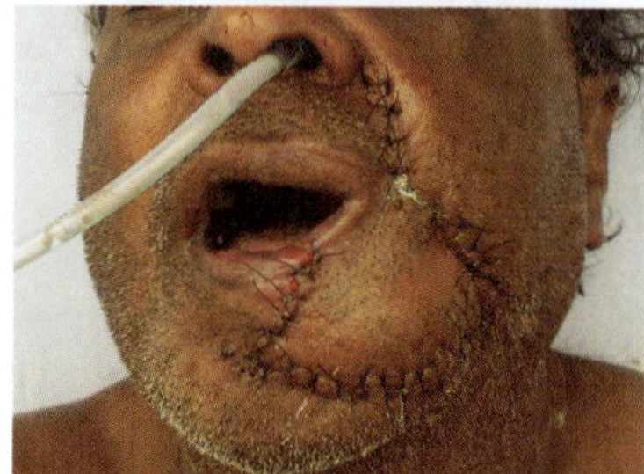

Figs 35.39 to 35.41: Wide excision of lip followed by reconstruction using nasolabial flap [*Courtesy:* Dr Biswas, Dr JK Jha, Dr SP Nayak, Chittaranjan National Cancer Institute (CNCI), Kolkata]

CARCINOMA MAXILLARY ANTRUM (Key Box 35.16)

It is rare in Western countries but common in Asia. The workers in furniture industries, chromic and nickel industries are more prone for the development of carcinoma maxillary antrum.

Ohngren's Line

- Antral carcinoma can be divided by a line joining medial canthus of eye to the angle of mandible. This line is called Ohngren's line.
- The region above the plane is suprastructure and one below is termed infrastructure.
- Poor prognosis in suprastructure because of proximity to skull base and pterygoid region.
- These suprastructure lesions as usually inaccessible and unresectable.

Key Box 35.16

Carcinoma Maxillary Antrum

- Majority are squamous cell carcinoma
- Most important method of spread is contiguous spread
- Early presentation is rare because maxillary antrum serves no important function
- Tissue diagnosis is by biopsy of the mass protruding through nasal cavity/oral cavity or transnasal needle through medial wall of the maxilla
- CT scan for bone involvement and MRI for soft tissue involvement are investigations of choice

Clinical Presentation (Table 35.3)

1. Growth originating on the **floor of antrum** may result in bulge of the hard palate. This results in pain in the teeth and they may become loose.
2. When **medial wall** is involved, nasal obstruction and epiphora occurs due to obstruction of the lacrimal duct. Bleeding from the nose can also occur, if there is ulceration.
3. **If anterolateral wall** is involved (Fig. 35.42), asymmetry of the face results in pain in the cheek. Anaesthesia over the skin of the cheek including upper lip occurs due to involvement of infra-orbital nerve, a branch of maxillary division of the trigeminal nerve.
4. If the **roof** is invaded, proptosis and diplopia occurs.
5. **Posterior extension of the growth** is difficult to assess clinically. When it involves the pterygoid muscles, it results in trismus. Paraesthesia over the cheek, gums, lower lip, postnasal discharge are the other features of these tumours. They carry poor prognosis because of late presentation.

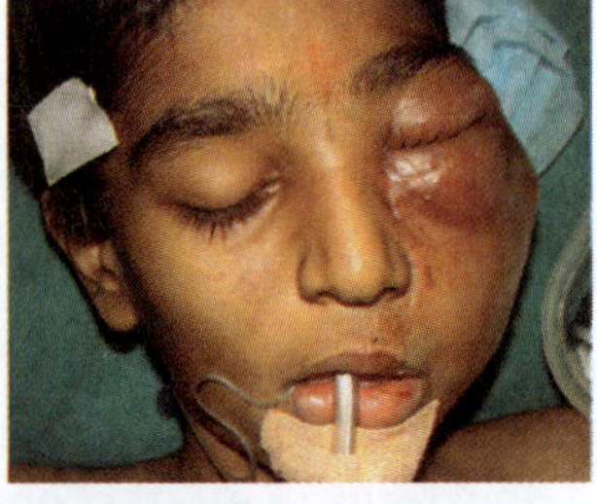

Fig. 35.42: Maxillary antral carcinoma

Lymphatic Spread

Nodal metastasis is uncommon in sinonasal malignancies.

Investigations

1. **Computed tomography** (CT scan) can define a lesion, its extent, bony destruction, posterior extension, etc. Hence, it is the first investigation of choice.
2. **Sinoscopy:** Fenestration will provide tissue for biopsy followed by curettage to reduce the tumour bulk and to drain necrotic contents outside.

Treatment

- **Radiotherapy is the main modality** of treatment in carcinoma maxillary antrum. Curative rate is around 70% in early cases. In advanced cases, radiotherapy is given first. This reduces the tumour bulk so that an unresectable lesion becomes resectable and maxillectomy can be done.
- Surgery can be done in the form of **total maxillectomy** when the growth involves entire maxilla or it is of **high grade** followed by postoperative radio-therapy.
- Tumours of the **lower half** of the antrum are treated by **partial maxillectomy**. It includes removal of the entire hard palate, alveolus and medial wall of the antrum up to and including middle turbinate.

Table 35.3 Clinical examination of a case of carcinoma maxillary antrum

Palatine bulge	→ Growth in the floor
Unilateral nasal obstruction (he is asked to breathe, closing the nostrils one by one)	→ Growth in the medial wall
Asymmetry of the face	→ Growth expanding anteriorly, superficial surface
Change in the level and sharpness of inferior orbital margin, proptosis	→ Growth on the roof (orbital surface)
Swelling (indurated) temporal region	→ Posterior extension into infratemporal region and then into temporal region
Hard, fixed or mobile submandibular nodes	→ Metastasis

- Indications and contraindications for surgery and radiotherapy are in similar lines as discussed earlier in this chapter.

NASOPHARYNX—CANCER

- Carcinoma arises in a small anatomic site bordered by nasal fossae, posterior wall continuous with posterior wall of oropharynx, body of the sphenoid and basilar part of occipital bone and soft palate.
- >90% are squamous cell carcinoma out of which 40–50% are **undifferentiated (lymphoepithelioma)** and 5% are lymphomas.
- Incidence is higher in Asia—Southern China, Malaysia, etc.
- May be associated with **Epstein-Barr virus (EBV)**
- Present as **high posterior cervical lymphadenopathy**
- **Cranial nerve syndromes** are common due to tumour invasion of base of skull.
  1. **Retrosphenoidal syndrome** from involvement of cranial nerves II through VI manifests as unilateral ophthalmoplegia, trigeminal neuralgia, ptosis, etc.
  2. **Retroparotid syndrome:** Occurs due to compression of cranial nerve IX through XII and causes various symptoms depending on nerve involvement including Horner's syndrome (*refer* Trotter's triad given in page 340).
- Diagnosis by endoscopy, biopsy, CT and MRI.
- Mainly managed by radiotherapy and chemotherapy.

BENIGN LESIONS IN THE ORAL CAVITY

DIFFERENTIAL DIAGNOSIS OF ULCER IN THE TONGUE

(Fig. 35.43 and Key Boxes 35.17 and 35.18)

1. Aphthous ulcer

- Small, multiple, very painful ulcers, can occur at any age group. More common in females at the time of menstruation. These are called **minor aphthous ulcers**.

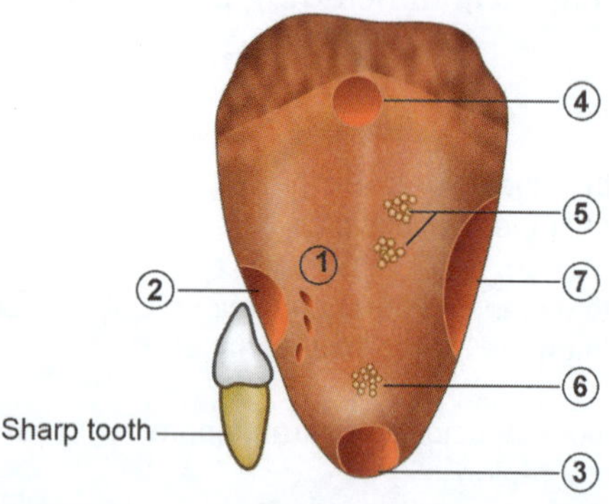

Fig. 35.43: Ulcers of the tongue—see text for numbers

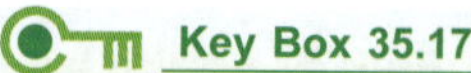

Key Box 35.17

Painful Ulcers in the Tongue

- Aphthous ulcers
- Dental ulcers
- Tubercular ulcers

Key Box 35.18

Painless Ulcers in the Tongue

- Carcinomatous ulcers
- Gummatous ulcers
- Systemic diseases

- When they are larger, deeper and painful, they are called **major aphthous ulcers.**
- They are due to viral infection. These ulcers are superficial ulcers with erythematous margin.
- They subside within a few days. Temporary relief can be obtained by applying **salicylate gel.**
- Vitamin B complex is usually given for the satisfaction of the patients.

2. Dental ulcer

- These ulcers occur due to broken tooth, sharp tooth, ill-fitting dentures, prosthesis, etc. They are very painful ulcers.
- Such ulcers are common on the lateral margin and they heal when the tooth is removed. This is an example for traumatic ulcer. It should not be confused with carcinomatous ulcer which commonly occurs on the lateral margin.

3. Tubercular ulcer of tongue

- Tuberculosis affects tip of the tongue. These ulcers are very painful with enlargement of regional nodes.
- It occurs in patients with fulminating pulmonary tuberculosis.
- Ulcers have undermined edges. These ulcers are sometimes multiple with serous discharge.

4. Gummatous ulcer

- Gumma is a complication of tertiary syphilis resulting in a firm swelling in the midline in the anterior 2/3 rds of the tongue. Induration is absent. Ulcer is nontender. Severe endarteritis obliterans results in the necrosis of gumma giving rise to gummatous ulcer. It has punched out edges and wash leather slough on the floor. Other sites of gumma include testis, palate, clavicle and liver. These ulcers are rare these days.

5. Systemic diseases

- Pemphigus
- Systemic lupus erythematosus (SLE)
- Lichen planus

6. Post-pertussis ulcer
- It occurs in children due to repeated coughing. Typical location of the ulcer on the under surface of the tongue and on the frenulum clinches the diagnosis.

7. Carcinomatous ulcer
- Lateral margin
- Nonhealing ulcer
- Everted edge
- Edge and base are indurated
- Bleeds on touch
- Fixity
- Significant lymph nodes in the neck.

MACROGLOSSIA

Diffuse painless enlargement of the tongue is described as macroglossia. It is a rare condition and can occur due to various causes.

1. **Lymphangioma:** In this condition, the tongue diffusely enlarges. Sometimes, it is a localised swelling. It may be associated with lymphangiomas elsewhere in the body such as cheek mucosa, lips, etc. The tongue becomes larger, indurated and gives rise to severe discomfort to the patients. Due to repeated trauma, the surface becomes ulcerated. It is treated by injecting sclerosants such as ethanolamine oleate, hypertonic saline. Partial excision may be necessary in cases of large lymphangioma.
2. **Haemangioma:** Cavernous haemangiomas occur in the tongue, lips, etc. It is present since birth but manifests during childhood. It presents with soft, cystic, fluctuant swelling and at times, pulsatile. Trauma due to teeth or food results in bleeding. Haemangioma of the tongue is treated on the same lines as lymphangioma. It is much more difficult to excise it, especially a large haemangioma. Preoperative angiography and ligation of lingual artery on both sides is necessary (Fig. 35.44).
3. **Neurofibroma:** It may be associated with von Recklinghausen's disease. It is treated by hemiglossectomy.

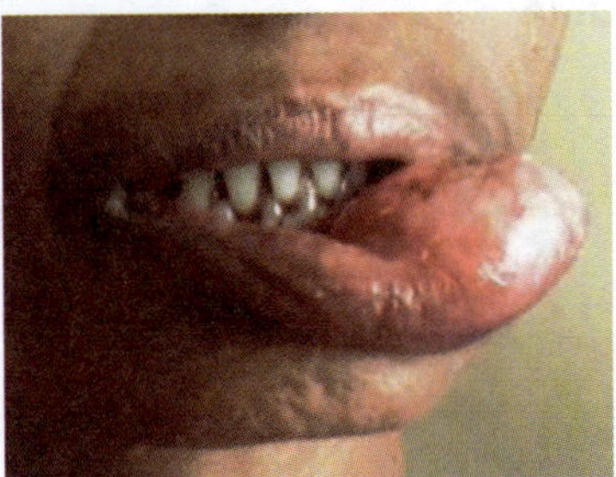

Fig. 35.44: Haemangioma. (*Courtesy*: Dr SV Mohan, Associate Professor, Shivamoga Institute of Medical Sciecnes, Shivamoga)

4. **Muscular macroglossia:** This condition, though rare, is seen in cretins. The tongue is thickened and cannot be held in place. Hence, it protrudes outside. It is treated by partial excision.

SYPHILITIC LESIONS OF THE TONGUE

1. **Primary syphilis:** Primary chancre that occurs in the tongue is highly contagious. It affects the tip of the tongue. It produces a painful ulcer with large significant enlargement of regional lymph nodes.
2. **Secondary syphilis** produces a white patch in the tongue, lips and on the anterior pillars of fauces. In the tongue, these are multiple which coalesce to form **snail track ulcers**. The ulcers heal with **fine tissue paper scar**. In some cases syphilitic organisms produce a flat, hypertrophied epithelium which is described as **condyloma.** This is called **Hutchinson's wart.**
3. **Tertiary syphilis:** It produces gumma. Syphilis also produces **chronic superficial glossitis**, which is characterised by bald tongue with loss of papilla and fissured tongue. **It is a precancerous condition.**

ODONTOMES

Definition: Odontomes are the cysts, malformations arising from epithelial or mesothelial elements of tooth resulting in swelling of the jaw. As a developmental anomaly, a few epithelial cells proliferate, persisting as **epithelial debris of Mallasez**. Three important odontomes have been given in Table 35.4.

DENTAL CYST: RADICULAR CYST/PERIAPICAL CYST

Pathogenesis

This arises from a normally erupted, chronically infected, pulpless caries tooth. The caries tooth produces a low grade, chronic inflammation which stimulates epithelial debris to proliferate. Later this brings about degeneration of epithelial and mesothelial cells resulting in a cyst within the maxilla.

Clinical Features

- Common in women around 3rd–4th decades.
- Commonly affects the upper jaw (maxilla).
- It presents as a slow-growing swelling in the maxillary region resulting in deformity of the face.

Diagnosis

- Presence of caries tooth with expansion of maxilla.
- X-ray—large, unilocular cyst in maxilla or orthopantomogram showing cyst in the mandible.
- Aspiration of the cyst demonstrates cholesterol crystals.

Table 35.4 Comparison of three common odontomes

	Dental cyst	Dentigerous cyst	Adamantinoma
1. Aetiology	Caries tooth	Unerupted tooth	True neoplasm—ameloblasts
2. Site	Maxilla	Mandible	Mandible
3. Age	30–50 years	20–30 years	40–50 years
4. Palpation	Smooth, thin bone-eggshell crackling	Smooth, expansion of the outer table of mandible	Expansion of mandible in the 3rd molar region, cystic areas
5. X-ray	Radiolucent unilocular cyst	Radiolucent unilocular cyst with unerupted teeth	Large radiolucent area with fine honeycombing
6. Treatment	Subperiosteal excision	Subperiosteal excision	Wide excision even though benign
7. Spread	Does not occur	Does not occur	Local spread, recurrence, late spread to the lung are the features

Treatment

Excision of cyst with its epithelial lining through intraoral approach. After excision of the epithelium, the cyst wall should be curetted, followed by soft tissue 'push-in' to obliterate dead space.

DENTIGEROUS CYST: FOLLICULAR ODONTOME

- Common in lower jaw (mandible) in women 30–40 years (Fig. 35.45).
- It occurs in relation to unerupted, permanent, molar tooth, most commonly the upper or lower third molar tooth.
- This unerupted tooth constantly irritates the cells, produces degeneration of the cells resulting in a dentigerous cyst. The cyst is lined by squamous epithelium surrounded by connective tissue. Within the cyst, the tooth lies obliquely or sometimes is embedded in the wall of the cyst. As it grows further, the cyst displaces the tooth to which it is attached. Thus, the tooth is displaced deeper and deeper and prevented from eruption.

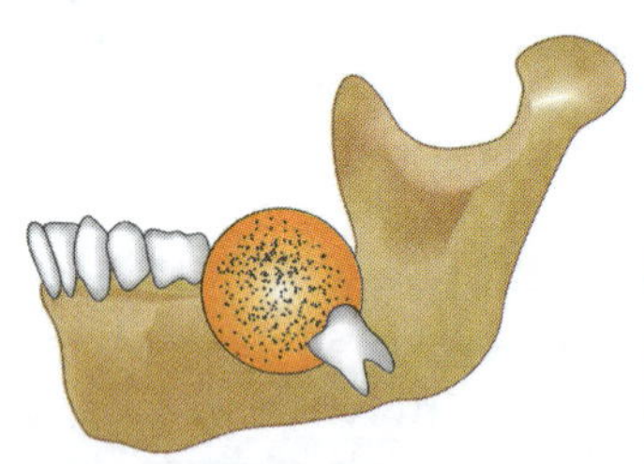

Fig. 35.45A: Dentigerous cyst

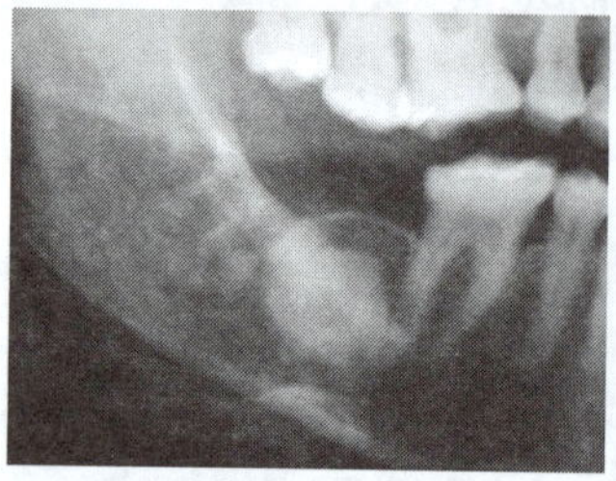

Fig. 35.45B: X-ray of the dentigerous cyst

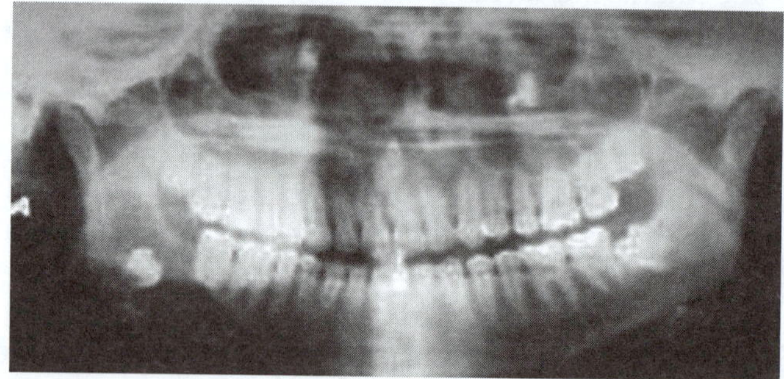

Fig. 35.46: Orthopantomogram showing unerupted tooth

Clinical Features

- Absence of molar tooth
- Expansion of mandible—since the inner table of the mandible is strong, the expansion mainly occurs in the outer aspect of mandible. The bone gets thinned out resulting in **egg-shell crackling**.

Diagnosis

X-ray mandible orthopantomogram (OPG) (Figs 35.45 and 35.46)

1. Tooth in the cyst
2. Soap-bubble appearance due to multiple trabeculations of the bone
3. Radiolucent well-defined swelling.

Treatment

- Small cyst—excision of the cyst by intraoral approach.
- Large cysts—managed by marsupialisation.

ADAMANTINOMA

- It is also called multilocular cystic disease, ameloblastoma, Eve's disease (Fig. 35.47).
- This tumour arises from ameloblasts (enamel forming cells).
- It is a benign tumour, very slow-growing and behaves like a basal cell carcinoma. Inadequate treatment results in local recurrence and later metastasis. Hence, even though the tumour is benign, it has to be treated like malignant tumour.

Images of Adamantinoma (Figs 35.47A to C)

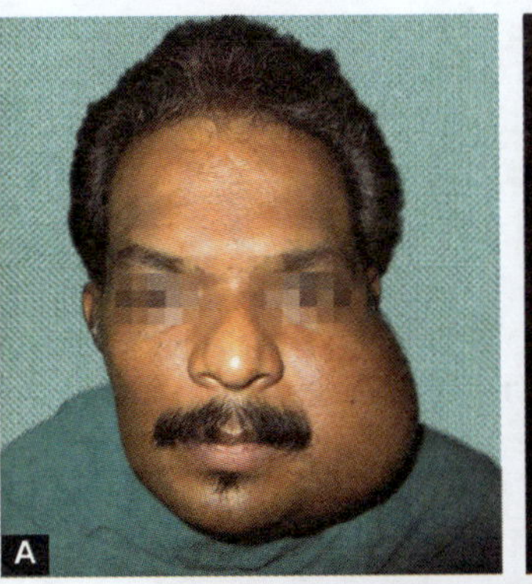

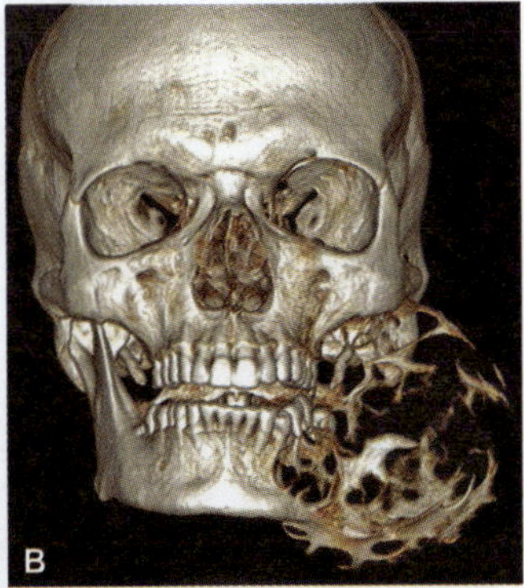

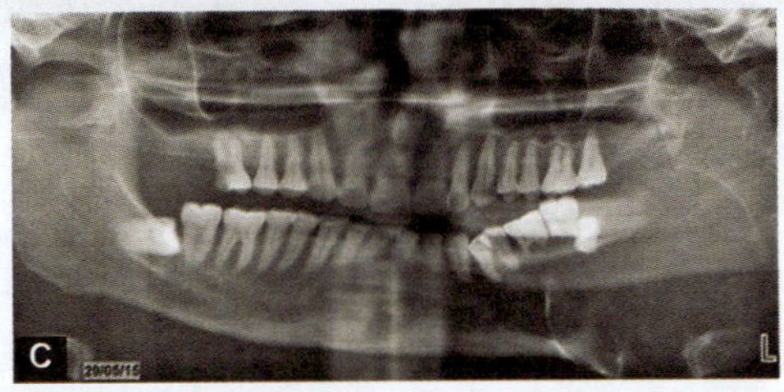

Figs 35.47A to C: Ameloblastoma. (A) Clinical presentation, (B) CT scan image, (C) OPG. (*Courtesy:* Dr Abhay Kamath, Head, Department of OFMS, College of Dental Sciences, Manipal)

Sites

- **Mandible** is the most common site.
- **Tibia** is the 2nd common site. It can be explained by inclusion of abnormal embryonic epithelium.
- **Pituitary** is another common site where adamantinoma can occur. **Both pituitary stalk and enamel arise from oral epithelium.**

Clinical Features

- Patients in 4th or 5th decade are commonly affected.
- This is a slow-growing jaw tumour in the region of angle of mandible and horizontal ramus of the mandible.
- As the tumour grows, it undergoes cystic degeneration resulting in multiple cystic spaces. Hence, it is called multilocular cystic disease.
- As it grows it causes expansion of the outer table of the mandible and causes fracture mandible.
- Patient may present with complaints of falling teeth.

Diagnosis

X-ray: A large cyst and small multiple cysts due to the trabeculations giving it a 'honeycomb' appearance.

Treatment

Even though it is **benign, simple curettage or enucleation may result in recurrence** and chances of recurrent adamantinoma turning into malignancy are high. Hence, wide excision with 1 cm of healthy normal tissue should be removed. It may amount to **segmental excision of the mandible or hemimandibulectomy** (Key Box 35.19 and Table 35.4).

Key Box 35.19

Adamantinoma

- Locally invasive solid tumour
- Nonfunctional, **intermittent in growth,** unicentric, **multilocular**
- Spreads within the medullary bone
- Invades soft tissues
- Should not fragment the tumour cells
- **Subperiosteal excision** should **not be done** as it may result in recurrence
- **Incomplete excision results in recurrence** and metastasis to the lung
- Hence, even though it is a **benign tumour** it is treated by wide **excision** or hemimandibulectomy.

Differential Diagnosis

1. Giant Celled Reparative Granuloma (Jaffe Tumour)

It is a benign tumour which occurs due to haemorrhage within the bone marrow.

Pathology

- It affects antral part of maxilla or mandible causing enlargement of the jaw.
- Stroma is vascular consisting of thin-walled blood vessels, scanty collagen, connective tissue cells.
- Microscopic features mimic giant cell epulis or brown tumour of hyperparathyroidism.

Clinical features

- Unlike an adamantinoma, this tumour affects females in the age group of 10–25 years.
- Painless enlargement of the jaw is the presenting feature. X-ray demonstrates radiolucent artery.

Treatment

- Calcitonin 0.5 mg (100 units) daily subcutaneous injection over a period of one year has been recommended as a first line of treatment. It has shown resolution of the tumour.
- Curettage is the surgical line of treatment.

2. Osteoclastoma

- This is a rare tumour seen in the lower jaw.
- Males between the age of 25 and 40 years are commonly affected.

- Unlike adamantinoma, it is a rapidly growing tumour.
- As the tumour enlarges, both tables of the lower jaw are thinned out.
- X-ray may show a large, radiolucent cyst with pseudo-trabeculation.
- Even though benign, it is radiosensitive.
- However, recurrence can occur and can turn into malignancy like that of adamantinoma.

EPULIS

- *Epulis* means "upon the gum". It refers to solid swelling situated on the gum (Key Box 35.20).
- It arises from alveolar margin of the jaw.
- Very often patients present with swelling on the gum which is painless.

Key Box 35.20

Epulis

○ Soft epulis	– Granulomatous
○ Firm epulis	– Fibrous
	– Giant cell
○ Hard epulis	– Carcinomatous
○ Malignant epulis	– Carcinomatous
○ Dangerous epulis	– Fibrosarcomatous

Types

Granulomatous Epulis (Fig. 35.48)

- Precipitating factors are caries tooth, dentures, poor oral hygiene.
- It manifests as a mass of granulation tissue around the teeth on the gums. It is a soft to firm, fleshy mass and bleeds on touch.
- Pregnancy epulis refers to this variety (gingivitis gravidarum).

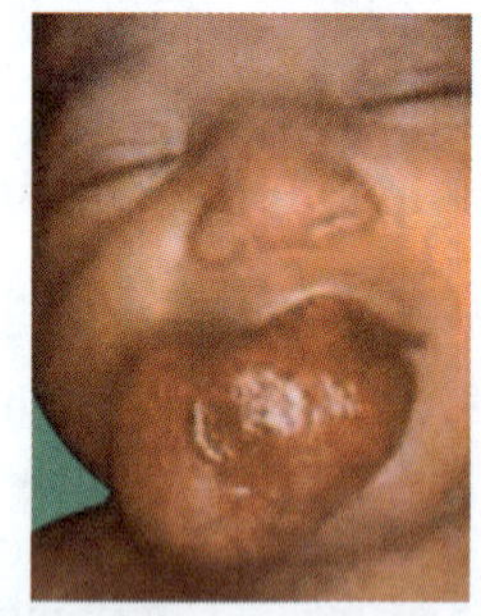

Fig. 35.48: Granulomatous epulis

Clinical Notes

65-year-old man was (Fig. 35.50) getting recurrent attacks of pain and swelling beneath the chin. Sometimes there was purulent discharge. He was treated with antibiotics and incision drainage had been done twice. Sinus persisted. Chief cause of his problems was his incisor teeth. Nobody had examined the oral cavity. He had caries teeth. Once these were removed, sinus healed. This case highlights the importance of clinical examination.

Fibrous Epulis (Fig. 35.49)

It is the commonest form. A simple fibroma arising from periodontal membrane, presents on the gum. It may undergo sarcomatous change. It is a firm polypoidal mass, slowly growing and nontender.

Giant Cell Epulis

- It is also called myeloid epulis.
- It is an osteoclastoma arising in the jaw. It presents as hyperaemic vascular, oedematous, soft to firm gums with indurated underlying mass due to expansion of the bone. It may ulcerate and result in haemorrhage. X-ray shows bone destruction with ridging of walls (pseudo-trabeculation).
- Small tumours are treated by curettage.
- Large tumours are treated by radical excision.

Carcinomatous Epulis

- This is an epithelioma arising from mucous membrane of the alveolar margin.
- Typically, it presents as a nonhealing, painless ulcer. It slowly infiltrates the bone.
- Hard regional lymph nodes are due to metastasis.
- Treated by wide excision which includes removal of segment of the bone.

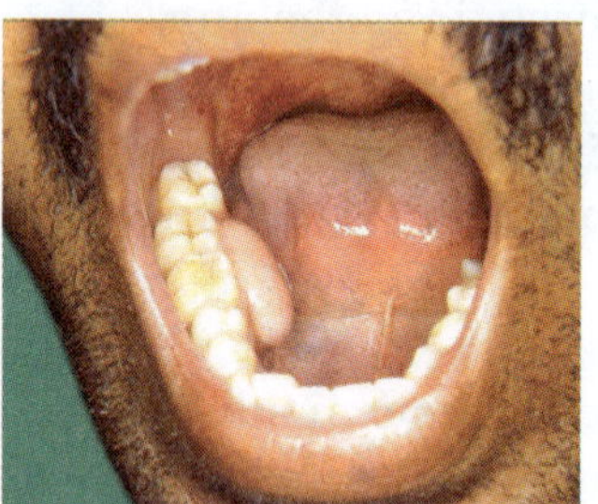

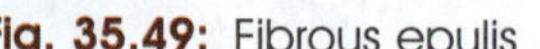

Fig. 35.49: Fibrous epulis

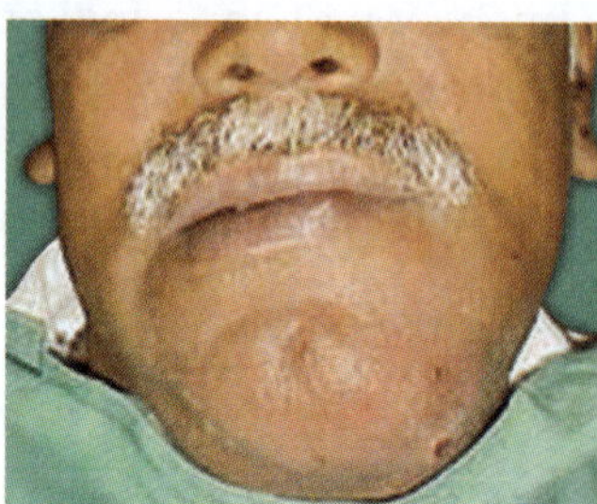

Fig. 35.50: Median mental sinus

MEDIAN MENTAL SINUS

This is a sinus in the midline just beneath the mentum.

Aetiopathogenesis

It is produced by an apical abscess of lower incisors which penetrate buccal cortical plate below the origin of mentalis muscle. This muscle takes origin from labial surface of alveolar process just above the labial sulcus. Hence, pus discharges through a sinus in the centre of chin.

Clinical Presentation (Fig. 35.50)

- Patients present with recurrent swelling in the sub-mental region which bursts open spontaneously discharging at times mucus and seropurulent fluid.

- Repeated history of swelling, discharge and healing are common presentations.
- Diagnosis is established by examination of the oral cavity, which reveals evidence of caries tooth.

Treatment

Once the caries tooth is extracted, sinus will heal spontaneously.

VINCENT'S ANGINA

It is an acute ulceromembranous stomatitis or acute ulcerative gingivitis and stomatitis. The disease is caused by Vincent's organisms—*Borrelia vincentii*, an anaerobic spirochaete and fusiformis. These are gram-negative rods which are the normal pathogens of oral cavity. However, streptococci and staphylococci are the common organisms involved here resulting in severe symptoms and toxicity.

PRECIPITATING FACTORS

- Malnutrition, diabetes mellitus, caries tooth, warm seasons, winter, etc.
- The disease starts in the intergingival defects as a deep penetrating ulcer which results in a **spontaneous gingival haemorrhage**. There is a thick membrane covering the ulcer.
- Once infection spreads to tonsillar region, it is called Vincent's angina—very severe painful condition.

Clinical Features

- Common in children and young adults between 20 and 40 years of age.
- It presents with very painful gums with fever, malaise and toxaemia.
- Gums are swollen, red, inflamed with or without slough.
- Difficulty in swallowing, painful swallowing (odynophagia), **foetor oris**, features of toxaemia and high grade fever are characteristic of this condition.

Treatment

- Improve nutrition. Mouthwashes with hydrogen peroxide help in washing away the membrane. Broad spectrum antibiotics such as Piperacillin-tazobactum combination are given, metronidazole 400 mg thrice/day for 7–10 days should be given.

CLEFT LIP AND CLEFT PALATE

Competency

SU19.1: Describe the etiology and classification of cleft lip and palate.

CLEFT LIP

- Cleft lip results from abnormal development of the median nasal and maxillary process.
- Cleft palate results from a failure of fusion of the two palatine processes.

Epidemiology and Etiology

Cleft lip-palate has a varied incidence of 1 in 500–2,500 live births depending on geographic location, maternal risk factors, prenatal exposure, ancestry, and socio-economic status. The latest CDC reported incidence is 1 in 940 live births, with the highest rates in Asians and Native Americans (1 in 500 births) and the lowest rate in Africans (1 in 2,500 births)

Cleft lip is seen in a Male:Female ratio of 2:1 and in contrast to cleft palate has a 1:2 ratio. It is postulated that maternal hormones may be involved in both sex determination and orofacial clefts.

The sporadic causes are multifactorial and involve genetics, environmental factors, and teratogens

- **Syndromes:** Most commonly van der Woude syndrome, Stickler syndrome, Hardikar syndrome, Treacher-Collins syndrome.
- **Genetics-IRF 6** which is commonly implicated in the syndromic forms, ch8q24, VAX1, FGFR2, BMP.
- **Maternal risk factors:** Smoking, alcohol consumption, pre-gestational and gestational diabetes, advanced maternal age, folate deficiency, zinc deficiency.
- **Teratogens:** Medications like anti-epileptics (valproate/phenytoin), retinoic acid, occupational exposure to pesticides/solvents etc.

Types of Cleft Lip (Figs 35.51 and 35.52)

I. **Central:** It is very rare and occurs due to failure of fusion of two median nasal processes.

II. **Lateral:** It is the commonest variety wherein there is a cleft between the frenulum and the lateral part of the upper lip. This is due to imperfect fusion of maxillary process with median nasal process. The lateral variety can be unilateral or bilateral.

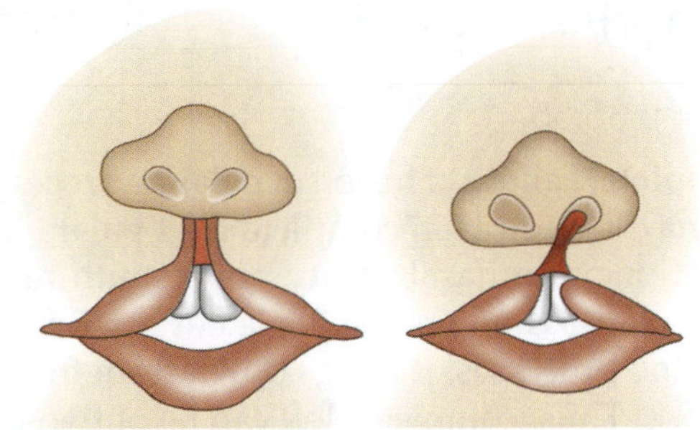

Figs 35.51 and 35.52: Types of cleft lip (I and II)

III. **Complete or incomplete:** In cases of complete variety, cleft lip extends to the floor of the nose. In cases of incomplete variety, the cleft does not extend up to the nostril.

IV. **Simple or compound:** Compound refers to cleft lip associated with a cleft in the alveolus.

Clinical Features (Figs 35.53 and 35.54)

1. In 80% of the cases, cleft lip is unilateral and in about 60% of the cases, it is associated with cleft palate.
2. In many cases, nostril is widened.
3. Maldevelopment or malalignment of the teeth in relation to the cleft is common.

Functional Effect

1. Presence of cleft lip does not interfere much with sucking. However, there may be some difficulty in bottle feeding.
2. Some degree of difficulty in speech (dysarticulation) is present.

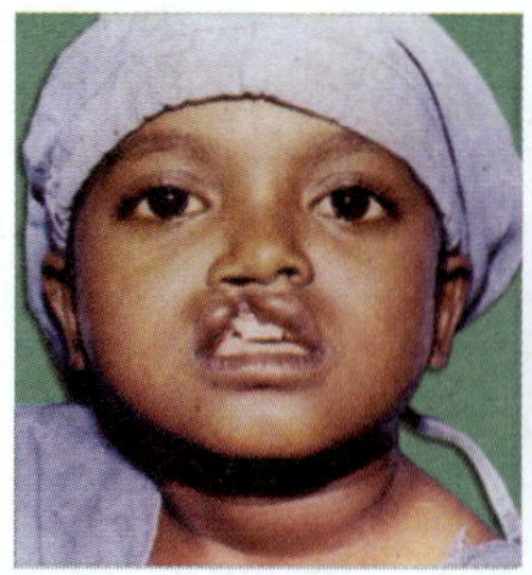
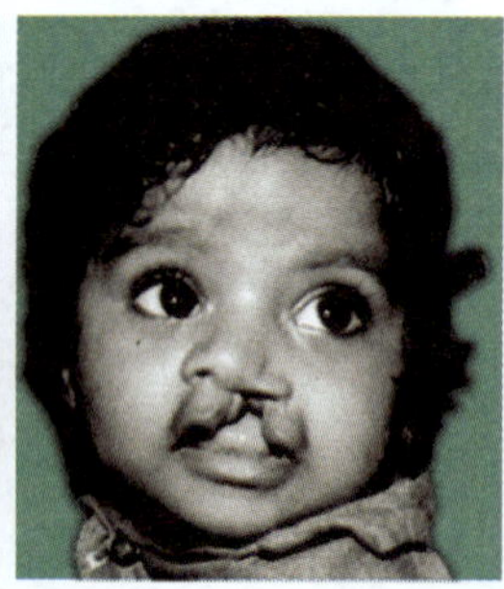

Figs 35.53 and 35.54: Cleft lip (*Courtesy:* Dr CG Narasimhan, Senior Consultant Surgeon, Mysore)

CLEFT PALATE

Development of Palate

- Palate is developed around 6–8 weeks of intrauterine life from **3 components**. The premaxilla is developed from the median nasal process and maxillary process contributes one palatine process on each side.
- The line of fusion of these processes is in the form of a letter Y.
- Imperfect fusion or developmental anomalies results in cleft palate.

Types (Fig. 35.55)

I. **Complete:** Failure of fusion of palatine processes and premaxilla results in complete cleft palate. In such situations, the nasal cavity and mouth are interconnected. When premaxilla is not fused with both palatine processes, it hangs down from the septum of nose. Thus, complete cleft can be of two types as shown below in the diagram.

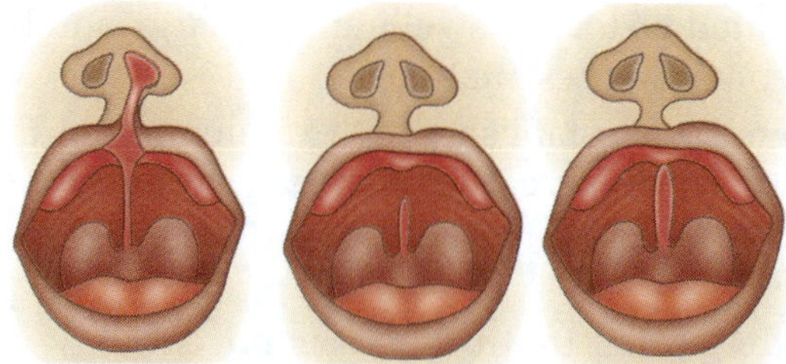

Fig. 35.55: Types of cleft palate (I, IIa and IIb)

II. **Incomplete:** When the fusion of three components of palate takes place, it starts from uvula and then backwards. Thus, various types of incomplete fusion result.
- Bifid uvula.
- The whole length of soft palate is bifid.
- The whole length of soft palate and the posterior part of hard palate are involved. On the other hand, anterior part of palate is normally developed. In about 25% of cases, cleft palate alone and in 50% of cases, both cleft palate and cleft lip are encountered.

Effects of Cleft Palate

1. Presence of cleft palate interferes with swallowing to some extent.
2. They are unable to pronounce the consonant sounds such as B, D, K, P, T.
3. **Teeth:** Upper lateral incisors may be small or even absent. The maxilla tends to be smaller. Teeth are crowded.
4. **Nose:** Oral organisms contaminate the upper respiratory mucous membrane through cleft palate.
5. **Hearing:** Even with repair, acute and chronic otitis media and hearing problems can occur.

Competency

SU19.2: Describe the principles of reconstruction of cleft lip and palate.

Management of Cleft Lip and Palate

- **A multidisciplinary approach** involving plastic surgery, orthodontics, speech pathology, ENT department, prosthodontics and paediatrics department is needed to rehabilitate the cleft palate cases. This approach to the problem results in aesthetically acceptable end result without much functional deficiencies.
- **Feeding advice:** Cleft palate babies are unable to suck mothers' milk because intraoral negative pressure cannot be created due to communication between oral and nasal cavity. Thus, expressed mother's milk is given by spoon with head end of baby elevated by

45 degrees. Swallowed air during feeding is released frequently by burping.

Cleft Lip Repair (Key Box 35.21)

Timing: Majority of surgeons follow "RULE OF 10" as a guide for timing of lip and anterior palate repair. At the time of repair, haemoglobin should be more than 10 g%, age approximately 10 weeks, weight more than 10 lb (4.54 kg) and total leucocyte count less than 10,000/cu mm (i.e. no infection).

Key Box 35.21

Rule of 10

- Hb >10 g%
- Age approx : 10 weeks
- Weight >10 lb (4.54 kg)
- TC <10,000/mm^3

Types of Cleft Lip Repair

- For unilateral cleft lip repair most commonly used methods are Millard rotation advancement flap and Tennison-Randall triangular flap method.
- Bilateral cleft lip can be repaired in single stage or in two stages at the interval of 3–6 months. For two-stage repair, any one of the methods described for unilateral cleft lip can be used. For bilateral repair in one stage, Veau III method is simple and gives satisfactory results. Other single stage methods which give good results are **Millard's single stage** procedure and Black procedure.

Basic Steps of Lip Repair

- Markings are made according to the method selected (e.g. Millard's repair, Fig. 35.56A and Tennison-Randall repair, Fig. 35.56B).
- Adrenaline-saline solution (1:200,000) is injected in the lip and labial sulcus for haemostasis.
- Full thickness of lip is incised along the marking.
- Lip repair is done in three layers—mucosa, muscle and skin. For better aesthetic result, Cupid's bow should become horizontal, **white line** continuity should be repaired and there should be no vermilion notching.

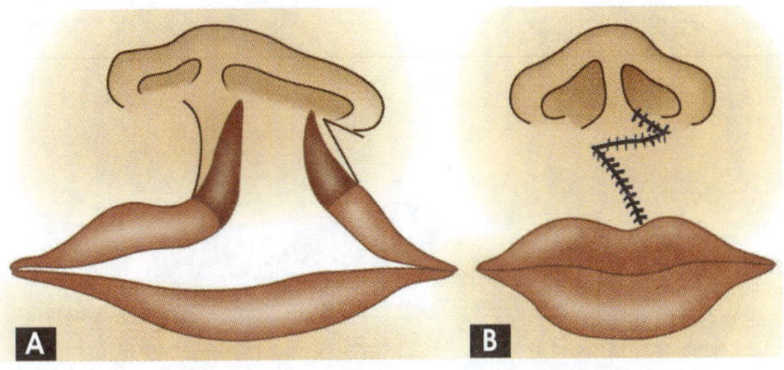

Figs 35.56A and B: Basic steps of lip repair

Cleft Palate Repair

Timing: Early repair results in retarded maxillary growth due to surgical trauma to growth centre and periosteum. Delay in repair results in speech defect. Best balanced result is achieved by repairing between one and a half years.

Types

- Palate repair: Palate is repaired by palatal shelves. **Mucoperiosteal flaps raised from various methods are available for palate repair.**
- Most commonly used method is V-Y, pushback palatoplasty.

Steps of 'V-Y' pushback palatoplasty (Fig. 35.57)

- Palate is infiltrated with 1:2 lakh adrenaline-saline solution.
- Two mucoperiosteal flaps are elevated, one from either side of palatal shelves. Then, nasal layers are mobilised.
- Palate is closed in three layers—nasal layer, muscle layer, oral layer.
- In V-Y pushback palatoplasty, palatal lengthening is achieved by V-Y plasty. Hook of hamulus can be fractured to relieve tension on suture line by relaxing the tensor palati muscle.

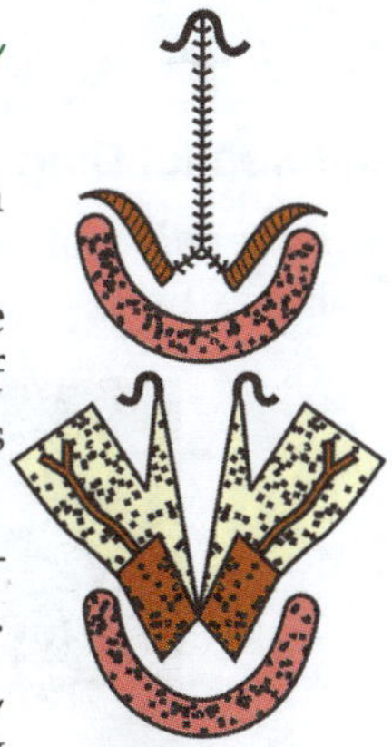

Fig. 35.57: V-Y palatoplasty

MISCELLANEOUS

ECTOPIC SALIVARY GLAND TUMOUR

- **Palate** is the most **frequent site.**
- These tumours can also occur anywhere in the mouth or pharynx.
- **It is a slow-growing and painless tumour.** At this stage, it may feel firm or hard without ulceration of mucous membrane.
- Slowly it **ulcerates.** Thus, it can have the shape of a **'verrucous'** carcinoma. Such lesions are ulcerated, hard, and painful with irregular margins.
- They are of **low-grade malignancy.**
- Neglected cases can invade base of skull and spread to lymph nodes.
- **Wide excision** with or **without reconstruction** is the treatment of choice.

MUCOUS CYSTS

- They are examples of retention cyst.
- They occur due to obstruction of the duct of many mucous secreting glands which cover the inner surface of the lips and whole of inside of mouth (Fig. 35.58).
- They are also a type of **extravasation** cyst.

Clinical Symptoms and Signs

- Painless, slow growing swelling on the inner side of lip or cheek.
- Most common on the lower lip.
- Typically round, soft, fluctuant, pale pink swelling or blue domed.
- Transillumination is positive but difficult to demonstrate as the cysts are small.
- Mucous membrane is free over the swelling.

Differential Diagnosis

- **Pyogenic granuloma:** It is red in colour, soft and bleeds. It may be associated with trauma or persistent infection.

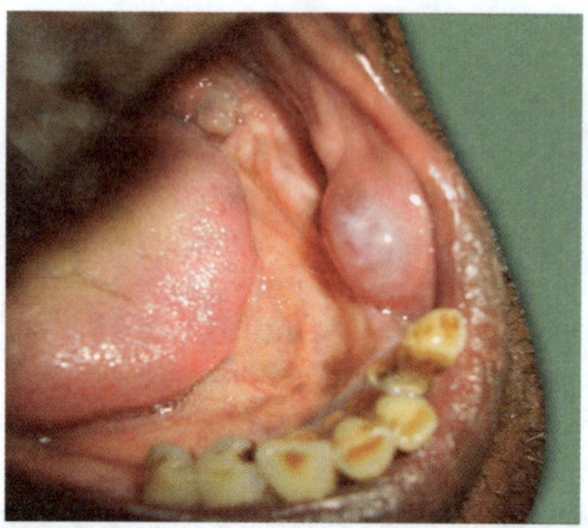

Fig. 35.58: Mucous cyst in the floor of the mouth

- **Ectopic salivary gland tumours:** They are firm and non-tender swellings.

Treatment

- Excision can be done under local anaesthesia.
- Once mucous membrane is incised, swelling can be dissected all around separating it from orbicularis oris/buccinator muscle and it is removed.
- The mucous membrane is closed with absorbable sutures.

MISCELLANEOUS

A case of malignant melanoma of the oral cavity
(see the clinical notes)

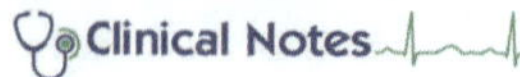

This 48-year-old man (Figs 35.59 and 35.60) presented with an innocent looking, painless submandibular lymph node enlargement. It was firm and nontender. Initially, it was thought to be due to dental caries. Examination of the floor of the mouth revealed an interesting melanomatous lesion. Diagnosis was malignant melanoma with metastasis in nodes. This is just to remind that melanoma can also occur in the oral cavity (mucosa and firm skin).

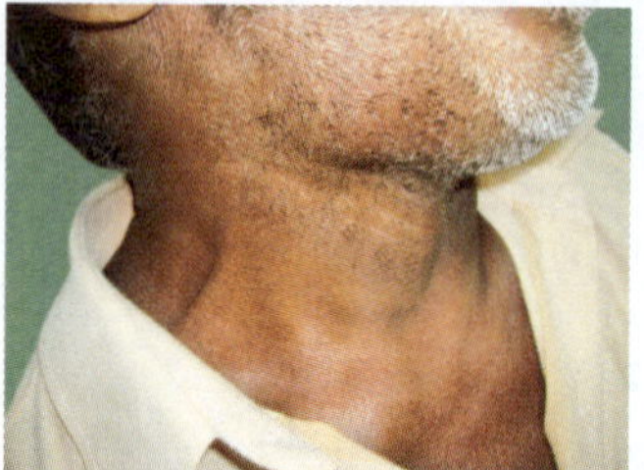

Fig. 35.59: This patient presented with right submandibular lymph node enlargement

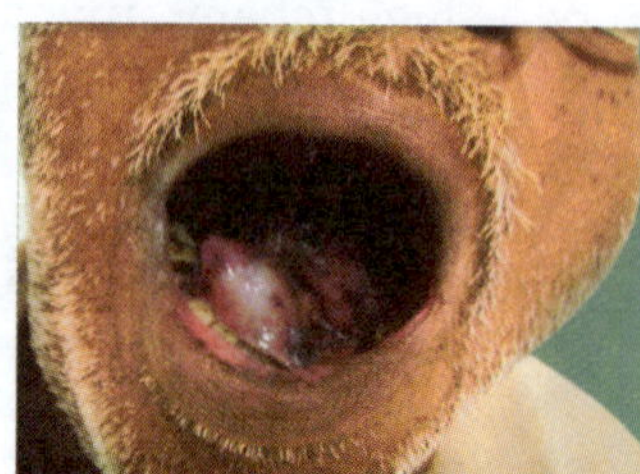

Fig. 35.60: Oral cavity examination reveals a pigmented ulcerated lesion

Multiple Choice Questions

1. **Which one of the following has highest chance of malignancy?**
   A. Acanthosis B. Dyskeratosis
   C. Leukoplakia D. Speckled leukoplakia

2. **Drug used to treat leukoplakia is:**
   A. Vitamin E B. Isonicotinic acid
   C. Isotretinoin D. Niacin

3. **Following are true for verrucous carcinoma *except:***
   A. Very slow-growing
   B. Poorly differentiated carcinoma
   C. Spread by lymphatics is not common
   D. Surgery is the best treatment

4. **Carcinoma tongue spreads to following lymph nodes *except:***
   A. Submandibular B. Submental
   C. Jugulo-omohyoid D. Supraclavicular node

5. **Following malignant lesions in the posterior third of the tongue can occur *except:***
   A. Squamous cell carcinoma
   B. Adenocarcinoma
   C. Lymphoepithelioma
   D. Sebaceous carcinoma

6. **The investigation of choice in oral cancer to find out the skull base involvement is:**
   A. CT scan
   B. Angiography
   C. MRI
   D. Ultrasound

7. **Which cancer in the oral cavity—T1 N0 M0—requires supraomohyoid block dissection?**
   A. Carcinoma buccal mucosa
   B. Verrucous carcinoma lower lip
   C. Carcinoma upper lip
   D. Carcinoma floor of the mouth

8. **Following are true for chronic hyperplastic candidiasis *except*:**
   A. Invasion of *Candida albicans*
   B. Antifungal treatment helps
   C. High malignant potential
   D. Floor of the mouth is affected

9. **Which one of the following conditions has high incidence of distant spread?**
   A. Carcinoma buccal mucosa
   B. Carcinoma tongue
   C. Carcinoma floor of the mouth
   D. Nasopharyngeal carcinoma

10. **Which is the most effective chemotherapeutic drug for head and neck cancers?**
    A. Carboplatins B. 5-Fluorouracil
    C. Bleomycin D. Cisplatin

11. **Best treatment of carcinoma buccal mucosa—T1 N0 M0 is:**
    A. Radiotherapy only
    B. Radiotherapy followed by surgery
    C. Surgery only
    D. Surgery followed by radiotherapy

12. **Khaini chewers more susceptible for development of which carcinoma?**
    A. Carcinoma lip
    B. Cracinoma tongue
    C. Carcinoma buccal mucosa
    D. Carcinoma floor of the mouth

13. **Estlander flap is used to cover:**
    A. Central defects of lip—lower lip
    B. Central defects of lip—upper lip
    C. Lateral defects of more than 50%
    D. Lateral defects up to 30%

14. **Following are true for precancerous lesions of lip/oral cavity *except:***
    A. Keratoacanthoma B. Leukoplakia
    C. Erythroplakia D. Submucous fibrosis

15. **Following are features of carcinoma maxillary antrum *except:***
    A. Can cause asymmetry of face
    B. Can cause proptosis
    C. Can cause infraorbital nerve paralysis
    D. Can cause buccal branch of facial nerve paralysis

16. **Following are the boundaries of nasopharyngeal space *except:***
    A. Nasal fossae
    B. Basilar part of occipital bone
    C. Body of sphenoid
    D. Cribriform plate of ethmoid bone

17. **Following are true for nasopharyngeal carcinoma *except:***
    A. Presents as high anterior cervical lymphadenopathy
    B. Can present as trigeminal neuralgia

C. Compression of IX and X cranial nerves
D. Can present as ophthalmoplegia

18. Following are painless ulcers in the tongue *except:*
A. Gummatous ulcers B. Carcinomatous ulcers
C. Systemic diseases D. Tuberculous ulcers

19. Following are painful ulcers in the tongue *except:*
A. Gummatous ulcers B. Tuberculous ulcers
C. Aphthous ulcers D. Dental ulcers

20. Following are true for syphilitic lesions of the tongue *except:*
A. Snail track ulcers B. Gumma
C. Hutchinson's wart D. Hunterian chancre

21. Following are true for dental cyst *except:*
A. Upper jaw is commonly involved
B. It is a large unilocular cyst
C. Cyst contains cholesterol crystals
D. Arises from unerupted tooth

22. Which one of the following swellings does not contain cholesterol crystals?
A. Branchial cyst B. Sebaceous cyst
C. Dental cyst D. Hydrocoele

23. Following are true for dentigerous cyst *except:*
A. Upper jaw is commonly involved
B. Produces egg shell crackling
C. X-ray shows soap bubble appearance
D. Arises from unerupted tooth

24. Adamantinoma of the jaw has following features *except:*
A. It is a malignant tumour
B. It spreads within medullary bone
C. It is treated by wide excision
D. Mandible is the most common site

25. Which of the following is unilocular cyst?
A. Adamantinoma B. Dentigerous cysts
C. Epididymal cyst D. Dental cyst

Answers

1. D	**2.** C	**3.** B	**4.** D	**5.** D	**6.** C	**7.** D	**8.** D	**9.** D	**10.** D
11. C	**12.** A	**13.** D	**14.** A	**15.** D	**16.** D	**17.** A	**18.** D	**19.** A	**20.** D
21. D	**22.** B	**23.** A	**24.** A	**25.** D					

CHAPTER

36

Salivary Glands

Competency

SU21.1: Describe surgical anatomy of the salivary glands, pathology and clinical presentation of disorders of salivary glands.

SU21.2: Enumerate the appropriate investigations and describe the principles of treatment of disorders of salivary glands.

INTRODUCTION

There are three pairs of salivary glands—parotid, submandibular and sublingual. In addition to these, there are many (450) minor salivary glands located in the cheek, mucosa, lips, palate and base of the tongue. Parotid, the "big brother of 3", suffers mainly from three diseases—infection, enlargement and tumour. Submandibular salivary gland suffers from mainly two diseases—sialoadenitis and tumours. Other salivary glands are of minor importance. However, it should be remembered that the commonest tumour of minor salivary glands is malignancy.

SURGICAL ANATOMY OF THE PAROTID GLAND

Parotid gland is present on the lateral aspect of the face, divided by the facial nerve into superficial lobe and deep lobe. Superficial lobe overlies the masseter and the mandible. Deep lobe is wedged between the mastoid process and the styloid process, ramus of the mandible and medial pterygoid muscle.

The superficial lobe also receives a duct from the accessory lobe which is in the region of zygomatic arch/zygomatic process. The **duct of parotid, Stensen's duct,** 2–3 mm in diameter, receives tributaries from superficial, deep and accessory lobes, passes through the buccinator muscle and opens in the mucosa of the cheek **opposite the upper 2nd molar tooth.** Parotid gland is covered by a true capsule which is a condensation of fibrous stroma of the gland and a **false capsule** formed by **parotid fascia**, a part of the deep cervical fascia.

Facial Nerve

After emerging from stylomastoid foramen, it hooks around the condyle of mandible, enters the substance of the parotid and divides into 2 major branches, **zygomaticotemporal** and **cervicofacial.** Facial nerve along with retromandibular vein (which is formed by the union of superficial temporal vein and maxillary vein, formed from branches of pterygoid plexus of veins) is present in this plane. This plane is called the **fasciovenous plane of Patey** (Figs 36.1 and 36.2 and

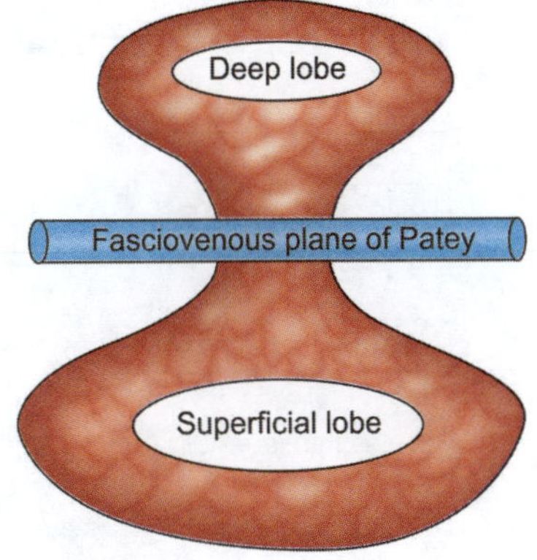

Fig. 36.1: Two lobes of parotid gland

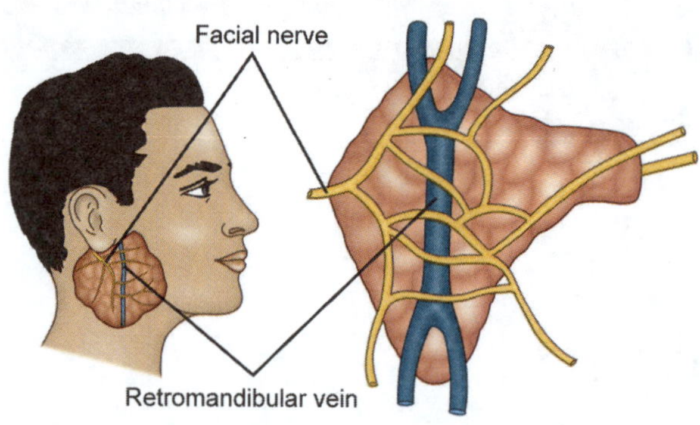

Fig. 36.2: Surgical anatomy of the parotid gland

Flowchart 36.1). The facial nerve then gives rise to 5 branches which are interconnected like the foot of a goose, called ***Pes anserinus***. Branches of facial nerve in the face and the muscles supplied by these nerves are given in Table 36.1.

Table 36.1 Facial nerve and its branches

Branches of facial nerve		Muscles supplied
1. Temporal	→	Auricularis anterior and superior portion of frontalis
2. Zygomatic		
Upper	→	Frontalis and upper half of orbicularis oculi
Lower	→	Lower half of orbicularis oculi and muscles below the orbit
3. Buccal	→	Buccinator, orbicularis oris and a few fibres of elevators of the lower lip
4. Mandibular	→	Muscles of the lower lip
5. Cervical	→	Platysma

Flowchart 36.1: Formation of retromandibular vein and its branches

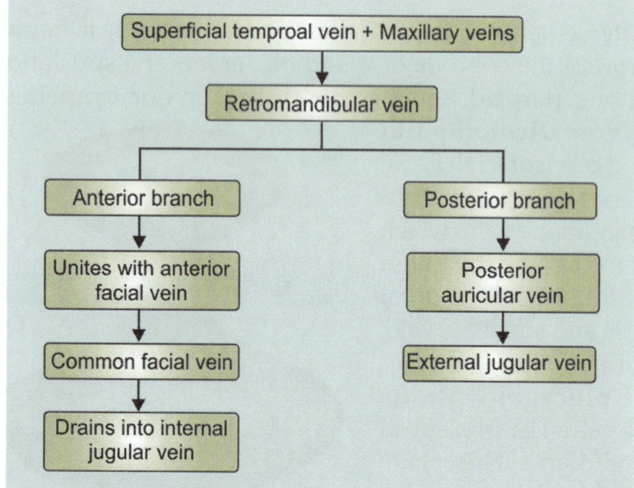

[1]It causes parotitis, orchitis and pancreatitis.

ACUTE PAROTITIS

Acute inflammation of the parotid can occur due to bacterial or nonbacterial causes. It can be unilateral or bilateral (Key Box 36.1). Three important causes and their treatment are given below:

Key Box 36.1

Causes of Acute Parotitis

1. Viral	:	**Mumps**—commonest Coxsackie A and B Parainfluenzae 1 and 3 Echovirus Lymphocytic choriomeningitis
2. Bacterial	:	Usually ascending infection *Staphylococcus aureus*
3. Recurrent parotitis of childhood	:	Recurrent, mistaken for mumps Resolves at puberty
4. Specific infections	:	Mycobacterial, cat-scratch disease, syphilis, toxoplasmosis
5. Allergic	:	Food and drugs
6. Sexual diseases	:	HIV-related
7. Postradiation	:	Reduction in the salivary juice
8. Postoperative	:	Due to dehydration

Mumps Parotitis

Mumps[1] is an acute generalised viral disease with painful enlargement of salivary glands, chiefly the parotids. The virus belongs to Paramyxoviridae family and only one serotype is known. The disease spreads from a human reservoir by direct contact, airborne droplets or fomites contaminated by saliva and possibly by urine.

Clinical Manifestation

- Incubation period is 10–24 days. Fever, headache and muscular pain are usually found. Both parotids are enlarged with pain and temperature.
- Swelling starts subsiding by 3–7 days of time.

Treatment

If symptomatic: Maintenance of good oral hygiene and hydration is useful. Antibiotics may be given to prevent secondary infection. One episode of infection confers lifelong immunity.

Acute Bacterial Parotitis

Staphylococcus aureus infection of parotid produces serious illness with marked engorgement of parotid.

Typically, it produces parotid abscess. Diabetes, malignancy, malnutrition increase the risk. Decreased salivary secretion is an important predisposing factor.

Suppuration occurs due to involvement of intra-parotid lymph nodes, peri-parotid lymph nodes or due to involvement of parenchyma of the gland.

Reduction in Salivary Juice

It can occur due to various factors mentioned in the box. **Postoperative parotitis** can be prevented by good mouth care and good oral hygiene. Due to poor oral hygiene, ascending infection occurs from the oral cavity resulting in parotitis (Key Box 36.2).

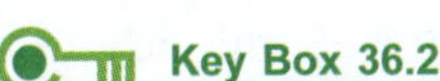

Key Box 36.2

Causes of ↓ Salivary Flow

- Postoperative
- Poor oral hygiene
- Dehydration
- Enteric fever, septicaemia
- Postradiotherapy, for oral cancer

Clinical Features

- A patient who is recovering in the postoperative period may complain of pain and swelling in the parotid region. Presence of severe pain with a very sick, toxic look and high grade fever, chills and rigors indicates parotid abscess. **Diffuse brawny swelling is characteristic.**
- The swelling is due to inflammation of parotid and since it is enclosed by parotid fascia, the swelling takes the shape of parotid gland. However, it is not common for a parotid abscess to raise the ear lobule. For the reason mentioned above, fluctuation is a late feature. **If the abscess is not drained, it is likely to rupture into the external auditory canal** (Key Box 36.3).
- The opening of the parotid duct may be inflamed and on gentle compression of the parotid gland, pus can be seen coming out of the parotid duct.

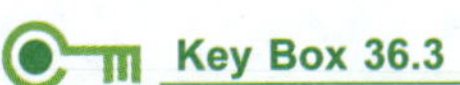

Key Box 36.3

Swellings wherein One should not Wait for Fluctuation

- Parotid abscess
- Breast abscess
- Ischiorectal abscess
- Pulp space infection
- Any deep-seated abscess

Investigations

Complete blood picture: Total count and neutrophils are elevated.

Blood sugars: Fasting and post-prandial sugar are done to rule out diabetes.

Ultrasound: It is the investigation of choice. It can differentiate parotid abscess from cellulitis with brawny induration. Abscess appear as hypo-anechoic lesions, with irregular margins.

Treatment

I. Conservative line of management

- Indicated in a stage of cellulitis with no abscess.
- Maintaining good hydration of the patient in the postoperative period.
- Improvement in the oral hygiene—mouthwashes with potassium permanganate ($KMnO_4$) solution.
- Appropriate antibiotics against staphylococci, such as cloxacillin, are administered in the dose of 500 mg, 6th hourly along with metronidazole 400 mg, 8th hourly to treat anaerobic infections.
- It takes about 3–5 days for the inflammation to settle down.

II. Surgical treatment when there is pus

- Under general anaesthesia, an adequate vertical incision is made in front of the tragus of the ear up to deep fascia. Open the deep fascia in two or three places and drain with blunt haemostat so as to avoid damage to facial nerve. This is described as **Blair's method** of drainage of parotid abscess. A drainage tube has to be kept which can be removed after 3–4 days (Key Box 36.4).

Key Box 36.4

Drainage of Parotid Abscess

- Should not wait for fluctuation
- High grade fever, and toxicity are indications
- Vertical incision
- **Hilton's method** is preferred to break multiple loculi

RECURRENT PAROTITIS OF CHILDHOOD

- Children between ages of 3 and 6 years are commonly affected.
- Aetiology is unknown, may be due to sialectasis (dilatation of branches of salivary duct).
- Recurrent pain and swelling of one or both parotids is common.
- Each attack may last for 3 to 7 days.
- It is **self-limiting** (if the attack is minor).

- Sialography shows **punctate sialectasis**, called **snowstorm** appearance.
- A short course of antibiotics has to be given to cover *Streptococcus viridans.*
- Rarely, superficial parotidectomy may be necessary.

SURGICAL ANATOMY OF THE SUBMANDIBULAR SALIVARY GLAND (Fig. 36.3)

- Submandibular salivary gland is located in the submandibular triangle. It lies partly below and partly above the mandible.
- It is in very close contact with the belly of the digastric muscle. At surgery, once the deep fascia is **opened, the intermediate tendon of digastric is located** and when it is retracted downwards, mobilisation of the gland becomes easy.
- Submandibular salivary gland is divided into a superficial part and a deep part by the mylohyoid muscle which forms the oral diaphragm. During excision of the gland, a few fibres of mylohyoid are also removed. When submandibular salivary gland enlarges, **it is bidigitally palpable** because the **deep portion is deep to mylohyoid** and it is in the floor of the mouth.
- Facial artery enters the gland from its posterolateral surface and **deeply grooves the gland.** It is ligated at this place first during excision of the gland. After grooving the gland, it ascends laterally and curls around the lower border of mandible to enter the face. It is ligated at this place also.
- Main duct of submandibular gland, **Wharton's duct** arises from deep part of gland and opens on a papilla beside the frenulum of the tongue in the oral cavity.

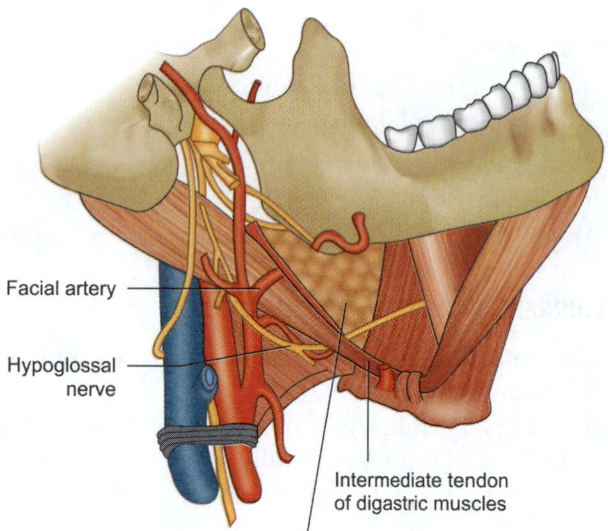

Fig. 36.3: Anatomy of the submandibular salivary gland

- In a deeper plane, the gland is related to **two nerves—lingual and hypoglossal.**

CHRONIC SUBMANDIBULAR SIALOADENITIS

- Obstruction is the most important cause of submandibular sialoadenitis. Trauma to the floor of the mouth is another cause.
- Obstruction can be due to stone, disease, stricture of the duct, or fibrosis of the papilla **(calculus—most common).**
- The causative organism is Staphylococcus.

SIALOADENITIS DUE TO CALCULI

- The disease starts with acute bacterial sialoadenitis which occurs secondary to obstruction. **The submandibular gland has a poor capacity for recovery following infection**. Despite control of acute symptoms with antibiotics, the gland becomes chronically inflamed.
- Calculi (80% of them occur in the submandibular salivary gland) commonly occur in the duct and also within the gland and produce recurrent sialoadenitis. Calculi are more common in the submandibular salivary gland than in the parotid gland because of the following reasons:
  1. **Higher mucin content** in the submandibular salivary gland secretions.
  2. **Calcium and phosphate** content in the secretion is high. Hence, 80% of them are radiopaque and are detected by plain X-ray (Fig. 36.4).
  3. **Nondependent drainage** of the secretions. Gland is in the neck and opening of the duct in the oral cavity.
  4. **Kinking or hooking** of submandibular duct by lingual nerve.

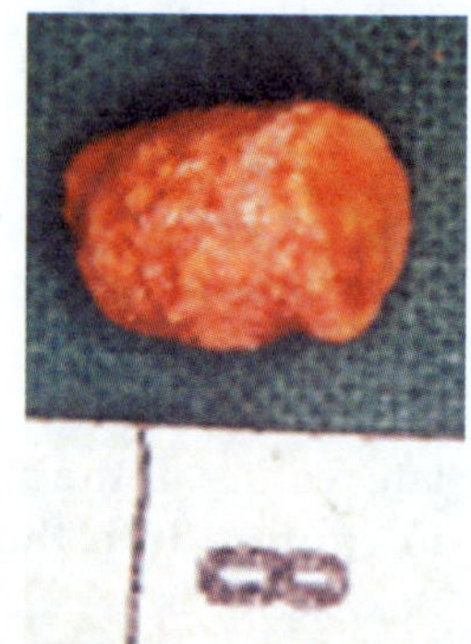

Fig. 36.4: Submandibular calculi in the duct—removed (intraoral approach)

Clinical Features (Key Box 36.5)

Key Box 36.5

Submandibular Salivary Gland Enlargement

- Location—submandibular region
- Lobular, firm swelling
- Bidigitally palpable
- Stone may be palpable within the duct, intraorally

- **Salivary colic:** It is a severe pricking type of pain which is exaggerated at the time of meals. Salivary secretions are induced by a meal or lemon (lemon juice test). As a result of blockage due to a stone, the tension within the gland increases, resulting in pain.
- **Lingual colic:** If a calculus is situated within the submandibular duct where it is hooked by lingual nerve, the pain can radiate to the tongue as a result of irritation to the lingual nerve.
- **Enlargement of salivary gland during meals is the characteristic feature of salivary calculus.** Classically submandibular salivary gland swelling is located in the submandibular region. It is firm in consistency with a lobular surface. It is tender and both lobes are enlarged. **It is bidigitally palpable (submandibular lymph node is palpable only in the neck)** both inside the oral cavity and in the neck. The swelling reduces in size once the stimuli are withdrawn (after meals).
- The stone may be palpable within the gland (in the neck), within the duct (intraorally), or sometimes it may be seen at the orifice of the submandibular duct on the side of lingual frenulum.
- It is not uncommon to get a severe septic sialoadenitis with gross swelling of the gland and inflammatory oedema almost like Ludwig's angina (Fig. 36.5).

Investigations

Ultrasound can easily detect the stone as hypoechoic areas, enlargement of gland and location of the stone. More common is stones are located in the distal part of the duct.

Treatment

- An oblique lateral or posterior oblique occlusal radiography may demonstrate a stone.
  1. **Stone in the submandibular duct:** This can be removed by incising the mucosa over the floor of the mouth, after stabilising the stone. Removal of the stone is followed by **gush of old dirty contents** of the submandibular gland (Fig. 36.6).

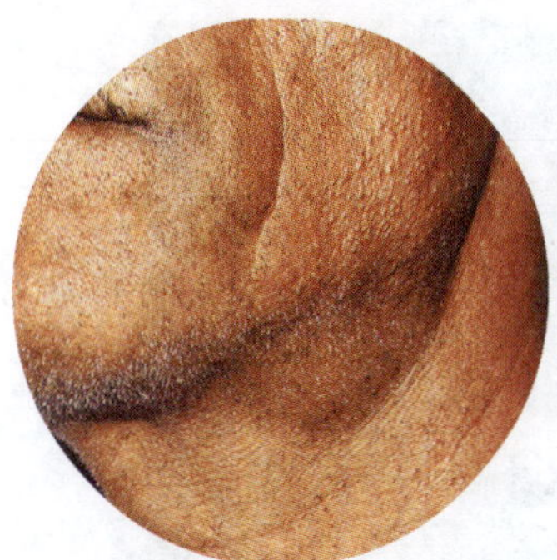

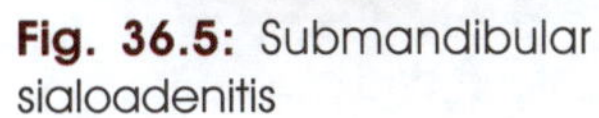

Fig. 36.5: Submandibular sialoadenitis

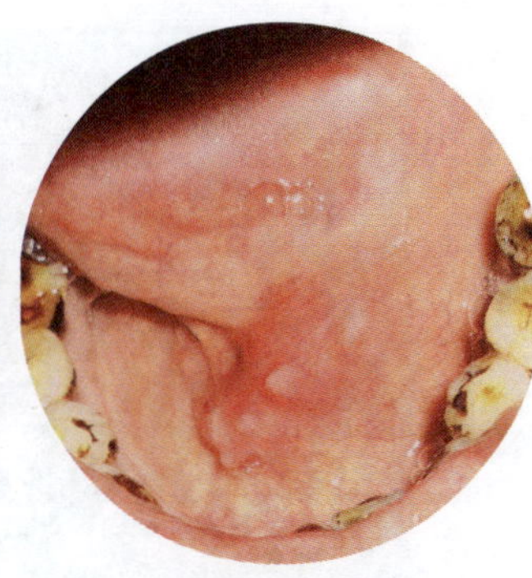

Fig. 36.6: Inflamed opening of submandibular duct

  2. **Chronic sialoadenitis:** This requires excision of submandibular salivary gland. Three steps of dissection of the gland include incision, mobilisation and excision (**Manipal Rule of 2**—Table 36.2).
- **Incision:** It should be a skin crease incision over the lower pole of the gland, the posterior limit of the incision should be at least 2 cm away from the angle of the mandible, to avoid damage to the cervical branch of facial nerve. The incision is deepened till the deep fascia is opened.
- **Mobilisation of the gland:** Division of the facial artery twice, once in a deeper plane on the posterolateral aspect and another at the superolateral aspect close to the lower border of the mandible is an important step which permits mobilisation of the gland. Separation of the gland from fibres of mylohyoid muscle by dividing small arteries completes the mobilisation (Fig. 36.7).
- **Excision of the gland:** It is done by ligating and dividing submandibular duct.

Complications

- Damage to lingual nerve, marginal mandibular nerve or even to hypoglossal nerve. Seroma and infection are the other complications.
- Transection of the nerve to mylohyoid muscle produces **anaesthesia of the submental skin.**

Table 36.2 Submandibular salivary gland excision—**Shenoy's Manipal rule of 2**

• 2 common indications	→ Stone and as a part of radical neck dissection
• 2" long incision	→ Curved incision over the swelling
• Protect 2 superficial nerves	→ Cervical and marginal mandibular branches of facial nerve
• Protect 2 deep nerves	→ Lingual and hypoglossal nerves
• Ligate facial artery 2 times	→ First at deeper plane and then at superficial plane
• Divide 2 muscles	→ Superficial—platysma; Deep—fibres of mylohyoid
• Remove 2 lobes	→ Superficial and deep lobe
• Incision is 2 cm medial to mandible, 2 cm anterior to angle of the mandible	→ To protect 2 superficial nerves

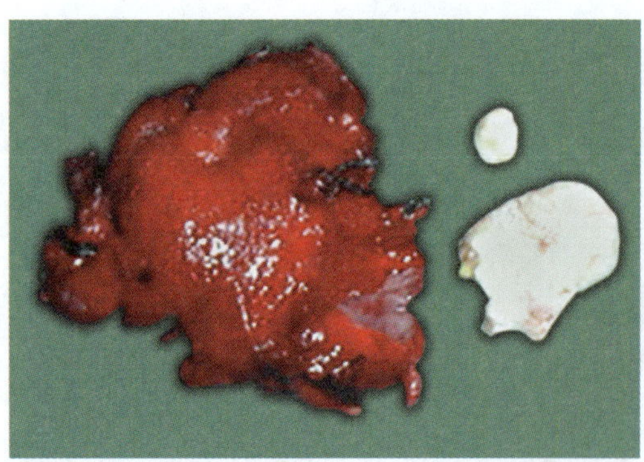

Fig. 36.7: Submandibular stone and gland

SALIVARY GLAND TUMOURS

INTERNATIONAL CLASSIFICATION

I. Epithelial tumours
II. Nonepithelial tumours.

I. Epithelial Tumours

A. Adenoma
   1. Pleomorphic adenoma
   2. Monomorphic adenomas
      - Adenolymphoma (Warthin's tumour)
      - Oxyphilic adenoma (oncocytoma)
      - Other types

B. Mucoepidermoid tumours
C. Acinic cell tumour
D. Carcinoma
   1. Carcinoma in pleomorphic adenoma
   2. Adenoid cystic carcinoma
   3. Undifferentiated carcinoma
   4. Adenocarcinoma
   5. Epidermoid carcinoma
   6. Acinic cell tumour
   7. Mucoepidermoid carcinoma
   8. Malignant mixed tumour

II. Nonepithelial Tumours

1. Lipoma
2. Lymphoma
3. Neurofibroma
4. Lymphangioma
5. Sarcoma

Salivary gland tumours are not uncommon. There are dozens of histological types of salivary gland tumours. However, pleomorphic adenoma and adenolymphoma are the common benign types. Carcinoma arising in pleomorphic adenoma, mucoepidermoid tumours and adenoid cystic carcinoma are important malignant tumours.

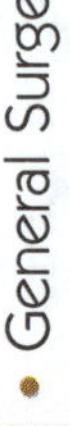

Incidence: 80% of salivary gland tumours are found in the parotid gland. Out of these, 80% are benign, of which 80% are pleomorphic adenomas.

In the submandibular salivary gland, 50% are benign and 50% are malignant.

In the minor salivary glands, 90% are malignant. Thus, the incidence of malignancy increases from major to minor salivary glands.

PLEOMORPHIC ADENOMA OF PAROTID GLAND (MIXED TUMOUR)

It is the most common benign salivary gland neoplasm.

Pathology

- Epithelial cells proliferate in strands, or may be arranged in the form of acini or cords.
- There are also myoepithelial cells which proliferate in sheets. They are called spindle-shaped cells.
- The tumour produces mucoid material, which displaces and separates the cells resembling cartilage in histological section.

Pearls of Wisdom

Because of the presence of epithelial cells, myoepithelial cells, mucoid material, pseudocartilage and lymphoid tissue, the tumour is called pleomorphic adenoma.

- As the tumour grows, it compresses the normal parotid tissue and the branches of the tumour penetrate the thin capsule and enter the substance of the parotid. Simple enucleation will result in a recurrence. Hence, superficial parotidectomy has to be done.

Clinical Features

1. Middle-aged women, around 40 years, are commonly affected (Fig. 36.8A) (female, fifth decade and fullness near ear lobule).
2. Typically, a history of a very slow-growing swelling (for a few years) is usually present.

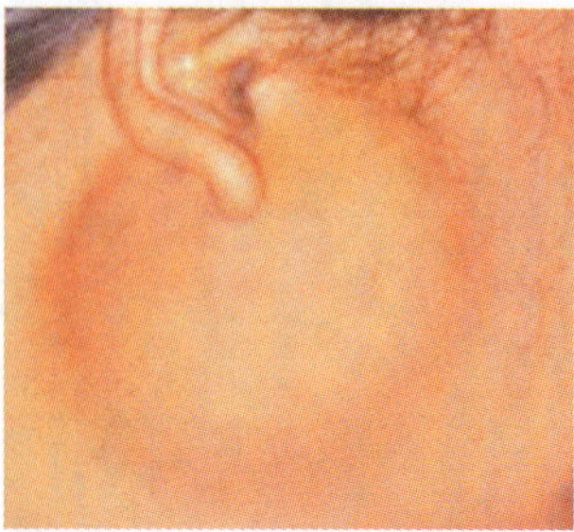

Fig. 36.8A: Pleomorphic adenoma—classical signs

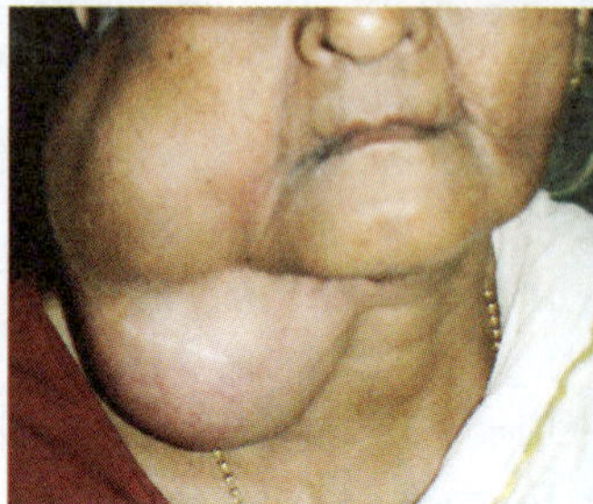

Fig. 36.8B: Gross enlargement of parotid gland of 30 years duration

3. The swelling is painless. **Any painless swelling near the ear is best assumed to be parotid gland neoplasm unless proved otherwise** (Fig. 36.8B).

Signs (Key Box 36.6)

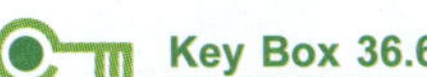

Key Box 36.6

Clinical Examination of Parotid Tumours

Benign	Malignant
Firm	Firm/hard
Nodular	Irregular/nodular
Not fixed	Restricted mobility (fixity to masseter)
No lymph nodes	Lymph nodes palpable
Facial nerve is not involved	Facial nerve paralysis

1. Parotid swelling has the following classical features:
   - It presents as a **swelling in front**, below and behind ear.
   - **Raises ear lobule** (Fig. 36.9)
   - **Retromandibular groove** is obliterated.
   - However, big is the parotid swelling, the upper border is confined (limited) to lower border of zygomatic process because of the attachment of parotid fascia. This is called **curtain sign** (Fig. 36.9).

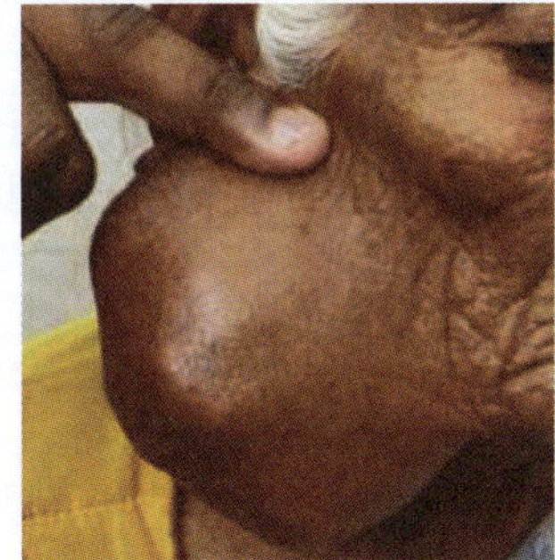

Fig. 36.9: Curtain sign. (*Courtesy:* Dr Haribabu, Dr Ramanayya, Dr G.V. Prakash, SVMC, Tirupathi)

2. It is rubbery or firm. Soft areas indicate necrosis. In long-standing cases, it can be hard. Surface can be nodular or sometimes bosselated. Skin is stretched and shiny. However, being a benign tumour, it is neither adherent to the skin nor to the masseter (Fig. 36.10).
3. After a few years, pleomorphic adenoma may show features of transformation into malignancy **(carcinoma expleomorphic adenoma)**.

   It should be suspected when
   - It starts growing rapidly
   - Skin infiltration occurs
   - Facial nerve paralysis occurs
   - Gets fixed to masseter muscle
   - Red, dilated veins over the surface
   - Presence of lymph nodes in the neck
   - Tumour feels stony hard.

Carcinoma ex Pleomorphic Adenoma (Ca ex PA)

- Presents as a firm mass
- Features of infiltration of facial nerve, masseter muscle, skin or bone may be present
- It occurs due to progressive change: Loss of heterozygosity (LoH) at chromosomal arms 8q, then 12Q and 17Q.
- Mutation of p53—a tumour suppressor gene is also implicated in the malignant transformations of Ca ex PA.
- In high grade Ca ex PAs, epidermal growth factor receptor (EGFR) is overexpressed. Thus, it may have a role in 'invasive' Ca ex PAs.

INTRAORAL EXAMINATION (Fig. 36.11)

- Approximately 10% of the parotid tumours are behind the facial nerve in the deep lobe.
- This is appreciated by intraoral examination wherein the tumour presents with a parapharyngeal mass which displaces the tonsil or soft palate medially.
- Deep lobe tumours present as dysphagia. Such tumours may not show gross swelling on the outer aspect but as they grow, they pass through the stylo-

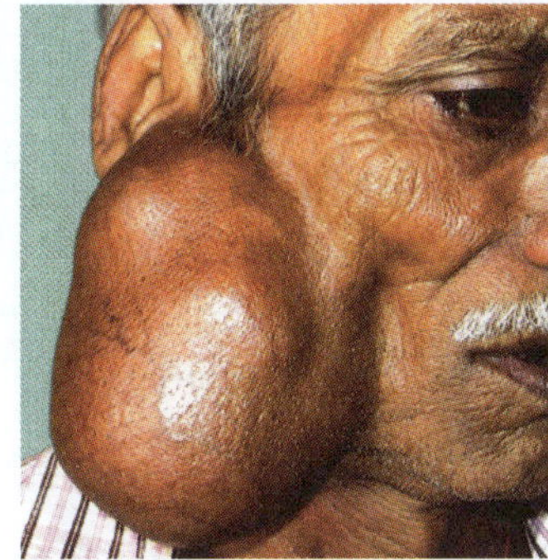

Fig. 36.10A: Lateral view. Note the upper extent limited up to zygomatic process, described as curtain sign positive.

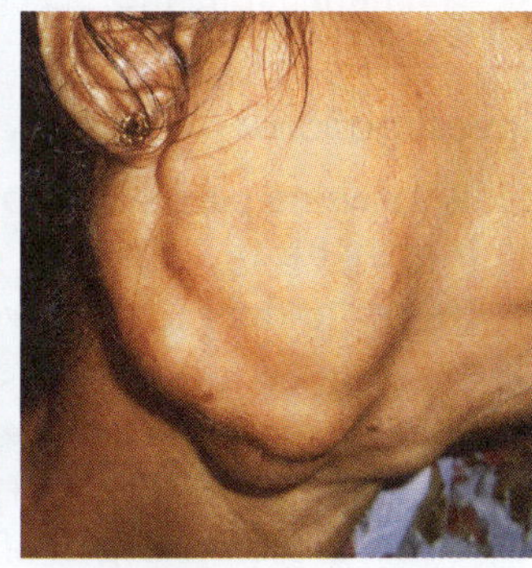

Fig. 36.10B: Lateral view showing nodular surface

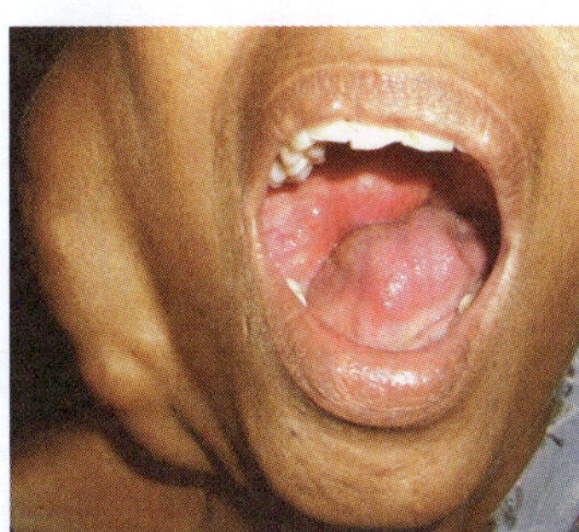

Fig. 36.11: Deep lobe tumour. Importance of intraoral examination (*Courtesy:* Dr Sreejayan, Professor, Department of Surgery, Calicut Medical College, Calicut, Kerala)

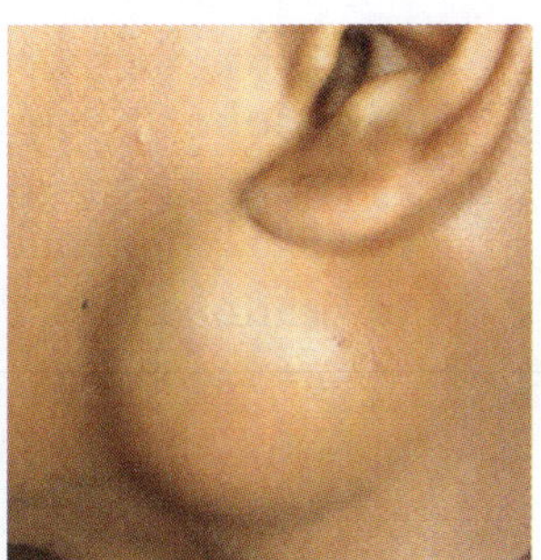

Fig. 36.12: Parotid cyst in a young boy—It was fluctuant and transillumination negative. It was a haemangioma

mandibular tunnel of Patey and push the pharyngeal wall, tonsil and soft palate. These tumours are called **dumb-bell tumours**.

Differential diagnosis of swelling in parotid region (Key Box 36.7)

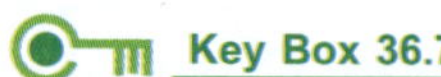

Key Box 36.7

Differential Diagnosis of Swelling in the Parotid Region

1. **When it involves the preparotid region and angle of mandible**
   - Preparotid lymph node enlargement: It may be enlarged due to tuberculosis, metastasis or in non-Hodgkin's lymphoma. Sebaceous cyst in pre-parotid region
   - Preauricular dermoid cyst (young patients)
   - Mesenchymal tumours such as lipoma, neurofibroma
   - Haemangioma, lymphangioma (Fig. 36.12)
2. **When it involves lower pole of parotid**
   - Upper jugular chain lymph node enlargement—metastatic or tubercular
   - Branchial cleft cyst
   - Epithelial inclusion cyst

Investigations

Slow growing parotid tumours **should not be subjected to biopsy** for two reasons:

- **Injury to the facial nerve.**
- **Seeding of tumour** cells in the subcutaneous plane which causes recurrence in about 40–50% of cases.

1. **Ultrasound is the first investigation.** It can recognise the organ of origin and can detect solid areas. It can assess neck lymph nodes also. Cystic areas represent necrosis. Thus ultrasound guided fine needle. **Fine needle aspiration cytology** (FNAC) is done to confirm the diagnosis and rule out malignancy.
2. **CT scan** is done when the tumour is arising from the **deep lobe**. It helps to define the **extraglandular spread**, the extent of parapharyngeal disease, cervical lymph nodes and bony infiltration.

   Indications for CT scan

   a. Suspected bone destruction at skull base
   b. Suspected involvement of mandible
   c. To assess neck nodes (Fig. 36.13)
3. **FNAC of the lymph nodes** that are palpable in the neck in cases of malignancy of the parotid gland.
4. **X-ray of the bones** (mandible and mastoid process) to look for bony resorption, if malignancy is suspected.

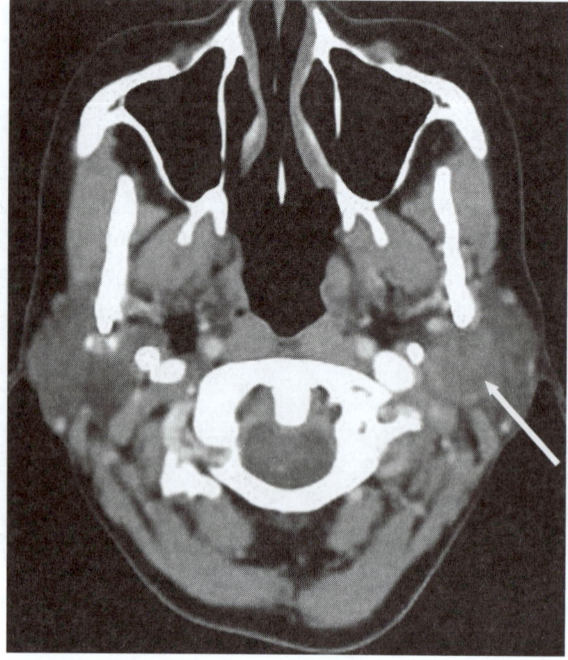

Fig. 36.13: CT scan showing parotid tumour

5. **MRI is a better investigation. However, it is expensive—CT scan and MRI lack specificity for differentiating between benign and malignant lesions.**

   Indications for MRI (Fig. 36.14)

   - Delineating the interface between tumour and normal salivary gland.
   - Better imaging of the parapharyngeal space.
   - Evaluating perineural spread, e.g. adenoid cystic carcinoma.
   - Facial nerve status may be better appreciated.

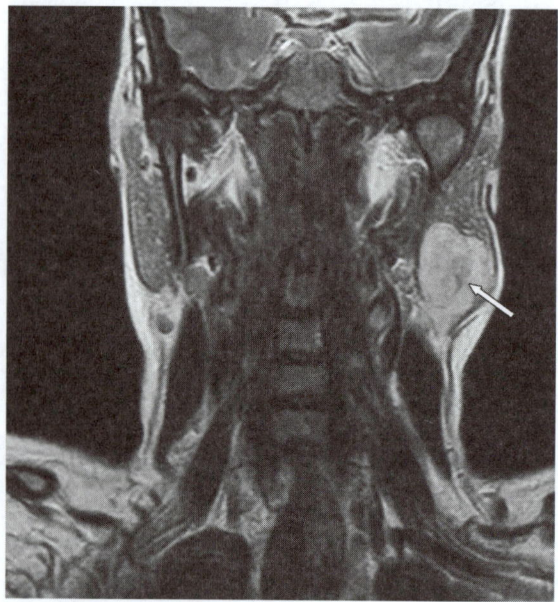

Fig. 36.14: MRI showing parotid tumour

Before we discuss treatment, let us study a few terminologies of parotidectomy.

Parotidectomy

- Superficial: When superficial lobe is removed (superficial to facial nerve).
- In cases of deep lobe enlargement, whole gland has to be removed—total parotidectomy.
- Superficial (partial) adequate: Only tumour with small portion of cuff of parotid gland is removed. Entire lobe is not removed.
- Total: Removal of the entire parotid gland.
- Radical: Total parotidectomy with or without removal of skin, petrous temporal bone, temporomandibular joint, facial nerve with selective neck dissection.
- Extended: Total parotidectomy + sacrifice facial nerve + removal of adjacent structures which are infiltrated such as mandible or masseter muscle, etc.

Extracapsular Dissection

- It is an alternative method of dissection of parotid gland
- Here, nerve is not dissected
- Hence, less invasive
- Temporary facial nerve paralysis is also very less—less than 10%
- Dissection is started in the plane just above parotid fascia (shining)
- After raising skin flaps, a cruciate incision is made over the surface of the tumour, flaps raised, tumour is dissected all around 2 mm.

Treatment of Pleomorphic Adenoma

- Superficial parotidectomy (Fig. 36.15 and Key Box 36.8).

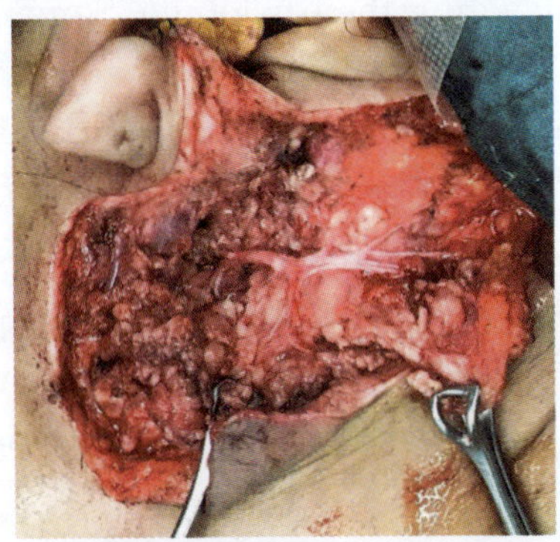

Fig. 36.15: Superficial parotidectomy: Facial nerve divides the gland into superficial and deep lobes. The entire superficial lobe is removed preserving the facial nerve

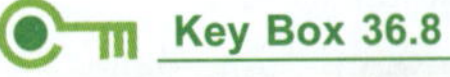

Key Box 36.8

Superficial Parotidectomy

- Indicated in pleomorphic adenoma and other benign neoplasms.
- Tumour along with the normal lobe is removed.
- Preserve the facial nerve, **even in malignant tumours unless grossly involved**.
- Avoid rupture of the gland.
- **Enucleation should not be done as it causes recurrence.**

- It is the standard surgery done for benign pleomorphic adenoma. It means removal of the entire lobe containing the tumour which is superficial to the facial nerve. **Facial nerve should always be preserved**. Enucleation should never be done as it causes recurrence and can injure facial nerve. It is difficult to remove a recurrent tumour.

Some Important Steps of Superficial Parotidectomy (Key Box 36.9)

1. **Adequate exposure** by an incision which starts in front of tragus of ear, vertically descends downwards, curves round the ear lobule up to the mastoid process and is carried downwards in the neck ('Lazy S' incision).
2. **Recognising the facial nerve at surgery**
   - Facial nerve lies **1 cm inferomedial to the bony cartilaginous junction of external auditory canal (Conley's pointer).**
   - In very difficult cases, identify styloid process and nerve is superficial to it.
   - **Trace the posterior belly of digastric** up to the mastoid process. Facial nerve is in between the muscle and tympanic plate (immediately above the muscle).
   - A **nerve stimulator** may be used.
3. **Developing a plane:** Facial nerve and retromandibular vein divide the parotid gland into superficial and deep lobes. Benign tumours do not invade this **faciovenous plane of Patey**.
4. **Gentle handling**, good suction and perfect haemostasis help in clear recognition of the nerve.
5. ***In toto* removal**—the tumour along with **the lobe** to avoid spillage (which is one of the causes of recurrence) (Fig. 36.16).
6. **Good suction drainage** of the wound is necessary to avoid haematoma, wound infection, etc.

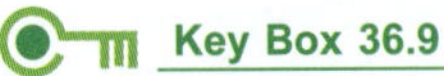

Key Box 36.9

What should be Done in Parotid Surgery?

- Wide exposure by an adequate skin flap.
- Always identify facial nerve (best way to avoid injury).
- Minimum surgery to be done is superficial parotidectomy (enucleation can cause recurrence and injury to facial nerve).
- Always try to preserve facial nerve even in malignancies unless it is directly infiltrated.
- If facial nerve is excised, try to reconstruct immediately by nerve graft—greater auricular or sural nerve.
- Always 'drain' the cavity.
- Buccal nerve can be excised without any repair.

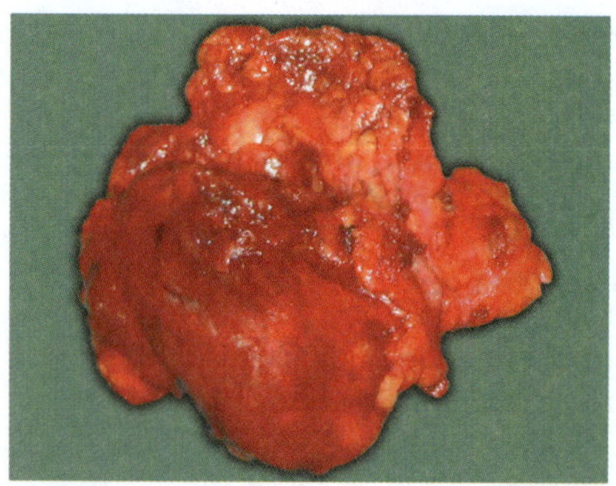

Fig. 36.16: Superficial parotidectomy specimen—avoid rupture of the gland at surgery

Total conservative parotidectomy: Excision of superficial and deep lobe of parotid gland while preserving the facial nerve.

Complications of Parotidectomy (Key Box 36.10)

Key Box 36.10

Complications of Parotidectomy

- **Flap necrosis**—avoid acute bending of the incision and to use gentle retraction
- **Facial nerve palsy**—careful identification
- **Fluid collection**: Blood or seroma—perfect haemostasis and drain should be used
- **Fistula salivary** duct should be ligated
- **Frey syndrome**—occurs in 10% of the cases

Observe **5 Fs**. "Details are given later"

Indications for Postoperative Radiotherapy

- If the deep lobe is involved
- If the lymph nodes are involved
- High grade tumours
- If margins are positive
- Perineural invasion
- Lymphovascular invasion

Postoperative Radiotherapy

T3/T4 cancer: Adenoid cystic carcinoma recurrent tumours.

ADENOLYMPHOMA (WARTHIN'S TUMOUR, PAPILLARY CYSTADENOMA LYMPHOMATOSUM)

- Adenolymphoma is not a lymphoma. It is a misnomer *(vide infra).*
- It is a benign parotid tumour and next common to pleomorphic adenoma. It constitutes about 10% of parotid tumours.
- **Origin of adenolymphoma:** During development, some parotid tissues get included within lymph nodes (preparotid) which are present within the parotid sheath.

Histology

- It is composed of double-layered eosinophilic epithelium. **The inner cells are columnar.**
- Presence of lymphatic tissue in the stroma and lymph follicles is characteristic of adenolymphoma (hence the name).

Clinical Features (Table 36.3)

- Middle-aged or elderly males are commonly affected—usually **they are smokers.**
- Can be **bilateral**, in some cases (10%).
- It has smooth surface, round border with soft, cystic consistency (Fig. 36.17).
- Classically, situated at the lower pole of parotid elevating the ear lobule. Sometimes it may be **multicentric.**
- **This tumour affects only parotid gland** (very, very rarely other glands may be affected).

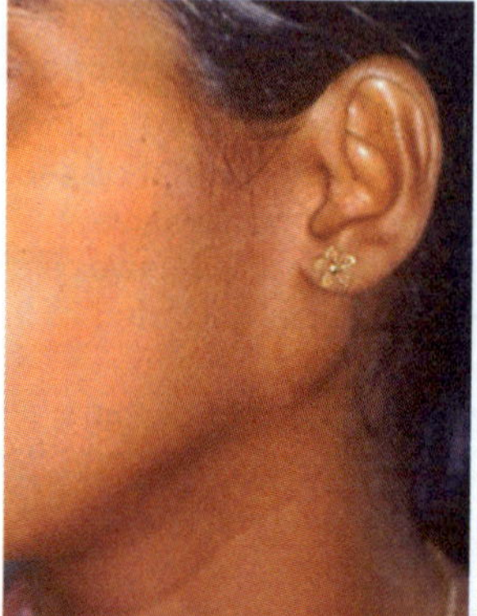

Fig. 36.17: Adenolymphoma

Table 36.3 Comparison between pleomorphic adenoma and adenolymphoma

Features	Pleomorphic adenoma	Adenolymphoma
1. Incidence	70–80%	10%
2. Sex	Common in females	Common in males
3. Number	Single	Sometimes multiple
4. Site	Unilateral	Bilateral
5. Clinical feature	Nodular, firm	Smooth, soft cystic
6. Histology	Pleomorphism	Double layer epithelium and lymphoid tissue
7. ^{99m}Tc-Pertechnetate scan	Cold spot	Hot spot
8. Treatment	Superficial parotidectomy	Superficial parotidectomy

Treatment

It has got a well-defined capsule. Hence, enucleation used to be done earlier **but not now. Superficial parotidectomy is the treatment of choice.**

MUCOEPIDERMOID TUMOUR

- As the name itself suggests, it consists of sheets of epidermoid cells and cystic spaces lined by mucus secreting cells (Fig. 36.18).
- **In childhood, it is the commonest parotid tumour.** It is benign, slow growing but hard in consistency. (Adenolymphoma and mixed tumours are firm but mucoepidermoid tumour is hard.) Parotid is the commonest site. In cases of minor salivary glands, palate is the commonest site.

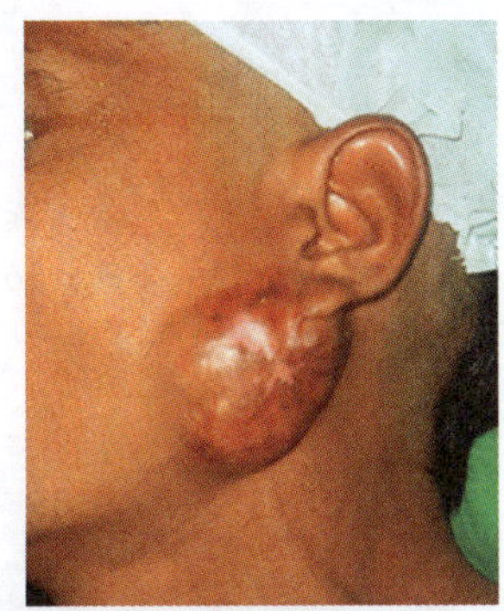

Fig. 36.18: Mucoepidermoid carcinoma

- Mucoepidermoid tumours can infiltrate local tissues, lymph nodes or skin. Hence, a few consider that **mucoepidermoid tumours are always carcinomatous.**
- **Well-differentiated** tumours behave like benign tumours, **intermediate ones** are aggressive and **undifferentiated** tumours metastasise early. Mucoepidermoid carcinoma is the most common malignant epithelial neoplasm of salivary gland.
- The **low grade** tumours are composed of predominantly **mucus secreting cells. High grade tumours** have predominantly **epidermoid cells.**
- Benign tumours need excision and malignant tumours need radical parotidectomy. Radiation is required in the postoperative period.

OTHER TUMOURS

Acinic Cell Tumour

- These are the uncommon parotid tumours. Commonly occur in women.
- The cells resemble those of serous acini and this tumour also has properties of invasion such as mucoepidermoid tumour. It tends to be soft and sometimes cystic.

Oxyphil Adenoma

Also called oncocytoma. It occurs exclusively in the parotid gland. It is a solid tumour and occurs in the sixth decade of life.

Adenoid Cystic Carcinoma

- It is a highly malignant tumour consisting of cords of dark staining cells with cystic spaces containing mucin. It also consists of myoepithelial cells and duct epithelium.
- Even though **slow growing,** it spreads along the **perineural tissue,** may invade periosteum or medullary bone at a distance. This bone resorption results in bony tenderness.
- These tumours have a **high incidence of distant metastasis** but in general **they display indolent growth**. Skin lesions are common as it spreads along the nerve tissue, which leads to treatment failure.
- Local infiltration, lymphatic and blood spread, and local recurrence are important features.
- It is **hard and fixed** and can produce **anaesthesia of the skin overlying the tumour.**
- Early cases are treated by radical parotidectomy with block dissection of the neck. However, many cases present late to the hospital. Thus, palliative radiotherapy is given to reduce pain and to arrest progress of the disease.

Summary of Malignant Salivary Gland Tumours

(Figs 36.19 to 36.23 and Table 36.4)

To find out the exact type of malignant tumour is of interest to pathologists. Clinically, one can suspect malignancy when a salivary tumour has one of the following features:

- Rapidly growing neoplasm.
- Change in consistency (the tumour tends to be hard).
- Fixity to underlying muscle such as masseter as in parotid tumours.
- Fixity to mandible as in parotid or submandibular tumour.
- Involvement of facial nerve as in 80% of cases of malignant parotid tumours.
- Resorption of adjacent bone such as mastoid, tenderness as in adenoid cystic carcinoma.
- Significant hard nodes in the neck.
- They are treated by radical sialoadenectomy with radical block dissection of the neck. Radiotherapy is used as a palliative treatment.

MALIGNANT PAROTID TUMOURS

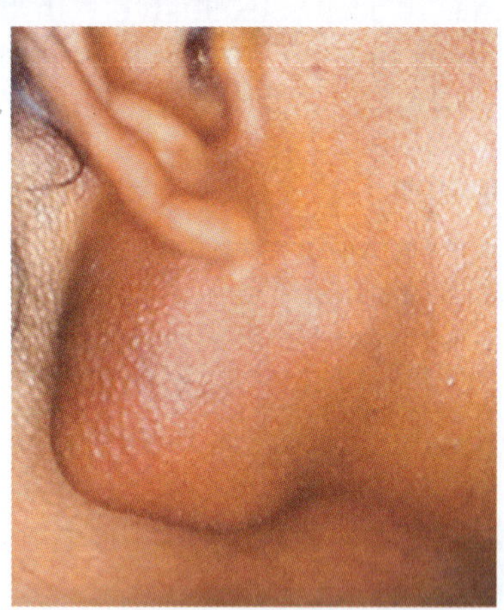

Fig. 36.19: Low grade mucoepidermoid carcinoma—had restricted mobility due to fixity to masseter

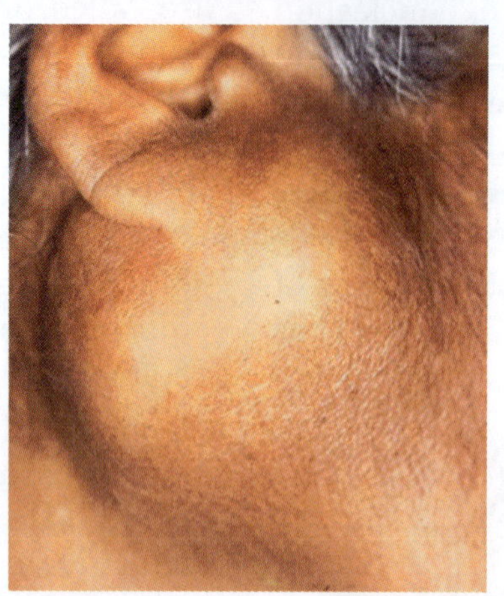

Fig. 36.20: Adenoid cystic carcinoma—perineural spread is common with this tumour

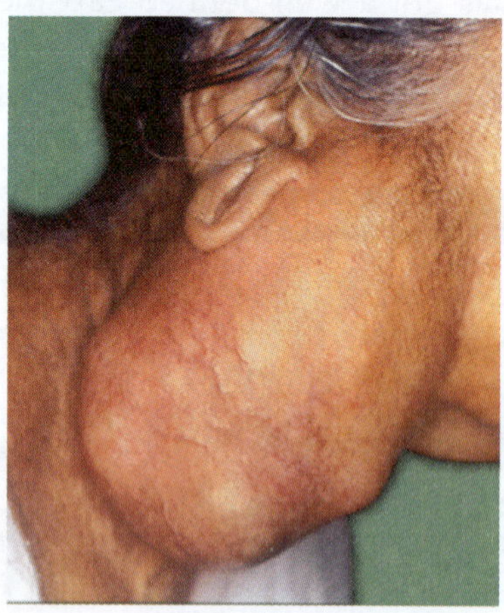

Fig. 36.21: High grade muco-epidermoid carcinoma—rapidly growing and dilated veins over the surface

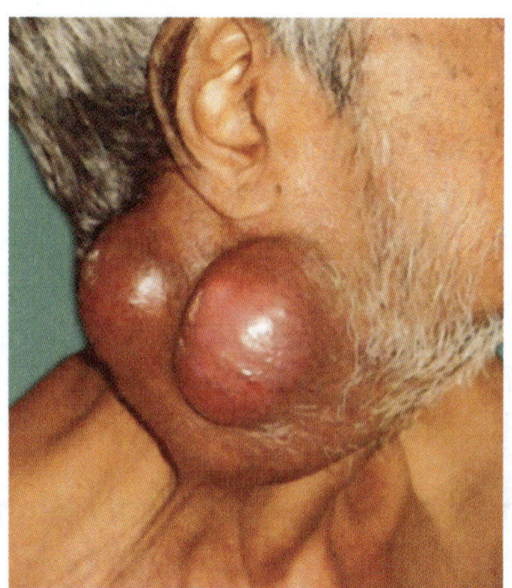

Fig. 36.22: Carcinoma parotid—late stage with involvement of platysma—**platysma sign**

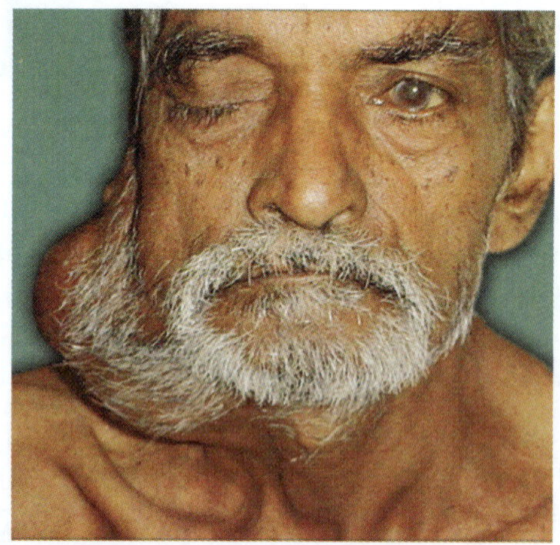

Fig. 36.23: Same patient in Fig. 36.22 also had facial nervé paralysis

Table 36.4 Comparison between submandibular and parotid tumours

	Submandibular tumour	Parotid tumour
• Incidence	Uncommon	Common
• Malignancy	50% of tumours	10–20%
• Location	Submandibular triangle	Parotid region
• Deep lobe involvement	Intraorally felt in the floor of mouth	Tonsillar shift, can also be felt in the lateral wall
• Surgical treatment of malignant tumour	Small tumours—intracapsular submandibular excision	Total conservative parotidectomy for malignant tumours
	Large tumours—radical excision with or without sacrifice of '2' nerves—lingual and hypoglossal	Facial nerve should always be preserved.
• Lymph nodes	Selective neck dissection—supraomohyoid neck dissection	Selective neck dissection (lateral) levels II, III, IV and V lymph nodes
• **Warthin's**	**Does not occur here**	**Exclusively occurs in the parotid gland**

OPERATIVE PHOTOGRAPHS (Figs 36.24 to 36.27)

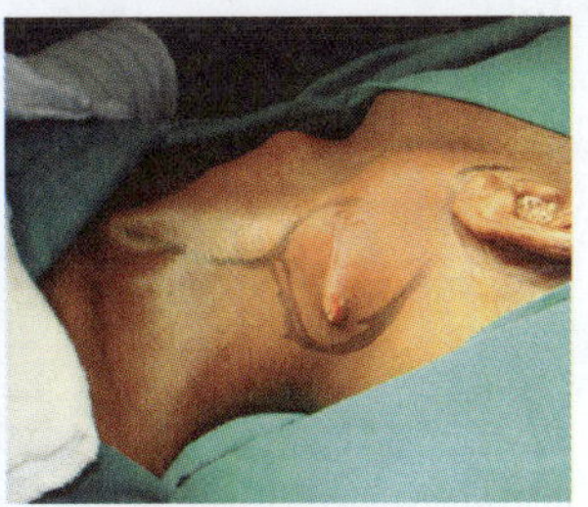
Fig. 36.24: Methylene blue is used to mark the site of incision and part to be raised

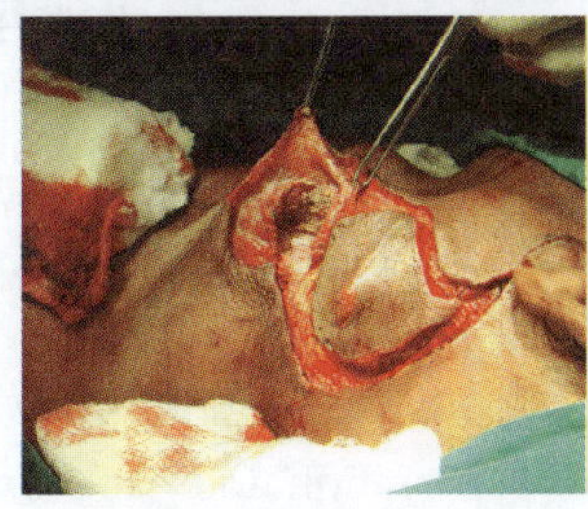
Fig. 36.25: Flaps are elevated

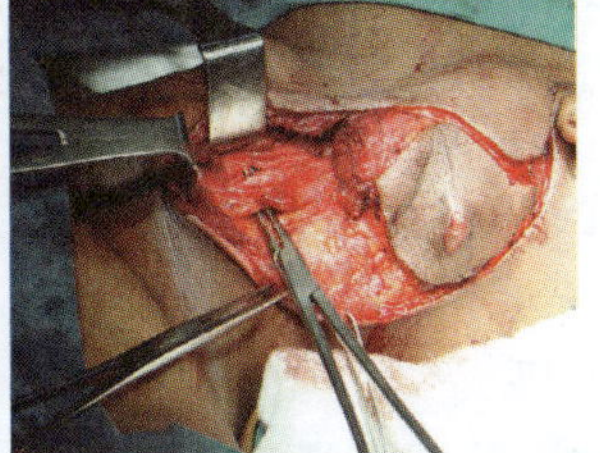
Fig. 36.26: Strap muscles are divided as a part of supraomohyoid block dissection

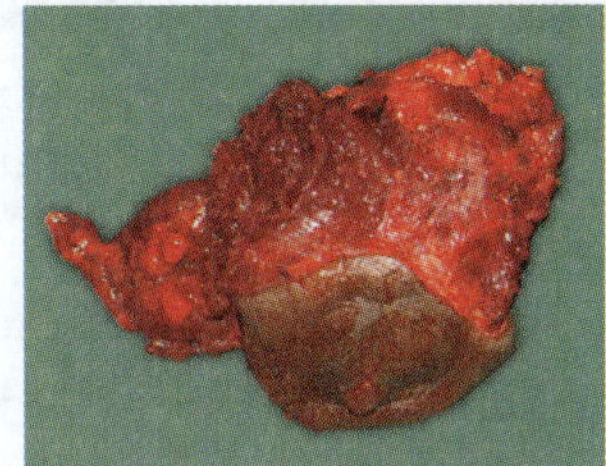
Fig. 36.27: Specimen of tumour with surrounding fat, fascia and lymphatic tissue

FREY'S SYNDROME—GUSTATORY SWEATING

- Auriculotemporal nerve passes through the fork of common carotid artery, passing between neck of the mandible and sphenomandibular ligament.

  Here it supplies parotid gland and ascends and supply auricle. Lastly, it crosses the root of zygomatic process of temporal bone. Kindly refer to Flowchart 36.2.

Flowchart 36.2: Trigeminal nerve and its branches

Trigeminal nerve (V)
↓
Mandibular nerve
↓ It comes out of skull through foramen ovale
→ Anterior
  ↓
  - Buccinator nerve
  - Lingual nerve
  - Inferior alveolar nerve
→ Posterior
  ↓ Pass through otic ganglion
  Two roots
  → Somatosensory root (superior)
    ↓
    1. Secretomotor thus to parotid gland
    2. Supplies auricle
    3. Internal acoustic meatus, outer part of tympanic membrane
  → Parasympathetic root
    ↓
    Carries postganglionic fibre to parotid glands

- Frey's syndrome occurs after surgery for parotid tumours, surgery in the region of temporomandibular joint or due to injury to the parotid gland. Injury to the auriculotemporal nerve can occur at a site where it turns around the neck of the mandible. The injury manifests at a later date, e.g. 2–3 months.
- Because of the injury, **postganglionic parasympathetic fibres from otic ganglion unite with sympathetic fibres of superior cervical ganglion** which **supplies the vessels** and sweat glands **over the skin overlying parotid region** (Key Box 36.11 and Fig. 36.28).

Key Box 36.11

Parts Supplied by Auriculotemporal Nerve

- Auricular part:
  - External acoustic meatus
  - Tympanic membrane surface
  - Skin of auricle above external acoustic meatus
- Temporal part: Hairy skin of the temple

- As a result of this, whenever the **act of chewing** or **mastication is started,** there is increased sweating and hyperaesthesia in the region supplied by auriculotemporal nerve **(cutaneous branch of mandibular division of trigeminal nerve).** Hence, it is called **auriculotemporal syndrome**.
- **Diagnosis: Starch iodine test**—paint the affected area with iodine and allowed it to dry before applying the dry starch.
- The starch turns blue on exposure to iodine in the presence of sweat.

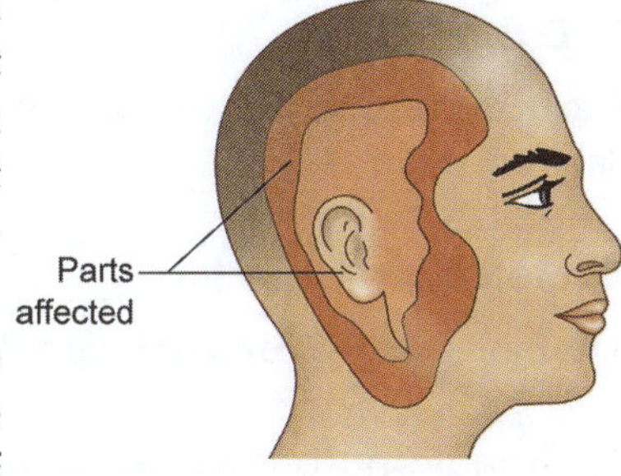

Fig. 36.28: Frey's syndrome

Prevention

Principle is to provide a barrier between the skin and parotid bed by using temporalis fascial flap or sternomastoid muscle flap.

Treatment

- **Reassurance, aluminium chloride—antiperspirant** which is a useful astringent
- Denervation by **tympanic neurectomy**
- Latest treatment includes injection of **botulinum toxin into the affected skin**.

RARE CAUSES OF SALIVARY GLAND ENLARGEMENT

1. Sjögren's Syndrome

It is the diffuse infiltration of salivary and lacrimal glands with lymphocytes resulting in enlargement of glands and slow destruction of acini. Thus, clinical features include dry eyes (keratoconjunctivitis sicca) and dry mouth (xerostomia). These along with a third component rheumatoid arthritis, form the triad of **Sjögren's syndrome (primary)**.

- 30% of patients with systemic lupus erythematosus and all patients with primary biliary cirrhosis develop Sjögren's syndrome. This is termed **secondary Sjögren's syndrome**.
- Other features: This disease is 10 times more common in females and presents with painful enlargement of the glands.
- **Complications**
  1. Lymphomatous transformation (high in primary).
  2. Oral candidiasis.

2. Mikulicz Disease

Due to autoimmune mechanism, symmetrical enlargement of all salivary glands and lacrimal gland enlargement occur. Dry mouth and narrow palpebral fissures are diagnostic of this condition.

3. Drugs

Carbimazole and **thiouracil** can cause enlargement of salivary glands.

4. Metabolic Disorders

Diabetes and **acromegaly** are the other causes.

5. Granulomatous Sialoadenitis

These are rare, painless swellings. Following are the causes:

- **Tuberculosis**
- **Sarcoidosis**—commonly affects parotid gland wherein it is called **pseudotumour**
- **Toxoplasmosis**
- **Cat-scratch** disease
- **Wegener's granulomatosis**

PAROTID FISTULA

It is an uncommon condition which commonly occurs after surgery on the parotid gland (Key Box 36.12).

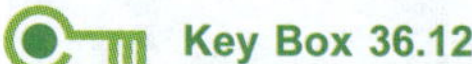

Key Box 36.12

Parotid Fistula

- Any surgery on the parotid gland—superficial parotidectomy, drainage of abscess, surgery for carcinoma cheek, facio-maxillary trauma are the causes.
- Discharging watery fluid, exaggerated by keeping lime in the mouth.
- Fistulogram confirms the diagnosis.
- Exploration and excision of fistula and ligation of duct is required.

MINOR SALIVARY GLAND TUMOUR (Fig. 36.29)

- Even though they are called minor, numberwise they are major (many), about 450 in number.
- They are mucus secreting.
- They can present as mucus retention cyst (common in lip) or as malignant tumour.
- 90% of minor salivary gland tumours are malignant.
- Since they are submucosal, they start as a submucous nodule (very important point in the history) to differentiate from carcinoma buccal mucosa/lip, etc.
- As they grow, they ulcerate. Ulceration is a feature of malignancy.
- Slowly lymph nodes get enlarged.
- Treatment of benign cyst/tumour is by simple excision and malignant tumour is by wide excision.

SURGERY FOR FACIAL NERVE PALSY

INDICATIONS FOR DIFFERENT TYPES OF SURGERY

1. Early immediate nerve repair, in case of injury to the nerve.
2. **Late nerve crossing** by suturing peripheral branches of facial nerve to one of the following nerves:
   - Hypoglossal nerve, spinal accessory nerve
   - Phrenic nerve.

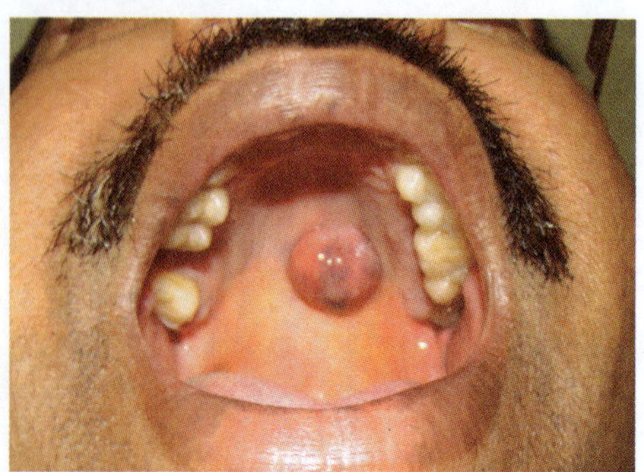

Fig. 36.29: Minor salivary gland tumour in the palate. Laser excision was done

3. Surgery to achieve movement in longstanding facial palsy (usually after 1 year).

A. Static Procedures

- Suspension of lips, cheek and angle of mouth to zygomatic bone or temporal fascia using fascia lata, palmaris longus tendon or other alloplastic materials.
- Medial canthoplasty to reduce epiphora.
- Lateral tarsorrhaphy (canthoplasty) to prevent exposure keratitis due to widened palpebral fissure.

B. Dynamic Procedures

- Muscle transfer with carefully preserved muscle nerve and vessel, e.g. temporalis muscle transfer, masseter muscle transfer.
- Cross face nerve transplantation using sural nerve. Using microscope, sural nerve is sutured to the two or three relatively insignificant branches of facial nerve (selected by intraoperative electric stimulation) on normal side. Other end of the sural nerve is sutured to distal end of the divided facial nerve on paralysed side.
- Free neurovascular gracilis muscle graft using microvascular techniques.

PERIPHERAL NERVE REPAIR AND TRANSFERS

PRINCIPLES OF NERVE REPAIR

1. Preoperative assessment of motor and sensory system.
2. Microsurgical tools should be available.
3. Tension-free repair should be done. If tension-free repair is not possible, then nerve graft can be used.
4. Primary repair when conditions permit.
5. Delayed repair should be done in case of extensive injury.

Microsurgical Techniques

- 4X magnification needed.
- 9–0/10–0 nylon is used for repair.
- Ends prepared with microscissors. First suture to be loose to ease the alignment of other sutures.
- Avoid postural manoeuvre to avoid tension. Nerve can be mobilised 1–2 cm proximally and distally for tension-free suturing but not more than that.

Conduits

- To place a polyglycolic acid tube to bridge the gap rather than to perform nerve grafting.
- **Indications**
  - Donor nerve harvest not possible due to availability and associated morbidity
  - Patients who decline autogenous nerve graft harvest
  - Nerve gap of not more than 3 cm.
- **Principle of conduits**
  - Nerve regeneration and proximal and distal axonal matching result from a combination of neurotropism and contact guidance.

TYPES

I. Nerve Grafting

- **Indications**
  - If a tension-free repair is not possible
  - If the nerve gap is more than 3 cm
  - Can be used in place of conduits
- **Principle**
  - The graft should be oriented in a reverse fashion from its native position so that the regenerating fibres are not diverted from the distal neurorrhaphy site and distal stump. Misalignment should be avoided.
- If the nerve gap is small, fascicular matching can be done
- If the nerve gap is long, techniques of awake stimulation or histochemical staining may be used.
- **Donor sources for nerve grafting**: Posterior interosseous nerve, medial antebrachial cutaneous nerve for small digital nerves, sural nerve for nerve gaps involving larger nerves, greater auricular nerve.

II. Nerve Transfer

- It is used for reconstruction of proximal nerve injuries.
- **Drawbacks** of nerve graft that become the merits of nerve transfer:
  - Grafting across a proximal nerve injury has poor functional outcomes.
  - Timely re-innervation may not be possible if the target muscle is too far from the regenerating site.
- A nerve transfer converts a high level nerve injury to a low level nerve injury by recruiting expendable nerve fascicles from the donor nerve to innervate critical nerves close to their target end organs.
- Donor nerves are preferentially selected according to their proximity to the target site.
- **Criteria for nerve transfers**
  - An expendable donor nerve
  - Donor nerve with a large number of pure axons
  - Donor nerve near the target organ
  - Donor motor nerve that innervates a muscle that is synergistic to the target muscle
- Nerve transfers are done for both motor and sensory nerves.

Intersting most common (Key Box 36.13)

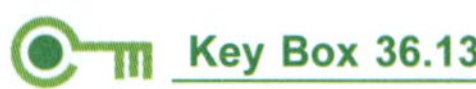

Key Box 36.13

Most Common for Salivary Gland Tumours

- Most common benign parotid tumour in adults—pleomorphic adenoma.
- Most common benign parotid tumour in children— haemangioma.
- Most common type of cancer arising in the parotid glands is mucoepidermoid cancer.
- Most common malignant tumour in submandibular gland—adenoid cystic carcinoma.
- Most common minor salivary gland tumour is adeno-carcinoma.
- Most common site of squamous cell carcinoma is sub-mandibular salivary gland.
- Most common response to radiotherapy among the malignant tumours is adenoid cystic carcinoma.

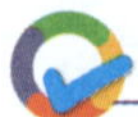

Multiple Choice Questions

1. Commonest tumour of minor salivary gland is:
A. Pleomorphic adenoma
B. Warthin's tumour
C. Malignant tumour
D. Mucoepidermoid tumour

2. Parotid duct opens opposite:
A. Upper canine tooth
B. Lower canine tooth
C. Upper 2nd molar tooth
D. Lower 2nd molar tooth

3. Chronic parotitis in children is pathognomonic of which infection?
A. HCV infection B. HBV infection
C. HIV infection D. Syphilis

4. Which is the common site of calculi in submandibular salivary gland?
A. Superficial lobe B. Deep lobe
C. Accessory lobe D. Duct

5. Deep lobe tumours of parotid gland present as following features *except:*
A. Dysphagia
B. Can push tonsils
C. Can push soft palate
D. Can block the external auditory meatus

6. The investigation of choice in deep lobe tumours of parotid gland is:
A. CT scan
B. Angiography
C. MRI
D. Ultrasound

7. Conley's pointer refers to:
A. Location of facial nerve in relation to tragal cartilage
B. Location of facial nerve in relation to posterior belly of digastric
C. Location of facial nerve in relation to retromandibular vein
D. Location of facial nerve in relation to pinna

8. Following are true for chronic hyperplastic candidiasis *except:*
A. Invasion of *Candida albicans*
B. Antifungal treatment helps
C. High malignant potential
D. Floor of the mouth is affected

9. Following benign tumours have high incidence of recurrence *except:*
A. Adamantinoma
B. Deep lobe tumours of parotid gland
C. Desmoid tumours
D. Diffuse lipomata

10. Recommended treatment of pleomorphic adenoma is:
A. Enucleation
B. Excision
C. Superficial parotidectomy
D. Wide excision

11. Which benign tumour of parotid produces hot spot in Technetium scan?
A. Pleomorphic adenoma
B. Adenoid cystic carcinoma
C. Mucoepidermoid tumour
D. Adenolymphoma

12. Commonest parotid tumour in children is:
A. Pleomorphic adenoma
B. Warthin's tumour
C. Mucoepidermoid tumour
D. Lymphangioma

13. Most common malignant tumour in submandibular salivary gland is:
A. Pleomorphic adenocarcinoma
B. Adenoid cystic carcinoma
C. Mucoepidermoid tumour high grade
D. Acinic cell tumour

14. Following are true for precancerous lesions of lip/ oral cavity *except:*
A. Keratoacanthoma
B. Leukoplakia
C. Erythroplakia
D. Submucous fibrosis

15. Following are features of carcinoma maxillary antrum *except:*
A. Can cause asymmetry of face
B. Can cause proptosis
C. Can cause infraorbital nerve paralysis
D. Can cause buccal branch of facial nerve paralysis

16. Following are the boundaries of nasopharyngeal space *except:*
A. Nasal fossae
B. Basilar part of occipital bone
C. Body of sphenoid
D. Cribriform plate of ethmoid bone

17. Following are true for nasopharyngeal carcinoma *except:*
A. Presents as high anterior cervical lymphadenopathy
B. Can present as trigeminal neuralgia
C. Compression on IX and X cranial nerves
D. Can present as ophthalmoplegia

18. Following are painless ulcers in the tongue *except:*
A. Gummatous ulcers B. Carcinomatous ulcers
C. Systemic diseases D. Tuberculous ulcers

19. Following are painful ulcers in the tongue *except:*
A. Gummatous ulcers B. Tuberculous ulcers
C. Aphthous ulcers D. Dental ulcers

20. Following are true for syphilitic lesions of the tongue *except:*
A. Snail track ulcers B. Gumma
C. Hutchinson's wart D. Hunterian chancre

21. Following are true for dental cyst *except:*
A. Upper jaw is commonly involved
B. It is a large unilocular cyst
C. Cyst contains cholesterol crystals
D. Arises from unerupted tooth

22. Which one of the following swellings does not contain cholesterol crystals?
A. Branchial cyst B. Sebaceous cyst
C. Dental cyst D. Hydrocele

23. Following are true for dentigerous cyst *except:*
A. Upper jaw is commonly involved
B. Produces egg-shell crackling
C. X-ray shows soap bubble appearance
D. Arises from unerupted tooth

24. Adamantinoma of the jaw has following features *except:*
A. It is a malignant tumour
B. It spreads within medullary bone
C. It is treated by wide excision
D. Mandible is the most common site

25. Which of the following is unilocular cyst?
A. Adamantinoma B. Dentigerous cysts
C. Epididymal cyst D. Dental cyst

Answers

1. C	**2.** C	**3.** C	**4.** D	**5.** D	**6.** C	**7.** A	**8.** D	**9.** D	**10.** C
11. D	**12.** C	**13.** B	**14.** A	**15.** D	**16.** D	**17.** A	**18.** D	**19.** A	**20.** D
21. D	**22.** B	**23.** A	**24.** D	**25.** D					

CHAPTER

37

Thyroid Gland

INTRODUCTION

Thyroid gland is an endocrinal gland present in the neck secreting T_3 and T_4 hormones. It is richly vascular and highly functional. Effects of hormonal changes affect every part of the body such as central nervous system, cardiovascular system, gastrointestinal system and reproductive system. It is also the site of various diseases—a simple enlargement, toxicity and malignant transformation.

Competency

SU22.1: Describe the applied anatomy and physiology of thyroid.

SURGICAL ANATOMY OF THYROID GLAND

Development and Anatomy

- It develops from **median downgrowth** (midline diverticulum) of a column of cells from the pharyngeal floor between first and second pharyngeal pouches.
- The descent is anterior to structures that form hyoid bone and larynx (Fig. 37.1).
- By 6 weeks of intrauterine life, the **central column,** which becomes the thyroglossal duct, gets reabsorbed.
- The duct bifurcates to form thyroid lobes.

Tubercle of Zuckerkandl: It is a posterolateral extension of thyroid gland. Incidence—30–40%. Arises

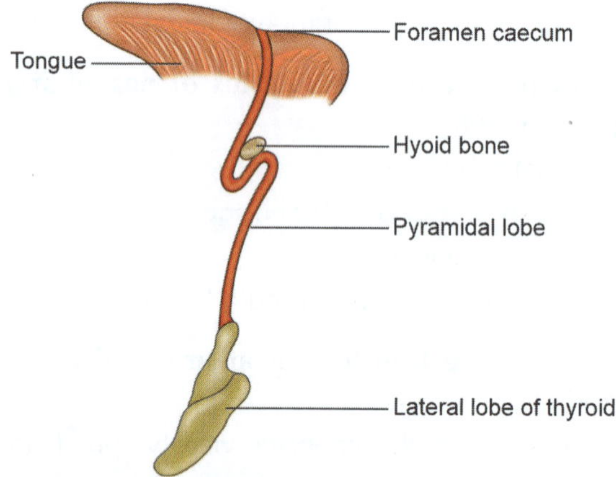

Fig. 37.1: Development of thyroid gland

from lateral anlage. It is closely related to recurrent laryngeal nerve at surgery. Tubercle points to the intersection between the nerve and inferior thyroid artery. It should be removed, if present specially in thyroidectomy for malignancies.

- **Pyramidal lobe** is formed by a portion of the duct.
- **Calcitonin** producing **parafollicular cells or C cells** originate from the fourth branchial pouch.
- Thyroid gland is present in the neck, enclosed by pretracheal fascia which is a part of deep cervical fascia. It has a right and left lobe joined by the

isthmus in front of **2nd, 3rd and 4th tracheal rings**. It weighs about 20–25 g. A projection from the isthmus usually on the left side is called pyramidal lobe. It is attached to the hyoid bone by a fibrous band or muscle fibres called levator glandulae thyroideae.

- Thyroid is covered by true capsule which cannot be separated. However, another layer (false capsule) which is surrounding thyroid gland can be separated.
- **Suspensory ligament of Berry:** This pair of strong condensed connective tissue binds the gland firmly to each side of cricoid cartilage and upper tracheal rings.
- **Pretracheal fascia,** which is part of deep cervical fascia splits to invest the gland. These structures (ligament of Berry and pretracheal fascia) are responsible for thyroid gland moving with deglutition.

Arterial Supply (Fig. 37.2)

- **Superior thyroid artery,** a branch of the external carotid artery, enters the upper pole of the gland, divides into anterior and posterior branches and anastomoses with ascending branch of inferior thyroid artery. Since the upper pole is narrow, ligation is easy.
- **Inferior thyroid artery** is a branch of thyrocervical trunk[1] and enters the posterior aspect of the gland. It supplies the gland by dividing into 4 to 5 branches which enter the gland at various levels (not truly lower pole).
- Inferior thyroid artery used to be ligated well away from the gland to avoid damage to RLN. However, ligation of these arteries on both sides will cause permanent hypoparathyroidism. Hence, *the current practice is to identify and ligate the branches of inferior thyroid artery (3–4) separately.*
- **Thyroidea ima artery** is a branch of either brachiocephalic trunk or direct branch of arch of aorta and enters the lower part of the isthmus in about 2 to 3% of the cases.

Venous Drainage

- **Superior thyroid vein**[2] drains the upper pole and enters the internal jugular vein. The vein follows the artery.
- **Middle thyroid vein** is single[3], short and wide and drains into internal jugular vein.
- **Inferior thyroid veins** form a plexus which drain into innominate vein. They do not accompany the artery.
- **Kocher's vein** is rarely found (vein in between middle and inferior thyroid veins).

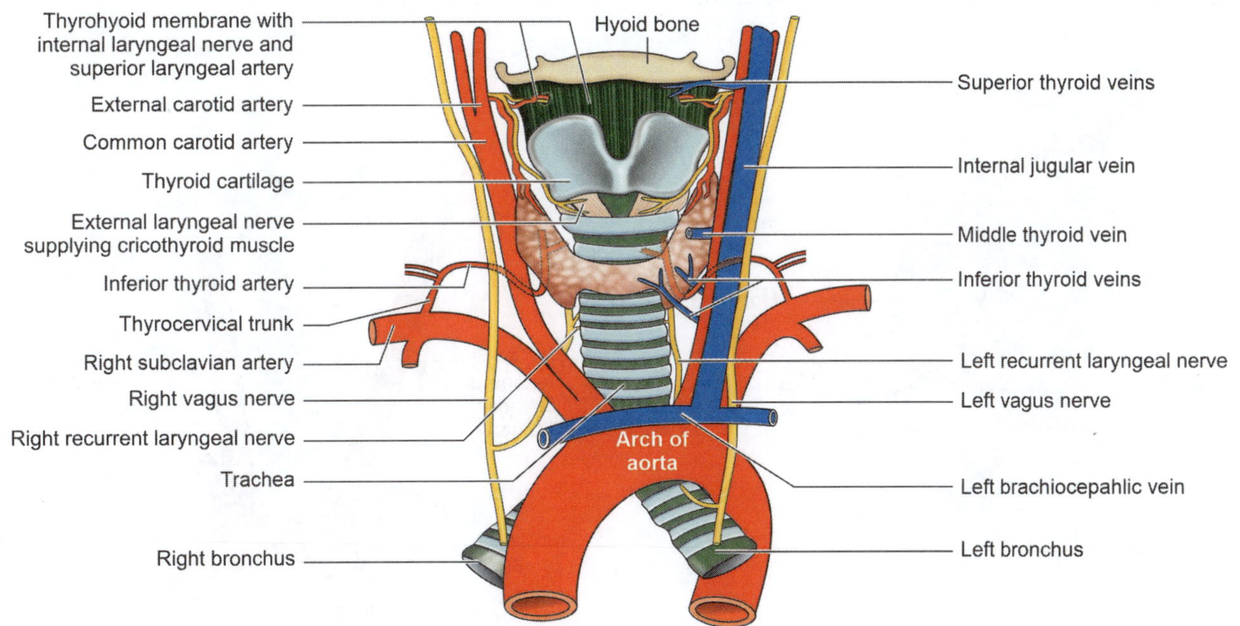

Fig. 37.2: Surgical anatomy of the thyroid gland. Arterial supply is shown on the right side and venous drainage is shown on the left side

[1]Branches of thyrocervical trunk can be remembered as SIT—suprascapular, inferior thyroid and transverse cervical artery.
[2]Superior thyroid artery and vein are like newly married couple, they go together, hand-in-hand.
[3]Middle thyroid vein is single, a bachelor and inferior thyroid artery and vein are a divorced couple.

Nerves in Relationship with Thyroid Gland

1. **Superior laryngeal nerve S(LN):** The vagus nerve gives rise to superior laryngeal nerve, which separates from it at skull base and divides into two branches. The larger **internal laryngeal nerve** is sensory to the supraglottic larynx. The smaller **external laryngeal nerve** runs close to the superior thyroid vessels and supplies cricothyroid. This nerve has been called as Amelita Galli-Curci nerve[1].
   - This nerve is away from the vessels near the upper pole. Hence, during thyroidectomy, the upper pedicle should be ligated as close to the thyroid as possible.
   - **Cricothyroid space of Reeves:** It lies between the cricothyroid muscle medially and upper pole of the thyroid lobe laterally. When we hold the upper pole of the thyroid gland with Babcock's forceps and retract the lobe infero-laterally, it opens up the space and SLN will be visible.
2. **Recurrent laryngeal nerve (RLN)** is a branch of vagus, hooks around ligamentum arteriosum on the left and subclavian artery on the right and runs in the tracheoesophageal groove near the posteromedial surface. Close to the gland, the nerve lies in between (anterior or posterior) branches of inferior thyroid artery (Figs 37.3 and 37.4 in the Riddle's triangle).
   - On the right side, it is 1 cm within the tracheo-esophageal groove (Key Boxes 37.1A and B).

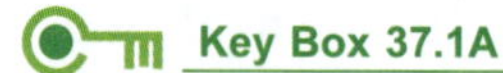

Key Box 37.1A

Recurrent Laryngeal Nerve at Surgery

- Lack of colour—white in colour
- Lack of elasticity
- Lack of pulsation
- Longitudinal vein on the surface
- Longitudinal course
- Location—**Riddle's triangle**—it is between inferior thyroid artery superiorly, carotid artery laterally and trachea medially. From here RLN runs upwards to enter larynx at greater cornu of thyroid cartilage, Riddle's triangle is also called Beahrs triangle

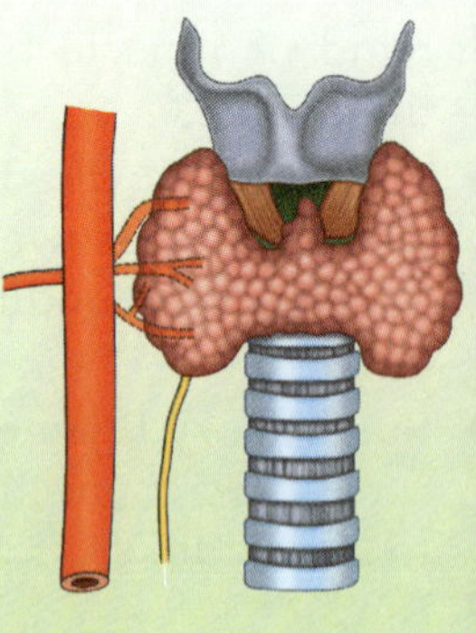

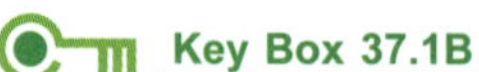

Key Box 37.1B

Recurrent Laryngeal Nerve Anomalies

- The nerve traverses through the gland in about 5–8% of cases.
- The nerve may be very closely adherent to the posteromedial aspect of the gland.
- Nerve not seen—may be far away in the tracheo-oesophageal groove.
- Nonrecurrent, recurrent laryngeal nerve is found in about 1 in 1,000 cases. The nerve has a horizontal course.
- In 25% of the cases, it is within the ligament of Berry.

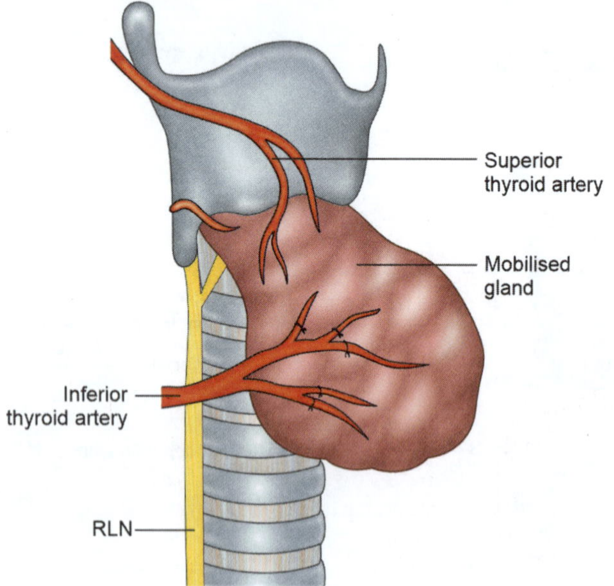

Fig. 37.3: Course of recurrent laryngeal nerve—gland is mobilised. The branches of inferior thyroid are ligated (not the main trunk)

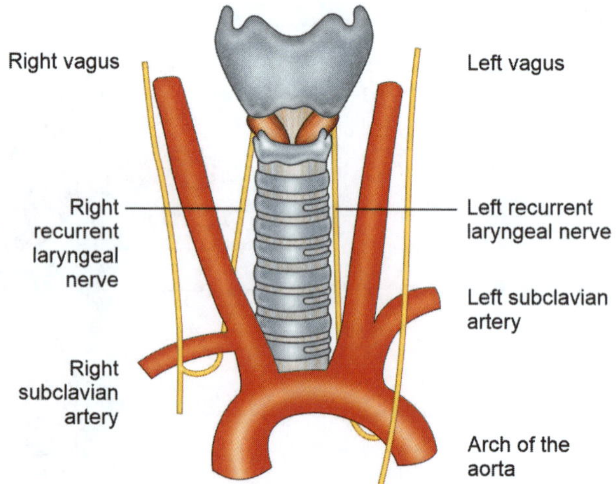

Fig. 37.4: Course of recurrent laryngeal nerve and origin

[1]Amelita Galli-Curci nerve was an opera singer whose SLN got injured resulting in voice changes. Often this nerve is referred to as Amelita Galli-Curci nerve.

Lymphatic Drainage of Thyroid

- Subcapsular lymphatic plexus drains into pretracheal nodes **(Delphic nodes means uncertain)** and prelaryngeal nodes which ultimately drain into lower deep cervical nodes and mediastinal nodes (Fig. 37.5).
- The chief lymph nodes are middle and lower deep cervical lymph nodes (Levels III and IV).
- Supraclavicular nodes and nodes in the posterior triangle can also be involved in malignancies of the thyroid gland, especially papillary carcinoma thyroid.

Histology (Fig. 37.6)

- Microscopically, it is divided into lobules.
- Each lobule has 20–40 follicles.
- Each follicle is lined by cuboidal epithelial cells.
- In the centre, colloid is present which is secreted from epithelial cells in response to calcitonin.
- Parafollicular cells are present in the interfollicular stroma.

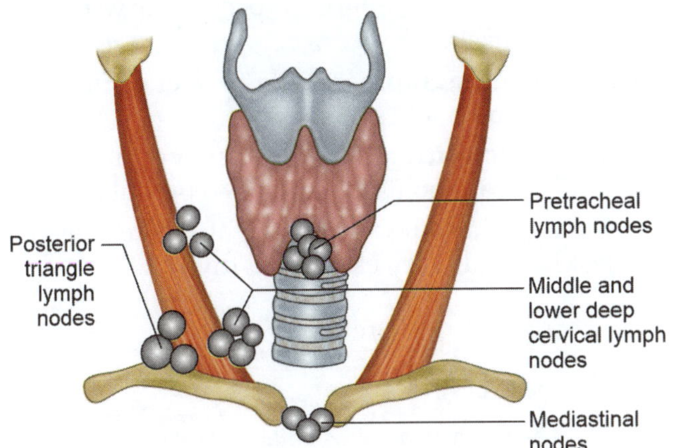

Fig. 37.5: Lymphatic drainage

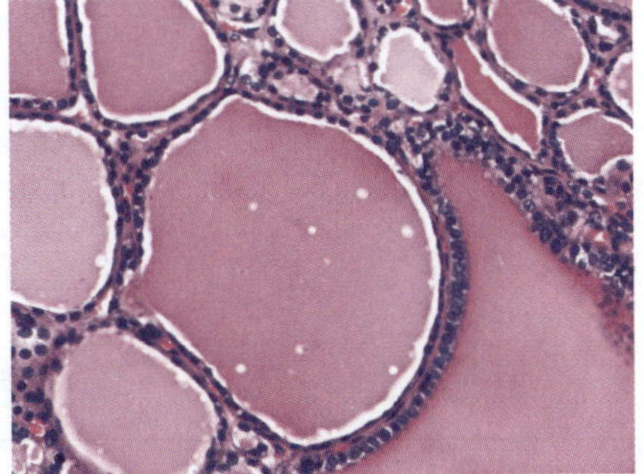

Fig. 37.6: Diffuse colloid goitre—acini lined by cuboidal follicular cells with luminal colloid (*Courtesy:* Dr Laxmi Rao, Head, Department of Pathology, KMC, Manipal)

PHYSIOLOGY

Tri-iodothyronine (T_3) and thyroxine (T_4) are the hormones secreted by the thyroid gland. Dietary requirement of iodine per day is 100–200 mg or 0.1 mg. Sources of iodine are milk, dairy products and sea food including fish.

Steps involved in the synthesis of these hormones

1. **Iodide trapping** from the blood into the thyrocyte is the first step in the formation of T_3 and T_4.
   - Thiocyanates and perchlorates block this step.
2. **Oxidation of iodide to inorganic iodine:** This step needs the enzyme peroxidase.
   - Drugs which block this stage (thioamides) are sulfonamide, PAS (para-amino-salicylic acid), carbimazole and propylthiouracil.
3. **Formation of iodotyrosines**
   - Iodine + Tyrosine = MIT (monoiodotyrosine) and diiodotyrosine (DIT)
   - This step is inhibited by thiourea group of drugs, i.e. carbimazole.
4. **Coupling reactions**
   - Coupling of two molecules of DIT results in T_4 and one molecule of DIT and MIT results in T_3.
   - This stage is blocked by carbimazole.
5. **Hydrolysis**
   - The hormones combine with globulin to form a colloid-thyroglobulin. They are stored in the thyroid gland and released as required by process of hydrolysis.
   - T_3 is an important physiological hormone and is fast-acting (few hours). T_4 is a slow-acting hormone and takes about 4–14 days to act.

THYROID FUNCTION TESTS

Serum T_3 and T_4 estimation is most commonly performed. Other tests are not commonly done and some of them are obsolete (Table 37.1).

1. **Serum T_3:** Normal levels—1.5–3.5 nmol/L
   - Most (80%) T_3 is produced by deiodination of T_4 in the liver, muscle, kidney and anterior pituitary.
   - T_3 is 3 to 4 times more potent than T_4.
   - The half-life of T_3 is approximately 24 hours, whereas half-life of T_4 is about 7 days.

Table 37.1 Levels of T_3, T_4 and TSH in some common conditions

Disease	T_3	T_4	TSH
• Thyrotoxicosis	↑	↑	Suppressed or undetectable
• T_3 toxicosis	↑↑	Normal	Suppressed
• Hypothyroidism	Low or normal	Low	↑

- Free T_3 (3 to 9 pmol/L) is most useful in confirming the diagnosis of early hyperthyroidism, especially in pregnancy wherein levels of free T_4 and free T_3 rise before total T_4 and T_3.

2. **Serum T_4:** Normal levels—55 to 150 nmol/L
   - They are measured by radioimmunoassay.
   - In euthyroid state, T_4 is the predominant hormone produced by the thyroid.
   - Total T_4 levels reflect output from the thyroid gland. Both T_3 and T_4 increase cell metabolism, normal growth, facilitate normal mental development and increase local effects of catecholamines.
   - Free T_3 (ref range 12–28 pmol/L) and free T_4 (3–9 pmol/L). Free T_4 estimates are not performed as a routine screening in thyroid disease. Use of this test is confined to cases of early hyperthyroidism Graves' disease where T_4 total may be normal but free T_4 is raised. In patients with end organ resistance to T_4, T_4 levels are raised but TSH is normal. Free T_4 is useful to confirm cases of early hyperthyroidism in which levels of both free T_3 and T_3 rise before total T_3 and T_4.
3. **Serum TSH (thyroid-stimulating hormone):** 0.3–5 IU/ml of plasma. Table 37.1 shows the levels of T_3, T_4 and TSH in a few common conditions.
4. **Serum thyroglobulin (TG)**
   - It is produced by thyroid tissue only. Hence, the levels should be low after total thyroidectomy.
   - The most important use of this test is to monitor patients after total thyroidectomy for well-differentiated carcinoma.
   - It is not normally released into circulation in large amount but increases suddenly in thyroiditis, Graves' disease or toxic multinodular goitre (MNG).
5. **Serum cholesterol:** It is increased in hypothyroidism and decreased in hyperthyroidism.
6. **Thyroid autoantibody levels:** More than 90% of the patients with Hashimoto's thyroiditis and 80% of patients with Graves' disease have antibodies which are called 'LATS' (long-acting thyroid stimulator). The detection of these antibodies helps in the diagnosis of such cases and also to suspect these diseases before clinical manifestation. These include anti-TG, antithyroid peroxidase and thyroid-stimulating immunoglobulin.
   - Anti-TPO levels >25 µ/ml and anti-thyroglobulin titres more than 1:100 are considered significant.
   - TSH receptor antibodies are also present in Graves' disease. They are largely produced within the thyroid itself.
7. **Thyroid scintigraphy** (Table 37.2 and Fig. 37.7): Uptake by both lobes.
8. **Serum calcitonin:** It is a sensitive marker for medullary carcinoma thyroid. (0–4 pg/ml basal)
   - CEA may also be used as an alternate screening test for medullary carcinoma thyroid.

Table 37.2 Thyroid scintigraphy

Substance	Dose	Half-life	Ideal case
^{131}I	High dose radiation (500 mrad)	Long 8–10 days	Lingual thyroid, retrosternal goitre; images are better.
^{123}I	Low dose radiation (30 mrad)	Shorter 8–10 hours	Well-differentiated carcinoma for bony metastasis.
^{99m}Tc (technetium)	Lowest radiation (5 mCi)	Shorter half-life 6–8 hours	Sensitive for nodal metastasis Lingual thyroid.

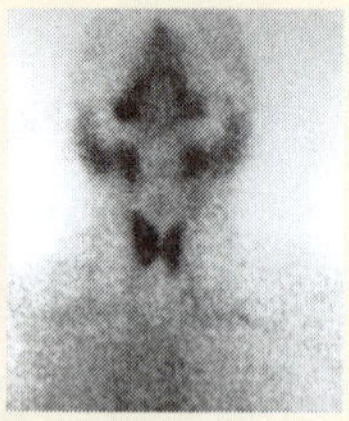

Fig. 37.7

A Few Terminologies of Thyroid Disorders (Table 37.3)

Table 37.3 Nomenclature of certain thyroid diseases

• **Ectopic thyroid** Diagnosis by isotope scan or CT scan	• Thyroid tissue along the line of descent Example: Floor of the mouth, submental region, mediastinum
• **Lingual thyroid** Diagnosis by isotope scan or CT scan	• Swelling in the region of foramen caecum in tongue
• **Dyshormonogenesis** It is familial.	• Autosomal recessive condition with deficiency of peroxidase or dehalogenase (enzymes)
• **Pendred's syndrome**	• Dyshormonogenesis with congenital deafness
• **Struma ovarii**	• Malignant ovarian teratoma containing thyroid tissue
• **Jod Basedow's disease** (German word)	• Excessive iodine given for hyperplastic goitre resulting in hyperthyroidism

CLINICAL EXAMINATION OF THYROID SWELLING

Diseases of the thyroid are very common and thyroid swellings are very often common cases in an undergraduate and postgraduate clinical examination. Hence, before discussing the various diseases of the thyroid gland, various aspects of the "CLINICS" are discussed in detail below.

COMPLAINTS—HISTORY TAKING

1. **Swelling:** Long duration of thyroid swelling indicates benign condition, e.g. multinodular goiter (MNG), colloid goitre. Short duration with rapid growth indicates malignancy, such as anaplastic carcinoma. Majority of thyroid swellings do not produce pain.
2. **Rate of growth:** Usually slow-growing in benign disease. If it is a rapid growth, it can be ***'de novo'* malignancy** or malignancy developing in a benign lesion, e.g. follicular carcinoma in MNG. Sudden increase in the size of swelling with pain indicates haemorrhage in the MNG (multinodular goitre).
3. **Dyspnoea:** Difficulty in breathing in a patient with goiter can be due to the following reasons (Key Box 37.2).
   - Small goitre, rapid growth—anaplastic carcinoma infiltrating the trachea.
   - When lower border is not seen, retrosternal goitre.
   - Hyperthyroidism causing arrhythmias leading to congestive cardiac failure can cause dyspnoea and orthopnoea.
   - Long-standing MNG compresses on the tracheal cartilages and produces **pressure atrophy** of tracheal cartilages. This is called **tracheomalacia**.

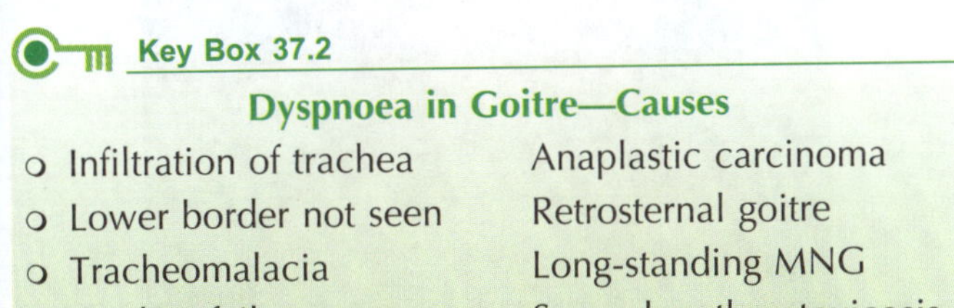

Key Box 37.2

Dyspnoea in Goitre—Causes

Infiltration of trachea	Anaplastic carcinoma
Lower border not seen	Retrosternal goitre
Tracheomalacia	Long-standing MNG
Cardiac failure	Secondary thyrotoxicosis

4. **Dysphagia** is relatively uncommon because oesophagus is a posterior structure and it is a fibromuscular tube.
5. **Hoarseness of voice** indicates malignancy. It always occurs in carcinoma thyroid infiltrating the recurrent laryngeal nerve (never in benign diseases of thyroid).
6. **Toxic features** suggestive of hyperthyroidism.

   A. ***CNS symptoms*** are predominantly seen in Graves' disease (primary thyrotoxicosis—Key Box 37.3)
   - Tremors of the hand
   - Sweating
   - Intolerance to heat
   - Preference to cold
   - Excitability
   - Irritability
   - Prominent eyes are observed by other persons. Double vision, oedema of the conjunctiva can be the presenting complaints in late cases.

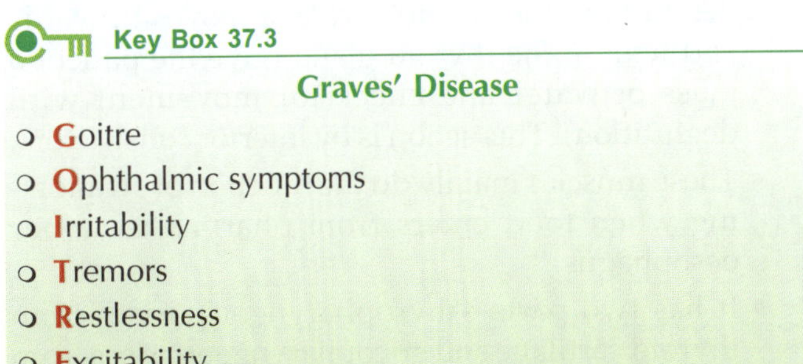

Key Box 37.3

Graves' Disease

- **G**oitre
- **O**phthalmic symptoms
- **I**rritability
- **T**remors
- **R**estlessness
- **E**xcitability

Remember as **GOITRE.**

   B. ***Cardiovascular symptoms*** (CVS) are predominantly seen in secondary thyrotoxicosis. Even though both forms of thyrotoxicosis produce palpitations, it is a significant complaint in multinodular goitre with thyrotoxicosis (secondary thyrotoxicosis). Precordial chest pain and dyspnoea on exertion are late manifestations of secondary thyrotoxicosis (Summary, Fig. 37.8).

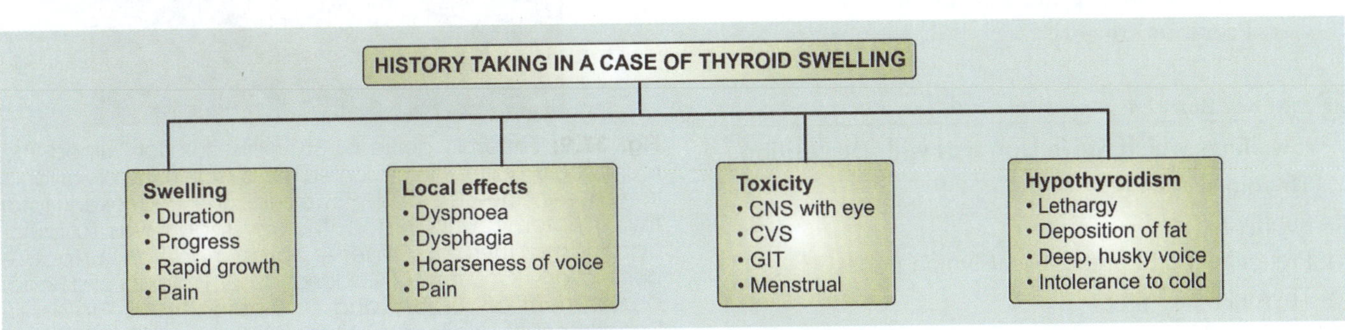

Fig. 37.8: Summary of history taking

ON EXAMINATION

Inspection

1. The location of the swelling is in front of the neck, extending from one sternomastoid to the other sternomastoid, vertically from suprasternal notch to the thyroid cartilage.
2. The size and shape have to be mentioned.
3. ***Surface:*** Thyroid swellings can have the following types of surfaces:
   a. Smooth—adenoma, puberty goitre, Graves' disease
   b. Irregular—carcinoma of the thyroid
   c. Nodular—multinodular thyroid
4. Borders are usually round.
5. Swelling moves up with deglutition because of the following reasons (Key Box 37.4):
   - Thyroid is enclosed by pretracheal fascia which is condensed to form a ligament posteromedially called **ligament of Berry**. These are pairs of ligaments attached above to cricoid cartilage. During deglutition, the cricoid cartilage moves upwards and with it, the thyroid gland (give the patient a glass of water and check for movement with deglutition). This action is by inferior constrictors.
   - These muscles mainly do the function of swallowing when food enters from pharynx to upper oesophagus.
   - It has two parts—thyropharyngeus arises from thyroid cartilage and cricopharyngeus arises from cricoid cartilage.
   - When these muscles act, thyroid and cricoid cartilage moves upwards. Thus, thyroid gland also moves upwards.
   - Inferior constrictors are supplied by vagus nerve. These are thickest constrictor muscles.
   - **If there is restriction of movement, it can be due to:**
     - Malignancy with fixity to the trachea
     - Retrosternal goitre
     - Large goitre because of the size
     - Previous surgery

Key Box 37.4

Swellings which Move Upwards with Deglutition

- Thyroid swellings
- Subhyoid bursitis
- Pretracheal and prelaryngeal lymph nodes
- Thyroglossal cyst
- Laryngocele

6. Movement on protrusion of the tongue suggests thyroglossal cyst. This test should be done when there is a nodule or a cyst in the region of isthmus of the thyroid gland. This test has no relevance in cases of MNG or other thyroid swellings.

Palpation

It should be done from behind. First mention what parts of thyroid gland are palpable.

1. Size, shape, surface and border should be confirmed. Local rise of temperature is a feature of toxic goitres. Very large nodular surface is described as bosselated surface (Fig. 37.9).
2. **Consistency:**
   - ***Soft:*** Graves' disease, colloid goitre.
   - ***Firm:*** Adenoma, multinodular goitre.
   - ***Hard:*** Carcinoma, calcification in the MNG.
3. Confirm the movement with deglutition by holding the thyroid gland.
4. **Intrinsic mobility** of the gland is very much restricted in carcinoma because of infiltration into prevertebral fascia behind or a malignant nodule which starts infiltrating trachea. Otherwise, thyroid gland has hardly any intrinsic mobility. When you try to move it moves with the trachea.
5. **Sternomastoid contraction test** is done when only one lobe is enlarged. In this situation, the examiner keeps the hand on the side of the chin, opposite the side of the lesion and asks the patient to push his hand against resistance. If the gland becomes less prominent (as with thyroid swellings), it indicates the swelling is deep to the sternomastoid muscle.

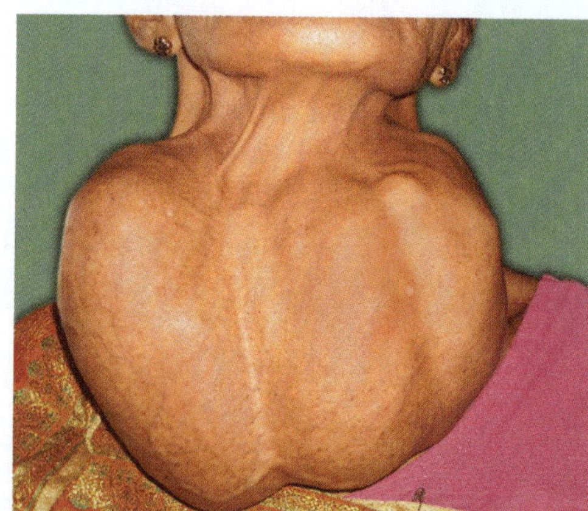

Fig. 37.9: Endemic goitre of 35 years duration turned into multinodular goitre. She presented with 3 months history of rapid increase in the size of the swelling. She underwent total thyroidectomy. Final histopathology report was follicular carcinoma thyroid. Observe large nodular surface—bosselations. (*Courtesy:* Dr Chidananda KV, Professor and Head, Department of surgery and Dr Gopinath Pai, Professor, Department of Surgery, KVG Medical College, Sullia, Dakshina Kannada, Karnataka. MBBS exam case 2007)

6. **Chin test (neck fixation test)** is classically done in multinodular goitre, wherein both lobes are enlarged. The patient is asked to bend the chin downwards against resistance. This produces contraction of both sternomastoids and strap muscles and the gland becomes less prominent (Fig. 37.10).
7. **Special tests** or methods of examination of thyroid gland:
   a. *Crile's method* is indicated when there is a doubtful nodule. Keep the thumb over the suspected area of the nodule and ask the patient to swallow. The nodularity is appreciated better with this test (Fig. 37.11).
   b. *Lahey's method* of examination of thyroid can be done from front as well as behind. In order to palpate the right lobe, push the gland to the right side and feel the nodules in the posteromedial aspect of the gland. The lobe becomes more prominent and thus nodules are appreciated better.
   c. *Pizzillo's method* **is indicated in obese patients especially short-necked individuals.** The patient is asked to clasp her hands and press against her occiput with head extended. Thyroid gland becomes more prominent and thus, palpation becomes better.
   d. *Kocher's test*: If gentle compression on lateral lobes produces stridor, it is described as positive. This is due to **scabbard[1] trachea**. Long-standing multinodular goitres causing tracheomalacia and collapse after thyroidectomy resulting in stridor.
8. **Position of trachea:** In cases of solitary nodule confined to one lobe, trachea is deviated to the opposite side. However, in cases of multinodular goitres, trachea need not be deviated because of symmetrical enlargement of both lobes.

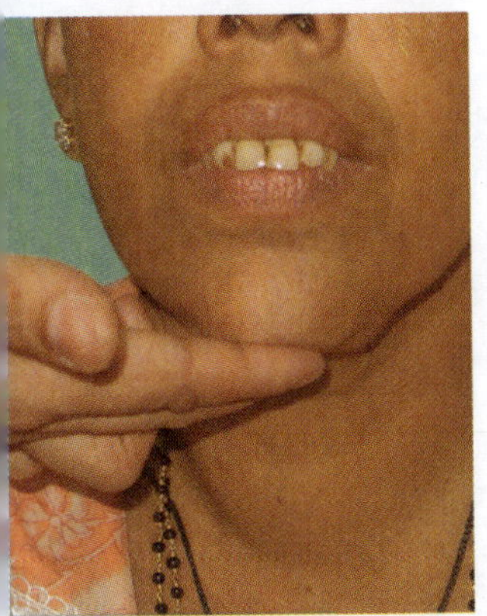

Fig. 37.10: Chin test—neck flexion test—thyroid swellings become less prominent

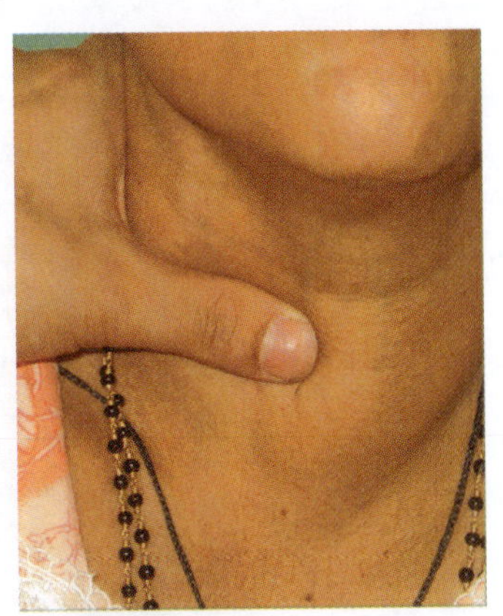

Fig. 37.11: Crile's method to detect nodule wherein thumb is used

9. **Palpation of lymph nodes** in the neck. If lymph nodes are significant, it indicates papillary carcinoma of the thyroid.
10. **Palpation of common carotid artery:** Draw a line from mastoid process to sternoclavicular joint. Then draw a horizontal line from upper border of thyroid cartilage. The point where these two lines meet is the site of bifurcation of common carotid artery. This artery should be palpated below this point, against tubercle on the transverse process of cervical 6th vertebra—called carotid tubercle or Chassaignac tubercle. ***The carotid artery can be massaged against this tubercle to relieve the symptoms of supraventricular tachycardia.***
    - In large multinodular goitres, the artery may be pushed laterally. Hence, pulsations are felt in the posterior triangle. Carcinoma of the thyroid engulfs the carotid sheath. Consequently, pulsations may be absent. Absent carotid artery pulsation is called **Berry sign positive**. Since the lumen is not narrowed, superficial temporal artery pulsations are felt normally.

Percussion

Percussion over the sternum gives a resonant note in normal cases. In retrosternal goitres, it gives a dull note.

Auscultation

- It should be done in the upper pole because of following reasons: Superior thyroid artery is a direct branch of external carotid artery. It is more superficial than inferior thyroid artery.
- Presence of thrill and bruit are the features of toxic goitre.

Systemic Examination

This includes CNS and eye signs, as in Graves' disease, examination of skeletal system to rule out metastasis as in carcinoma of the thyroid, and examination of cardiovascular system in cases of toxic goitre. These have been dealt with in detail in the corresponding topics. Deep tendon reflexes also have to be elicited—there is a slow relaxation phase in hypothyroidism.

Diagnosis

You need to confirm it is thyroid gland (Key Box 37.5) and to mention the disease and functional status. It should be noted that the neural tumours arising from vagus nerve can present in the same location, but it will not move with deglutition.

[1]Scabbard is a sheath for holding a sword or other large blade (it is narrow and curved).

Key Box 37.5

Anatomical Features of the Thyroid Gland

1. Thyroid gland is in front of the neck
2. Deep to pretracheal fascia
3. Moves up with deglutition
4. Butterfly-shaped when whole gland is enlarged

GOITRE

DEFINITION

Diffuse enlargement of the thyroid gland is described as goitre. (It is derived from the Latin word, Guttur = the throat.)

Classification of Goitre

I. Simple goitre

- Puberty goitre
- Colloid goitre, iodine deficiency goitre (Fig. 37.12)
- Multinodular goitre

II. Toxic goitre

- Graves' disease; diffuse toxic goitre
- Secondary thyrotoxicosis in multinodular goitre
- Toxic nodule; other causes.

III. Neoplastic goitre

- Benign adenoma (follicular adenoma)
- Malignant tumours: They are further classified as follows:

A. *Primary*

- Well-differentiated carcinoma
  – Papillary carcinoma, follicular carcinoma
- Poorly differentiated carcinoma
  – Anaplastic carcinoma
- Arising from parafollicular cells
  – Medullary carcinoma
- Arising from lymphatic tissue
  – Non-Hodgkin's lymphoma.

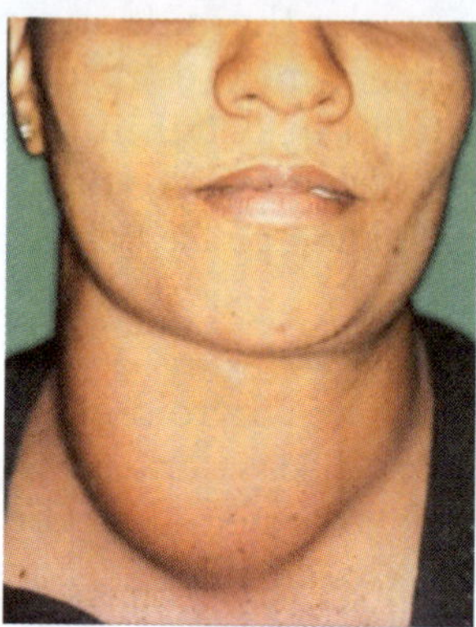

Fig. 37.12: Observe smooth surface—colloid goitre of 15 years duration

B. *Secondary (Metastasis)*

- Malignant melanoma, renal cell carcinoma breast carcinoma produce secondaries in the thyroid, due to blood spread.

IV. Thyroiditis

- Granulomatous thyroiditis
- Autoimmune thyroiditis
- Riedel's thyroiditis.

V. Other rare causes of goitre

- Acute bacterial thyroiditis
- Thyroid cyst
- Thyroid abscess
- Amyloid goitres

Pearls of Wisdom

Multinodular goitre, solitary thyroid nodule, malignant goitres, and puberty goitres are common causes of goitre. Bacterial thyroiditis is rare. Riedel's thyroiditis is very rare.

MULTINODULAR GOITRE

- A multinodular goitre is the end-stage result of diffuse hyperplastic goitre. Excessive metabolic demands cause an excessive enlargement of the thyroid. Therefore, it is common in women.
- Metabolic demands increase during puberty. A goiter appearing during that period is called puberty goitre. A goitre can develop during pregnancy and is called pregnancy goitre. Both of them are physiological but may eventually develop into multinodular goiter (MNG) (Fig. 37.13).

Competency

SU22.2: Describe the etiopathogenesis of thyroidal swellings.

Aetiopathogenesis

Multinodular goitre occurs due to continuous stimulation by TSH secreted from the anterior pituitary.

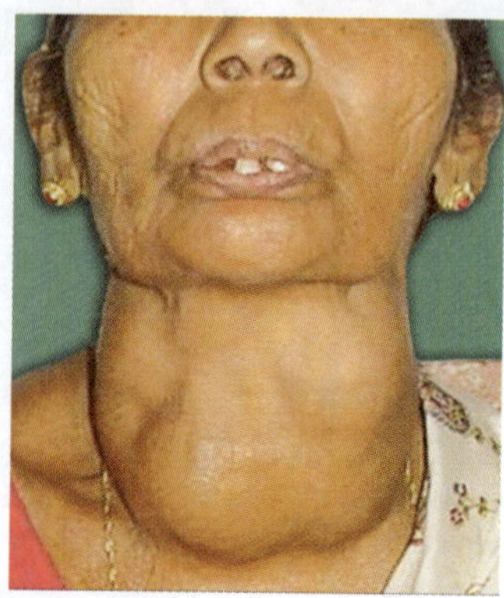

Fig. 37.13: Multinodular goitre showing nodules

1. **Puberty goitre, pregnancy goitre**
   - It is seen in girls at puberty or during pregnancy when the metabolic demands are high and the production of T_3, T_4 are comparatively normal. Due to feedback mechanism, TSH levels increase, which stimulates thyroid gland and causes diffuse hypertrophy and hyperplasia.
   - This is also called physiological goitre and can be treated by giving tablet thyroxine (T_4) 50 to 100 micrograms/day to suppress TSH.
   - Goitre may disappear, if treatment is given in the stage of diffuse hypertrophy.
2. **Iodine deficiency goitre**
   - Daily iodine requirement is about **100–125 µg.**
   - Common in hilly/mountainous or low-lying areas because of decreased iodide content of water. This causes iodine deficiency goitre mediated by the same feedback mechanism.
   - This is treated with iodised salt (which is used in food) and iodine—containing preparations.
   - If the iodine deficiency status continues for a long time, it results in accumulation of colloid material in the gland and causes colloid goitre.
   - All these three types of goitre, if left untreated, will change to multinodular goitre (Fig. 37.14).
     - **Stage I:** Stage of diffuse hypertrophy and hyperplasia of thyroid.
     - **Stage II:** Due to fluctuating levels of TSH because of pregnancy, lactation, menstruation, etc. Some areas in thyroid are overstimulated and are converted to active follicles.
     - **Stage III:** The active follicle ultimately undergoes necrosis and many such necrosed follicles join to form a nodule. Many such nodules form a multinodular goitre. Nodules contain necrosed tissue, i.e. inactive tissue. The internodular tissue is active.
3. **Goitrogens** such as cabbage (contains thiocyanates), drugs such as amiodarone and sulfonamides, cause goiter by preventing oxidation of iodide to iodine. Excess iodides inhibit organic binding of iodine and produce goitre.
4. **Dyshormonogenesis** (*see* Table 37.3)

Clinical Features

- Common in females. Female: male ratio is 10 : 1. Seen in the age group of 20–40 years.
- Long duration of swelling in front of the neck, dyspnoea due to tracheomalacia and dysphagia are the presenting features. The gland is nodular, firm in consistency and both the lobes are enlarged. Hard areas may suggest calcification and soft areas, necrosis.
- Sudden increase in size with pain is mainly due to haemorrhage in a nodule.

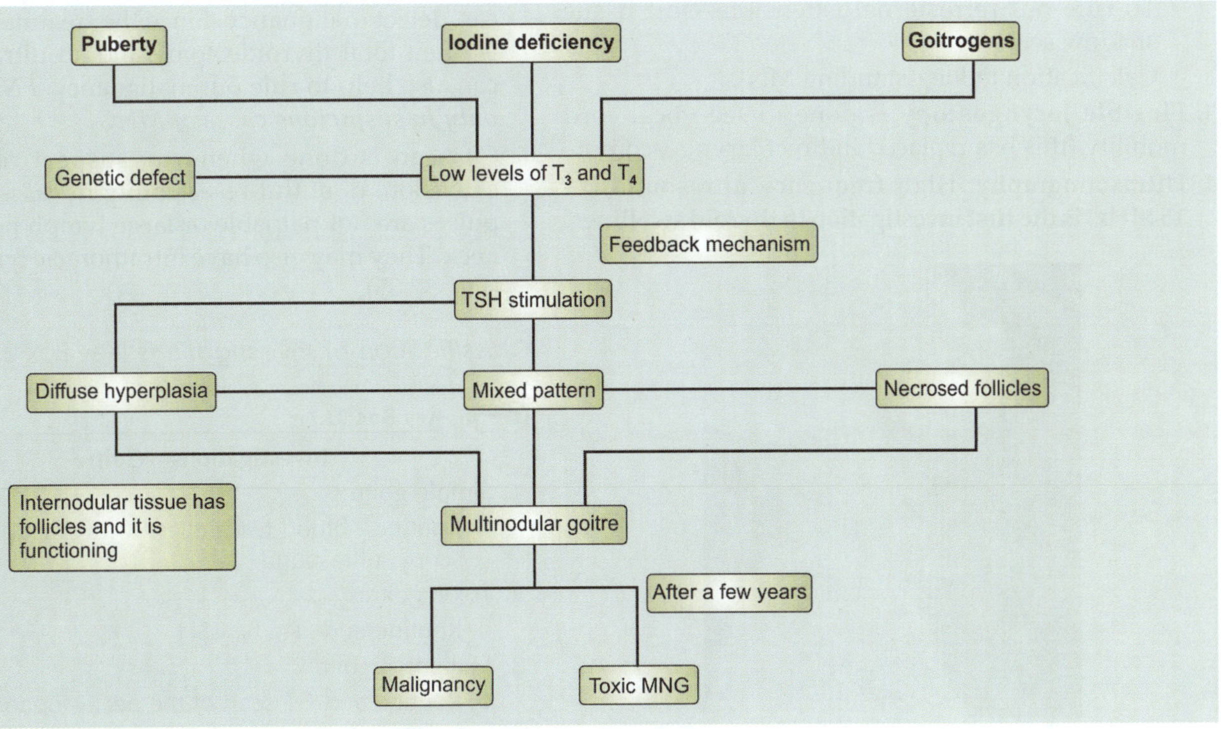

Fig. 37.14: Pathogenesis of MNG

Pearls of Wisdom

The most common site of a nodule is at the junction of isthmus with one lobe.

Complications of Multinodular Goitre

1. Calcification in long-standing MNG.
2. Sudden haemorrhage in one of the nodules causes dyspnoea.
3. In 10–20% of cases, patients can develop secondary thyrotoxicosis with CVS involvement. Palpitation is the predominant symptom. Toxic multinodular goitre is also called **Plummer's disease**.

Tachycardia can be graded as follows—**Crile's** grading

Grade I	<90/min—mild
Grade II	90 to 100/min—moderate
Grade III	>110/min—severe

4. Follicular carcinoma in a long-standing goitre 8 to 15%.

Management of Multinodular Goitre

Investigations

1. **Complete blood picture (CBP)**, and a few investigations for fitness including baseline ECG and echo cardiography more so in toxic goitres.
2. **X-ray of the neck:** Anteroposterior and lateral view.
   - To look for compression of trachea—to check feasibility of intubation during anaesthesia (Fig. 37.15).
   - To rule out retrosternal extension—soft tissue shadow seen.
   - Calcification in long-standing MNG.
3. **Flexible laryngoscopy** is done to see vocal cord mobility (this has replaced indirect laryngoscopy).
4. **Ultrasonography: High frequency ultrasound (7–15 MHz) is the first investigation in thyroid swellings.**

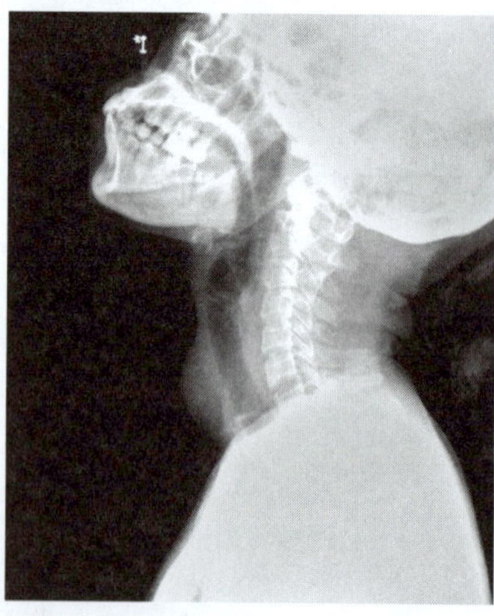

Fig. 37.15: X-ray of the neck—lateral view

(TIRADS—More details are given on page 417). In multinodular goitres, ultrasound guided FNAC can be done. It can also detect clinically impalpable lymph nodes in the neck (suggest malignancy) (Key Box 37.6). Like in the breast, ultrasound examination of the thyroid gland has been categorised into TIRADS—Thyroid Imaging Reporting and Data Systems. 5 categories have been identified. It is applicable in all nodules more than 1 cm or more in diameter.

- Ultrasound examination is inexpensive, easily done and has more advantages than disadvantages. Thus, it is often the first investigation in thyroid swellings (Refer to clinical notes).

Key Box 37.6

Ultrasound

- It can distinguish solid from cystic lesions.
- It can measure the size of the nodule.
- It can reveal multicentric nature of the goitre.
- It can detect lymphadenopathy and can guide FNAC.
- It can detect microcalcification—a feature of malignancy-peripheral punctate calcification in the cervical nodes.
- ↑ echogenicity means ↑ chances of tumour/malignancy.
- ↑ sonolucent means ↑ chances of cyst (benign).

5. **Fine needle aspiration cytology (FNAC):** It can be done in suspected **hard** nodule of multinodular goitre. It is a simple and useful investigation which can detect malignancy. Since the treatment of MNG is often total thyroidectomy and an ultrasonogram can also help to rule out malignancy, ***FNAC is done only in suspicious cases of MNG.***
6. CT scan is done when you suspect retrosternal extension, doubtful resectability in cases of carotid pulses are not palpable or large lymph nodes in the neck. They may also have intrathoracic lymph nodes (Fig. 37.55).

Classification of Investigations (Key Box 37.7)

Key Box 37.7

Investigations—Goitre

1. Simple goitres
   - Routine—blood tests, chest X-ray, flexible laryngoscopy, ultrasound
2. Toxic goitres
   - Routine and T_3, T_4, TSH
3. Malignant goitre
   - Routine and CT scan of the neck—optional
   - FNAC: Ultrasound guided is a must

Clinical Notes

1. A 22-year-old lady was referred to us for a nodule in the right side of neck in the thyroid region that was moving with deglutition. She also had epigastric pain since 6 months. Clinical diagnosis of solitary thyroid nodule with hyperacidity was made. An ultrasound examination of the neck was requested and the report was a surprise. She was having a parathyroid adenoma with calcific pancreatitis and nephrocalcinosis. You know the diagnosis now—a case of hyperparathyroidism.
2. We sent a case of MNG to thyroid scan. The scan detected jugular lymphadenopathy on both sides. The diagnosis changed from MNG (benign) to malignancy (papillary carcinoma because of lymph nodes). Lymph nodes were not palpable on clinical examination in this patient.
3. A 21-year-old lady had a multinodular goitre with the entire gland replaced by nodules. Case was posted for a total/near total thyroidectomy. A senior experienced Professor asked one question, 'what is the duration of this swelling?' It was 10 years. He said postpone the surgery, and do FNAC. As per his advice, FNAC was done. FNAC report was lymphocytic thyroiditis. Surgery was cancelled. She was put on T-Eltroxin 0.1 mg, 2 tablets/day. She is on follow-up now. Gland size is reduced to 30% in the last 2 years.

Prevention of MNG

Prevention is mainly important in endemic area and is done by supplementing iodine (Key Box 37.8).

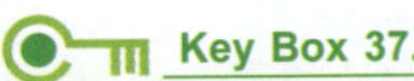
Key Box 37.8

Prevention of MNG

- *Puberty goitre*: 0.1 g to 0.2 mg of thyroxine.
- *Iodine deficiency goitre*: Use iodised salt, sea food, milk, egg, etc.
- *Goitrogens*: Avoid cabbage, drugs.

Treatment

Three choices are given to patients.

1. **Total thyroidectomy is the choice today provided** complications such as recurrent laryngeal nerve, paralysis and hypocalcaemia due to removal of parathyroid glands can be avoided. Thus, it is desirable to do a total thyroidectomy, if **experience of the surgeon is good** and in a **high volume centre**. It gives permanent quick cure to the patient (Fig. 37.16).
2. **Subtotal thyroidectomy:** In this operation, parts of right and left lobes and entire isthmus are removed in flush with tracheal surface leaving behind a small amount of tissue in the tracheoesophageal groove to protect recurrent laryngeal nerve and parathyroid gland. Subtotal thyroidectomy is not done nowadays. Students should study Fig. 37.17 first. Details of management of MNG are given in Fig. 37.17.

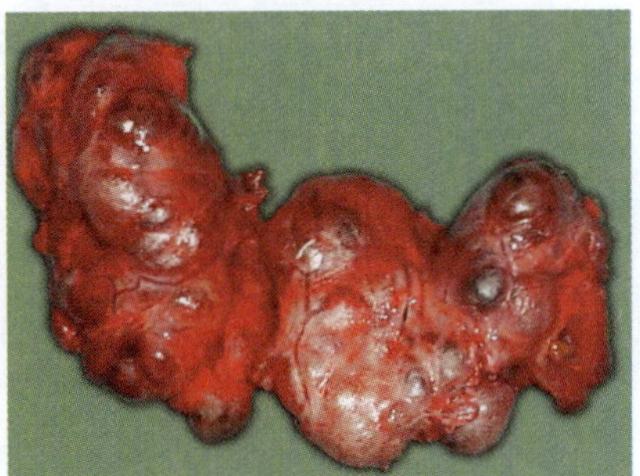

Fig. 37.16: Total thyroidectomy specimen

3. **Dunhill procedure:** In a few cases, one lobe is completely replaced with nodules and a few nodules on the other side. In such cases total lobectomy on one side and subtotal lobectomy on the other side can be done.
   - Some surgeons treat these patients with 0.1 mg of thyroxine to suppress the TSH stimulation in the postoperative period, for a period of 2–5 years.
   - However, it should be remembered that risk of osteoporosis, atrial fibrillation and increased morbidity and mortality from cardiovascular disease can occur. Hence, patients should be told about these complications.

RETROSTERNAL GOITRE

Definition: When more than 50% of goitre is below suprasternal notch, it is called retrosternal goitre. Very often, it is a multinodular goitre that develops in the neck and is slowly pulled down behind the sternum due to the following reasons.

1. Negative intrathoracic pressure
2. Pretracheal muscles are strong in men
3. Short neck, obesity

Rarely, it arises from an ectopic thyroid tissue.

Classification

I. **Primary:** It arises from ectopic thyroid tissue in the mediastinum. It also derives blood supply from mediastinum. It is rare (1%).

II. **Secondary:** It is the common variety—it is MNG which gets pulled down into thorax.

Clinical Types

- **Substernal:** The most common type where the lower border of the gland is behind the sternum.
- **Intrathoracic:** No thyroid is seen in the neck, diagnosed by radio-iodine scan.

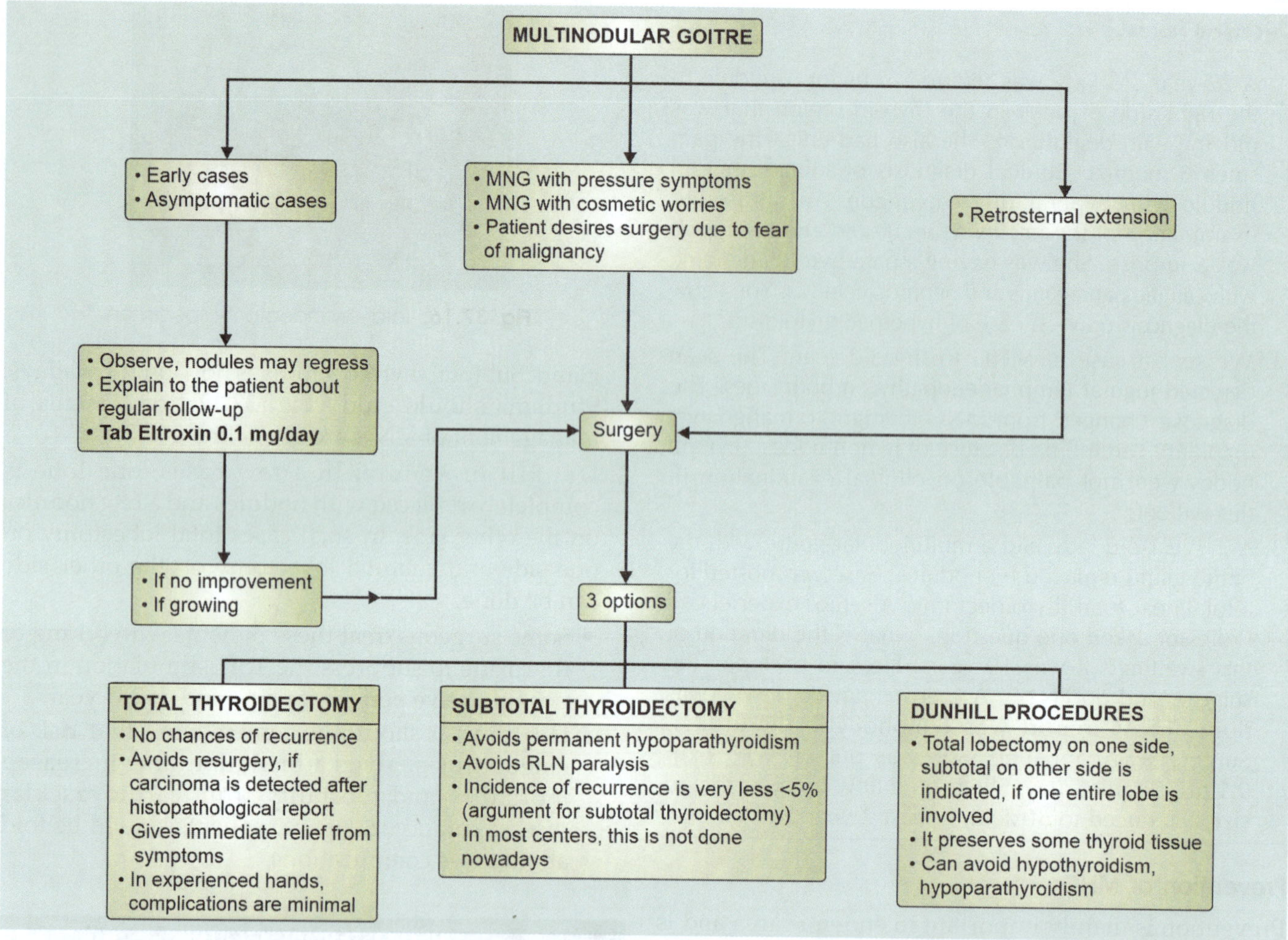

MULTINODULAR GOITRE

- Early cases
- Asymptomatic cases

→
- Observe, nodules may regress
- Explain to the patient about regular follow-up
- **Tab Eltroxin 0.1 mg/day**

→
- If no improvement
- If growing

→ Surgery

- MNG with pressure symptoms
- MNG with cosmetic worries
- Patient desires surgery due to fear of malignancy

→ Surgery

- Retrosternal extension

→ Surgery

Surgery → 3 options

TOTAL THYROIDECTOMY
- No chances of recurrence
- Avoids resurgery, if carcinoma is detected after histopathological report
- Gives immediate relief from symptoms
- In experienced hands, complications are minimal

SUBTOTAL THYROIDECTOMY
- Avoids permanent hypoparathyroidism
- Avoids RLN paralysis
- Incidence of recurrence is very less <5% (argument for subtotal thyroidectomy)
- In most centers, this is not done nowadays

DUNHILL PROCEDURES
- Total lobectomy on one side, subtotal on other side is indicated, if one entire lobe is involved
- It preserves some thyroid tissue
- Can avoid hypothyroidism, hypoparathyroidism

Fig. 37.17: Management of multinodular goitre—for diagrams see operative surgery chapter on thyroid diseases

- **Plunging goitre:** When patient is asked to cough, intrathoracic pressure increases. As the thyroid plunges out, the lower border of gland is clearly seen in the neck.

Clinical Features

- It can be suspected when the lower border of the swelling is not seen.
- Most of the patients have difficulty in breathing or even stridor.
- Dysphagia is more common.
- Engorgement of neck veins and superficial veins. These become more prominent when the hands are raised above the head, and the arms touch the ears with congestion and cyanosis of the face—**Pemberton's sign** (Fig. 37.18).

Investigations

- They are similar to MNG. However, isotope scan is very useful in the diagnosis of intrathoracic goitres.
- CT scan to localise and to know the size and extent.
- CT scan classification of retrosternal goitre is important because depending upon the extent of intra-thoracic extension, treatment is planned.

Treatment

- **No conservative line of treatment.**
- It can be easily explored through the neck incision and removed, with gentle dissection with the finger specially when the intra-thoracic part has narrow apex.
- Very rarely, a sternal split may be necessary.

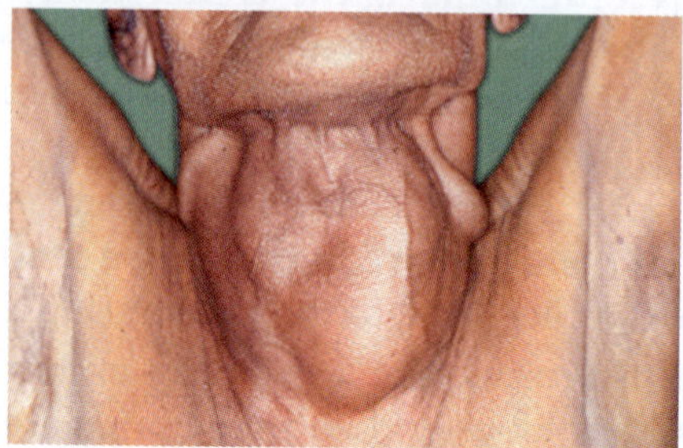

Fig. 37.18: Observe the engorged veins due to retrosternal goitre. Such veins are also seen when mediastinal nodes are enlarged as in papillary carcinoma thyroid

Summary (Key Box 37.9)

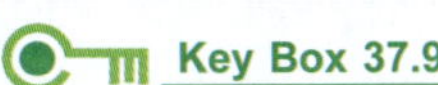

Key Box 37.9

Retrosternal Goitre

- Very often, it is an MNG with the lower border unseen
- Rarely from ectopic thyroid tissue
- Severe breathlessness even though small
- Drugs should not be given, if it is toxic
- Pressure effects diagnosed by **Pemberton's sign**
- Excision is the treatment
- No radioiodine therapy

TOXIC GOITRE—THYROTOXICOSIS

It is a complex disorder which occurs due to increased levels of thyroid hormones (hyperthyroidism) and manifests clinically with various signs and symptoms involving many body systems. Following are the causes of thyrotoxicosis.

1. **Primary thyrotoxicosis** (Graves' disease, exophthalmic goitre, diffuse goitre).
2. **Secondary thyrotoxicosis:** Secondary to nodular goitre (multinodular) (Plummer's disease).
3. **Solitary toxic nodule:** Autonomous nodule which is not under the influence of TSH but occurs due to hypertrophy and hyperplasia of gland (tertiary thyrotoxicosis).
4. **Other causes of thyrotoxicosis**
   - **Thyrotoxicosis factitia:** False thyrotoxicosis occurs due to overdosage of thyroxine, given for puberty goitre.
   - **Jod-Basedow's thyrotoxicosis:** Jod means iodine in the German language, Basedow means toxic goitre. Iodine-induced thyrotoxicosis (iodine given for hyperplastic endemic goitres).
   - Initial stage of **thyroiditis:** Hashimoto's thyroiditis, viral thyroiditis can produce temporary thyrotoxicosis features.
   - Very rarely, malignant goitres can be toxic (differentiated carcinoma).
   - **Neonatal thyrotoxicosis** occurs in babies born to thyrotoxic mothers.
   - TSH-secreting **tumours of pituitary**
   - **Struma ovarii**
   - ***Drugs:*** Amiodarone is an iodine-containing preparation given as antiarrhythmic drug.

GRAVES' DISEASE

- Also called diffuse toxic goitre.

Aetiopathogenesis

The exact aetiological factors responsible for the disease are not clear. Following are considered as possible aetiological factors:

1. **Autoimmune disorder** is the first possible cause due to the demonstration of autoantibodies in the circulation. *Example:* TSH receptor antibodies. It can be associated with other autoimmune disorders like vitiligo, type 1 diabetes mellitus, Addison's disease, myasthenia gravis and pernicious anaemia.
2. **Familial/genetic:** The disease can run in families. Familial/genetic Graves' disease has been documented in identical twins.
   - Graves' disease is associated with certain HLA haplotypes, like HLA-B8, DR3, DQA1. Here a few triggering factors can result in Graves' disease. (Key Box 37.10).
   - HLA-DRB1*0701 is protective against Graves' disease.
   - Polymorphism of cytotoxic T lymphocyte antigen-4 (CTLA-4) is also associated with Graves' disease.
3. **Thyroid-stimulating immunoglobulins** (TSI) and long-acting thyroid stimulator (LATS) are responsible for pathological changes in the thyroid gland in Graves' disease. They stimulate thyrocytes to grow and synthesize excess thyroid hormones.
4. **Exophthalmos producing substance (EPS)** is responsible for 'ophthalmopathy' seen in Graves' disease.
5. **Female sex**, emotions, stress, young age also have been considered as other factors responsible for the disease.

Key Box 37.10

Triggering Factors for Graves' Disease

- Postpartum state
- Iodine excess
- Lithium therapy
- Infection—bacterial and viral

Pathology

As a result of continuous stimulation, acinar hypertrophy and hyperplasia take place. The acinar cells which are normally flat, become tall columnar. The normal colloid disappears and the cells are empty. However, rich vascularity is seen. Thus, small follicles with hyperplastic columnar epithelium is characteristic (Flowchart 37.1).

Flowchart 37.1: Aetiopathogenesis

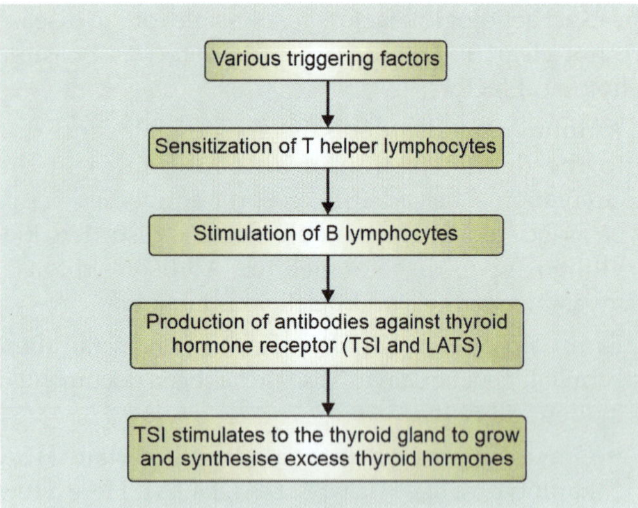

Clinical Features

- Primary thyrotoxicosis is 8 times more common in females than in males, especially in the age group of 15–25 years. Thyroid swelling, features of thyrotoxicosis and exophthalmos are considered as triad of Graves' disease. **Symptoms, signs and swelling appear simultaneously.**
- Very often young women present with unexplained loss of weight in spite of good appetite and insomnia is brought with diarrhoea. Diarrhoea occurs due to increased smooth muscle activity of small intestines. Intolerance to heat, preference to cold, fine tremors, excitability, hyperkinetic movements, excessive sweating are the other features. **Free steroid hormone levels decrease Graves' disease. This results in decreased effective oestrogen at the cell level which in turn causes oligomenorrhoea. Never forget to examine pulse rate specially in young patients who are losing weight unintentionally. Tachycardia is a feature.**

Pearls of Wisdom

Sleeping pulse rate is counted after the patient is sedated with 30 mg of phenobarbitone. In a case of toxic goitre, the pulse rate remains high even during sleep because of increased metabolism. This is a simple bedside investigation in cases of toxic goitre. In anxiety states, pulse rate may be high in the waking hours and it comes back to normal during sleep.

Clinical Notes

Following are three case reports which highlight the clinical symptomatology of primary thyrotoxicosis.

1. An 18-year-old girl visited many doctors for her complaint of loss of weight. She was investigated for tuberculosis (common disease in India), malignancy, etc. She was given unnecessary tonics. After nearly 6 months, when eye-signs started developing, it was proved to be Graves' disease.
2. A bank clerk's only complaint was that he could not sign the cheque because of excessive sweating. Thyroid gland was not palpable. His pulse rate was very high, investigations revealed that it was a case of primary thyrotoxicosis. On careful questioning, he admitted that he was a "nervous character".
3. A 24-year-old lady was being asked by her friends every day why her eyes were prominent. Her only complaint was prominent eyes. On careful questioning, she admitted having anxiety, tension, excitability.

Signs of Primary Thyrotoxicosis

I. Signs of Thyroid Gland in Graves' Disease

- Uniformly enlarged (mild degree)
- Smooth surface—no nodules (treated cases may have nodularity)
- Gland is soft or firm in consistency.
- It is warm—highly vascular and can be pulsatile
- Auscultation—a bruit can be heard.

II. Central Nervous System (CNS) Signs

- Tremors of the tongue when the tongue is within the oral cavity and tremors of the outstretched hands are characteristics. A piece of paper may be placed on the fingers in doubtful cases for demonstrating the tremors of the hand. Extensor surface of the hand is used because extensors are weak when compared to flexors.
- Hyperkinetic movements
- Always a moist, warm hand (shake hands with the patient).

III. Cardiovascular System (CVS) Signs

- Pulse rate is always raised and rapid indicating tachycardia. Depending upon the pulse rate, thyrotoxicosis can be classified as follows: Mild—90–100/min, moderate—100–110/min, severe—more than 110/min.
- Palpitation and extrasystoles can also be found in primary thyrotoxicosis even though other cardiac features, such as fibrillation and cardiac failure, are rare.

IV. Eye Signs

- Prominent eyeballs and retraction of the eyelid result in thyrotoxic exophthalmos. This is due to retrobulbar deposition of inflammatory cells and round cells with venous congestion resulting in oedema (Figs 37.19 and 37.20).

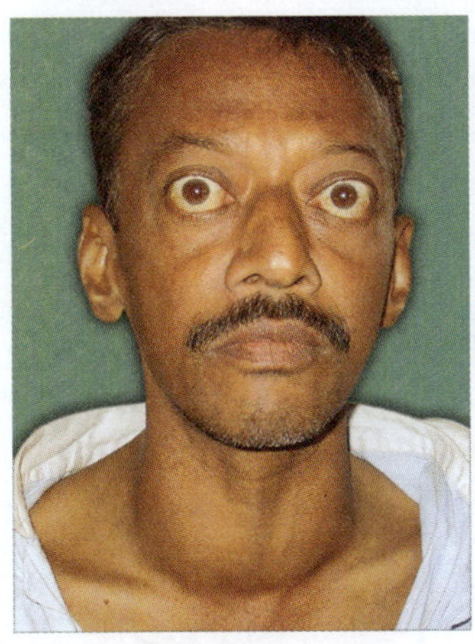

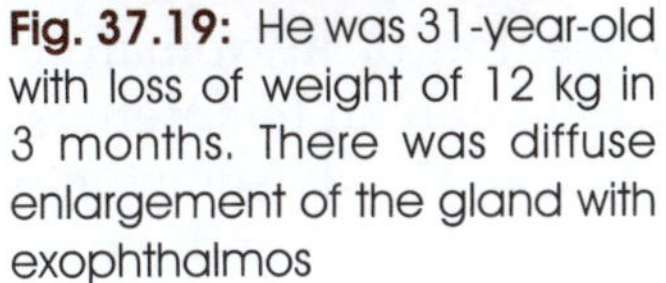

Fig. 37.19: He was 31-year-old with loss of weight of 12 kg in 3 months. There was diffuse enlargement of the gland with exophthalmos

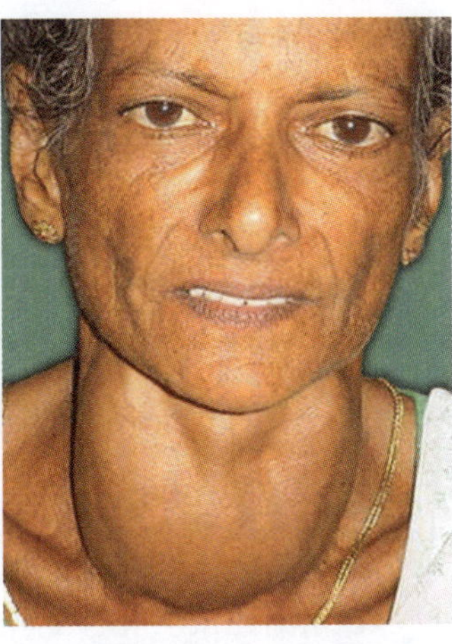

Fig. 37.20: She was 48-year-old lady who had multinodular goitre of 10 years duration. She also had lid-lag sign (rare in toxic MNG)

- **Levator palpebrae superioris** muscle is innervated by **oculomotor nerve** which also carries sympathetic fibres derived from cavernous plexus for the smooth muscle part of the levator. Contraction of this muscle produces lid spasm.
- This is aided by **spasm of Müller's muscle**, a sympathetic muscle which lies adjoining the levator palpebrae superioris muscle. This is responsible for keeping the eyeball forwards. All these factors together produce a classical stare.

1. **Assessment of exophthalmos**
   - Upper sclera is seen above the limbus (upper margin of the cornea and conjunctiva—**Dalrymple's sign**.
   - **Naffziger's method:** Stand behind the patient and look at the supraciliary arch, by tilting the patient's head backwards. In normal cases, eyeball is not seen. In cases of exophthalmos, eyeball is protruded outside and hence it is seen.
2. **Moebius' sign:** Loss of convergence of eyeball occurs due to muscle paresis as a part of thyrotoxic ophthalmoplegia. Diplopia is due to weakness of extraocular muscles (inferior oblique-elevators).
3. **Stellwag's sign:** Infrequent blinking and widening of palpebral fissure is due to spasm of sympathetic fibres in the levator palpebrae superioris.
4. **Joffroy's sign:** Absence of wrinkling of the forehead when the patient is asked to look upwards. This occurs due to increase in the field of vision due to exophthalmos.
5. **von Graefe's sign (lid-lag sign):** When the patient is asked to look up and down, upper eyelid cannot cope up with the speed of movement of the finger because of the lid spasm. Hence, the lid lags behind.
6. **Enroth sign:** Oedema of eyelids and conjunctiva.
7. **Gifford's sign:** Difficulty in everting the upper eyelid.
8. **Kocher's sign:** When an attempt is made to lift the eyes higher, upper eyelid springs up more quickly than the eyebrows.

Pearls of Wisdom

How to differentiate proptosis form exophthalmos? In thyrotoxicosis the upper eyelid cannot be everted or inverted easily but in cases of proptosis due to intra-orbital mass upper eyelid can be everted easily.

Summary (Table 37.4 and Key Boxes 37.11 to 37.13)

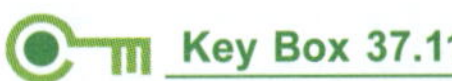

Key Box 37.11

Thyrotoxic Exophthalmos

- Proptosis and lid retraction result in exophthalmos
- Sclera is visible beyond limbus
- Naffziger's method to examine
- Staring look
- Typically seen in Graves' disease
- Rarely seen in secondary thyrotoxicosis

Key Box 37.12

Interesting 6 Ps of Graves' Ophthalmopathy

- **P**rominent eyes
- **P**eriorbital oedema
- **P**apilloedema
- **P**roptosis
- **P**alpebral fissure widening
- **P**rogression to blindness

Table 37.4 Symptoms of thyrotoxicosis

Symptoms of hyperthyroidism	Symptoms of increased adrenergic stimulation	In females	In children
Heat intolerance Increased sweating, thirst Weight loss in spite of good caloric intake	Palpitations Nervousness, fatigue Emotional lability Hyperkinesis, tremors Prominent stare is due to catecholamine excess	Amenorrhoea Decreased fertility Miscarriages	Rapid growth

Key Box 37.13

Grading of Thyroid Eye Diseases

Grade 0	No signs or symptoms
Grade 1	Only signs, no symptoms
Grade 2	Both signs and symptoms
Grade 3	Proptosis
Grade 4	Extraocular muscle involvement
Grade 5	Corneal involvement
Grade 6	Loss of vision with optic nerve atrophy

Malignant Exophthalmos

- This occurs in untreated cases of Graves' disease.
- If the disease continues, infrequent blinking secondary to exophthalmos results in constant **exposure of the cornea to the atmosphere**. This results in keratitis, corneal ulcer, conjunctivitis, chemosis and may even lead to blindness. This is called malignant exophthalmos.
- Malignant exophthalmos is probably due to **autoimmune disease**.
- In late stages, **optic nerve damage and blindness** can occur.

Treatment of thyrotoxic ophthalmopathy

1. Massive doses of steroids—methylprednisolone and metronidazole
2. Lateral tarsorrhaphy
3. Orbital decompression may be necessary in late cases.
4. Guanethidine eyedrops are useful to decrease lid spasm and lid retraction.
5. Head end elevation and disease control.
6. Dark spectacles, 7% methylcellulose eye drops.

Important causes of exophthalmos

1. Thyrotoxicosis
2. Primary CNS tumours: Meningioma, optic nerve glioma, haemangioma, lymphoma, etc.
3. Metastatic tumours: Neuroblastoma, central carcinoma.
4. Vascular: Cavernous sinus thrombosis—aneurysm of ophthalmic artery.

Causes of pulsating exophthalmos

1. Cavernous sinus thrombosis
2. Carotid—cavernous sinus, A-V fistula
3. Orbital vascular tumour
4. Ophthalmic artery aneurysm

V. Thyrotoxic Myopathy

- **Mild weakness of proximal limb muscles,** ocular and frontalis muscles is not uncommon. On careful questioning, patient may admit difficulty in climbing steps.
- Weakness of extraocular muscles results in double vision (diplopia).
- Features suggestive of myasthenia gravis, periodic paralysis can be found.
- **Myopathy improves with treatment.**

VI. Thyrotoxic Dermopathy (Key Box 37.14)

- Popularly called pretibial myxoedema—is seen in thyrotoxicosis patients treated with surgery or antithyroid drugs. It is always associated with exophthalmos. It is seen in 1–2% of patients.
- Bilateral symmetrical deposition of myxomatous tissue (glycosaminoglycans) mainly in the pretibial region, may also affect the foot and ankle, sometimes the entire leg below knee. Skin is dry and coarse (thickening of skin by mucin—like deposits). **Swelling is due to the obliteration of initial lymphatics by mucin** (*see* page 125).
- Pretibial myxoedema (misnomer) is nonpitting in nature and may be associated with clubbing of fingers and toes called thyroid acropachy. Responds to topical steroids and thyroid disorder treatment (Key Boxes 37.15 and 37.16).

Interestingly following 4 important features are seen only in primary thyrotoxicosis, not in secondary thyrotoxicosis (Key Box 37.17).

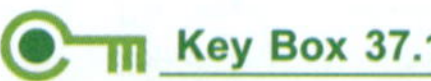

Key Box 37.14

Skin Changes

- Pretibial myxoedema
- Pruritis
- Palmar erythema
- Thinning of hair
- Dupuytren's contracture

Key Box 37.15

Pretibial Myxoedema—Misnomer

- **A**cropachy—clubbing of fingers and toes
- **C**oarse hair
- **R**ed shiny skin
- **O**bliteration of initial lymphatics by mucin, oedema non-pitting
- **P**retibial region, foot and ankle
- **A**fter a few years of toxicosis, it develops
- **C**yanotic when cold
- **H** • Hyaluronic acid deposition in dermis
- **Y** • Bilateral and symmetrical

Remember as **ACROPACHY**

Key Box 37.16

Some Misnomers

- Pretibial myxoedema – Not seen in myxoedema
- Mycosis fungoides – Not a fungal infection
- White bile – Not white, not bile
- Adenolymphoma – Not a lymphoma
- Sternomastoid tumour – Not a tumour
- Malignant hydatid – Not malignant

Key Box 37.17

Extrathyroidal Manifestations of Graves' Disease

- Pretibial myxoedema
- Proximal myopathy
- Pachy (acropachy)
- Progressive ophthalmoplegia

At the end of clinical examination, commonly asked question is, how will you differentiate primary thyrotoxicosis from secondary thyrotoxicosis (Table 37.5).

Management of Primary Thyrotoxicosis

Routine isotope scanning has been abandoned in toxic goitres except when toxicity is associated with nodularity.

Investigations

- Routine investigations such as complete blood picture, **flexible laryngoscopy and X rays are done.**
- Serum T_3, T_4 and TSH are measured. T_3 or T_4 levels are high and TSH levels are low in thyrotoxicosis. The normal level of T_3 is 1.3–3.5 nmol/L and normal level of T_4 is 55–150 nmol/L.
- Thyroid stimulating antibodies are elevated (TSHRAbs). Measurement of IgG immunoglobulins (TSHRAbs) is not essential to make the diagnosis of thyrotoxicosis.
- As a first line investigation, ultrasound is done to rule out nodularity (seconadry thyrotoxicosis).

Treatment of Primary Thyrotoxicosis

Aim of treatment

I. To restore patient to euthyroid state
II. To reduce the functioning thyroid mass to a very critical level (about 6–8 g of thyroid tissue)
III. To minimise complications

I. To Restore the Patient to Euthyroid State (Table 37.6)

- Other drugs such as **potassium perchlorate** are given in the dose of 200 to 400 mg daily. Propylthiouracil in the dose of 200 mg three times a day can also be given in patients **who develop neutropaenia due to carbimazole.**
- Propranolol inhibits peripheral conversion of T_4 to T_3. This results in rapid control of tachycardia and surgery can be scheduled in a few days (within one week). It should be continued for one week after surgery because it does not interfere with synthesis of hormones.

Please note

- Iodine containing **antiarrhythmic drug amiodarone** may worsen thyrotoxicosis.
- **Propyl thiouracil is safe in pregnancy** with Graves' disease.
- Role of Lugol's iodine is doubtful.
- **Antithyroid drugs will not cure** the disease. In selected patients (30–40%), remission is possible with regular intake of drugs. They may be continued for a maximum period of 2 years. If toxicity persists or recurs on stopping drugs, surgery is recommended.+ However, majority of the patients ultimately require surgery or radioiodine.

Table 37.5 Differences between primary and secondary thyrotoxicosis

	Primary thyrotoxicosis (Graves)	Secondary thyrotoxicosis (toxic MNG)
1. Age	20–40 years	35–50 years
2. Symptoms and signs	Appear simultaneously, duration is short	Long duration of a swelling and short duration of signs
3. Skin over thyroid	Warm	Not warm
4. Consistency	Soft or firm	Firm or hard
5. Surface	Smooth	Nodular
6. Auscultation	Bruit is common	Bruit uncommon
7. Eye signs	Commonly found	Rarely found (lid lag)
8. Predominant symptoms	CNS	CVS
9. Pretibial myxoedema	Seen in 1–2% patients	Never seen
10. Proximal myopathy	Seen in 5% patients	Never seen
11. Malignant exophthalmos	Can be seen	Never seen

Table 37.6 Antithyroid drugs: Routine preoperative preparation

Drugs and mode of action	Dose	Precautions/side effects
• Carbimazole: It blocks oxidation of iodide to iodine and coupling reactions, thus reducing T_3 and T_4 levels. It is metabolised to methimazole after ingestion	10 mg, 6th hourly and maintenance dose of 10 mg two to three times a day	Takes 12 weeks for its action It should be given 6–8 hourly interval Dangerous agranulocytosis can manifest as sore throat. Skin rashes and toxic hepatitis are not uncommon. Aplasia cutis is another side effect if carbimazole is given in the first trimester.
• Propranolol is a nonselective β-blocker, reduces tachycardia.	20–40 mg, two or three times a day depending on the pulse rate	Congestive cardiac failure Can precipitate bronchial asthma. T_3 and T_4 levels are not decreased

Corticosteroids

- They can be used as reserve drugs in severe, uncontrolled or resistant hyperthyroidism cases.
- They act by two ways—one by suppressing pituitary thyroid axis and another by inhibiting peripheral conversion of T_4 to T_3.
- Action is rapid
- They are used along with other antithyroid drugs.

Block and replace treatment

- If a small dose of T_3 (20 mg up to 4 times/day) or T_4 (0.1 mg/day) is given along with antithyroid drugs, there is less incidence of development of hypothyroidism and increase in the size of goitre.

II. To Reduce the Functioning Thyroid Mass

1. *Total thyroidectomy* can be offered to young patients with a small-sized gland. This is the choice of treatment today. It controls the toxicity very faster. Hypothyroidism occurs but it is easy to treat. However, it should be done by an experienced surgeon.
2. *Radioiodine therapy:* This is a suitable alternative to surgery in cases of primary thyrotoxicosis in patients above the age of 30 (Key Box 37.18).

III. To Minimise Complications

Good preoperative preparation of the patient, good anaesthetic and surgical techniques, and good post-operative care will reduce the complications of surgery. Thus, antithyroid drugs, subtotal thyroidectomy and radioiodine therapy are the three different modalities available for the treatment of primary thyrotoxicosis. The indications, merits and demerits of each treatment are given in Fig. 37.21.

Key Box 37.18

Radioiodine Therapy

- Today there is **'no restriction of age and gender'**. (However, this is preferred in children only after completion of growth and in adults only after family is complete.)
- Absolute contraindication is pregnancy.
- Conception must be avoided for a period of 4 months after radioiodine therapy.

Treatment of Secondary Thyrotoxicosis (Plummer Disease)

- Patients with severe cardiac damage entirely or partly due to hyperthyroidism are middle-aged or elderly with secondary thyrotoxicosis and the hyperthyroidism is not very severe. These patients develop atrial fibrillation and cardiac failure, if left untreated (Key Box 37.19). In elderly patients, when the operative risk is unacceptable, radioiodine is given. Treatment with antithyroid drugs is started 48 hours later and continued until radioiodine has had its effect (6 weeks).
- If the cardiac symptoms are controlled well and anaesthesia risk is acceptable, subtotal thyroidectomy/total thyroidectomy is done. However, the gland that is left behind should be equal to the distal phalanx of the thumb of the patient.

Secondary Thyrotoxicosis Effects on CVS (Key Box 37.19)

Key Box 37.19

Secondary Thyrotoxicosis Effects on CVS

- Tachycardia
- Wide pulse pressure
- Systolic scratch (Means-Lerman scratch)*
- Extrasystoles
- Atrial fibrillation
- Cardiac failure

*Means-Lerman scratch is occasionally heard in left 2nd ICS during expiration due to hyperdynamic circulation in thyrotoxicosis (Described by J. Lerman and J. H. Means of Massachusetts' General Hospital)

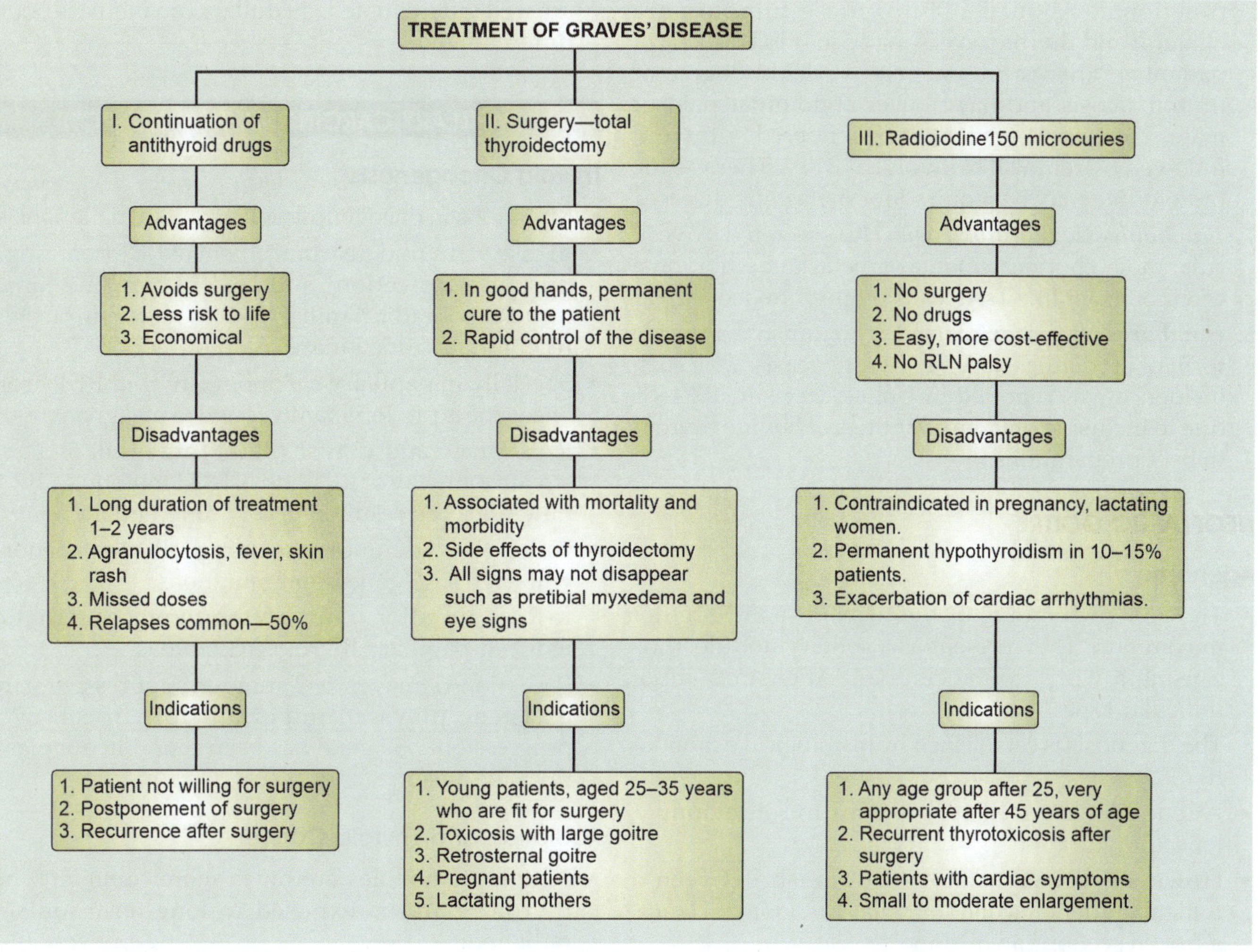

Fig. 37.21: Indications, merits and demerits of different modalities of treatments for primary thyrotoxicosis

SOLITARY TOXIC NODULE

Treatment

- This is not under control of TSH. It is an autonomous nodule.
- The control of toxicity is in the usual manner—carbimazole and propranolol.
- This is an indication to do I^{131} scan or preferably ^{99}mTc scan. Hot nodule takes up isotope (also in carcinoma). Rest of the gland does not.
- Treatment is either by hemithyroidectomy or radioactive iodine therapy—I^{131} (details will be given later).
- More details about solitary thyroid nodule and how to evaluate has been given later.

A Few Specific Thyroid Conditions Causing Thyrotoxicosis

1. *Thyrotoxicosis in children:* Initially antithyroid drugs are given for 10–15 years followed by surgery.
    - Radioiodine is absolutely contraindicated as there is a fear of carcinoma and growth retardation (Key Box 37.21).
2. *Thyrocardiac:* It refers to a condition wherein cardiac damage has resulted due to hyperthyroidism. Classically, it happens in secondary thyrotoxicosis. It is usually seen in middle-aged or old-aged patients. Propranolol controls the disease very well. Radioiodine therapy is the treatment of choice.
3. *Hyperthyroidism in pregnancy:* Invariably, it occurs in Graves' disease. In the first trimester, surgery and radioiodine are contraindicated. Carbimazole and propylthiouracil cross the placenta. Surgery, if necessary, can be done in 2nd trimester.
4. *Apathetic thyrotoxicosis:* Thyrotoxicosis in elderly wherein pulse rate is low, they appear to be hypothyroid rather than hyperthyroid. Thyroid gland is rarely palpable. Lethargy and behaviour changes.
5. *Graves' disease in postpartum period:* Postpartum thyroiditis with transient thyrotoxicosis due to thyroid cell dysfunction may occur in 5 to 10% patients during the first 4 to 12 months after delivery.
6. *Struma ovarii:* Thyroid tissue is present in 5 to 10% of teratomas and occasionally such foci are hyper-

functional. About 5–10% of these tumours are bilateral and thyrotoxicosis may occur in 8 to 10% of patients. Patients present with variable degree of thyrotoxicosis and have lower abdominal pain or mass. Treatment—patient to be rendered euthyroid followed by removal of involved ovary. Therapeutic radioiodine may be required for metastatic disease.

7. ***Trophoblastic thyrotoxicosis:*** HCG secreted by vesicular mole, choriocarcinoma or metastatic embryonal carcinoma act like TsAb causing thyrotoxicosis.
8. ***Hamburger thyrotoxicosis:*** It is an unusual and rare form of epidemic exogenic thyrotoxicosis. One such incidence was reported in United States in 1984–85 due to inclusion of large quantities of bovine thyroid in beef preparations.

NEOPLASTIC GOITRE

Adenoma

- The benign tumours of the thyroid gland are not uncommon. They present as a solitary nodule, thus causing a worry to the clinician. Adenomas are of follicular type.
- The diagnosis is established by histological examination.
- Adenomas are treated by hemithyroidectomy/lobectomy.
- However, FNAC cannot distinguish between a follicular adenoma and follicular carcinoma. Hence, a frozen section can be done.

Competency

SU22.4: Describe the clinical features, classification and principles of management of thyroid cancer.

MALIGNANT TUMOURS[1]

- Thyroid is the only endocrine gland wherein malignant tumours are easily accessible to clinical examination.
- Thyroid is the only endocrine gland wherein malignant tumours occur in children, young age, middle age, old age, and in both sexes.
- Thyroid is the only endocrine gland wherein malignant tumours spread by all possible routes—local, lymphatic and blood spread.
- Thyroid is the only endocrine gland wherein malignant tumours are usually nonfunctional. Malignant tumours of the thyroid are common. They are interesting tumours, having good prognosis, if diagnosed early. Papillary and follicular carcinomas are well differentiated, medullary carcinoma is poorly differentiated.

PAPILLARY CARCINOMA THYROID (PCT)

Thyroid Oncogenesis

- Mutations in oncogenesis will result in malignancies.
- In case of thyroid, rearrangement of RET (rearranged during transfection) and NTRKI tyrosine kinase result in sporadic papillary carcinoma (neurotrophic receptor, tyrosine kinase receptor)
- Specially in papillary carcinoma thyroid RET proto-oncogene is predominantly found in malignant tissue.
- RAS, kinase and 13 type (BRAF) are result of downstream pathway of RET and NTRKI mutations. BRAF mutations can result in poorly differentiated cancer.
- 40% of thyroid tumour including follicular adenoma will have RAS gene point mutations.
- K-RAS mutations more often found in radiation induced-papillary thyroid carcinomas
- Radiation damages p53 tumour suppressive gene. p53 gene plays an important role in cell cycle progression. p53 gene has been found in anaplastic thyroid cancer.

Radiation and Thyroid Cancer

- Neoplastic nodules are much more common when thyroid gland is exposed to long-term ionising radiation.
- High amount of radiation causes increased incidence of thyroid cancers.
- Risk of cancers in adults is high when they had contacted low or moderate doses of irradiation during childhood as found in survivors of Hiroshima and Nagasaki.
- Generally after 5 years of radiation exposure (radiation to head and neck for childhood lymphoma or too many CT scans for head and neck malignancy), papillary carcinoma thyroid can occur.

Aetiology

- Irradiation to the neck during childhood: In olden days, ***radiotherapy was given for benign conditions such as acne in teenagers or enlarged tonsils or thymus gland. Those children had increased risk of papillary carcinoma thyroid. These indications are obsolete now.*** However, accidental radiation to the neck or radiation given to Hodgkin's lymphoma can precipitate the development of papillary carcinoma thyroid.

[1]These were the teachings or sayings of Late Prof Sharath Chandra, FRCS, Department of Surgery, Madras Medical College, Chennai (conveyed to me by Late Prof Subbu, MMC, Chennai, when for the first and last time, I sat with Prof Subbu as a co-examiner at Govt. Medical College, Coimbatore, 1998).

- It can be a complication of Hashimoto's thyroiditis.
- Papillary cancer of thyroid occurs more often in patients with Cowden's syndrome, Gardner's syndrome or Carney's syndrome.
- **Associated mutations:** Chromosomal translocation involving RET proto-oncogene (tyrosine kinase) chromosome 10q11.

Pathology

- It is made up of colloid-filled follicles with papillary projections. In some cases, concentric, lamellated calcific structures are found which are called ***psammoma bodies***. (Psammoma bodies are also found in meningioma, and papillary serous cystadenoma of the ovary.) These are suggestive of papillary carcinoma of thyroid. **Nuclear grooving and intranuclear cytoplasmic inclusion (INCI) are diagnostic of papillary carcinoma thyroid.** Characteristic pale, empty, nuclei are present in a few cases which are described as ***Orphan Annie-eye nuclei***. Thyroid gland has very rich intrathyroidal lymphatic plexus. Papillary carcinoma can be unifocal or multifocal (Figs 37.22 and 37.23).
- **Papillary microcarcinoma:** They measure 1 cm or less in diameter. Distant metastasis is extremely rare. **Hence, a simple hemithyroidectomy is the treatment of choice**.

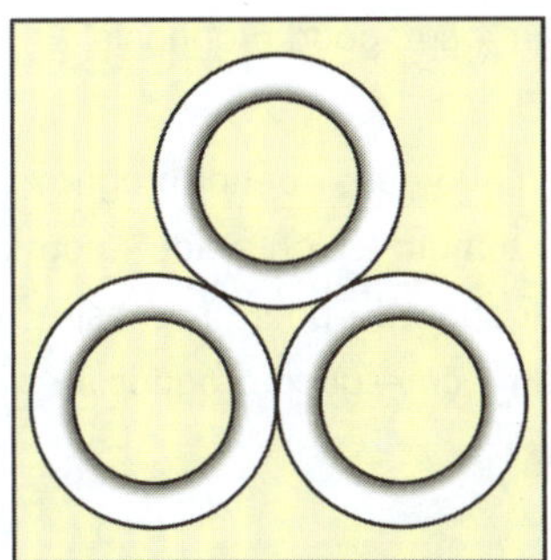

Fig. 37.22: Orphan Annie-eyed nuclei

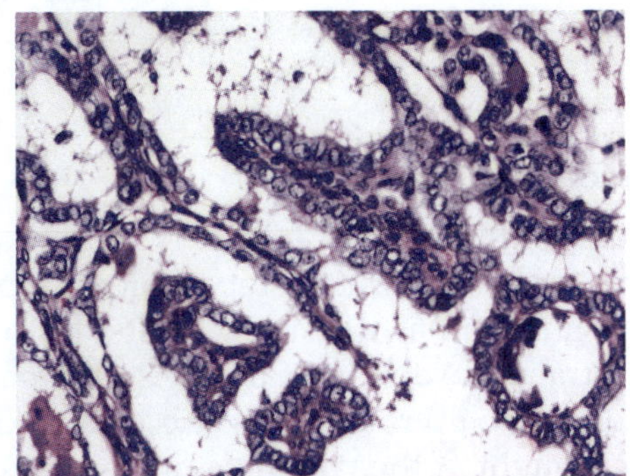

Fig. 37.23: PCT showing papillae with fibrovascular cores lined by follicular cells with Orphan Annie nucleus (*Courtesy:* Dr Laxmi Rao, Head, Department of Pathology, KMC, Manipal)

- **Follicular variant of papillary cancer:** This is a mixed lesion with a predominance of follicles over papillae. These are treated by total thyroidectomy. It is called **Lindsay tumour**.
- **Tall cell papillary cancer:** This is an aggressive and rapidly growing tumour. It occurs in elderly patients and should be treated by total thyroidectomy.
- Other details are given in Key Box 37.20.

Key Box 37.20

Pathology of Papillary Carcinoma Microscopy

- Calcification
- Cystic changes/necrosis
- Cuboidal pale cell with grooving
- Crowded nuclei
- Cytoplasmic inclusions—intranuclear
- Cartoon character—Orphan Annie
- Calcified laminated, basophilic, spherical concretions—Psammoma bodies

Observe **7 Cs**

Types—Woolner classification

- Minimal/occult/microcarcinoma: Tumour of 1 cm or less in size with no invasion/no lymph node metastasis
- Intrathyroidal: Confined to thyroid gland
- Extrathyroidal: Invasion of adjacent structures.

Clinical Presentation

- **As solitary nodule:** Young females are commonly affected (in the age of 20–40 years). It can present as a solitary nodule (Fig. 37.24) Nodule can be firm or hard. Unlike a nodule of anaplastic malignancy, nodule of papillary carcinoma is usually mobile in vast majority of cases. However, when it occurs in elderly patients, it can be rapidly growing. Ulceration and fungation is rare but can occur only in neglected cases as in Fig. 37.25.
- **As enlarged lymph node:** Very often, the lymph nodes in the lower deep cervical region—level 3 and level 4 are involved and they can be huge size also as in Figs 37.26 and 37.27.
- **As occult primary with palpable nodes:** In these cases thyroid gland may or may not be palpable. When thyroid gland is not palpable, it is called occult (hidden). However, papillary carcinoma less than 1.5 cm in diameter is also called 'occult'.
- Interestingly a few patients present as lateral aberrant thyroid or even a cystic swelling which is misdiagnosed as even a lymphatic cyst (Key Box 37.21).
- Tracheal fixity, common carotid artery engulfment and recurrent laryngeal nerve infiltration are very uncommon features of papillary carcinoma thyroid. But can occur in advanced cases more so in elderly patients.

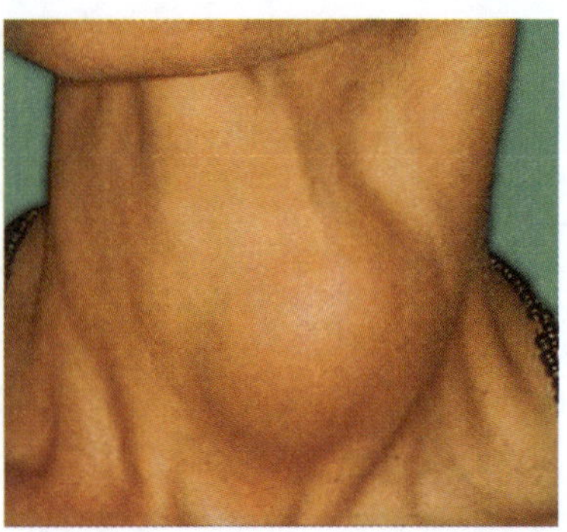

Fig. 37.24: Papillary carcinoma thyroid presenting as solitary nodule. FNAC gave the correct diagnosis. Total thyroidectomy was done in this patient

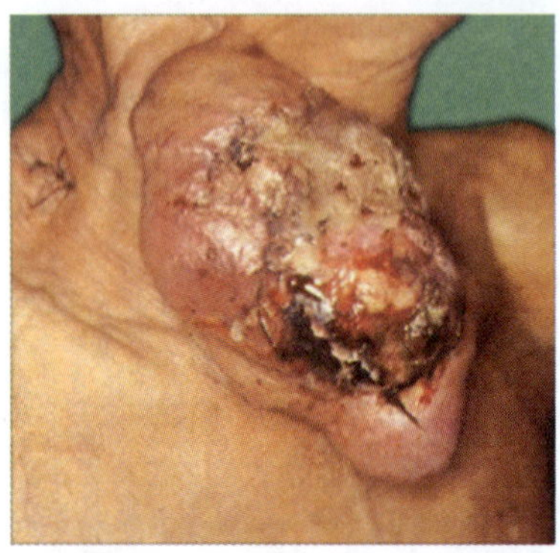

Fig. 37.25: Papillary carcinoma thyroid in a 75-year-old lady—it behaves aggressively in elderly patients. Total thyroidectomy was done (uncommon presentation)

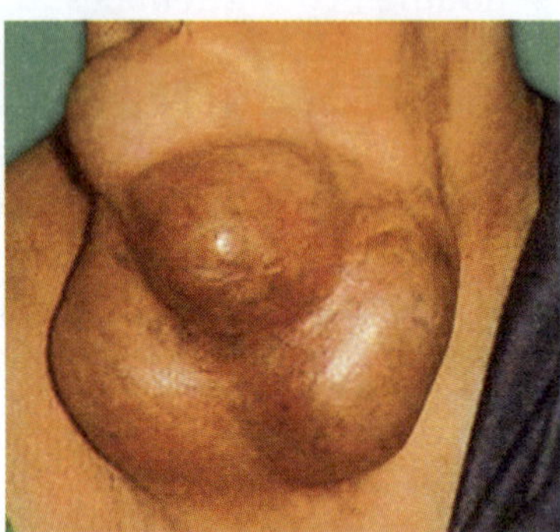

Fig. 37.26: Another case of papillary carcinoma thyroid with huge lymph node secondaries—advanced, neglected case

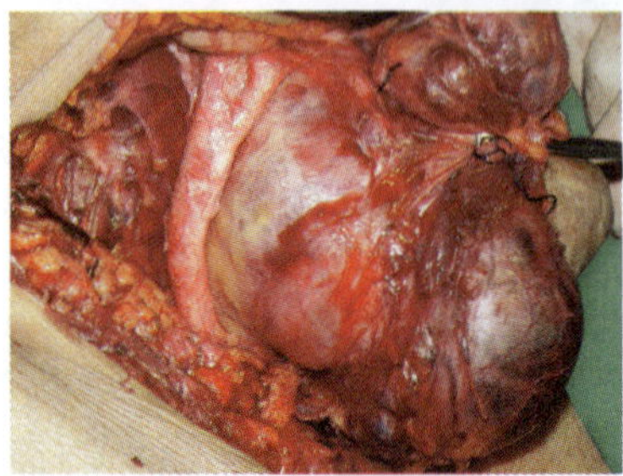

Fig. 37.27: Same patient as in Fig. 37.26—underwent total thyroidectomy with functional block dissection of the neck. *See also* exposed common carotid artery

Key Box 37.21

Papillary Carcinoma—Lymph Node Metastasis—Peculiarities

1. They may be palpable even when thyroid gland is not palpable—occult primary
2. Very slow growing
3. Very often, they are intracapsular
4. They need not be hard, are often cystic and firm in consistency
5. At operation, they are bluish in colour because of rupture of the papillae
6. Presence of lymph node metastasis does not affect the prognosis
7. Mostly central neck nodes and jugular chain of lymph nodes are cleared. Dissection of posterior triangle and suprahyoid dissection is not necessary.

Prognostic Criteria

There are many prognostic criteria that have been used in cases of well-differentiated carcinoma. Various scoring systems are available for well-differentiated carcinomas. Some examples are given below.

AMES scoring

A: Age less than 40 years—better prognosis
M: Distant metastasis—poor prognosis
E: Extent of tumour extracapsular spread—poor prognosis
S: Size less than 4 cm, good prognosis

AGES scoring

A: Age less than 40 years—better prognosis
G: Grade of the tumour—high grade—poor prognosis
E: Extracapsular spread—poor prognosis
S: Size less than 4 cm—good prognosis

MACIS scoring

M: Metastasis
A: Age
C: Completeness of resection
I: Invasion
S: Size

Histological Surprise

If a patient undergoes hemithyroidectomy for suspicious adenoma and histopathology reported is papillary carcinoma, dilemma exists as to how to proceed. Straightaway, one can advise the patient for completion (total) thyroidectomy. According to another school of thought, if the patient is in low-risk category with intrathyroidal malignancy and other factors favoring good prognosis, then 'wait and watch' policy can be undertaken.

Investigations

- **Ultrasound imaging and image guided FNAC: It is the first investigation of choice. As in breast imaging (BIRADS) in thyroid diseases also various findings have been classified depending upon composition, echogenecity, shape, margin and echogenic focus. Imaging by ultrasound has been described as TIRADS** (Fig. 37.28). Hypoechoic lesion with solid components, taller than wide, richly vascular/microcalcification and with or without jugular lymphadenopathy are suggestive of malignancy. In all such cases, ultrasound guided FNAC is done. Intranuclear inclusion bodies and nuclear grooving confirm diagnosis of papillary carcinoma thyroid.
- **Image-guided FNAC:**

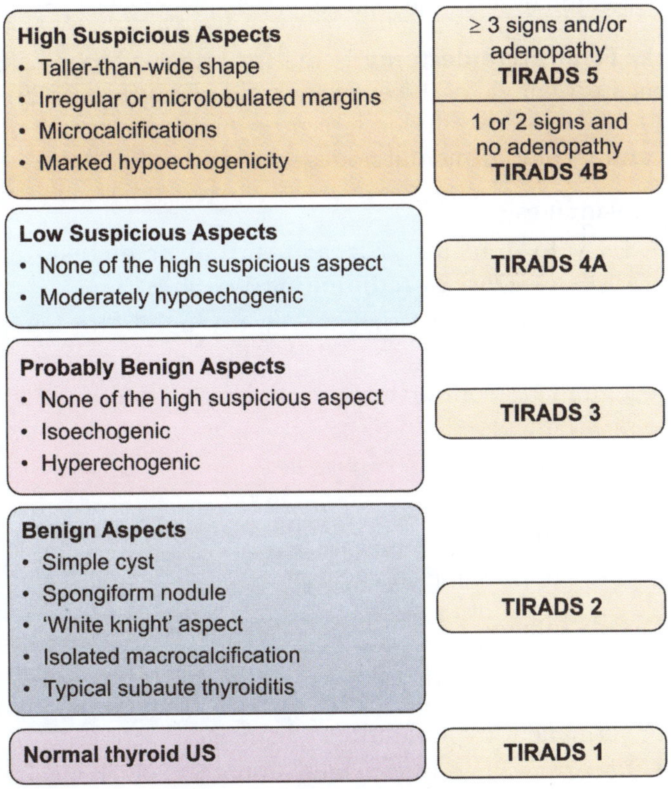

Aspects	TIRADS
High Suspicious Aspects • Taller-than-wide shape • Irregular or microlobulated margins • Microcalcifications • Marked hypoechogenicity	≥ 3 signs and/or adenopathy **TIRADS 5** 1 or 2 signs and no adenopathy **TIRADS 4B**
Low Suspicious Aspects • None of the high suspicious aspect • Moderately hypoechogenic	**TIRADS 4A**
Probably Benign Aspects • None of the high suspicious aspect • Isoechogenic • Hyperechogenic	**TIRADS 3**
Benign Aspects • Simple cyst • Spongiform nodule • 'White knight' aspect • Isolated macrocalcification • Typical subaute thyroiditis	**TIRADS 2**
Normal thyroid US	**TIRADS 1**

Fig. 37.28: TIRADS imaging

- **Hemithyroidectomy** (if done for solitary nodule) may reveal histological surprise with orphan Annie eyed nuclear and psammoma bodies (calcified clumps of cells with the papillary projections).
- **CECT scan:** It is routinely not done. Indications are: Advanced lesions to know the distorted anatomy of neck, infiltration into carotid sheath, retrosternal extension/doubtful fixity.

STAGING AJCC, 8th edition, 2018, TNM definitions

Primary tumour (pT) for papillary, follicular, poorly differentiated, Hürthle cell and anaplastic thyroid carcinomas:

- **TX:** Primary tumour cannot be assessed
- **T0:** No evidence of primary tumour
- **T1:** Tumour <2 cm in greatest dimension limited to the thyroid
- **T2:** Tumour >2 cm but <4 cm in greatest dimension limited to the thyroid
- **T3:** Tumour >4 cm limited to the thyroid or gross extrathyroidal extension invading only strap muscles
  - **T3a:** Tumour >4 cm limited to the thyroid
  - **T3b:** Gross extrathyroidal extension invading only strap muscles (sternohyoid, sternothyroid, thyrohyoid or omohyoid muscles) from a tumour of any size
- **T4:** Includes gross extrathyroidal extension into major neck structures
  - **T4a:** Gross extrathyroidal extension invading subcutaneous soft tissues, larynx, trachea, oesophagus or recurrent laryngeal nerve from a tumour of any size
  - **T4b:** Gross extrathyroidal extension invading prevertebral fascia or encasing carotid artery or mediastinal vessels from a tumour of any size

Primary tumour (pT) for medullary thyroid carcinomas:

- **TX–T3:** *Definitions are similar to the above*
- **T4:** Advanced disease
  - **T4b:** G
  - **T4a:** Moderately advanced disease; tumour of any size with gross extrathyroidal extension into the nearby tissues of the neck, including subcutaneous soft tissue, larynx, trachea, oesophagus or recurrent laryngeal nerve
  - **T4b:** Very advanced disease; tumour of any size with extension toward the spine or into nearby large blood vessels, invading the prevertebral fascia or encasing the carotid artery or mediastinal vessels

Regional Lymph Node (pN)

- **NX:** Regional lymph nodes cannot be assessed
- **N0:** No evidence of regional lymph node metastasis
- **N1:** Metastasis to regional nodes
  - **N1a:** Metastasis to level VI or VII (pretracheal, paratracheal, prelaryngeal/Delphian or upper mediastinal) lymph nodes; this can be unilateral or bilateral disease
  - **N1b:** Metastasis to unilateral, bilateral or contralateral lateral neck lymph nodes (levels I, II, III, IV or V) or retropharyngeal lymph nodes

Distant Metastasis (M)

- **M0:** No distant metastasis
- **M1:** Distant metastasis

AJCC Prognostic Stage Grouping			
Differentiated Thyroid Cancer			
	Age at diagnosis <55 years		
Stage I:	any T	any N	M0
Stage II:	any T	any N	M1
	Age at diagnosis ≥55 years		
Stage I:	T1	N0 / NX	M0
	T2	N0 / NX	M0
Stage II:	T1	N1	M0
	T2	N1	M0
	T3a / T3b	any N	M0
Stage III:	T4a	any N	M0
Stage IVA:	T4b	any N	M0
Stage IVB:	any T	any N	M1
Medullary Thyroid Cancer			
Stage I:	T1	N0	M0
Stage II:	T2	N0	M0
	T3	N0	M0
Stage III:	T1-3	N1a	M0
Stage IVA:	T4a	any N	M0
	T1-3	N1b	M0
Stage IVB:	T4b	any N	M0
Stage IVC:	any T	any N	M1
Anaplastic Thyroid Cancer			
Stage IVA:	T1–T3a	N0 / NX	M0
Stage IVB:	T1–T3a	N1	M0
	T3b	any N	M0
	T4	any N	M0
Stage IVC:	any T	any N	M1

Aims or Goals of Treatment of Papillary Carcinoma Thyroid

- Excise primary tumour → Total thyroidectomy
- Remove clinically significant/palpable lymph node → Functional neck dissection (no prophylactic neck dissection)
- Minimal complications of surgery—preserve internal jugular vein, accessory nerve.
- Once surgery is done—stage the disease
- Postoperative radioablation for residual thyroid tissue (usually it is present).
- Long-term follow-up with ultrasound of the neck and thyroglobulin for recurrence.
- Postoperative supplementary and suppressive dose of thyroxine.
- Look for metastasis.

Treatment

It can be discussed under three headings. Treatment of the primary, treatment of the secondaries in the **lymph nodes and suppression of TSH.**

I. Treatment of the Primary: Papillary Carcinoma Thyroid without Lymph Nodes. Stage I

(A) Total thyroidectomy, (B) Lobectomy and (C) Radio-remnant ablation.

Indications for total thyroidectomy

- Age older than 45 years
- Contralateral nodules
- Prior irradiation
- Familial—differentiated thyroid carcinoma (DTC)
- DTC >1 cm in size
- Extra thyroidal extension
- Regional/local metastasis

A. Total thyroidectomy is the treatment of choice. It means removal of the entire thyroid gland (Fig. 37.29). No role for prophylactic lymph node dissection of central compartmental nodes—level 6.

Advantages

- Easy to detect and treat residual or metastatic disease—**Dose of radioiodine 30–100 mCi**.
- Easy to assess recurrence by thyroglobulin level estimation.
- Eliminates contralateral occult cancer (multifocal in 80% patients).
- Eliminates re-surgery.
- Eliminates risk of recurrence, thus improving survival.
- TSH suppression can be done.

Disadvantages

- Total thyroidectomy has high complication rates such as RLN paralysis, permanent hypothyroidism, permanent hypoparathyroidism, etc.
- Recurrence in opposite lobe is only 5% which means in 95% of the cases, removal of the opposite lobe is unnecessary.
- Even if it occurs later, since it is not dissected at the time of initial surgery, the lobe can be removed easily.

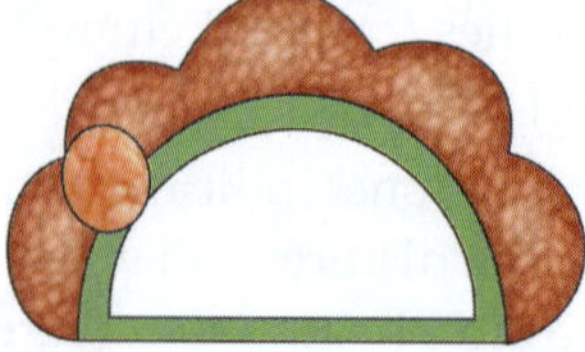
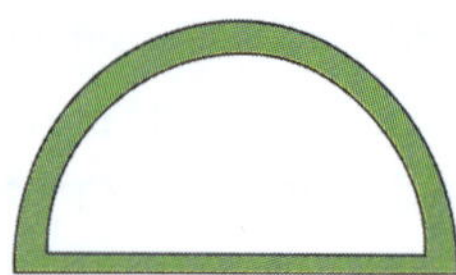

Fig. 37.29: Total thyroidectomy—in majority of cases

- **Tumour multicentricity has a little prognostic significance.** Thus in a few selected cases, lobectomy can be done.

B. Lobectomy (hemithyroidectomy) means removal of one lobe and entire isthmus (Fig. 37.30).

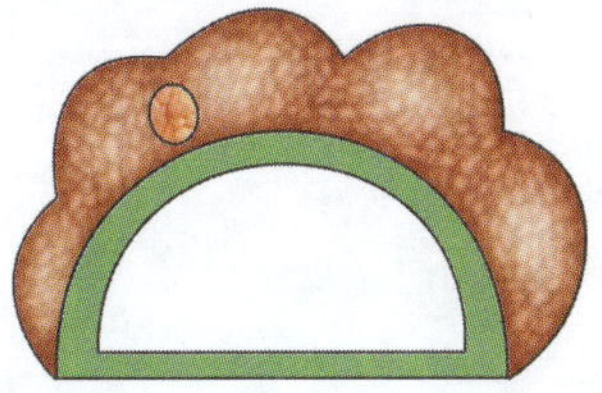
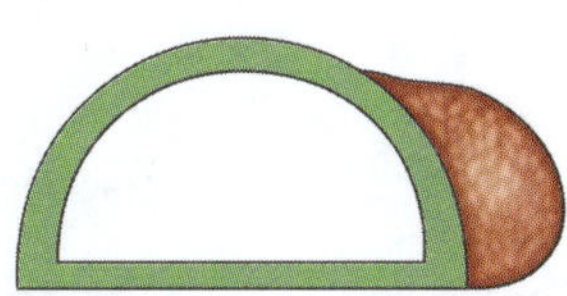

Fig. 37.30: Lobectomy—low-risk groups (hemithyroidectomy)

Indications for lobectomy

- Papillary carcinoma thyroid (PCT) less than 1 cm (called microcarcinoma)—no clinically palpable nodes, no extrathyroid extensions.

Advantages of lobectomy

- No hormone replacement
- No hypoparathyroidism
- Need not test thyroid function regularly.

II. Treatment of Papillary Carcinoma Thyroid with Secondaries in the Lymph Nodes (Figs 37.31 to 37.33)

- This is therapeutic not prophylactic lymph nodes dissections. At surgery, one has to carefully look for central compartment nodes—for enlargement. If palpable and enlarged, they should be removed. If nodes are enlarged in the anterior triangle, they are dissected and removed *en bloc* along with fat and fascia. This is called **functional block dissection** (**Berry picking** means removal of enlarged lymph nodes only. **It is no longer followed**).
- Level 2, 3, 4 and 5 nodes are removed when they are enlarged.
- Structures, such as **internal jugular vein, sternomastoid muscle, accessory nerve are not removed** because lymph nodes are slow growing and they rarely spread/outside the capsule of the lymph node. However, in exceptional cases of papillary carcinoma with infiltration to these structures, there should not be hesitation to remove these structures, this is called lateral neck dissection. In children, prophylactic/direct lymph node dissection is done.

C. Radio remnant ablation: After surgery, thyroxine is not given for a period of 4 weeks. Patient should be hypothyroid and TSH is around 30 mU/L. At this stage, radioisotope scan is done to look for residual thyroid gland. Even after total thyroidectomy, it is possible that some part of thyroid tissue may be present near the trachea esophageal groove or Berry ligament area. This needs to be ablated with 50 to 150 mCi of radioiodine.

- To avoid hypothyroidism for 4 weeks, patients can be given T_3 because it acts quickly and it can be stopped and restarted quickly. Dose of T_3 is 40–60 mg/day. It is very costly; not freely available.

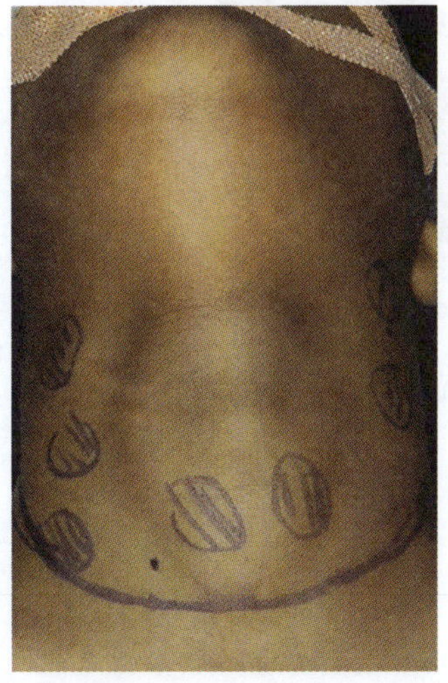

Fig. 37.31: Papillary carcinoma thyroid in an 18-year-old young patient with lymph node metastasis at levels 2,3,4 and 6. This patient was diagnosed as non-specific lymphadenitis for about 1 month with various antibiotics

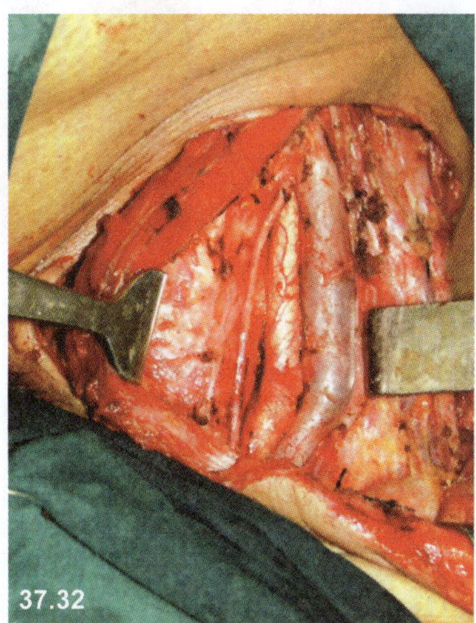

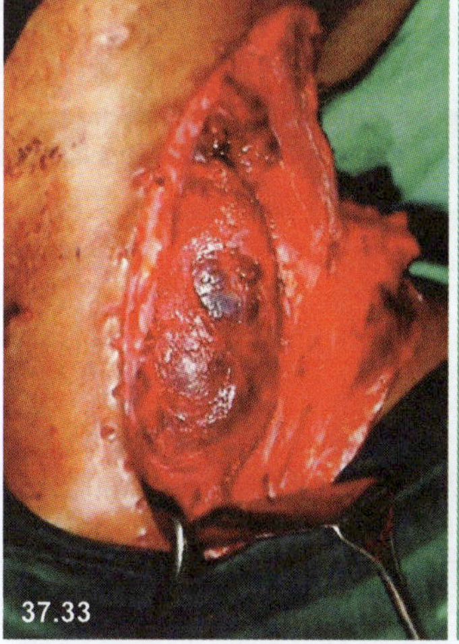

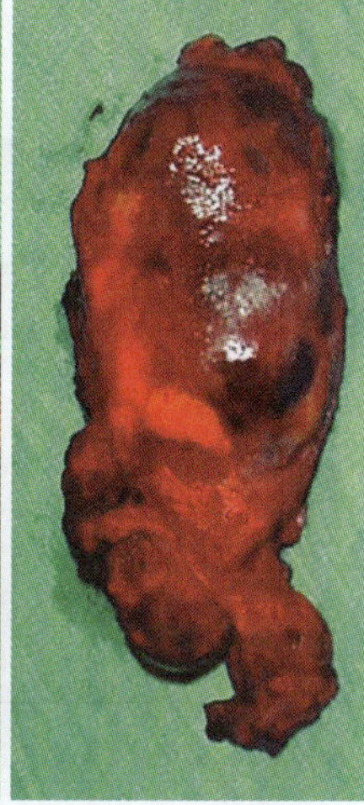

Figs 37.32 and 37.33: Functional neck dissection is done for papillary carcinoma thyroid. Routine central compartment dissection is not required. Figure shows vagus nerve, carotid artery and internal jugular vein. Sternocleidomastoid is retracted. All these structures are preserved. Hence, the name functional neck dissection. Observe bluish colour lymph nodes at surgery and specimen of lymph nodes. (*Courtesy:* Dr Gabriel Rodrigues, Professor, Department of Surgery, Dr Suresh BP, Assistant Professor, Department of Surgery, KMC, Manipal).

III. Suppression of the TSH

- This is an important aspect in the postoperative period because papillary carcinoma is a TSH dependent tumour. To prevent the patient developing hypothyroidism in the postoperative period and to suppress TSH, thyrotoxine (T4) 100 to 200 micrograms are given. This need to be monitored—increase or decrease depending upon the levels of TSH and toxicity.
- Failure of suppression of TSH to a level <0.1 mU/L suggests inadequate dose of thyroxine or noncompliance. Summary of papillary carcinoma thyroid is given in Key Box 37.22.

Key Box 37.22

Summary of Papillary Carcinoma Thyroid

- Most common histological type of thyroid cancer (60 to 65%).
- Most often it is multifocal (80%).
- Commonly it spreads by lymphatic spread.
- Psammoma bodies are suggestive and nuclear grooving is diagnostic of papillary carcinoma of thyroid.
- Most often it presents as solitary nodule and with or without lymph node metastasis.
- Most commonly done procedure for papillary carcinoma thyroid is total thyroidectomy with or without functional neck dissection.
- Radioactive iodine ablation and thyroxine 0.2 mg are important post-operative.
- Most of the patients (>95%) have 10-year survival rate.

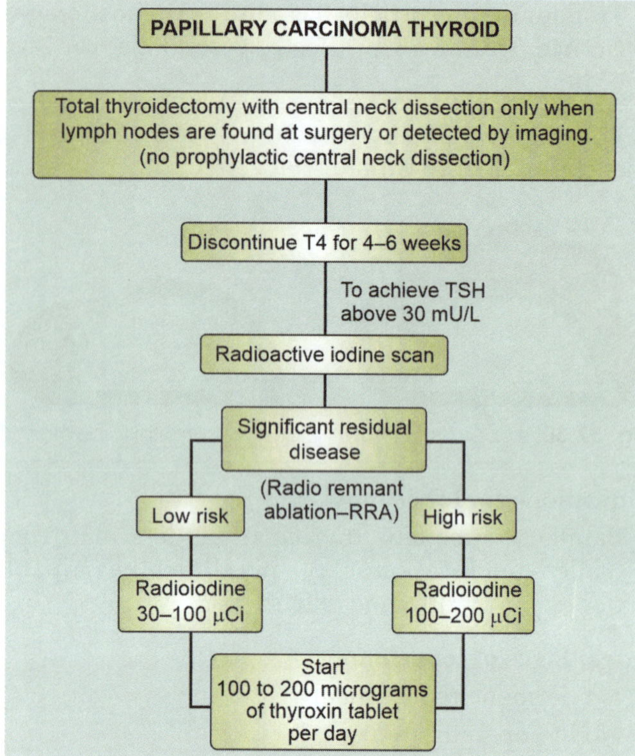

Fig. 37.34: Management protocol of papillary carcinoma

Management Protocol of Papillary Carcinoma of the Thyroid (Fig. 37.34)

Figure 37.34 depicts management protocol of papillary carcinoma of the thyroid.

FOLLICULAR CARCINOMA

- *Incidence:* Constitutes 17% of cases (Key Box 37.23).
- Follicular adenoma 20% are malignant and 80% are benign.

Aetiology

- Follicular carcinoma usually arises in a multinodular goitre, especially in cases of endemic goitre. It should be suspected when MNG starts growing rapidly (Fig. 37.35).

Key Box 37.23

Incidence of Thyroid Malignancy

Papillary carcinoma	60–65%
Follicular carcinoma	15–20%
Anaplastic carcinoma	10–12%
Medullary carcinoma	5–10%
Others	10%

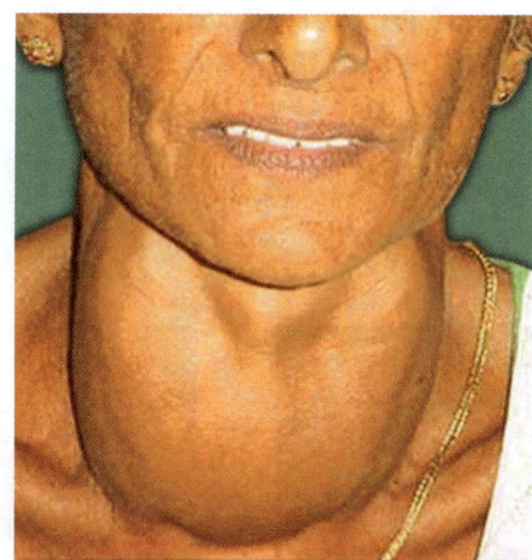

Fig. 37.35: Follicular carcinoma thyroid—clinically suspected—ultrasound showed microcalcification—FNAC revealed follicular cells. She underwent total thyroidectomy. Final report was follicular carcinoma thyroid

Pathology

Depending upon the property of invasion, it is classified into:

- **Non-invasive** which means minimal invasion.
- **Invasive** refers to angioinvasion and capsular invasion, necessary for the diagnosis of follicular carcinoma of thyroid. The tumour cells line the blood vessels and get dislodged into the systemic circulation producing secondaries in the bones. Microscopically, most of the tumours are well encapsulated (Fig. 37.36).

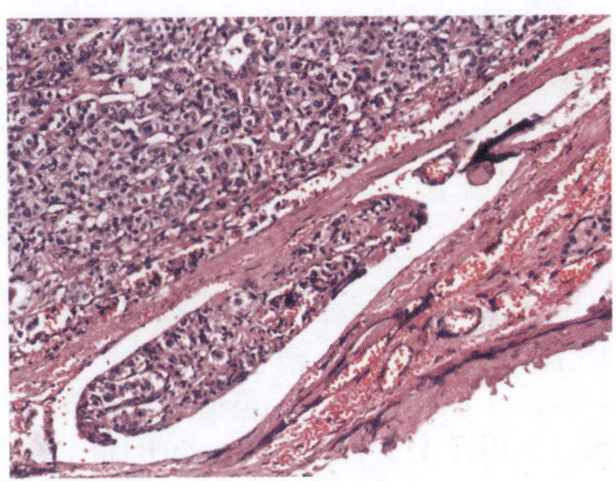

Fig. 37.36: Follicular carcinoma thyroid showing well-differentiated follicles invading the capsule and capsular veins. Please remember follicular carcinoma cannot be diagnosed by FNAC but by histopathology only (*Courtesy:* Prof Laxmi Rao, Head, Department of Pathology, KMC, Manipal)

Clinical Presentation

- It can present as a solitary nodule. The diagnosis is considered only after an ultrasound scan reveals some features of malignancy, such as **microcalcification**. Peak age group is around 40 years.
- In case of long-standing multinodular goitres, if the goitre is rapidly growing, hard or has restricted mobility, follicular carcinoma can be considered.
- **Metastasis in the flat bones:** The only clinical situation wherein a follicular carcinoma can be considered as the diagnosis is when a patient with a thyroid swelling presents with metastasis in the bone in the form of bony swelling or pathological fractures. Commonly, secondaries develop in the flat bones such as skull, ribs, sternum, vertebral column because the flat bones retain red marrow for a longer time. **When bony swelling is obvious and thyroid is not palpable clinically, it is called occult primary site** (Figs 37.37 to 37.40).
- **The clinical features of secondary in the skull are:**
  - They are rapidly growing.
  - They are warm.
  - Vascular and pulsatile
  - Underlying bony erosion may be present.

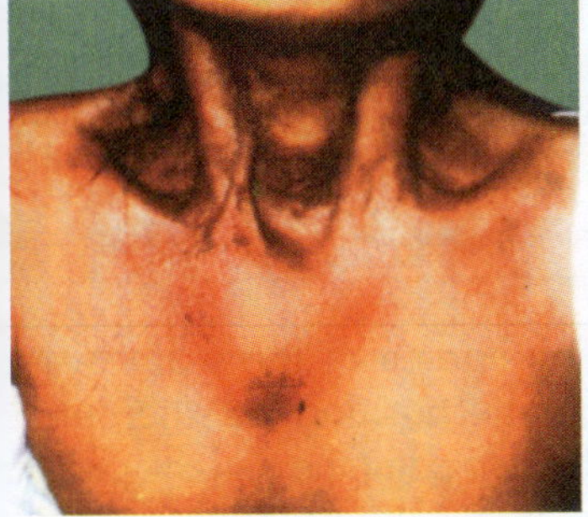

Fig. 37.37: Secondary deposit in the sternum in a patient who underwent near-total thyroidectomy for follicular carcinoma 5 years back

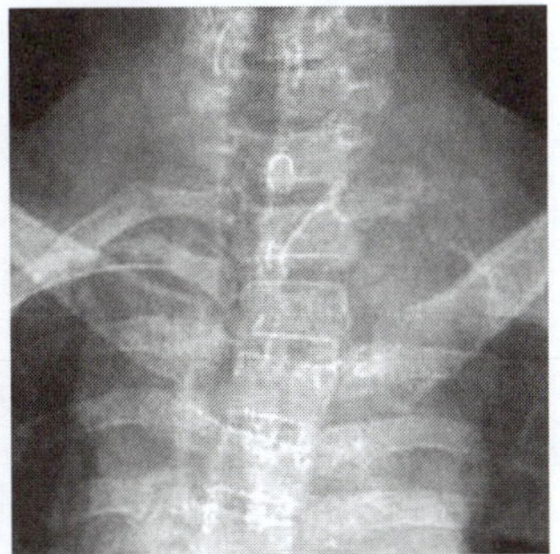

Fig. 37.38: Chest X-ray showing osteolytic lesion in the left clavicle

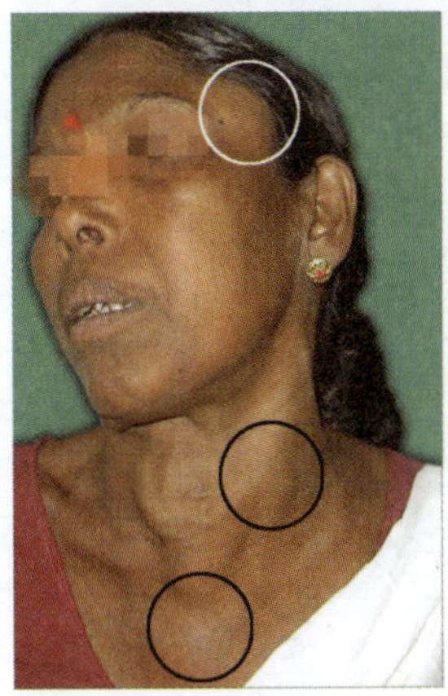

Fig, 37.39: This lady presented with thyroid swelling of 5 years' duration with swelling in the scalp and sternum of 2 months duration. Bony swellings were painful—it was a case of follicular carcinoma of thyroid with multiple bony metastasis: **Lady with three swellings**

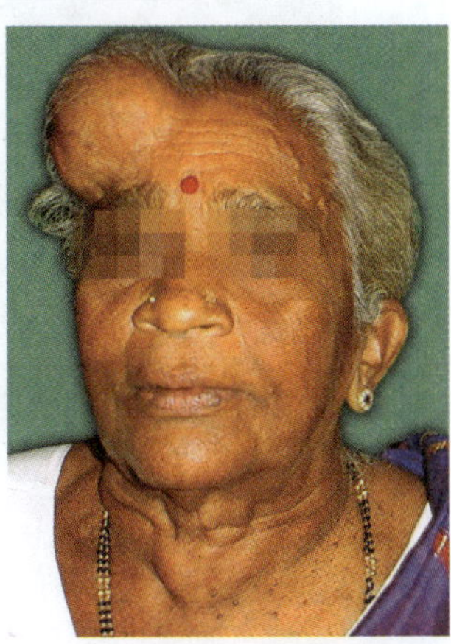

Fig. 37.40: Ulcerated secondary in the scalp bone from follicular carcinoma thyroid. See dilated veins in the neck. No other differential diagnosis in such patients. Initially it was diagnosed as lipoma. Neck examination for thyroid enlargement was not done.

Key Box 37.24

Reasons why Bone Metastasis Grow Rapidly from Follicular Carcinoma Thyroid—Seed and Soil Hypothesis

1. Tumour cells secrete angiogenesis compounds
2. Tumour cells secrete factors which enhance bone resorption
3. Increase production of IL-1, IL-6 which increase osteolytic activity
4. Maliganant cells synthesise adhesive molecules because of which they get attached to bone matrix

Investigations

- High frequency **ultrasound scan** is done (Figs 37.41 and 37.42) to demonstrate nature of the nodule, whether solid or cystic and to guide FNAC. It should be remembered that FNAC cannot differentiate a follicular adenoma from follicular carcinoma. Hence, if FNAC reports as follicular cells, **overtreat the patient** by total thyroidectomy. Some follow with frozen section and proceed. If frozen section is follicular carcinoma, total thyroidectomy is done. No role for open biopsy except in inoperable advanced carcinoma thyroids specially anaplastic carcinoma thyroid.

Pearls of Wisdom

Open biopsy is also not taken in cases of parotid tumors for the fear of damage to fascial nerve, in testicular tumors for the fear of dissemination of the tumor.

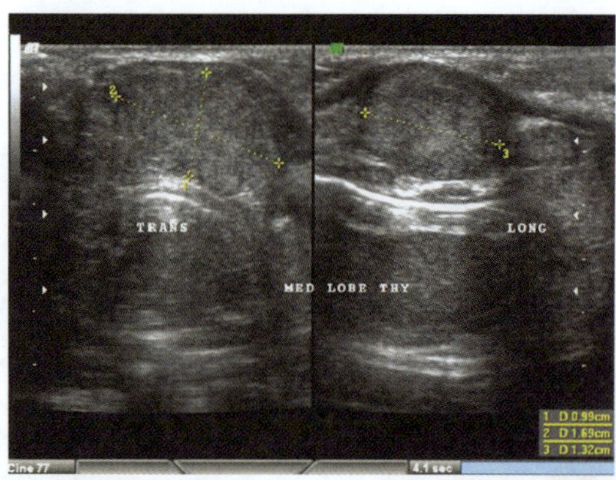

Fig. 37.41: Ultrasound revealing recurrence (nodules) in both lobes of the thyroid gland (*Courtesy:* Dr Chandrakanth Shetty, Professor, Department of Radiodiagnosis, KMC, Manipal)

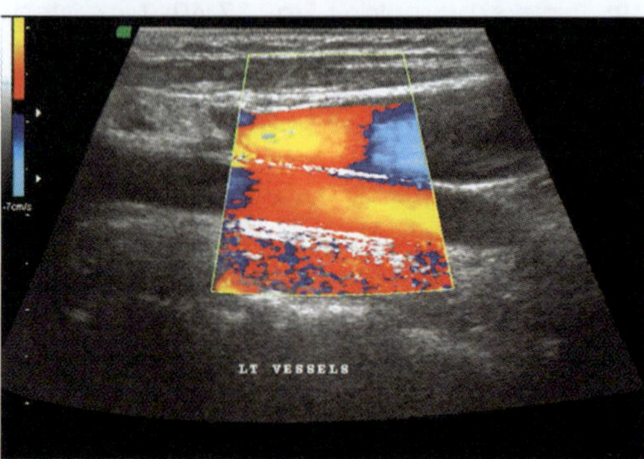

Fig. 37.42: Colour Doppler showing the relationship of the gland to major vessels of the neck (*Courtesy:* Dr Chandrakanth Shetty, Professor, Department of Radiodiagnosis, KMC, Manipal)

- **Plain X-ray** of the involved bone can reveal **osteolytic lesions** (Fig. 37.43).

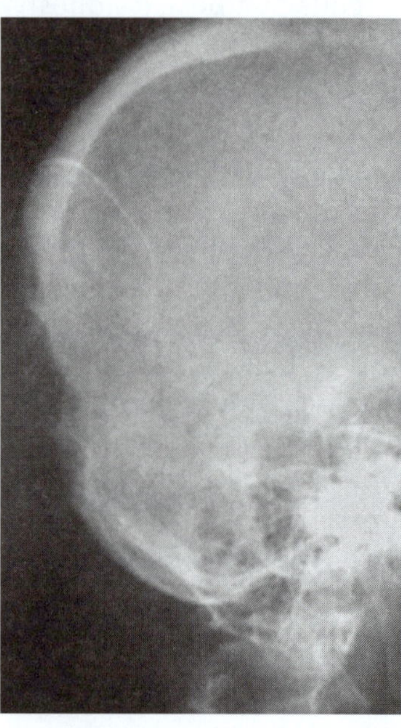

Fig. 37.43: Erosion of skull bone

- Whole body bone scan-I131 is done to rule out multiple osseous metastasis. Flat bones are commonly involved. They retain the red marrow for a longer period. Because of increased angiogenesis, secondaries grow more rapidly than primary tumors in follicular carcinoma thyroid. A few differential diagnoses of secondaries in the skull bones are given below in the Key Box 37.25.
- Whole-body MRI (91% diagnostic accuracy) to be superior to PET-CT (78% diagnostic accuracy) in detecting bone metastases. MRI is excellent in detecting marrow component and osseous and extra skeletal extent of the disease.

Key Box 37.25

Causes of Secondary in the Skull

1. Follicular carcinoma of thyroid
2. Renal cell carcinoma
3. Hepatocellular carcinoma
4. Prostatic carcinoma
5. Bronchogenic carcinoma

- **CT scan** in appropriate cases such as very large tumours adherent to trachea, vessels in the neck and mediastinal extension (Fig. 37.44).
- When primary is not found, **bone biopsy** is required to find out the site of the primary.

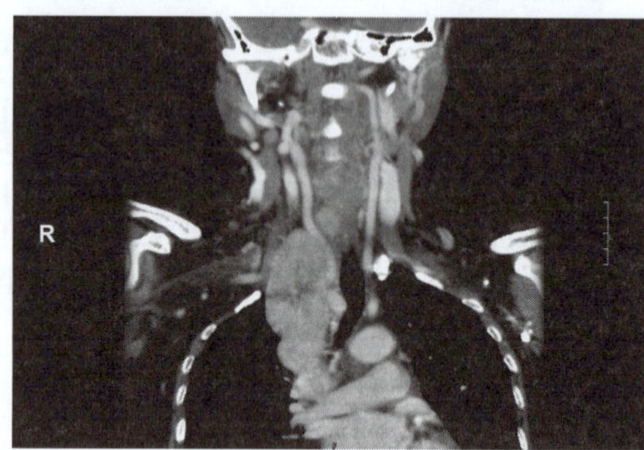

Fig. 37.44: CT neck and chest showing the large mass displacing the carotid artery, internal jugular vein thrombosis and mediastinal lymph nodes. Lymph nodes were cleared after sternotomy

Clinical Notes

A patient with a diagnosis of 'lipoma of the scalp' was posted for excision in the prone position. As the chief surgeon scrubbed and was about to paint the part, he could see the pulsatile nature of the swelling, which he had missed in the outpatient department. Fortunately, it was not excised. A needle was introduced and frank blood was aspirated. Surgery was cancelled. X-ray skull showed osteolytic lesion. She had a small thyroid nodule (Fig. 37.40).

TREATMENT OF FOLLICULAR CARCINOMA OF THYROID

I. Treatment of the Primary

- ***Situation I:*** When a patient has enlarged thyroid gland and scalp swelling, total thyroidectomy is the treatment of choice. Secondaries do not take up the radioisotope (^{131}I) in the presence of primary tumour. Hence, lobectomy or hemithyroidectomy should not be done.
- ***Situation II:*** A patient undergoes subtotal thyroidectomy for MNG and final report is follicular carcinoma thyroid. In such cases, it is better to do **completion thyroidectomy within 7 days** or **after 4 weeks.**
- If done, within 7 days, or after 4 weeks, it is relatively easy to do. Between 7 days and 4 weeks, the inflammatory process would have produced dense fibrosis, chances of injuring RLN, parathyroids are high.
- ***Situation III:*** A patient with solitary nodule—high suspicion of malignancy after sonography and FNAC reported as follicular cells, it is better to go ahead with total thyroidectomy.

II. Treatment of the Metastasis

- After total thyroidectomy, a whole body bone scan is done to look for metastasis in the bone. Bone metastasis occur in about 15% of patients with follicular carcinoma thyroid. A single secondary can be treated by oral radioiodine therapy, followed if necessary by external radiotherapy depending upon the response of the tumour. Multiple secondaries, if present, can best be detected by CT-PET scan and are treated by oral radioiodine therapy. Dose may be around 100 to 200 micro Ci.

III. Postoperative Thyroxine

- In the postoperative period, patients should receive thyroxine 100 to 200 mg/day to suppress TSH and to supplement thyroxine. The dose may have to be adjusted based on toxicity (tachycardia) and level of TSH.

Prognosis: 15% mortality in 10 years.

HÜRTHLE CELL CARCINOMA

- Hürthle cell carcinoma is a **variant of follicular carcinoma** (Key Box 37.26). It is more aggressive than follicular carcinoma.
- These tumours are defined by the presence of more than **75% of follicular cells** having oncocytic features.
- Tumour contains sheets of eosinophilic cells packed with mitochondria.

Key Box 37.26

Hürthle Cell Carcinoma

- More aggressive follicular carcinoma
- More than 75% malignant cells
- More chances of lymphatic spread
- More chances of distant spread
- More chances of mortality

- **They secrete thyroglobulin.**
- Even if Hürthle cell adenoma is well encapsulated, it is **potentially malignant**.
- It does not take up ^{131}I. Hence, it is less likely to respond to ^{131}I ablation.
- Higher mortality (20% at 10 years).
- ^{99m}Tc—sestamibi scan can detect Hürthle cell carcinoma.

Criteria to Diagnose Hürthle Cell Carcinoma

- Capsular/vascular invasion, distant metastasis.
- Higher chance of spread to lymph nodes compared to follicular thyroid carcinoma.
- Higher chances of spread to distant sites also.

Treatment

- Total thyroidectomy is the treatment of choice. In many cases of Hürthle cell carcinoma, lymph nodes are enlarged. Hence, modified radical neck dissection is done (MRND).
- TSH suppression and follow-up are regularly required.

Pearls of Wisdom

All Hürthle cell neoplasms are almost malignant and all adenomas are almost follicular. In all suspicious solitary nodules of follicular cell origin, it is better to overtreat them by total thyroidectomy than relying upon the frozen section, to avoid second surgery.

Follow-up of patients with papillary and follicular carcinoma thyroid—differentiated thyroid cancer

- **Serum thyroglobulin (Tg):** Thyroid is the only organ which produces thyroglobulin. Levels greater than 10 ng/ml in patients receiving replacement thyroxine therapy indicates presence of metastasis. Hence, assess the serum Tg response to injected recombinant human TSH every year. In thyrotoxicosis and thyroiditis, thyroglobulin levels may be increased (Key Box 37.27).
- **Ultrasonography or MRI** scans of the neck for localisation of residual or recurrent tumour.

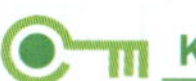

Key Box 37.27

Serum Thyroglobulin

- Normal value: The normal value for thyroglobulin is **3 to 40 nanograms per milliliter**.
- Above 50 nanogram/ml suggests malignancy.
- Above 100 nanogram/ml suggests pulmonary or skeletal metastasis.
- It is produced by follicular cells of the thyroid. Hence elevated in well-differentiated carcinoma. Not in medullary carcinoma thyroid.
- Hence, it is a tumour marker of well-differentiated carcinoma.
- Anti-thyroglobulin antibodies (ATA-TgAb) are found in Hashimoto's thyroiditis and in Graves' disease.

ANAPLASTIC CARCINOMA

Incidence: 10–12% of cases.

Clinical Features (Key Box 37.28)

Key Box 37.28

Anaplastic Carcinoma Thyroid

- The most rapidly growing thyroid malignancy
- Advanced age group at presentation
- Advanced nature of presentation
- Gross local infiltration—Berry's sign positive
- No form of treatment is successful.
- Intrinsic carcinoma of larynx spreading outside and infiltrating the skin should be considered as a differential diagnosis.

- Common in elderly women around 60–70 years of age.
- Majority of the patients present with rapidly growing thyroid swelling of short duration. The surface is **irregular,** and consistency is **hard**.
- **Early infiltration of the trachea** results in stridor (scabbard trachea).
- Infiltration of carotid sheath: In such cases, common carotid artery pulsation will not be palpable. This is described as **'Berry sign positive'**. However, superficial temporal artery pulsations will be palpable. It means the lumen is not blocked but common carotid artery is engulfed.
- **Early fixity** is characteristic. Thus, the respectability rate is almost nil (Fig 37.45).
- Pathologically highly pleomorphic malignant cells are seen (Fig. 37.46).

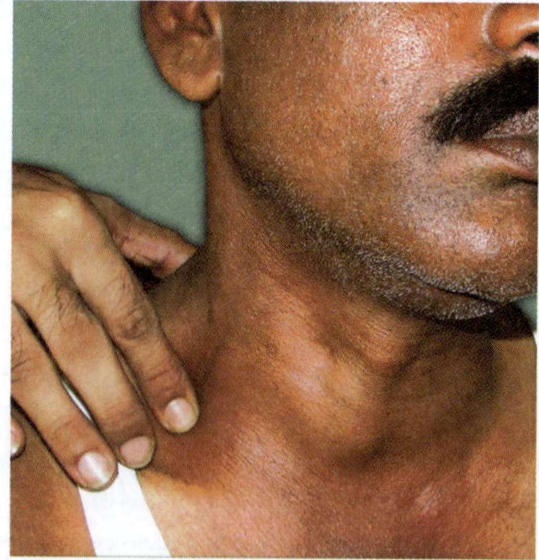

Fig. 37.45: A 40-year-old male with 3 cm hard, fixed nodule with recurrent laryngeal nerve paralysis. FNAC—anaplastic carcinoma

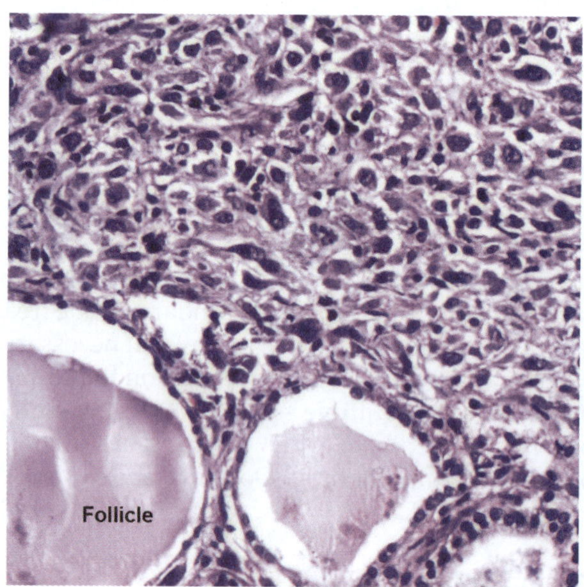

Fig. 34.46: Highly pleomorphic malignant cells. (*Courtesy:* Prof Laxmi Rao, Head, Department of Pathology, KMC, Manipal)

Diagnosis

It is established by FNAC, other investigation being CT scan.

Treatment

- Due to the gross local infiltration into the vital structures in the neck, such as common carotid artery and trachea, the respectability rate is low.
- However, very rarely, a surgeon will get an opportunity to excise isthmus so as to relieve compression of the trachea.
- Postoperative radiotherapy is given as a palliative treatment.
- In many cases, death occurs within 6 to 8 months.

MEDULLARY CARCINOMA OF THE THYROID (MCT)

These tumors arise from parafollicular 'C' cells which are derived from ultimobranchial bodies and not from thyroid follicle. Parafollicular cells are pale-staining cells found in the thyroid gland. They are always situated within the *basement membrane*, which surrounds the entire follicle.

These tumors present in two different ways.

1. Sporadic is common, seen in about 80–90% of cases.
2. Familial variety presents as a part of multiple endocrine neoplasia (MEN).

MEN Type I

Pituitary adenoma
Parathyroid adenoma
Pancreatic adenoma

MEN Type IIa

Parathyroid adenoma
Phaeochromocytoma
Medullary carcinoma of thyroid

When it is associated with mucocutaneous neuromas involving lips, tongue, eyelids, it is called ***Sipple syndrome***, with an occasional marfanoid habitus (MEN type IIb) (Fig. 37.47).

Pathology: It has got a characteristic ***amyloid stroma*** (Fig. 37.48).

These tumours are not TSH-dependent and do not take up radioactive iodine.

Hormones Produced by MCT

Calcitonin (Key Box 37.29)
Prostaglandins
Serotonin (5-HT), ACTH

Spread

- Both by lymphatics and blood, thus worsening the prognosis.

Key Box 37.29

Calcitonin and Medullary Carcinoma Thyroid

- Not measurable in normal persons
- MCT produces very high levels
- It is the tumour marker of MCT
- Level decreases after thyroidectomy
- Level increases in case of recurrence
- Prophylactic thyroidectomy in relatives, if calcitonin levels are high

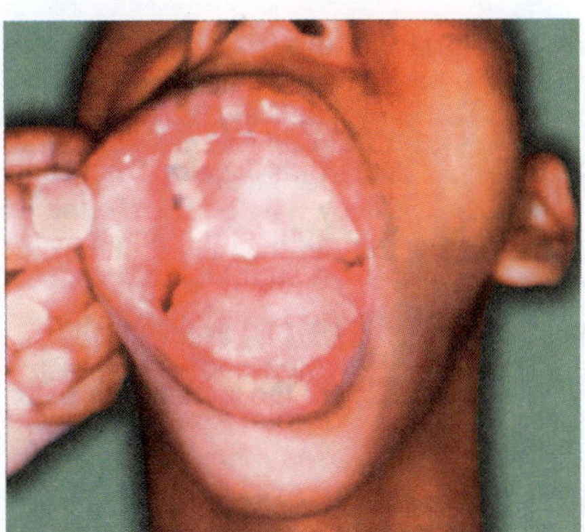

Fig. 37.47: FNAC proved medullary carcinoma with mucocutaneous neuroma—MEN type IIb

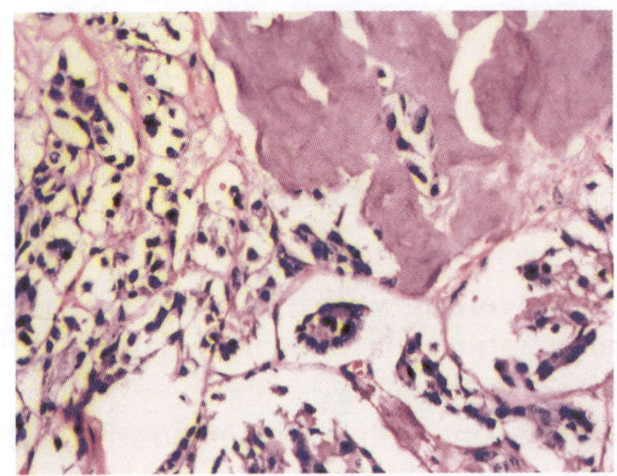

Fig. 37.48: Medullary carcinoma thyroid—characteristic amyloid stroma

Treatment

1. Total thyroidectomy with modified radical dissection
   - Before proceeding with surgery, **look for an associated phaeochromocytoma**.
2. The lymph nodes are treated by radical block dissection because they are fast-growing, when compared to papillary carcinoma.

Pearls of Wisdom

If there are multiple secondaries in the bone, oral 131I has no role because this tumour does not arise from thyroid cells. Only palliative radiotherapy can be given.

Clinical Criteria for the Diagnosis of Carcinoma of Thyroid: Summary

1. A thyroid swelling which is rapidly growing.
2. Thyroid swelling with lower deep cervical lymph nodes and lymph nodes in the posterior triangle (papillary carcinoma thyroid) involved.
3. Hard gland, fixed to the trachea—anaplastic carcinoma of the thyroid.
4. Thyroid swelling with a rapidly growing, vascular, pulsatile swelling, commonly in the skull (follicular carcinoma).

Table 37.7 Summary of the malignant tumours of thyroid gland

	Papillary	Follicular	Anaplastic	Medullary
1. Aetiology	Irradiation	Endemic goitre	Unknown	Sporadic or familial
2. Incidence	60%	17%	13%	6%
3. Age (years)	20–40	30–50	50 and above	Middle age
4. Diagnosis	Thyroid swelling with lymph node metastasis	Thyroid swelling with bony metastasis	Thyroid swelling, local fixity, stridor	Difficult to diagnose clinically
5. Microscopy	Orphan Annie-eye nuclei, psammoma bodies	Angioinvasion, capsular invasion	Poorly differentiated cells	Amyloid stroma-like carcinoid
6. Spread	Lymphatic	Blood	Local infiltration	Lymphatic, blood
7. Investigation	FNAC	Frozen section	FNAC, incision biopsy	FNAC, calcitonin
8. Treatment of the primary	Near total/total thyroidectomy	Near total/total thyroidectomy	Isthmusectomy, external RT	Total thyroidectomy
9. Treatment of metastasis	Functional neck dissection	Radioiodine ^{131}I or external RT	Palliative external radiotherapy	Radical block dissection
10. TSH dependence	Yes	Yes	No	No
11. Hormone production	Very rare	Very rare	No	Calcitonin, 5-HT, ACTH
12. Prognosis	Excellent	Good	Worst	Bad

5. Thyroid swelling with hoarseness of the voice indicating infiltration of recurrent laryngeal nerve is a feature of malignancy.
6. Thyroid swelling with Berry sign positive (anaplastic carcinoma of the thyroid).
7. Kocher's test positive may be an indication of infiltration into trachea. Summary of the malignant tumours of the thyroid gland is shown in Table 37.7.

LYMPHOMA

- It is rare. Hashimoto's thyroiditis can predispose to lymphoma.
- Older patients are commonly affected.
- The tumour can present as rapidly-growing, large thyroid swelling (primary lymphoma).
- Sometimes, it can appear as a part of generalized lymphoma (non-Hodgkin's variety).
- FNAC may give the diagnosis—**Tru-cut biopsy is ideal.**
- It is interesting to note that lymphomas of the thyroid respond very well to chemotherapy and radiotherapy (Fig. 37.49A and B).

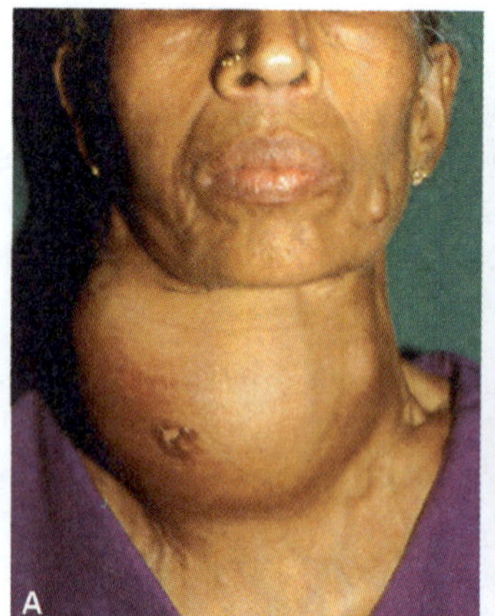

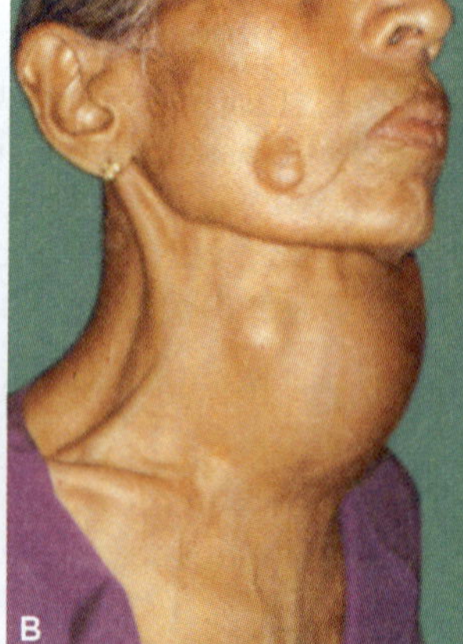

Fig. 37.49A and B: Lymphoma of the thyroid gland wit mediastinal lymph nodes and superior vena caval obstructior Watch dilated veins and also three cutaneous nodules

SOLITARY NODULE OF THE THYROID GLAND

Definition: Solitary nodule (SN) is a clinical term denoting presence of a single palpable nodule in the thyroid gland **(no other part of thyroid gland is palpable)** (Fig. 37.50A).

- Almost all the thyroid swellings initially can present as a solitary nodule. However, puberty goitres, colloid goitres, diffuse toxic goitres produce uniforn enlargement of the thyroid gland. Multinodula goitre (MNG) presents as multiple nodules. However very often a solitary nodule on clinical examination may turn out to be a multinodular goitre at exploration. **The solitary nodule has a higher incidence o malignancy when compared to MNG.**
- It is a **common surgical problem** encountered by general surgeons. By definition, one can call it a solitary nodule **when only the nodule is clinically palpable** but rest of the gland is not palpable.
- However, when a nodule is palpable and the opposite lobe or any other part of the thyroid is palpable, it is a **'dominant' nodule.** It may probably be a case o multinodular goitre (Fig. 37.50B).

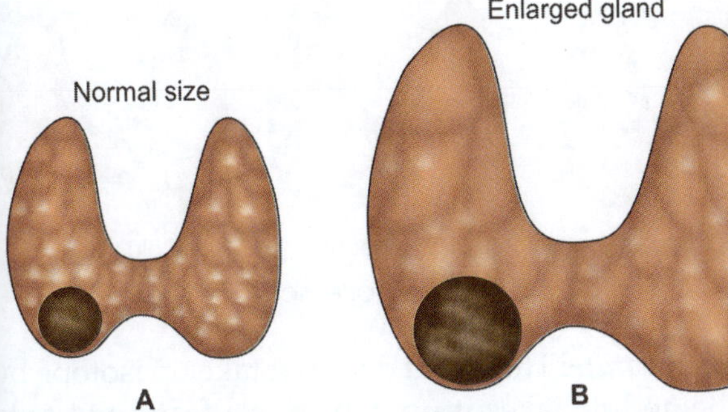

igs 37.50A and B: (A) Solitary nodule. Rest of the gland is normal; 3) Solitary nodule. Rest of the gland is enlarged—mostly it is MNG

ntroduction

It is the **most common surgical disease** of the thyroid gland. Incidence is about 4%. It is 4 times more common in women than men. About 20 to 30% of patients may have nodules on the other side when detected by ultrasound, thus the diagnosis changes to multinodular goitre. Risk of malignancy is more in a solid nodule and in men. It is about 48%. However, in females it is about 12%. In general, incidence of malignancy is 8–10%. Ultrasonography followed by FNAC is the first line of investigations. Aim is to identify a solitary nodule which has **high risk**, e.g. **male, solid, solitary nodule is a nodule which has features suggestive of malignancy** (Key Box 37.30).

Key Box 37.30

High Risk Solitary Nodule

- **Male** patients with **'solid'** nodule
- Rapid growing nodule of short duration
- Nodule which has **restricted** mobility
- Nodule with jugular **lymphadenopathy** on ultrasound
- Nodule which is **hard in consistency**
- Nodule with **hoarseness of voice**

Causes of Solitary Nodule of the Thyroid Gland

(Figs 37.51 and 37.52)

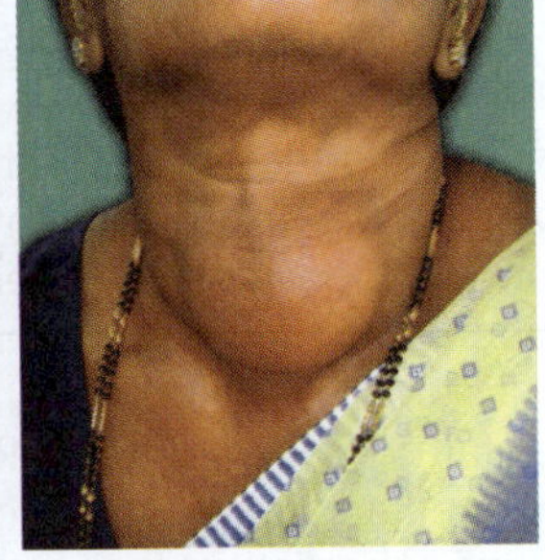

Fig. 37.51: A 45-year-old female with solitary nodule. FNAC revealed thyroid cyst

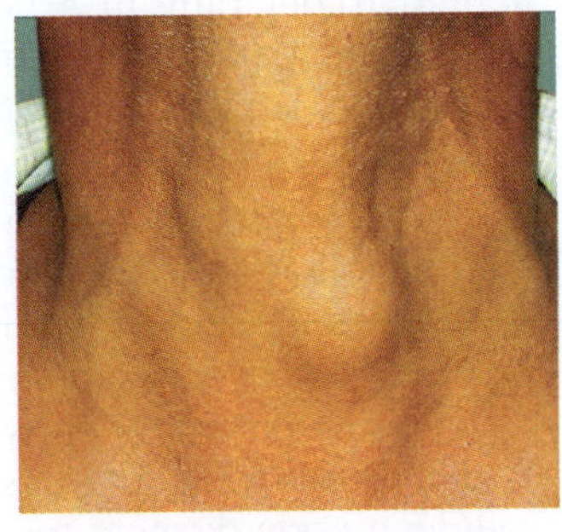

Fig. 37.52: A 45-year-old male presented with solitary nodule. Hormone levels were elevated. He underwent hemithyroidectomy—solitary toxic nodule

1. In about 30 to 40% of the cases, a clinically palpable solitary nodule is a part of multinodular goitre
2. Toxic autonomous nodule
3. Adenoma
4. Carcinoma
5. Cysts

Pearls of Wisdom

About 2 to 3% of solitary nodules are associated with hyperthyroidism. Chances of malignancy in a hyperthyroid nodule is very low.

Indications for Surgery

- Malignant cytology: Refer to Bathesda Criteria for FNAC thyroid
- Suspicious cytology
- Large size
- Pressure effect, substernal extension
- Clinical suspicion of malignancy
- Cosmesis
- Male sex
- Cyst—recurs after aspiration and bloodstained fluid

Investigations

1. Blood investigations

- T_3, T_4 and TSH: Free thyroxine—better indicator of thyroid status than total T_4. T_3 is useful when T_4 level is borderline (T_3 toxicosis). TSH is needed when there is no clinical manifestation of hyper- (or) hypothyroidism.
- Thyroid autoantibodies—when Hashimoto's thyroiditis is suspected.
- Serum thyroglobulin (STG)—tumour marker
  a. Normal value is <1–35 nanog/L
  b. STG level above 50 nanog/L—suggests residual (or) recurrent tumour
  c. STG level goes above 100 nanog/L suggests pulmonary (or skeletal metastasis)
  d. Increased in hyperthyroidism, thyroiditis and tumour
  e. Serum calcitonin—useful for screening medullary carcinoma when a patient has history of thyroid cancer and presents with a solitary nodule.

2. 24 hours collection of urine for catecholamine to exclude phaeochromocytoma (MEN II syndrome) because of association with medullary carcinoma (Rare).

3. Ultrasonography (USG): It is noninvasive, cheap and it has become the investigation of choice in solitary nodule. Totally sonolucent unilocular lesions, sonolucent cyst with internal echoes, septae, nodule with homogeneous echogenicity (hyper or hypo), mixed echogenicity and microcalcification enlargement of jugular lymphadenopathy are a few features suggestive of malignancy. With increasing use of high frequency ultrasound probe, radionuclide scan is rarely used or almost not used in the evaluation of solitary nodule thyroid gland.

4. **Ultrasound guided fine needle aspiration cytology (FNAC):** Using a 22 or 23 gauze needle attached to a 10 ml syringe, under ultrasound guidance, needle is introduced within the gland while maintaining negative pressure and about 4 to 6 passes are done within the gland and syringe and needle are withdrawn. Contents are pushed into slides and about 6 slides are prepared and are air dried. Most popular criteria used for FNAC thyroid is Bathesda criteria (Table 37.8). (Bathesda is name of the pool in Jerusalem and it is a City in central Maryland).
5. **CT scan:** Specific indications are: Doubt about the origin of the swelling, large lesion with local infiltration into vascular structures and intrathoracic extension.
6. **Isotope scan** (not routinely done nowdays): Most commonly used isotope—^{99m}Tc. ^{131}I should not be used for evaluation of nodule. ^{123}T will not detect nodules of 1 cm size. However, it is indicated in a 'toxic nodule' which is 'hot'. Rest of the gland is suppressed, so that such patient can be managed easily by radioiodine. It can demonstrate three different patterns as follows Fig. 37.53).

Table 37.8 Bathesda criteria for FNAC thyroid

Bathesda category	Implied malignancy rate	Usual management
1. Non-diagnostic or unsatisfactory	1–4%	Repeat FNAC with image guidance
2. Benign	0–3%	Clinical follow-up
3. Atypia of Undetermined Significance/ Follicular lesion Of undetermined Significance (AUS/FLUS)	5–15%	Repeat FNAC or lobectomy
4. Follicular neoplasm or suspicious of follicular neoplasm	15–30%	Lobectomy
5. Suspicious of malignancy	60–75%	Lobectomy or total thyroidectomy
6. Malignant (specific type)	97–99%	Total thyroidectomy

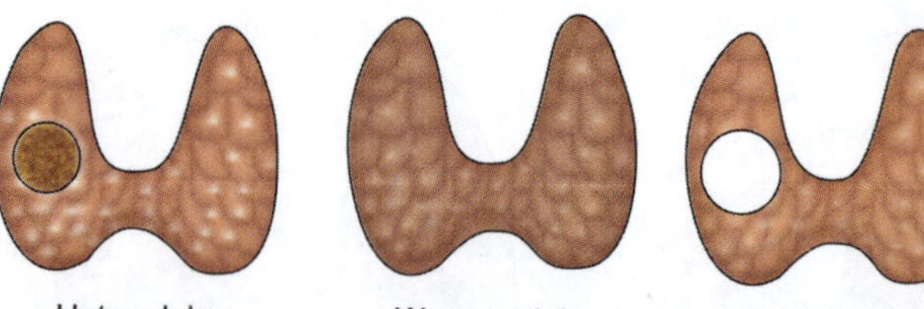

Fig. 37.53: Radioisotope scan findings

- ***Hot nodule:*** The gland does not take up isotope bu the nodule takes it up, which is a feature of **auto nomous solitary toxic nodule**. Here, the norma thyroid tissue is suppressed. Localisation of ove activity in a nodule with suppression of remainde of the gland is characteristic of solitary toxic nodul In toxic MNG, multiple areas show overactivity.
- ***Warm nodule:*** The entire gland takes up isotope. Thi is typical of Graves' disease (primary thyrotoxicosis wherein each cell is active and equally stimulatec
- ***Cold nodule*** is a nodule which does not take u isotope. It should be remembered that only 10% c the cold nodules are malignant. Keeping this i mind, surgeons do not investigate MNG wit isotope scan. The assessment of malignancy is don clinically (Key Box 37.31).

Key Box 37.31

Cold Nodule—Differential Diagnosis

1. Haemorrhage
2. Carcinoma
3. Thyroiditis
4. Thyroid cyst

Please read the clinical notes of a case of thyroid swelling

Clinical Notes

Case of Thyroid Swelling

A 31-year-old female with solitary nodule (2 cm) underwent FNAC—reported as adenoma. She underwent hemithyroidectomy in a peripheral hospital which was reported as papillary carcinoma thyroid (PCT). It was a histological surprise. How to proceed now?

- At our hospital, ultrasound neck was done again which could not reveal any abnormality. She underwent completion thyroidectomy (of the opposite lobe) after 4 weeks (re-exploration is done within 7 days or after 4 weeks once tissue oedema subsides completely). Thus, the patient underwent total thyroidectomy. HPR of opposite lobe did not show papillary carcinoma. No lymph node dissection was done. The patient was not given T4 for 4 weeks.
- After 6 weeks, ^{131}I scan was done giving 1 mCi, residual thyroid tissue was found in neck. It was ablated with 100 mCi of ^{131}I.

Section II • General Surgery

- ☞ Even though the aim of surgery is to remove the entire thyroid gland (total thyroidectomy), some parts of gland might have been left behind by the surgeon, specially in the region of ligament of Berry. Hence, a routine postoperative radionuclide scan is advisable.
- ☞ After ablation, she was put on T_4 0.3 mg/day to be taken in the morning on an empty stomach.
- ☞ She came after 6 months with pain in the neck for which ultrasound was done. It revealed suspicious residual thyroid tissue.

What to do now?

- ☞ Serum thyroglobulin was estimated. It was <0.2 (almost undetectable limits; Normal 0.2–55). So, the suspicious lesion could have been some fibrous tissue due to surgery. As thyroglobulin was normal, we did not investigate her further.
- ☞ Now it is 3 years since completion of thyroidectomy and the patient has no disease but is on T_4 0.3 mg/day.

What are the annual tests to be done?

- ☞ Serum TSH, calcium, thyroglobulin, ultrasound, thyroglobulin antibody and, if necessary, nuclear scan of neck.

COMMENTS

I have heard in a few surgical meetings, the following statement made by a surgeon, 'I have done total thyroidectomy, how can residual thyroid tissue be present in the neck?' Remember, it is always possible that some thyroid tissue is left behind especially in the region of ligament of Berry, tracheoesophageal groove and posteromedially.

Treatment

The final decision about treatment of solitary nodule depends upon the clinical findings, sonography findings and FNA cytology results. Depends upon Bathesda criteria, decision is taken. A few examples of treatment when diagnosis is established are given below:

- Papillary carcinoma: Total thyroidectomy
- Follicular neoplasm: Bethesda 3 or 4 : Lobectomy 5 or 6 : total thyroidectomy
- Medullary carcinoma: Total thyroidectomy with the modified radical neck dissection
- Adenoma: Lobectomy (hemithyroidectomy)
- Toxic nodule in young: Lobectomy
- Toxic nodule in elderly: Lobectomy or ^{131}I ablation
- Simple cyst: If it resolves after aspiration, wait and watch. If it recurs, do a lobectomy
- Refer to Key Box 37.32, 37.33 and Fig. 37.54.

Key Box 37.32

'Most Common' for Solitary Nodule Thyroid

- Most common surgical disease of thyroid gland is solitary nodule.
- Most of the thyroid diseases begin as solitary nodule.
- Most common investigation of choice for solitary nodule is ultrasonography.
- Most common cause of a solitary nodule is multinodular goitre.
- Most common cause for solid solitary nodule in a male is malignancy.
- Most commonly used investigation of choice for tissue diagnosis is FNAC.

Key Box 37.33

What should not be Done in a Nodule

- Nodule should never be enucleated.
- Male solitary solid nodule should never be left alone for observation.
- Suppression therapy should never be attempted for a solitary nodule without a definitive diagnosis.
- Radioablation/suppression therapy should never be given to a nodule causing compression on the trachea.
- FNAC should not generally be done to a nodule, if it is a post-irradiated gland or there is familial thyroid cancer.

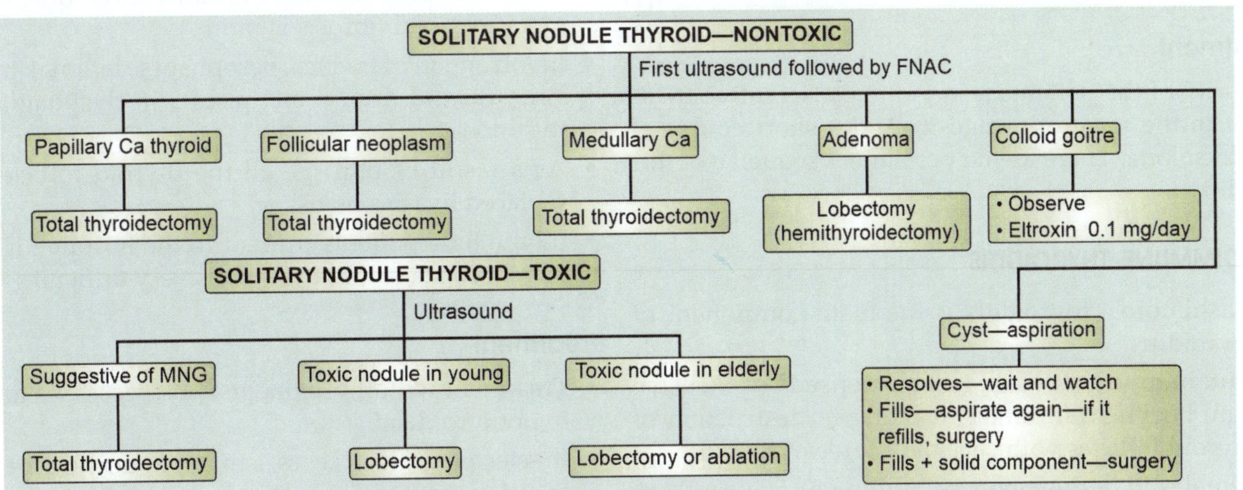

Fig. 37.54: Algorithm of treatment plan in solitary thyroid nodule

THYROID INCIDENTALOMA

- As the name suggests, these are incidentally detected during head and neck ultrasonography done for some other problems. In western countries with increasing obesity, and short neck, it is not surprising to see many such cases of incidentaloma detected by ultrasound.
- In such situations, the management is similar to that of a solitary nodule.
- Any lesion more than 1 cm and lesion which is solid should be subjected to sonography-guided FNA.
- Depending on the results of the FNA, treatment is recommended.
- If it is <1 cm, just follow-up with annual sonogram.

THYROIDITIS

- Viral and autoimmune thyroiditis are more common in the thyroid gland infection of thyroid is very rare because of its rich blood supply.
- Thyroiditis is broadly classified into granulomatous, autoimmune and Riedel's thyroiditis (Table 37.9).

GRANULOMATOUS THYROIDITIS

- It is also called subacute thyroiditis or de Quervain's disease.
- This occurs due to viral infection. It usually follows sore throat (mumps virus has been incriminated in a few cases).
- Patients present with fever, body ache and painful enlargement of thyroid gland. The gland is enlarged, tender to touch, soft to firm and a few symptoms of hyperthyroidism occur initially.
- ESR is increased.

Treatment

Majority of the patients respond to conservative treatment in the form of analgesics and a short course of prednisolone. There are no permanent sequelae of this condition.

AUTOIMMUNE THYROIDITIS

- Hashimoto's thyroiditis is the main component of thyroiditis.
- Autoimmune aetiology is characterised by extensive lymphocytic infiltration resulting in destruction of thyroid follicles with variable degree of fibrosis.
- Females in perimenopausal group (40–50 years) are commonly affected. Initially, symptoms of mild hyperthyroidism (Hashitoxicosis) may be present. Later, extensive intrathyroidal fibrosis results in permanent hypothyroidism. Transient hyperthyroidism is due to destruction of cells resulting in thyrotoxicosis.
- The thyroid follicles are destroyed by significant fibrosis. The deep eosinophilic-staining thyroid follicular cell, Askanazy cell, is characteristic of Hashimoto's thyroiditis.
- The gland can be firm to hard and sometimes rubbery in consistency, smooth or irregular and can involve a lobe or the entire gland.
- In many cases, thyroid antibodies are raised, suggesting an autoimmune disorder.

Treatment

- Thyroxine 0.2 mg/day is given as a supplementary dose.
- If there is compression on the trachea, isthmusectomy is done to relieve compression.
- If the goitre is big and causing discomfort, subtotal thyroidectomy can also be done.

COMPLICATIONS OF HASHIMOTO'S THYROIDITIS

- Permanent hypothyroidism
- Papillary carcinoma of the thyroid
- Lymphoma

RIEDEL'S THYROIDITIS

- This is a very very rare cause of a goitre which is supposed to be a collagen disorder.
- It can be associated with **mediastinal fibrosis, retroperitoneal fibrosis and sclerosing cholangitis**.
- In this condition, there is intrathyroidal fibrosis but extrathyroidal fibrosis is more.
- Involvement of trachea, oesophagus, internal jugular vein, carotid artery, etc. results in dysphagia and dyspnoea.
- As a result of fibrosis, all the thyroid follicles are replaced by fibrous tissue.
- By the time patients present to the hospital, it is an advanced stage and excision is very difficult.

Treatment

- Treatment with thyroxine may be necessary to treat hypothyroidism.
- In selected difficult cases, isthmusectomy can be tried to relieve compression on the trachea. Three types of thyroiditis are compared in Table 37.9.

Table 37.9 Comparison of three forms of thyroiditis

	Granulomatous	Hashimoto's	Riedel's
1. Aetiology	Virus	Autoimmune	Collagen disorder
2. Age group	Young	Woman at menopause	Old age
3. Pathology	Inflammatory cells	Lymphocytes, fibrosis	Extensive fibrous tissue
4. Clinical	Painful, tender, smooth, sudden goitre	Irregular or nodular, firm nontender	Hard, irregular, fixed, nontender
5. Toxicity	Initial toxicity, later normal	Initial toxicity, later hypothyroidism	Hypothyroidism
6. Laboratory tests	ESR is increased	Antithyroid antibodies	No biochemical test
7. Treatment	Symptomatic	Thyroxine, surgery	Thyroxine, surgery
8. Differential diagnosis	Acute bacterial thyroiditis	Multinodular goitre	Anaplastic carcinoma

COMPLICATIONS OF THYROIDECTOMY

1. **Haemorrhage** can be a primary haemorrhage which occurs during surgery.
   - Reactionary haemorrhage is more dangerous and occurs within 6–8 hours after surgery. This is due to slipping of ligature because of straining, coughing, hypertension, etc.
   - It is a tension haematoma which develops deep to deep fascia, compressing the larynx. Reexploration of neck under GA, control of bleeding points and evacuation of haematoma should be done immediately.
   - Without evacuating haematoma, an attempt to intubate the patient may result in cardiac arrest (as such patient will be struggling).
2. **Respiratory obstruction** can be due to tension haematoma resulting in compression of the larynx, collapse, tracheal cartilage softening (tracheomalacia).
   - Endotracheal intubation and a short course of steroid therapy is necessary.
3. **Laryngeal nerve paralysis** (Tables 37.10 and 37.11).
   A. ***Unilateral recurrent laryngeal nerve (RLN) palsy*** produces a whispering voice. The opposite vocal cord compensates. There will not be problems of aspiration or airway obstruction (Fig. 37.55A).
   B. ***Bilateral recurrent laryngeal nerve palsy:*** It is also known as bilateral abductor paralysis. Both the vocal cords come to be in median or paramedian position (Table 37.10), the airway is inadequate causing dyspnoea and stridor but the voice is good (Fig. 37.55B).

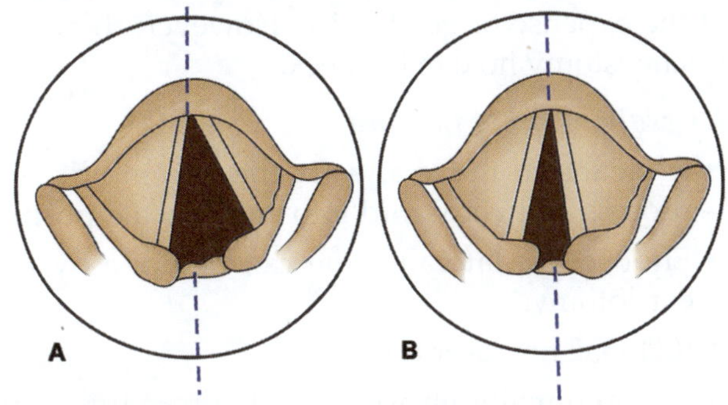

Figs 37.55A and B: Vocal cord position in unilateral and bilateral recurrent laryngeal nerve paralysis

Table 37.10 Various positions of vocal cord in laryngeal nerve paralysis (Fig. 37.56)

Position	Inference	Distance from the midline
1. Median	Seen in phonation	Nil
2. Paramedian	Bilateral RLN palsy	Distance: 1–2 mm
3. Intermediate (cadaveric)	Bilateral, combined paralysis of RLN and superior laryngeal nerve	Distance: 3–4 mm
4. Full abduction	Forceful inspiration	Distance: 8–9 mm

Fig. 37.56

Table 37.11 Causes of recurrent laryngeal nerve paralysis

Left RLN lesions	Right RLN lesions
• Ca bronchus	• Ca apex of the lung
• Ca oesophagus	• Ca oesophagus
• Ca thyroid	• Ca thyroid
• Operative injury	• Operative injury
• Peripheral neuritis	• Peripheral neuritis
• Aortic aneurysm	• Subclavian aneurysm
• Mediastinal mass	
• Left atrial enlargement	

Treatment: Tracheostomy is required as an emergency procedure. Following tracheostomy, the patient is followed up on an outpatient basis for a period of 8–9 months. This period is required for any spontaneous recovery. If no recovery occurs after this period, it requires a permanent solution. The choice is between a permanent tracheostomy with a speaking valve or a surgical procedure to lateralise the cord which can be done by endoscopic method. The former relieves stridor and preserves good voice but has the disadvantage of a tracheostomy hole in the neck. The latter relieves airway obstruction but at the expense of good voice. However, there is no tracheostomy hole in the neck.

Lateralisation of the cord

- It means to move and fix the arytenoid, vocal process and vocal cord into an abducted position.
- Endoscopic lateralisation can be done by laser cordotomy.
- KTP-532 nm laser is used.
- It is minimally invasive, single procedure, quick recovery.

C. ***Superior laryngeal nerve (SLN):*** It is a branch of vagus, gives a 'motor' branch—external laryngeal nerve. Dissection and retraction of the upper pole of the right thyroid lobe to reveal the external branch of the superior laryngeal nerve in **the cricothyroid space of Reeves**. This nerve supplies cricothyroid which is adductor of the cord. Paralysis causes weak and husky voice and inability to raise the pitch of voice. **This is of particular importance in singers. Amelita Galli Curci, an Italian opera singer lost her voice following thyroidectomy due to damage to SLN.**

- Large internal laryngeal nerve supplies whole supraglottic larynx—sensory innervation to the epiglottis, pyriform sinus and larynx as far down as vocal folds.

D. ***Combined (complete paralysis):***

- ***Unilateral:*** This results in paralysis of all muscles of larynx on one side. Vocal cord will be in cadaveric position. The healthy cord is unable to approximate the paralysed cord, thus causing glottic incompetence. This results in hoarseness of voice and aspiration of liquids through glottis. Cough is ineffective due to air wastage.

  Treatment includes procedures to medialise the cord and speech therapy.
- ***Bilateral:*** This is an uncommon condition. This results in paralysis of all the intrinsic muscles of the larynx. Both vocal cords assume cadaveric position. There is also a total anaesthesia of larynx.

Pearls of Wisdom

It is better to identify RLN in all cases of thyroidectomy—specially total thyroidectomy and lobectomy.

4. **Permanent hypothyroidism** can develop slowly after thyroid surgery especially after subtotal thyroidectomy for Graves' disease. It takes 2–3 years for manifestation of hypothyroidism to become apparent.
5. **Permanent hypoparathyroidism** is managed with calcium tablets or with 1, 25-dihydroxy cholecalciferol.
6. **Thyrotoxic crisis (storm)**
   - Thyrotoxic storm occurs in patients with primary thyrotoxicosis who are improperly treated or prepared for surgery. At surgery, due to handling of the gland, sudden release of thyroxine into the systemic circulation results in thyrotoxic crisis (Key Box 37.34).
   - Hyperpyrexia—above 105°F, severe sweating, gross dehydration, hypovolaemic shock and tachycardia are the diagnostic features.
   - It is treated by following measures:
     - ICU admission and resuscitation: O_2, correction of dehydration by rapid IV fluids.
     - Cold tepid sponging, to control the temperature.
     - IV and oral propranolol 2–4 mg and as necessary.

Key Box 37.34

Thyrotoxic Storm Prevention

- Euthyroid before surgery
- β-blockers, carbimazole
- Lugol's iodine
- Good anaesthesia
- Perfect haemostasis
- Gentle manipulation

- Hydrocortisone 100 mg, thrice daily.
- Carbimazole or propyl thiouracil
- In spite of the above treatment, mortality is high.

What is Wolff-Chaikoff effect?

- On ingestion of a large amount of iodine, there will be reduction of thyroid hormones.
- It is an autoregulatory mechanism which inhibits organification in the thyroid gland.
- This principle is used to treat hyperthyroidism (especially thyroid storm by infusion of iodine—large quantities).

Pearls of Wisdom

Prevention is better than 'cure'. With adequate preparation, thyrotoxic storm can be prevented.

7. **Wound infection:** It is not common to get wound infection after thyroid surgery. However, antibiotics are started, if there is evidence of local erythema, tenderness and if the patient has fever.
8. Scar hypertrophy and keloid.
9. **Stitch granuloma:** May occur with/without sinus formation and is seen after the use of nonabsorbable suture material. Absorbable ligatures and sutures (vicryl) can be used throughout thyroid surgery except for skin closure where silk is still appropriate.

MISCELLANEOUS

LINGUAL THYROID

- Occasionally, a patient presents with a small swelling in the middle of the tongue at the junction of anterior 2/3rd and posterior 1/3rd of the tongue.
- It could be lingual thyroid—an aberrant thyroid tissue found in the region of foramen caecum on the tongue.
- Foramen caecum represents the junction of epithelial floor of the mouth with proximal portion of thyroglossal duct.
- Even though lingual thyroid is rare, it can give rise to significant complications (Fig. 37.57).

Clinical Features

- Common in females (3:1)
- Swelling in the tongue in the classical location, firm in consistency, can be irregular. Impairment of speech, haemorrhage, dysphagia, airway obstruction may be the presenting features.
- Majority of patients have hypothyroidism (70%) and 10% are cretins.

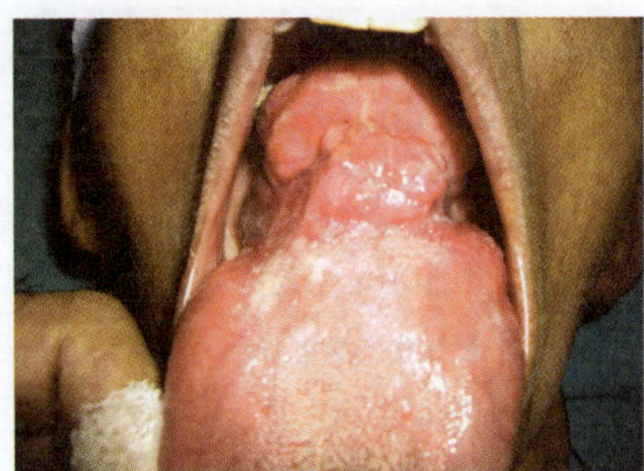

Fig. 37.57: Four centimetre lingual thyroid in the classical location causing dysphagia—successfully removed with LASER

Diagnosis

- Usually made on clinical grounds.
- Thyroid scan—ultrasound of neck is done to find out whether thyroid tissue is present or not (often it is absent).
- ^{99m}Tc (technetium) scan will detect ectopic thyroid tissue (Fig. 37.58).

Differential Diagnosis

1. **Ectopic salivary gland tumour:** Tongue is the commonest site. To begin with, mucosa is normal, starts as a submucosal swelling.
2. **Gumma:** Rare nowadays. It is a midline, indurated, firm, smooth swelling, painless.
3. **Lymphangioma and haemangioma:** These are present since birth, more diffuse, fluctuant cystic swellings. Haemangioma is compressible and lymphangioma is transilluminant.

Treatment

- Small dose of thyroxine may decrease the size of the swelling (similar to a puberty goitre) as a treatment of hypothyroidism or to suppress TSH
- Large swelling with significant symptoms needs to be excised. Laser excision is better.
- Radioactive iodine to suppress/destroy can be given.

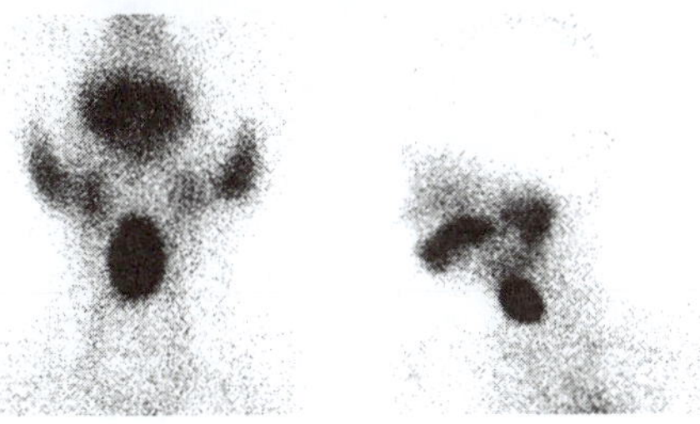

Fig. 37.58: ^{99m}Tc (Technetium) scan showing lingual thyroid

Pearls of Wisdom

Lingual thyroid may be the only thyroid tissue present in a patient. Hence, a thyroid scan is done to confirm the presence of normal thyroid tissue.

ECTOPIC THYROID

- It occurs due to failure of median thyroid anlage to descend normally. Hence, thyroid tissue can be found anywhere from the tongue to mediastinum (Key Box 37.35 and Figs 37.59 and 37.60).
- Ectopic thyroid tissue can have the diseases similar to normal thyroid tissue, such as solitary nodule, multinodular goitre, malignancies, etc.

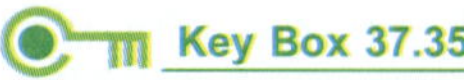

Key Box 37.35

Ectopic Thyroid Tissue

- Lingual thyroid
- Thyroglossal ectopic thyroid in the upper part of the neck
- Adjacent to aortic arch, aortopulmonary window, within upper pericardium, etc.
- Struma ovarii—malignant ovarian teratoma containing thyroid tissue.

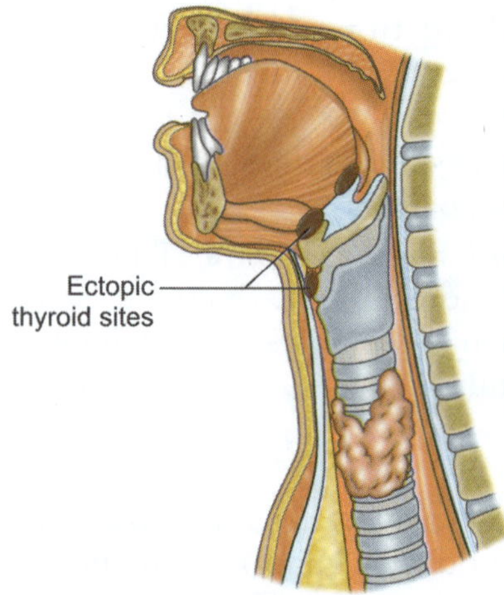

Fig. 37.59: Ectopic thyroid sites

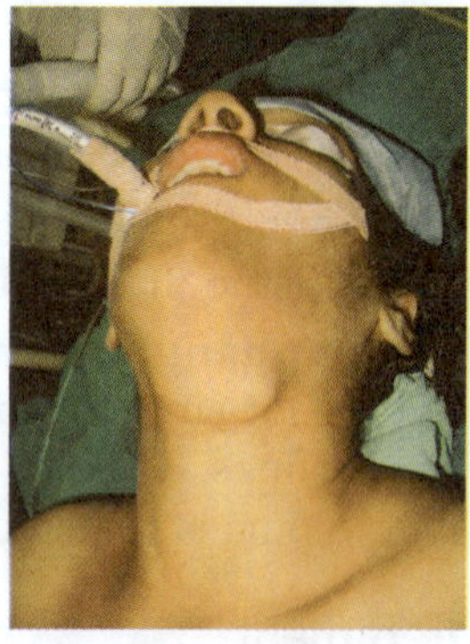

Fig. 37.60: Ectopic thyroid tissue in the submandibular region turned out to be papillary carcinoma thyroid

- Diagnosis is by ultrasound, CT scan. FNAC to confirm the diagnosis.
- Treatment depends upon the pathology.

INTERESTING 'MOST COMMON' FOR THYROID GLAND

- Most common surgical disease of the thyroid gland is solitary thyroid nodule.
- Most common site of thyroid nodule is at the junction of isthmus and lobe.
- Most commonly used drug for thyrotoxicosis is carbimazole.
- Most commonly used investigation for thyroid diseases is ultrasonogram.
- Most commonly done surgery for well-differentiated carcinoma thyroid is total thyroidectomy.
- Most common thyroid cancer in children is papillary carcinoma thyroid.
- Most common thyroid cancer following exposure to ionising radiation is papillary carcinoma thyroid.
- Most common solitary nodule of thyroid gland is multinodular goitre.

MOST DIAGNOSTIC FEATURES IN THYROID GLAND

- Most diagnostic feature of medullary carcinoma thyroid is amyloid stroma.
- Most diagnostic feature of papillary carcinoma thyroid is presence of psammoma bodies.
- Most diagnostic feature of Hashimoto's thyroiditis is Askanazy cell.
- Most diagnostic investigation for lingual thyroid is ^{99m}Tc (technetium) scan.
- Most diagnostic feature of anaplastic carcinoma is early fixity
- Most diagnostic feature of Graves' disease is exophthalmos

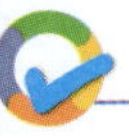

Multiple Choice Questions

1. **Superior thyroid artery is a branch of:**
   A. Common carotid artery
   B. Internal carotid artery
   C. External carotid artery
   D. Thyrocervical trunk

2. **Following are true for T3 hormone *except:***
   A. It is more important physiologic hormone
   B. It can be produced by peripheral conversion of T4
   C. It is more quickly acting
   D. It is given once a day for suppressive dose

3. **Following are true for primary thyrotoxicosis *except:***
   A. 8 times more common in women than men
   B. Gland is vascular and smooth
   C. Cardiac failure is common
   D. Proptosis is a feature

4. **Replacement dose of thyroxin—T4 is:**
   A. 0.1 mg B. 0.2 mg
   C. 0.3 mg D. 0.01 mg

5. **Papillary carcinoma thyroid spreads to which lymph nodes?**
   A. Submental
   B. Submandibular lymph nodes
   C. Scalene nodes
   D. Jugular chain of lymph nodes

6. **Following is not the common sign of Graves' disease:**
   A. Proptosis
   B. Pretibial myxoedema
   C. Proximal myopathy
   D. Cardiac failure

7. **The widely used first investigation of choice in solitary nodule thyroid is:**
   A. X-ray neck B. CT scan
   C. MRI D. Ultrasound

8. **Which one of the following is not the treatment for Graves' disease?**
   A. Carbimazole
   B. Propranolol
   C. Massive doses of steroids in ophthalmopathy
   D. Digoxin

9. **Following are true for treatment options for toxic goitre *except:***
   A. Thyroidectomy
   B. Antithyroid drugs
   C. Radioiodine treatment
   D. Radiotherapy

10. **Which one of the following is the treatment of choice for toxic goitre in a child?**
    A. Radioiodine
    B. Thyroidectomy
    C. Antithyroid drugs
    D. Radiotherapy

11. **Which is the most effective drug for thyrotoxic storm?**
    A. Steroids B. Noradrenaline
    C. IV propranolol D. Carbimazole

12. **Which one of these operative steps is not done routinely in thyroidectomy?**
    A. Ligation of middle thyroid vein
    B. Ligation of superior thyroid artery
    C. Ligation of inferior thyroid artery
    D. Ligation of inferior thyroid veins

13. **A few landmarks for identification of recurrent laryngeal nerve include following *except:***
    A. Parallel to tracheo-oesophageal groove on the left side
    B. Below the inferior thyroid artery on the right side
    C. Between branches of the inferior thyroid artery
    D. Between the branches of inferior thyroid veins

14. **Following are true for external branch of superior laryngeal nerve *except:***
    A. It is close to superior thyroid artery
    B. Paralysis of this nerve leads to loss of tension in the vocal cord
    C. Paralysis of this nerve diminishes power and range in the voice
    D. It supplies adductors of the vocal cord

15. **Following are true for papillary carcinoma thyroid *except:***
    A. Childhood irradiation is an important cause
    B. Orphan Annie-eyed nuclei is characteristic
    C. Multiple foci are common in the same lobe
    D. It spreads predominantly by blood spread

16. Single most important aetiological factor in papillary carcinoma is:

A. Endemic goitre
B. Childhood irradiation
C. Autoimmune thyroiditis
D. Multiple endocrine neoplasia syndromes

17. Following are the important steps of surgery for well-differentiated thyroid cancers of more than 2 cm in size *except:*

A. Lobectomy
B. Total thyroidectomy
C. Selective neck dissection
D. Removal of all macroscopic diseases

18. Following are true after total thyroidectomy before radioiodine scan *except*:

A. If T_3 is given, only one week of stopping of hormone is enough
B. Otherwise minimum 4 weeks stoppage of T4 is required
C. Alternative to thyroxine withdrawal is to administer synthetic TSH over 48 hours
D. TSH administration is not at all effective

19. Following are true about thyroglobulin *except*:

A. Normal levels are not detectable
B. Increasing levels indicate metastasis in papillary carcinoma thyroid
C. Increasing thyroglobulin prompts surgeon to get ultrasound of the neck
D. Useful in medullary carcinoma thyroid

20. Following are true for medullary carcinoma thyroid *except:*

A. Calcitonin is the tumour marker
B. It arises from parafollicular cells
C. It has amyloid stroma
D. It can be treated by lobectomy

21. Following is an indication for core needle biopsy of thyroid swellings:

A. Lymphoma
B. Papillary carcinoma thyroid
C. Follicular carcinoma thyroid
D. Medullary carcinoma thyroid

22. Following are pathological features of papillary carcinoma *except:*

A. Microcarcinoma
B. Orphan Annie-eyed nuclei
C. Tall cell cancer
D. Hürthle cell cancer

23. Following are true for medullary carcinoma thyroid *except:*

A. It arises from parafollicular cells
B. Cells are like carcinoid tumour
C. Does not spread by lymphatics
D. Tumours are not TSH dependent

24. Follicular carcinoma thyroid is diagnosed by:

A. Orphan Annie-eyed nuclei
B. Askanazy cell
C. Angioinvasion and capsular invasion
D. Amyloid stroma

25. Non-operative treatment can be offered in a solitary nodule *except:*

A. Cyst less than 1 cm size
B. Colloid goitre less than 1 cm in size
C. Retrosternal goitre
D. Hashimoto's thyroiditis

26. Parafollicular cells are located in which part of thyroid gland?

A. Upper pole
B. Lower pole
C. Isthmus
D. Organ of Zuckerkandl

27. About recurrent laryngeal nerve (RLN) following are true *except:*

A. RLN crosses medial to inferior thyroid artery
B. Superior parathyroid is posterior to RLN
C. Inferior parathyroid is 1 cm away from RLN
D. RLN passes immediately medial to tubercle of Zuckerkandl.

Answers

1. C	**2.** D	**3.** C	**4.** A	**5.** D	**6.** D	**7.** D	**8.** D	**9.** D	**10.** C
11. C	**12.** C	**13.** D	**14.** D	**15.** D	**16.** B	**17.** A	**18.** D	**19.** D	**20.** D
21. A	**22.** D	**23.** C	**24.** C	**25.** C	**26.** A	**27.** C			

CHAPTER

38

Parathyroid and Adrenals

- Surgical anatomy
- Congenital anomaly
- Physiology—calcium and action of PTH and calcitonin
- Tetany
- Hyperparathyroidism
- Cryopreservation
- Acute hypercalcaemic crisis
- Adrenal glands—anatomy, physiology
- Disorders of adrenal cortex
- Neuroblastoma
- Phaeochromocytoma
- Incidentalomas

Competency

SU22.5: Describe the applied anatomy of parathyroid.

PARATHYROID GLANDS

SURGICAL ANATOMY

- These are the endocrinal glands situated in the neck and secrete the hormone parathormone (PTH). Their secretion is **not dependent on pituitary gland.**
- They are 4 in number; 2 on the right and 2 on the left.
- **Superior parathyroids** are *derived* from endoderm of **4th branchial arch** and thus, they develop along with the thyroid gland. Superior parathyroids are found in relation to inferior thyroid artery in the middle of posterior aspect of thyroid gland. They are situated in the fat above inferior thyroid artery, close to cricothyroid artery and cricothyroid articulation. They are constant in position. They are smaller (30–40 mg). They are **dorsal to recurrent laryngeal nerve** (RLN).
- **Inferior parathyroids** develop from endoderm of **3rd branchial arch** (with thymus) and are not constant in position. They may be seen in the lower pole, within fascial sheath of thyroid gland, low down in the neck (rarely in the mediastinum), outside the fascial sheath or even within thyroid gland. They are large (30 to 50 mg). They are **ventral to RLN** (Fig. 38.1).

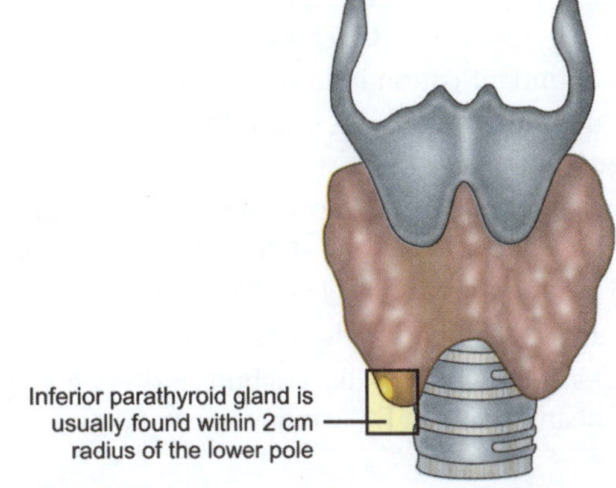

Fig. 38.1: Location of inferior parathyroid gland

- Parathyroids appear golden-yellow to light brown in adults. In children, they are pinkish in colour.

Blood Supply

Inferior thyroid artery supplies both the parathyroids in about 95% of cases by a leash of vessels. Ligature of both inferior thyroid arteries **may not result in hypoparathyroidism** because there is adequate collateral circulation and a few branches of superior thyroid artery also supply 20% of upper glands.

Histology

Principal cells (chief cells) are the cells which secrete PTH (parathormone). Water clear cells (rich in glycogen) are found in hyperplastic and neoplastic glands.

CONGENITAL ANOMALY AND SYNDROME

DiGeorge syndrome: Congenital absence of the parathyroid glands and thymus. Neonatal hypoparathyroidism along with absence of thymus-dependent lymphoid system.

PHYSIOLOGY—CALCIUM AND ACTION OF PTH AND CALCITONIN

PTH is a peptide containing 84 amino acids. It is secreted in response to increase in calcium or decrease in magnesium. Actions of PTH are:

1. Resorption and mobilisation of calcium from the bone (Key Box 38.1).
2. Increased reabsorption of calcium from kidney prompting excretion of phosphate.
3. Enhances absorption of calcium from the gut.
   - Thus, PTH increases serum calcium level.
   - Normal serum calcium level 9–11 mg/dl (total).
   - In normal persons, the PTH is balanced by calcitonin, secreted from *C cells* of the thyroid glands.

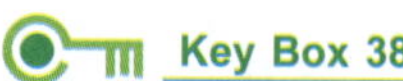

Key Box 38.1

Calcium

- Most abundant cation in human beings
- 50% of calcium is in the ionised form, which can be measured
- 50% of calcium is bound to albumin. Hence, total calcium levels will be low when albumin levels are low
- Total calcium levels: 9–11 mg/dl
- Calcium is absorbed in the small intestines
- Sources of calcium: Milk, yoghurt and cheese, green peas, beans, oranges. Daily requirement: 1000–1300 mg/day
- Calcium is an important ion for blood coagulation, cellular activity, bone density and neuromuscular activity

CALCITONIN

- It is released from 'C' cells—parafollicular cells of the thyroid gland.
- Normal values are unmeasurable less than 10 pg/ml.
- It reduces calcium levels by inhibiting activity of osteoclasts. Thus its action is opposite that of PTH.
- It also increases excretion of calcium in the urine.

Competency

SU22.6: Describe and discuss the clinical features of hypo- and hyperparathyroidism and the principles of their management.

TETANY

Tetany is a condition wherein there is hyperexcitability of peripheral nerves.

Causes of Tetany

1. **Hypoparathyroidism:** It results from surgical removal of parathyroids. Subtotal thyroidectomy and near-total thyroidectomy are the most common causes of tetany. Hypoparathyroidism may be 'familial' variety or neonatal variety. It may be temporary after thyroidectomy or permanent, if all the 4 parathyroids are removed or deprived of their blood supply. The incidence is around 1–2%.
2. **Severe respiratory alkalosis** can cause tetany as in ***hyperventilation.***
3. Low calcium levels can occur due to dietary factors or poor absorption from the gut or ***acute pancreatitis, chronic renal failure,*** etc.
4. **Osteomalacia** and **rickets** due to deficiency of ***vitamin D.***
5. **Hypokalaemic alkalosis** of pyloric stenosis.
6. Following massive transfusion (citrate overload).

Signs and Symptoms (Key Box 38.2)

Key Box 38.2

Tetany—Clinical Features

- Creaking or grating sound (stridor)
- Circumoral pallor
- Carpopedal spasm—Trousseau's sign
- Chovstek's sign
- Clonic seizure
- Convulsions (rare)

Observe 6 'Cs'

1. Tingling and numbness of the fingers, toes, lips (circumoral paraesthesia) and occasionally, with circumoral pallor.
2. Cramps of the hands and feet.
3. In severe hypocalcaemia, there may be ***carpopedal spasm.*** **Metacarpophalangeal (MP)** joints are flexed, **interphalangeal joints** are extended and the thumb is adducted. This is called *thumb in palm deformity* **(obstetrician's hand)**. In the foot, extension in the ankle joints and flexion of the toes are seen (Fig. 38.2).

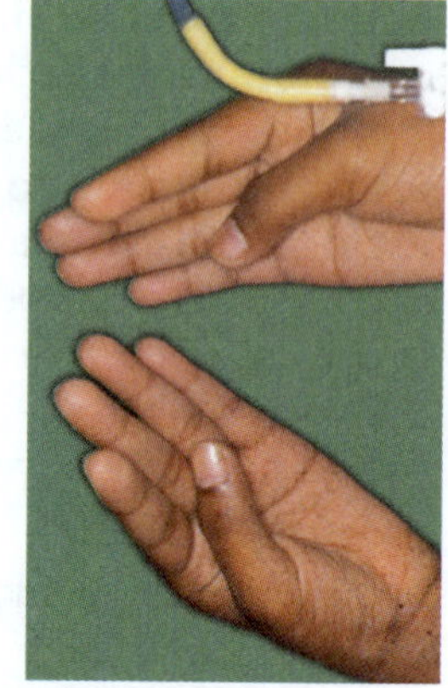

Fig. 38.2: Severe tetany following removal of the parathyroid adenoma requiring calcium infusion

4. **Stridor** is a dangerous complication of severe tetany due to spasm of muscles of respiration.
5. *Latent tetany* can be diagnosed by:
   - Tapping the facial nerve at the angle of jaw. This produces twitching of eyelids, corner of the mouth, etc. It is called **Chvostek's sign**. It indicates facial nerve hyperexcitability.
   - **Trousseau's sign:** When a blood pressure cuff applied to the arm is inflated above the systolic pressure (200 mm of Hg), the hands and feet go into spasm (obstetrician's hand, carpopedal spasm).
6. Spasm of intraocular muscles results in blurring of vision.
7. **Convulsions**, even though rare, can occur in infants.

Diagnosis

This is established by estimating **serum calcium level** which is usually <7 mg%.

Treatment

1. Oral calcium such as calcium lactate, calcium gluconate may relieve mild symptoms.
2. In **acute cases, injection calcium gluconate** 10% (10 ml) should be given *slowly intravenously* over 10 minutes to avoid cardiac arrhythmias.
3. If any precipitating cause is detected, it needs to be corrected.

HYPERPARATHYROIDISM (HPT)

Hyperparathyroidism is an uncommon disease and occurs due to an increased activity of parathyroids and manifests as hypercalcaemia.

Types of Hyperparathyroidism

- **Primary hyperparathyroidism:** It refers to hyperactivity of parathyroids due to an adenoma or primary hyperplasia of parathyroid glands.
- **Secondary hyperparathyroidism:** It occurs due to persistently low levels of calcium as in chronic renal failure and malabsorption, which results in decreased levels of calcium and increased levels of hyperphosphataemia.
- **Tertiary hyperparathyroidism:** This is seen in patients who undergo dialysis and transplantation for chronic renal failure. After a few years of prolonged stimulation, autonomy develops and the secondary hyperparathyroidism changes into tertiary hyperparathyroidism. They can also have problems similar to primary hyperparathyroidism.

PRIMARY HYPERPARATHYROIDISM

Incidence

0.50 to 1 per 1000 population in United States. More common in postmenopausal women.

Aetiology

- Exact cause of primary hyperparathyroidism (PHPT) is unknown.
  1. **Familial/genetic:** Can be a part of MEN syndrome I and MENII A or familial PHPT with jaw tumour syndrome. Both occur due to genetic mutation.

Pearls of Wisdom

Primary HPT is the earliest and most common manifestation of MEN type I and develops in 80–100% of these patients by 40 years of age.

  2. Low dose therapeutic ionising radiation is also one of the causes.
  3. Lithium is associated with parathyroid hyperplasia and primary HPT. Interestingly there is no hypercalciuria and bone mineral density is not affected.
  4. Renal leak of calcium and declining renal function with age may also be causative factors for primary HPT.

Pathology (Key Box 38.3)

- Single chief cell adenoma is the most common cause (80%). It can be due to **diffuse hyperplasia** involving all 4 glands (5–10% of cases).
- Very rarely, it can be due to carcinoma arising in the parathyroid glands (1%).
- Adenoma can be a part of **multiple endocrine neoplasia** (MEN) syndrome.

Clinical Features

- Common in *females:* Female to male ratio is 4:1.
- Age: 30–60 years, the most common age group is 5th decade—middle aged
- Incidence is 1:1000 patients.

Key Box 38.3

Pathology

- Adenoma—reddish brown, only 1 gland is enlarged
- Chief cell hyperplasia—reddish brown, >1 gland is enlarged
- Water cell hyperplasia—chocolate brown, >1 gland is enlarged
- Multiple gland enlargement is a feature of familial disease

- **The most common** presentation is **asymptomatic hypercalcaemia** in about 50% of the patients and **renal stones** in 25% of the patients. The clinical features are as follows.

1. Bone Disease—Painful Bones

Due to increasing levels of PTH, extensive *skeletal* decalcification occurs. This results in bony pains, *pathological fractures* due to brittle bones, *subperiosteal* erosions, cysts in the phalanges, mandible, skull, etc. They are called **pseudotumours**. The changes are similar to that seen in ***osteitis fibrosa cystica*** (von Recklinghausen's disease). Thus, osteopenia, osteoporosis and osteitis fibrosa cystica are found in 15% of PHPT.

2. Renal Disease—Renal Stones

- Increased calcium levels result from increased calcium absorption from the kidneys. Hence, patients are prone to develop **renal stone and nephrocalcinosis** (calcification of kidney), hypertension.
- Calcium also **increases the tone of the vessels** which adds to the hypertension. Primary hyperparathyroidism is the cause of stones in 1–3% of all patients with kidney stones and in 10% of those who have recurrence of stones.
- **Calculi** are specially composed of **calcium phosphate or oxalate.**

3. Abdominal Groans

- Calcium stimulates **gastrin** which is a powerful stimulator of acid. This may result in pain abdomen due to peptic ulcer. The patient can present with dyspeptic symptoms.
- Calcium can cause **pancreatitis**, resulting in pain radiating to the back.
- Metastatic calcification is also a feature.
- Increased incidence of gallstones has been reported as a consequence of increase in secretion of calcium in the bile-calcium bilirubinate stone.
- All these factors result in abdominal pain, which has been called abdominal groans.

4. Psychiatric Moans

- Hypercalcaemia can result in depression, fatigue, anxiety, psychosis and even coma.
- These patients, more often women, mostly middle age, having bony pains, backaches and behavioural abnormalities are thought to have a psychiatric illness. They are referred to mental institutions, orthopaedic department, gynaecology department and are shunted from doctor to doctor.

5. Fatigue Overtones

Many patients present with weakness and fatigue.

Pearls of Wisdom

PHPT is a disease of stones, painful bones, abdominal groans, psychiatric moans and fatigue overtones.

Acute Presentation of Hypercalcaemia

- Abdominal pain
- Oliguria
- Dehydration
- Vomiting
- Coma

Symptoms

• Asymptomatic	50–60% of cases
• Renal stones	25–30%
• Bone disease	8–10%
• Joint pains	3–5%
• Abdominal pain (peptic ulcer)	3–5%
• Hypertension	3–5%

Other Features (Key Box 38.4)

- Corneal calcification/band keratopathy (inside iris) may be seen in the eye on **slit-lamp examination**.
- **Proximal myopathy,** muscle wasting is also seen.
- Interestingly, clinical examination of the neck *may not reveal* any parathyroid enlargement. Hence, the diagnosis should be suspected by the various symptoms. High index of suspicion is necessary in arriving at a proper diagnosis.

Key Box 38.4

Primary Hyperparathyroidism and Calcinosis

- Nephrocalcinosis and renal stones
- Cholelithiasis
- Chondrocalcinosis
- Calcification at ectopic sites such as blood vessels, cardiac valves, skin, etc.—metastatic calcification

Note: Soft tissue calcification and tumoural calcinosis occur in secondary hyperparathyroidism.

Pearls of Wisdom

When a patient develops multiple urinary calculi, reduced bone density, high serum calcium, symptomatic hypercalciuria and pathological fractures, suspect primary HPT and request for PTH assay.

Investigations

Investigations can be classified as follows:

I. **To prove hyperparathyroidism**
- Serum calcium, phosphate, albumin
- **Serum PTH assay**
- Alkaline phosphatase
- X-ray of bones.

II. **To localise parathyroid glands**
- Ultrasound of neck
- Thallium and technetium subtraction scan
- Selective venous sampling with PTH assay. This is most reliable but more difficult.
- Sestamibi scanning.

I. To Prove Hyperparathyroidism

1. Serum **calcium** levels are always raised above normal limits (9–11 mg%). There are many causes of hypercalcaemia which are depicted in Key Box 38.5. Hence, estimation of serum calcium alone will not give the diagnosis.
2. **Albumin is the main calcium binding protein** in the plasma. Hence, it should also be measured.
3. Serum **PTH** level which is estimated by immunoassay is the *diagnostic investigation.* It is called **tumour marker** for hyperparathyroidism. Estimation of PTH is difficult, costly and needs sophisticated set up.
4. Serum **phosphorus** levels are decreased.
5. **Alkaline phosphatase** is increased when bones are involved.

Key Box 38.5

Causes of Hypercalcaemia

Endocrinal	Primary hyperparathyroidism Thyrotoxicosis Phaeochromocytoma
Malignancy	Multiple bone secondaries[1]—(Ca breast, prostate, kidney, follicular carcinoma thyroid) Multiple myeloma, oat cell carcinoma[2]
Renal failure	Secondary and tertiary hyperparathyroidism
Nutritional	Vitamin D intoxication
Chronic disease	Tuberculosis sarcoidosis
Skeletal	Paraplegia, quadriplegia patients also are immobilised—hypercalciuric hypercalcaemia

[1]The common causes are carcinoma breast, prostate, kidney, bronchus, follicular carcinoma of the thyroid.

[2]It produces PTH-like polypeptide (pseudohyperparathyroidism).

6. **X-ray of the hand** may reveal decalcification cysts in the phalanges, telescoping of fingertips, etc. **X-ray of the skull** may reveal subperiosteal erosions, hazy outline of the skull **and pepper pot** appearance (Key Box 38.6) (Figs 38.3 to 38.5).

Key Box 38.6

Interesting Radiological Changes

Osteopenia	Bone density loss in cortical bone—radius
Bone cysts and brown tumours	Aggregation of osteoclasts (osteoclastoma)
Rugger Jersey spine	Generalised loss of bone density
Pepper pot skull	Demineralised bone—mottled appearance
Subperiosteal resorption **(pathognomonic)**	Seen in radial aspect of middle phalanges of 2nd and 3rd fingers, bone cysts and tufting of the distal phalanges

II. To Localise Parathyroid Glands

1. **High frequency ultrasound** of the neck can be very accurate in the hands of an experienced sonologist. It can also detect renal disease, pancreatic disease, etc. It cannot scan behind sternum and cannot pick up lesions less than 0.5 cm. Specially useful in detecting intrathyroidal parathyroid adenoma (sensitivity is about 75%) (Figs 38.6 and 38.7).
2. **Thallium-technetium isotope scan:** First the thyroid is outlined with ^{99m}Tc and then isotope ^{201}TICl (thallium chloride) is administered. This is taken up by both the thyroid and parathyroid. By computer subtraction of the two and enlargement of images, the parathyroid appears as a hot spot.
3. **Technetium 99m (^{99m}Tc)–labelled sestamibi (MIBI) scanning:** MIBI (methyl-isobutyl-isonitrile radionuclide—sestamibi is concentrated in tissues rich in mitochondria)
   - Heart
   - Salivary glands
   - Thyroid glands
   - Parathyroid glands

   This test has proved to be superior to thallium and technetium subtraction scanning.
   - Sestamibi is a protein labelled with technetium 99m that localises diseased gland—most widely used and is an accurate modality.
   - It is **very sensitive to identify adenomas** (90%) than hyperplasia.

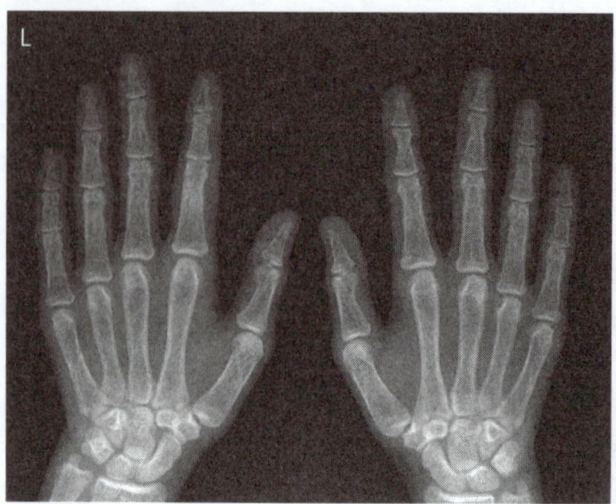

Fig. 38.3: Generalised osteopenia and subperiosteal resorption of the radial aspect of middle phalanx—tunnelling of the cortex (double lines) is seen

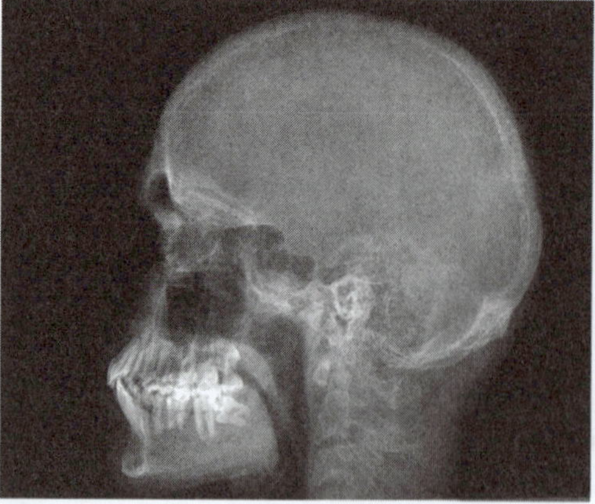

Fig. 38.4: X-ray skull showing multiple lytic sclerotic lesions—pepper pot appearance

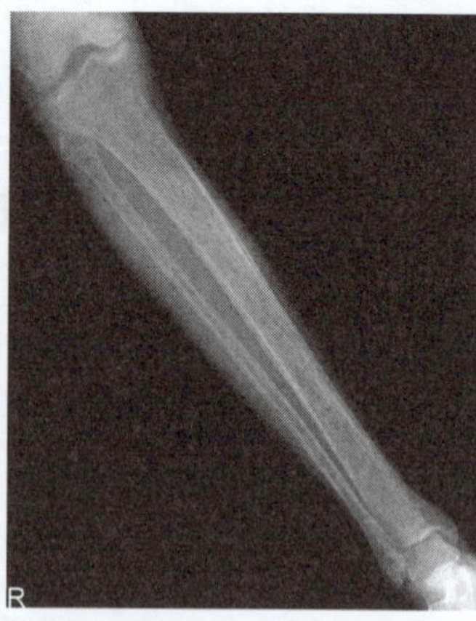

Fig. 38.5: X-ray forearm bones showing osteopenia

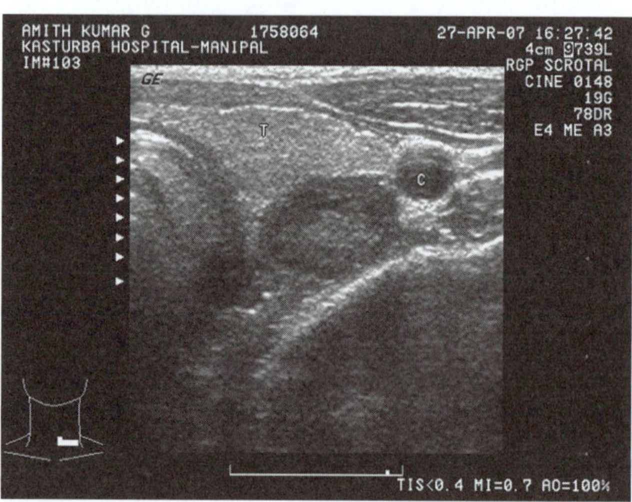

Fig. 38.6: Ultrasonography of the neck reveals heterogeneous nodule predominantly echogenic

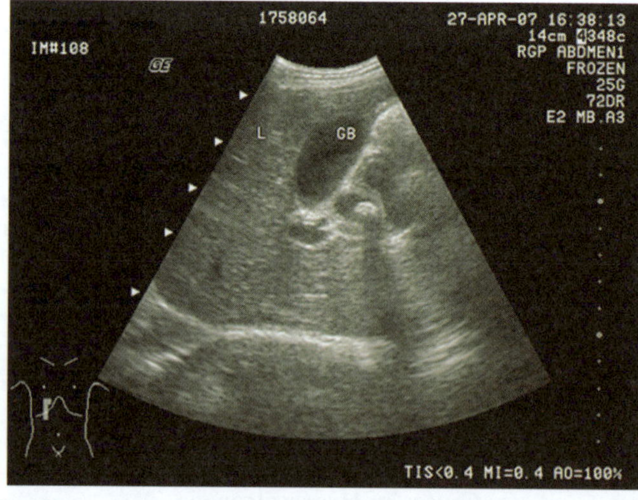

Fig. 38.7: Ultrasonography of the abdomen shows gallstone with posterior acoustic shadow

(*Courtesy:* Figs 38.3 to 38.7 Dr Rajgopal KV, Head, Department of Radiology, KMC Manipal)

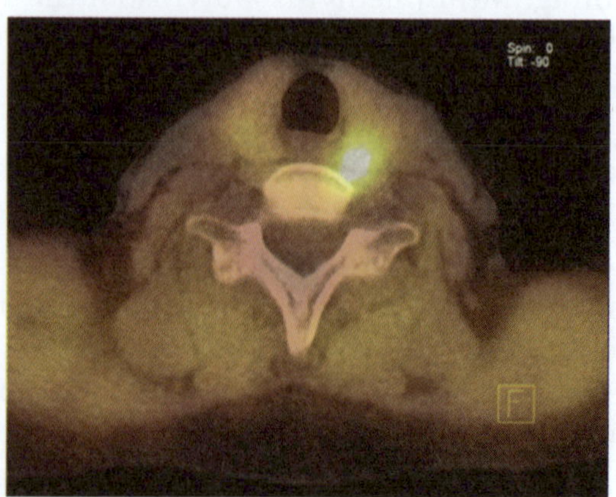

Fig. 38.8: Sestamibi scan shows bright spot—parathyroid adenoma. He also had hypercalcaemia (Key Box 20.10)

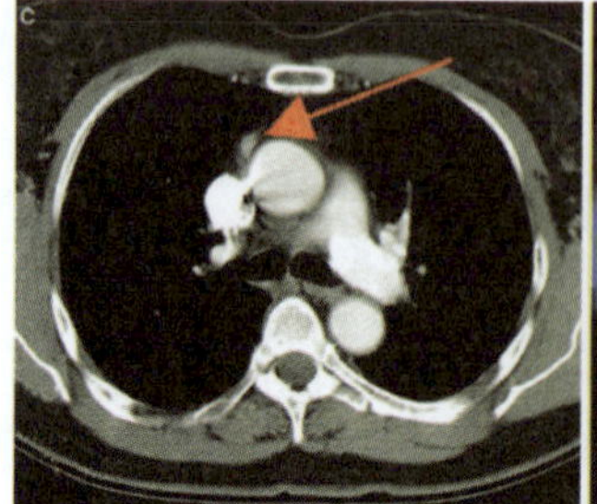

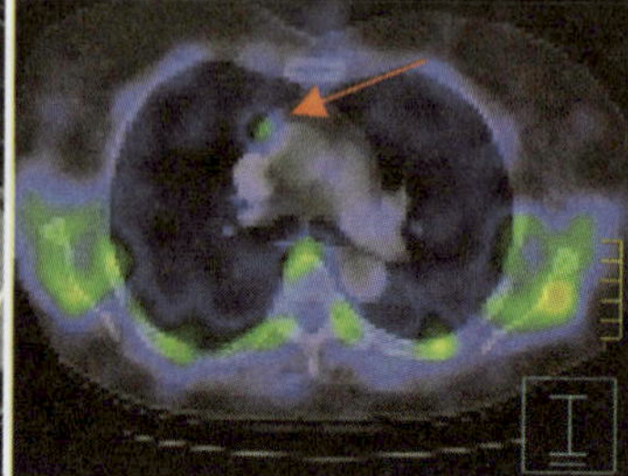

Figs 38.9 and 38.10: Fusion of single-photon emission computed tomography (SPECT) and computed tomography data, shows the site of ectopic parathyroid adenoma

- However, it is very expensive. Hence, it can be used in **'Re-exploration of neck'** for parathyroidectomy.

4. **SPECT: Single Photon Emission Computed Tomography** when used with sestamibi is useful in evaluation of ectopic parathyroid adenomas—deep in the neck or mediastinum (Figs 38.8 to 38.10).

Pearls of Wisdom

CT scan, PET scan and MRI are not indicated prior to first time surgery.

Indications for Surgery

1. Symptomatic hyperparathyroidism
2. Serum calcium greater than 20 mg%
3. Renal stones
4. Hypercalciuria (>400 mg/day)
5. Decreased creatinine clearance by 30%
6. Reduced cortical bone density

Treatment

A. Intraoperative recognition of parathyroid

1. Radioguided parathyroidectomy—it is possible if there is a preoperative MIBI scan.
2. Frozen section has failure rates about 2–3%.
3. Intraoperative tissue aspirate PHT—in primary HPT.
4. Methylene blue is not recommended because of the risk of **toxic encephalopathy.**

B. Surgery: The surgery of the parathyroid glands needs **patience, skill** and **expertise**. The neck is explored with a collar neck incision (3–4 cm) caudal to cricoid cartilage. Parathyroid gland, when it is enlarged can be dark-brown or chocolate brown colour. Occasionally, the surgeon is lucky to encounter a single adenoma usually located on the posterior surface of the thyroid gland, when it arises from superior parathyroid (Key Box 38.7). Very often, identification of the parathyroid may be difficult because they may be intrathyroidal or within the mediastinum (Key Box 38.8).

Key Box 38.7

Identification of Parathyroid at Surgery

- Bloodless field is necessary.
- Ligate middle thyroid vein. Then, retract thyroid gland medially and anteriorly.
- Identify inferior thyroid artery and recurrent laryngeal nerve.
- Parathyroids are covered by fat.
- Incise fat lobule.
- Parathyroid 'pops out'.

Key Box 38.8

When you cannot Identify at Surgery?

- Divide thyrothymic ligament.
- Search in tracheoesophageal groove.
- Call for intraoperative ultrasound to rule out intrathyroidal gland.
- Incise and look inside carotid sheath.
- Remove thymus—send it for frozen section.
- Sometimes parathyroid can be more than 4.
- Do sternotomy—last step.

- **Frozen section** of parathyroid glands is essential to confirm whether it is an adenoma or hyperplasia because treatment depends upon the pathology of the gland (Key Box 38.9).

1. **Single adenoma:** Excision of the gland. **However, one other normal parathyroid gland is also removed for histopathological study** (Fig. 38.11).

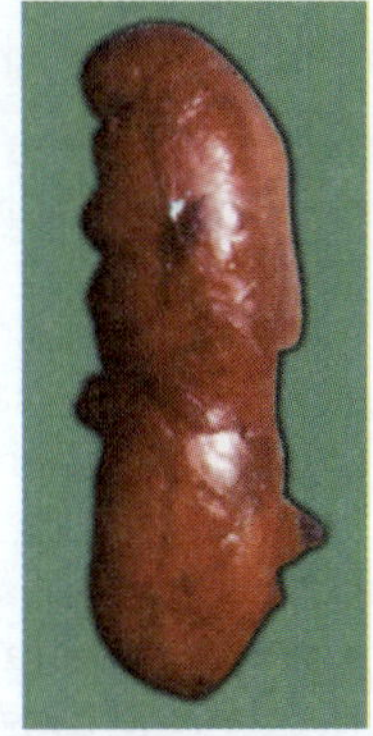

Fig. 38.11: Proved to be adenoma—rest of the glands not enlarged (*Courtesy:* Prof. L Ramachandra, Dr S Prasad, Dr Chethan, Department of Surgery, KMC, Manipal)

Pearls of Wisdom

Single adenoma is more common cause of PHPT in about 80% of patients. Multiple adenomas are more common in older patients.

2. **Diffuse hyperplasia:** 3½ or 3¾ parathyroids are removed and **small pieces are autotransplanted into the forearm muscle tissue.** In case there is hyperactivity of this parathyroid tissue, surgical exploration becomes easy. At the same time, if this functions normally, patient will not develop hypoparathyroidism (13–14 pieces of 1 mm each in brachioradialis)

Parathyroid autotransplantation

- Indicated after removal of all four parathyroids and in HPT with renal failure.
- 1 mm × 1 mm × 2 mm pieces are made from parathyroid tissue and placed in sterile iced saline.
- It is transplanted in patient's nondominant forearm within fibres of brachioradialis.
- 4 to 5 pieces (about 100 mg) are transplanted.
- Sutured with silk.
- It will take 14–21 days for parathyroids to function.

Cryopreservation of parathyroid glands

- Patients who became a parathyroid after re-explorations specially in MEN syndrome, are candidates for cryopreservation.
- Here 200 mg of cut parathyroids tissue is frozen in solutions containing 10% dimethyl sulfoxide, 10% autologous serum and 80% Weymouth solution.

Exploration of the neck and parathyroidectomy

- Preoperative localisation of gland is preferable.
- Rapid intraoperative PTH measurement after minimally invasive parathyroidectomy should be done.
- Fall in PTH is highly indicating of the success.
- More often it is a single adenoma—it is removed and rest normal glands are left undisturbed.
- If one cannot identify parathyroids glands, look for ectopic glands—posterior and deep to thyroid gland, in the tracheoesophageal grooves, posterior to inferior thyroid vessels between carotid artery and oesophagus.

3. **Carcinoma:** All four glands should be removed along with ipsilateral thyroid lobe with modified radical neck dissection in the presence of lymph node metastasis (Key Box 38.9)—radical parathyroidectomy.

Key Box 38.9

Preoperatively Suspect Parathyroid Carcinoma when

- Severe symptoms
- Serum calcium levels greater than **14 mg/dl**
- Significantly elevated PTH levels
- Swelling of parathyroid gland.

Follow-up

- Estimation of calcium should be done in the postoperative period to assess the functioning of the parathyroid tissue. Very often, after surgery for adenoma, there is a sudden drop in the levels of calcium because of absorption of the calcium by the bones. This is described as '**hungry bone syndrome**'. **This is seen in patients who have generalised bone disease**. In one of our patients, calcium levels dropped down to 4 mg% with severe tetany. It took 7–10 days for it to return to the normal levels. She required 24 hr constant infusion of calcium (Fig. 38.12).
- Absorption of calcium can be enhanced by **oral administration of 1,25-dihydroxycholecalciferol**, which is the most active metabolite of vitamin D. Vitamin D stimulates the absorption of calcium and phosphate.

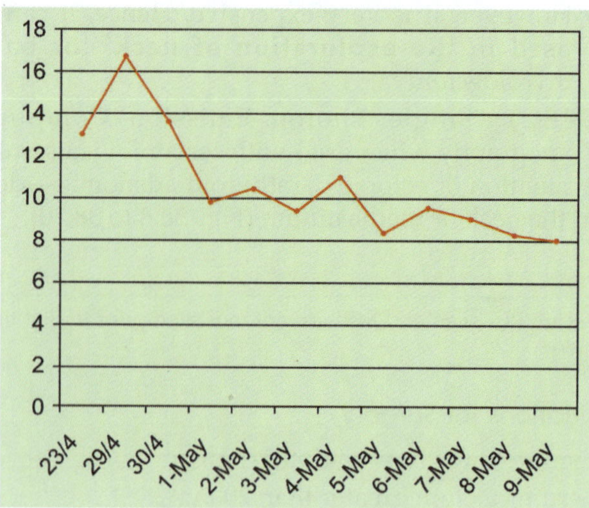

Fig. 38.12: Hypercalcaemia responding after excision of parathyroid adenoma

RECENT ADVANCES IN PARATHYROID SURGERY

Cervicoscopy

1. **Minimally invasive endoscopic parathyroidectomy (MIP)**
   - This is possible today because of localisation by ultrasound/sestamibi combined with SPECT
   - Popularised by Gagner
   - Indicated for a single adenoma
   - Can be done under general anaesthesia or regional—cervical block by using xylocaine (1%) with adrenaline
   - **3–4 trocars** are required
   - CO_2 insufflation is required
2. **Video-assisted parathyroidectomy—minimally invasive**
   - It is popularised by Parlo Miccoli from Italy
   - Ideal for a single adenoma **without thyromegaly**
   - No previous neck surgeries
   - It can be done without CO_2 insufflation—**gasless**
   - Bleeding, recurrent laryngeal nerve injuries are not uncommon
   - Can be done for bilateral cases
   - **No trocars**, a small 2–3 cm incision
3. **Totally endoscopic parathyroidectomy** by lateral approach by Henry, et al. It is the choice for adenoma deeper to thyroid gland. **Not for bilateral cases**. 10 mm endoscope is required. Require CO_2 insufflation.
   - Refer to Key Box 38.10 and clinical notes.

Key Box 38.10

Primary Hyperparathyroidism (PHPT)—Interesting 'Most'

- Mostly it is sporadic.
- Mostly it is due to single adenoma.
- Most abundant cation in the body is calcium.
- Most common and earliest manifestation of MEN type I is PHPT.
- Most common presentation of PHPT is asymptomatic hypercalcaemia.
- Most widely used and accurate investigation for localising parathyroid gland is sestamibi scan.
- Most commonly done surgery for PHPT is excision of adenoma.

Clinical Notes

A 20-year-old boy attended dental outpatient department for a loose tooth. He was diagnosed to have a loose tooth and a cyst in the lower jaw as confirmed by X-ray. Patient also had genu valgus deformity with backache (Fig. 20.5). An ortho opinion was sought for. Investigations revealed high calcium levels. An ultrasound neck revealed a parathyroid adenoma of 6 cm. At exploration a single adenoma was found arising from right inferior parathyroid and was excised. Incidentally, X-ray abdomen also revealed bilateral nephrocalcinosis. This case illustration has been given to highlight the various presentations of hyperparathyroidism. High degree of suspicion is necessary for a clinician to consider the possibility of hyperparathyroidism.

ACUTE HYPERCALCAEMIC CRISIS

- Also called parathyroid crisis.
- It presents with severe abdominal pain and effortless vomiting. Dehydration, oliguria, renal failure follow soon. Drowsiness and confusion are other features.
- Untreated cases develop coma and cardiac arrest.
- Profound muscular weakness is characteristic.

Causes

1. **Hyperparathyroidism**
   - Sudden increase in PTH levels occur due to spontaneous bleeding in a parathyroid tumour or rupture of a cystic parathyroid tumour. Severe dehydration also precipitates a crisis.
2. **Disseminated carcinoma** with bony metastasis (usually from carcinoma of the breast).
3. **Parathyroid carcinoma.**

Investigations

- Hypercalcaemia (16 to 20 mg/dl)
- Azotemia abnormal high level of urea, cratinine, etc.

Treatment

1. Restore fluid volume urgently: 300 to 500 ml/hr of 0.9% sodium chloride (normal saline) 5 to 10 L/day IV should be given. It not only helps in volume restoration but also helps in renal excretion of calcium. Inj. furosemide (80 to 100 ml) can be given after volume restoration.
2. **Bisphosphonates**—disodium pamidronate slow 15–60 mg single IV infusion or over 2–4 days. Maximum dose is about 90 mg. This drug stops mobilisation of calcium from the bone.
3. **Mithramycin:** It is produced by *Actinomyces*, *Streptomyces plicatus*. Given in high doses of 20–25 µg/kg/IV over 4 to 6 hours/day for 3 to 4 days. Can have beneficial effects. However, effect seems to be temporary. Used in all cases of **malignant hypercalcaemia.**

   Avoid thiazide diuretics. Cases which do not respond to corticosteroids can be treated with mithramycin.
   - Mithramycin rapidly controls hypercalcaemia of malignant disease in most of the patients. This control sometimes is temporary, and intermittent administration of the antibiotic was required.
4. Steroids (in cases of vitamin D intoxication and sarcoidosis).
5. **Gallium nitrate therapy** is highly effective and superior to maximally approved doses of calcitonin for acute control of cancer-related hypercalcaemia. It inhibits bone resorption increasing calcium containing bone in majority of patients.

CALCIPHYLAXIS

Etiopathogenesis

It is also called calcific uremic arteriolopathy. It is seen in end stage kidney disease patients or patients with secondary hyperparathyroidism who are undergoing parathyroidectomy. A few other conditions which can predispose to calciphylaxis are inflammatory bowel diseases, autoimmune diseases, etc. Obesity, diabetes, corticosteroids, chronic liver disease are a few risk factors. It occurs due to extensive disseminated calcification of vessels and skin necrosis.

Clinical Features

Patients develop expanding painful cutaneous lesions which are purpuritic. Extremities and areas wherein fat contents are more such as breast, buttocks and abdominal wall, gets affected often. Due to high levels of calcification, ischemic necrosis occurs, and it results in gangrene. Once gangrene sets in sepsis and death occur.

Diagnosis

It is based on the clinical features and high levels of calcium, phosphate and with or without high levels of PTH.

Treatment

Renal transplantation is the definite treatment for secondary hyperparathyroidism. A few drugs used to treat this are calcimimetic drugs. They reduce the stimulation of parathyroid glands and thus lower the PTH levels. If it is associated with persistent high levels of PTH—more than 500 pg/ml total parathyroidectomy with autograft in the nondominant forearm brachioradialis muscle or subtotal parathyroidectomy wherein three and half parathyroid are removed.

ADRENAL GLANDS/SUPRARENAL GLANDS

Competency

SU23.1: Describe applied anatomy of adrenal glands.

Anatomy

- Weight of a normal gland is 4 g.
- Yellowish in colour.
- Surrounded by perinephric pad of fat.
- **Right side** / **Left side**

Right side	Left side
Pyramidal in shape	Crescent shaped
More apical	More medial to superior half of the kidney
Anterolateral to right crus	Related to spleen, tail of pancreas and left crus of diaphragm

- **Parts:** Two parts—cortex and medulla.

Blood Supply

- Superior suprarenal arteries arise from **inferior phrenic** arteries.
- Middle suprarenal arteries arise from **abdominal aorta.**
- Inferior suprarenal arteries arise from renal artery.
- Suprarenal arteries branch before entering the gland so that **50 to 60 arteries** penetrate the capsule.
- **Venous drainage is through a single large suprarenal vein.** On the right side, it is short and drains into IVC. On the left side, it is longer and joined by inferior phrenic vein and empties into left renal vein.

Surgical Importance

One has to clearly identify and ligate suprarenal vein especially on the right side because of its short course. **Avulsion of right suprarenal vein** can be catastrophic.

Physiology (Table 38.1)

Table 38.1 Histology and function

Cortex	Hormone	Functions
1. Cells of zona glomerulosa	• Aldosterone	• Regulates sodium and potassium haemostasis
2. Cells of zona fasciculata and reticularis	• Cortisol (corticosteroids)	• Gluconeogenesis • Lipolysis, fat distribution, immunological response
Medulla	• Adrenaline (epinephrine) • Noradrenaline (norepinephrine) • Dopamine	• Activation of CVS • Bronchodilatation • Increases BP • Splanchnic vasoconstriction • Vasodilatation in skeletal muscle • Increases heart rate

Cortex

- Derived from mesoderm
- Secretes corticosteroids, androgens, aldosterone.

Medulla

- Derived from neural crest cells.
- It is a mass of nervous tissue associated with sympathetic system.
- Chromaffin cells of the medulla are related to sympathetic system.
- These cells secrete catecholamines (mostly epinephrine).

Lymphatics

Drain into caval or aortic lymph nodes.

Competency

SU23.2: Describe the aetiology, clinical features and principles of management of disorders of adrenal gland.

DISORDERS OF ADRENAL CORTEX

PRIMARY HYPERALDOSTERONISM (PHA)

- Triad of PHA is hypertension, hypokalaemia and hypersecretion of aldosterone (Key Box 38.11).
- PHA can be due to a **single adrenocortical adenoma** wherein it is called **Conn's syndrome.**
- It can also be due to bilateral micronodular hyperplasia.
- Clinical features are headache, hypertension, hypokalaemia and weakness, commonly in women.
- Polyuria, polydypsia, nocturia are other features.
- The diagnosis is established by measuring potassium level and aldosterone to plasma renin activity ratio.
- CT scan is the most important test to locate the lesion (usually it is 1–2 cm).
- Treated by spironolactone and antihypertensive medications in bilateral hyperplasia.
- **Laparoscopic adrenalectomy** is an effective treatment in unilateral cases.

Key Box 38.11

Aldosterone

- Angiotensin II increases aldosterone secretion.
- Hyperkalaemia is another **potent stimulator of aldosterone.**
- It functions mainly to increase sodium reabsorption and potassium and hydrogen ion excretion.
- It acts at distal convoluted tubules.

CUSHING'S SYNDROME

- Refers to various clinical manifestations resulting from increased secretion of corticosteroids.
- When it is due to pituitary adenoma secreting large amount of ACTH—it is called Cushing's disease.
- **Ectopic ACTH producing tumours causing Cushing's syndrome** are:
  - Small cell lung cancers
  - Foregut carcinoid
  - Medullary carcinoma thyroid
  - Neuroendocrine pancreatic tumour.

Classification

- ACTH—dependent (70% pituitary or ectopic ACTH producing tumours).
- ACTH—independent: Adrenal adenoma or hyperplasia.

Clinical Features (Key Box 38.12)

They are mainly due to increased corticosteroids, aldosterone and androgens. The net result is typical cushingoid facies—with facial plethora, buffalo hump and moon face.

Key Box 38.12

Clinical Features

- **C**entral obesity
- **U**nusual site obesity: Supraclavicular space, posterior neck
- **S**econdary osteoporosis: Buffalo humps
- **H**ypertension, Hyperglycaemia, Hypokalaemia, Hirsutism
- **I**rregularity in menstruation
- **N**eurological: Depression, mania
- **G**ain in weight
- **S**kin changes: Abdominal striae, ecchymosis, acne, plethora due to thinning of subcutaneous tissues

Remember as **CUSHINGS**

Investigations

1. Morning and midnight plasma cortisol levels are increased.
2. Serum ACTH levels: If increased, it is from pituitary source or ectopic ACTH.
3. CT chest and abdomen to assess not only adrenals but also to detect ectopic sites.

Treatment

1. **Medical:** Ketoconazole or metyrapone can reduce steroid synthesis. Thus, symptoms can be controlled. They are also indicated if surgery is not possible.
2. **Trans-sphenoidal resection** of ACTH producing pituitary tumours.
3. **Unilateral adenoma:** Adrenalectomy.
4. **Bilateral tumours:** Bilateral adrenalectomy. Postoperatively cortisol should be given.

Pearls of Wisdom

Stereotactic radiosurgery, which uses CT guidance to deliver high doses of radiotherapy to the tumour (photon or gamma knife) is being increasingly used to treat pituitary adenomas.

ADRENAL INSUFFICIENCY

***Definition*:** Loss of function of adrenal cortex is also called Addison's disease.

- Diseases associated with Addison's disease include:
  1. After bilateral adrenalectomy
  2. Tuberculosis
  3. Metastases
  4. Haemorrhage
  5. Amyloidosis, Wilson's disease
  6. HIV infection

Types

1. Acute adrenal insufficiency

- Shock
- Fever
- Abdominal pain, vomiting confused for acute abdomen

  Waterhouse-Friderichsen syndrome. It is a bilateral adrenal infarction associated with meningococcal sepsis.

2. Chronic adrenal insufficiency

- Anorexia, weakness and nausea
- ACTH and POMC—pro-opiomelanocortin levels increase—resulting in hyperpigmentation of skin and oral mucosa
- Hypotension, hypercalcaemia and hyponatraemia.

Diagnosis

- Basal ACTH levels are increased
- Cortisol levels are decreased
- ACTH tests: No rise in cortisol levels following administration of ACTH.

Treatment

- **Acute cases:** IV hydrocortisone 100 mg 6th hourly, saline transfusion, control of infections and cardiac care.
- **Chronic cases:** Oral hydrocortisone (10 mg/m^2 body surface area) and fludrocortisone (0.1 mg).
- Lifelong treatment with glucocorticoid and mineralocorticoid replacement.

Competency

SU23.3: Describe the clinical features, principles of investigation and management of adrenal tumours.

TUMOURS OF THE ADRENAL GLAND

I. Classification of the tumours of the adrenal cortex

A. Cortical carcinoma,
B. Cortical adenoma,
C. Sex cord stromal tumours,
D. Adenomatoid tumour, mesenchymal and
E. Stromal tumours (myelolipoma and schwannoma),
F. Haematological tumours, and secondary tumours.

II. Tumours of the adrenal medulla and extra-adrenal paraganglia:

A. Pheochromocytoma,
B. Paraganglioma (head and neck paraganglioma and sympathetic paraganglioma),
C. Neuroblastic tumours (neuroblastoma, nodular ganglioneuroblastoma, intermixed ganglioneuroblastoma, and ganglioneuroma),
D. Composite pheochromocytoma, and composite paraganglioma.

Adrenocortical carcinoma, neuroblastoma and phaeochromocytoma are discussed in more details here.

ADRENOCORTICAL CARCINOMA

- Incidence: One in 1,000,000 cases.
- Age: Bimodal with a first peak in childhood and second between fourth and fifth decades.
- **60%** of patients present with Cushing's syndrome.
- Diagnosis of malignancy is (>6 cm) by size of the tumour, presence of necrosis or haemorrhage, capsular or vascular invasion.
- CT—heterogeneous tumour, irregular margins, haemorrhage, lymphadenopathy, metastasis in liver.
- MRI—angiography to exclude tumour thrombus in vena cava.
- Open radical tumour resection (R_o)—*en bloc* removal of tumour lymph nodes and involved organs is the treatment of choice.
- Adjuvant chemotherapy—**mitotane** alone (derivative of insecticide DDT) is used. It has **adrenolytic** activity.
- Etoposide, cisplatin and doxorubicin are also used.
- **Steroid hypertension** is managed by **ketoconazole**.

I. Neoplasm of the sympathetic neurons

1. **Ganglioneuroma:** It is a benign neuronal tumour, commonly arising from retroperitoneal lumbar sympathetic trunk. FNAC, ultrasound followed by surgical excision is the management.
2. **Neuroblastoma**

II. Neoplasm of the chromaffin cells

- Phaeochromocytoma

NEUROBLASTOMA

- It is a malignant tumour, derived from sympathetic nervous system and adrenal medulla.
- Since it originates from the neural crest, it may be found from **orbit to pelvis** where sympathetic nervous tissue is found.

- It occurs in 1 in 10,000 live births.
- It is the **most common solid tumour** of infancy in childhood.
- Adrenal gland is **the most common** site of neuroblastoma.
- As the name suggests, the tumour occurs due to **malignant proliferation of the neuroblasts** or failure of maturation of primitive sympathetic nerve cells, the neuroblasts (Key Box 38.13).

Key Box 38.13

Neuroblastoma

- Most common solid tumour in infancy and childhood.
- Adrenal gland is the most common site.
- Mass abdomen and metastasis are common presenting features.
- Surgical excision is the best treatment.
- Younger the child, better the prognosis.
- Highest incidence of spontaneous remission.

Pathology

- Characterised by presence of immature cells derived from neuroectoderm of sympathetic nervous system.
- It is pale with grey surface and well-encapsulated.
- A few areas of calcification are seen (Key Box 38.14).
- Necrosis and haemorrhage are late features.
- Microscopically, uniform round cells containing hyperchromatic speckled nucleus, **Homer-Wright rosettes** with central fibrillar core.

Clinical Features

- 50% of children present to the hospital **under the age of one year** and 80–90% are less than 3 years of age.
- An **abdominal mass** is the most common presenting feature. The mass has all the features of a renal mass but location is slightly higher. It is firm to hard, nodular and fixed.
- The child is **sick** with weight loss, fever, abdominal distension, anaemia, etc.

Key Box 38.14

Tumours with Calcification

- Neuroblastoma
- Chondrosarcoma
- Papillary carcinoma thyroid
- Phaeochromocytoma (10%)

- Functional tumours produce diarrhoea and hypokalaemia due to release of **vasoactive intestinal polypeptide** (VIP), sweating and flushing due to release of **catecholamines**.
- **Proptosis** and **periorbital swellings** are due to bony metastasis and subcutaneous nodules are quite common (Key Box 38.15).
- Secondaries in retro-orbital region result in infra-orbital ecchymosis—**Raccoon's eye sign.**
- Posterior mediastinal neuroblastomas can produce cord compression and even paraplegia due to protrusion within the spinal canal **(dumbbell tumours).**

Key Box 38.15

Types of Neuroblastoma

1. Pepper type: Right-sided tumours with secondaries in the liver.
2. Hutchinson's type: Left-sided tumour with metastasis in bones—orbit and skull.

Investigations

- **Vanillylmandelic acid (VMA)** and homovanillic acid (HVA) are the byproducts of catecholamines passed in the urine. 24-hour urinary excretion of catecholamines and these two metabolites will be very high.
- **Plain X-ray** abdomen shows fine stippled calcification. X-ray chest is done to rule out cannonball secondaries.
- Abdominal **ultrasound** and **computed tomography (CT)** can define the mass, nature and extent of the tumour and can detect hepatic metastasis.
- **Magnetic resonance imaging (MRI)** is better than CT scan in detecting the mass as well as bony metastasis. CT-/MRI-guided core biopsy can be done.
- **Bone marrow aspiration** is positive in around 60–70% of cases.

Treatment

- **Intermediate- and high-risk** cases can be managed by chemotherapy followed by surgery.
- **Early cases** respond very well to surgical excision.
- However, many children present with metastasis, and chemotherapy and radiotherapy are given first to control the disease followed by surgical excision. **Autologous bone marrow transplantation** has improved the outlook for patients with advanced disease.

PHAEOCHROMOCYTOMA

Definition: These are catecholamine producing tumours arising from adrenal medulla and sympathetic ganglia which are derived from chromaffin cells (Key Box 38.16).

- As the name suggests, phaeo (dusty) chromo (chromaffin cells)—phaeochromocytoma is a neoplasm arising from chromaffin cells.
- 90% of the tumour occurs in adrenal glands.
- When phaeochromocytoma occurs in extra-adrenal sites, it is called paraganglioma.
- Extra-adrenal sites include organ of Zuckerkandl (the most common site), urinary bladder, renal hilum, chest, neck, etc. These are the sites of paraganglionic system.
- In about 5% of cases, the tumour can be a component of multiple endocrine neoplasia (MEN) type IIa or type IIb.
- Other syndrome associated with **phaeochromocytoma is von Hippel-Lindau syndrome** (Key Box 38.17).
- The clinical manifestations are due to release of adrenaline and noradrenaline. When the level of noradrenaline is high, symptoms are severe.

Pathology

- It is a soft, highly vascular tumour consisting of large sympathetic ganglionic cells. Most of the cells are differentiated.

Key Box 38.16

Phaeochromocytoma

10%	Bilateral
10%	Malignant
10%	Extra-adrenal
10%	Multiple
10%	Familial
10%	Children

This 10% rule has been challenged

Key Box 38.17

Other Neuroectodermal Anomalies with Phaeochromocytoma

- Neurofibromatosis (NF) type I
- Acoustic neuroma
- Meningioma, glioma, haemangioblastoma (von Hippel-Lindau (vHL)) syndrome
- Astrocytoma
- MEN type II—hereditary phaeochromocytoma
- Familial paraganglioma syndrome along with carotid body tumours

- Usually, it is small in size and well-encapsulated.
- Sometimes, it can present as a large abdominal mass.
- Microscopic features are **polygonal** or spheroidal chromaffin cells within a vascularised fibrous stroma.
- Presence of high number of Ki-67 positive cells, vascular invasion or breached capsule and PASS—phaeochromocytoma of the adrenal gland scale score suggests metastasis.

Clinical Features

- Sporadic cases peak at 40–50 years, whereas familial tend to occur early.
- The most common presenting feature is paroxysmal or persistent hypertension (80–90%). It is associated with palpitation (50–70%), fever, pallor, tremors, sweating and severe headache (60–90%).
- The paroxysmal attack may last for a few minutes to a few hours (Key Box 38.18).
- **The factors which stimulate an attack are**
  - Surgery
  - Anaesthesia
  - Invasive procedure
  - Late pregnancy
  - Drugs—histamine, glucagon, etc.
  - Palpation of the mass
  - **Classical triad** consisting of headache, diaphoresis and palpitations is seen in only a few patients.
- **A high index of suspicion is necessary to diagnose phaeochromocytoma in a hypertensive patient.**

Investigations

1. **Urinary levels of free catecholamines,** vanillylmandelic acid (VMA) in excess of 7 mg/24 hours and meta-adrenaline 1–3 mg/24 hours are suggestive of phaeochromocytoma.

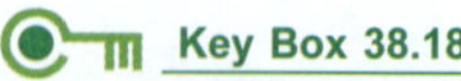

Key Box 38.18

Hypertension in Phaeochromocytoma

- **P**aroxysmal
- **P**ersistent
- **P**alpitations
- **P**allor
- **P**rofuse sweating
- **P**ain abdomen
- **P**alpation of the mass

Observe **7 Ps**

2. **Plasma metanephrines:** A fractionated plasma-free metanephrine level may be measured. Blood sample drawn after 15–20 minutes of IV catheter insertion (not immediately).
3. **Computed tomography**
   - Noninvasive, safe investigation
   - It has a high degree of accuracy
   - It can pick up lesions of less than 1 cm in size.
4. **MRI** is preferred because **contrast media used for CT scan can provoke paroxysms.**
5. ^{131}I Metaiodobenzylguanidine (MIBG) scan
   - Iodine labelled MIBG (radionuclide) scan is found to be very specific for phaeochromocytoma. This radionuclide scan locates only abnormal adrenal tissue and is **more useful in detecting ectopic sites of phaeochromocytoma** (Fig. 38.13).

Treatment (Figs 38.14 and 38.15)

- Surgical removal is the treatment.[1] However, a good preoperative preparation is essential before doing surgery. It includes control of blood pressure and tachycardia, by α- and β-blockers (Key Box 38.19).
- **Contraction of vascular bed which occurs due to catecholamines results in hypovolaemia which must be corrected with IV fluids.**

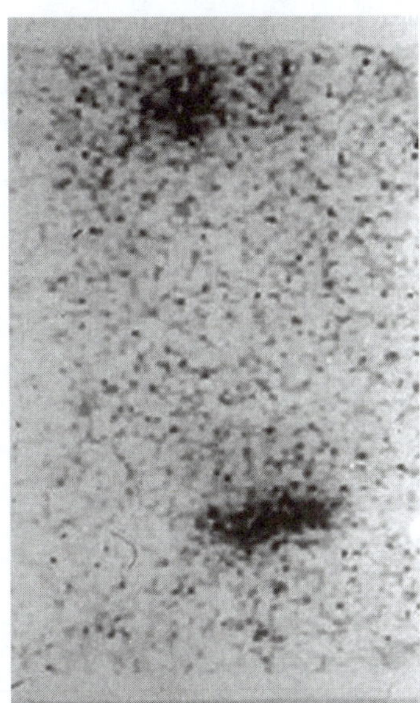

Fig. 38.13: MIBG scan showing extra-adrenal phaeochromocytoma

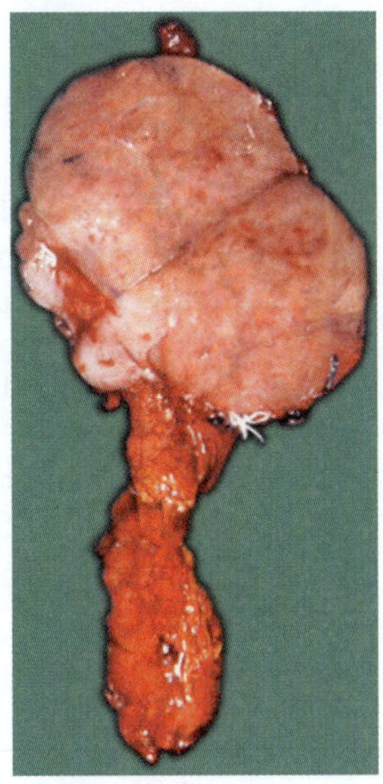

Fig. 38.14: Phaeochromocytoma excised

(*Courtesy:* Prof. MG Shenoy, Senior Consultant in Surgery, KMC, Manipal)

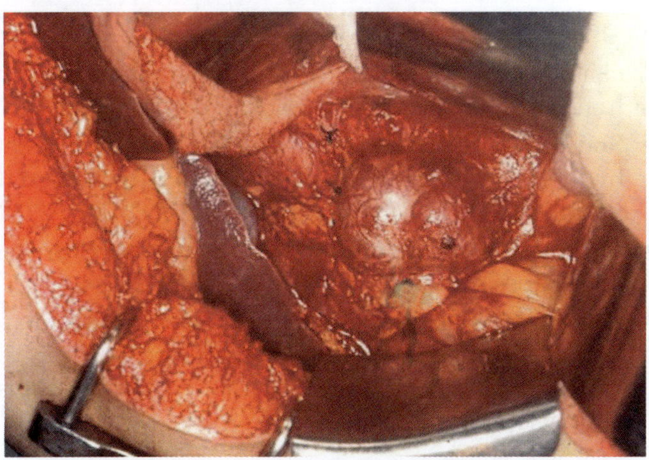

Fig. 38.15: Phaeochromocytoma at surgery

Key Box 38.19

Hyperte Phaeochromocytoma (Preoperative Preparation)

- **Phenoxybenzamine:** 20–60 mg/day for 3–4 weeks before surgery to control **hypertension**—increased to 10 mg/day—total of 100–160 mg.
- **Propranolol:** 20–60 mg/day for 5–7 days before surgery to control **tachycardia** and **arrhythmias**.
- Plenty of **fluids** before surgery to correct **hypovolaemia**.

- **First**, alpha-adrenergic blockers such as phenoxybenzamine is given to control hypertension and to permit **re-expansion of intravascular volume. Only after the complete alpha-adrenergic blockade, beta-adrenergic blockade may be added.**

TEN COMMANDMENTS OF PHAEOCHROMOCYTOMA

1. MRI is better because CT scan provokes paroxysm
2. MIBG—^{123}I single-photon emission CT will diagnose about 90% of cases
3. Should not do FNAC/biopsy of adrenals
4. α-**adrenergic blockers** should be started first
5. β-blockade is always given **after** α-**blockade**
6. CVP and intra-arterial monitoring is a must, as they may hold a large volume of fluids
7. Should also look on the contralateral side for phaeochromocytoma
8. Ligate adrenal vein first
9. Never allow vaginal delivery in patients who have phaeochromocytoma
10. Laparoscopic adrenalectomy is the 'Gold standard'

[1]Surgery for phaeochromocytoma is like going to a war. Without proper preparation, going to war is a sure failure.

Surgery (see ten commandments given above)

Excision is the treatment. Certain steps of excision (adrenalectomy) are as follows (Key Box 38.20):

- **Sodium nitroprusside** must be kept ready to treat hypertension during surgery as it is a **direct arterial vasodilator** (0.5 to 10 µg/kg/minute).
- Thorough search in the abdomen **for other sites**, due to the possibility of multiple tumours.
- **Postoperative hypotension** can be a serious problem which needs to be treated with large volume of plasma expanders, blood transfusions, corticosteroids and vasopressors.

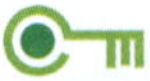 Key Box 38.20

Precautions during Surgery

- Midline incision for familial cases
- Anterior or posterior approach for sporadic cases
- Careful positioning
- **Ligation of adrenal vein first**
- Gentle handling
- Haemodynamic monitoring—CVP, arterial monitoring
- Avoid rupture of the tumour to prevent recurrence
- Laparoscopic adrenalectomy is very popular now

METASTATIC PHEOCHROMOCYTOMA

It was called malignant phaeochromocytoma earlier.

- 10% of phaeochromocytomas are malignant.
- Rate is higher in extra-adrenal tumours.
- Malignancy is suspected when metastasis or vascular invasion is present or when a capsule is breached.
- Open adrenalectomy is the choice for excision.
- Debulking should be done even if metastasis is present, so as to decrease tumour burden and to control catecholamine excess.

MISCELLANEOUS

INCIDENTALOMAS

- Incidentally detected adrenal masses.
- Detected by ultrasound or CT scan (1 to 5% of patients undergoing CT abdomen for evaluation of abdominal pain).
- Some patients may have subclinical Cushing's syndrome or aldosteronism.
- Nonfunctioning situations may be metastatic cancer (primary from breast, kidney, melanoma, lung).
- Myelolipoma
- Adrenal cysts
- Majority of such tumours are **nonfunctioning cortical adenomas of no clinical significance**.
- Indication to do adrenal gland biopsy is to rule out/ diagnose metastasis.
- Absolute contraindication to do adrenal biopsy in phaeochromocytoma.
- Any nonfunctioning adrenal incidentaloma should be resected.
- Majority of incidentalomas are nonfunctional adenomas.

Refer to clinical notes.

Clinical Notes

An 18-year-old girl was admitted for tonsillectomy. This girl suffered from occasional headache. She was diagnosed to have migraine. Preoperative blood pressure showed mild elevations which were thought to be due to anxiety. During tonsillectomy, there was a rise in BP, which was controlled well. However, in the postoperative period, there was severe tachycardia, hypertension, arrhythmias and hypovolaemia. Within 8 hours of surgery, the patient died even as the diagnosis of phaeochromocytoma was being considered.

Multiple Choice Questions

1. Superior parathyroids derive blood supply from:

A. Common carotid artery
B. Internal carotid artery
C. Inferior thyroid artery
D. Superior thyroid artery

2. Superior parathyroids are found:

A. Above inferior thyroid artery
B. Below inferior thyroid artery
C. Above superior thyroid artery
D. Below superior thyroid artery

3. Following are true for primary hyperparathyroidism *except:*

A. Majority are due to a single adenoma
B. Majority are sporadic
C. Hypercalcaemia with decreased PTH levels are often seen
D. Rarely it can be due to carcinoma also

4. Following are true for inferior parathyroid glands *except:*

A. Derived from 3rd pharyngeal pouch
B. It is inferior to inferior parathyroid artery
C. It is superior to inferior parathyroid artery
D. Inferior parathyroids are less constant in position

5. Following are functions of parathyroid gland *except:*

A. Activates osteoclasts to resorb bone
B. Increased calcium reabsorption from urine
C. Renal activation of vitamin D
D. Decrease renal excretion of phosphate

6. Following is not the feature of primary hyperparathyroidism:

A. Hypercalcaemia
B. Most common manifestation of MEN type I
C. Band keratopathy in cornea
D. Dystrophic calcification

7. The best investigation of choice to localise parathyroid gland is:

A. ^{99m}Tc-labelled sestamibi scan
B. CT scan
C. MRI
D. Ultrasound

8. Which one of the following is not the site of inferior parathyroid gland?

A. Thyrothymic axis
B. Mediastinum
C. Within carotid sheath
D. Cricothyroid articulation

9. Following are true for parathyroid hyperplasia *except:*

A. It affects all 4 glands
B. It is not the common cause of hyperparathyroidism
C. Total parathyroidectomy is the treatment of choice
D. Thymectomy need not be done

10. Which one of the following is the treatment of choice for acute hypercalcaemic crisis?

A. Steroids B. Diuretics
C. Vasopressors D. Bisphosphonates

11. Which is the first drug to be used in the preoperative preparation of a patient with phaeochromocytoma?

A. Steroids
B. Noradrenaline
C. Propranolol
D. Phenylbenzamine

12. Which one of these operative steps is done first in excision of phaeochromocytoma?

A. Ligation of adrenal vein
B. Ligation of inferior phrenic artery
C. Ligation of branch of renal artery
D. Isolation from kidney

13. A few landmarks for identification of ectopic sites of phaeochromocytoma include following *except:*

A. Urinary bladder
B. Along 5th cranial nerve
C. Organ of Zuckerkandl
D. Superior para-aortic region—below the diaphragm and renal poles

14. Following are true for management of phaeochromocytoma *except:*

A. Phenoxybenzamine is given prior to propranolol
B. Intra-arterial monitoring is a must
C. It is dangerous to infuse large volumes of fluid after ligation of adrenal vein
D. Laparoscopic resection is the gold standard

15. Following are true for right adrenal gland *except:*

A. Right adrenal gland drains into renal vein
B. Right adrenal gland is partly behind inferior vena cava
C. Right adrenal gland is pyramidal in shape
D. Right adrenal gland is anterolateral to the right crus

16. The majority of the sporadic primary hyperparathyroidism is due to:

A. Hyperplasia B. Adenoma
C. Carcinoma D. Cystic degeneration

17. Severe bone disease due to primary hyperparathyroidism is called:

A. Sipple syndrome
B. Werner syndrome
C. von Recklinghausen's disease
D. Paget's disease

18. Superior parathyroid gland can be found by:

A. Ligating the middle thyroid vein and dividing the lobe
B. Ligating inferior thyroid artery and mobilising the gland
C. Ligating superior thyroid pedicle and mobilising the gland anteriorly
D. Ligating inferior thyroid veins and diving isthmus

19. Following are locations of inferior parathyroid gland *except:*

A. Upper horn of thymus
B. Within carotid sheath
C. Within thyroid lobe
D. Behind superior thyroid pedicle

20. Following are causes of secondary hyperparathyroidism *except:*

A. Malabsorption
B. Vitamin D-deficient rickets
C. Pseudohypoparathyroidism
D. Acute renal failure

21. Parathyroids can be autotransplanted to:

A. Brachioradialis muscle
B. Biceps
C. Coracobrachialis
D. Flexor digitorum superficialis

22. Which of the following drugs is not used in treating acute hypercalcaemic crisis due to primary hyperparathyroidism (benign)?

A. Mithramycin
B. Bisphosphonates
C. Furosemide
D. Normal saline

Answers

1. C	**2.** A	**3.** C	**4.** B	**5.** D	**6.** D	**7.** A	**8.** D	**9.** D	**10.** D
11. D	**12.** A	**13.** B	**14.** C	**15.** A	**16.** B	**17.** C	**18.** C	**19.** D	**20.** D
21. A	**22.** A								

CHAPTER

39

Breast

- Congenital anomalies
- Surgical anatomy
- Cystic swellings of breast—classification
- Acute bacterial mastitis
- Antibioma
- Retromammary abscess
- Aberrations of normal development and involution
- Fibroadenoma
- Duct ectasia—plasma cell mastitis
- Idiopathic granulomatous mastitis
- Macrocysts
- Galactocele
- Galactorrhoea
- Duct papilloma
- Gynecomastia
- Phyllodes tumours
- Carcinoma breast
- Effects of lymphatic obstruction from carcinoma of breast
- Breast reconstruction
- Male breast carcinoma
- Mondor's disease
- Angiosarcoma of the breast
- Disorders of augmented breast
- Rare breast cancers
- A case of carcinoma breast
- Oncoplastic breast conservation surgery

Competency

SU25.1: Describe applied anatomy and appropriate investigations for breast disease.

EMBRYOLOGY

- The breast is a modified sweat gland and it is derived from a downward growth of ectoderm into the underlying mesenchyme.
- At 5th or 6th week of intrauterine life, two ventral bands of thickened ectoderm, called mammary ridge/milk line or line of Schultz, appear. The line extends from axilla to the groin. Thus, accessory nipples can appear along the milk line from axilla to groin (Fig. 39.1).
- Persistent part of mammary ridge is converted into a pit. Placental sex hormones enter fetal circulation during 3rd trimester of pregnancy. They induce canalizations of branched epithelial tissues.
- Secondary buds develop, divide and form more lobes.
- The nipple is everted at the site of original position.

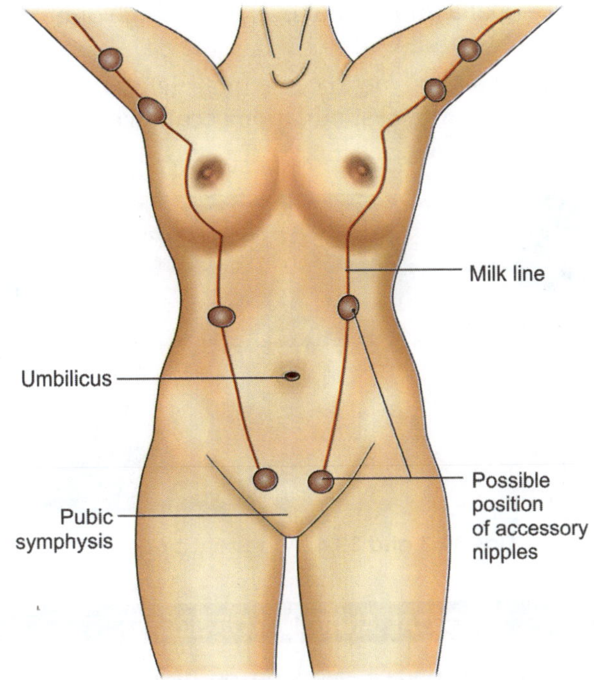

Fig. 39.1: Milk line with possible positions of accessory nipples

- Oestrogens cause enlargement of mammary glands at puberty and progesterone stimulates development of secondary alveoli.

CONGENITAL ANOMALIES OF BREAST

I. **Amazia:** Congenital absence of breast is very rare. It can be unilateral or bilateral.

II. **Poland's syndrome**
   - Amazia
   - Absence of sternal portion of pectoralis major
   - Occurs commonly in males

III. **Supernumerary nipples:** Accessory nipples, polythelia (Fig. 39.2)

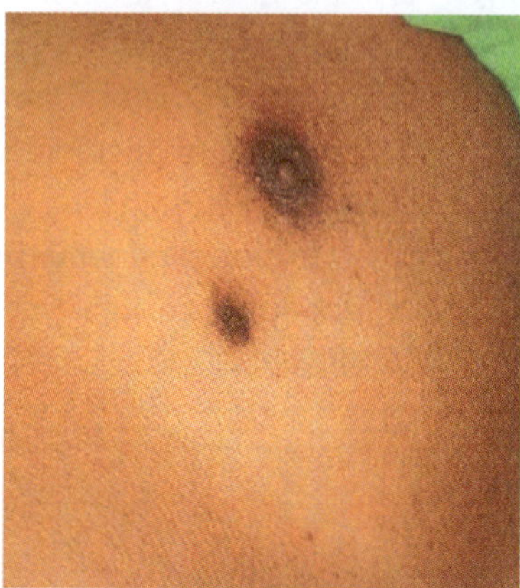

Fig. 39.2: Accessory nipple

IV. **Athelia:** Absence of nipple.

V. **Polymastia:** Accessory breasts occur along the milk line—axilla (most common), groin, thigh or buttock (Figs 39.3 and 39.4).

VI. **Micromastia:** Due to congenital defects of ovary, lack of hormonal stimulation occurs which results in small breast.

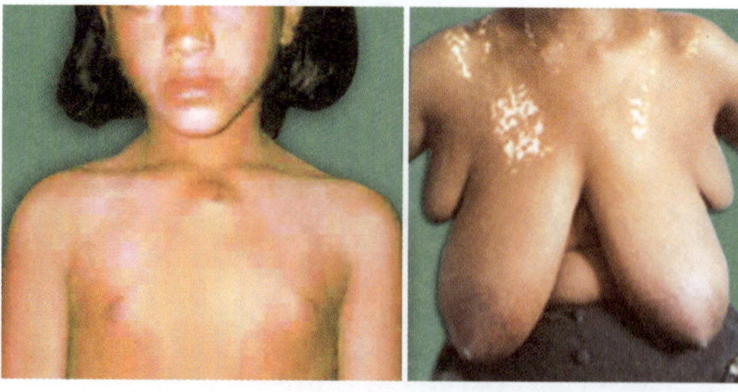

Figs 39.3 and 39.4: Accessory breasts

SURGICAL ANATOMY OF BREAST

- Breast, a modified sweat gland, occupies the pectoral region from the 2nd to the 6th rib vertically, and from the lateral border of sternum to the midaxillary line, horizontally. It is hemispherical, and lies in the superficial fascial planes.
- It is composed of fatty tissue and does the function of secreting milk. **The axillary tail of Spence is the part of the breast which is in the axilla and is deeper to the deep fascia**, whereas the entire breast is a *sub-cutaneous structure*.
- The opening in the axillary fascia, through which outer quadrant breast tissue enters into axilla is called foramen of **Langer**.

Structure of the Breast (Fig. 39.5)

1. **Nipple and areola complex:** The **nipple** is located in the 4th intercostal space, in the midclavicular line. It is the erectile structure of the breast, and is directed forwards and laterally for the convenience of feeding the child. **Areola** has modified sweat glands and sebaceous glands. These enlarge during pregnancy and are called **glands of Montgomery**. Both nipple and areola are pigmented due to melanin deposition which increases during pregnancy. Hair is absent in the areola of women (present in males).
2. **Parenchyma** of breast.
3. **Stroma** gives support to the glandular structure. Therein lie **ligaments of Cooper** which are cone-shaped fibrous bands. Their apex is attached to overlying skin, and base to the fascia over pectoralis major. **Puckering of the skin is due to infiltration of the ligaments of Cooper**.

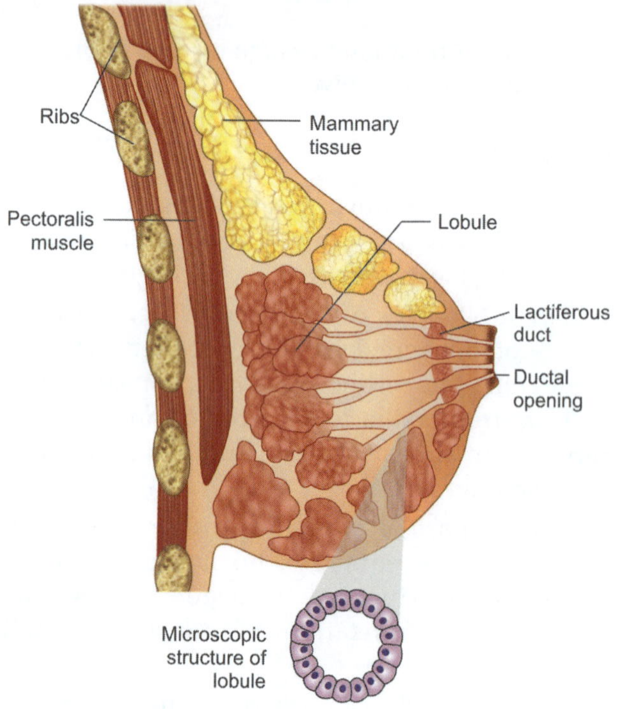

Fig. 39.5: Structure of the breast

. **Lobule** is the chief functional and structural unit of breast. Many lobules join to form a lobe. There are **15–20 lobes and** each lobe is drained by a **lactiferous duct**. They are 15–20 in number arranged radially, lined by myoepithelial cells, which converge into the nipple. Diameter of a lactiferous duct is 2–4 mm.

. **Skin:** The skin of the breast is thin and contains hair follicles, sebaceous glands and eccrine sweat glands.

ymphatic Drainage

They can be divided into lymph nodes and lymphatics Fig. 39.6).

. *Lymph Nodes*

. Anterior or pectoral: They are under the pectoralis major which forms anterior fold of axilla.

. Central group: These lymph nodes are present in the centre of axilla (armpit). One has to dip the examining fingers slightly deeper into axilla to detect the enlargement.
   - Anterior and central group of nodes are commonly involved in carcinoma breast.

. Lateral group are felt against humerus. They are also called brachial group.

. Apical: They are found at apex of the axilla. It is the space between pectoralis minor and clavicle. They are also called infraclavicular nodes, situated very high in the axilla. They are difficult to feel clinically.

. Posterior: They are also called subscapular group of lymph nodes. They are felt along the posterior fold of the axilla. These five groups together form the axillary group of lymph nodes.

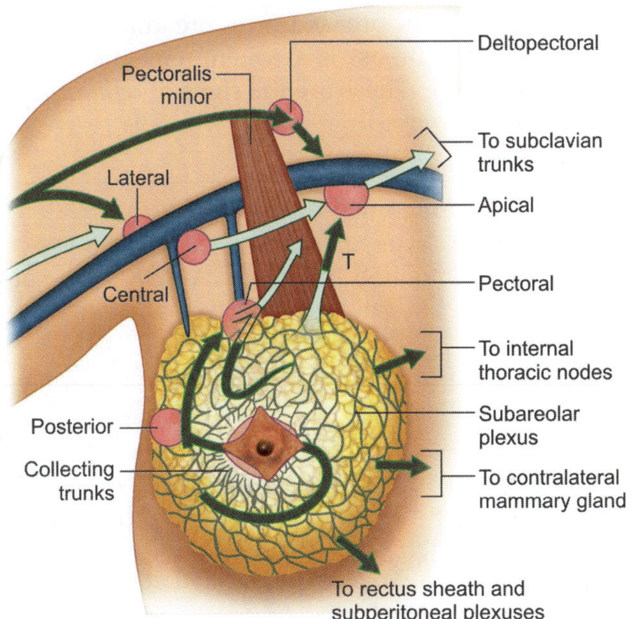

Fig. 39.6: Lymph nodes and lymphatic spread from breast

6. Internal mammary lymph nodes: Also called parasternal nodes. They lie along internal mammary vessels. They are located in the 2nd, 3rd and 4th space.
7. Supraclavicular lymph nodes: Spread to supraclavicular lymph nodes indicates advanced stage of the disease. It indicates poor prognosis.

Miscellaneous lymph nodes/plexus

1. Cephalic nodes—deltopectoral nodes
2. Interpectoral nodes—Rotter's nodes
3. Posterior intercostal nodes—in front of heads of ribs
4. Intra-abdominal—subdiaphragmatic/retroperitoneal.

II. *Lymphatic Vessels*

1. **Superficial lymphatics:** Drain skin over the breast except nipple and areola. Superficial lymphatics of one breast communicate with the contralateral breast across midline.
2. **Deep lymphatics:** Drain parenchyma of the breast. They also drain nipple and areola.

Important key points about lymphatics and spread

- The first **lymph nodes** draining the tumour-bearing area is called **sentinel node**.
- 75% of the lymph from the breast drains into axillary nodes.
- 20% drains into the internal mammary nodes.
- 5% of lymph drains into posterior intercostal lymph nodes.
- Most of the lymphatics eventually drains into central to apical and then to supraclavicular lymph nodes.
- Internal mammary nodes receive lymphatics not only from inner quadrant but also from outer quadrant.
- Lymphatics from inner quadrant of the breast penetrate rectus sheath and thus spread into coelomic cavity. It results in ascites, rectovesical deposits and Krukenberg tumours.
- Krukenberg tumours are bilateral bulky ovarian metastasis in premenopausal women. During ovulation, raw surface develops over the ovary into which malignant cells drop and develop into large tumours (transcoelomic spread).

Blood Supply of the Breast
(Branches of Axillary Artery)

Arterial Supply

1. **Lateral thoracic artery** gives many branches which penetrate through the pectoralis major and supply the breast.
2. **Internal mammary artery** gives branches which perforate intercostal spaces.
3. **Pectoral branches of thoracoacromial artery** supply upper part of the breast.
4. **Lateral branches of posterior intercostal arteries.**

Venous Return

Breast is drained by perforating branches of internal mammary veins, tributaries of axillary veins and perforating branches of posterior intercostal veins. Venous return follows the arteries but drain into large veins that also receive blood from vertebrae and thoracic cage, e.g. posterior intercostal veins joining paravertebral plexus of veins **(Batson's venous plexus)**. This explains the occurrence of metastasis in the vertebrae and pelvic bones from carcinoma of the breast.

Physiology (Key Box 39.1)

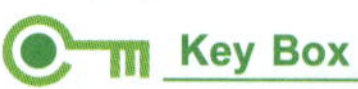

Key Box 39.1

Physiology of the Breast

- ***Oestrogen:*** Initiates ductal development.
- ***Progesterone:*** Differentiation of epithelium and lobular development (glandular development)
- ***Prolactin:*** Lactogenesis in late pregnancy and post-partum period. It also upregulates hormone receptors and stimulates epithelial development.

Competency

SU25.2: Describe the etiopathogenesis, clinical features and principles of management of benign breast disease including infections of the breast.

CYSTIC SWELLINGS OF BREAST

Classification

1. **Inflammatory:** Acute bacterial mastitis with abscess*
2. **Neoplastic:**
   a. ***Benign:*** Phyllodes tumour*
   b. ***Malignant:*** Intracystic carcinoma*
3. **Non-neoplastic cyst**
   a. Fibroadenosis—cyclical mastalgia
   b. Simple cysts of the breast
   c. Cyst of Bloodgood—blue domed cyst
4. **Retention cyst of the breast:** Galactocele
5. **Other rare causes of cysts of the breast**
   a. Tuberculous mastitis with cold abscess*
   b. Lymphatic cyst of the breast (congenital)
   c. Hydatid cyst of the breast
   d. Haematoma of the breast

ACUTE BACTERIAL MASTITIS (BREAST ABSCESS—PYOGENIC MASTITIS)

Aetiopathogenesis

1. **Lactational mastitis:** It is most commonly encountered during **lactation**. Hence, it is called lactational mastitis.

*These swellings may give rise to fluctuation in a 'small' part of the swelling. Truly, they are not cystic swellings.

Precipitating factors

- Crack/fissure in the nipple
- Retracted nipple. Hence, cleaning of the breast is a problem.
- Oral cavity infection in the child

2. **Haematoma**

- Infection in a haematoma can result in an abscess—rare cause.
- *Staphylococcus* produces many enzymes/toxins such as catalase, coagulase, hyaluronidase which result in an abscess. It also inhibits phagocytosis because of type 'A' protein on its surface. *Staphylococcus aureus*, which enters through the nipple, proliferates intraductally and produces *clotting of the milk*. Within the clot, the organisms multiply, which results in a **cellulitic stage of the breast** (mastitis) and in untreated cases, it may give rise to a breast abscess. Initially, only one lobule and duct get affected. Later other lobules get infected, giving rise to an intramammary abscess.

3. **Nonlactational breast abscess:** It occurs in patients with duct ectasia and periductal mastitis. When such an abscess ruptures, it results in a mammary duct fistula. It classically drains at the junction between the areola and breasts skin. **Anaerobic bacteria** are the cause in majority of cases.
4. **Other factors:** Diabetes, AIDS and chronic illness also can give rise to breast abscess (Key Boxes 39.2 and 39.3).
5. **MRSA and breast abscess**

Clinical Features

- Severe pain in the breast due to spreading inflammatory exudate. Breast is swollen, tense, tender and warm to touch. These are the signs of *cellulitic stage*.

Key Box 39.2

MRSA and Breast Abscess

- Methicillin resistant *Staphylococcus aureus* (MRSA) or community acquired MRSA or CA-MRSA can cause breast abscess in patients who have no traditional risk factors
- Hospitals, nursing homes (patients with open wounds) are the risk areas
- Co-amoxyclav 1000 mg 2 times/day—7–10 days
- Erythromycin 500 mg 3 times/day—7–10 days
- Vancomycin 1.5 g vial 12th hourly × 7–10 days
- Suspect MRSA infection when abscesses recur, abscess persists and is nonlactational.

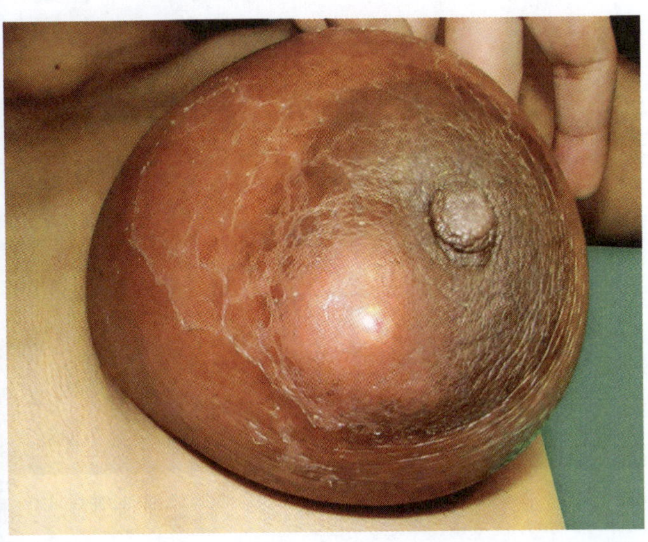

Fig. 39.7: Large breast abscess presented late to the hospital. Managed by incision and drainage (I and D), not aspiration

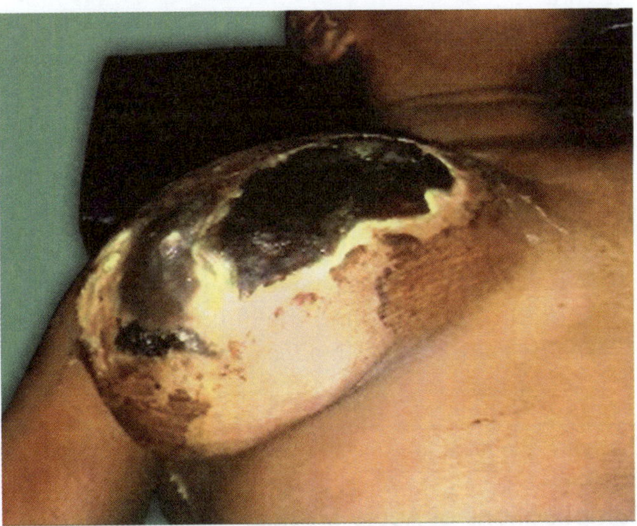

Fig. 39.8: Extensive necrosis of skin due to severe mastitis (*Courtesy:* Dr CG Narasimhan, Surgeon, Mysore, Karnataka)

- Once *breast abscess* develops, there is high grade fever with chills and rigors and a soft, cystic fluctuant swelling can be felt in the breast. In untreated cases, abscess may rupture through the skin resulting in *necrosis of the skin of the breast, ulceration* and discharge (Figs 39.7 and 39.8).
- In deep-seated abscess, it is difficult to elicit fluctuation and often fluctuation is a late sign. Hence, if **throbbing pain and fever with chills and rigors** are present, immediate drainage is mandatory. If not done, significant amount of breast tissue will be destroyed.

Treatment

1. Stage of cellulitis

- Not to feed the child on the affected side.
- Cloxacillin 500 mg, 6th hourly, orally for 7–10 days.
- Anti-inflammatory drugs, such as ibuprofen 400 mg, three times a day.

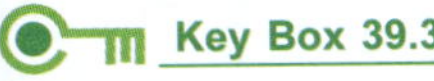

Key Box 39.3

Breast Abscess

- Common organism—*Staphylococcus aureus*
- Retracted nipple is one of the causes
- Commonly seen during **lactational period**
- Very painful condition
- Do not wait for fluctuation
- Ultrasound-guided aspiration should be done **(Fig. 39.9)**
- Cloxacillin is the drug of choice
- Nonlactational abscess—Metronidazole is drug of choice
- Abscess confined to one sector—aspiration is the treatment of choice. It can also be repeated.

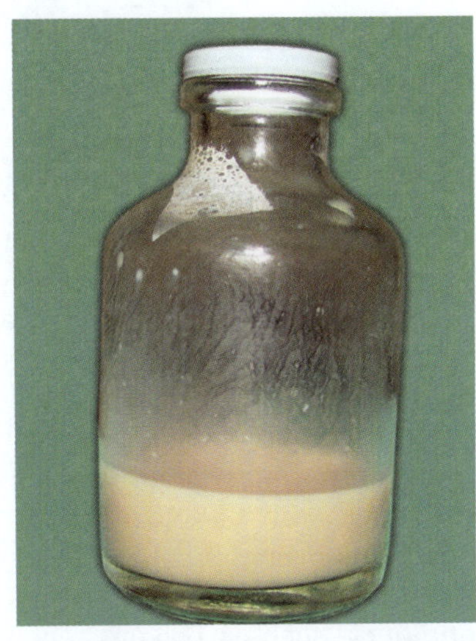

Fig. 39.9: Breast abscess aspirated. Current thinking is that repeated aspiration of the breast abscess can also be an alternative treatment to incision and drainage

- Good support to the breast.
- For nonlactational breast abscess, add metronidazole 400 mg, 3 times a day for 5–7 days.

Advice given to mothers in cases of breast abscess:

- Pus is frequently expressed from nipple.
- Breast feeding is stopped.
- Antibiotics are started.
- Milk is expressed and is boiled and can be given to baby in cases of absolute requirement.
- Never feed the baby when there is active breast abscess.

2. Stage of abscess

- The abscess should be drained—incision and drainage (I and D) under antibiotic cover.

– If the abscess is situated in any quadrant of breast, other than lower quadrant, it is drained by **radial incision**.
– Abscess in lower quadrant is drained by **infra-mammary** incision placed in the inferior aspect of breast (*refer to* breast abscess drainage under operative surgery section).
– When both the breasts have an abscess, the breasts should be emptied and the milk that is expressed *can be boiled and given to the child.*

Pearls of Wisdom

Currently, the initial treatment policy is USG-guided drainage.

Complications of Acute Mastitis

- Abscess
- Toxaemia
- Skin
- Antibioma (Fig. 39.10)

MRSA and Breast Abscess

- Postpartum MRSA infections among young, immuno-competent women lacking risk factors for MRSA have surfaced in the past few years. CA-MRSA are susceptible to multiple non-beta-lactam antibiotics. **Although they are sensitive to vancomycin, it should be given to patients with signs of systemic septicaemia, hence routine admission for intravenous vancomycin is not necessary**. Patients with MRSA infections should be evaluated based on their culture sensitivity results and treated accordingly. Many may respond to beta-lactam antibiotics, such as penams, cephalosporins and even many other drugs, such as cotrimoxazole and erythromycin.
- All patients should be tested for swabs from nostril, axilla and groin for MRSA.
- Unilocular abscess or even multilocular abscess without toxicity can be managed with ultrasound-guided aspiration followed by drugs according to the culture sensitivity.
- However, when patients have toxicity, tachycardia, immunocompromised status, they need to be admitted and aspirations can be done. However, if tachycardia does not subside, better to do open drainage.
- Recent trails have shown superior results to open drainage than aspiration.
- Abscess: Patients with severe infections with sepsis should be admitted and are treated with injectable antibiotics.

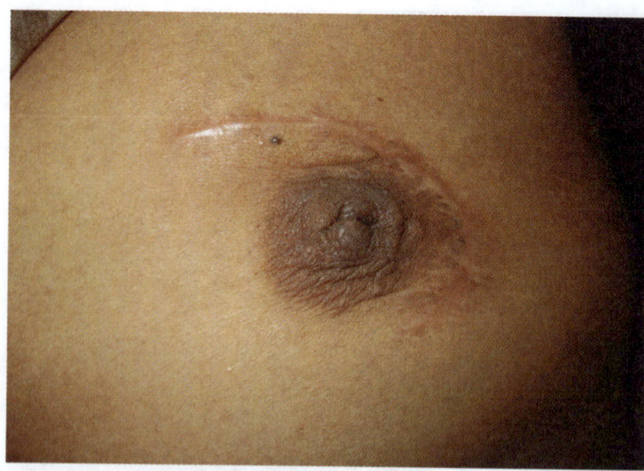

Fig. 39.10: Nipple retraction—she also had a lump-antibioma. Observe previous drainage incision

ANTIBIOMA

- It means an antibiotic-induced swelling. [Oma = Tumour (swelling)].
- When an abscess occurs in the breast and antibiotics are given, without draining the abscess, the abscess cavity may become fibrous and it results in **firm to hard lump** in the breast. It gives rise to vague **ill health of the patient**.
- This hard lump can be confused for *malignancy*.
- It is treated by excision.

OTHER TYPES OF BREAST ABSCESSES

RETROMAMMARY ABSCESS

It is collection of pus behind the *pectoralis major* (Fig. 39.11).

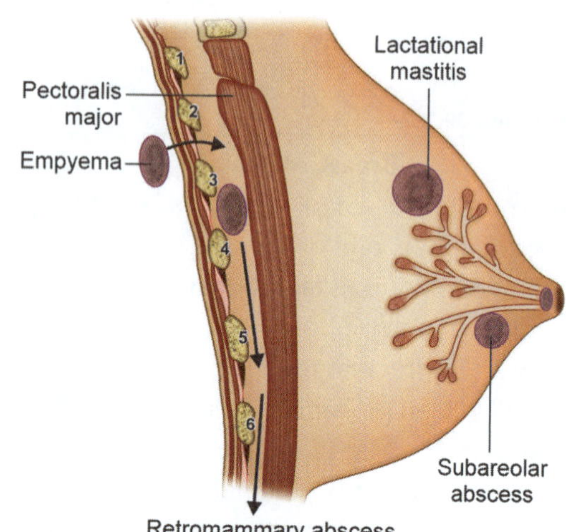

Fig. 39.11: Different types of breast abscesses

Common Causes

1. Haematoma with secondary infection
2. Tuberculosis of ribs with cold abscess
3. Cold abscess arising from lymph node
4. **Empyema necessitans:** Empyema of lung, if left untreated, tracks out and the pus collects in the subcutaneous plane posteriorly and retromammary region anteriorly, thereby forming retromammary abscess. There may be a tense, tender and cystic lump palpable which can be confused with breast abscess.

Management

- Chest X-ray to rule out pulmonary tuberculosis.
- It is treated by draining the abscess by means of submammary (Galliard-Thomas) incision.

SUBAREOLAR ABSCESS

- It is common in nonlactating women.
- It communicates with lactiferous duct resulting in mammary fistula.
- In chronic cases, retraction of the nipple can occur which is partial or slit-like.
- It can also be due to an infected sebaceous cyst.

TUBERCULOUS MASTITIS

- Incidence is 1 to 4% in India.
- Poor socioeconomic conditions
- Presents as a lump, which can be hard and mimics carcinoma.
- More common in the reproductive age group—mainly in lactating women.
- Clinical features may include multiple tender abscesses, sinuses and matted nodes in the axilla (need not always be present).
- Involvement of nipple and areola is very rare.
- It is almost secondary to a pulmonary lesion—retrograde lymphatic spread via paratracheal and internal mammary lymph nodes.
- **Few types:** Nodular, sclerosing, disseminated type, TB mastitis obliterans and miliary form.
- FNAC, care biopsy will help in the diagnosis—caseating granuloma with Langhan type of giant cells.
- Aspiration of pus, lumpectomy, excision/even mastectomy may be required along with concurrent antitubercular treatment (Fig. 39.12).

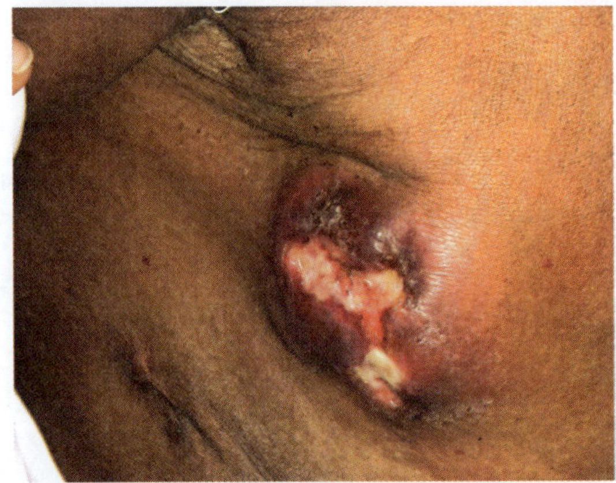

Fig. 39.12: Tuberculous mastitis *(Courtesy:* Dr Maruthu Pandyan, Government Medical College, Madurai)

ABERRATIONS OF NORMAL DEVELOPMENT AND INVOLUTION OF THE BREAST

The concept of aberrations of normal development and involution (ANDI) of the breast was first published by **LE Hughes,** et al. of **Cardiff Breast Clinic** in **1987**. The ANDI classification is based on pathogenesis, and recognises that a spectrum exists from normal, through mild abnormality to disease. This has resulted in a radical change in attitude to the understanding and management of breast disorders. Changes previously regarded as disease are so common that they must be regarded as lying within the spectrum of normality (Fig. 39.13).

This concept is of value in dispelling the supposed association between the benign conditions and cancer. Most patients with lumps and mastalgia are concerned that they may be harbouring cancer (the result of a successful information campaign!!), and once a definite opinion of the benign nature of the lump is conveyed and the patient is informed that no further treatment is required, most would be reassured.

Having noted the above, a word of caution is due here—it is preferable to overtreat a benign breast disease rather than miss or delay treatment of an early carcinoma of the breast (Fig. 39.13). So following the clinical dictum "in a patient who is above the age of 40, with a recently detected lump in the breast, it should be considered to be carcinoma breast until proved otherwise" may prove to be a wrong answer in many but the correct management in most.

From the above, it follows that, in case of doubt (where there is a high-risk patient or doubtful signs of malignancy), it would be prudent on the part of the treating surgeon to rule out malignancy by triple assessment (physical examination, mammography and cytology).

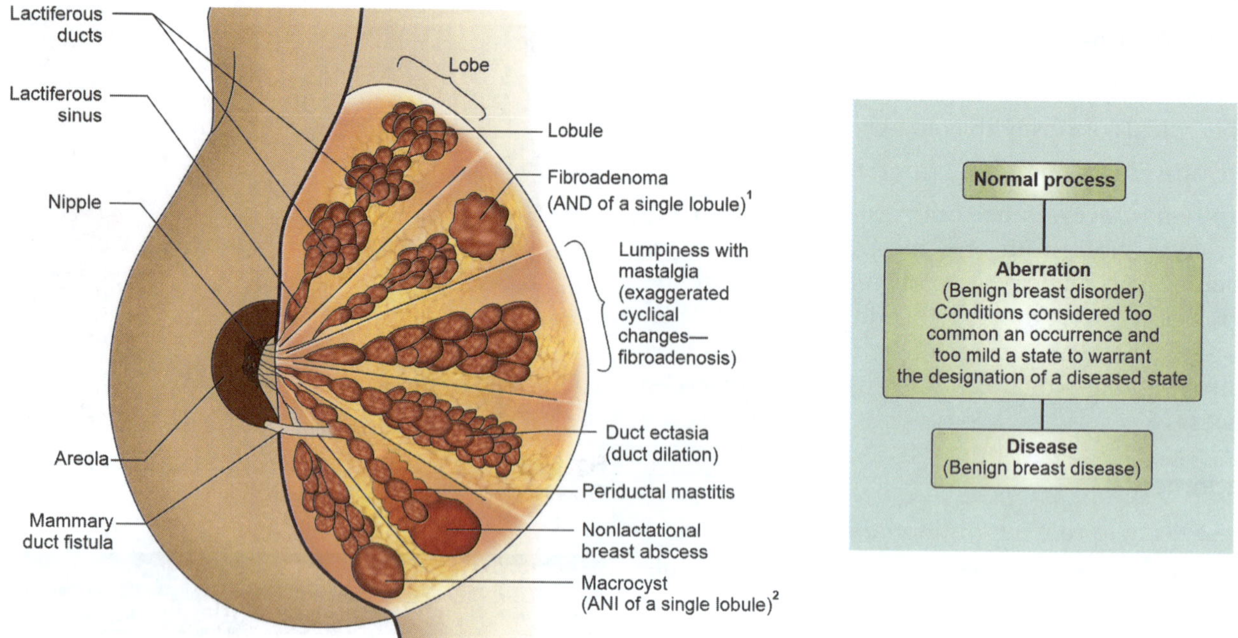

Fig. 39.13: Benign breast disorders and diseases (*Courtesy:* Dr Stanley Mathew, Professor, Department of Surgery, KMC, Manipal)
Note:[1] *Fibroadenoma is an **AND** (Aberration of Normal Development) of a lobule.*
[2]*Cyst (macrocyst) is an **ANI** (Aberration of Normal Involution) of a lobule.*

If it is not possible to conclusively rule out the possibility of malignancy, then the patient would be best advised a lumpectomy.

The term ANDI should not be confined to imply fibroadenosis (now termed mastalgia with nodularity).

ANDI includes several aberrations and disorders (Table 39.1). Table 39.1 includes all the aberrations, disorders and disease entities originally included under the ANDI classification as proposed by LE Hughes, et al.

Table 39.1 Aberration of the **N**ormal **D**evelopment and **I**nvolution **(ANDI)** of the breast

Stage (Peak age in years)	Normal process	Aberration: Underlying condition	Aberration: Clinical presentation	Disease state
Early reproductive period (15–25 years)	Lobule formation	Fibroadenoma	Discrete lump	Giant fibroadenoma (more than 5 cm).
	Stroma formation Nipple eversion	Juvenile hypertrophy Nipple	Excessive breast development	Multiple fibroadenomas Submammary abscess/ mammary fistula
Mature reproductive period (25–40 years)	Cyclical hormonal effects on glandular tissue and stroma	Exaggerated cyclical effects. Bloody discharge per nipple	Generalised or discrete lump	Cyclical mastalgia and nodularity (incapacitating)
Involution (25–55 years)	Lobular involution (including microcysts, apocrine changes, fibrosis, adenosis)	Macrocysts Sclerosing lesions Adenosis	Discrete lumps X-ray abnormalities	Cystic diseases
	Ductal involution (including periductal round cell infiltrates), dilate with scleroma	Duct dilatation Periductal fibrosis	Nipple discharge Nipple retraction	Periductal mastitis with bacterial infection and nonlactational breast mammary duct fistula
	Epithelial turnover	Mild epithelial hyperplasia	Histological report	Epithelial hyperplasia with atypia

Terms to be avoided: Fibroadenosis—replace with mastalgia and nodularity.
Cystosarcoma phyllodes—replace with phyllodes tumour.
Instructions to the students: Carefully go through Tables 39.1, 39.2 and Fig. 39.1
References: British Medical Bulletin: Volume 47, Number 2, April 1991.

Table 39.2 Classification of benign breast diseases

Nonproliferative disorders	Proliferative breast disorders	Atypical
• Cysts, apocrine metaplasia • Duct ectasia • Calcification • Fibroadenoma and other related lesions	• Sclerosing adenosis • Intraductal papilloma • Ductal epithelial hyperplasia • Radial scar • Complex sclerosing lesions	• Atypical ductal hypoplasia (ADH) • Atypical lobular hypoplasia (ALH)

Breast Pain

- It is for mastalgia that many women attend breast clinic. It can be classified as given in Table 39.3.
- If painful nodularity is present for more than one week, it is significant (more than normal discomfort).
- Cyclical mastalgia pain is bilateral, located in the upper quadrant of the breast, poorly localised, radiation to the axilla and patient also complains of the heaviness of the breast.

CYCLICAL MASTALGIA WITH NODULARITY

Also called **mammary dysplasia**, fibrocystic disease, ***Schimmelbusch disease,*** hormonal mastopathy, or fibroadenosis.

The term ANDI should not be confined to imply fibroadenosis (now termed mastalgia and nodularity). In fact fibroadenoma is an AND of a lobule and cyst (macrocyst) is an ANI of a lobule.

Definition

- It is an aberration of physiological changes that occur in the breast from menarche till menopause. It is an ANDI (aberration in normal development and involution).
- Women around the age of 40 are the usual sufferers.

Table 39.3 Mastalgia

Cyclical	Noncyclical
• Related to monthly cycles • Associated with premenstrual nodularity and breast discomfort	• Less common • Pain can be due to periductal mastitis or costochondritis (Tietz's disease)
• Excessive prolactin release from pituitary gland may be the cause	• Simple measures, such as well supported brassieres
• Premenopausal women are affected (35 years age) • Reassurance • Drugs • Excision—last resort	• Analgesics may be beneficial • Injection with local anaesthetic on a trigger point

Pathology (Key Box 39.4)

1. **Fibrosis** results in increased connective tissue growth. Fat and elastic tissue become less, and chronic inflammatory cells, such as plasma cells, can be present.
2. **Cyst formation:** Fibrosis compresses the ductules, which is responsible for cyst formation. Hence, it is a retention cyst. The cyst contains dark mucoid material and it may discharge serous fluid or green coloured fluid through the nipple. Hence, it is called ***fibrocystic disease*** of the breast. Cyst may be single or multiple confined to one lobe or many lobes. These are microcysts.
3. **Adenosis:** Proliferation of the acini and gland is an important feature of fibroadenosis.
4. **Epitheliosis:** Fibroadenosis is not a precancerous condition but if the degree of **epitheliosis** is more, it can be considered as **premalignant** condition. Epithelial hyperplasia mainly occurs in the acini.
5. **Papillomatosis** and **apocrine metaplasia** of the epithelium lining cystic spaces are the other features. These changes are not considered premalignant.

Key Box 39.4

Pathology

- Fibrosis
- Cyst formation
- Adenosis
- Epitheliosis
- Papillomatosis
- Apocrine metaplasia

Clinical Features

- Females around the age of 30–40 are the victims—spinsters, married childless women and women who have not suckled their babies are the usual sufferers.
- Severe pain in the breast in the premenstrual period and during menstruation. **It is called cyclical mastalgia.** Upper outer quadrant, bilaterally is affected.

- Clinical examination of the breast reveals a coarse, nodular, tender, lumpiness which is better felt with the finger and the thumb. Often, there are multiple, irregular, firm, nodularities palpable bilaterally, especially in the upper outer quadrants. Nipple discharge which is serous or green coloured may occur.

Treatment

It can be discussed on the following headings:

- Reassurance
- Lifestyle modifications
- Evening primrose oil
- Bromcryptine
- Antioxidants
- Topical NSAID
- Danazol
- Tamoxifen
- Non-steroidal SERM
- Goserelin

1. **Reassurance is the most effective treatment for mastalgia:** Breast pain may be cyclical (worse before a period) or non-cyclical, originating from the breast or the chest wall, and occurs at some time in 70% of women. Cyclical breast pain resolves spontaneously in 20 to 30% of women, but tends to recur in 60% of women. Non-cyclical pain responds poorly to treatment but tends to resolve spontaneously in half of women. Sometimes so serious disturbs routine activities. Support to the breast, reassurance, a few drugs. Surgeon should have good communication skills in these cases. Just to assure the lady that this is not a cancer, this is not a serious disease, it is just an aberration of normal physiology, related to hormonal changes and it may disappear. Vast majority of patients can be managed by reassurance only. However, in a few patients, it will not work. They require pharmacotherapy.
2. **Lifestyle modifications:** Decrease use of coffee, cigarettes, calories, chocolates. Caffeine restriction is an effective means of management of breast pain associated with fibrocystic disease. Smoking might increase breast pain by increasing epinephrine levels.
3. **Evening primrose oil (EPO):** Basis: Cyclical mastalgia patients have abnormal fatty acid profiles and decreased levels of essential fatty acids. EPO contains 7% linolenic acid and 72% linoleic acid. 1000 mg 3 to 6 times per day. 3 to 4 months period. No side effects.

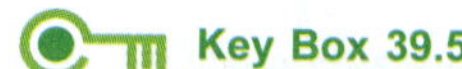
Key Box 39.5

Evening Primrose Oil

- First choice of treatment of cyclical mastalgia is evening primrose oil (EPO)
- Useful to treat mild to moderate cyclical mastalgia
- EPO contains 7% linolenic acid and 72% linoleic acid
- Dose is 1000 mg capsule—6 per day
- EPO can be taken with oral contraceptive pills
- No side effects

Initially proved to have a role in treating cyclical mastalgia, but no trials have been able to prove the benefit over and above the control oils, placebo oils and antioxidants (Key Box 39.5).

4. **Bromocriptine** which decreases the prolactin levels, 1.25 mg, twice a day, may reduce the pain and may be increased to 2.5 mg twice a day. It is useful for cyclical mastalgia.
5. **Danazol** is a gonadotrophin releasing hormone inhibitor. 200–400 mg/day, thrice a day is given. It acts by reducing FSH and LH levels.
6. **Tamoxifen** 10 mg, twice a day, is a better alternative to danazol.
7. **Other drugs:** Antioxidants, non-steroidal SERM and Goserelin also have been used rarely.

Treatment may have to be continued for some months (Table 39.4).

Pearls of Wisdom

- Diuretics have no role. Topical NSAID application may help.
- Danazol is the best drug in cases of noncyclical mastalgia but it is teratogenic. Hence, the patient should take precautions against pregnancy.

Surgery

Indications for surgery:

- FNAC suggests **epitheliosis**
- A very **painful lump**
- A hard lump about which the patient is worried and anxious.

1. **Excision of the lump.** Surgery for fibroadenosis ends up in removing some breast tissue and the lump. As it has no capsule of its own, it is a messy surgery unlike fibroadenoma surgery (Figs 39.14 to 39.16).
2. Is there a role for **subcutaneous mastectomy?** In patients with family history of breast carcinoma, if they have lumps in the breast with severe degree of epitheliosis, it may be worthwhile doing subcutaneous mastectomy.

Table 39.4 Drug treatment of cyclical mastalgia

Drug	Mechanism of action	Dose	Maintenance dose	Side effects
1. Evening primrose oil	• Contains essential fatty acids which correct abnormal prostaglandin synthesis • Natural form of gamolenic acid	• 1000 mg/day 6 capsules • First choice in cyclical mastalgia • 4 months treatment	• Can be reduced to 3 capsules/day • Mild to moderate mastalgia	No side effects
2. Danazol	Interfere with FSH and LH	• 50 mg/day—increased to 100 mg/day	• 50 mg/day for 3 months • Severe breast pain with nodularity	Amenorrhoea Weight gain Acne, hirsutism
3. Bromocriptine	It lowers prolactin by blocking its release from pituitary	• 2.5 mg/day—slowly increased to 2.5 mg twice/daily	• 2.5 mg/day • Inferior to danazol	Nausea, vomiting, dizziness
4. Tamoxifen	Antioestrogen	• 10 mg/day for 3 months	• Only for 3 months • Start if relapses occur	Minimal when used for short period.
5. Goserelin	Luteinising hormone Releasing hormone analogue	• 98% success in cyclical mastalgia	• Reserved for refractory cases	Reversible postmenopausal symptoms

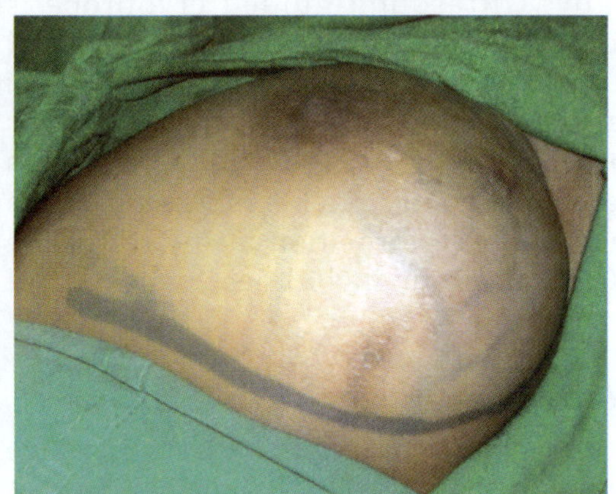

Fig. 39.14: Submammary incision is given to excise a large lump in the breast

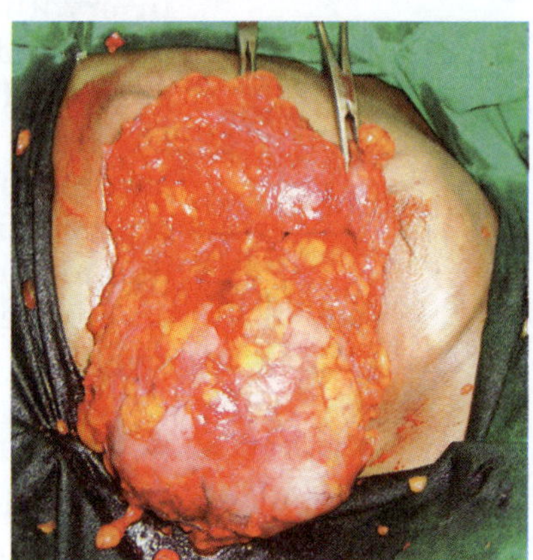

Fig. 39.15: Observe the nodularity of the lump

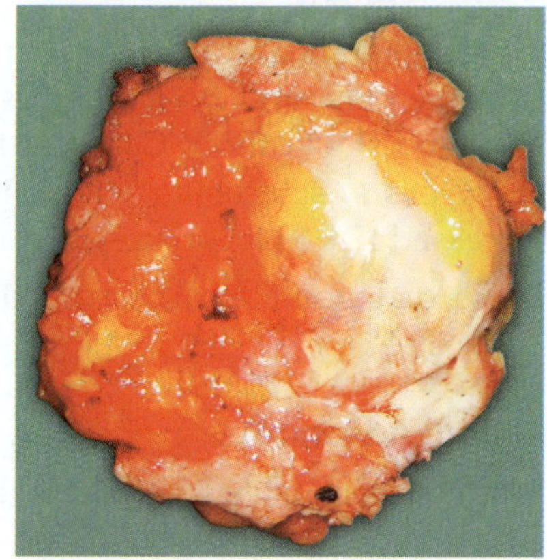

Fig. 39.16: Excised specimen having nodularity and cystic changes

Competency

SU25.3: Describe the etiopathogenesis, clinical features, investigations and principles of treatment of benign and malignant tumours of breast.

Benign tumour of the breast is fibroadenoma—given here. Malignant tumours are: Phylloides and carcinoma breast are given in page ...

FIBROADENOMA

It is a benign tumour in which the epithelial cells are arranged in a fibrous stroma. It is an **AND** (**A**berration of **N**ormal **D**evelopment) of a single lobule.

Types

1. Pericanalicular type in which fibrosis is more.
2. Intracanalicular type in which fibrosis is less.

Pearls of Wisdom

- Small fibroadenomas (1 cm in size or less) are considered normal.
- Larger fibroadenomas (up to 3 cm) are disorders.
- Giant fibroadenomas (more than 3 cm) are a disease.

Clinical Features

- Peak age of incidence is at 20 years.
- Patients present with painless lump in the breast.
- It is smooth, round bordered, firm to hard in consistency, and freely mobile within the breast.
- Due to its free movement within breast tissue, it is known as **breast mouse**.
- However, when fibroadenoma occurs in elderly patients, it may not have characteristic features because of fibrosis.

Treatment

- Excision of the lump
  1. In **intracanalicular** type, the lump is deeper and peripheral. It is removed by submammary incision.
  2. In **pericanalicular** type (Figs 39.17 and 39.18), the lump is superficial. It is removed by periareolar incision.

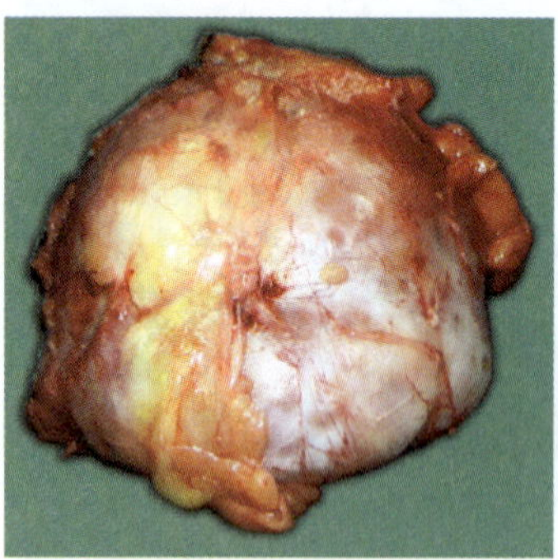
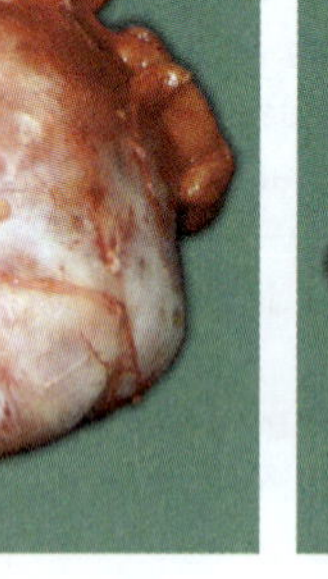

Fig. 39.17: Fibroadenoma excised—external view

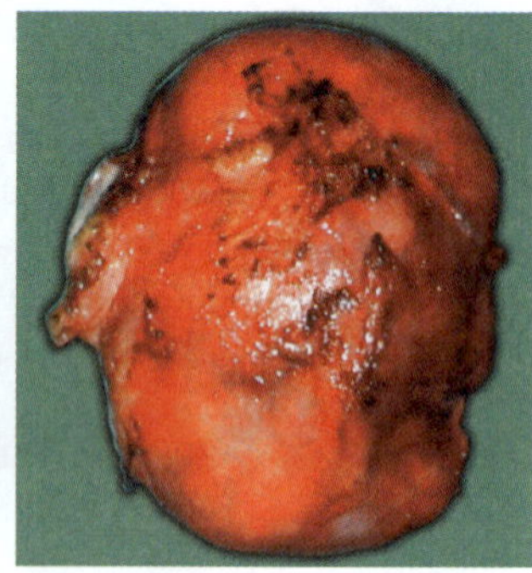

Fig. 39.18: Fibroadenoma—excised specimen

Complications

Fibroadenoma and malignancy: Patients with **simple** fibroadenoma and no family history of breast cancer have no risk of cancer. **Complex** fibroadenomas which show cysts, sclerosing adenosis, calcification have increased risk (3 to 4 times) of cancer.

Fibroadenoma and fibroadenosis are compared in Table 39.5.

Recent Advances

Minimally invasive techniques are becoming popular. Advantages being breast preservation, no scarring and cosmesis is better. Four types of treatment is followed.

1. Surveillance and no Treatment

Basis: 40% of fibroadenoma remain stable at the end of 2 years and 20% of fibroadenoma resolve without treatment. Hence women under 40 years of age, conservative treatment of reassurance, surveillance and observation. Automated breast volume scans are available to detect even a minute increase in fibroadenomas—useful specially in multiple fibroadenomas.

2. High Intensity Focused Ultrasound

Non-invasive treatment which ablates the tissues. It uses the **piezoelectric transducer** inside a ultrasound machine and generates a high frequency high intensity ultrasound beam. This beam is directed towards the specific target area of fibroadenoma. It results in **increase in local temperature**, denaturation of protein, cell death and results in tissue necrosis due to temperature. A few reports say about 50% reduction of maximum diameter of the fibroadenoma and also with significant reduction in the discomfort or pain. However, takes about **more than 2 hours**.

3. Cryotherapy

Localized destruction of the target tissue happens in cryotherapy. Ultrasound-guided cryoprobe is introduced into the fibroadenoma after making a **small skin incision**. Cooling temperature is **–170°C.** Different varieties of systems are available such as argon-gas-based system, using liquid nitrogen as cryogen. Irreversible damage to fibroadenoma occurs due to **intracellular ice** formation at the tip of the cryoprobe. Complications include **ecchymosis and swelling**.

4. Vacuum-Assisted Excision

Small incision is made in the breast and 8 or 11 gauge probe is inserted through the lesion. Small amount of tissue is aspirated. **Probe is inserted into different parts** of the tissue and aspirated again. Procedure will take about 30 to 60 minutes. Compression is applied at the site of puncture. Haematoma, recurrence and post-procedure pain are complications.

Table 39.5 Differences between fibroadenoma and fibroadenosis

	Fibroadenoma	Fibroadenosis
• Incidence	Less common	More common
• Nature	Benign tumour of one lobule	Aberration of normal changes in the breast
• Pain in the breast	Not a feature	Very common, premenstrual
• Location	Unilateral	Usually bilateral
• Lump	Well-defined, firm, mobile	Irregular, ill-defined, tender lump
• Capsule	Well-defined	No capsule
• Discharge	No	Serous or green coloured
• Malignancy	Rarely–sarcoma	Carcinoma (if epitheliosis is present)
• Treatment	Excision	Excision or drugs

DUCT ECTASIA/PERIDUCTAL MASTITIS—PLASMA CELL MASTITIS

- Common in middle-aged women.
- There is primary dilatation in one of the lactiferous ducts.

Aetiology

- Actual cause is not known. **Mild low-grade infection** (anaerobic bacteria) has been considered as one of the factors. Enterococci, staphylococci, bacteroids are also found.
- The toxic substances in cigarette smoke may damage ducts directly or cause local hypoxia.
- Increased in **smokers:** Smoking increases the **virulence** of commensal bacteria.

Pathology

- There is dilatation of one of the lactiferous ducts.
- Due to dilatation, the contents tend to undergo stasis. The epithelial debris, and serous fluid collectively form a thick paste-like material rich in lipid.
- It may cause discharge per nipple
- There is **intense periductal inflammation with lymphocytes and plasma cells** (Fig. 39.19). Hence, it is called plasma cell mastitis (Key Box 39.6).
- Fibrosis causes nipple retraction.

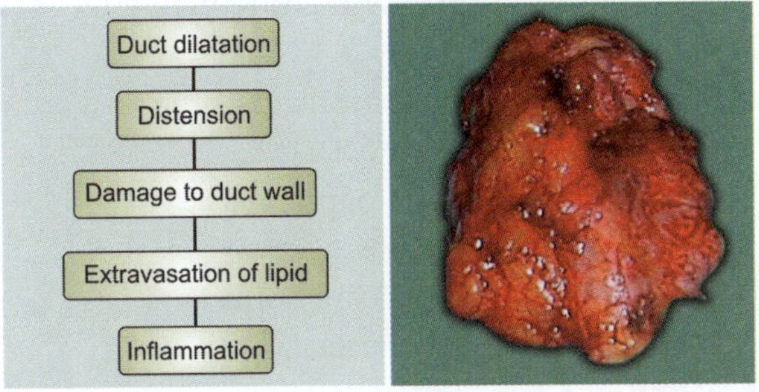

Fig. 39.19: Excised specimen. Observe the fibrosis due to periductal inflammation

Key Box 39.6

Summary of the Treatment of Periductal Mastitis

Periductal infiltration of plasma cells, lymphocytes
Excision of all major ducts (Hadfield's operation)
Retraction of nipple (partial)
Infection by anaerobes/irritation by smoking
Dilatation of breast /ducts
Untreated—abscess/fistula/lump
Creamy/paste-like discharge
Treated by co-amoxiclav and metronidazole
Remember as **PERIDUCT**

Clinical Features

- Middle-aged woman
- **Paste-like material** discharge per nipple.
- After some time, because of fibrosis, a lump can be felt, which can be confused for carcinoma of breast.
- **Bilateral slit-like retraction of nipple** of long duration.
- Recurrent abscess and recurrent fistula are other complications.
- Routine mammogram—microcalcification
- Palpable subareolar mass

Management

- FNAC to confirm diagnosis.
- Antibiotics, drainage, excision of all major ducts.

IDIOPATHIC GRANULOMATOUS MASTITIS (IGM)

- IGM is a rare, inflammatory noncaseating chronic granulomatous benign disease occurs within 5 years of parturition. It is an autoimmune localised response.
- Often patients present with features of mastitis (non-lactating) with pain, nipple retraction, lump in the breast.
- Some of them are treated with antituberculous treatment with FNAC, tru-cut or even biopsy findings of granuloma but they are nontuberculous.
- When tuberculosis, sarcoidosis, diabetes and Wegener's granulomatosis are excluded, the diagnosis of idiopathic granulomatous mastitis is made.
- Aetiology is not known. However, a few factors responsible can be autoimmune disease, undetected organisms, reaction to childbirth, use of oral contraceptives, hyperprolactinaemia?
- To begin with damage to ductular epithelium by infection, trauma or chemically induced inflammation. As a result of which, luminal secretion to escape into the lobular connective tissue. It stimulates a granulomatous response. Further damages the lobular structures. Hence, it is also called idiopathic lobular granulomatous mastitis.
- Characteristic histological features include multinucleated giant cells, epithelioid histiocytes—noncaseating.
- Recurrent bouts of mastitis and or chronic discharging sinuses. Core biopsy is done to rule out malignancies and tuberculosis or sarcoidosis. Organisms, if any, to be treated—*Corynebacterium kroppenstedtii* infection. The diagnosis of IGM is established via core needle biopsy of a solid mass. The biopsy should be sent for Gram stain, bacterial culture, acid-fast bacilli stain and culture, fungal stain and culture, and histopathology.

- Many diseases may cause granulomatous response in the breast including cryptococcosis, actinomycosis, filariasis, autoimmune diseases, plasma cell mastitis, etc.
- IGM is a self-limiting inflammatory condition that resolves slowly; complete resolution may take 9 to 12 months. Steroids, oral and topical, can be used. **Steroids with methotrexate—10 to 15 mg/week found to be successful. 80% success rates.**
- ***Corynebacterium* infection**—amoxicillin-clavulanate (875 mg orally every 12 hours); for penicillin-allergic patients, doxycycline (100 mg orally twice daily) may be used.

MACROCYSTS

- They occur due to excessive secretion of thin fluid within the lobules which enlarge to produce a cyst. Clinically, they present as firm swelling in the breast. It is an ANDI of a single lobule (firm because it is tense).
- They can be single or multiple. One of them can have huge dimension having a thin bluish capsule—***blue-domed cyst of Bloodgood*** (Figs 39.20 to 39.21 and Key Box 39.11).

Treatment

Excision of cyst in the following situations:

1. Recurrence after 2 aspirations
2. Blood-stained aspirate
3. Residual lump after aspiration.

GALACTOCELE (Fig. 39.22)

- It is a solitary, subareolar retention cyst filled with milk. It occurs and dates back to the lactational period.
- It occurs due to inadequate drainage of the milk added by epithelial debris which blocks the lactiferous duct. Once the duct is blocked, proximally, the milky fluid accumulates resulting in a huge enlargement of breast.

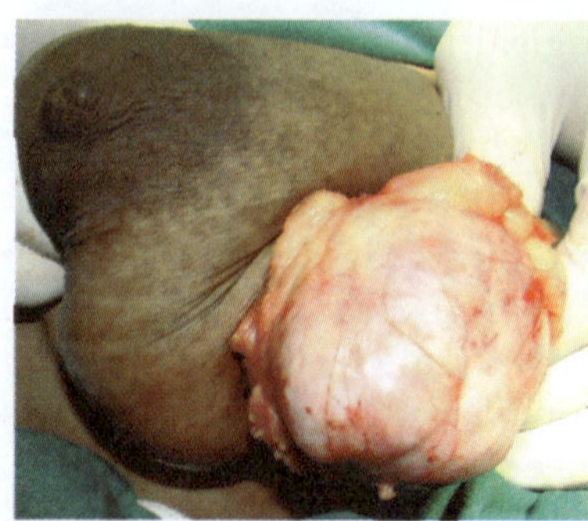
Fig. 39.20: Submammary incision—cyst delivered

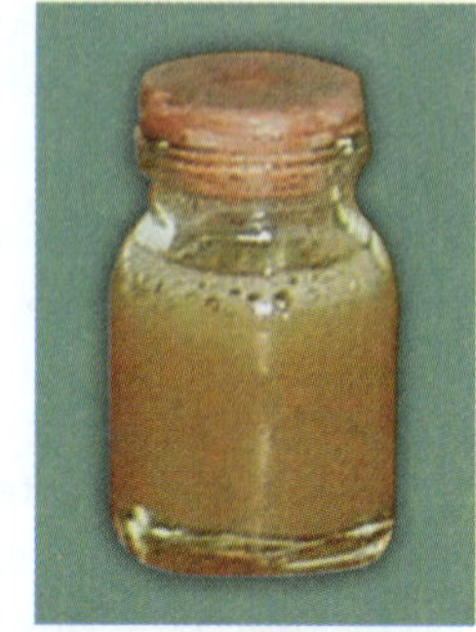
Fig. 39.21: Fibrocystic disease—nature of fluid

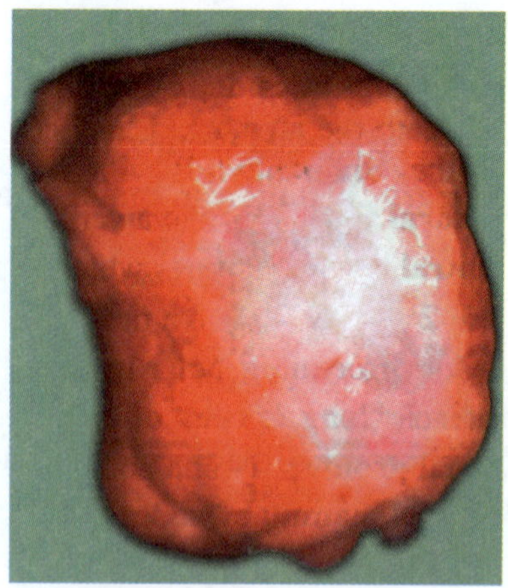
Fig. 39.22: Galactocele

- Rarely, they undergo calcification.
- It is treated by repeated aspirations. Duct patency can be restored by using 4-0 nylon.
- Excision is the last choice.

DISCHARGE PER NIPPLE

Nipple Discharge

- It is a common problem encountered in the outpatient department. It can be physiological, such as lactational and/or pathological from various causes.
- The clinical evaluation of the case of nipple discharge consists of the following history examination.

1. **Nature of the discharge:**

• Serous	Fibrocystic disease Duct ectasia
• Bloody	Duct papilloma Duct ectasia Duct carcinoma
• Greenish	Duct ectasia
• Milk	Lactational Non-lactational—Hyperprolactinaemia Oestrogen replacement therapy
• Yellow (purulent)	Breast abscess

2. **Unilateral or bilateral:** Duct papilloma is unilateral; fibrocystic disease and hyperprolactinaemia are bilateral.
3. **Single or multiple ducts:** Duct carcinoma/duct papilloma involves single duct, but fibrocystic disease affects multiple ducts.
4. **Spontaneous discharge** is typical of duct papilloma. Blood-stained discharge on pressing the mass may be seen in carcinoma breast.

5. **Related to menstruation:** This is seen in fibrocystic disease and patients who are taking oestrogen replacement therapy.
6. **Discharge with mass:**
   - Tender mass—fibrocystic disease breast abscess
   - Nontender mass—carcinoma

Localisation

- Mammogram and ultrasound to detect any mass, any cystic lesions. Very often they do not help in the diagnosis.
- Prolactin levels, thyroid hormone profile (rarely hypothyroidism can cause discharge per nipple)
- Cytological examination of bloody discharge for malignancy.
- Ductoscopy has been done but not very successful.

Treatment

- Rule out carcinoma—first
- Watery/serous discharge needs reassurance after ruling out fibrocystic disease
- A duct papilloma requires microdochectomy
- Discharge from multiple ducts or origin of the discharge is not clear—'core excision' of major ducts should be done (Hadfield's operation).

GALACTORRHOEA

Secretion of milk unrelated to breastfeeding.

Causes

Physiological

- Stimulation during sexual activity.
- Extremes of reproductive age (puberty and menopause)

Drugs

- Oral contraceptive agents and oestrogen
- Antihypertensive agents, such as methyldopa, atenelol, clonidine
- Dopamine receptor blocking agents, such as chlorpromazine, haloperidol, metoclopramide.
- H_2 receptor antagonists, such as ranitidine

Pathological

- Pituitary adenoma/microadenoma

Miscellaneous

- Ectopic prolactin secretion
- Hypothyroidism
- Chronic renal failure

Treatment

- If the cause is identified, such as drugs mentioned above, stop them.
- If any other reason is detected, then treat the cause.
- Often no cause is identified, reassure the patient.

DUCT PAPILLOMA

- It is a benign lesion of the breast, usually single and, unilateral, rarely multiple.
- Middle-aged women are affected and present with bleeding per nipple (Fig. 39.23).
- The tumour is situated in one of the larger lactiferous ducts.
- It presents as a small swelling just beneath the areola, palpation of which results in **discharge of blood**.
- Since, it is a *premalignant condition*, it is treated by microdochectomy.
- **Microdochectomy:** The opening of the lactiferous duct discharging blood is identified. It is probed with lacrimal probe or a straight needle. A small triangular piece of skin, along with the needle, and a wedge of breast tissue to a depth of about 4–5 cm is removed (Figs 39.24 and 39.25).
- **Hadfield's operation:** Cone excision of the lactiferous ducts is done when duct of origin of nipple bleeding

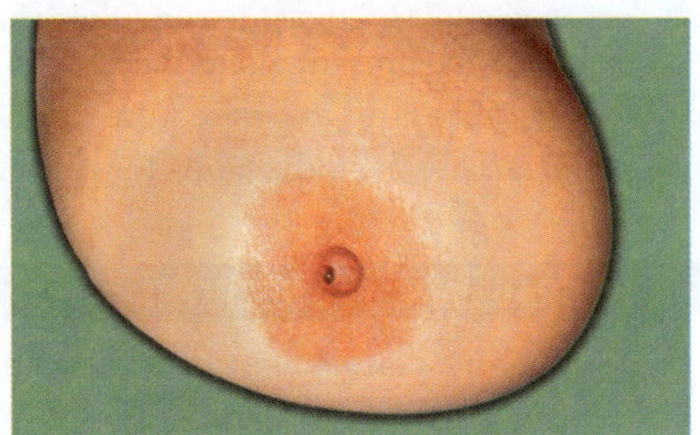

Fig. 39.23: Bleeding per nipple

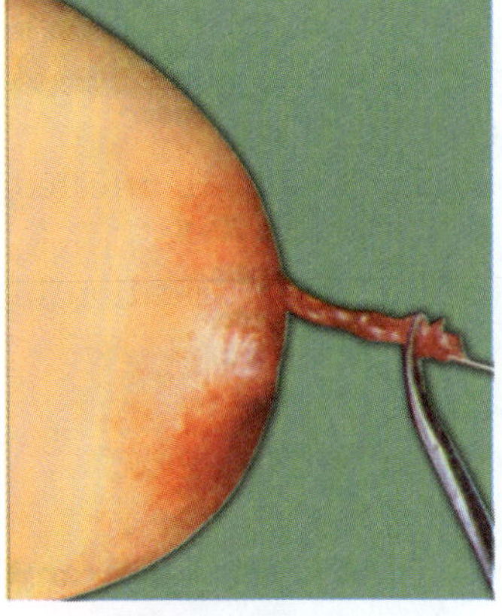

Fig. 39.24: Papilloma excision

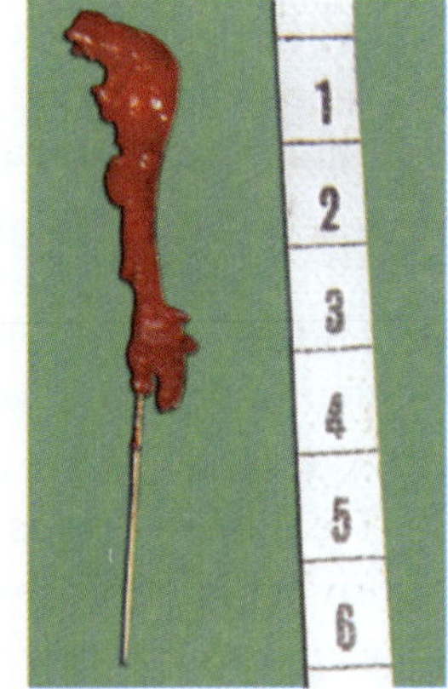

Fig. 39.25: Specimen of papilloma

is uncertain. A circumareolar incision confined to one-third of the circumference is given and deepened. The flap is better not raised to avoid necrosis of areola. A core or cone of breast tissue from nipple to pectoral fascia or about 5 cm length is removed. **Most of the ductal papilloma will be located within 5 cm from the nipple.**

- **Nipple ductoscopy:** Fibreoptic—less than 1 cm diameter with 0.2 mm secondary channel attachment. Ductoscopy—dilatations can be done—sterile saline is used for distension. Minimally invasive, scarless. According to the findings, it can be classified as polypoidal, epithelial, suspicious, normal. Excision of papilloma/lesions can be done. It is not possible to remove lesions that are more than 10 mm.

AXILLARY TAIL HYPERTROPHY

- More commonly it is the enlargement of axillary tail of Spence.
- It is usually bilateral and feels like fatty tissue, lobular, soft to firm. This is how it is differentiated from lymph nodes in the axilla.
- Causes can be physiological at puberty or during premenstrual/menstruation period or can be a part of 'ANDI'.
- Pregnancy is also one of the causes of enlargement.
- Rarely 'ectopic' axillary breast tissue other than tail of the breast may be present along the milk line.
- Usually reassurance is all that is required.
- *Pain* and *cosmesis* are the indications for removal.

TRAUMATIC FAT NECROSIS

T: Trauma either by a direct blow or by a seat belt or trivial contraction of pectoralis major. Sometimes no history of trauma.

R: Retraction of nipple, palpable hard lump, tethering of skin mimic carcinoma.

A: Acids—fatty acids and glycerol released due to injury to the fat causes saponification.

U: Unusually large, pendulous breasts are affected more often.

M: Middle-aged women with microcalcification in mammography—mimics carcinoma.

A: Age around 40 to 50 years

T: Treatment—biopsy/excision of the lumps

I: Immediate reconstruction is possible

C: Can develop after tamoxifen therapy and, after any type of breast surgery

You can *remember as* **TRAUMATIC**

GYNAECOMASTIA

This is an *unphysiological enlargement of the male breast.*

Causes

Physiologic causes

- Neonatal period, adolescence, senescence
- Idiopathic is the most common wherein no cause can be identified. However, there are many other causes of gynaecomastia which can be summarised as "**MASTIA**" (Key Box 39.7).

Key Box 39.7

MASTIA

- **M**alignant tumour: Teratoma, bronchogenic carcinoma.
- **A**norchism: Absent testis
- **S**ex chromosome anomaly: Klinefelter's syndrome (XXY).
- **T**ablets: Cimetidine, stilboesterol, digitalis, spironolactone
- **I**diopathic: No cause is found
- **A**trophy of the testis: Liver cell failure, leprosy, etc.

Clinical Classification of Gynaecomastia

Grade I	Mild grade enlargement
Grade IIa	Moderate grade enlargement
Grade IIb	Moderate grade enlargement with skin redundancy
Grade III	Marked grade enlargement with skin redundancy and ptosis (simulates a female breast)

Clinical Features

- In idiopathic variety, gynaecomastia is bilateral. In other cases, it may be unilateral.
- A 'disk' like tender lump is palpable, with smooth surface.
- Examination should also include palpation of testis and to look for liver cell failure.

Treatment

Lumpectomy or mastectomy with preservation of nipple and areola (subcutaneous mastectomy).

Complications

Rarely, gynaecomastia can predispose to male breast carcinoma (Fig. 39.26).

Pearls of Wisdom

- However, innocent looking the breast lump may be, it can be malignant unless proved otherwise.
- Multicentricity refers to occurrence of a second *in situ* breast cancer outside the breast quadrant of primary *in situ* carcinoma.

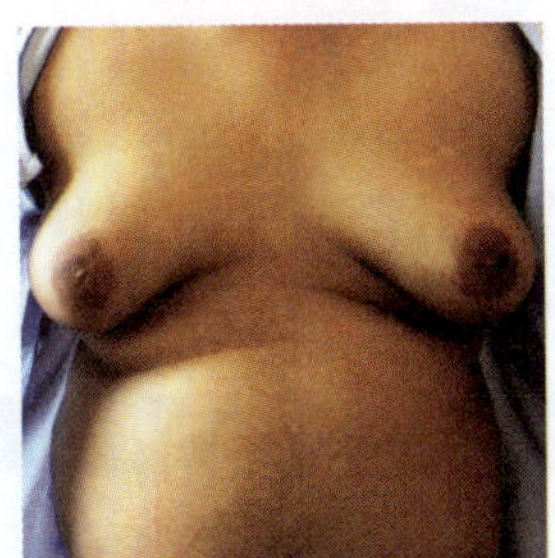

Fig. 39.26: Gynaecomastia (*Courtesy:* Dr Satish Deshmukh and Dr Murtaza Akhthar, NKP Salve Institute of Medical Sciences, Nagpur)

Competency

SU25.3: Describe the etiopathogenesis, clinical features, investigations and principles of treatment of malignant tumours of breast.

PHYLLODES TUMOURS

- They are fibroepithelial tumours composed of an epithelial and cellular stromal component.
- Earlier known as cystosarcoma phyllodes and mistakenly labelled as a giant intracanalicular fibroadenoma. They are tumours of the breast, with a predilection to attain massive size and recur locally after lumpectomy (Figs 39.27 and 39.28).
- It is considered as potentially malignant tumour of the breast.
- Account for less than 1% of all breast neoplasms.

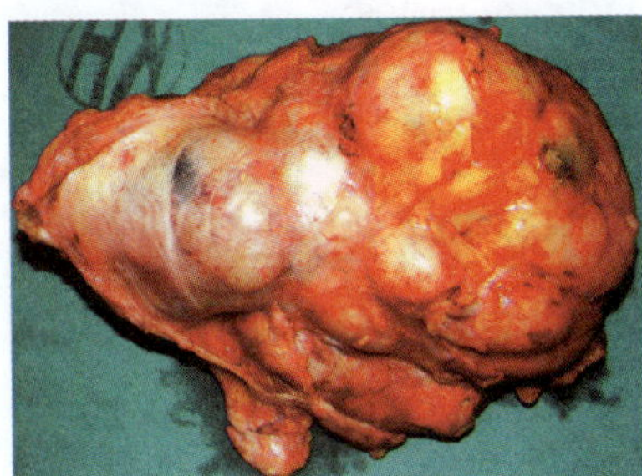

Fig. 39.27: Phyllodes tumour of the left breast at surgery (*Courtesy:* Dr Hartimath B, Associate Professor, KMC, Manipal)

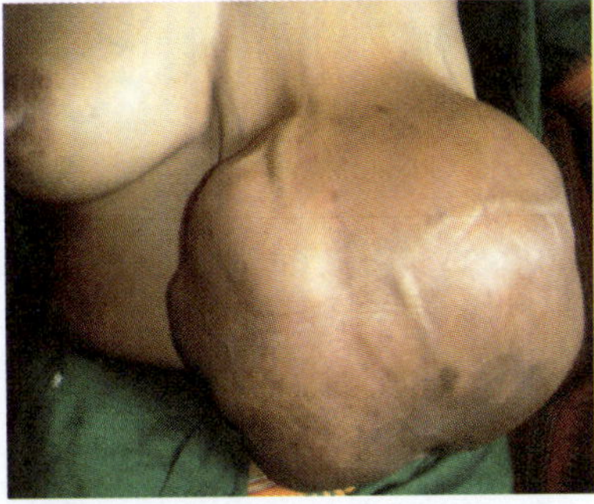

Fig. 39.28: Phyllodes tumour with dilated veins (*Courtesy:* Dr Sreejayan, Professor, Department of Surgery, Calicut Medical College, Kerala)

Types of Phyllodes

- Benign: **More than 60% younger women**
- Borderline Depends upon mitotic activity, cellularity
- Malignant and infiltration at the edge of the tumour

Clinical Features (Key Box 39.8)

- Age group—30 to 40 years—premenopausal
- Rapid growth
- Stretched, shiny skin
- Red, dilated veins over surface, warm to touch
- Bosselated surface (big nodules), a few cystic areas.

It is differentiated from carcinoma by:

- No fixity to the skin
- No fixity to the pectoralis—mobile on the chest wall
- Lymph nodes will not be involved.
- No nipple retraction.
  - As the tumour grows very fast, it undergoes necrosis in various places resulting in cystic areas within the breast. It discharges serous fluid. Hence, the name *serocystic disease of Brodie. However, it rarely feels cystic.*
  - Histologically, the tumour cells have a branching pattern, penetrating the cystic cavity (*phyllus* means leaf-like pattern). Fibrous stromal proliferation is a feature.

Diagnosis

- Very often, it is a clinical diagnosis.
- Ultrasound will help to detect the size of the tumour, solid and cystic areas.
- Tru-cut biopsy may reveal mitotic figures suggestive of malignancy.

Treatment of Phyllodes

I. Report after FNAC/excision:

A. Those who undergo, excision and report is fibroadenoma, just wait and watch.

B. If after excision report is phyllodes—benign and borderline—if 1 cm margin is adequate, just watch. If margin is not adequate—re-excise with 1 cm margin.

C. If it is invasive carcinoma or *in situ* carcinoma—treat accordingly.

Key Box 39.8

Bosselated Surface—Conditions

- Phyllodes tumour
- Polycystic kidney
- Polycystic liver
- Large nodular goitre

II. Report after core needle biopsy:

A. Excision if it is fibroadenoma, or indeterminate.

B. Phyllodes—benign and borderline and malignant wide local excision with 1 cm margin. Enlarged nodes should be subjected for biopsy (like carcinoma-sentinal node) and treat accordingly.

C. If it is invasive carcinoma or *in situ* carcinoma—treat accordingly.

D. When whole breast is involved as in advanced cases, simple mastectomy and re-construction.

Summary of Phyllodes Tumour

- Median age of presentation is 45 years.
- Rapid growth and large size can also be a feature of benign phyllodes tumour.
- Large lump with dilated veins, shiny skin is typical of phyllodes tumour.
- No nipple retraction, no skin fixation, no axillary nodes.
- High resolution ultrasound will reveal well-circumscribed lesion with smooth walls. Intramural septations can be defined better with MRI.
- Core biopsy can give more details about cellular pleomorphism, hypercellularity and nuclear hyperchromatism (Refer below).
- Distant metastasis rare—sites are lungs, bone, heart, liver.
- Adjuvant radiotherapy for phyllodes with recurrence with invasion to chest wall or inadequate margin, can be given.
- Chemotherapy, hormonal manipulations have proven no role.

Azzopardi and Salvadori criteria for diagnosis of nature of phyllodes tumour

	Histological type		
Criteria	**Benign**	**Borderline**	**Malignant**
Tumour margins	Pushing	—	Infiltrative
Stromal cellularity	Low	Moderate	High
Mitotic rate (per 10 hpf)	<5	5–9	>10
Pleomorphism	Mild	Moderate	Severe

Complications

- Pressure necrosis—secondary infection
- Distant spread—lungs and long bones

Intracystic Carcinoma of Breast: Reeclin's Disease

Rapidly growing carcinoma of the breast can undergo cystic degeneration resulting in a cyst, called intracystic carcinoma of the breast. Aspiration reveals haemorrhagic fluid, containing malignant cells and which refills after aspiration. Other features of carcinoma of the breast may be present.

Competency

SU25.3: Describe the etiopathogenesis, clinical features, investigations and principles of treatment of benign and malignant tumours of breast.

CARCINOMA BREAST

Incidence

Breast cancer is a major global public health concern for women in the 21st century. Worldwide it is leading cause of cancer in women and the leading cause of cancer-related mortality. In India as of 2018 ICMR statistics obtained from Indian Cancer Registries, it is the number one cancer afflicting women, also the leading cause of cancer-related mortality. In the United States, breast cancer remains the most frequent cancer in women and the second most frequent cause of cancer death. Better understanding of tumour biology, genetics and availability of advanced multimodality treatment options is gradually increasing survival.

RISK FACTORS FOR BREAST CANCER

The aetiology of breast cancer is multifactorial. A combination of risk factors appears to have a role in its causation. Majority of these factors carry a small to moderate increase in risk for any individual woman. We cannot identify risk factors in least half of women who develop breast cancer. These factors can be divided into two broad categories:

A. Non-modifiable

B. Modifiable

A. Non-Modifiable Risk Factors

Female sex: Women are 100 times more likely to have breast cancer as compared to men.

Age: Increasing age is a strong risk factor. Carcinoma breast is very rare below 20 years of age. More common in 35 to 75 years of age. Indian women tend to get carcinoma breast a decade earlier than western women.

Race: Highest in whites, rare in Japanese and Taiwanese population.

Breast Cancer and Hereditary Factors

- A family history of breast cancer has long been recognized as a risk factor for the disease, but only 5 to 10% of women who develop breast cancer have a true hereditary predisposition. Overall, the risk of developing breast cancer is increased 1.5- to 3-fold, if a woman has a mother or sister with breast cancer.
- **BRCA I and BRCA II genes** have been found in long arm of chromosome 17 and 13 respectively in women

with a family history of carcinoma of the breast. BRCA I and BRCA II are the genes associated with increased risk. BRCA I and II mutations are more common in Ashkenazi Jews. They are more prone to ovarian cancer also. Hence all patients with BRCA I and BRCA II mutations should consider a prophylactic bilateral oophorectomy after child-bearing is completed, with bilateral mastectomy.

- **Cowden's disease** (multiple hamartoma syndrome): It is associated with reduced tumour suppressor gene PTEN. 30–50% of patients will develop breast cancer by 50 years of age. The lesions found in this syndrome are multiple facial trichilemmoma (pathognomonic), oral papilloma, bilateral breast cancer, haemangiomas, lipomas, thyroid tumours, etc.
- **Ataxia telangiectasia:** It is associated with haemangioma and carcinoma breast.
- **Li-Fraumeni syndrome** is a rare disease with familial breast cancer and is associated with inherited mutation of tumour suppressor P53 gene. It is a rare autosomal dominant disorder. 90% of carriers will develop breast cancer by the age of 50. They also can have other tumours in childhood, such as soft tissue sarcoma, osteosarcoma, and leukaemia.

Patient which Requires Genetic Evaluation

Diagnosis of DCIS (ductal carcinoma *in situ*) or invasive breast cancer + one or more of the following:

- Diagnosed at 50 years and younger
- Triple-negative breast cancer diagnosed at 60 years and younger
- At any age:
  - A known mutation in a cancer susceptibility gene within the family
  - An additional breast cancer primary
  - ≥1 close blood relative (first to third degree) with breast cancer 50 years and younger
  - ≥1 close blood relative with ovarian cancer at any age
  - ≥2 close blood relatives with breast cancer, pancreatic cancer, or prostate cancer (Gleason score ≥7 or metastatic) at any age
- An individual of Ashkenazi Jewish ancestry
- Male breast cancer

Patients without diagnosis of cancer should consider further genetic risk evaluation, if they have:

- Close relative with a known mutation in a cancer susceptibility gene; 2 or more breast primaries in a single individual; 2 or more individuals with breast cancer on the same side of the family with at least one diagnosed at age of 50 years or younger; ovarian cancer
- Male breast cancer
- A first- or second-degree relative with cancer at age of 45 years or younger.
- A family history of 3 or more of the following: Breast cancer, pancreatic cancer, prostate cancer (Gleason 7 or higher or metastatic), melanoma, sarcoma, adrenal cortical carcinoma, brain tumours, leukaemia, diffuse gastric cancer, colon cancer, endometrial cancer, thyroid cancer, kidney cancer, dermatologic manifestations, and/or macrocephaly, or hamartomatous polyps of GI tract.

History of Breast Cancer

Risk of developing second breast cancer is about 0.5 to 0.7% in women with previous invasive breast cancers. Breast cancer is 3 to 4 times more likely to develop in women with a first degree relative who had breast cancer. **This risk is further increased, if they had premenopausal and bilateral cancer.** Women with ductal carcinoma *in situ* (DCIS) are at an increased risk of developing ipsilateral and contralateral breast cancers (4.1% after 5 years).

Hormonal Factors

The development of breast cancer in many women appears to be related to female reproductive hormones, particularly endogenous oestrogens. Early age at menarche, nulliparity or late age at first full-term pregnancy, and late age at menopause increase the risk of developing breast cancer.

Benign Breast Disease

Benign breast lesions are classified as proliferative or nonproliferative. Nonproliferative disease is not associated with an increased risk of breast cancer. Proliferative disease without atypia results in a small increase in risk, whereas proliferative disease with atypical hyperplasia is associated with a greater risk of breast cancer.

B. Modifiable Risk Factors (Table 39.6)

- Breastfeeding, particularly for longer duration, lowers the risk of breast cancer.
- Postmenopausal hormone replacement therapy (HRT) particularly when a combination of oestrogen and progesterone is used.
- Diet: Increased risk has been found in postmenopausal obese women and is due to increased synthesis of oestrogen (oestradiol) in the body fat. As a result of aromatisation of androgens in adipose tissue, circulatory oestrogen levels are increased. Increased intake of saturated fats and reduced intake of phyto-

[1]It means spread of individual cell proliferation in the upper level of dermis

Table 39.6 Lifetime risk factors and relative risk factors

Relative risk <2	Relative risk (2–4)	Relative risk >4
Early menarche	One first-degree relative with breast-cancer	Mutation BRCA I or BRCA II
Late menopause	CHEK2 mutation	Lobular carcinoma *in situ*
Nulliparity	Age older than 35 y for first birth	Ductal carcinoma *in situ*
Oestrogen plus progesterone	Proliferative breast disease	
Hormone replacement therapy	Mammographic breast density	Atypical hyperplasia
Alcohol use		Radiation exposure before age of 30 years
Postmenopausal obesity		

oestrogens increase risk. Decreased intake of nutrients such as vitamin C, folate, and β-carotene increases the risk (Fig. 39.29).

- Obesity is associated with both an increased risk of breast cancer development in postmenopausal women and increased breast cancer mortality.
- Smoking is risk factor for carcinoma breast.
- Alcohol intake is associated with a 1.5-fold increased risk of breast cancer.

Environmental Factors

Exposure to ionizing radiation at a young age increases risk of breast cancer. There is marked increased risk of breast cancer development has been reported in women who received mantle irradiation for the treatment of Hodgkin lymphoma before age of 15 years.

PATHOLOGY

Non-Invasive Breast Cancers (Precursor Lesions)

- These are lesions which may or may not turn into invasive breast cancer.
- They do not invade the basement membrane and survive by assimilation.
- They are diagnosed by screening mammogram or biopsy.

Ductal Carcinoma in Situ (DCIS)

- Proliferation of malignant-appearing mammary ductal epithelial cells without evidence of invasion beyond the basement membrane.
- A comedo-type ductal carcinoma *in situ*, also known as comedo-carcinoma *in situ* is the high grade subtype of ductal carcinoma *in situ* (Figs 39.30 and 39.31 shown here to compare with infiltrative carcinoma).
- It completely fills and dilates the ducts and lobules in terminal ductal-lobular unit with plugs of high grade tumour cells with central necrosis "comedonecrosis".
- Common presentation
  - Mammographically detected calcifications
  - Mass on mammogram (no palpable mass)
  - Palpable lump
  - An incidental finding at biopsy
  - Paget disease of the nipple

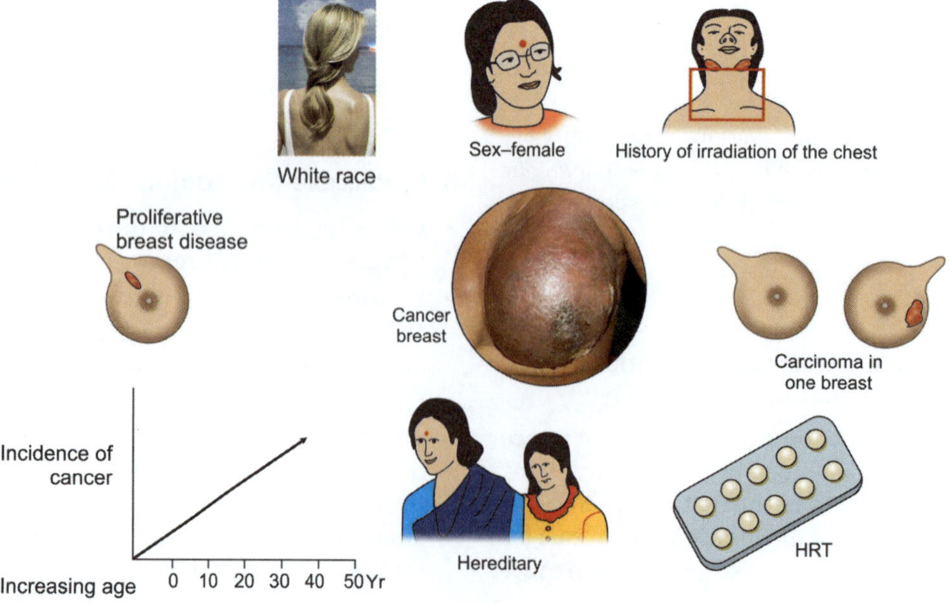

Fig. 39.29: Carcinoma breast—probable risk factors

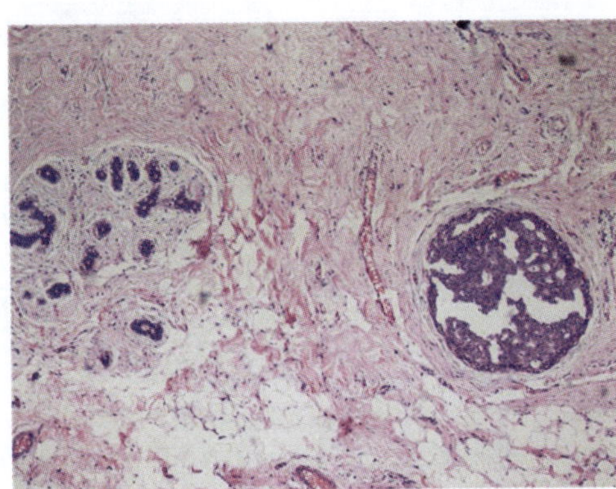

Fig. 39.30: Normal *vs* carcinoma *in situ*: Here you can see normal breast lobule (left) and *in situ* carcinoma (right) (*Courtesy:* Dr Laxmi Rao, Head, Department of Pathology, KMC, Manipal)

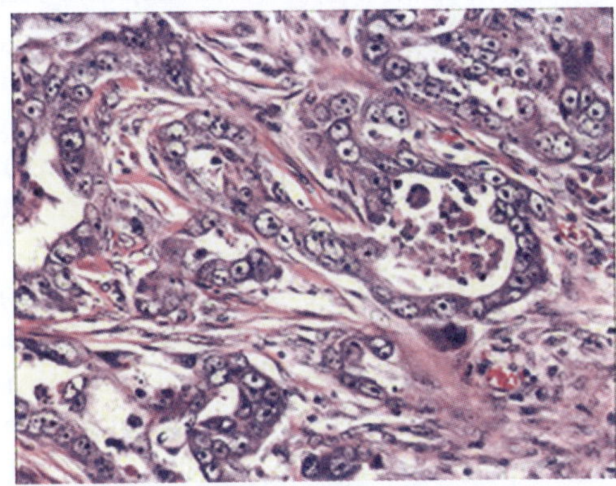

Fig. 39.31: Infiltrative ductal carcinoma: Infiltrating islands of malignant cells forming glands and trabeculae surrounded by desmoplastic stroma (*Courtesy:* Dr Laxmi Rao, Head, Department of Pathology, KMC, Manipal)

- There is no regional lymphadenopathy or distant metastasis
- **Treatment**
  - Breast conserving surgery followed by whole breast radiotherapy is the treatment of choice.
  - Alternatively simple mastectomy with sentinel lymph node biopsy should be done because mastectomy alters the lymphatic drainage pattern and makes future SLNB unfeasible.
  - **There is no role for chemotherapy.**
  - Premenopausal women receive tamoxifen.
  - Postmenopausal women receive letrozole.

Van Nuys Prognostic index for DCIS (Table 39.7)

- The Van Nuys Prognostic Index (VNPI) classifies patients with DCIS to guide decisions on the best treatment option. The index uses patient age, tumour size, tumour growth patterns (histological grade) and the amount of healthy tissue surrounding the tumour after removal (resection margin width) to predict the risk of cancer returning.
  - Low-risk (total VNPI score of 4–6)
    - Breast conserving surgery (BCS) without radiotherapy is recommended.
  - Intermediate-risk (total VNPI score of 7–9)
    - BCS with radiotherapy is recommended.
  - High-risk (total VNPI score of 10–12)
    - Mastectomy is recommended.

Table 39.7 Lobular carcinomas *vs* ductal carcinoma *in situ*

Score	1	2	3
Size (mm)	Less than 16	16–40	More than 40
Margin width (mm)	Greater than 10	1–9	Less than 1
Histological grade	1–2, no necrosis	1–2, necrosis	3
Age	More than 60	40–60	Less than 40

Lobular Carcinoma in Situ (LCIS)

- Proliferation of generally small and often loosely cohesive cells originating in the terminal duct-lobular unit, with or without pagetoid[1] involvement of terminal ducts.
- It does not present clinically and is diagnosed on biopsy or surgery for other lesions.
- It cannot be detected usually by imaging like mammogram.
- There are two types: Classic and pleomorphic
  - Enlargement and distension of acini making up the terminal duct lobular unit (TDLU).
  - Proliferation of monomorphic, dyshesive, small, round, or polygonal cells with loss of polarity and inconspicuous cytoplasm.
  - Essentially, groups of round, almost identical looking cells that fill and expand the lobule spaces, occasionally extending into the adjacent terminal ducts.
  - Pleomorphic LCIS
    - One or multiple distended lobules
    - Enlarged and dyscohesive cells
    - Irregularly shaped nuclei and abundant eosinophilic cytoplasm
    - Regularly associated with comedo necrosis and calcification and hence is often mammographically detectable.
- Classic LCIS requires no surgical treatment and since there is a risk of carcinoma breast which may be

[1]It means spread of individual cell proliferation in the upper level of dermis

Table 39.8	Lobular carcinomas *vs* ductal carcinoma *in situ*	
Origin	**Terminal duct lobular unit (TDLU)**	**Epithelium that lines minor breast ducts**
Incidence in males	None	5%
Multicentricity	60–90%	40–80%
Bilateral occurrence	High 50–70%	Low 10–20%
Precursor lesion for	Both invasive lobular and invasive ductal carcinoma	invasive ductal carcinoma
Age	44–47	54–58
Incidence	2–5%	5–10%
Clinical sign	None	Mass, nipple discharge
Mammogram	Classic LCIS	Microcalcifications not seen Only pleomorphic variant is seen

bilateral and hence patients should be followed up closely. Patients should be informed of this risk.

- Pleomorphic LCIS requires an approach just like DCIS. Comparison of DCIS and LCIS is given in Table 39.8.

Invasive Breast Cancer

The most widely used classification is that of the World Health Organization. It is based on the growth pattern and cytological features of the invasive tumour cells. Most invasive breast cancers arise in the terminal duct lobular unit regardless of histologic type.

WHO classification (the list is not complete but a list of important histological subtypes).

Invasive breast carcinoma (This term is used when cancer cells invade through basement membrane).

Foot-Stewart Classification of Invasive Breast Cancer

I. Paget's disease of the nipple
II. Invasive ductal carcinoma: 85% (Fig. 21.47)
   a. Adenocarcinomas [scirrhous, simple, NST (80%)]
   b. Medullary carcinoma 4%
   c. Mucinous (colloid) carcinoma 2%
   d. Papillary carcinoma 2%
   e. Tubular carcinoma 2%
III. Invasive lobular carcinoma 10%
IV. Rare types: Adenoid cystic, squamous cell, apocrine.

Invasive Carcinoma of No Special Type (NST) (Commonest)

- Invasive lobular carcinoma
- Tubular carcinoma
- Cribriform carcinoma
- Mucinous carcinoma (colloid carcinoma)
- Medullary carcinoma
- Papillary carcinoma
- Paget's disease of the breast/nipple
- Inflammatory breast cancer

Invasive (Infiltrating) Ductal Carcinoma

- The most common histologic type of breast cancer is invasive (infiltrating) ductal carcinoma, composing 70 to 80% of cases.
- Since it is diagnosed after excluding all other types of breast cancer, it is classified as infiltrating carcinoma of no special type (NST). The older terminology was infiltrating ductal carcinoma, not otherwise specified (NOS).
- Scirrhous carcinoma was a term previously used as it presents as a hard lump and produces grating sound when it is cut. Atrophic scirrhous is an infiltrating duct carcinoma seen in elderly patients when there is atrophy of the breast.
- Tumor cells induce **desmoplastic reaction in stroma causing excessive fibrosis** and less cellular reaction.
- Depending on the grade the tumour may form glands and tubules and shows stromal desmoplasia. Well-differentiated tumours show gland/tubule formation in >75% of the invasive component. Malignant cells are round to polygonal with round to oval dark nuclei with a few mitoses. Perivascular and perineural space infiltration is common (Fig. 39.32).

Invasive Lobular Carcinoma (ILC)

- Comprises approximately 10% of breast cancers.
- Incidence of this type of breast cancer is increasing, especially among postmenopausal women.
- Characterized by small, round cells that are bland in appearance and have scant cytoplasm, which

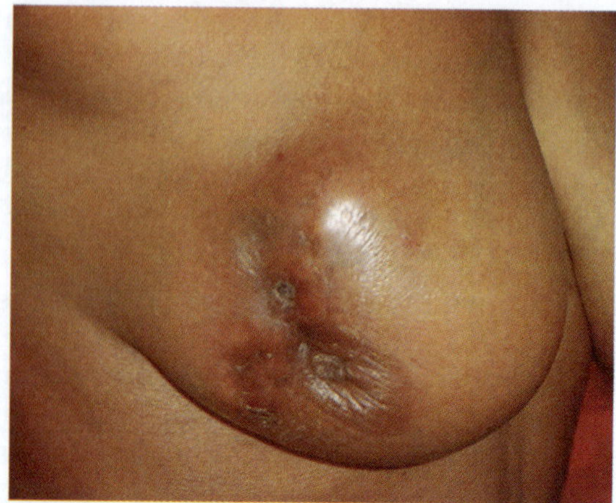

Fig. 39.32: Scirrhous carcinoma—with nipple retraction

infiltrate the stroma in single file and surround benign breast tissues in a targeted manner.

- Infiltration typically does not destroy anatomic structures or incite a substantial connective tissue response.
- They do not form distinct masses or have mammographic findings and hence are difficult to diagnose.
- They tend to **be multifocal and multicentric** and have a propensity for bilaterality.

Special Types

Medullary Carcinoma

- Accounts for less than 5% of all breast cancers (Fig. 39.33).
- Medullary breast cancer is more common carriers of BRCA-I mutation.
- It is commonly a triple-negative breast cancers: ER-ve PR-ve HER2/neu negative.
- Occurs in younger women breasts in the reproductive age group.
- It feels more soft than hard.
- Medullary growth of large cells with a high histological grade (particularly high mitotic count), circumscribed edges, central fibrosis and necrosis, and is often accompanied by lymphocytic infiltration. This is thought to represent a good host response.
- Despite its aggressive histological features (such as the lack of hormonal receptors and grade of 3), medullary carcinoma has a better prognosis than non-medullary carcinoma.

Inflammatory Carcinoma

- The word inflammatory is a misnomer and given because of the physical findings of erythema and warmth.
- It constitutes less than 1% of all cases of carcinoma breast.
- It may be misdiagnosed as breast abscess.
- Predominantly seen during pregnancy and lactation.

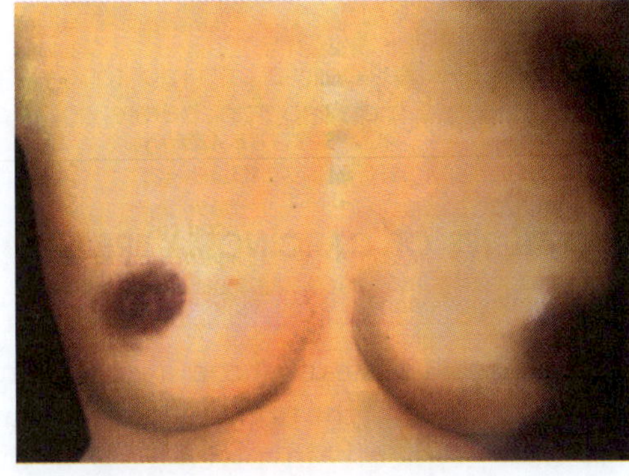

Fig. 39.33: Medullary carcinoma—common in middle age

- Malignancy grows so rapidly that it invades more than half of the breast tissue.
- It is classified as a type of locally advanced breast cancer (LABC).
- Dermal lymphatic invasion is characteristic. Redness, pain and enlargement appear so suddenly that it is diagnosed as mastitis. Hence the name, mastitis carcinomatosa.
- It is differentiated from breast abscess by absence of fever and a classic 'peau d'orange' or 'orange peel' appearance of the affected breast. Presence of gross peau d'orange due to blockage of subdermal lymphatics.
- This variety has the worst prognosis as it has high angiogenic and angioinvasive capability. **Most of them are ER negative** (Figs 39.34 and 39.35).

Paget's Disease of the Nipple

- Paget's disease of the breast has been recognized as a distinct clinical entity for over 120 years.
- It is rare (1–4.3% of all the breast carcinomas).
- It is a misnomer as it is not a disease of the nipple but is often associated with underlying ductal carcinoma *in situ* and/or invasive ductal cancer (Fig. 39.36).

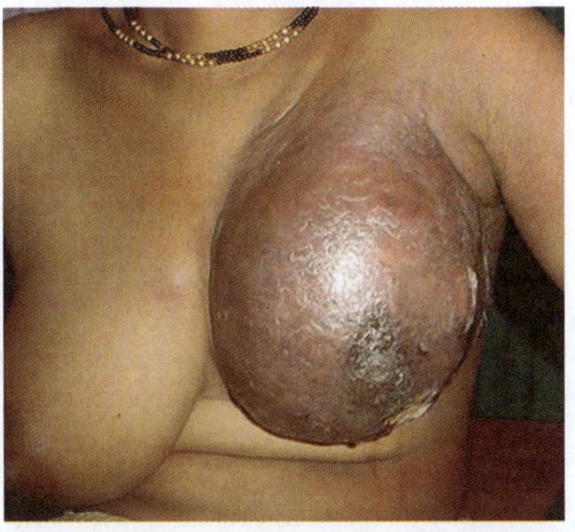

Fig. 39.34: Inflammatory carcinoma—stage T4D

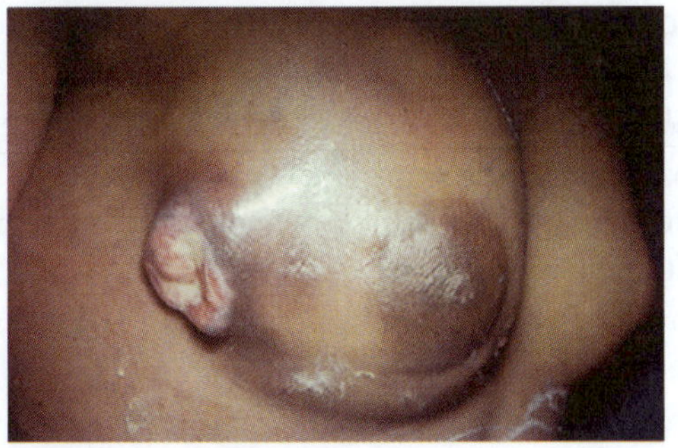

Fig. 39.35: Another case of inflammatory carcinoma. It has been incised mistaking it for an abscess

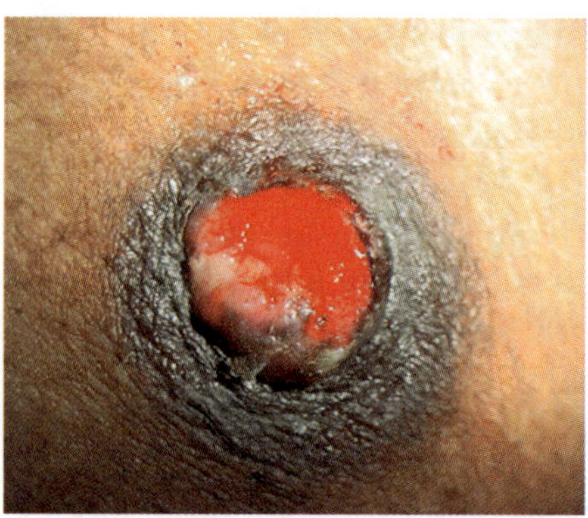

Fig. 39.36: Paget's disease of the nipple—totally destroyed nipple

- It is usually a thickened, sometimes pigmented, eczematoid, erythematous weeping or crusted lesion with irregular borders. Usually, the lesion is limited to the nipple or extended to the areola, and in advanced cases, it also may involve the surrounding skin. The surface of the lesion is occasionally slightly infiltrated.
- Complaints of pain or itching are frequent. The nipple may be retracted or deformed.
- Early changes including scaling and redness may be mistaken for eczema or some other inflammatory conditions.
- Advanced lesions present as a round, ovoid or polycyclic eczema—like plaque with a pink or red hue but it is sharply demarcated from the adjacent normal skin. These stages of the Paget's disease may result in ulceration and destruction of the nipple–areola complex. In these stages, serous and bloody discharge may occur.
- Retraction of the nipple can be seen.
- Lump appears much later than changes in the nipple.
- It characterized by the invasion of epidermis by Paget's cells, malignant glandular epithelial cells with enlarged pleomorphic and hyperchromatic nuclei, with discernible but not prominent nucleoli, with abundant pale, clear cytoplasm, which often contains mucin. The cytoplasm may also contain melanin pigment.

Mucinous Carcinoma (Colloid Carcinoma)

- It accounts for about 2% of breast cancers and tends to occur in older women above 75.
- If palpable, it tends to manifest as soft masses.
- At pathological examination, the dominant feature is the presence of mucin within and surrounding cancer cells.
- A core biopsy specimen usually gives a gelatinous appearance.
- Microscopically, it is formed by large mucin lakes surrounded by mucus-producing cancer cells.
- It has a good prognosis.

Comedocarcinoma of Breast (Fig. 39.37)

Comedos means cast or plug. It is a peripheral carcinoma wherein the tumour cells block the ductules by forming a case or plug producing a small cystic lesion. It is an example for intracystic carcinoma.

Multicentric and Multifocal

Multifocality refers to occurrence of a second *in situ* breast cancer within same breast quadrant as the primary *in situ* cancer (Figs 39.38 and 39.39).

Upper and outer quadrant is commonly involved (60–65%) because breast tissue is more there.

Pearls of Wisdom

Multicentricity refers to occurrence of a second *in situ* breast cancer outside the breast quadrant of primary *in situ* carcinoma.

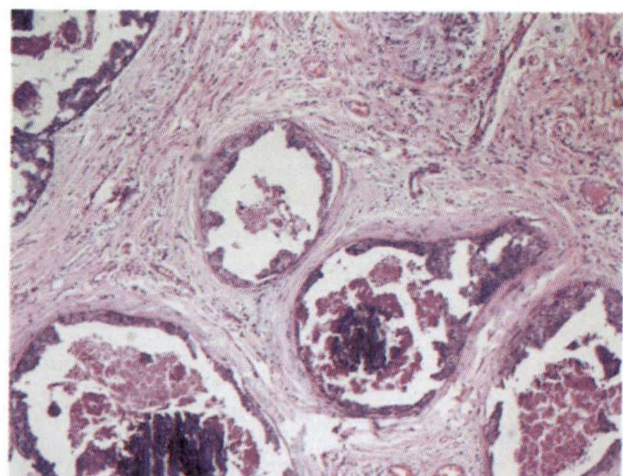

Fig. 39.37: Comedocarcinoma *in situ*—it is a DCIS—dilated terminal duct lobular units (TDLU) lined by malignant epithelial cells with luminal necrosis. No invasion into stroma. Slowly, the lumen gets occluded, can present as cyst and later calcification

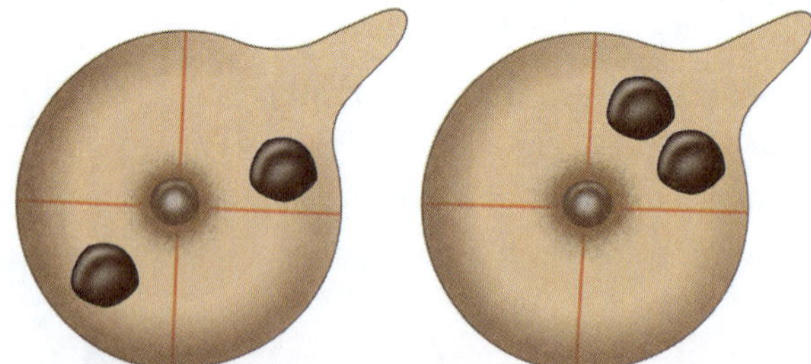

Figs 39.38 and 39.39: Multicentric and multifocal—this is the reason behind getting a mammogram before doing a breast conservative surgery

CLINICAL FEATURES OF CARCINOMA BREAST

Symptoms

- Lump in the breast is the most common presentation. It is the breast tissue in the upper and outer quadrant which is most frequently involved (65%) as this area has the most amount of tissue.

- Bleeding per nipple is an uncommon symptom of carcinoma of the breast. It involves multiple ducts and is unilateral.
- Pain is a late sign in carcinoma breast.
- About 5% of patients present with bony metastasis give rise to bony pains, i.e. pathological fractures, paraplegia, quadriplegia.

Signs (Figs 39.40 to 39.48)

- Important signs are described here first, later clinical methods are described.
- The nipple may be elevated and retracted. It is a centrally retracted nipple: Recent retraction indicates malignancy. It is due to fibrosis caused by extension of growth along the lactiferous duct. Fixation to the

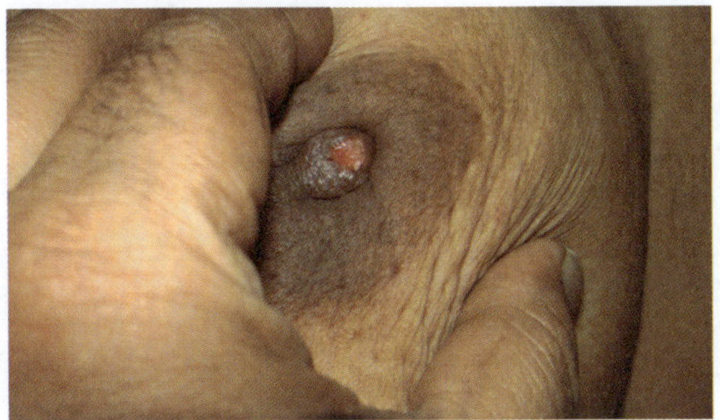

Fig. 39.40: Scirrhous carcinoma presenting as hard lump with *peau d'orange*

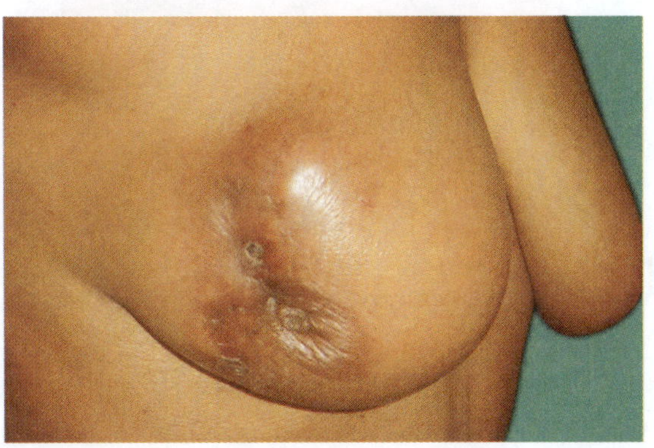

Fig. 39.41: Carcinoma breast presenting as lump and ulceration

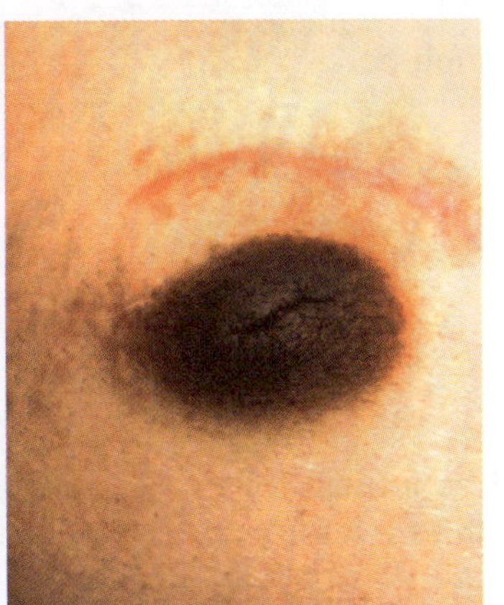

Fig. 39.42: Slit-like retraction

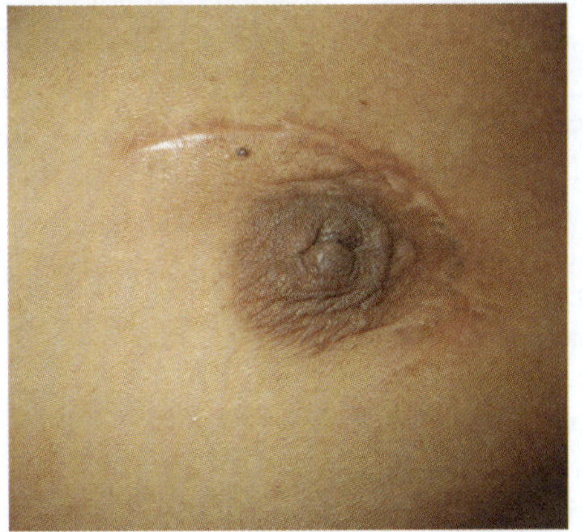

Fig. 39.43: Another case of nipple retraction—chronic abscess

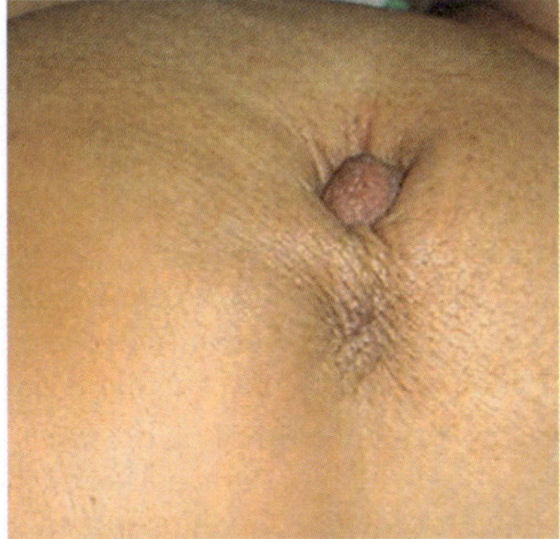

Fig. 39.44: Retraction of the nipple—classical feature of intraductal carcinoma

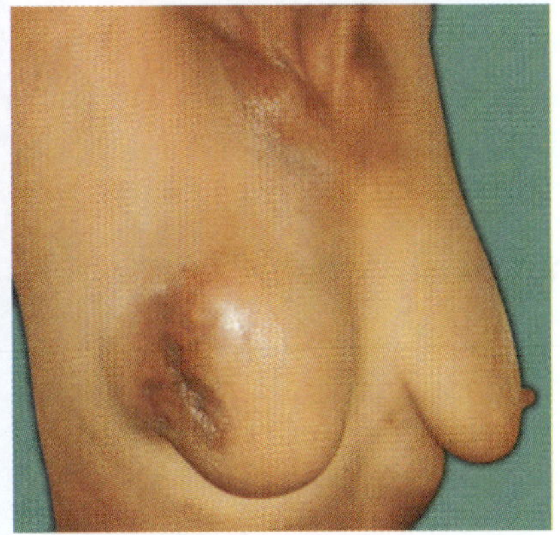

Fig. 39.45: Large lump with ulceration and bleeding

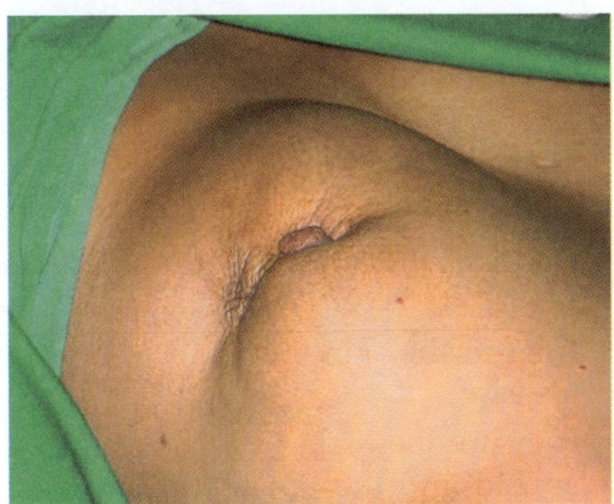

Fig. 39.46: Retracted nipple

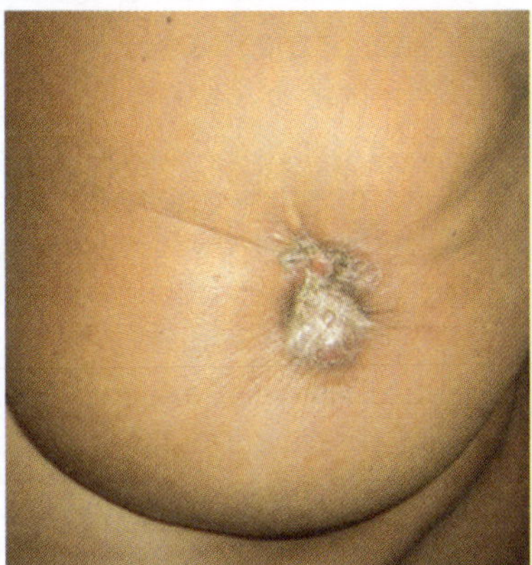

Fig. 39.47: Paget's disease of the nipple (*Courtesy:* Dr Sreejayan, Professor, Department of Surgery, Calicut Medical College, Calicut, Kerala)

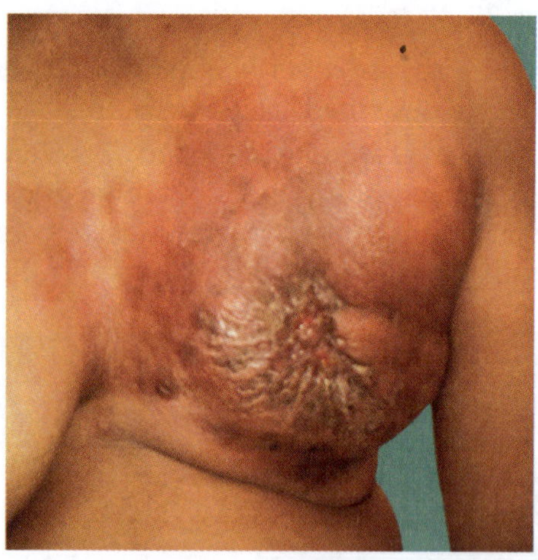

Fig. 39.48: Cancer en cuirasse (*Courtesy:* Dr Sreejayan, Professor, Department of Surgery, Calicut Medical College, Calicut, Kerala)

skin, ulceration, peau d'orange, fixation to pectorals and chest wall occurs late.

- Destruction of the nipple is a feature of Paget's disease of the nipple.
- The lump is usually hard and irregular but it can also be firm and in some subtypes—soft.

  It gets fixed to breast tissue and cannot move independent of the breast. In the later stages, it can get fixed to the pectoralis major muscle (lumps which are located in the upper outer and inner quadrants and lower inner quadrants). The lower outer quadrants tend to get fixed to the seratous anterior muscle (part of chest wall). In advanced cases, the ribs and intercostal muscles are involved (chest wall).
- Puckering or dimpling of skin is due to thin fibrous bands which are embedded in the subcutaneous fat and are attached to the skin and pectoral fascia called ligaments of Cooper which are infiltrated by the malignancy. It is not considered as skin involvement and, therefore, is not a late sign.
- Oedema of the breast is involvement of the skin and is, therefore, a late sign.
- Peau d'orange: Literally means orange peel appearance. It is due to obstruction of the subdermal lymphatics by malignant cells, sparing the sweat glands and hair follicles, therefore, giving an orange peel-like appearance.
- Satellite nodules are multiple nodules in the skin. Their presence indicates advanced disease.
- Ipsilateral axillary lymph nodes: They are the first station of regional lymph node spread and they should be examined for enlargement, size, consistency and fixity.
- Ipsilateral supraclavicular nodes are the next station of involvement.

Signs which do not Affect Staging

- Nipple retraction
- Dimpling
- Involvement of pectoralis major muscle

Signs of Locally Advanced Breast Cancer (Important for Staging)

Skin Involvement

- Peau d'orange
- Oedema of the breast
- Ulceration of the skin
- Satellite nodules in the skin

Fixity to the Chest Wall

- Seratous anterior
- Ribs
- Intercostal muscle

Pectoralis major is not a part of chest wall.

Inflammatory Breast Cancer

- 2/3rds of the breast have oedema.
- 1/3rd of the breast has Peau d'orange.

Regional Lymph Nodes

- Fixed axillary group of lymph nodes
- Internal mammary group of lymph nodes are involved.
- Ipsilateral supraclavicular group of lymph nodes.

Distant Metastasis

- The carcinoma can spread to the contralateral axilla and supraclavicular nodes. They should be always examined.
- Bony tenderness should be looked for in the spine, long bones, skull, etc. (axial skeleton).
- The respiratory system can be involved by secondaries and pleural effusion.
- The abdomen is examined for:
  - Hepatomegaly with nodular liver
  - Ascites due to peritoneal deposits
  - Bilateral ovarian involvement Krukenberg's tumour.
  - Per vaginal and per rectal examination for deposits in the pouch of Douglas (rectouterine pouch).

Spread of Carcinoma Breast

Local Spread

Infiltration into skin causing ulceration, fungation, bleeding, secondary infection and foul smelling discharge/subsequently it invades the pectoralis major and minor muscles, the serratus anterior and chest wall.

Lymphatic Spread

- Axillary group of lymph nodes: Central group, pectoral, lateral, subscapular.

- The internal mammary lymph nodes: Drain the medial quadrant tumours may involve in the upper three or four intercostal spaces, close to the sternum.
- Ipsilateral supraclavicular lymph nodes.
- Earlier considered as distant metastasis, now is included under regional lymph nodes.
- Lymphatics from inner medial quadrant of the breast penetrate the rectus sheath and join the intraperitoneal lymphatics, thus producing ascites, Krukenberg's tumour (in premenopausal patients, ovary is vascular and fertile), rectovesical deposits, secondaries in the liver.
- Blood spread
  - Liver
  - Lung parenchyma
  - Secondaries in flat bones are common (vertebral column, femur, ribs, scalp, etc.).
  - Secondaries in brain result in headache, vomiting and blurring of vision.
  - Malignant pleural effusion is the common cause of death in carcinoma of breast.

Triple Assessment

The breast triple assessment is a hospital-based assessment that allows for the early and rapid detection of breast cancer. **Triple assessment test is used as Gold standard in diagnosing all palpable breast lumps.**

It includes:

- Clinical examination
- Radiological imaging (ultrasonography and mammography)
- Biopsy of the lump

Combining the three modalities increases the overall accuracy of diagnosis to nearly 99%.

CLINICAL EXAMINATION OF A CASE OF CARCINOMA BREAST

Inspection should be done only in two positions: Bending forward is no longer required as the same information can be obtained by palpation. Detailed examination is given in *Manipal Manual of Clinical Methods, 1st edition*.

1. Hands by the Side of the Patient

A. Examine the nipples:

- Compare the level of the nipples
  - A tumour may push the nipple in the opposite direction.
  - Inspect the nipple of the side with tumour for
    - Destruction: This indicates Paget's disease of nipple
    - Retraction
- If it is present, ask the patient, if this was recent in origin: This indicates malignancy.
- The retraction of nipple in carcinoma breast is usually central
  - Nipple discharge
- Bloody discharge indicates duct carcinoma.

B. Areola: Peau d'orange may occur in the areola because of subdermal lympatic obstruction leading to oedema, sparing the hair follicles.

C. Examine the skin of the breast for:

- Ulcerations
- Satellite nodules
- Dimpling
- Peau d'orange
- Oedema
- Erythema
- Scars
- Dilated veins

D. Inspect the breast to see whether a lump is visible:

- If a lump is seen, it is described in detail.
- If it is not seen, ask the patient to press against her hip on the ipsilateral side, this contracts the pectoralis major and makes the lump more visible allowing its description.

2. Hands above the Head Prominent

- The effected breast may get lifted sometimes indicating fixity to pectoral fascia.
- Peau d'orange gets noticed better by this manoeuvre.
- Any lesions in the inframammary fold and inferior quadrant of the breast is better visualized.

Palpation

- Local rise of temperature and tenderness are usually not found in cases of carcinoma of the breast. However, rapidly growing carcinoma and inflammatory carcinomas do exhibit local rise of temperature, redness and tenderness.
- Describe the lump: The lump is the commonest presentation of carcinoma of the breast. The upper and outer quadrant is the commonest site of carcinoma of the breast because of more breast tissue in that quadrant. Typically, the lump is hard and irregular. However, very often carcinoma breast can present as a firm lump. In mastitis carcinomatosa, the lump can be soft due to tumour necrosis.

- Intrinsic mobility may be present but it moves with the breast tissue (fibroadenoma moves independent of breast tissue).
- Plane of the swelling
  - Lift the skin. If it is not possible, it indicates that the tumour is fixed to skin.
  - Pectoralis major contraction test: Ask the patient to keep the hands on the flanks and press against the hip. If the lump cannot be moved after contraction, it indicates fixity to pectoralis major.
- Fixity to the chest wall
  - A tumour which is fixed to the chest wall will not be mobile when pectoralis major is relaxed.
  - Serratus anterior contraction test by pressing the hand against the wall. The test has to be done when the tumour is situated in the outer and inferior quadrant.

Axillary Lymph Nodes Examination

- There are 5 groups of nodes in the axilla which are described under lymphatic drainage of the breast. However, very often, central group of nodes and pectoral nodes are enlarged. It is very difficult to feel the apical group of nodes.
- If the axillary nodes are hard, with or without fixity, they are significant.
- Soft to firm nodes need not be malignant but can be due to secondary infection because of fungating, ulcerating growth.

Examination of Supraclavicular Lymph Nodes: Presence of these nodes indicates it is a N3C-stage III

Examination for distal metastasis, opposite breast for any mass, opposite axilla, abdomen, skull and spine and respiratory system.

Workup for a carcinoma breast case

Assessment of general health status	• History • Menopausal status • Physical examination • Full blood count • LFT • RFT • Cardiac evaluation
Assessment of primary tumour	• Physical examination • Breast ultrasound • Mammogram • MRI (when indicated only) • Core biopsy: Histology, grade, ER, PR, HER2, Ki67
Assessment of lymph nodes	• Physical examination • Ultrasound • Ultrasound-guided FNAC
Assessment of distant metastasis	• CT scan chest and abdomen • Bone scan when symptoms of bone pain are present and in all stage III cases

INVESTIGATIONS (Figs 39.49 to 39.59)

Laboratory

- Full blood count: Hb% may be lowered. Planning for neoadjuvant chemotherapy requires the TLC and DLC.
- Liver function test: Elevated serum alkaline phosphatase indicates metastasis in the liver or bone.
- Renal function test is required when planning a chemotherapy regimen.

Local Imaging Studies

- These include ultrasound of breasts, bilateral mammogram and ultrasound of lymph nodes. All three are mandatory in assessment.
- Ultrasound of the breast is the first investigation
  - It accurately measures the lump size.
  - More accurate for lymph node assessment.
  - It can differentiate between cystic and solid lesions.
  - It is more accurate in assessment of breast lump in younger women.
- Mammogram
  - Detects any multifocal and multicentric lesions.
  - It is done before the biopsy as biopsy of any type will introduce artefacts and obscure its interpretation.
- Breast MRI: It is an optional investigation (not mandatory). Indications are:
  - BRCA associated carcinoma breast
  - Bilateral tumours
  - Reconstructed breasts
  - Breast implants
  - Assessment of neoadjuvant chemotherapy

Mammography

Details are given below.

- The process of using low-energy X-rays (usually around 30 kVp) to examine the human breast for diagnosis and screening.
- Diagnostic accuracy is about 90–95%.
- **Procedure:**
  - A selenium coated X-ray plate is used directly in contact with the breast.
  - The breast is compressed using a dedicated mammography unit.
  - Parallel-plate compression evens out the thickness of breast tissue to increase image quality by reducing the thickness of tissue that X-rays must penetrate, decreasing the amount of scattered, reducing the required radiation dose, and holding the breast still (preventing motion blur).
  - In screening mammography, craniocaudal view and mediolateral oblique images of the breast are taken.

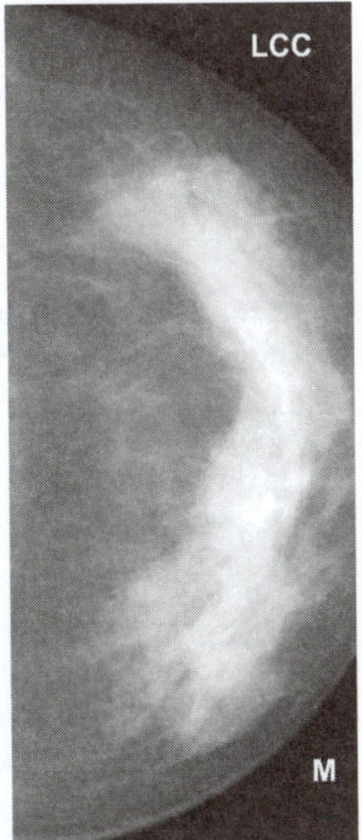

Fig. 39.49: Architectural distortion

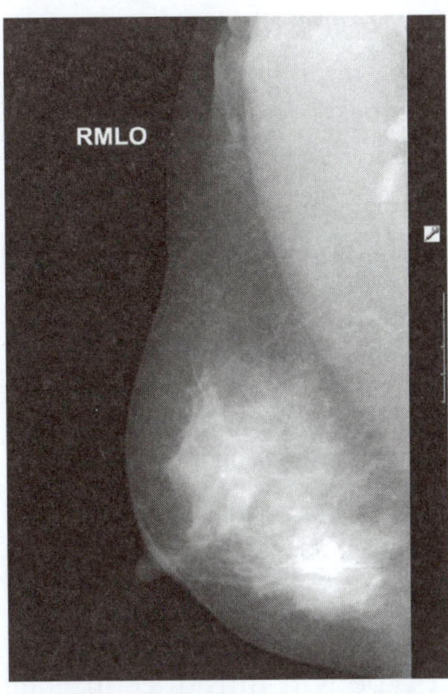

Fig. 39.50: Spiculation—mediolateral view—right side

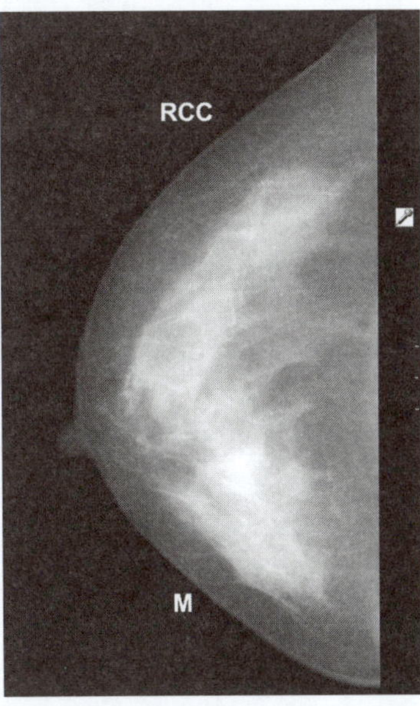

Fig. 39.51: Spiculation—craniocaudal view—right side

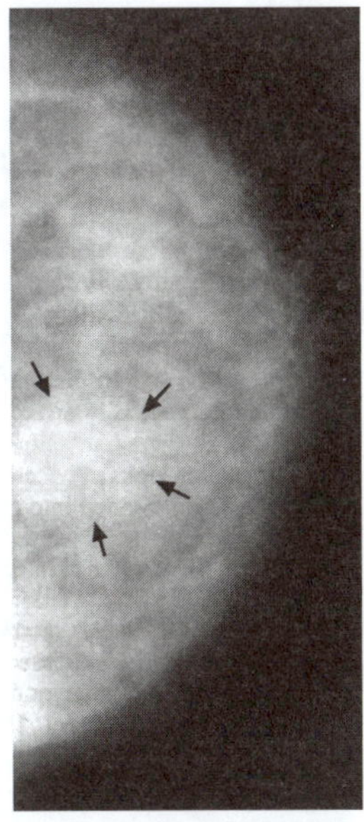

Fig. 39.52: Mammography showing a cystic lesion

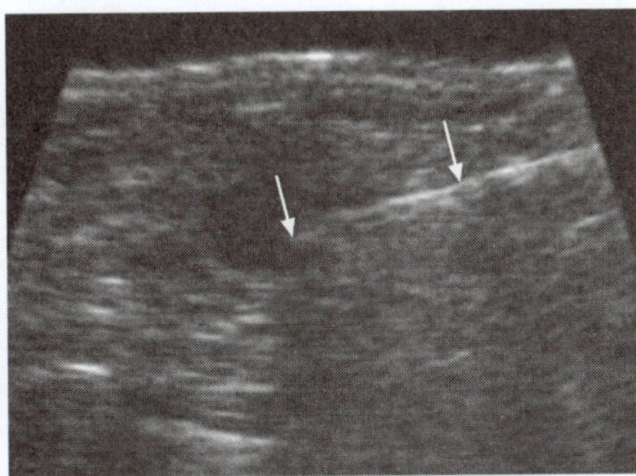

Fig. 39.53: Ultrasound detecting a lump in the breast and a wire is being introduced within

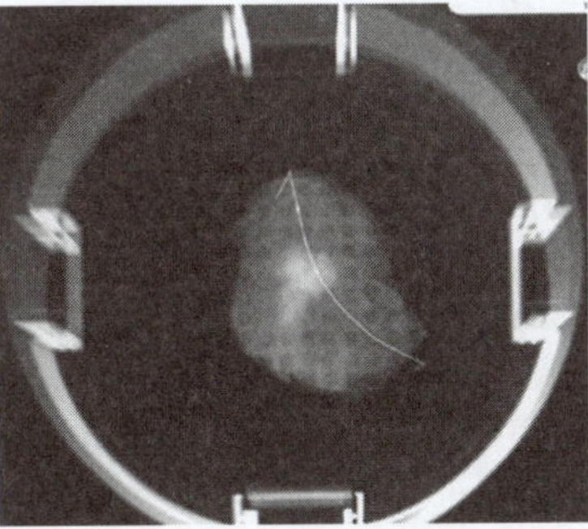

Figs 39.54 to 39.56: Mammography directed wire localisation (*Courtesy:* Dr Sampath Kumar, Professor, Department of Surgery, Dr Chandrakant Shetty, Professor, Department of Radiology and Imaging, Dr Poornima, Resident, Department of Surgery, KMC, Manipal)

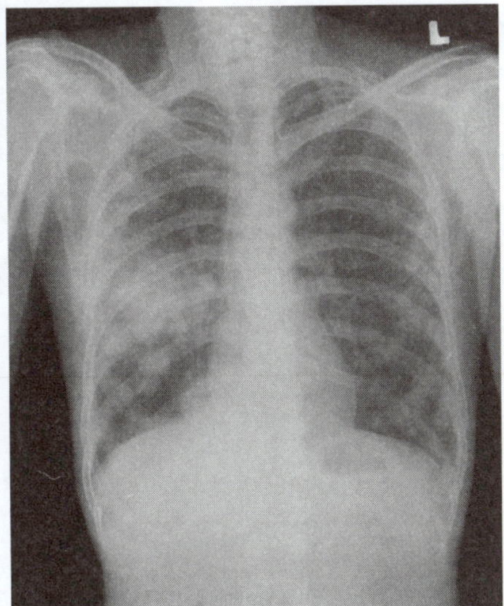

Fig. 39.57: Cannonball secondaries

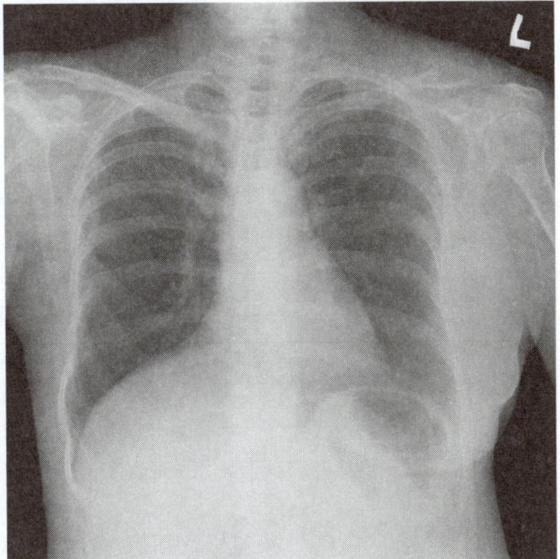

Fig. 39.58: Carcinoma breast with metastasis in the left clavicle

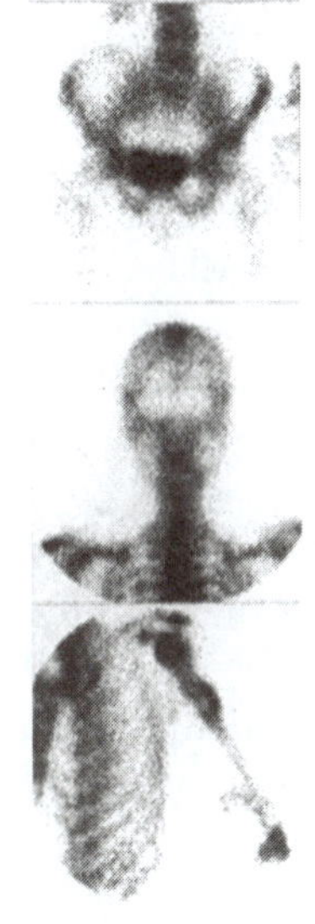

Fig. 39.59: Bone scan Ca breast

- Diagnostic mammography may include these and other views, including geometrically magnified and spot-compressed views.
- A mammogram is reported using BI-RADS (breast imaging-reporting and data system) (Key Box 39.9)

Key Box 39.9

Mammography

- **Screening:** Asymptomatic women of more than 40 years.
- **Diagnostic:** Women with pain in the breast, mass, discharge, family history of breast cancer.
- Two views—mediolateral oblique view is for outer quadrant and axilla. Craniocaudal view is for medial quadrants.
- Radiation dose is 0.1 centigray (cGy)—4 times that of chest X-ray dose but no side effects.
- Benign lesions are round, punctate, popcorn-like, etc.
- Highly suspicious—pleomorphic, heterogeneous
  - Solid mass with **irregular edges, spiculation**
  - Long tentacles—tentaculation
  - Fine scattered calcification—**microcalcification**
  - **Distortion of architectural pattern** of the breast
  - Asymmetrical thickening of breast tissues

BI-RADS SCORES RANGE FROM 0 TO 6

0: This score identifies a mammogram study that is still incomplete. The X-ray may have been cloudy, making it difficult to read the images. This can happen, e.g. if the patient moved at the precise moment the picture was taken.

1: This score means that mammogram is negative (i.e. no evident signs of cancer were found).

2: This score also means that mammogram is normal, with no apparent cancer, but that other findings (such as cysts) are described in the report.

3: A score of 3 means that mammogram is probably normal but **that there is an approximately 2% chance of cancer**. Hence, follow-up with a repeat mammogram in 6 months. And if there is a family or personal history of breast cancer, the radiologist may opt to do more tests at this stage rather than wait.

4: This score means that the findings on the mammogram are suspicious and that there is an approximately **20 to 35%** chance that a breast cancer is present. Core biopsy is a must in such cases for tissue sample.

5: This score means that the mammogram results are highly suspicious, **with a 95%** chance of breast cancer.

6: This means that patients have already been diagnosed with breast cancer and the pathologist has confirmed the diagnosis.

Screening Mammogram

- Mammogram done for detection of breast cancer in breasts with no lumps
- Always bilateral
- Indications:
  - Women above 40. Below this age, women tend to have more fat in the breast so lesion can be missed.
  - Women who have a family history of breast cancer begin screening after the age of 30.

Diagnostic Mammogram

- When it is performed in a palpable lump as a part of triple assessment.
- Always bilateral.
- It is always done before biopsy as biopsy of any type will introduce artefacts and obscure the BI-RADS.
- Done to detect multicentricity and multifocality especially when breast conservation is planned.
  - Multicentricity
    - Multicentricity is defined by presence of carcinoma in a breast quadrant other than the one containing the dominant mass more than one quadrant.
  - Multifocality
    - Multifocality is defined as the extension of a single carcinomatous focus within ducts and lobules limited to one region or quadrant (limited to one quadrant).

Biopsy

- The presence or absence of carcinoma can only be reliably determined by a tissue biopsy.
- Biopsy techniques include fine-needle aspiration cytology (FNAC), core needle biopsy, and excisional biopsy.

A. Fine Needle Aspiration Cytology (FNAC)

- No longer the investigation of choice.
- Is easily performed and results are obtained quickly.
- False positive rates are low (1%) but higher false negative rates (15%) can occur.
- Requires a trained cytopathologist for accurate specimen interpretation.
- Does not reliably distinguish invasive cancer from DCIS.
- Biological markers are difficult to obtain.
- Currently used in superficial tumours and for assessing lymph nodes.

B. Core Biopsy (Tru-cut Biopsy)

- It is the investigation of choice with clear advantages over FNAC.
- It can differentiate between invasive breast cancers and carcinoma *in situ*.
- Allows for placement of a clip to mark the area of interest in the event that subsequent surgical excision or definitive breast cancer treatment is indicated.
- Using vacuum-assisted biopsy (VAB) device increases amount of lesion sampled and reduces false negative rates to less than 1%.
- **Biological markers** which have become a critical component of multidisciplinary treatment planning are determined using the core biopsy samples therapy.
  1. **Estrogen receptors:** Estrogen receptors (ER) are overexpressed in around 70% of breast cancer cases, referred to as 'ER-positive', and can be demonstrated in such tissues using immunohistochemistry. Normal value of ER is <10 fmol/mg proteins. It is considered positive >10 fmol/mg proteins. Upper levels as high as 1000 fmol/mg proteins may be there. The overexpression means hormonal therapy will be an option in treatment of carcinoma breast.
  2. Progesterone receptors: Progesterone receptors (PR/PgR).
  3. HER2/neu (human epidermal growth factor receptor 2):
     - It is a membrane tyrosine kinase receptor and a marker of cellular proliferation, expressed in up to 50% of cases. It is usually associated with ER negativity and high grade tumour, poor prognosis but **there is a better response to adriamycin** (Key Box 39.10).
  4. Ki-67: Proliferative index: Antigen Ki-67 is a nuclear protein that is associated with and may be necessary for cellular proliferation (Key Box 39.11).

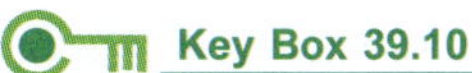

Key Box 39.10

HER2

- Measured by immunohistochemistry
- Test for gene amplification—fluorescent *in situ* hybridisation (**FISH**) is gold standard
- 25% of all breast cancers overexpress HER2
- It is a transmembrane tyrosine kinase receptor
- High grade tumours usually express this
- ER negative—poor prognosis
- Responds to 'TRASTUZUMAB'

Thus 'FISH' is done only when HER2/neu is 2+

Key Box 39.11

Ki-67

- Also known as MKI67
- It is a marker for cellular proliferation
- It depicts growth fraction of all proliferation
- Higher values suggest aggressive tumour
- A cut-off value of <14% is generally used to denote low and high values

Based on the biological markers Ca breast is classified into intrinsic subtypes which is given in Tables 39.9 to 39.11.

Table 39.9 Association of clinicopathologic features of breast cancer with intrinsic subtype

	Luminal A	Luminal B1	Luminal B2	HER2 enriched	Basal (triple negative)
ER	Positive	Positive	Positive	Absent	Absent
PR	High	Low	Any level	Absent	Absent
HER2	Negative	Negative	Positive	Positive	Absent
Ki-67	Low	High	Any level	Any level	Any level

Table 39.10 Adjuvant treatment approaches in breast cancer based on biological markers

	Tumour hormone receptor status	
Tumour HER2/neu status	Positive	Negative
HER2 negative/normal	Endocrine therapy ± Chemotherapy	Chemotherapy
HER2 positive/overexpressed	Endocrine therapy ± Chemotherapy + Trastuzumab	Chemotherapy + Trastuzumab

Table 39.11 Treatment based on breast cancer intrinsic subtype

Luminal A (lymph node negative)	Luminal A (lymph node positive)	Luminal B1	Luminal B2 (HER2/neu rich)	HER2 enriched	Basal (triple negative)
Hormonal therapy only	*Sequential chemotherapy plus hormonal therapy	Sequential chemotherapy plus hormonal therapy	Sequential chemotherapy plus hormonal therapy plus trastuzumab	Sequential chemotherapy plus hormonal therapy plus trastuzumab	#Dose dense regimen chemotherapy

*Sequential chemotherapy: 21-day cycles

#Dose dense regimen: 15-day cycles. High risk of febrile neutropenia due to bone marrow suppression. Always give granulocyte colony stimulating factor (GCSF)

Gene Expression Profiling

- Expensive
- Individualized treatment
- Requires core biopsy sample or the excised tumour
- **MammaPrint**
  - 70-gene breast cancer assay which is a prognostic and predictive diagnostic test for early stage breast cancer patients that assess the risk that a tumour will metastasize.
  - Divides patients into low-risk and high-risk groups.
  - Determines whether or not a patient will benefit from chemotherapy.
  - High risk will get chemotherapy and low risk can avoid it without a risk of recurrence.
- **Oncotype DX**
  - 21 gene assay
  - It is done usually in oestrogen receptor positive tumours.
  - Results are reported as a recurrence score (RS), where a higher RS is associated with a worse prognosis and will benefit from chemotherapy.

Image-guided Biopsy in Indeterminate Lesions

- Done when lesions cannot be palpated or there is repeated inconclusive reports.
- Ultrasound guided.
- Wire localisation
  - When lesions cannot be palpated.
  - Under mammogram guidance, a hooked wire is placed in the vicinity of a suspicious lesion or microcalcifications.
  - The patient is then shifted to the OT.
  - In the theatre, the area around the hook is excised along with hook and the tissue is sent for histopathology.
- Mammogram-guided stereotactic biopsy
  - It is the choice in case of microcalcifications or non-palpable lesions seen only on mammogram.
  - The coordinates of the lesion are calculated digitally and the patient is positioned accordingly.
  - Any of the methods of biopsy can then be done including FNAC, CORE biopsy or vacuum assisted core biopsy (VACB).
  - Mammotome™ VACB is a hand held device which consists of a control unit which maintains aspiration at constant values (23–25 mmHg) and of a driver where a 11–14 G needle is placed.
- MR guided

Excision Biopsy

- Seldom performed
- Incision is placed in planned manner
- Complete haemostasis
- No drains are placed
- Indications after core needle biopsy
  - Imaging abnormalities that cannot be targeted for core biopsy
  - Atypical ductal hyperplasia
  - LCIS
  - Lack of concordance between imaging findings and histologic diagnosis
  - Radial scar
  - Complex sclerosing lesions
  - Papillary lesion
- Incisional biopsy with frozen section
  - Frozen section is no longer proven very reliable in decision making in carcinoma breast
  - However, some centres practice this method where an incisional biopsy is taken and on receiving a report of malignancy definitive surgery, i.e. mastectomy is performed.

Investigations for Metastasis

- Chest X-ray
  - Pleural effusion
  - Lung secondaries: They look like 'cannonballs' due to the lung compliance
  - Mediastinal widening

- Abdominal ultrasonography is done to rule out secondaries in the liver, ascites, rectouterine deposits. Incidence of liver metastasis in Ca breast is 6%.
- **Contrast-enhanced CT scan of thorax and abdomen is gradually replacing ultrasound of abdomen and chest X-ray in investigating carcinoma breast as it is more accurate.**
- Bone scan: Incidence of bone metastasis in stage IIb and stage III is high, hence recommended in these settings.
- CT scan of brain is not recommended unless there are symptoms.
- PET-CT scan is used only in locally advanced breast cancer and inflammatory breast cancer.

After the surgery, pathological assessment of carcinoma breast is done.

Pathological Assessment of the Tumour

- Size: The maximum diameter of tumour removed.
- Assessment of entire specimen of breast for any other tumours.
- The resected margins, especially the deep margins should be evaluated.
- The distance of the margins of tumour from resected margins should be evaluated.
- Vascular invasion should be noted.
- Tumour grade
  - Originally was used Scarff-Bloom-Richardson (SBR) grading system
  - **Now the Elston-Ellis modification of the SBR grading system (Nottingham grading system) is preferred.**
  - Depends upon three factors:
    - Nuclear pleomorphism
    - Tubule formation
    - Mitotic rate
  - Tumours are given scores and graded (Table 39.12).

Table 39.12 Elston-Ellis modification of the SBR grading system

Score	1 point	2 points	3 points
Nuclear pleomorphism	Uniform cells with small nuclei	Large cells with moderate variations in nuclei	Large cells with marked variations in nuclei
Tubule formation	More than 75% of tumour	10–75% of tumour	Less than 10% of tumour
Mitotic rate (per high power field)	Less than 7	8–15	Above 16

- The scores for each of these three criteria are added together to give a final overall score and a corresponding grade as follows:
  - 3–5 grade 1 tumour (well-differentiated). Best prognosis.
  - 6–7 grade 2 tumour (moderately differentiated). Medium prognosis.
  - 8–9 grade 3 tumour (poorly differentiated). Worst prognosis.

Lymph Node

- Number of lymph nodes removed (a minimum of 10 is mandatory in axillary dissection).
- Number of positive nodes should be mentioned.

Biological markers should be assessed:

- Oestrogen receptor (ER)
- Progesterone receptor (PR/PgR)
- HER2
- Ki-67 index

TNM STAGING **American Joint Committee on Cancer Staging: Breast cancer**

Primary Tumour (T)+

TX	Primary tumour cannot be assessed
T0	No evidence of primary tumour
Tis	Carcinoma *in situ*
Tis (DCIS)	Ductal carcinoma *in situ*
Tis (LCIS)	Lobular carcinoma *in situ*
Tis (Paget's)	Paget's disease of the nipple NOT associated with invasive carcinoma, DCIS and LCIS
T1	Tumour <20 mm in greatest dimension
T1mi	Tumour <1 mm in greatest dimension
T1a	Tumour >1 mm but <5 mm in greatest dimension (round any measurement >1.0–1.9 to 2 mm)
T1b	Tumour >5 mm but <10 mm in greatest dimension
T1c	Tumour >10 mm but <20 mm in greatest dimension
T2	Tumour >20 mm but <50 mm in greatest dimension
T3	Tumour >50 mm in greatest dimension
T4	Tumour of any size with direct extension to the chest wall and/or to skin (ulceration or skin nodules); invasion of the dermis alone does not qualify as T4
T4a	Extension to chest wall; invasion or adherence to pectoralis muscle in the absence of invasion of chest wall structures does not qualify as T4
T4b	Ulceration and/or ipsilateral macroscopic satellite nodules and/or edema (including peau d'orange) of the skin that does not meet the criteria for inflammatory carcinoma are present
T4c	Both T4a and T4b
T4d	Inflammatory carcinoma

Regional Lymph Nodes—Clinical (cN)

cNXb	Regional lymph nodes cannot be assessed (e.g. previously removed)
cN0	No regional lymph node metastases (by imaging or clinical examination)
cN1	Metastases to movable ipsilateral level I, II axillary lymph node(s)
cN1mic	Micrometastases (approximately 200 cells, larger than 0.2 mm, but none larger than 2.0 mm)
cN2	Metastases in ipsilateral level I, II axillary lymph nodes that are clinically fixed or matted or in ipsilateral internal mammary nodes in the absence of axillary lymph node metastases
cN2a	Metastases in ipsilateral level I, II axillary lymph nodes fixed to one another (matted) or to other structures
cN2b	Metastases only in ipsilateral internal mammary nodes in the absence of axillary lymph node metastases
cN3	Metastases in ipsilateral infraclavicular (level III axillary) lymph node(s) with or without level I, II axillary lymph node involvement; or in ipsilateral internal mammary lymph node(s) with level I, II axillary lymph node metastases; or in ipsilateral supraclavicular lymph node(s) with or without axillary or internal mammary lymph node involvement
cN3a	Metastases in ipsilateral infraclavicular lymph node(s)
cN3b	Metastases in ipsilateral internal mammary lymph node(s) and axillary lymph node(s)
cN3c	Metastases in ipsilateral supraclavicular lymph nodes

Regional Lymph Nodes—Pathologic (pN)

pN0	No regional lymph node metastasis identified or ITCs only
pN0(i+)	ITCs only (malignant cell clusters no larger than 0.2 mm) in regional lymph node(s)
pN0(mol+)	Positive molecular findings by RT-PCR; no ITCs detected
pN1a	Metastases in 1–3 axillary lymph nodes, at least one metastasis >2.0 mm
pN1b	Metastases in ipsilateral internal mammary sentinel nodes, excluding ITCs
pN1c	pN1a and pN1b combined
pN2	Metastases in 4–9 axillary lymph nodes; or positive ipsilateral internal mammary lymph nodes by imaging in the absence of axillary lymph node metastases
pN2a	Metastases in 4–9 axillary lymph nodes (at least one tumour deposit >2.0 mm)
pN2b	Metastases in clinically detected internal mammary lymph nodes with or without microscopic confirmation; with pathologically negative axillary nodes
pN3	Metastases in 10 or more axillary lymph nodes; or in infraclavicular (level III axillary) lymph nodes; or positive ipsilateral internal mammary lymph nodes by imaging in the presence of one or more positive level I, II axillary lymph node(s); or in more than 3 axillary lymph nodes and micrometastases or macrometastases by SLNB in clinically negative ipsilateral internal mammary lymph nodes; or in ipsilateral supraclavicular lymph nodes
pN3a	Metastases in 10 or more axillary lymph nodes (at least one tumour deposit >2.0 mm); or metastases to the infraclavicular (level III axillary lymph) nodes
pN3b	pN1a or pN2a in the presence of cN2b (positive internal mammary nodes by imaging); or pN2a in the presence of pN1b
pN3c	Metastases in ipsilateral supraclavicular lymph nodes

Distant Metastases (M)

M0	No clinical or radiographic evidence of distant metastases
cM0(i+)	No clinical or radiographic evidence of distant metastases in the presence of tumour cells or deposits no larger than 0.2 mm detected microscopically or by molecular techniques in circulating blood, bone marrow, or other non-regional nodal tissue in a patient without symptoms or signs of metastases
cM1	Distant metastases detected by clinical and radiographic means
pM1	Any histologically proven metastases in distant organs; or if in non-regional nodes, metastases greater than 0.2 mm

Stage Group

0		
Tis	N0	M0
IA		
T1	N0	M0
IB		
T0	N1mi	M0
T1	N1mi	M0
IIA		
T0	N1	M0
T1	N1	M0
T2	N–	M0
IIB		
T2	N1	M0
T3	N–	M0
IIIA		
T0	N2	M0
T1	N2	M0
T2	N2	M0
T3	N1	M0
T3	N2	M0
IIIB		
T4	N–	M0
T4	N1	M0
T4	N2	M0
IIIC		
ANY T	N3	M0
IV		
ANYT	ANYN	M1

TREATMENT OF BREAST CANCER

Introduction

Breast cancer is a heterogeneous disease. This means no two breast cancers will have similar biological behaviour. Therefore, patient's clinical progression cannot be predicted. When William Halsted pioneered the radical mastectomy procedure in the later part of the 19th century (circa 1889). **According to the Halsted-Meyer theory, the major pathway for breast cancer dissemination was through the lymphatic ducts.** Therefore, it was thought that performing wider and more mutilating surgeries that removed a greater number of lymph nodes would result in greater chances of cure. His results encouraged other surgeons to perform the radical mastectomy. However, the surgery had significant morbidity and had both a physical and psychological impact on the patients.

Bernard Fisher in 1977 proposed that breast cancer was a systemic disease in that tumour cells were likely to have been disseminated throughout the body by the time of diagnosis and that more extensive loco regional therapy was unlikely to improve survival. His work led to the development of less invasive surgery and incorporation of adjuvant treatment in the form of chemotherapy. The most common surgery performed is modified radical mastectomy.

1. Radical mastectomy was the procedure in Asia till 5 decades back. It is given here to understand the concepts. It is no longer done.
2. The most common surgery performed is modified radical mastectomy.
3. However, breast conservative surgery—local wide excision is done in selected patients. It is already popular now.

In the 21st century, breast cancer has evolved from the mutilating radical mastectomy proposed by Halstead and others to breast conservation therapy. The availability of gene assays, like MammaPrint and oncotype DX, has allowed doctors to individualise treatment.

Treatment for carcinoma breast is based on the TNM stage of the tumour.

For the purposes of treatment protocol, breast carcinoma is arbitrarily classified based on the TNM staging as:

I. Early breast carcinoma: TNM stage I and II

II. Locally advanced breast carcinoma
- Operable LABC: TNM stage III A
- Inoperable LABC: TNM stage III B and C

III. Metastatic breast carcinoma: TNM stage IV

I. Treatment Modalities for Early Breast Carcinoma: TNM Stage I and II

Breast cancer treatment has a multidisciplinary approach. The treatment involves more than one modality. The modalities available to treat breast carcinoma are classified as:

- Local treatment
- Systemic treatment
- Targeted treatment

Local Treatment

- Surgery
- Radiotherapy

Systemic Treatment

- Chemotherapy
- Hormonal therapy

Targeted Treatment

- Directed towards HER2/neu receptors.

Surgery

Radical Mastectomy (it is mentioned here to understand why it was done and why major changes have happened since 1889)

- The traditional surgery for carcinoma breast was a radical mastectomy proposed by William Halsted in 1889.
- What made it radical?
- Removing all the breast tissue
- Skin was removed because the disease involved the skin, which was often ulcerated.
- The two muscles—the pectoralis major and the pectoralis minor muscles. The pectoralis muscles were removed not only because the chest wall was involved, but also because it was thought that removal of the transpectoral lymphatic pathways were necessary.
- All the axillary lymph nodes (axillary clearance).
- Three important structures were preserved:
  1. Axillary vein
  2. Bell's nerve (long thoracic nerve which supplies serratus anterior)
  3. Cephalic vein
- Disadvantages of radical mastectomy: Significant morbidity
  1. Mutilating surgery
  2. Poor cosmetic results
  3. Lymphedema of arm
  4. Injury to the Bell's nerve and nerve to serratus anterior
- The surgery was performed for nearly a century and is not performed in the 21st century.

Note: This should not be told in the examination. It is given here to understand the concepts.

Patey's Modified Radical Mastectomy (Table 39.13)

- The entire breast tissue including axillary tail is removed with at least level II lymph nodes. The modification was to preserve the pectoralis major to maintain the contour of the chest wall.
- Pectoralis minor was removed to clear all the axillary nodes (axillary clearance).
- It had results equivalent to the radical mastectomy with significantly lesser morbidity.
- It was cosmetically better accepted as axillary fold is maintained.
- The function of the shoulder was better, and it gave a stronger and more useful arm.
- Different levels of axillary lymph nodes are broadly classified into level I, II and III nodes.
- Level I axillary lymph nodes are the nodes located lateral to pectoralis minor muscle.
- Level II axillary lymph nodes are the nodes located beneath or over the pectoralis minor muscle.
- Level III axillary lymph nodes are the nodes located medial to pectoralis minor muscle.

Scanlon's Modified Radical Mastectomy

Pectoralis minor muscle is divided but not removed to clear all the axillary nodes (axillary clearance).

Auchincloss' Modified Radical Mastectomy

- Pectoralis minor is retracted but not divided.
- Axillary lymph node clearance is NOT done.
- Axillary lymph node dissection (ALND) is done.
- **It is the current surgery technique practiced for an MRM.**

TABLE 39.13 Various types of mastectomy

Surgery	Pectoralis major	Pectoralis minor	Axillary clearance	Axillary lymph node dissection
1. Radical mastectomy (Patey's)	Removed	Removed	All levels	Not done
2. Modified radical mastectomy	Spared	Removed	All levels	Not done
3. Scanlon's modified radical mastectomy	Spared	Detached	All levels	Not done
4. Auchincloss' modified radical mastectomy	Spared	Retracted	Not done	Levels I and II

Complications of MRM

1. **Seroma/lymph collection** (30 to 50%): In spite of adequate drainage of the chest wall and axilla, drainage occurs for about 5–10 days. Just patiently reassure the patient.
2. **Secondary infection:** It manifests as redness, discharge, fever, etc. Appropriate antibiotics are necessary.
3. **Flap necrosis:** True mastectomy requires elevation of both upper and lower flaps (almost skin thin). Thus it predisposes to flap necrosis. This requires debridement, antibiotics, suturing and rarely skin grafting also.
4. **Haemorrhage:** Not common. If infection is severe especially in the axillary tissue, it is possible that the blood vessels may get eroded and bleeding can occur. This usually stops with pressure but may require ligation of bleeders in the operating theatre.
5. **Pain and numbness in the axilla,** medial side of arm. It is usually due to irritation of intercostobrachial nerve. Generally subsides by a few days of time. They require simple analgesics.
6. **Shoulder dysfunction** can occur especially when pectoral muscles are injured or retracted resulting in haematoma or when pectoralis muscles are removed. It improves over a period of time. Incidence is about 8–10%.
7. **Injury/thrombosis of axillary veins.** It manifests as severe pain in the hand and swelling. Treated by low molecular weight heparin.
8. **Injury to axillary vein** needs to be repaired by 5 or 6–0 Prolene sutures.
9. **Winging scapula** is due to injury to long thoracic nerve of Bell. The good anatomical knowledge is essential to prevent this complication.
10. **Lymphedema of the arm** appears a few months later (Figs 39.60 to 39.65).

Treatment of the Axilla

- The status of the axillary lymph nodes is one of the strongest prognostic factors in women especially in early stage breast cancer.
- Lymph nodes of the axilla have to be addressed.

Different Levels of Axillary Lymph Nodes

Axillary lymph nodes are broadly classified into level I, II and III nodes.

- Level I axillary lymph nodes are the nodes located lateral to pectoralis minor muscle.
- Level II axillary lymph nodes are the nodes located beneath or over the pectoralis minor muscle.
- Level III axillary lymph nodes are the nodes located medial to pectoralis minor muscle.

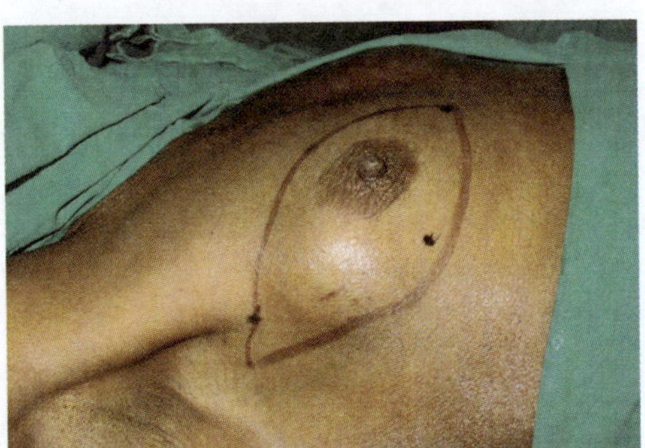

Fig. 39.60: Classical MRM incision which includes nipple areola complex and slightly extending into axilla to facilitate axillary block dissection

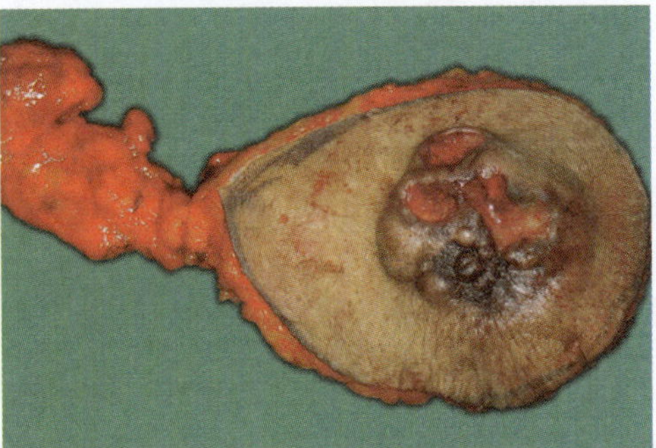

Fig. 39.61: Patey mastectomy specimen: In this operation, entire breast including axillary tail with all the axillary group of lymph nodes and pectoralis minor are removed

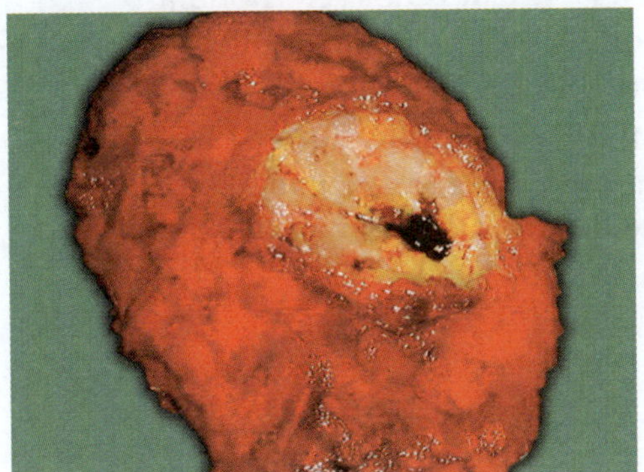

Fig. 39.62: Tumour with degeneration

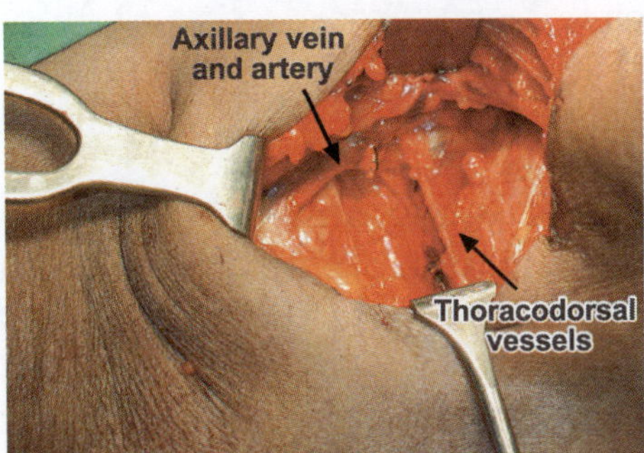

Fig. 39.63: You can see the axillary vein and thoracodorsal nerve as the axillary dissection is in progress

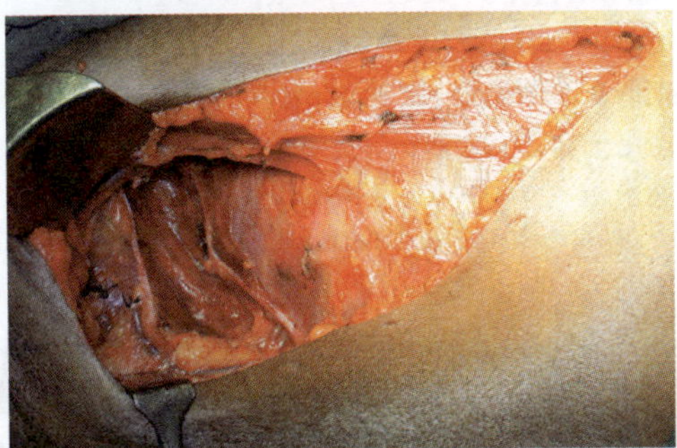

Fig. 39.64: Same patient as shown in Fig. 39.63. Axillary block dissection is complete

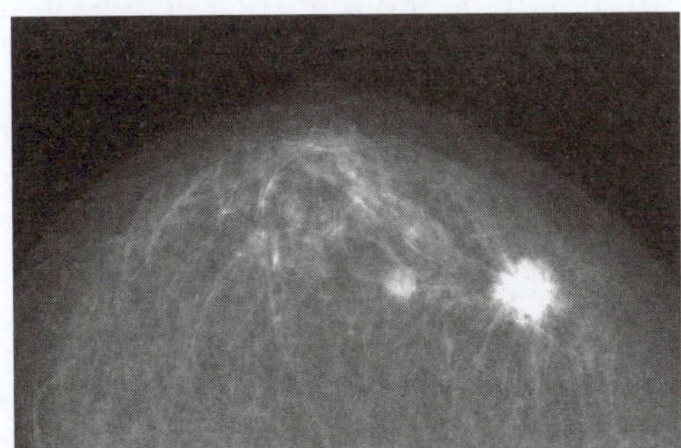

Fig. 39.65: Initially local wide excision was planned in this patient. Mammogram revealed multicentricity. Hence, MRM was done

Axillary Clearance vs Axillary Lymph Node Dissection

- Axillary clearance is removal of all levels of axillary lymph nodes. It is no longer recommended and can have significant morbidity with upper limb oedema and injury to the nerve to latissimus dorsi and nerve to serratus anterior.
- Axillary lymph node dissection (ALND) is removal of a minimum of 10 axillary lymph nodes without baring the axillary vein. Levels I and II dissection are sufficient.
- Currently we practice ALND
- Indications for ALND
  - T3 lesions
  - Patients with clinically positive axillary nodes.
  - Ultrasound-guided fine needle aspiration of an axillary lymph node proving metastasis.

Sentinel Lymph Node Biopsy (SLNB)

- The sentinel lymph node is frequently the first node in the lymphatic basin that receives drainage from an anatomic region.
- Sentinel means guard.
- SLNB has become the standard over the axillary lymph node dissection (ALND) in the staging of the axilla for clinically node negative disease.

- **Procedure:**
  - Preoperative is better and followed more commonly.
  - Patent blue (Isosulfan vital blue dye 2.5–7.5 ml) or ^{99m}Tc radioisotope labelled albumin is used.
  - Where to inject? Near the tumour: Peritumour area: Into subdermal plexus around nipple.
  - Detection: By visually blue staining after making an incision and a handheld gamma camera.
  - The node is biopsied and sent for frozen section biopsy or imprint cytology.

Where exactly to detect the sentinel lymph node (SLN)?

- A 2–4 cm incision is made in between the pectoralis major and latissimus dorsi, 5–7 minutes after the injection.
  - Blue-stained lymphatics are identified.
  - 2–3 lymph nodes have to be removed.
- **Interpretation**
  - If sentinel lymph node (SLN) is negative for malignant cells, no axillary block dissection is required.
  - If SLN is positive for malignant cells, ALND is done.
- **Detection rates**
  - Blue dye: 90%
  - Radioisotope: >95%.
- **Indications for SLNB**
  - Early T1–T2 invasive breast cancer and clinically negative axillary nodes irrespective of surgical therapy on the breast.
  - Women with DCIS undergoing mastectomy.
  - Ipsilateral recurrent breast cancer following breast conservative therapy.
- **Contraindications for SLNB**
  - Inflammatory breast disease
  - Patients with clinically positive axillary nodes
  - Ultrasound-guided fine needle aspiration of an axillary lymph node proving metastasis
  - Prior axillary sampling
  - Post-chemotherapy
  - Post-radiotherapy to axilla
  - Multifocal breast carcinoma
  - Allergy to blue dye localisation (procedure)

Breast Conserving Surgery (BCS)/Breast Conservative Therapy (BCT)

- The goal of breast conserving surgery (BCS) is to combine a conservative surgery like lumpectomy with postoperative radiotherapy and providing a result equivalent with MRM with preservation of appearance of the breast and a low rate of recurrence in the treated breast.
- Wide local excision (lumpectomy) is indicated in tumour less than 4 cm in size and with well-differentiated histology.
- It includes removal of the tumour with a rim of at least 1 cm of normal breast tissue.
- Axilla is treated with either ALND, if nodes are palpable or SLNB, if axilla is negative for nodes.
- **QUART therapy by Veronesi:** It includes Quadrantectomy (the entire segment of the breast containing tumour is removed), axillary block dissection and radiotherapy to the breast or axilla.
- However, quadrantectomy, by removing large amount of breast tissue, gives rise to poorer cosmetic results. It seems unnecessary to remove entire segment of the breast, when in reality breast cannot be strictly divided into quadrants (unlike hepatectomy). Hence, it is not very popular.
- Radiotherapy is mandatory following breast conserving surgery (BCS)
- **Absolute contraindications of BCS**
  - Diffuse suspicious or malignant appearing microcalcifications throughout the breast
  - Multicentricity
  - Inflammatory breast cancer
  - Pregnancy (radiotherapy cannot be given)
  - Previously irradiated breast
- **Relative contraindications**
  - Active connective tissue disease involving the skin (especially scleroderma and lupus)
  - Tumours >5 cm
  - Positive pathologic margins
  - Women with a known or suspected genetic predisposition to breast cancer may have an increased risk of ipsilateral breast recurrence (likely new primary development in conserved breast tissue).

TEN COMMANDMENTS

A few important tips about local wide excision—lumpectomy

1. Incision is made directly over the tumour.
2. Pectoral fascia is usually not opened unless the tumour is adherent.
3. Perfect haemostasis
4. Tumour removed with 2–5 cm margin all around.
5. Ideally specimen mammogram and frozen section is done to look for clearance.
6. Cavity should not be closed or obliterated by sutures as small seromas get absorbed.
7. For better orientation of the tumour, a long silk is tied on the lateral side. Remember a **long lateral, short suture short superior**.
8. Metal clips or coloured beads can be applied.
9. Drain should not be kept.
10. Anterior and posterior margins are less important, if a full thickness of breast tissue is removed.

Radiotherapy

- It is a form of local therapy.
- It is an adjuvant to surgery and is utilised only when indicated.
- **Indications**
  - Breast conservation surgery
  - All T3 and T4 lesions
  - T1 and T2 lesions
    - Positive resected margins after surgery
    - Inadequate axillary lymph node dissection
    - Positive axillary lymph nodes
    - Involvement of pectoralis major muscle
    - Inner quadrant tumours
- **Radiation field after MRM**
  - The chest wall
  - Internal mammary lymph nodes
  - Supraclavicular nodes
  - Axilla is not irradiated after ALND
- **Radiation field after BCS**
  - Whole breast radiation (WBRT)
  - WBRT with boost radiation is required in
    - Age below 50
    - Grade 3 tumours
    - Vascular invasion
  - Accelerated partial breast irradiation
    - More than 50 years
    - Unicentric unifocal non-lobular breast cancer
    - Less than 3 cm
    - No vascular invasion
- **Radiation dosage**
  - 45–50 gray in 25–28 fractions 1.8–2 Gy with a boost of 10–16 Gy in 2 Gy doses
  - Radiation can be given with external beam radiotherapy (EBRT) or brachytherapy

Chemotherapy

- Chemotherapy is the mainstay of treating carcinoma of the breast.
- It is because all invasive breast cancers spread even before they are palpable as they invade the basement membrane. Tumours which are more than 0.5 cm (10^5 cells) cannot survive without blood supply, hence have to invade the basement membrane to get blood supply and in the process the carcinoma breast becomes a systemic disease.

  When given postoperatively, it is called adjuvant chemotherapy. Adjuvant chemotherapy has to be given within 6 weeks of the surgery and it is given before radiotherapy. Beyond a period of 12 weeks postoperatively, it is of no benefit to the patient.

  When given preoperatively, it is called neoadjuvant chemotherapy. Chemotherapy is mandatory in all cases of carcinoma breast, except: Carcinoma *in situ*, node negative luminal A subtype of carcinoma breast.
- Chemotherapy regimens and decision making is governed by intrinsic subtypes based on the biological markers.

Pharmacological Agents Used for Chemotherapy

A combination of agents is usually given as single agent has poorer results.

- **First-line regimens**
  1. Anthracycline based
     - 5-fluorouracil. Adriamycin. Cyclophosphamide (FAC)
       - Adriamycin is the anthracycline and is cardiotoxic.
     - 5-fluorouracil. Epirubicin. Cyclophosphamide (FEC)
       - Epirubicin is the anthracycline and is less cardiotoxic.
       - 6 cycles every 21 days
  2. Anthracycline combined with Taxane
     - Adriamycin. Cyclophosphamide with taclitaxel or docetaxel
       - Paclitaxel or docetaxel is the Taxane.
       - Given with granulocyte colony stimulating factor
       - 4 cycles of AC every 21 days followed by 4 cycles of paclitaxel every 21 days (total 8 cycles)
  3. Cyclophosphamide. Methotrexate. 5-fluorouracil (CMF)
     - This is the older regimen and still effective.
     - It is economical compared to other regimens.
  4. Second-line regimens
     - Carboplatin
     - Capecetabine
     - Gemcitabine
     - Eribulin

Adjuvant Hormonal Therapy

- Also called endocrine therapy.
- It is indicated in all patients whose tumours are ER +ve irrespective of the use of chemotherapy, radiotherapy or targeted therapy.

- *Pharmacological agents* used for hormonal therapy:
  A. *Premenopausal*
  - Tamoxifen: The standard treatment is 20 mg daily for 5–10 years. Giving it for 10 years drastically reduces recurrence rates.

  B. *Postmenopausal*
  - Tamoxifen is the first option.
  - Aromatase inhibitors (Key Box 39.12)
    - They prevent synthesis of endogenous oestrogens/steroids by blocking the aromatase enzyme which converts androstenedione to oestradiol in the adrenals.
    - Drugs include anastrozole, letrozole, etc.
      - More expensive than tamoxifen
      - Reduces oestrogen levels by 98%
      - Slows down oestrogen sensitive, breast cancers.

        It is given in a dose of 2.5 mg per day.
      - Side effects include vaginal bleeding, vaginal dryness, night sweats, hot flushes, osteoporosis
    - Exemestane

Anti-HER2/neu Targeted Treatment

- Also called adjuvant trastuzumab therapy.
- Trastuzumab: A monoclonal antibody against tyrosine kinase receptor (HER2 receptor)
  - It is administered in patients with HER2 +ve patients since it has been shown to improve disease-free survival (DFS) by 50%.
  - It is cardiotoxic and should not be combined with anthracyclines.
  - It potentiates the action of Taxane, hence can be combined with them.
  - It is given over a period of 1 year.
  - Loading dose: 4 mg/kg body average and maintenance 2 mg/kg/week for a week.

Key Box 39.12

Aromatase Inhibitors

- Aromatase is an enzyme which synthesizes oestrogen.
- It converts androgens into oestrogen by process of aromatisation.
- Aromatase inhibitors inhibit this process.
- Thus in premenopausal women—it can be used to decrease production of oestrogen by ovary. However, tamoxifen is better.
- In postmenopausal woman—oestrogen is produced in peripheral tissues, such as fat, liver and muscle.
- Hence, drug of choice in postmenopausal patients is an aromatase inhibitor.
- Anastrazole, letrozole, exemextane are the drugs.
- Cardiac problems, osteoporosis are side effects.

Summary of Treatment for Early Breast Carcinoma: TNM Stage I and II

- Goal of the treatment is to the cure patient, improve survival and prevent recurrence.
- Surgery is the primary treatment either MRM or BCS.
- Axilla can be addressed either by ALND or SLNB.
- Evaluate the pathology report of the specimen.
- Chemotherapy is given within 6 weeks of surgery and is of no benefit after 12 weeks except in node negative Luminal A.
- Tumours that expressed HER2/neu require trastuzumab for a year.
- Hormonal therapy with either tamoxifen (premenopausal) or letrozole (postmenopausal) is given for 5 years.
- Radiotherapy 50 gray over 25 fractions is given after chemotherapy (Flowchart 39.1).

II. Locally Advanced Breast Carcinoma

- Operable LABC: TNM stage III A: T3N1 M0
- Inoperable LABC: TNM stage III A, B and C
- Goal of treatment is local control with a cure, if possible
- The treatment of operable LABC is similar to early breast carcinoma

Flowchart 39.1: Treatment of early breast carcinoma

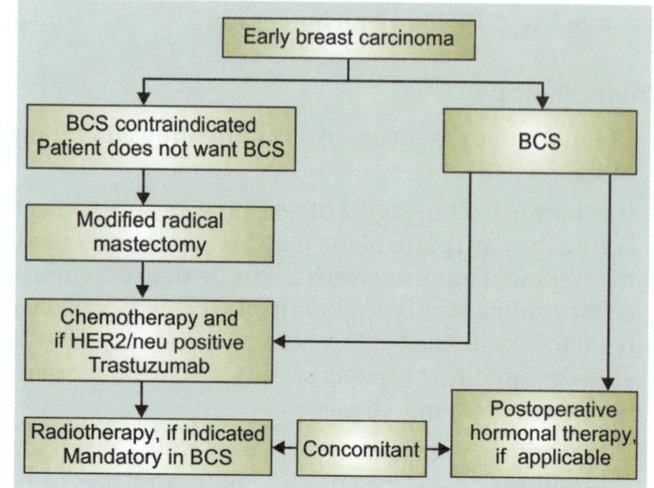

- Mandatory chemotherapy
- Mandatory radiotherapy
- Trastuzumab therapy, if indicated
- Hormonal therapy, if indicated

Inoperable LABC

- Patients who undergo surgery in this group do not have very good survival rates and have high local recurrence rates. Hence a different approach is adopted for treatment of these cases.
- A core biopsy with biological markers is mandatory before the chemotherapy is given as it can help us decide the chemotherapy regimen to be given.
- Percutaneous placement of marker clips within the primary tumour prior to the initiation of chemotherapy will provide a landmark for localization and excision should a clinical and radiographic complete response occur (Figs 39.66 to 39.68 and Key Box 39.13).
- These patients first receive preoperative chemotherapy.
- Neoadjuvant chemotherapy is also called preoperative chemotherapy or induction chemotherapy or primary chemotherapy.

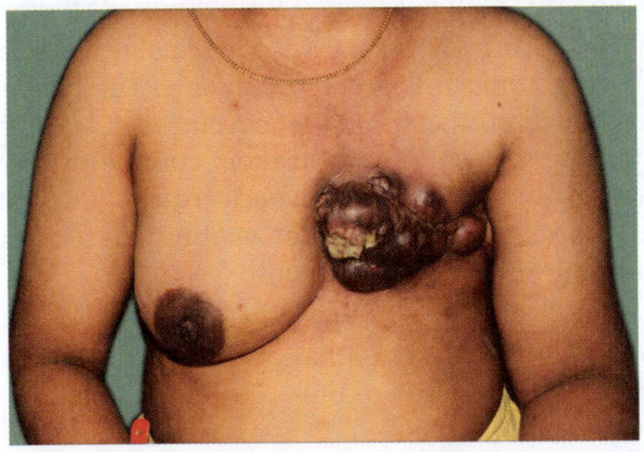

Fig. 39.66: LABC—tumour was fixed to chest wall with fungating ulcer and oedema arm. (*Courtesy:* Dr Ankur Sharma, Assistant Professor, Department of Surgery, KMC, Manipal)

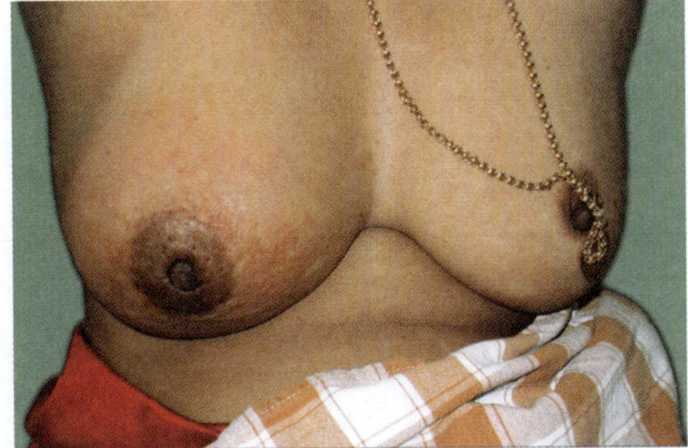

Fig. 39.67: LABC—tumour was fixed to skin with *peau d'orange*, tumour was 8 cm in size (*Courtesy:* Dr Basavaraj Patil, Associate Professor, Department of Surgery, KMC, Manipal)

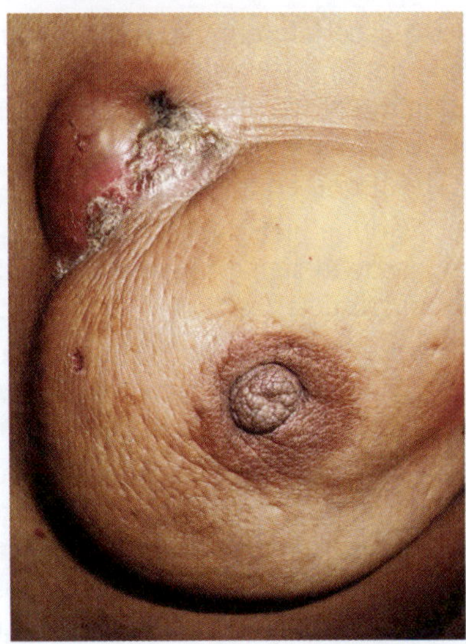

Fig. 39.68: LABC (*Courtesy:* Dr Satish Deshmukh and Dr Murtaza Akhthar, NKP Salve Institute of Medical Sciences, Nagpur)

Key Box 39.13

Summary of LABC

- Tru-cut or open biopsy is done to confirm the diagnosis followed by **identification of receptor** status.
- Neoadjuvant chemotherapy is given first which will **shrink the tumour**.
- **Surgical resection** is carried out to achieve a clear margin (mastectomy or breast conservation surgery).
- **Radiotherapy** is given to chest wall and supraclavicular area.
- **Additional chemotherapy** can also be given (adjuvant).
- If the tumour is fungating/bleeding and the surgeon feels adequate cancer clear margin can be achieved, toilet mastectomy can be done first followed by chemoradiotherapy.

Neoadjuvant Chemotherapy (NACT/Preoperative Chemotherapy)

- It is the chemotherapy which is given before any surgery.
- The goal being to make an inoperable LABC into an operable LABC.

- **Advantages of neoadjuvant chemotherapy:**
  - It allows an earlier systemic treatment, even before local care.
  - Since the index tumour is *in vivo* (in the body), the NACT may induce a reduction in the size of the tumour. This phenomenon is called a clinical response. It is evident that the NACT regimen is working on the tumour and, therefore, working on micrometastasis in the rest of the body. It is not

possible to ascertain clinical response after surgery as there is no tumour. If the size does not reduce, it means that the NACT regimen is not working hence patient should be given second-line agents or surgery should be done.
- If surgery is done first, the indolent micrometastasis may get a growth signal to have a growth and may become macrometastasis.
- In some patients, after complete clinical response occurs, BCS can be done.
- In cases receiving the NACT followed by surgery, it is possible for a pathologist to tell the surgeon the response of the tumour to the NACT by studying the operative specimen; this is called pathological response. Patients with pathological response do better than those who do not have the pathological response.

- **Preoperative chemotherapy regimens:**

  A. Adriamycin. Cyclophosphamide with paclitaxel or docetaxel
  - 4 cycles of AC every 21 days followed by 4 cycles of paclitaxel every 21 days (total 8 cycles)
  - Given with granulocyte colony stimulating factor
  - All 8 cycles are given (the full course) and no further chemotherapy is required after the surgery. This has the advantage of studying the pathological response of the entire regimen.
  - However, if only 2–3 cycles are given before the surgery and then patient is operated, then the chemotherapy should be completed.

  B. Trastuzumab is started with the taxane and continued after the surgery for 1 year.
- After completion of 8 cycles, surgery is done.
- **Surgery**
  - Done following the chemotherapy.
  - MRM is the preferred surgery. Only ALND is done, there is no role for SLNB.
  - BCS can be done in selected cases.
- **Radiotherapy** is mandatory.
- **Neoadjuvant hormonal therapy**
  - Patients whose tumours are ER positive.
  - Above 70 years of age
  - Patients who are ER positive and who cannot tolerate chemotherapy.
  - Either tamoxifen or letrozole is the drug of choice.

Terminology

- **Clinical responders**
  - Complete clinical response (cCR): Disappearance of the primary tumour and its reduction in size of lump in short axis to <10 mm.
  - Partial clinical response (cPR): At least a 30% decrease in the sum of diameters of the primary tumour, taking as reference the baseline sum diameters.
- **Non-responders:** Progressive disease (PD)—at least a 20% increase in the sum of diameters of the primary tumour, taking as reference the baseline sum diameters.
- **Complete pathological response:** No evidence of residual tumour in the breast or axillary lymph node.
- **Partial pathological response**
  - Only residual *in situ* carcinoma,
  - Residual tumour evidently modified by treatment,
  - Histologically unmodified tumour (Flowchart 39.2).

III. Metastatic Breast Cancer

- Breast cancer is a systemic disease at the onset. Even at early stages, patient may harbour micrometastasis at some sites, which may remain dormant for years together or may get treated with adjuvant therapy.
- **Metastatic breast cancer (MBC)** may be seen in almost all organs but some organ involvement is seen more frequent than others. Soft tissue recurrence, bone, liver and lung metastasis is seen more commonly. Metastasis to brain, pleura and pericardium, altogether less common, may have devastating consequences and require specific treatment.
- It is defined as TNM stage IV.
- Goal of treatment is palliation, to prolong survival and improve quality of life

  I. General treatment
  - Palliative hormonal therapy (ER +ve patients)
    - Tamoxifen
    - Letrozole
    - Exemestane
  - Palliative chemotherapy (ER –ve patients)
  - In HER2/neu expressive tumours trastuzumab can be added.
- Even if the tumour disappears, surgery should not be done.

  II. Palliative surgery (simple mastectomy)
  - No axillary dissection required
  - Indications are
    - Bleeding
    - Fungating tumours
    - Ulcerative tumours
    - Pain

Flowchart 39.2: Summary of treatment of LABC

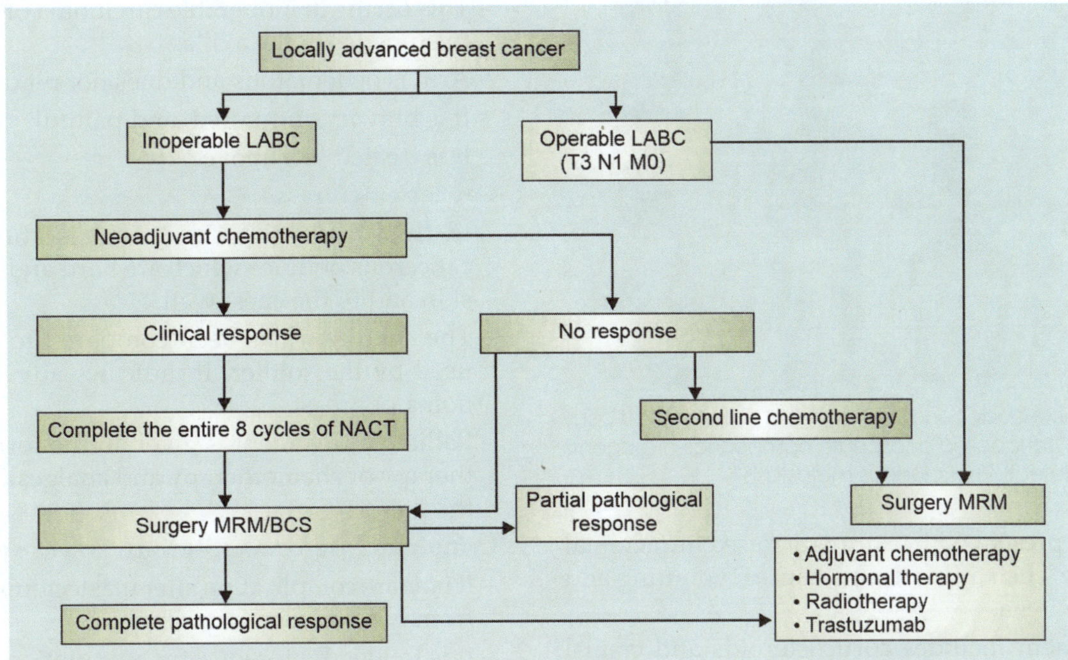

III. Palliative radiotherapy is an option to palliative surgery.

IV. Patients with bone secondaries

- Very common in stage IV breast cancer
- Problems are:
  - Severe pain
  - Pathological fractures
  - Paraplegia
  - Quadriplegia
- Localised radiotherapy is given to spine secondaries
- Spinal decompression may be required in a few patients.
- Bisphosphonates inhibit osteoclast formation and decrease bone resorption
  - Osteolytic lesions benefit the most.
  - Contraindicated, if creatinine levels are more than 3 mg/100 ml
  - Zolendronic acid—4 mg intravenously over 15 minutes every 12 weeks

• Supplement with calcium 1500 mg daily

• Supplement with vitamin D_3 400–800 international units daily
  - Pamidronate—90 mg IV over 2 hours every 4 weeks (Key Box 39.14 and Figs 39.69 and 39.70)

• Calcium and vitamin D_3 are supplemented
- Denosumab
  - Monoclonal antibody
  - Newer drug
  - Cerebral metastasis

Key Box 39.14

Bisphosphonates

- Important drugs in addition to radiotherapy to treat bone metastasis in malignancies
- Used to treat hypercalcaemia
- Inhibits osteoclast formation
- Decreases bony resorption and induces apoptosis of osteoclasts
- Decreases bony pain, increases mobility
- Helps in recalcification of lytic bone metastasis
- IV—pamidronate or zoledronic acid 4 mg IV monthly for 10 courses are used

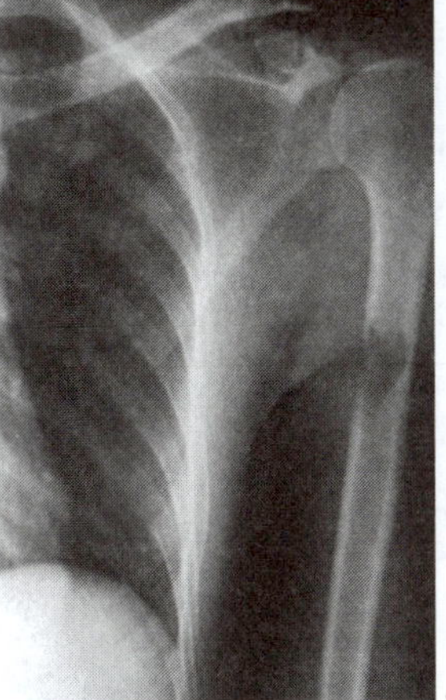

Fig. 39.69: Pathological fracture—humerus—treated by internal fixation followed by radiotherapy

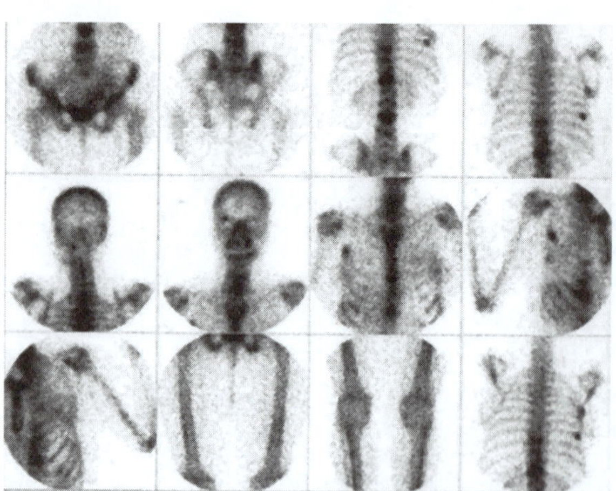

Fig. 39.70: Whole body bone scan showing disseminated bony metastasis—^{99m}Tc-labelled phosphate compounds are agents of choice for detection of osseous metastasis

V. Patients present with features of raised intracranial pressure, such as headache, nausea, vomiting and papilloedema.
   - Treatment includes corticosteroids and cranial radiotherapy.

VI. Malignant pleural effusion
   - Once effusion is confirmed by aspiration and cytology, an intercostal drain is left in place for a few days.
   - Once the drainage is nil or completely dry.
   - Talc insufflation is done, to achieve pleurodesis.
   - Talc is the most effective agent, followed by tetracycline or bleomycin, etc. In selected cases, effective pleurodesis has given an asymptomatic period up to 1–2 years.

EFFECTS OF LYMPHATIC OBSTRUCTION FROM CARCINOMA OF BREAST

1. **Peau d'orange:** It occurs due to lymphoedema due to subareolar lymphatic obstruction and fixation of hair follicle to the underlying malignancy.
2. **Oedema of the arm**
   - Also called elephantiasis chirurgens
   - It is a complication of radical mastectomy when all the nodes in the axilla are removed, especially when postoperative radiotherapy is given in the axilla.
   - It occurs due to destruction of all lymphatics and lymph nodes.
   - It does not pit on pressure. Some amount of infection also plays a role.
   - Treatment
   - Difficult
   - Elastic bandage, exercise, massages and antibiotics may help.
3. **Brawny oedema of the arm**
   - This occurs in inoperable carcinoma of breast with fixed nodes in the axilla.
   - Arm is oedematous and does not pit on pressure.
   - It is brawny, indurated, and painful.
   - It is treated like above.
4. **Cancer-en-cuirasse**
   - In this, the entire chest wall is studded with cancerous nodules which are hard and fixed to the skin and to the chest wall.
   - The condition has been compared to an armour used by the soldier. It indicates advanced carcinoma of breast.
   - Palliative treatment is given in the form of radiotherapy or chemotherapy and analgesics to relieve the pain.
5. **Lymphangiosarcoma (Stewart-Treves syndrome)**
   - It is a rare complication after mastectomy and arises from lymphoedematous limb.
   - It is treated by forequarter amputation (Figs 39.71 to 39.73).

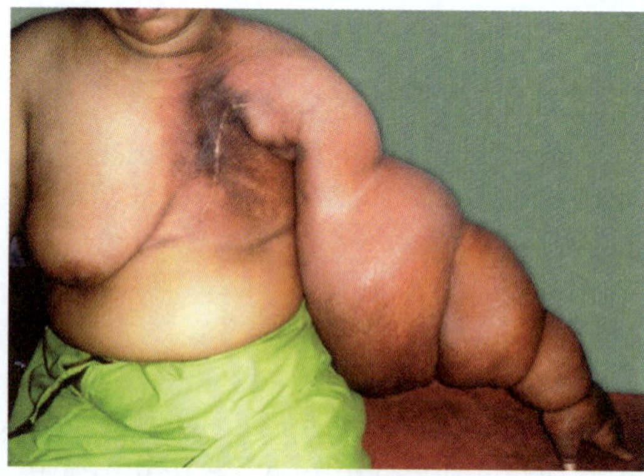

Fig. 39.71: Postmastectomy lymphoedema (*Courtesy:* Dr Sreejayan, Professor, Department of Surgery, Calicut Medical College, Calicut)

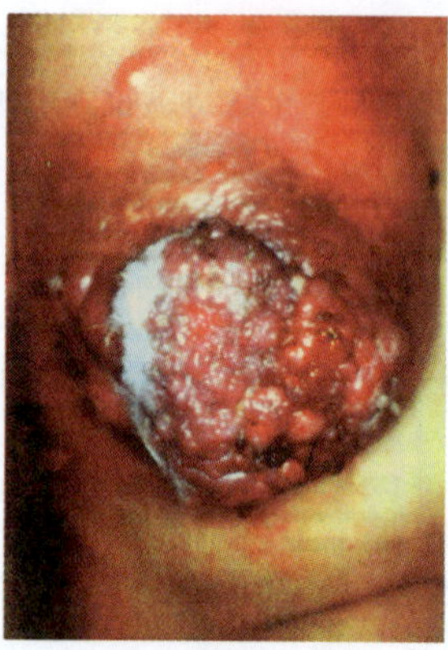

Fig. 39.72: Cancer-en-cuirasse—chest wall studded with cancerous nodules—very painful bleeding lesion

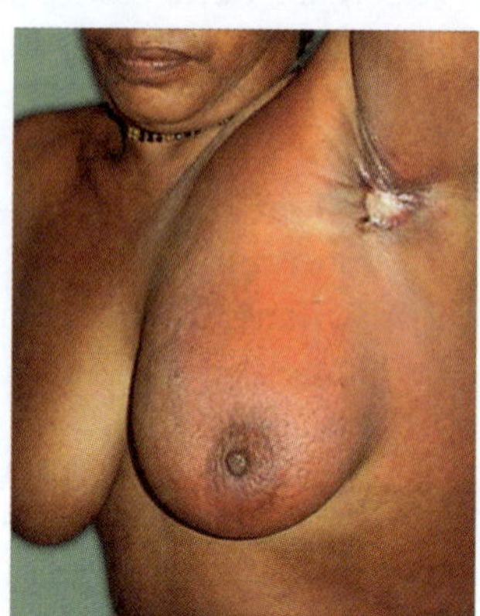

Fig. 39.73: Extensive lymphoedema and lymphangitis due to carcinoma axillary tail of the breast

ANGIOSARCOMA OF THE BREAST

- They are uncommon malignant tumours of the breast.
- Aetiology is not clear.
- Breast is one of the sites of angiosarcoma.
- Clinically, it presents as rapidly growing lump in the breast with infiltration of the skin producing ulceration.
- On careful observation, the edges are not everted and the lesion is very vascular.
- It is difficult to make a clinical diagnosis of angiosarcoma of the breast (Fig. 39.74). However, with careful examination, it is possible to suspect because of increased vascularity of the tumour and the features mentioned above.
- Confirmation of the diagnosis is by FNAC or by biopsy from the lump. Chest X-ray and CT scan of the chest are other helpful investigations.
- Treated by course of chemotherapy followed later by mastectomy.

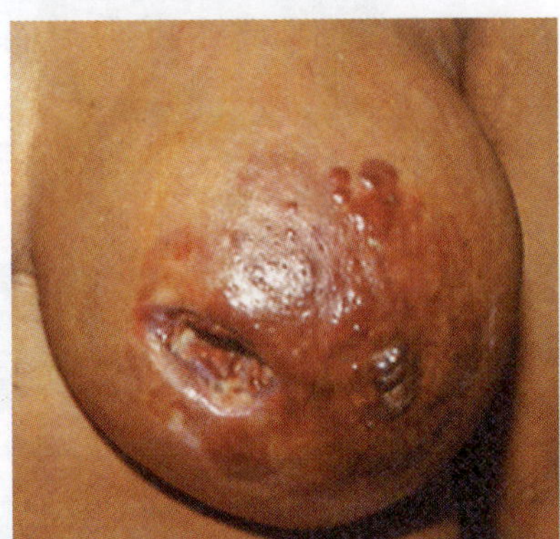

Fig. 39.74: Angiosarcoma of the left breast

BREAST RECONSTRUCTION

The ideal candidate for breast reconstruction is a patient who has undergone modified radical mastectomy.

Mastectomy results in following changes in a woman such as:

- Psychological stress
- Mood disturbances and anxiety
- Increased consciousness about clothes
- Decreased sexual interest and satisfaction
- Negative body image

Reconstruction

- Improves self-confidence
- Better social life
- Decreases concern about cancer
- Better sex life
- Feel 'whole again'

Timing

Immediate vs delayed

- Immediate reconstruction should be done, if no contraindications.
- Immediate reconstruction has the advantages of avoiding the need for a second major operative procedure and the psychological morbidity of the loss of the breast.
- It has proven psychological benefits and patient satisfaction.
- It is cost-effective.
- It does not delay adjuvant treatment and recurrence detection.

Reconstruction Options

Myocutaneous Tissue Flaps

- Flap reconstructions allow more flexibility in the size and shape of the reconstructed breast.
- Pedicled flaps
  - Latissimus dorsi myocutaneous flap (with implant)
  - Tram flap (transversely oriented rectus abdominis myocutaneous flap)
- Free flaps
  - Tram flap
  - Gluteus maximus myocutaneous flap
  - Anterolateral thigh flaps

Implant Reconstructions

- Small-to-moderate-sized breasts with minimal ptosis
- Using silicon compound gel/saline
- Expandable
- Adjustable
- Lesser risk of complications

Breast Reconstruction with TRAM Flap

- Transversely oriented rectus abdominis myocutaneous flap popularly known as TRAM flap is the most common reconstructive option in post-mastectomy breast reconstruction.
- This flap can be pedicled based on the superior pedicle or based on inferior pedicle.
- It can be used for breast reconstruction as a free flap using microvascular technique.
- Superior epigastric artery is the artery supplying the flap. If it is used as a pedicled flap for breast reconstruction, the contralateral side is used for reconstruction.
- If TRAM flap is taken with inferior pedicle using microvascular technique, deep inferior epigastric artery forms the main vascular basis of the flap (Key Box 39.15 and Figs 39.75 to 39.80).

BREAST RECONSTRUCTION WITH TRAM FLAP

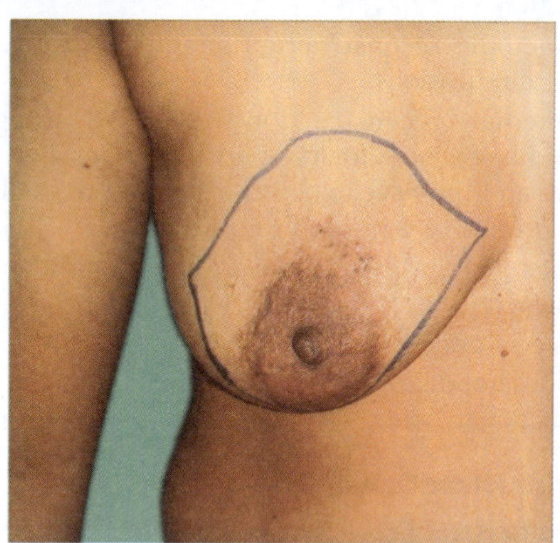

Fig. 39.75: Mastectomy site is marked

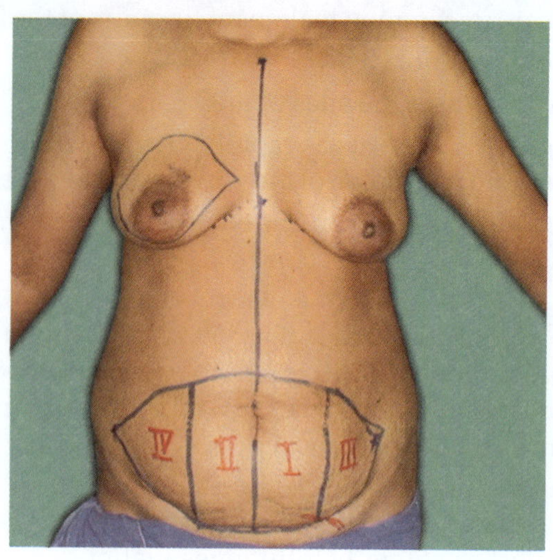

Fig. 39.76: TRAM flap marking is done

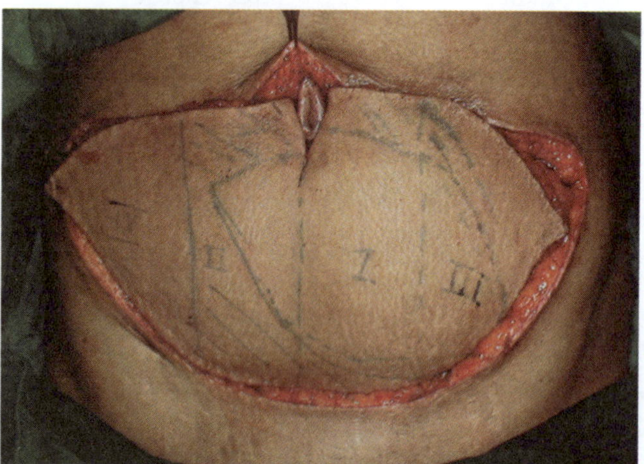

Fig. 39.77: TRAM flap is raised—flap design: Zone I–IV

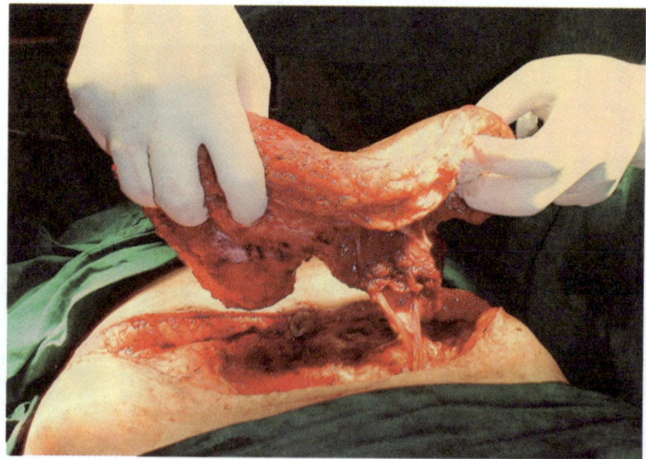

Fig. 39.78: TRAM flap is shown with its blood supply

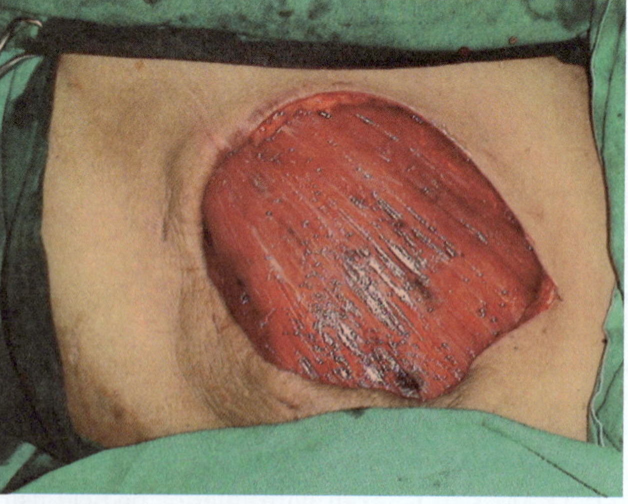

Fig. 39.79: Mastectomy bed—pectoralis muscle fibres

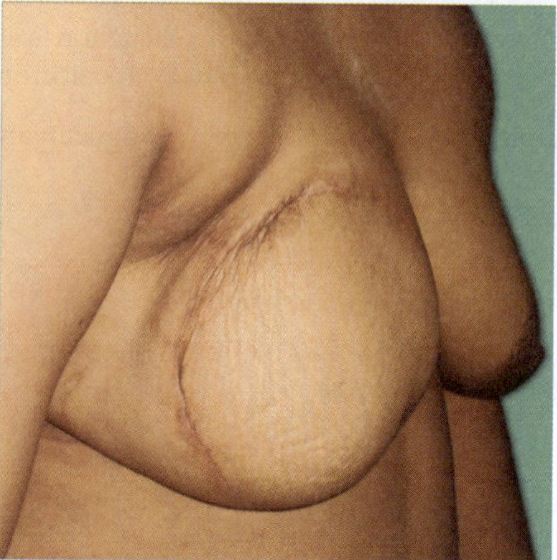

Fig. 39.80: Healing after 20 days

[*Courtesy:* Dr Bhaskar KG, Senior Consultant, Plastic Surgeon, Medical Trust Hospital, Cochin, Kerala (next page photos also)]

Key Box 39.15

Components of Breast Reconstruction

- **Chest wall reconstruction:** This can be achieved by using latissimus dorsi musculocutaneous flap or contralateral transversus abdominis muscle (TRAM) flap.
- **Creation of a mould:** A silicone gel implant is inserted under pectoralis major muscle (subpectoral pocket).
- **Reconstruction of nipple and areola:** This can be achieved by skin taken from inner thigh, labia minora or from opposite breast (nipple sharing). However, this reconstruction is done 4–6 weeks later, once the implant settles down.
- **Symmetry with the opposite breast:** It is achieved by doing reduction mammoplasty of the other breast.

Breast Reconstruction with Latissimus Dorsi Musculocutaneous Flap (Table 39.14 and Figs 39.81 to 39.87)

Indications

Breast or skin reconstruction, post-mastectomy or wide excision of large chest wall.

Contraindications

- Previous lateral thoracotomy.
- Very large breast in patient who does not desire reduction.
- Planned postoperative radiation therapy (Figs 39.81 to 39.82).

Table 39.14 Breast reconstruction

Type	Advantage	Disadvantage
Implant	• Single stage procedure • Less hospital stay • Lesser cost	• Poor symmetry, if skin removed • Capsular contracture • Leakage • Rupture
Latissimus dorsi flap	• Very low risk of flap loss • Natural contour	• Donor site scar • Usually requires an implant • Moderate prolongation of hospitalization
TRAM flap	Natural contour Good match for large or ptotic breasts	• Donor site scar • Fat necrosis • Flap loss possible • Abdominal wall weakness plus hernia • Significant prolongation of hospitalization

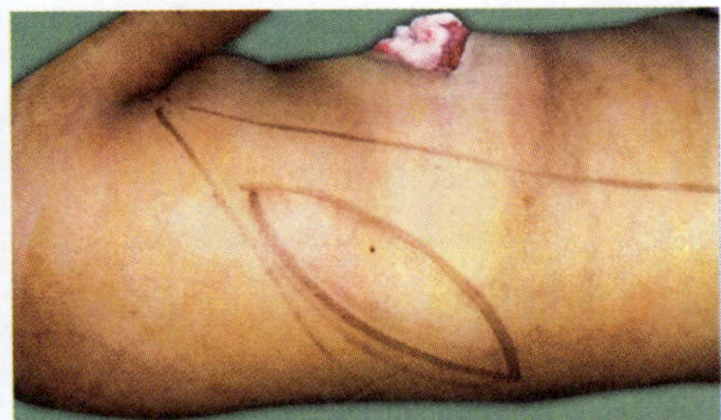

Fig. 39.81: Latissimus dorsi (LD) flap is marked

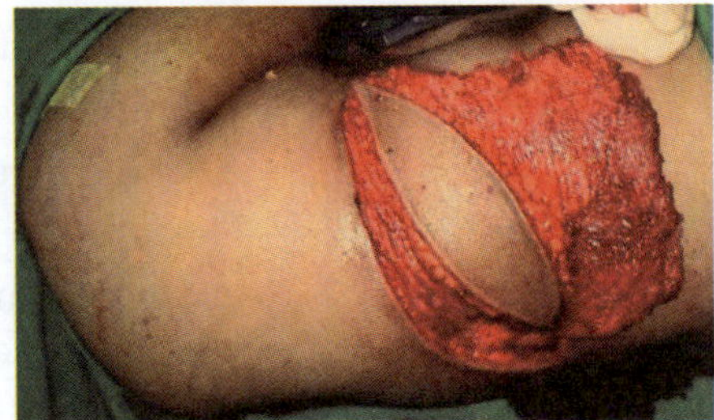

Fig. 39.82: LD flap is raised

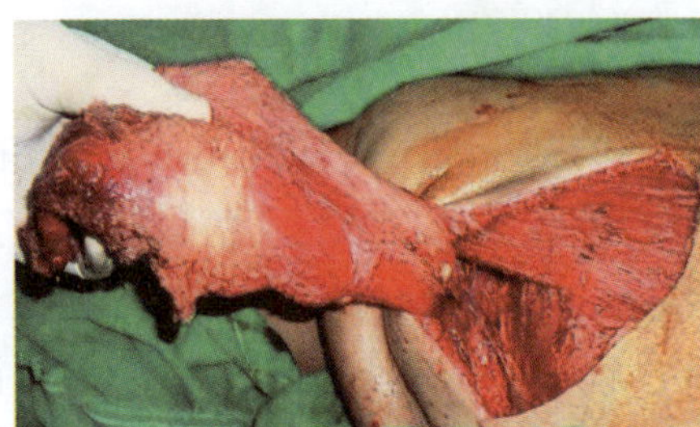

Fig. 39.83: LD flap is brought to the mastectomy site

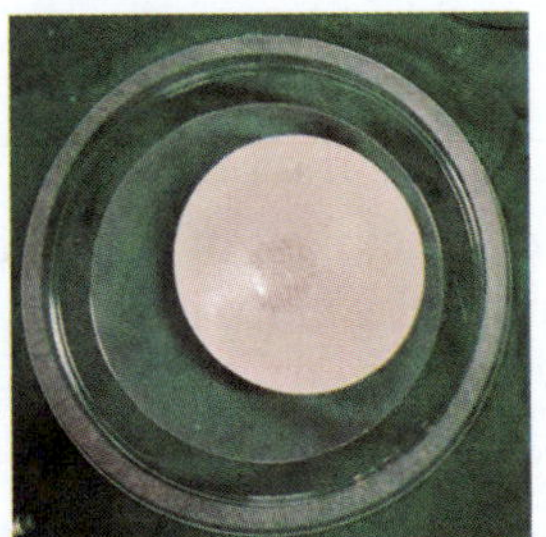

Fig. 39.84: Silicone implant

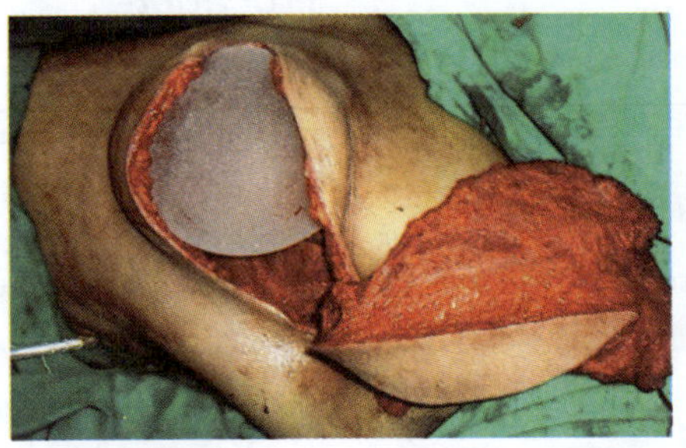

Fig. 39.85: Silicone implant placed

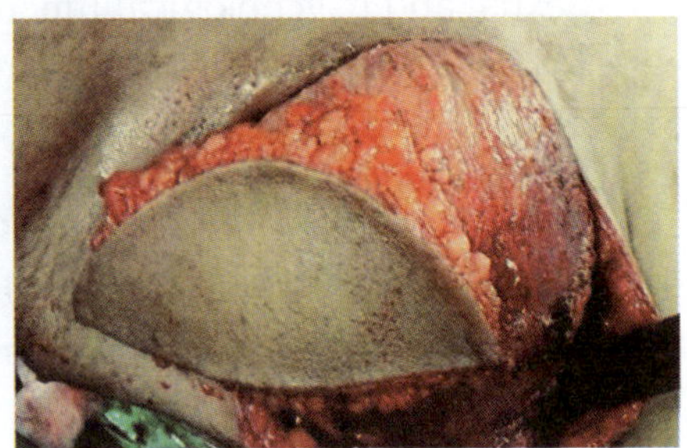

Fig. 39.86: Silicone implant placed in the subpectoral pocket

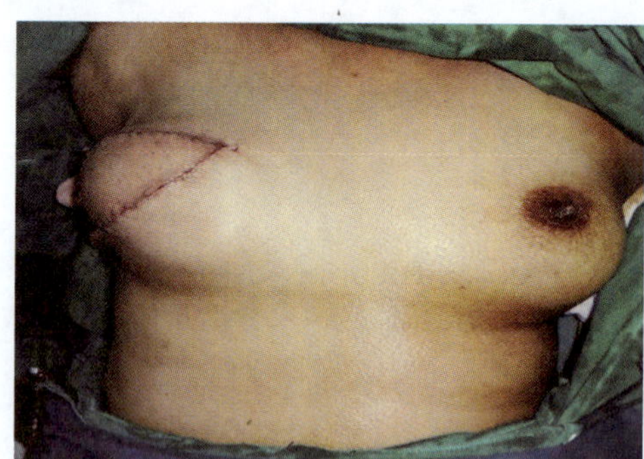

Fig. 39.87: Wound closed after implant

Positioning

- Lateral decubitus position
- Marked before mastectomy
  Vasculature/blood supply: Thoracodorsal pedicle

Procedure

- Skin island of about 5–6 cm wide, outlined transversely.
- Divide the paraspinal origins of the muscle preserving the pedicle.
- Rotated on its humeral insertion towards the anterior chest wall beneath a bridge of thoracic skin below the axilla.
- Breast implant can be placed in a submuscular pocket.

Advantages

- Proximity to the breast
- Reliable/robust circulation (rich blood supply)

Disadvantages

- Large scar on the back.
- Cannot be used, if there is an injury to thoracodorsal pedicle.

Prophylactic Mastectomy

- Also called risk reduction mastectomy.
- Breast reconstruction is done in all cases.
- Counselling is a prerequisite because:
  - Loss of breast is irreversible.
  - Sexual and psychological function.
  - Reconstruction has its own complications.
  - Does not guarantee 100% safety against cancer.

Cancer Risks in BRCA Mutation Carriers

- BRCA I: 65 to 85% (long arm of chromosome 17)
- BRCA II: 40–85% (long arm of chromosome 13)
- BRCA mutations:
  - Highest incidence in Ashkenazi Jews
  - High risk of ovarian cancer
  - High risk of contralateral breast cancer
  - Multiple ipsilateral primaries
  - Adenocarcinoma of invasive type
  - High grade
  - BRCA I—ER, PR, HER2/neu negative
  - High risk for a recurrence.

Aim

To decrease the risk of developing invasive cancer and subsequently reducing mortality.

Risk Assessment

Two specific genes—BRCA I and BRCA II are responsible for 5% of all breast cancers.

Why Prophylactic Mastectomy

- BRCA I associated cancers are invasive, high grade, ER, PR and HER2/neu negative.
- Hence, more aggressive and carry poor prognosis.

Other Risk Reduction Strategies

- Lifestyle modification: Exercises, decrease alcohol intake, avoid HRT.
- Early detection by annual mammogram.
- Tamoxifen as a primary chemoprevention drug.

Types of risk reduction mastectomy

- Total mastectomy
- Subcutaneous mastectomy.

Indications

- Biopsy proved
  - Non-invasive intraductal carcinoma *in situ*
  - A single focus of lobular carcinoma *in situ*
  - Florid cystic disease
- A mammogram that is suspicious of moderate-to-severe mammary dysplasia.
- Persistent breast nodules that do not vary with menstrual cycles and are of concern to the patient and physician.
- Familial or hereditary breast carcinoma.

Procedure

- Submammary incision is given.
- Breast tissue is dissected from the pectoral muscles.
- Skin flap along with even thickness of subcutaneous fat which is retained under the skin, is raised (helps in retaining vascularity of the flap).
- Haemostasis is obtained.
- Immediate reconstruction or reconstruction at a later date can be done.
- Skin sparing mastectomy

- Remove entire breast including axillary tail.
- Flaps should be thin.
- Axillary block dissection is not necessary.

Results

Prophylactic mastectomy reduces incidence of breast cancer by 90%.

MALE BREAST CARCINOMA

Introduction

- Rare in males
- Less than 1% of all cancer in men.
- Minimum age is around 65 years
- Many males with breast cancer have inherited a BRCA mutation.

Probable Aetiological Factors

- Genetic BRCA mutation
- Radiation exposure
- Oestrogen therapy
- Gynaecomastia
- Klinefelter's syndrome XXY
- Testicular feminising syndrome
- Obesity
- Increased incidence in prostate cancer patients.

Pathogenesis

- Male breast cancers tend to be more advanced at the time of presentation because of less subcutaneous fat.
- More than 90% cases are infiltrating duct carcinoma, about 10% are ductal carcinoma *in situ* (DCIS).

Clinical Features

- Lump in the breast which is hard and irregular.
- Nipple retraction (Fig. 39.88)

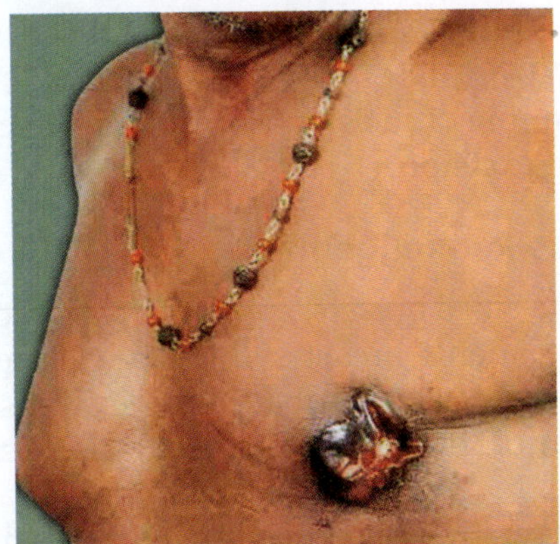

Fig. 39.88: Male breast carcinoma—tends to ulcerate and infiltrate chest wall early (*Courtesy:* Dr Surya Prakash Saxena, District Surgeon, Durg, Chhattisgarh)

- Early skin involvement
- Metastatic axillary nodes.

Differential Diagnosis

- Chest wall sarcoma
- Bony lesions, other bony metastasis
- Tuberculosis
- Gynaecomastia

Investigations

- Core biopsy
- CT scan of chest and abdomen

Treatment

- MRM with radiation to the chest wall.
- 80% of these cases are ER positive, hence role for tamoxifen.
- *Goserelin 3.6 mg/28 days for 2 years—it is an LHRH agonist. It causes reversible chemical castration.*

MONDOR'S DISEASE

Mondor's disease is spontaneous thrombophlebitis of the superficial veins of the breast and anterior chest wall. The common causes of thrombophlebitis, such as injury or infection, are not found in these cases.

Signs

1. Indurated subcutaneous thrombophlebitic cord about 3 mm diameter of varying length is situated in the subcutaneous plane with an attachment to the skin. Consistency is like that of vas deferens.
2. When the skin over the breast is stretched by raising the arm, a narrow, shallow subcutaneous groove along the side of the cord becomes apparent.

Treatment

Restricted arm movements (otherwise it is very painful). Spontaneous recovery is expected within a few days.

DISORDERS OF AUGMENTED BREAST

- This is called augmentation mammoplasty.
- Implant used is outer silicone shell filled with silicon gel, saline or a combination of both.
- **Site of implant**

  A. *Subpectoral*: More often this is the side. Even if a cancer develops in this breast, mammography can detect early lesion. After mastectomy—if recurrence develops, easy to detect if it is subpectoral.

B. *Subcutaneous:* Not many advantages: Easy to keep and easy to remove. It interferes with detection of malignancy. Easy to rupture.

- **Complications:**

1. Implant rupture: 5 to 10%
2. Bleed

RARE BREAST CANCERS

1. **Squamous cell (epidermoid) carcinoma**
   - Rare cancer from metaplasia within duct system and devoid of distinctive clinical/radiological characteristics.
   - Regional metastasis occurs in 25% of patients
   - Distant metastasis is rare.
2. **Adenoid cystic carcinoma**
   - Rare, less than 0.1%.
   - Well circumscribed and usually 1–3 mm in diameter.
   - Axillary lymph node metastasis is rare.
   - Death usually occurs from pulmonary metastasis.
3. **Apocrine carcinoma**
   - Well-circumscribed cancers have rounded vesicular nuclei and prominent nucleoli.
   - Usually aggressive.
4. **Sarcomas**
   - Large painless breast mass with rapid growth
   - Diagnosis: Core/open biopsy.
   - Sarcomas graded on—eccentricity, degree of differentiation, nuclear atypia, mitotic activity
   - Axilla is addressed only if palpable lymph nodes are present.
   - Usually in patients with history of adjuvant RT.
5. **Lymphomas:** Two variants (good prognosis)
   a. Women <39 years—bilateral, associated with Burkitt's lymphoma. Axillary dissection is done for staging and clearance of the disease. Recurrence is treated with CT/RT.
   b. Women >40 years—B cell type. Rarely Hodgkin's lymphoma

AN EXAMPLE OF A CASE OF CARCINOMA BREAST

A 59-year-old postmenopausal lady complains of lump in the right breast of 3 months duration. Lump was hard in consistency. Sonomammogram revealed ill-defined hypoechoic lesion with spiculations seen in the superolateral quadrant of the breast. FNAC was suggestive of malignancy. Whole body bone scan after 3 hours IV inj. of 20 mCi of Tc 99m MDP showed a few osteoblastic lesions—so degenerative changes.

Treatment: She underwent local wide excision followed by axillary block dissection. Final report was tubular carcinoma—30% arising in a background of proliferative breast disease (70%). All margins were free. Lymph nodes were free from metastasis.

Immunohistochemistry: Tumour cells are ER positive, PR positive quick score 2. HER2/neu 1+ Ki-67: 12%—hormone responsive.

Next plan: External beam radiotherapy of 60 Gy in 30 fractions over 6 weeks, including boost to the lumpectomy side.

- She also received tablet letrozole 2.5 mg HS and 6 monthly zoledronate—zoledic acid.

ONCOPLASTIC BREAST CONSERVATION SURGERY

- **Aims:** Complete removal of lesion and to get clear margins, thus to have R-0 resection/excision and with one surgery to do a definite procedure.
- **Introduction:** More and more women with carcinoma breast undergo wide excision—breast conservative surgery (BCS) for carcinoma breasts now. Various treatment modalities have affected the disease free survival to many years. Thus, the thought of oncoplastic surgery to give a better quality of life to a women is considered. Excisions over 5–15% of breast tissue are generally associated with unsatisfactory outcome.
- **Indication:** Breast tissues with severe ptosis and resection >20% of breast tissue.
- **Contraindications:** Previously radiated breast tissue and small breasts without ptosis.
- **Skin incisions for favourable oncoplastic outcomes:**
  - For upper pole tumours: Crescent incision or Batwing incision (Fig. 39.89)
  - For lower pole tumours: Triangle or trapezoid
  - Inframammary: Reduction
  - Any segment: Radial-ellipse (most versatile), Circumareolar with flap advancement
- One example of incision and details are given here. **Batwing excision.**

Local Tissue Rearrangement

- Moderate-sized breasts, small tumors, grade 1 ptosis. In such patients breast symmetry can be obtained by raising of skin/subcutaneous flaps to allow mobilisation of underlying glandular tissue to fill defect. Here advantage of subcutaneous fat and skin is also taken. Full thickness breast parenchyma plus skin are rotated or transposed *en bloc*. It is not for large defects because scarring and nipple distortion are the side effects if done in such cases.

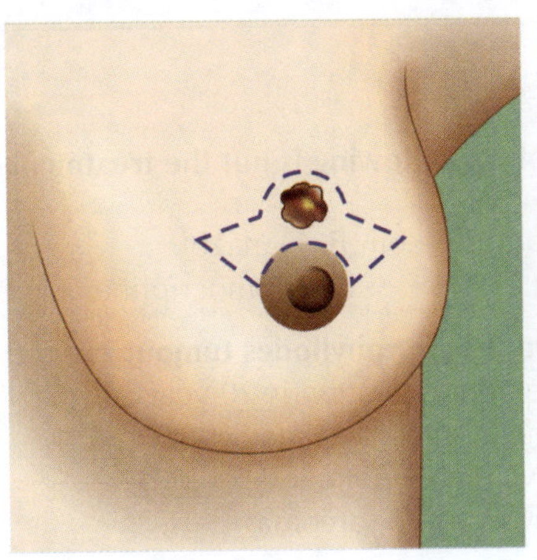
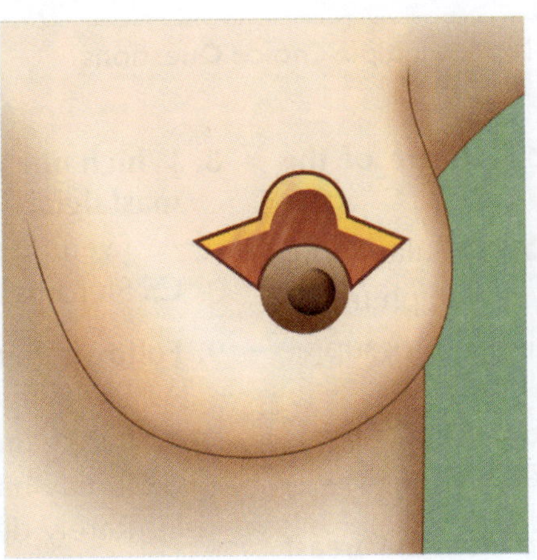
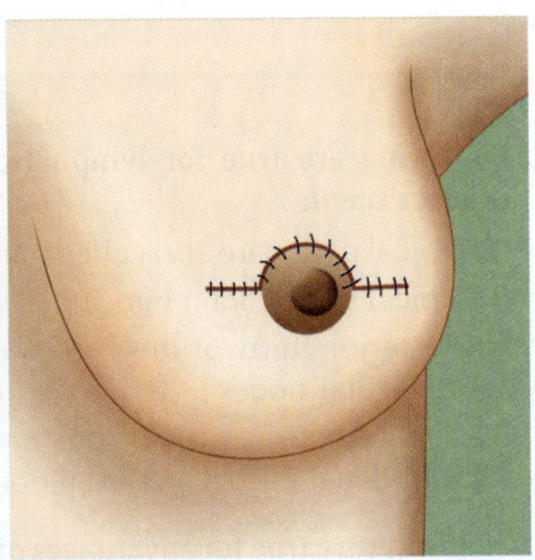

Fig. 39.89: One example of oncoplastic breast surgery—Batwing excision

Regional Flaps

- When insufficient tissue for local arrangement is present and large defect results after index surgery, few flaps can be used, e.g. latissimus dorsi flap or intercostal perforator flap. These are ideal after mastectomy.

Oncoplastic Reduction Mammoplasty

- Ideal for patients with preoperative macromastia. Based on tumour location, a skin pattern and NAC pedicle designed preoperatively to allow for tumour resection with margins and fill the defect with remaining breast tissue. Once adequate resection is done on ipsilateral side, contralateral breast is reduced to match. Incision pattern is such that it maintains viability of skin flaps while giving adequate access and exposure for partial mastectomy to be performed. The dermoglandular pedicle vascularises the NAC. Pattern used depends on tumour location.

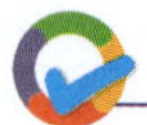

Multiple Choice Questions

1. **Following are true for lymphatic drainage of the breast *except*:**
   A. Apical nodes are also called infraclavicular nodes
   B. Apical nodes drain into subclavian lymph trunk
   C. Posterior third of the breast drain into supraclavicular nodes
   D. For detection of sentinel node, ideal site is subdermal plexus around nipple

2. **Following are true for advantages of MRI in the breast *except:***
   A. It is the best modality for women with breast implants
   B. Screening in women with strong family history
   C. It is also better than ultrasound to image axilla
   D. It can distinguish scar from recurrence in women who have undergone breast conservative surgery

3. **Following are true for retraction of the nipple *except:***
   A. Slit-like retraction is seen in duct ectasia
   B. Circumferential retraction is seen in carcinoma breast
   C. Extension of the growth along lactiferous duct causes retraction of the nipple
   D. Horizontal retraction can occur at puberty suggests fibroadenosis

4. **Following are true lactational mastitis *except:***
   A. Retracted nipple is one of the causes
   B. Majority of the cases are due to anaerobic infection
   C. Repeated aspiration is recommended treatment
   D. Fluctuation is a late sign

5. **Smoking is associated with which of the following breast diseases?**
   A. Tuberculosis B. Breast abscess
   C. Duct ectasia D. Mondor's disease

6. **Following is not the common sign of periductal mastitis:**
   A. Discharge per nipple
   B. Indurated mass
   C. Fistula
   D. Circumferential retraction of the nipple

7. **The widely used first investigation of choice in a lady of 25 years with lump breast is:**
   A. Ultrasonography B. CT scan
   C. MRI D. FNAC

8. **Which one of the following is not the treatment for mastalgia?**
   A. Evening primrose oil B. Danazol
   C. Steroids D. Bromocriptine

9. **Following are true for phyllodes tumour *except:***
   A. Usual age of presentation is 20 years
   B. Large tumour with bosselated surface
   C. It may have high mitotic index
   D. Rarely develop into sarcoma

10. **Which one of the following is the treatment of choice for early breast cancer in a 30-year-old lady who is 4 months pregnant?**
    A. Chemotherapy
    B. Tamoxifen
    C. Local wide excision
    D. Modified radical mastectomy

11. **Which is the drug used in a patient to prevent breast cancer with positive family history but unlikely carrier of breast cancer gene?**
    A. Adriamycin B. Tamoxifen
    C. Letrozole D. Trastuzumab

12. **Which one of the operative steps is not done in modified radical mastectomy?**
    A. Total mastectomy
    B. Axillary block dissection
    C. Removal of pectoralis major
    D. Removal of pectoralis minor

13. **Following are the components of breast conservative surgery *except:***
    A. Excision of tumour plus a rim of 1 cm of normal breast tissue
    B. Axillary block dissection
    C. Routine removal of the skin over the tumour
    D. Sentinel node biopsy in selected patients

14. **Following are true for radiotherapy in carcinoma breast *except:***
    A. It should be given after breast conservative surgery
    B. Large tumours after surgery require radiotherapy
    C. Extensive lymphovascular invasion is an indication
    D. Routinely given to axilla after a complete block dissection

15. **Following are true for aromatase inhibitors *except:***
    A. Maximum use in the premenopausal patients
    B. Relapse free survival is prolonged
    C. Reduction in the contralateral disease
    D. Increase in the bone density loss

16. Which of the following is the most important aetiological factor for carcinoma breast?
A. Oral contraceptive pills
B. Childhood irradiation for Hodgkin's lymphoma
C. Duct ectasia
D. Racial factors

17. Following are true for ductal carcinoma *in situ* (DCIS) *except:*
A. It is usually unilateral
B. Multifocal
C. Excision with or without radiotherapy is the treatment of choice
D. No role for chemotherapy

18. Following are true for inflammatory carcinoma *except:*
A. It results in blockage of dermal lymphatics
B. It is considered as locally advanced breast cancer
C. Neoadjuvant chemotherapy is the treatment of choice
D. Severe degree of inflammation present pathologically

19. Following are true for lobular carcinoma *in situ except:*
A. It is usually unilateral
B. Multifocal
C. Excision with or without radiotherapy is the treatment of choice
D. 20% will develop into invasive carcinoma

20. Following are true about internal mammary lymph nodes *except:*
A. They drain posterior part of the breast
B. They communicate with subdiaphragmatic lymph nodes
C. They are included in the staging system now
D. Their involvement indicates metastatic disease

21. Following are true for sentinel node biopsy in carcinoma breast *except:*
A. Injection of patent blue localises the sentinel node
B. Injecting into subdermal plexus around the nipple is ideal
C. Hand held gamma camera detects this
D. It is ideal in clinically node positive axilla

22. Following is an indication for radiotherapy to chest wall in carcinoma breast *except:*
A. Extensive lymphovascular invasion
B. Large number of positive nodes in the axilla
C. Base is involved by the tumour
D. Skin is infiltrated

23. Following are true for tamoxifen *except:*
A. It is widely used as hormonal treatment in premenopausal patients
B. It decreases the annual recurrence by 25%
C. It also has benefit in preventing contralateral breast cancer
D. It is not recommended in patients who have family history of carcinoma breast but unlikely carriers of breast cancer gene

24. Treatment option for carcinoma breast in pregnancy is:
A. Local wide excision B. Radiotherapy
C. Chemotherapy D. Mastectomy

25. Which one of the following is not true in male breast cancer?
A. Most commonly it is infiltrating duct carcinoma
B. Mostly it presents as bleeding per nipple
C. Mostly mastectomy is required
D. Gynaecomastia is a predisposing factor

26. When do you use vancomycin in breast abscess due to MRSA?
A. All cases
B. Breast abscess in pregnant patients
C. Stage of mastitis to prevent progression to abscess
D. Breast abscess with systemic toxicity

27. Following are true for ductal carcinoma *in situ except:*
A. Wide excision and radiotherapy is given
B. Pre-menopausal women are treated with tamoxifen postoperatively
C. Comedocarcinoma *in situ* requires chemotherapy
D. It can present as mammographically detected microcalcification

Answers

1. C	**2.** C	**3.** D	**4.** B	**5.** C	**6.** D	**7.** A	**8.** C	**9.** A	**10.** D
11. B	**12.** C	**13.** C	**14.** D	**15.** A	**16.** B	**17.** B	**18.** D	**19.** A	**20.** D
21. D	**22.** D	**23.** D	**24.** D	**25.** B	**26.** D	**27.** C			

Section

III

Gastrointestinal Surgery

CHAPTER

40

Oesophagus and Diaphragm

- Surgical anatomy
- Physiology
- Gastro-oesophageal reflux disease (GORD)
- Barrett's oesophagus
- Motility disorders of the pharynx and oesophagus
- Achalasia cardia
- Nutcracker oesophagus/Jackhammer oesophagus
- Carcinoma of the oesophagus
- Corrosive oesophageal stricture
- Oesophageal perforations
- Diverticulum of oesophagus
- Differential diagnosis dysphagia
- Surgical anatomy of the diaphragm
- Diaphragmatic hernia
- Tracheo-oesophageal fistula

Competency

SU28.5: Describe surgical anatomy of oesophagus.

SURGICAL ANATOMY

- Oesophagus is 25 cm in length, extending from the cricopharyngeal sphincter to the cardio-oesophageal junction (Fig. 40.1).
- Cardio-oesophageal junction lies to the left of T11 vertebra. It is identified at endoscopy by a Z-line.
- It is a jagged line where the oesophageal mucosa changes to gastric mucosa.
- **Collar of Helvetius:** It is the site at which the circular muscles of oesophagus turns to oblique muscles of the stomach at the incisura.
- It runs in the posterior mediastinum as a continuation of pharynx. 2 cm of this tube lies below the diaphragm.
- **Physiological constrictions** (Table 40.1).

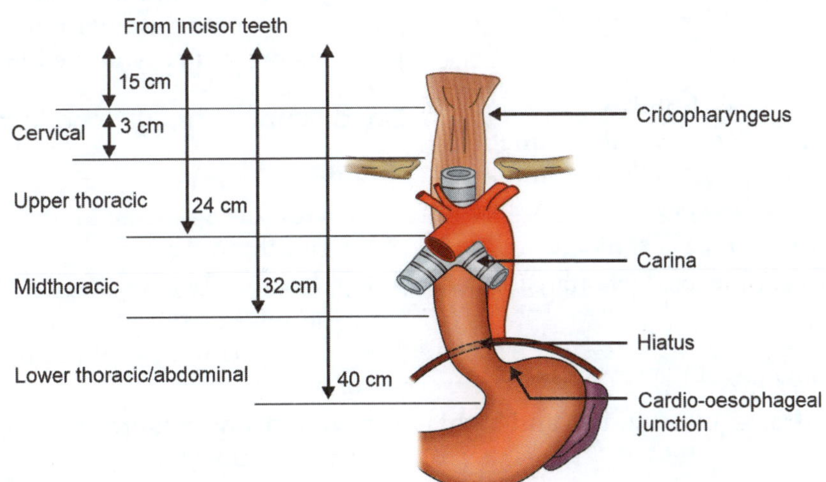

Fig. 40.1: Division of oesophagus into 4 parts based on distance from incisor teeth

Table 40.1 Physiological constrictions			
Constrictions	**Distance from incisor teeth**	**Diameter of oesophagus**	**Problems**
1. Cricopharyngeal	15 cm	14 mm	Foreign body lodgement
2. Aortic and bronchial	25 cm	15–17 mm	Perforations during endoscopy
3. Diaphragmatic sphincter	40 cm	16–19 mm	Malignancy

Muscle Layers (Figs 40.2 and 40.3)

- It has an inner circular layer and an outer longitudinal layer.
- Upper 1/3rd has striated muscle fibres.
- Lower 2/3rd has smooth muscle fibres.

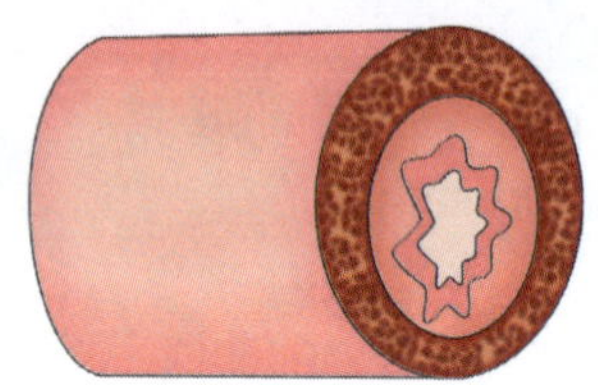

Fig. 40.2: You can see the multilayered structure. Endosonography detects all these layers

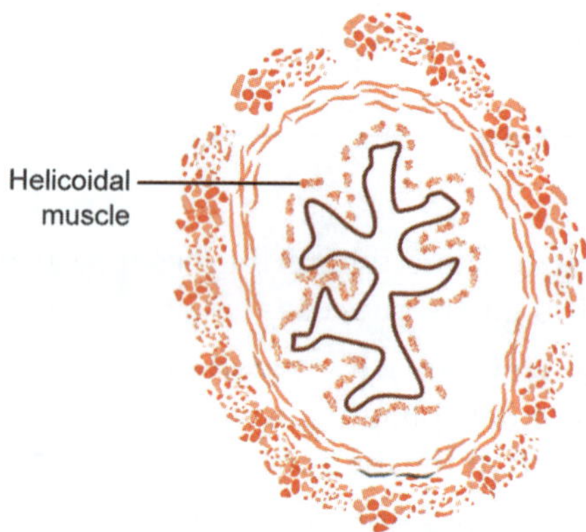

Fig. 40.3: Helicoidal muscle

Pearls of Wisdom

Clinically significant motility disorders affect lower two-thirds (smooth muscle) of oesophagus.

Mucosa

- The entire oesophagus is lined by squamous epithelium except last 3 cm which is lined by columnar cells. The columnar cells are similar to gastric mucosa but oxyntic and peptic cells are absent.
- **Mucosa is the toughest coat of oesophagus.**
- The smooth oesophageal mucosa gets transformed into rugal folds.

Lymphatic Drainage (Key Box 40.1)

- Upper oesophagus drains into the left and right supraclavicular nodes.
- Middle oesophagus drains into the tracheobronchial nodes and paraoesophageal nodes.

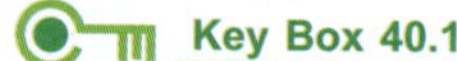 Key Box 40.1

Lymphatic Drainage of Oesophagus

- Extensive lymphatic plexus in the submucosa which explains the easy spread
- Like in the colon they are classified as perioesophageal, paraoesophageal and lateral oesophageal lymph nodes
- Thus, throughout the entire length of oesophagus various groups of lymph nodes are enlarged such as deep cervical, mediastinal, subcarinal, hilar, diaphragmatic, para- and peri-oesophageal, gastric, coeliac, etc.
- Presence of coeliac nodes indicates inoperability
- **Longitudinal lymphatics are 6 times more than transverse**. Hence, distant spread occurs fast—satellite nodules occur proximal and distal to the growth. This is the reason why 10 cm margin must be given in resection of the oesophagus
- These are advantages of transhiatal resection over Ivor-Lewis operation (*see* page 533)

- Lower oesophagus drains into lymph nodes along the lesser curvature of stomach and then into coeliac nodes. Involvement of coeliac nodes indicate inoperability.

Nerve Supply

The parasympathetic nerve supply is by vagus nerve through extrinsic and intrinsic plexuses. The intrinsic plexus has **no Meissner's network** and **Auerbach's plexus is present only in the lower two-thirds.**

Blood Supply (Figs 40.4 and 40.5)

Arterial

- **Cervical oesophagus:** Mainly from branches of the inferior thyroid artery.
- **Upper thoracic oesophagus:** Mainly from branches of the inferior thyroid artery and less consistently from anterior oesophagotracheal branch from aorta.
- **Mid and lower thoracic oesophagus:** Supplied by bronchial arteries.
- **Lower oesophagus:** Small branches of the left gastric artery.

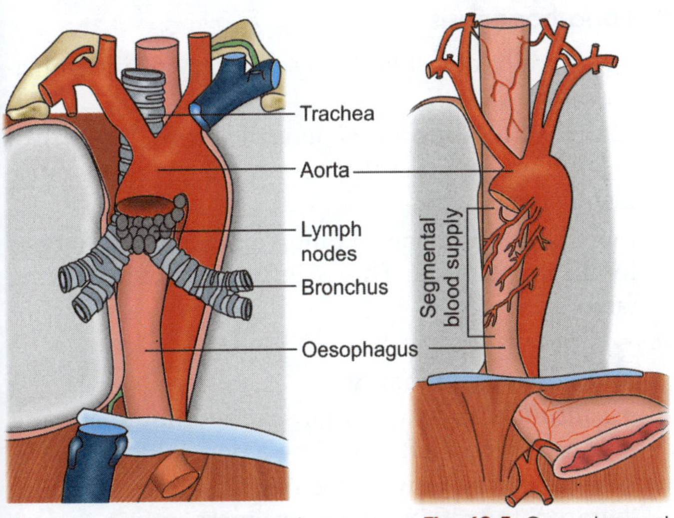

Fig. 40.4: Oesophageal anatomy—relationships

Fig. 40.5: Oesophageal anatomy—segmental blood supply

Rich internal arterial anastomosis is present in the oesophagus and in the stomach. Hence, extensive mobilisation of oesophagus can be done without compromising viability.

Venous Drainage

Veins accompany corresponding arteries. Importantly, thoracic oesophagus drains into azygos and hemiazygos veins. Key points of surgical anatomy are given in Table 40.2.

PHYSIOLOGY (Deglutition–Swallowing)

The main function of the oesophagus is to transfer food from the mouth to the stomach. Voluntary contraction of the oropharynx pushes food into the upper oesophagus through a relaxed cricopharyngeal sphincter (Key Box 40.2). Then, due to primary and secondary peristalsis, the food bolus is transferred to the stomach (Fig. 40.6).

- **Cricopharyngeal sphincter** is closed at rest. It helps in preventing regurgitation of oesophageal contents into the respiratory passage. Killian's dehiscence (also known as Killian's triangle) is **a triangular area in the wall of the pharynx between the cricopharyngeus and thyropharyngeus** which are the two parts of the inferior constrictors—site wherein Zenker's diverticulum can occur (Table 40.2).

Key Box 40.2

The Pharyngeal Stage—Reflex

- Food stimulates mechanoreceptors
- Soft palate is pulled upwards so that food will not enter nasal cavities
- Vocal cords adduct and larynx is pulled upwards against epiglottis so that food will not enter trachea
- Cricopharyngeal sphincter opens
- Muscular wall of the pharynx then contracts from above downwards

Table 40.2 Surgical anatomy of the oesophagus—key points

Surgical anatomy	Significance	Surgical points of interest
1. Upper oesophageal sphincter	Dense cricopharyngeus muscle	Zenker's diverticulum through Killian triangle.
2. Lower oesophageal sphincter	High pressure zone at gastro-oesophageal junction	Weakness causes reflux oesophagitis
3. Oesophageal mucosa	Toughest coat of oesophagus	Important in oesophageal anastomosis
4. No serosa, no mesentery	Requires mobilisation	Leak rate is high, easy spread of carcinoma
5. Helicoidal muscle	Helps in peristalsis but it recoils due to elasticity	Hence, once resection takes place—specimen 'shortens' or retracts—anastomosis may become difficult especially in abdominal anastomosis
6. Segmental arterial supply	Extensive mobilisation can be done without compromising blood supply	Hence, transhiatal esophagectomy (THE) is done with ease
7. Lower end of oesophagus—veins	Rich intercommunicating veins between portal and systemic veins	Oesophageal varices occur here
8. Azygos vein crossing oesophagus in thorax	Can get injured and bleed	Resection of midoesophageal tumours
9. Mucosal and submucosal lymphatics out number capillaries	Oesophageal tumours extend over a long distance within oesophageal wall	Need for total oesophagectomy and cervical anastomosis + lymph node clearance

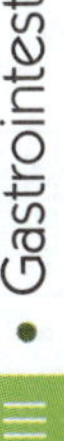

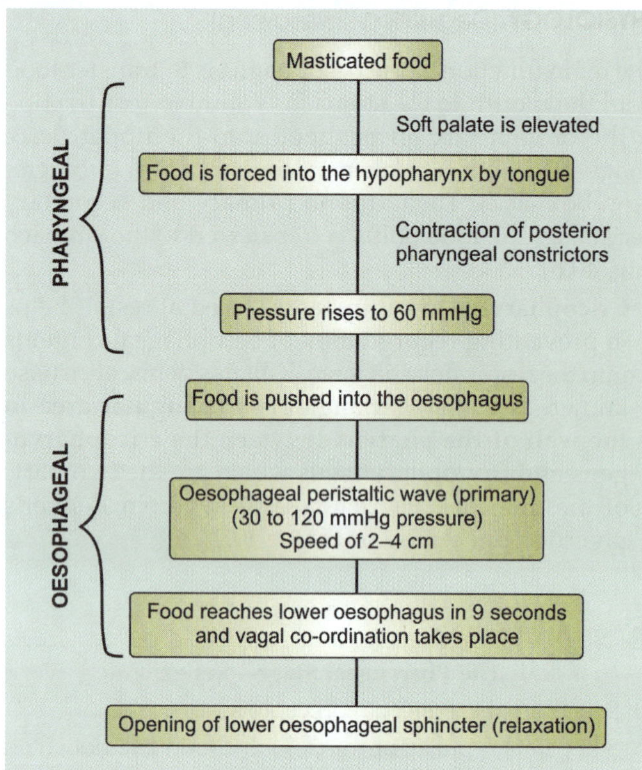

Fig. 40.6: Mechanism of swallowing—two phases

- **Lower oesophageal sphincter (LOS):** It is a physiological sphincter at the gastro-oesophageal junction. It is 3–4 cm long with a resting pressure of 20–25 mmHg. Hence, it is known as **high pressure zone (HPZ)**.
- This HPZ prevents reflux of gastric contents into the oesophagus. Cigarette smoking affects this zone and so, smokers have a high incidence of reflux oesophagitis.

Competency

SU28.5: Describe etiopathogenesis, clinical features, investigations, principles of management and complications of GERD and Barrett's oesophagus.

GASTRO-OESOPHAGEAL REFLUX DISEASE

- Loss of competence of LOS leads to gastro-oesophageal reflux disease (GORD). The competence of LOS can be affected by obesity, smoking, excessive eating, etc. Sliding hernia is associated with GORD.
- As a result of reflux of gastric acid, extensive inflammation of the lower oesophagus occurs which results in various forms of oesophagitis.

Types

1. **Acute:** Following alcohol, burns, stress.
2. **Chronic:** It is associated with hiatus hernia or following oesophagojejunostomy.

Aetiopathogenesis

1. Structurally defective LOS secondary to inflammatory injury.
2. Inadequate abdominal length (short length) of oesophagus—precipitates a reflux when gastric distension occurs.
3. Ineffective oesophageal pump affecting clearance of food into stomach. This is influenced by following factors:
   - Gravity
   - Oesophageal motility
   - *Salivation*—saliva neutralises the minute amount of acid that is left following a peristaltic wave.

   When salivary flow is decreased (following radiotherapy), the reflux can get exaggerated.
4. **Increased gastric pressure:** Can occur due to pyloric stenosis and diabetic gastroparesis. Following vagotomy, loss of receptive relaxation occurs resulting in increased intragastric pressure.
   - Acid refluxes into the lower oesophagus and produces diffuse inflammation with multiple ulcers.
   - The symptoms are worse when the patient lies down.
   - Due to vagal hyperactivity, inflammation and ulcers develop which produce severe longitudinal muscle spasm. Consequently, the cardia is drawn up into the thorax, leading to an increase in the oesophagocardiac angle. This increases the reflux.

     Later, fibrosis causes shortening of the oesophagus.
   - Thus, it becomes a vicious circle of *oesophagitis—longitudinal muscle spasm—displacement of oesophagus—increased regurgitation.*

Clinical Features

Most common presentation of GORD is history of heartburn and regurgitation. Heartburn is confined to epigastrium and retrosternal areas, does not radiate to the back. Clinical presentation of the GORD can be classified as follows: Atypical symptoms can be so many and can thus confuse the picture.

Oesophageal	: Dysphagia, regurgitation, heartburn
Gastric	: Early satiety, belching, bloating, nausea
Pulmonary	: Asthma, wheezing, aspiration, cough, dyspnoea, bronchitis, hoarseness of voice due to damage to vocal cords, etc.
Ear, nose, throat	: Waterbrash, globus, hoarseness
Cardiac	: Chest pain

What is globus? Sensation of a substernal lump (globus). When this occurs during fasting, it is termed 'globus hystericus'. It is a neurotic symptom in patients with emotional instability.

- **Retrosternal pain:** It is burning in nature and becomes worse on lying down. The pain reduces in the sitting position. The pain is described as *heartburn and can be confused for angina pectoris.* It is relieved on taking antacids.
- **Heartburn** is otherwise called **pyrosis**.
- **Occult blood in stools** and streaks of blood in the vomitus are common.
- **Anaemia** and weakness are uncommon features.
- **Dysphagia:** Transient difficulty in swallowing results from spasm due to inflammation of the lower end of oesophagus. Late dysphagia is due to stenosis or stricture of the oesophagus. Belching is not uncommon.

Complications

- **Benign:** Oesophageal ulcers, bleeding and peptic strictures. Peptic strictures are not common nowadays due to the treatment of aid peptic disease with proton pump inhibitors.
- **Barrett's oesophagus and adenocarcinoma:** Chronic reflux will bring metaplasia in the lower and mid-oesophagus resulting in Barrett's oesophagus which progresses to adenocarcinoma oesophagus (Fig. 40.7).

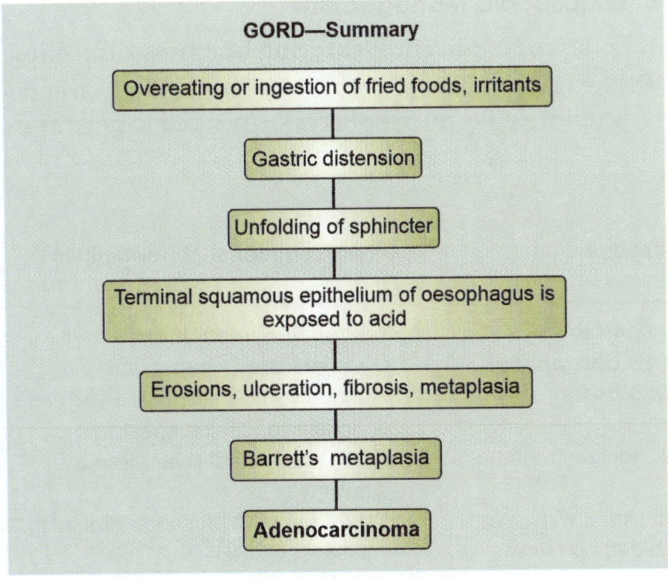

Fig. 40.7: Carcinogenesis due to GORD

Scoring Systems/Classification of GORD

Johnson-DeMeester Scoring System

Three important symptoms are taken into consideration.

Grade	Features
	Heartburn
0	None
1	Minimal—occasional episodes
2	Moderate—medical therapy visits
3	Severe—interferes with daily activities
	Regurgitation
0	None
1	Minimal—occasional episodes
2	Moderate—on position or straining
3	Severe—features of aspiration
	Dysphagia
0	None
1	Minimal
2	Needs fluid to clear
3	Causes food impaction

Modified Savary-Miller Classification of Reflux Oesophagitis

Grade I: Single or isolated erosion at or above GE junction

Grade II: Multiple non-circumferential erosions above GE junction

Grade III: Circumferential erosions above GE junction

Grade IV: Chronic lesion—stricture, ulceration/short oesophagus

Grade V: Columnar epithelium in continuity with Z line (Barrett's oesophagus)

Investigations (Table 40.3, Key Boxes 40.3 and 40.4)

- **Barium swallow**[1] in the Trendelenburg's position (head down position) can demonstrate the reverse flow of barium into the lower end of the oesophagus (from the stomach).
- **Oesophagoscopy** may reveal red, angry looking mucosa in the lower end of the oesophagus.
- **Oesophageal manometry** to detect motility disorders. A thin catheter is passed through the nose which contains pressure sensors.
- **24-hour pH monitoring is the gold standard.**

[1]Barium swallow: Thick paste to see the oesophagus. Barium meal: A thin paste to see the stomach. Both are radio-opaque.

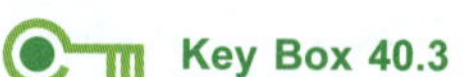

Key Box 40.3

Oesophageal Manometry

- Information about LOS
  - Resting pressure
  - Length
  - Relaxation
- Quality of oesophageal peristalsis
- **Manometry is essential. To place the pH probe 5 cm above upper border of LOS for ambulatory pH monitoring.**

Key Box 40.4

24-hour pH Monitoring is the Gold Standard

- Indications: When symptoms are certain but endoscopy is normal, atypical symptoms
- It involves the transnasal placement of a pH measuring electrode in the lower oesophagus. The pH electrode monitors the changes in intra-oesophageal pH over 24-hour
- A 24-hour pH profile is thus obtained that provides information on frequency, duration and pattern of reflux
- A reflux episode is defined as a pH drop to below pH 4
- Thus, identification, type and duration of reflux is noted

Summary of the investigations and the utility of these have been summarized in Table 40.3.

Treatment

It can be classified as medical, endotherapy and surgical line of management. Conservative treatment or medical line of treatment should be attempted in all these patients. Majority of the patients respond to conservative line of treatment.

A. Medical Management

Treatment of uncomplicated GORD can be discussed under the following headings:

I. Lifestyle modification

- Stop smoking
- Stop alcohol
- Control obesity
- Small meals
- Avoid coffee, chocolate and coke
- Head up—propped-up position
- Avoid stooping
- Avoid tight garments

II. Drugs

- Antacids with alginate—antireflux floating alginate.
- **Proton pump inhibitors:** Pantoprazole 40 mg, esomeprazole till 20 mg may have to be given for one or two months or full symptoms are controlled. These are antisecretory drugs.
- **Prokinetics:** Itopride 50 mg can be given 2–3 times a day for 8 weeks on empty stomach. Prokinetics enhance motility. Cisapride and mosapride are not favoured because they can cause cardiac arrhythmias.

III. Mucosa protective agents

- Sucralfate colloidal bismuth—cytoprotective agent.
- It is a sucrose sulphate–aluminium complex which binds to the mucosa. Thus, it protects mucosa of GI tract against hydrochloric acid.
- Colloidal bismuth compounds.

B. Endoscopic Management

I. Endoscopic plication/suturing or enteryx injection

- **Plexiglass microspheres (PMMA):** Through an endoscopic needle, microspheres suspended in gelatin are

Table 40.3 Investigations of GORD

To detect structural abnormalities	To detect increased exposure to gastric juice	To detect functional abnormalities
A. Barium swallow • Detects hiatus hernia (prone position) • Detects stricture or any rings • Extrinsic compression can be detected • Can also detect small carcinoma ***B. Flexible endoscopy*** • Can detect hiatus hernia or diverticulum, etc. • Can detect oesophageal abnormalities	***A. Flexible endoscopy and to biopsy—the Barrett's oesophagus*** ***B. Grading of oesophagitis by endoscopy*** Grade I: Small, circular, nonconfluent erosions Grade II: Linear erosions lined with granulation tissue that bleeds on touch Grade III: Erosions with circumferential loss of the epithelium—cobblestone oesophagus Grade IV: Stricture	***A. Oesophagus manometry*** • It is indicated when motor abnormality is suspected such as achalasia, diffuse spasm • Can also detect scleroderma polymyositis • Average LOS pressure <6 mmHg, suspect GORD • High resolution manometry is more accurate

injected. Gelatin is absorbed and spheres cause tissue bulking.

II. Endoscopic treatment of GORD: Three types:

1. **Radiofrequency energy to LES:** It changes sphincter compliance.
2. **Barrier at GE junction:** An ethylene vinyl alcohol copolymer is injected into submucosa 1–2 mm caudal to Z line.
3. **Direct endoscopic suturing and tightening of LES:** To summarise, quit smoking, decrease alcohol intake, avoid overweight and start walking. Do not drink coke and do not eat chocolates, take mucosa protective agents (Key Box 40.5).

Key Box 40.5

Medical Management of GORD

- **A**lcohol to be minimised
- **L**ose weight
- **C**offee/tea to be minimised
- **O**esophageal mucosa protectors—antacids, H_2 receptor blockers
- **H**ead—up tilt
- **O**ily and spicy food must be avoided
- **L**arge meal to be avoided at night times

Remember as **ALCOHOL**

C. Surgery: Indications

- Intractable pain—heartburn and dysphagia
- Complications such as haemorrhage or stricture
- The results of antireflux surgery are good with a small mortality rate (0.1 to 0.5%). However, careful selection of patients depending upon their symptoms and lifestyle are important factors.

Types of Surgery

1. **Nissen's total fundoplication** (Figs 40.8A and B): The aim is to restore 2–4 cm of intra-abdominal oesophagus by reducing the hernia, followed by repair of the hiatus.

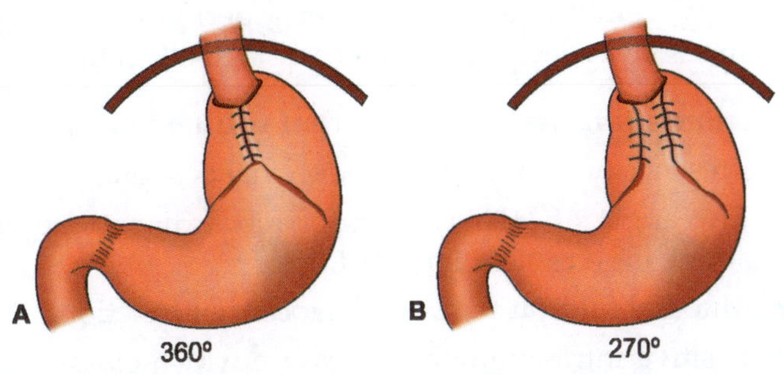

Figs 40.8A and B: Nissen's fundoplication

- In this operation, fundus of the stomach is mobilised by dividing short gastric arteries.
- Fundus is brought behind the oesophagus and wrapped in front of oesophagus. It is a ***loose wrap (Floppy Nissen).***
- Diaphragmatic defect is repaired by using nonabsorbable sutures such as nylon or silk. This is the operation which serves all aims.
- Mortality and morbidity should be minimised.

Laparoscopic fundoplication

- Most popular today
- Minimal morbidity and mortality
- Early discharge, within 1–2 days
- Early recovery
- All operative steps that are performed in open surgery are carried out here with a 'better vision' in laparoscopic method.

Principles of fundoplication

- 360° gastric fundoplication should be no longer than 2 cm.
- It should be constructed over a 60°F bougie.
- Fundoplication should be placed in the abdomen without tension.
- Only 'fundus' should be used to wrap (fundus relaxes—body does not relax on swallowing).
- Vagus should not be damaged because it may result in failure of sphincter to relax.
- Lengthen the oesophagus with a Collis gastroplasty (in cases of short oesophagus).
- Patients with normal peristaltic contractions do well with 360° Nissen's fundoplication—for others, two-thirds partial fundoplication may be the procedure of choice.

Complications

- Too tight a plication may result in dysphagia or gas bloat syndrome wherein belching is prevented.

2. **Partial fundoplication (Toupet)** solves the above problem wherein fundus is sutured around the back of oesophagus (Fig. 40.9) or Dorr's, where fundus is sutured anterior to the oesophagus.
3. **Linx device treatment**

- It is a ring of interlinked titanium beads with magnetic cores.
- It is indicated in patients who have **GORD but without hiatus hernia.**
- These are magnetic beads placed around oesophagogastric junction.
- These beads will stretch with increased pressure in the oesophagus.
- This is called magnetic sphincter augmentation.

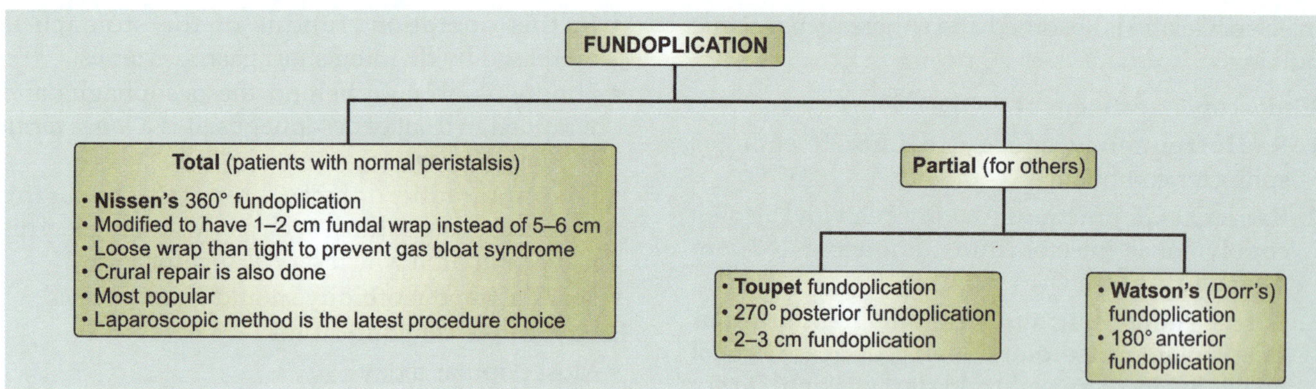

Fig. 40.9: Types of fundoplication

HIATUS HERNIA

Definition

Abnormal protrusion of abdominal viscus through the oesophageal hiatus into the chest.

Types (Key Box 40.6)

I. **Sliding hernia or oesophagogastric hernia:** It is the commonest type of hiatus hernia, accounting for about 80% of cases (Fig. 40.11). It may be associated with GORD.

II. **Rolling or paraoesophageal hernia**

III. Mixed hernia

IV. Massive herniation.

Key Box 40.6

Types

I	:	H^0	:	Normal
II	:	H^1	:	Sliding
III	:	H^2	:	Paraoesophageal
IV	:	H^3	:	Mixed
V	:	H^4	:	Massive herniation

1. **Type I** hernias are sliding hiatal hernias, where the gastroesophageal junction migrates above the diaphragm. The stomach remains in its usual longitudinal alignment and the fundus remains below the gastroesophageal junction.
2. **Type II** hernias are pure paraoesophageal hernias (PEH); the gastroesophageal junction remains in its normal anatomic position but a portion of the fundus herniates through the diaphragmatic hiatus adjacent to the esophagus, through a defect in the phrenooesophageal membrane.
3. **Type III** hernias are a combination of Types I and II, with both the gastroesophageal junction and the fundus herniating through the hiatus. The fundus lies above the gastroesophageal junction.
4. **Type IV** hiatal hernias are characterized by the presence of a structure other than stomach, such as the omentum, colon or small bowel within the hernia sac.

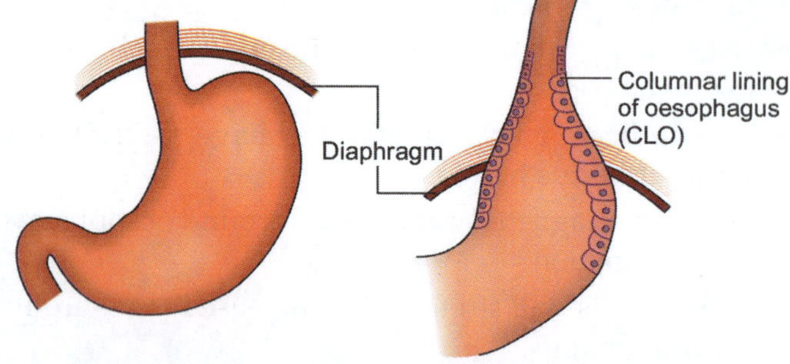

Fig. 40.10: Normal position

Fig. 40.11: Sliding hernia

Common Symptoms

1. **Symptoms due to reflux:** Regurgitation and heart burn are the two most common symptoms.
2. **Symptoms due to complications:** They are dysphagia, odynophagia, haematemesis and melaena.
3. **Nonoesophageal symptoms:** They are asthma and chest pain.

SLIDING HERNIA

In this variety, squamocolumnar junction or Z line is at a higher place resulting in loss of angle of His. Due to loss of angle of His and lower oesophageal sphincter activity, reflux takes place. Over a period of time, it changes into columnar-lined oesophagus (CLO).

Anatomical factors which prevent sliding hernia

- Presence of 2 cm of intra-abdominal oesophagus.
- **The angle of His:** The oesophagocardiac angle of about 45° has valvular effect.
- Mucosal folds at the oesophagocardiac junction.
- Positive intra-abdominal pressure which closes the abdominal oesophagus.

- **Lower oesophageal sphincter (LOS):** It is a functional sphincter which increases the pressure during coughing, straining, etc.

Causes of Sliding Hernia[1]

- Deposition of **fatty tissue** in the hiatus leads to weakening of the hiatus in obese individuals.
- Advancing **age** resulting in muscular degeneration can predispose to hernia.
- Raised intra-abdominal pressure due to lower **abdominal tumours**, pregnancy, etc.
- **Saint's triad:** Gallstones, diverticulosis and hiatus hernia can occur together in a patient.

Clinical Features

- In many patients, there may not be any symptoms. Symptoms are like that of reflux oesophagitis—heartburn, chest pain, bloating sensation.
- More common in women, especially if obese.
- Symptoms are exaggerated after a heavy meal or binges of alcohol.

Investigations

- **Oesophagoscopy** reveals varying degree of inflammation. During oesophagoscopy, when the patient is asked to strain (Valsalva's manoeuvre), the sphincter is seen to be more patulous and herniation of gastric mucosal folds can be seen. **Reflux of the gastric acid is the most valuable sign. Biopsy should be taken from suspicious areas of metaplasia.**
- **Barium meal** demonstrates gastroesophageal reflux in the Trendelenburg position.
- **Ultrasound** of abdomen to rule out gallstones. Reflux can be due to some extraluminal pathology compressing GE junction such as retroperitoneal or pancreatic tumours.

Treatment

Conservative Treatment

In all cases of GORD, conservative treatment has to be tried first. The results of surgery are appreciated only when the symptoms are significant and conservative treatment fails.

Principles—You can remember pneumonic LORD

1. **Lifestyle changes**
   - Decrease in weight
   - Diet control with increased intake of proteins and decreased consumption of fat and sugar.
   - Decreased alcohol and tobacco consumption.
2. **Oesophageal mucosa protection**
   - *Antacids:* Preparations containing alginates, cytoprotective agents.
   - H_2 blockers: Ranitidine.
   - Proton pump inhibitors: Omeprazole or esomeprazole.
3. **Reflux prevention**
   - Oesophageal reflux: Cisapride, metoclopramide
   - Gastric reflux: Domperidone, metoclopramide
4. **Decision of surgery:** When all measures fail, surgery should be done—reduction of hernial sac, repair of hiatus and reduce reflux by fundoplication—laparoscopic fundoplication

Pearls of Wisdom

Oh LORD, save me from GORD!

ROLLING HERNIA

- This is also called as paraoesophageal hernia. A Paraoesophageal hernia is characterized by an ascend of the gastric fundus through a defect in the phreno-esophageal membrane. In this condition, cardio-oesophageal junction is normal. Thus, there are no features of reflux oesophagitis but the sac containing stomach in the thorax causes compression of the heart and lung.
- Volvulus of the stomach is a dangerous complication in this variety.
- It is an uncommon type of hiatal hernia that mainly affects older adults, with a median age of presentation between 65 and 75 years. Loss of elastic fibres as in advancing age or raised increased intra-abdominal pressure or multipara are the few causes mentioned.
- As the hernia enlarges, the greater curvature of the stomach rolls up into the thorax. Because the stomach is fixed at the GE junction, the herniated stomach tends to rotate around its longitudinal axis, resulting in an organoaxial volvulus. Infrequently, rotation occurs around the transverse axis resulting in a mesenteroaxial volvulus.

Clinical Features

- No retrosternal burning pain because no reflux
- Discomfort after a small meal
- Feeling of fullness after a meal or dysphagia due to large sac
- Palpitations due to compression on the heart
- Respiratory tract infection and hiccough due to irritation of phrenic nerve.

[1]Causes can be remembered as FATTY (F: fat, A: age, T: tumour, T: triad (Saint's triad), Y: yielding hiatus.)

Investigation

- Barium meal shows the sac in the thorax containing stomach. Sometimes, it can be upside down.
- Contrast CT scan is the investigation of choice. Patients who come with features of volvulus with obstruction are evaluated with plain X-ray and CT scan as shown in Fig. 40.12—grossly dilated stomach and duodenum showing a large gas fluid level on the right side with partial volvulus.

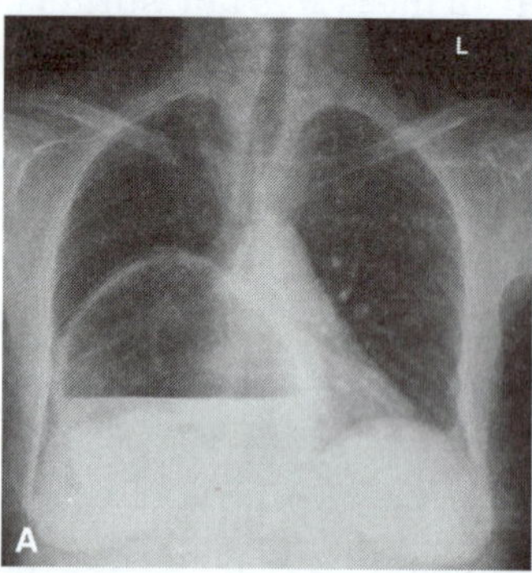

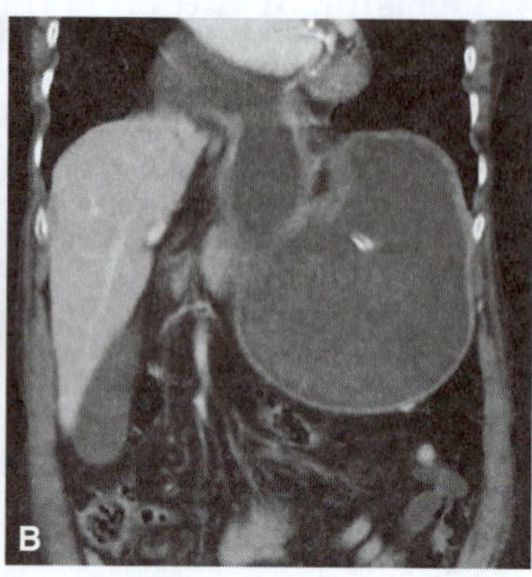

Fig. 40.12: (A) A large gas fluid level on the right side caused by obstruction of the duodenum by the defect in the diaphragm through which stomach is herniated and with partial volvulus. (B) CT scan showing grossly dilated stomach and duodenum showing with partial volvulus.

Treatment

- Reduction of the sac and repair of the hiatus by using nonabsorbable suture material to approximate the right crus of the diaphragm.
- When the defect is large nonabsorbable mesh, such as prolene, is used to cover the defect.

MIXED HERNIA

- In this, both sliding and rolling hernias are present. Symptoms are mixed—features of reflux esophagitis and compression on the mediastinal structures. Treatment is also mixed and is done for both sliding and rolling hernias.

Complications of GORD

1. **Stricture oesophagus:** It is seen in middle-aged and elderly patients. Due to repeated reflux, ulcers, fibrosis and stricture develop in the lower end of the oesophagus. Early diagnosis by endoscopy followed by **frequent dilatation** and **proton pump inhibitors** will help the situation.

   Peptic strictures are difficult to manage surgically. Surgery is indicated in refractory cases of dilatation, in the form of **gastroplasty**.
2. **Oesophageal shortening** is also treated by Collis gastroplasty by using stomach (short oesophagus).
3. **Barrett's oesophagus:** Also known as columnar-lined oesophagus (**CLO**) (details are given below).
4. **Gastric/oesophageal ulcers**—can give rise to bleeding. **Cameron ulcers** are the ulcers in the stomach of a patient with haitus hernia. They are seen in about 3 to 5% of the patients. These ulcers occur at the site of extrinsic compression of the diaphragm on the stomach in patients with large hiatal hernias. It can be easily missed. Cameron ulcer is one of the causes of occult upper GI tract bleeding.
5. Aspiration pneumonitis, asthma and pneumonia are common features. Chronic aspiration can result in fibrosis of lung and bronchiectasis.

BARRETT'S OESOPHAGUS

Definition

- When columnar mucosa extends at least 3 cm into oesophagus or when it shows intestinal metaplasia, it is described as Barrett's oesophagus.
- Ulcer in the Barrett's CLO is called **Barrett's ulcer**.

Pathogenesis

Repeated reflux results in shifting of the esophagogastric junction upwards, which further increases the reflux resulting in intestinal metaplasia of **middle and lower oesophagus.**

Pathological Types

- **Gastric type** with chief and parietal cells.
- **Intestinal type** with ***goblet cells*** is a marker of intestinal metaplasia. This mucosa is smooth (unlike gastric folds).
- **Junctional type:** It has mucus glands and resembles gastric cardia.

Prague classification for Barrett's oesophagus

- The lower measurement boundary is formed by the proximal cardiac notch (optimally with moderate insufflation), and the two upper measurement boundaries are marked by the proximal limit of the circumferential Barrett's segment (C) and the longest tongue of Barrett (M).

  In Fig. 40.13, the circumferential segment (C) is 3 cm and the tongue an additional 2 cm, so that M is 5 cm (3 cm circumferential + 2 cm tongue = 5 cm maximum Barrett's extent, M). The length of the Barrett is thus C3M5. A short Barrett segment only forming a 1 cm tongue is reported as C0M1. A circular Barrett's that is 2 cm long without tongues, i.e. with a relatively straight proximal boundary is reported as C2M2.

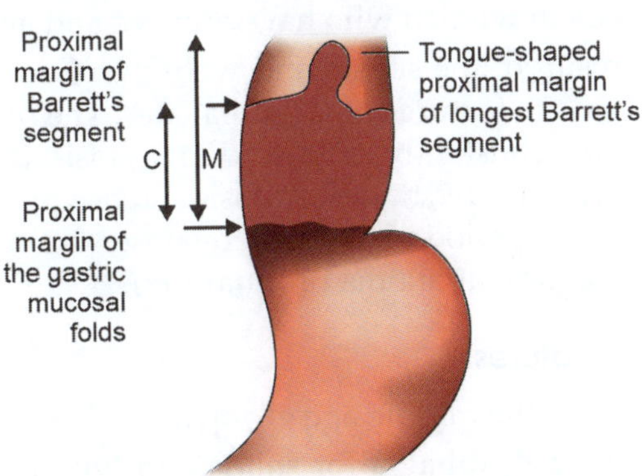

Fig. 40.13: Prague classification

Clinical Types

- **Long segment:** Metaplastic changes involving more than 3 cm.
- **Short segment:** Metaplastic changes involving less than 3 cm.

Incidence of Malignancy

40 times more prone to carcinoma of the **lower and middle oesophagus** as compared to the general population (Key Boxes 40.7 and 40.8).

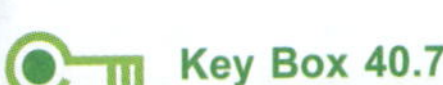
Key Box 40.7

Risk Factors for Carcinoma

- CLO >8 cm
- Smoking
- Reflux due to previous gastric surgery
- High grade dysplasia—indication for oesophagectomy

Key Box 40.8

Carcinoma in Barrett's Oesophagus

- It will be invasive
- It is more proximal
- Carries poor prognosis
- 40 times increased risk compared to general population

Types of Dysplasia

- Low grade: Negligible risk of carcinoma
- High grade: Very high-risk of carcinoma

Endoscopy and Screening Programme

It is important to screen these patients regularly with **repeat endoscopies and multiple biopsies to find dysplasia. Few endoscopy pictures are given here** (Figs 40.14 to 40.17).

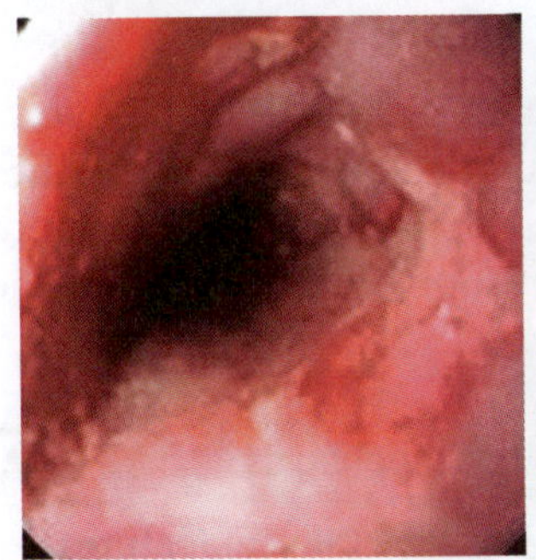
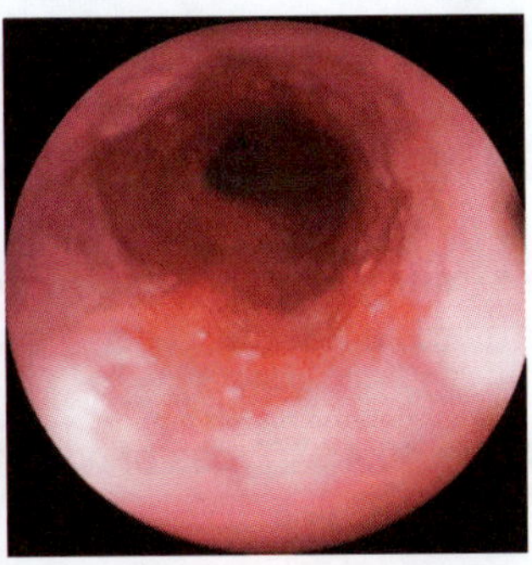

Figs 40.14 and 40.15: Endoscopic view of reflux oesophagitis and Barrett's oesophagus

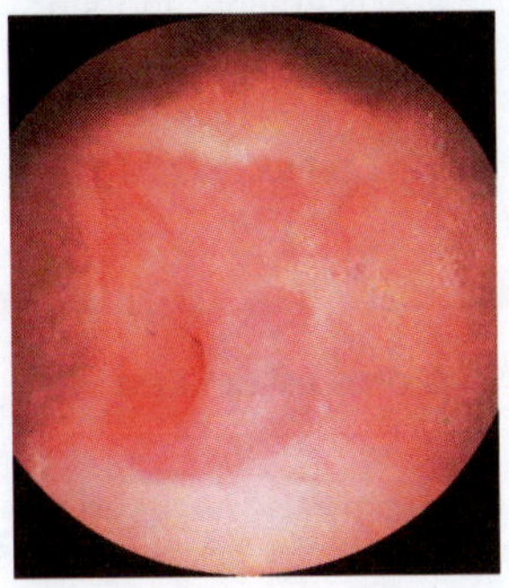
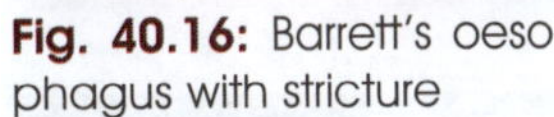

Fig. 40.16: Barrett's oesophagus with stricture

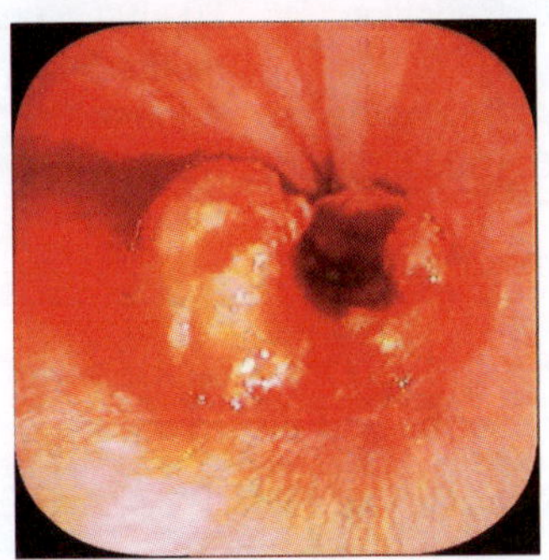

Fig. 40.17: Carcinoma GE junction in Barrett's oesophagus

Treatment

- High dose proton pump inhibitors for 8 weeks.
- Radiofrequency ablation (RFA) is better than photodynamic therapy and very effective. RFA produce heat and destroys superficial tissue. Ablation pulses of two double pulses of 125/cm^2.
- Laser photodynamic therapy.
- Argon beam plasma coagulation
- Asymptomatic, symptomatic Barrett's oesophagus responds well to laparoscopic antireflux surgery. Antireflux surgery also prevents progression to high grade dysplasia or adenocarcinoma.
- Endoscopic mucosal resection for Barrett's oesophagus with low grade dysplasia.
- Oesophagectomy in cases of high grade dysplasia.

Pearls of Wisdom

Antireflux surgery may protect mucosa against development of dysplasia in patients with Barrett's oesophagus.

Complications of Barrett's Oesophagus

1. **Oesophageal ulcers:** Barrett's ulcer—pain, bleeding and perforation.
2. **Oesophageal stricture:** Usually located in the middle or upper oesophagus.
   - **Peptic stricture occurs in the distal oesophagus.**
3. Dysplasia and adenocarcinoma.

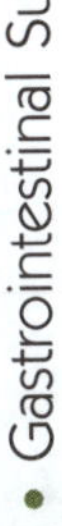
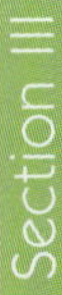

Nonreflux Oesophagitis

This is also a condition which occurs due to several factors such as corrosives, drugs, chemoradiation, AIDS, etc. They are summarised in Table 40.4. Basic treatment is similar to that of reflux oesophagitis and avoid the causative agents.

Table 40.4 Types of nonreflux oesophagitis

	Agents causing	Clinical features
1. Corrosive:	Lye, acid, alkali	Burns, stricture
2. Infective:	Candida, herpesvirus	Chronic illness, AIDS
3. Radiation:	20–40 Gy units to mediastinum	Ulceration and stricture
4. Chemotherapy:	Adriamycin	–
5. Drug induced:	NSAID, doxycycline	↑ reflux

Competency

SU28.5.4: Describe the various symptoms associated with oesophageal disorders.

SU28.5.5: Describe the various investigations used in evaluation of oesophageal disorders.

MOTILITY DISORDERS OF THE PHARYNX AND OESOPHAGUS

Introduction: Motility disorders of the oesophagus is an important chapter for postgraduate students. There are many classifications. However, Chicago classification has been widely accepted. Few important lesions have been discussed here.

Classification:

A. **Disorders affecting lower oesophagus (oesophagogastric junction)**
   - Achalasia
   - Diffuse oesophageal spasm
   - Nutcracker oesophagus or Jackhammer oesophagus

B. **Disorders affecting upper oesophagus and pharynx**
   - Plummer-Vinson syndrome

C. **Disorders affecting body**
   - Diffuse oesophageal spasm.

PLUMMER-VINSON SYNDROME

Introduction: It is also called Paterson-Kelly syndrome. It is a precancerous condition in which there is a severe spasm of circular muscle fibres at the cricopharyngeal sphincter level or pharyngo-oesophageal junction, and it is associated with **development of postcricoid web.**

Aetiopathogenesis

- Aetiology is not known.
- It is seen in women who have worries and anxiety.
- As a result of the spasm and web, dysplasia occurs and leads to features of anaemia later. The proximal mucosa is constantly irritated due to stasis. It undergoes hypertrophy, hyperkeratosis and desquamation. This, over a period of years, predisposes to carcinoma oesophagus (carcinoma oropharynx).

Clinical Features

- Women in the middle age group are affected.
- Increasing **dysphagia** for solids and liquids due to spasm.
- Features of **anaemia**—pallor, stomatitis, ulcerations, bald tongue (without papillae), koilonychia, splenomegaly and microcytic hypochromic anaemia.
- As a result of obstruction, the fluid tends to spillover into the larynx giving rise to recurrent aspiration, respiratory tract infection, cyanosis or choking.

Treatment

- Reassurance
- Improving anaemia: Iron tablets or blood transfusion and correction of nutritional deficiencies.
- Regular dilatation by using gum elastic bougies.

Summary: Refer Key Box 40.9.

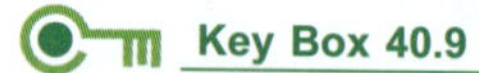

Key Box 40.9

Summary

Post cricoid web
Low haemoglobin–anaemia–correction by iron supplements
Upper cricopharyngeal sphincter spasm
Middle aged woman
Malignancy is a complication
Elastic bougie—dilatation
Respiratory complications
You can remember as PLUMMER

ACHALASIA CARDIA

- Achalasia means failure to relax.
- It is a primary oesophageal motility disorder.
- It is also called cardiospasm because of severe spasm of the circular muscle fibres of the lower end of the oesophagus. The contracted segment does not relax during the act of swallowing (achalasia = failure of relaxation). As a result of this, there is dilatation, tortuosity and hypertrophy of the oesophagus above.
- Incidence: 6 in 1,00,000 population/year.
- Importantly it is a pre-cancerous condition for carcinoma oesophagus.

Achalasia and Carcinoma Oesophagus

- 8% chances of carcinoma over 20 years period.
- Squamous cell carcinoma is the most common due to prolonged stasis and irritation.
- Sometimes adenocarcinoma can occur in the middle third.
- Long-term surveillance program is required.

Aetiopathogenesis

1. **Idiopathic:** This occurs due to absence or degeneration of Auerbach's plexus throughout the body of the oesophagus leading to improper integration of the parasympathetic impulse. This is called primary achalasia.
2. **Acquired variety** is seen in South American countries caused by *Trypanosoma cruzi* (sleeping sickness)—**Chagas disease**. This organism destroys the ganglion cells of the Auerbach's plexus.

Pearls of Wisdom

Trypanosoma cruzi causes megaoesophagus, megaduodenum, megacolon and megaureter. Can we call it a 'mega'organism?

3. Stress and emotional factors and vitamin deficiencies are also associated with this disease.

Pathophysiology

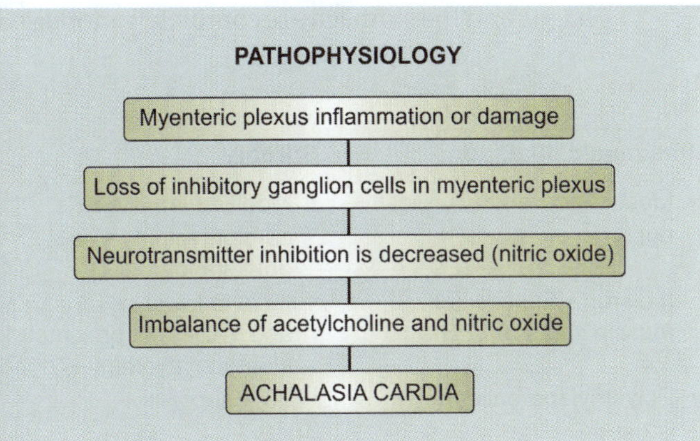

Types of Achalasia Cardia

- Classical achalasia: Loss of ganglion cells and neural fibrosis occurs (**Type I—classic**)
- Achalasia with oesophageal compression (**Type II**)
- Vigorous achalasia: No loss of ganglion cells but ganglionitis occurs **(Type III/spastic achalasia)**

Clinical Features

- Women around 30–40 years of age are commonly affected. The ratio of affected females to males is 3:2.
- Most patients find eating slow and the drink large volume of fluid. As a result when peristalsis starts retrosternal pain develops.
- **Dysphagia** develops slowly, and it is progressive. Solids, by forming a bolus and aided by gravity, as they touch the contracted segment, may partially open up the sphincter. Thus, there is no dysphagia for solids. Dysphagia for liquids is an important feature and it results in **regurgitation** (oesophageal pseudovomiting). The regurgitant material contains foul-smelling oesophageal contents. Malnourishment, ill health and weight loss follow soon. **Dysphagia, regurgitation and weight loss form the triad of achalasia cardia.**
- **Recurrent respiratory tract infection** due to spillage of liquids can also occur.
- **Features of anaemia**—glossitis, stomatitis, pallor, bald tongue.
- **Retrosternal discomfort** and radiation of pain to the interscapular region may be present.
- **Pseudoachalasia:** Tumours of cardia mimicking achalasia. Often patients present with features of recent achalasia (dysphagia). During endoscopy, some difficulties are encountered and once the scope enters the GE junction, growth will be seen.

Pearls of Wisdom

Inhalation of amyl nitrite leads to sphincter relaxation in achalasia but not in pseudoachalasia.

Investigations

1. **Barium swallow**
   - Uniformly dilated oesophagus above, with a smooth tapering segment below—**cucumber oesophagus**.
   - In chronic cases, it may be sigmoid-shaped (Figs 40.18 and 40.19).

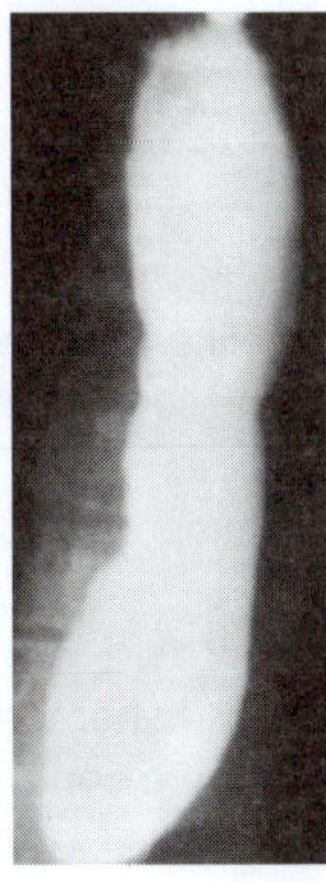

Fig. 40.18: Barium swallow showing dilated oesophagus

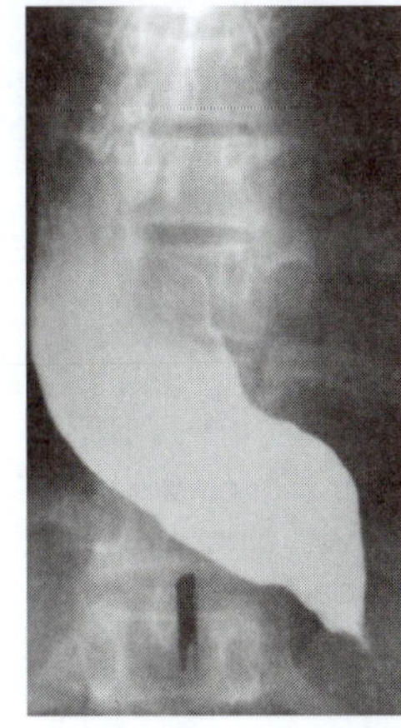

Fig. 40.19: Barium swallow showing sigmoid oesophagus

2. **X-ray chest**
   - Mediastinal mass (pseudotumour)[1] produced by dilated oesophagus can be seen (Fig. 40.20).
   - **Retrocardiac air-fluid level is seen in the lateral view.**
   - Aspiration pneumonitis can be diagnosed.
3. **Plain X-ray abdomen erect:** Fundic air bubble is absent because of the stasis of fluid in the oesophagus.
4. **Oesophagoscopy:** It reveals a dilated sac containing stagnant food and fluid due to stasis which splashes out with each heartbeat and with each respiratory movement.

   LES: Lower oesophageal sphincter is closed, with air insufflation. It has a 'rosette' appearance (Fig. 40.21).
   - Oesophagoscopy is also done to rule out proximal malignancy.

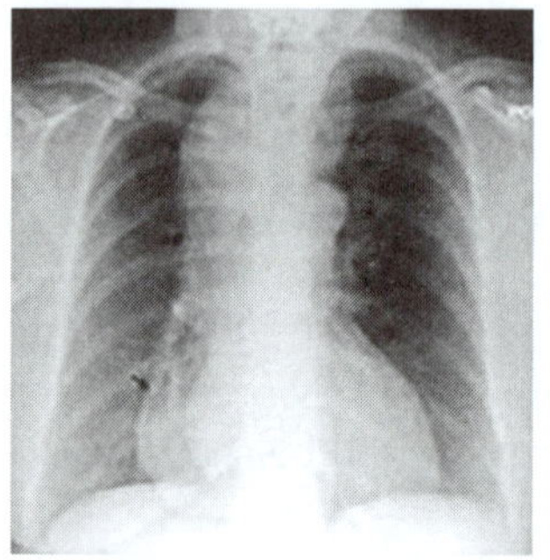

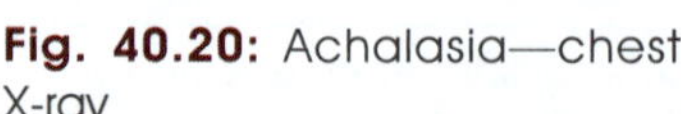

Fig. 40.20: Achalasia—chest X-ray

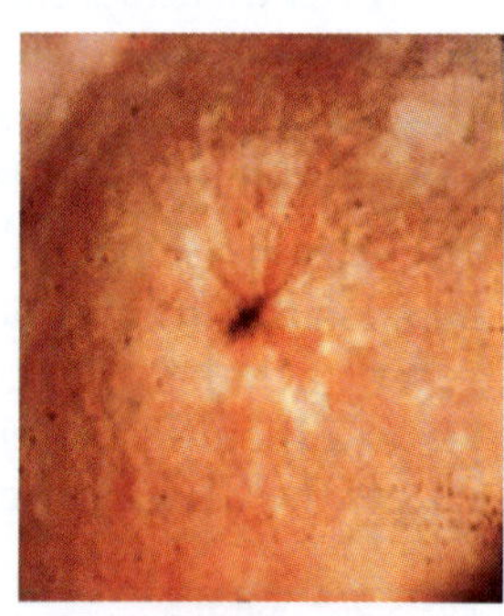

Fig. 40.21: Endoscopy showing rosette appearance

   - Also done to evaluate oesophagitis, stricture or a tumour at cardia.
5. **Oesophageal manometry:** Following features are characteristic of achalasia cardia:
   - Hypertensive lower oesophageal sphincter (LOS): It does not relax on swallowing.
   - **Aperistalsis in the body** of oesophagus
   - Increased resting pressure in the oesophagus
6. **Ultrasound:** It may detect subepithelial tumour infiltration in secondary achalasia due to a distal carcinoma.

Pearls of Wisdom

You suspect of achalasia by clinical features
You support achalasia by barium swallow
You confirm achalasia by manometry
You exclude carcinoma by UGI scopy
You treat by dilatation or POEM or surgery

Treatment (Table 40.5—four choices)

- Aim of the treatment is to cure the disease.
- **More importantly, the obstruction at the lower end of oesophagus must be relieved.**
- **Modified laparoscopic Heller's cardiomyotomy is the choice of surgery now.**

  1. **Heller's cardiomyotomy:** The aim is to reduce outflow resistance at the lower oesophageal sphincter.
     - With a left thoracoabdominal incision, the oesophagus and the stomach are completely mobilised.

Table 40.5 Treatment of achalasia cardia

Pharmacological therapy	Botulinum toxin injection	Pneumatic dilatation	Surgery
• Sublingually used	• BoTx A 80–100 units are injected in one sitting	• Most effective nonsurgical option	• Modified lap. Heller's cardiomyotomy is the gold standard
• Nitrates and calcium channel blockers	• 20–25 IU are injected into each quadrant	• It disrupts the circular muscle fibres of LES	• 6 cm of lower oesophagus and 1–2 cm of proximal stomach myotomy is done
• Nitrate 5–20 mg before meal and calcium channel blockers 10–30 mg before meal	• Use 5 mm sclerotherapy needle	• Polyethylene balloon is used	• 90% success
• They relax smooth muscle	• It acts by blocking acetylcholine release	• Dilators are 3, 3.5 and 4 cm	• 3% reflux oesophagitis
• Nitrates have more intense effect and more side-effect vice versa with calcium channel blocker	• Repeat injections are necessary as effect is temporary	• 70% permanent relief	**POEM: Per Oral Endoscopic Myotomy is popular now**
• Headache is the side-effect	• Pregnancy, hypersensitivity to albumin are contraindications	• Side-effect is perforation, gastro-oesophageal reflux, haemorrhage	

[1]Aortic aneurysm, cold abscess (paravertebral), scoliosis are the other pseudotumours in the chest X-ray.

- The contracted segment is felt between the fingers.
- A 7–10 cm long incision is made through the lower end of the oesophagus and carried over to the stomach. The muscles are cut till the mucosa bulges out. **The myotomy should extend proximally up to the aortic arch and distally up to the stomach to 1–2 cm below the junction.** Success rate is around 90%. 3 to 5% of the patients develop reflux oesophagitis which needs to be treated conservatively.

2. **Forceful dilatation:** By using **pneumatic balloon**—the balloon is positioned under fluoroscopic control within LOS. It should be rapidly inflated to a pressure of 300 mmHg for 15 seconds. Success rate is around 70%. 20% chances of reflux are present. Oesophageal perforation can also occur. Recurrences are common (Figs 40.22 and 40.23).

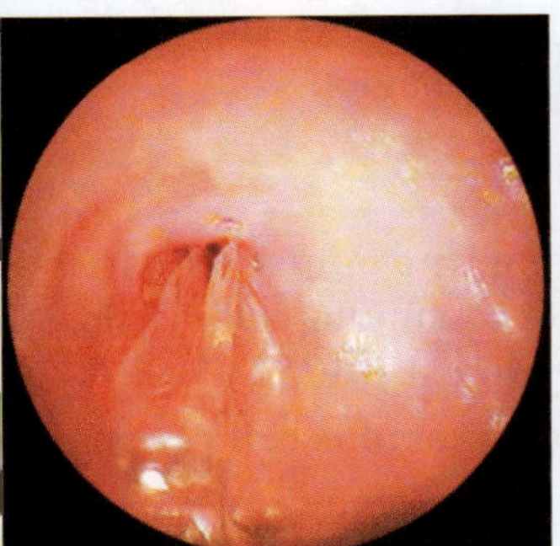

Fig. 40.22: Oesophageal balloon dilators

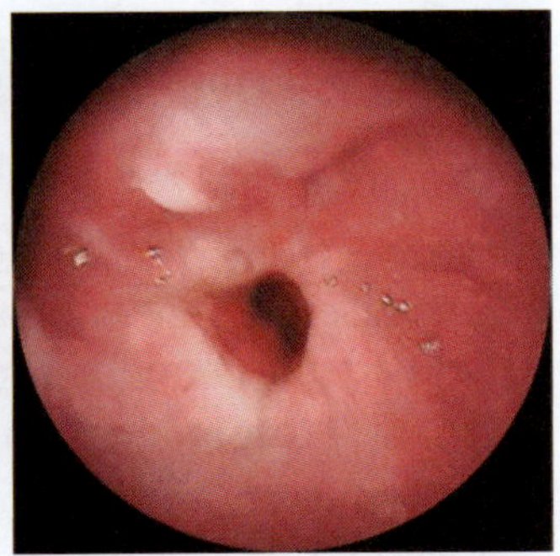

Fig. 40.23: Oesophageal narrowing of lower end

3. **Injection treatment: Inj. botulinum toxin A** is injected into the lower oesophageal sphincter (LOS) endoscopically. It is temporary and repeat injections are necessary (Key Box 40.10).
4. **Drugs:** Sublingual nifedipine can produce short-term relief.

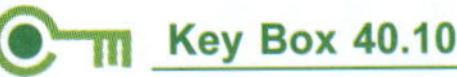

Key Box 40.10

Injection Botulinum Toxin A

- Endoscopic botulinum toxin is the most common initial treatment of achalasia cardia in USA.
- It is a neurotoxin.
- 8 different types of toxin are available. Most common being type A.
- Injection acts by interfering with cholinergic excitatory neural activity at LOS and blocking acetylcholine release from nerve terminals.
- It is an excellent endotherapy for short-term treatment of achalasia cardia.
- In about more than 50% cases, relapse occurs within few months and repeat injections are necessary.

5. **Endoscopic myotomy—popularly called POEM:** In this, through endoscope, a submucosal injection of a mixture of indigo rouge, epinephrine, and saline is done. A 2 cm long incision is made and submucosal tunnel is created. Then circular muscle bundle is cut slowly, beginning from 7 to 8 cm above GE junction to 2–3 cm below GE junction. Mucosa is sutured with absorbable sutures.

Complication of Achalasia Cardia

- Reflux is the most common complication. As a result of which recurrent aspirations and lung complications including pneumonia are the features.
- Due to prolonged stasis and chronic irritation, it can predispose to **carcinoma** of the mid and lower oesophagus (due to metaplasia). Hence, it is a precancerous condition. Squamous cell carcinoma is the most common type identified in a patient with achalasia.
- Nutritional deficiencies—anaemia and weight loss.

DIFFUSE OESOPHAGEAL SPASM

- An entity of unknown aetiology, presents with dysphagia and chest pain. It is a hypermotility disorder of the oesophagus.
- Motor abnormality affects body of the oesophagus.
- Degeneration of branches of vagus nerve has been documented.

Aetiology

Exact cause is not known. *Stress* may be one of the factors.

Symptoms and Signs

- Discomfort in the chest (chest pain) or spasmodic pain, dysphagia, weight loss.
- Regurgitation is common. But no acid reflux is found.

Investigations

1. **Barium swallow:** It is typically described as cork-screw oesophagus—segmental spasms, area of narrowing and irregular uncoordinated peristalsis.
2. **Manometry:** It is the diagnostic test. Findings are normal lower oesophageal sphincter, alteration of oesophageal peristalsis and contractions. Contractions of high amplitude >120 mmHg of long durations (>2.5 seconds) are findings.
3. **Ambulatory 24-hour pH monitoring:** This is an important test to rule out GORD.

Treatment

- It is directed in the similar lines of achalasia cardia—medical therapy, pneumatic dilatation intrasphincteric botulinum toxin injection, Heller's myotomy and partial fundoplication.

- Long oesophageal myotomy may be required.
- These patients need counselling. Depression, anxiety status to be ruled out.
- Sedation, nitrates, calcium channel blockers are used.

NUTCRACKER OESOPHAGUS OR JACKHAMMER OESOPHAGUS

- Aetiology is not known.
- Chest pain is the most common symptom followed by painful dysphagia (odynophagia).
- Barium swallow is usually normal. An epinephric diverticulum is usually present.
- Majority of the patients have normal propagation of peristaltic waves. However, in the distal oesophagus, peristaltic waves have very high amplitude (>180 mmHg) and duration (>6 seconds).
- Dilatation, myotomy, proton pump inhibitors, calcium channel blockers are used with limited success.
- Requrgitation and reflux are uncommon.

Competency

SU28.6: Describe the clinical features, investigations and principles of management of benign and malignant disorders of oesophagus.

CARCINOMA OF THE OESOPHAGUS

Introduction

- Majority of oesophageal cancers are squamous cell carcinomas, worldwide. However, in most Western countries, more than 70% are adenocarcinomas. This shift is mainly due to smoking, alcohol and Barrett's oesophagus. More than 50% of patients present with locally advanced carcinomas. Some improvement has taken place now because of early diagnosis, detection and multimodality treatment.
- **Oesophageal cancers have poor prognosis because of the following reasons**
  1. More lymph vessels are present in the submucosa than blood capillaries and hence, spread is fast.
  2. Lymph flow in submucosal plexus runs in a longitudinal direction. Hence, primary tumour can extend for a considerable length both superiorly and inferiorly.
- Cervical oesophagus has direct spread to regional nodes and there are less lymphatics in the submucosa. Hence, prognosis is better.

What is the 'Change' in Carcinoma Oesophagus?

- Squamous cell carcinoma is more common in Africans and Asians. Adenocarcinoma is more common in whites and Americans. Adenocarcinoma is increasing.
- Survival is improving.
- There is improvement in detection and staging.
- Detected more frequently in younger patients.
- Detected at an early stage also.

AETIOPATHOGENESIS

I. Precancerous/Predisposing Conditions

A. GORD with Barrett's oesophagus (*see* page 514). Malignancy in Barrett's oesophagus is curable if detected at an early stage. Hence, endoscopic surveillance is recommended.

B. Plummer-Vinson syndrome with squamous metaplasia (*see* page 522)—upper oesophagus.

C. Achalasia cardia (*see* page 522)—lower oesophagus.

D. Corrosive strictures (*see* page 536). **Lye strictures up to 30%:** Squamous cell carcinomas may arise in lye strictures, often developing 40–50 years after caustic injury. The majority of these cancers are located in the middle third of the oesophagus.

II. Carcinogens

A. Tobacco, heavy smoking and abuse of alcohol increase incidence of both squamous cell carcinoma and adenocarcinoma by almost 20–25%.

B. **Dietary carcinogens and squamous cell carcinoma**
  - Elevated nitrates in drinking water.
  - Food (pickles, corn) containing fungi—*Geotrichum candidum* as in endemic areas of China.
  - Baked bread

III. Viral

Human papillomavirus (HPV) infection increases squamous cell carcinoma. This oncogenic virus has been associated with cervical and oropharyngeal cancers also.

IV. Hereditary

A. Hovels-Evans syndrome or tylosis—40–60% of the patient develops cancers. Also called familial keratosis plantaris.

Tylosis (focal nonepidermolytic palmoplantar keratoderma) is a rare disease inherited in an autosomal dominant manner that is characterised by hyperkeratosis of the palms and soles and oesophageal papillomas. Patients with this condition exhibit abnormal maturation of squamous cells. They also cause inflammation within the oesophagus and are at extremely high risk of developing oesophageal cancer.

B. Patients with head and neck cancers—field cancerisa tion.

V. Bacterial

Helicobacter pylori infection: Infection with *Helicobacter pylori*, and particularly with cag A+ strains, is inversely associated with the risk of adenocarcinoma of the oesophagus. Mechanism is not clear. In fact, it should not have been a factor responsible because *H. pylori* infection can cause chronic atrophic gastritis leading to decreased acid production, which negates the effects of chronic reflux, including the potential for development of Barrett's oesophagus.

VI. Miscellaneous

Factors for adenocarcinoma

- **Obesity:** Increased body mass index is a risk factor for adenocarcinoma of the oesophagus, and individuals with the highest body mass index have up to a seven-fold greater risk of oesophageal cancer than those with a low body mass index. Probably, the linkage between obesity and gastro-oesophageal reflux disease is presumed to be a chief factor.
- **Economic status:** Low socioeconomic status as defined by income, education, or occupation is associated with increased risk for oesophageal squamous cell carcinoma, and adenocarcinoma to a smaller extent.

SITES

- 50%—middle 1/3rd of oesophagus
- 33%—lower 1/3rd of oesophagus
- 17%—upper 1/3rd of oesophagus.

TYPES

I. Squamous Cell Carcinoma

- Epitheliomatous ulcer (carcinomatous) with raised edges and flat base.
- Proliferative growth (cauliflower) with surface ulcer which commonly bleeds.
- Infiltrative variety or annular stenosing variety with a 5-year survival of 10%, gives rise to early dysphagia due to circumferential and longitudinal spread.
- Polypoidal lesions (5 years survival 70%).

II. Adenocarcinoma

Mostly lower end and middle oesophagus (in Barrett's oesophagus).

Comparison of squamous cell carcinoma and adenocarcinoma is given in Table 40.6.

CLINICAL FEATURES

- Men more than 60 years.
- **Dysphagia** which is **progressive** and mainly for solids (it takes 18 months for dysphagia to develop). It means 60% of the circumference of the lumen is involved by the growth. By the time, the patient presents with dysphagia, the disease is fairly advanced. Hence, it has a poor prognosis. **Dysphagia is a late symptom because smooth muscle of oesophageal wall can dilate with ease due to lack of serosal layer on the oesophagus.**
- **Regurgitation** of the food contents. Haematemesis is not very common. Vomitus may contain streaks of blood and melaena is rare.
- Loss of appetite, loss of weight and cachexia
- Backache indicates enlarged lymph nodes (coeliac).

SPREAD

1. Local Spread or Direct Spread

- To start with, it is a mucosal ulceration which spreads to the submucosa. Later, it causes fibrosis and the

Table 40.6 Comparison of two types of oesophageal cancer

	Squamous cell carcinoma	Adenocarcinoma
Site	Upper two-thirds	Lower one-third
Predisposing factors	Smoking alcohol	Barrett's oesophagus—GORD
Behaviour	Less aggressive	More aggressive
Incidence	Less common	More common
Achalasia cardia	Is the predisposing factor	Does not give rise to adenocarcinoma
Chemoradiation	It can be an alternate treatment	Not alternate to surgery
Surgery	Can be the first choice or chemoradiation	Surgery is the first choice—unfit patient, chemotherapy
Dietary carcinogens	A. Elevated nitrates in drinking water B. Food containing fungi—*Geotrichum candidum*—pickles, corn C. Baked bread	Consumption of meat Alcohol

lumen gets narrowed. The spread occurs transversely and longitudinally. Once it spreads to all the layers, the structures in the vicinity are involved. Factors Responsible for Early Spread and Aggressive Behaviour of Carcinoma Oesophagus are lack of serosal layer, proximity of vital structures, extensive mediastinal lymphatic drainage and late presentation.

- When the trachea is involved, tracheo-oesophageal fistula develops from carcinoma upper 1/3rd of oesophagus.
- Broncho-oesophageal fistula from carcinoma middle 1/3rd.
- Oesophagoaortic fistula results in massive bleeding (one of the causes of death).
- All these complications are contraindications for surgery and radiotherapy.

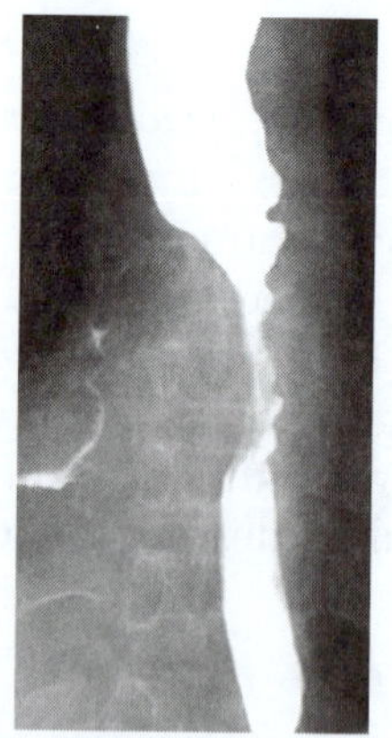

Fig. 40.24: Barium swallow—carcinoma middle oesophagus

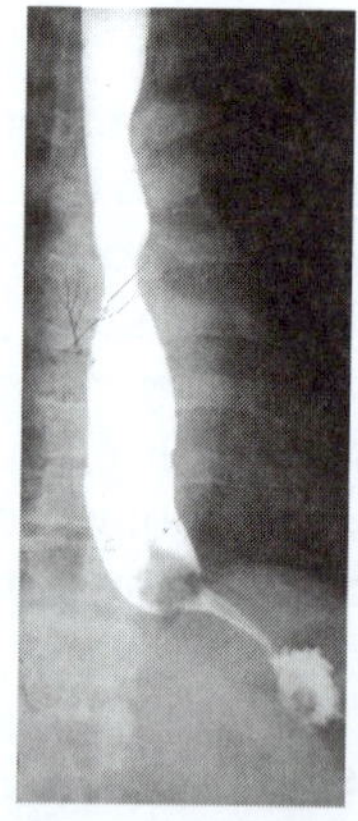

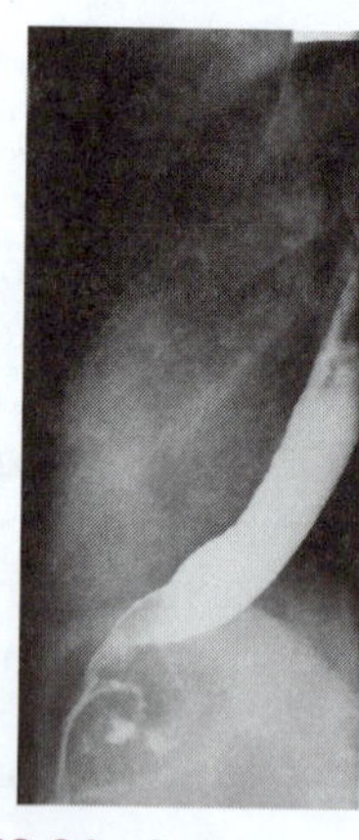

Figs 40.25 and 40.26: Carcinoma lower end of the oesophagus. Observe proximal shouldering

2. Lymphatic Spread

Studies have showed that **patients having metastasis to 5 or fewer lymph nodes** have a better outcome. Palpable left supraclavicular nodes indicate advanced disease. This sign is described as **Troisier's sign.**

3. Blood Spread

It results in secondaries in the liver, which clinically appear as nodular enlarged liver. Later, ascites and rectovesical deposits occur.

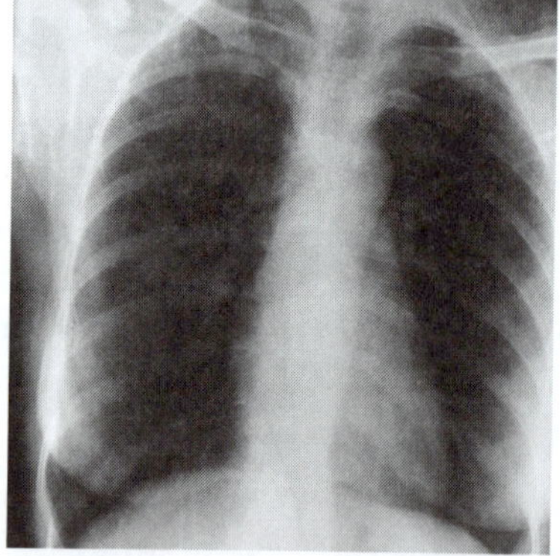

Fig. 40.27: Barium swallow showing straight axis—inoperable sign

INVESTIGATIONS

1. **Hb%** is low, which is the cause of generalized weakness.
2. **Liver function test (LFT)** is affected, if secondaries in liver occur (increased ALP).
3. **Ultrasound** is done to rule out liver secondaries, lymph nodes in the porta hepatis, coeliac nodes, etc.
4. **Barium swallow** demonstrates irregular, persistent, intrinsic filling defect (Figs 40.24 to 40.27)—**shouldering is characteristic**. Barium can also detect abnormal 'axis'. It can also demonstrate fistula. Both these features suggest that 'CURE' is not possible.
5. **Oesophagoscopy** to visualise the growth and to take biopsy (Figs 40.28, 40.29 and Key Box 40.11).
   - **Multiple biopsies** may be necessary. In high-risk areas like China, **endoscopic staining with supravital dyes** (indigocarmine) is done to identify dysplastic epithelium. If found, some advocate endoscopic mucosal resection.
6. **Chest X-ray** to rule out aspiration pneumonia, mediastinal widening and posterior tracheal indentation.
7. **Bronchoscopy** to rule out involvement of bronchus, as in carcinoma middle 1/3rd. If involved, it can confirm that tumour is locally unresectable.

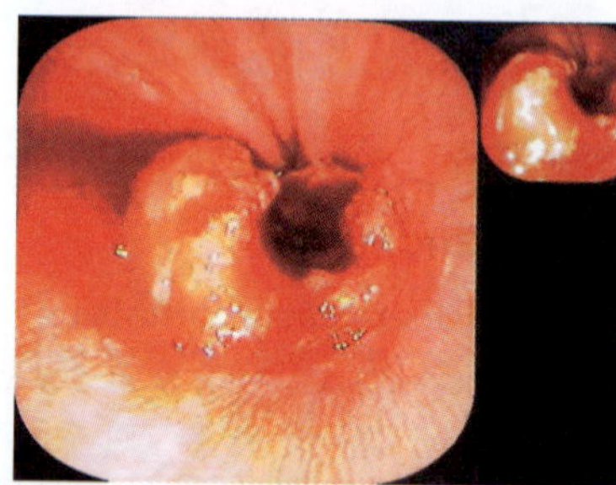

Fig. 40.28: Biopsy taken—observe the bleeding—friable growth

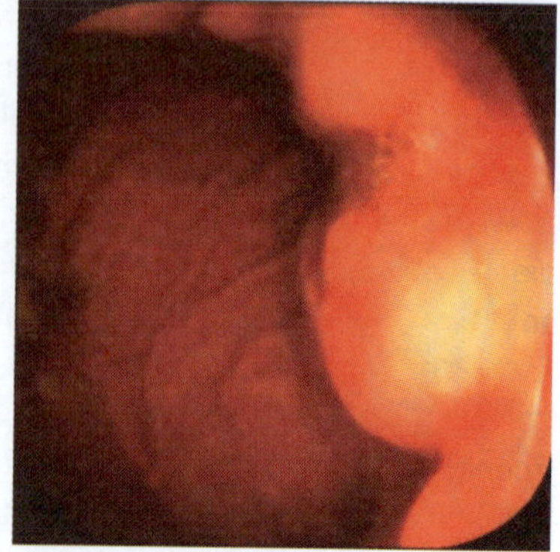

Fig. 40.29: Polypoidal growth at GE junction—patient presented with reflux

Key Box 40.11

Chromoendoscopy

- Chromoendoscopy involves the topical application of stains or pigments to improve tissue localisation, characterisation, or diagnosis during endoscopy.
- Several agents have been described that can broadly be categorised as absorptive (vital) stains, contrast stains, and reactive stains.
- Absorptive stains (e.g. Lugol's solution and methylene blue) diffuse or are preferentially absorbed across specific epithelial cell membranes.
- Contrast stains (e.g. indigocarmine) highlight surface topography and mucosal irregularities by permeating mucosal crevices.
- Reactive stains (e.g. Congo red and phenol red) undergo chemical reactions with specific cellular constituents, resulting in a colour change.

8. **CT scan** (Figs 40.30 and 40.31) of the chest and abdomen to detect local infiltration and to stage the disease. It is a very useful investigation before contemplating for total oesophagectomy. It is useful to assess involvement of vital structures such as bronchus, airway, pericardium, aorta, etc. Obliteration of fat planes gives the clue.
9. **Endoscopic ultrasound** to know the depth of wall involvement, to detect mediastinal lymph nodes, etc. (Fig. 40.32 and Key Box 40.12).
10. **Positron emission tomography (PET)/computerized tomography scanning:** PET scan is based on the principle that metabolically active tumour cells can be visible once radiopharmaceutical agent 18F-fluorodeoxyglucose (FDG) is given intravenously. These lymph nodes, if malignant, are clearly visible thus differentiating them from nonmalignant enlargement (Fig. 40.33). Applying the same principles, PET can be used to know the 'response' after radiotherapy or chemotherapy.

Key Box 40.12

Endoscopic Ultrasound (Endosonography)

- It relies on a high frequency (5–30 MHz) transducer
- To determine the depth of spread of a malignant tumour through the oesophageal wall
- Involvement of adjacent organs
- Metastasis to lymph nodes
- Also detects contiguous spread **downward into cardia**
- Can detect metastasis in the liver
- Can also detect small lymph nodes which are less than 5 mm (which cannot be detected by CT scan also)
- If 'endosonography' detects more than **5 lymph nodes,** it is not a case for curative resection.

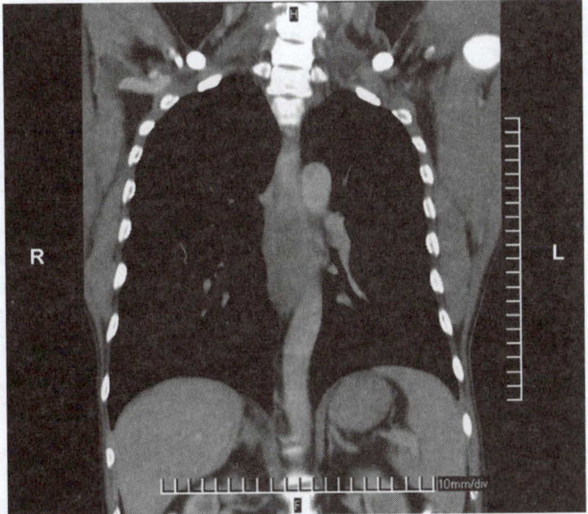

Fig. 40.30: Contrast CT showing a large midoesophageal growth

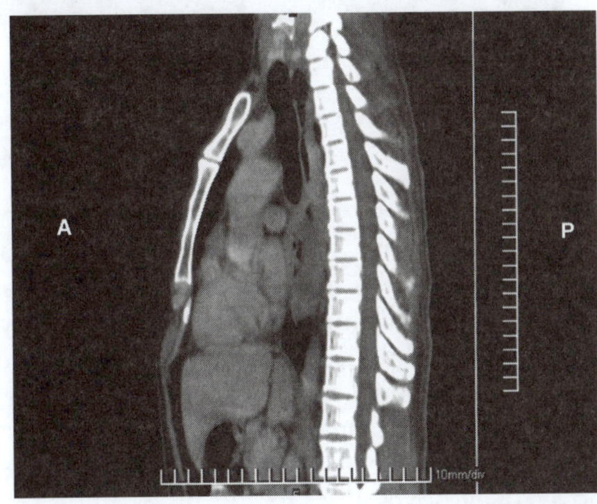

Fig. 40.31: Contrast CT lateral picture showing total occlusion of midoesophagus

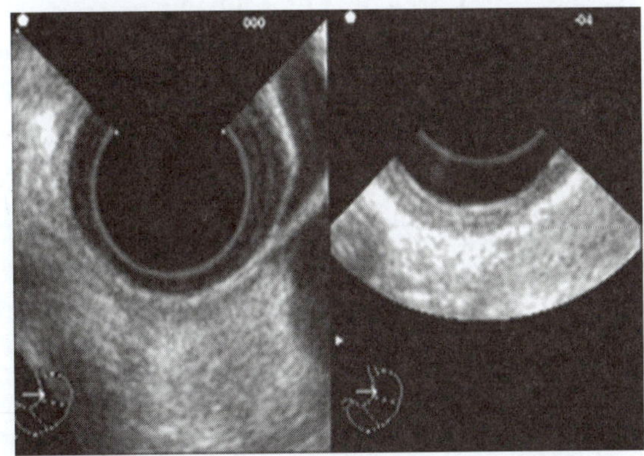

Fig. 40.32: Endosonography showing oesophagus and stomach layers. (*Courtesy:* Prof Ganesh Pai, Head, Department of Medical Gastroenterology, KMC, Manipal)

CECT—PET SCAN OF CARCINOMA OESOPHAGUS

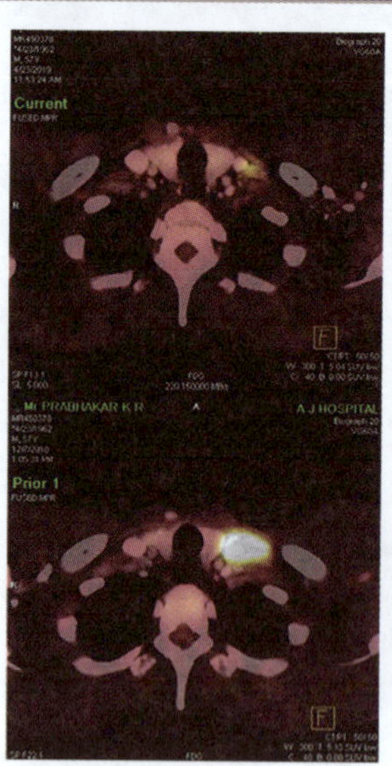
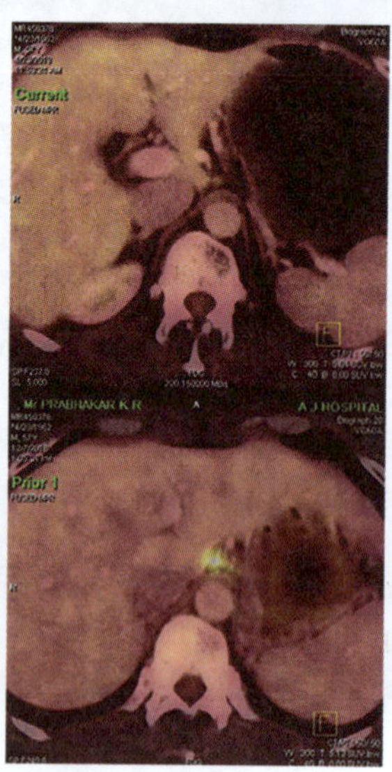
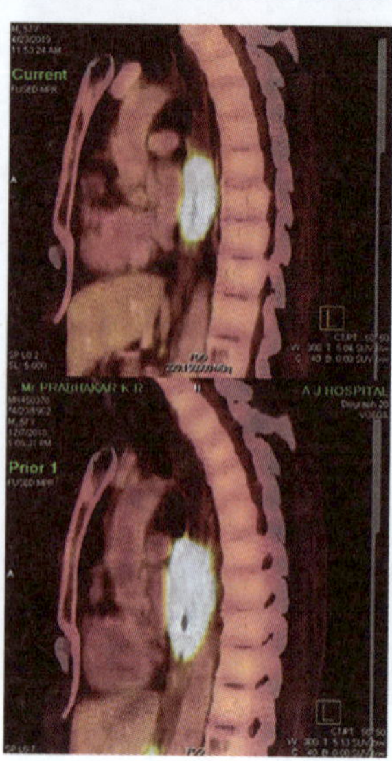
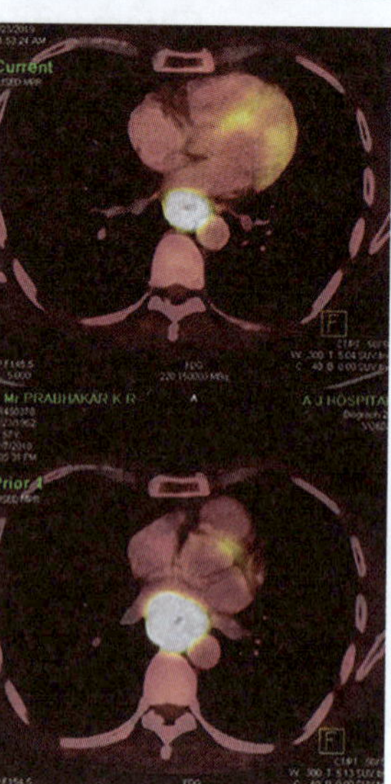

Fig. 40.33: CECT—PET scan of carcinoma oesophagus. Increased FDG uptake is noted in the circumferential wall thickening involving the mid and lower oesophagus (max wall thickness 1.9 cm, length 6.6 cm, SUVmax 24.43) causing near total occlusion of lumen and dilatation of proximal oesophagus. Increased FDG uptake is noted in the left supraclavicular nodal mass measuring 3.1 × 2.2 cm, SUVmax 13.12. (*Courtesy:* Dr Anant Pai, Associate Professor, Medical Oncologist, KMC, Manipal).

11. **Thoracoscopy and laparoscopy:** At the end of all investigations, it is important to decide, whether one can resect this tumour or not? Is it worthwhile resecting? Can patient tolerate the procedure? Is palliative majoe resections worth doing? Even in the absence of systemic spread, some features will suggest surgical cure is unlikely. Check these key boxes (Key Boxes 40.13 to 40.15).

Key Box 40.13

Investigations and their Importance in Carcinoma Oesophagus

- **Haemoglobin:** If it is low, wound healing is delayed
- **Albumin:** If it is low, anastomotic leak rates are high
- **Barium studies:** Straight axis of oesophagus indicates inoperability
  Fistula can be detected
- **Chest X-ray:** If it shows coin lesions, it is an advanced disease
- **Bronchoscopy:** Infiltration of bronchus indicates inoperability
- **CT scan:** Investigation of choice, helps in deciding the type of treatment
- **Endosonography:** To know the involvement of different layers of oesophagus for TNM staging
- **PET scan:** Is not done in the initial stage for evaluation, done for recurrent disease.
- **Diagnostic laparoscopy** before radical surgery, if peritoneal metastases are present—avoid radical surgery

Key Box 40.14

Thoracoscopy and Laparoscopy

- Staging tools in oesophageal cancer.
- More accurate in determining nodal status than non-invasive techniques and helpful in evaluating the extent of local invasion and metastatic disease.
- Thoracoscopy is accurate in 93% and laparoscopy in 94% of patients in identifying metastatic disease.
- Studies have proved that 6 cases of unsuspected coeliac nodal disease were identified in 19 patients despite preoperative CT and EUS.

Key Box 40.15

Unlikely Surgical Cure in the Absence of Systemic Spread

- **L**oss of weight more than 20%
- (O)**E**sophageal 'axis' is abnormal on barium test
- **N**odes—multiple on CT scan
- **G**rade—invasive, poorly differentiated
- **T**umour length more than 8 cm
- **H**orner's syndrome

Remember as **LENGTH**

12. **Laparoscopic ultrasound:** It is an extended investigation (Key Box 40.16).

Key Box 40.16

Laparoscopic Ultrasound (LUS)

- LUS is also a staging modality and may provide improved accuracy in T and N staging.
- LUS may also be more accurate for staging coeliac nodes because EUS probe is more distant and does not provide direct inspection.

Depth of invasion

- For T1 lesions, conservative oesophageal resection such as vagal-sparing, transhiatal or minimally invasive oesophagectomy can be opted.
- For localised intramucosal tumours of limited extent, EMR or ESD are an acceptable alternative.
- There is almost no role for chemoradiotherapy for treatment of T1 lesions.
- Surgical or endoscopic resection alone carries a good long-term survival, as high as 88% in some series.

Depth of tumour vs lymph node involvement (LNI)

1. T1 lesion (intramucosal)	18% LNI
2. T1 lesion (submucosal)	55% LNI
3. T2 lesion	60% LNI
4. T3 lesion	80% LNI

General Assessment for Staging

- Once the diagnosis is confirmed and staging (TNM) is done by metastatic work-up, performance status is done by using ECOG (Eastern Cooperative Oncology Group) criteria.
- General health of the patient, co-morbid conditions, fitness for anaesthesia—all these factors decide the choice of therapy.

TREATMENT WITH CURATIVE INTENT

- Once diagnosis and accurate staging is done, the histological diagnosis is also considered for treating carcinoma oesophagus.
- Incidence of lymph node positivity is around 5% even when the disease is confined to submucosal region—early cases.
- Tumour location is also important because of close proximity of oesophagus to pleura, pericardium azygos vein, aorta, etc.

While treating, cancers in the oesophagus can be broadly classified as follows (Fig. 40.34):

- **Cervical oesophagus:** It is from hypopharynx to thoracic inlet (at sternal notch), upper, thoracic oesophagus is from thoracic inlet to azygos vein.
- **Midthoracic oesophagus** tumours arise from lower border of azygos vein to inferior pulmonary vein (IMV).
- Lower oesophageal tumours distal (IMV) to gastro-oesophageal junction.

TNM STAGING AJCC, 8th edition

Tumour

T0	No primary tumour
Tis	Carcinoma *in situ*—high-grade dysplasia
T1a	Tumour invades lamina propria, muscularis mucosa
T1b	Tumour involving submucosa
T2	Tumour involving muscularis propria
T3	Tumour with paraoesophageal spread
T4	Involvement of recurrent laryngeal nerve, phrenic nerve, sympathetic chain, azygos vein; malignant effusion (adjacent structures)
T4a	Resectable structure
T4b	Tumor invades unresectable structure

Nodal Status

Nx	Lymph nodes cannot be assessed
N0	No regional lymph node metastasis
N1	Regional lymph node metastasis—1 to 2 nodes
N2	Metastasis in 3–6 regional nodes
N3	Metastasis in 7 or more regional nodes

Metastasis

M0	No distal spread
M1	Upper thoracic oesophageal carcinoma with spread to other nonregional nodes or distant spread. Middle thoracic oesophageal carcinoma with spread to neck nodes/coeliac nodes or other nonregional nodes. Lower thoracic oesophageal carcinoma with spread to other nonregional nodes or distant spread.
Mx	Distant metastasis cannot be assessed.

TNM Stage Grouping

Stage 0	: Tis N0 M0
Stage I	: T1 N0 M0
Stage IIA	: T2 N0 M0, T3 N0H0
Stage IIB	: T1N1N0, T2N1, M0
Stage III	: T3N1M0, T4 and N1N0
Stage IV	: A—Any T and N, M1a B—Any T1 and N, M1b

GX	Grade cannot be assessed—stage grouping as G1
G1	Well differentiated
G2	Moderately differentiated
G3	Poorly differentiated
G4	Undifferentiated—stage grouping as G3

A. Carcinoma Cervical and Upper Thoracic Oesophagus

- In vast majority of cases, treatment of carcinoma oesophagus is aimed at to relieve dysphagia by palliative resection/palliative radiotherapy/metallic stenting.
- **Tumours that have not penetrated** through oesophageal wall and have not metastasised to regional lymph nodes are **potentially curable.**

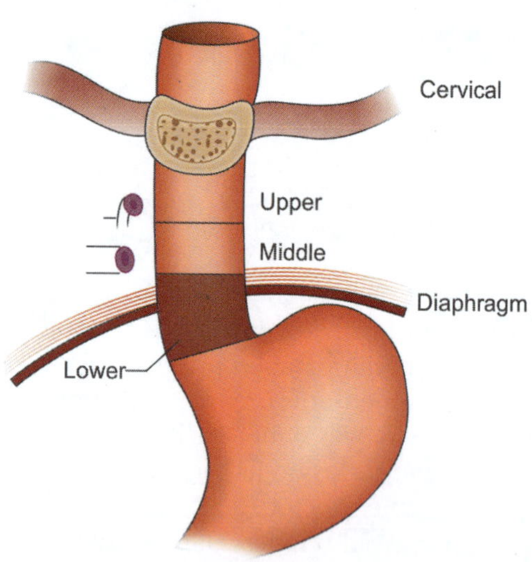

Fig. 40.34: Division of oesophagus for resection purposes

- **Decision of surgery/radiotherapy** also depends upon location of the tumour, histology, site of the tumour, staging and cardiopulmonary reserve. Nutritional status has to be improved to raise albumin levels from 3 to 3.4 g/dl to decrease complications such as anastomotic leak.
- **Cervical oesophageal cancers** (Fig. 40.35) are almost always squamous cell carcinomas. Usually they are postcricoid in a female patient. It is very unusual for this malignancy to involve intrathoracic nodes. Upper thoracic is also squamous cell carcinoma. Involvement of thoracic nodes, early spread to trachea, bronchus and great vessels is common.

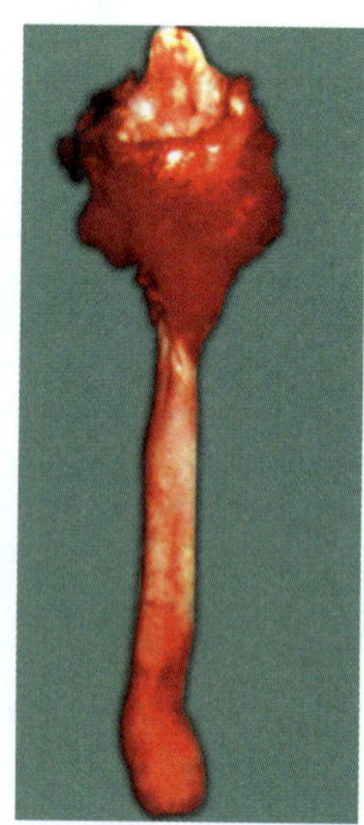

Fig. 40.35: Total pharyngolaryngo-oesophagectomy—followed by gastric pull-up

- Surgery followed by radiotherapy is the treatment of choice. Local recurrence is high and they succumb to local disease.
- If adjacent structure is not involved, total oesophagectomy with or without laryngectomy can be done. Preoperative neoadjuvant chemotherapy can also be given first (2–3 cycles followed by 3–5 Gy of radiation therapy).
- This is followed by total laryngectomy with bilateral neck dissection and reconstruction using gastric pull-up.
- Tumours in the upper thoracic oesophagus are removed by posterolateral thoracotomy, excision of the tumour and lymph nodes followed by gastric pull-up requiring laparotomy and pharyngogastric anastomosis in the neck. This is the three-stage oesophagectomy.

B. Tumours of the Thoracic Oesophagus and Cardia

They are usually **adenocarcinomas**. These tumours have a tendency to spread for long distances submucosally and the lymphatic flow is in the longitudinal direction.

Two Choices (Table 40.7)

I. Ivor Lewis operation

- In this operation, abdomen is opened first, stomach is mobilised and the wound is closed. The patient is put in left lateral position, and right thoracotomy is done through 6th intercostal space. **The growth is removed and oesophagogastric anastomosis is done inside the thorax, above the level of aortic arch.** Hence, it is described as a two-stage Ivor Lewis approach (Figs 40.36 to 40.38).

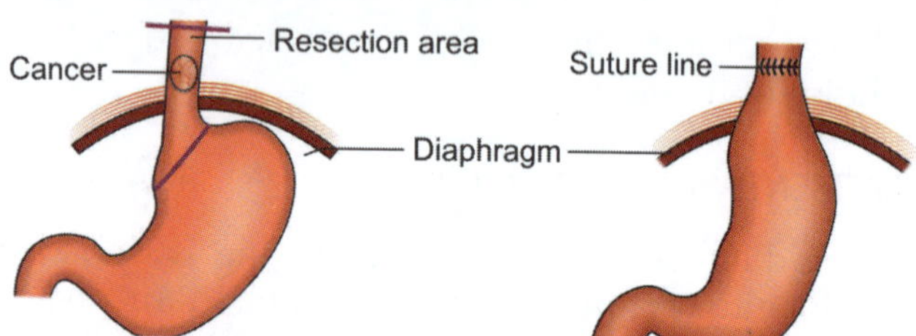

Fig. 40.36: Ivor Lewis operation

Fig. 40.37: Anastomosis in the thorax

Table 40.7 Total oesophagectomy—comparison of two types (*see* next page for figures)

***En bloc* oesophagectomy—McKeown**	**Transhiatal resection—Orringer**
First choice	**Alternate choice**
• Three incisions: Consequently, mobility is restricted and postoperative pain is more. Hence, morbidity and mortality are higher	• Two incisions: Abdominal and cervical. Hence, mobility is better and postoperative pain is less
• Under vision all lymph nodes in the thorax, neck and the abdomen can be removed	• Pulmonary complications are less as chest is not opened. Hence, mortality and morbidity are less than *en bloc* resection
• Surgery takes longer period of time	• Some mediastinal lymph nodes get cleared if proper dissection is done through hiatus
• However, long-term survival is not much compared to THE	• Surgery takes much shorter period of time
• When lymph nodes involved are less than 8 in number, survival is better than THE	

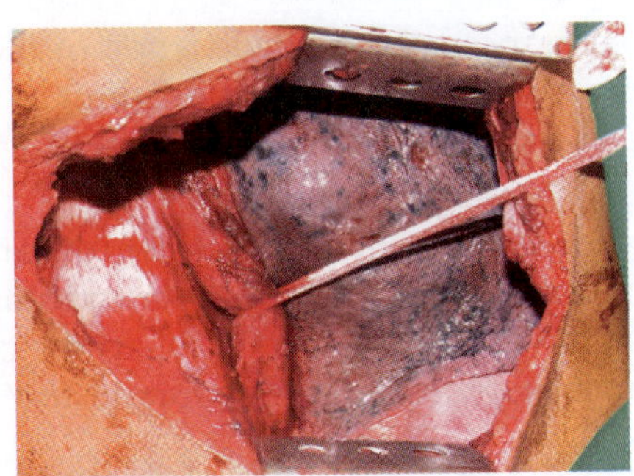

Fig. 40.38: Oesophagus is mobilised in the thorax

- However, a few surgeons do not advocate this surgery because of the following reasons:
  1. Higher incidence of **pulmonary complications**.
  2. Higher morbidity associated with **anastomotic leak**.
  3. Higher incidence of **oesophagitis**.
  4. Higher chances of **local recurrence** due to inability to resect long length of oesophagus. Hence, the alternate procedure (McKeown) is a better choice.

II. McKeown's three-stage *en bloc* oesophagectomy

En bloc resection is the best treatment with removal of all lymph nodes (abdominal and thoracic). Hence, three incisions are required: (1) Abdominal, (2) right postero-lateral thoracotomy through the fifth space, and (3) left cervical incision. Local recurrence at the anastomosis is not a problem because of wide clearance (by obtaining a 10 cm margin of normal oesophagus above the tumour). Gastrointestinal continuity is obtained by **gastric tube anastomosis to cervical oesophagus.**

C. Carcinoma Lower Oesophagus and Cardia

- They are adenocarcinomas.
- Surgery is the best method of treatment and palliation.
- *En bloc* resection is the best treatment with removal of all lymph nodes (abdominal and thoracic).
- An alternative method is **transhiatal oesophagectomy** (THE) without thoracotomy. Figure 40.39 shows various types of oesophageal surgery done for carcinoma oesophagus.

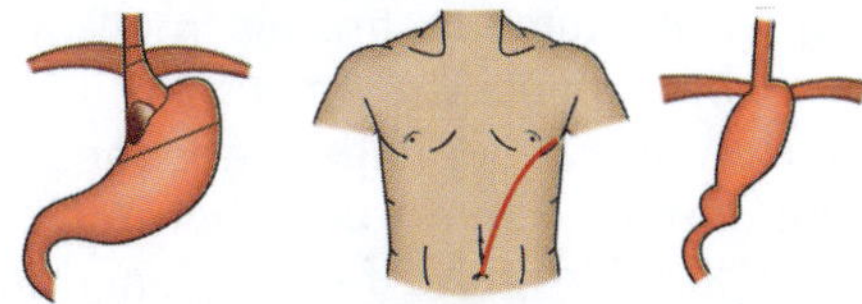

Left thoracoabdominal incision for carcinoma GE junction growth

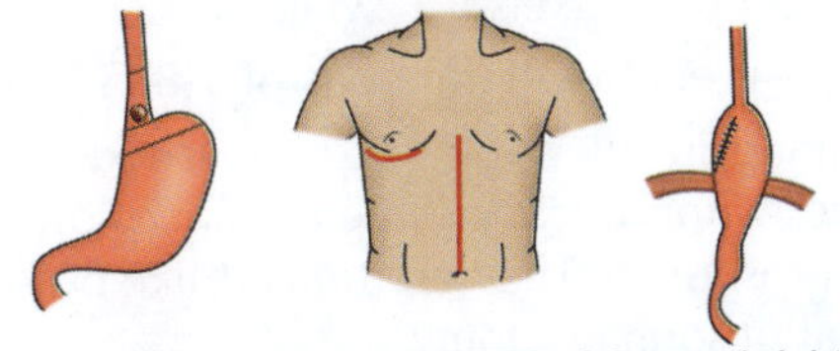

Ivor Lewis operation—upper midline incision and right thoracotomy

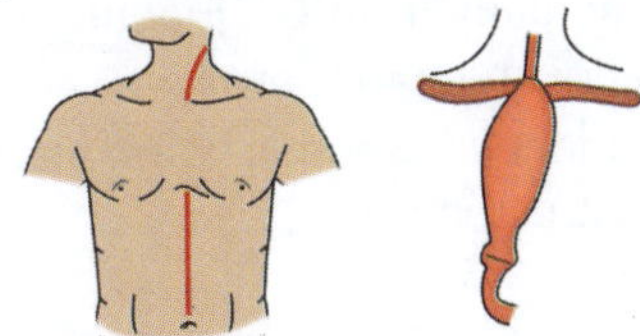

Orringer's transhiatal oesophagectomy—upper midline incision and incision in the left side of the neck along the sternocleidomastoid muscle and anastomosis at cervical oesophagus to stomach.

Fig. 40.39: Various incisions for oesophageal surgery

TRANSHIATAL OESOPHAGECTOMY (THE)—WITHOUT THORACOTOMY—ORRINGER (Figs 40.40 to 40.42)

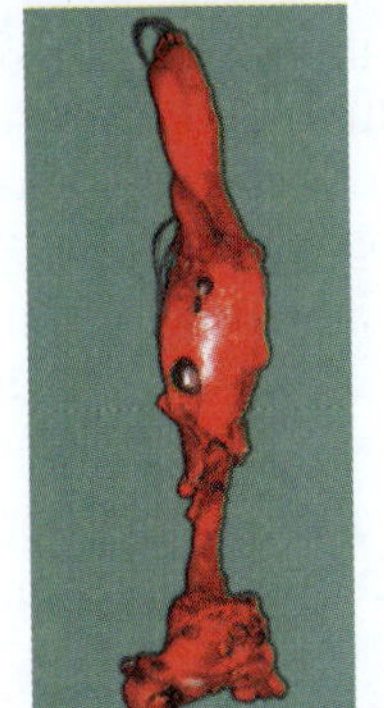

Fig. 40.40: THE for mid-oesophageal cancer

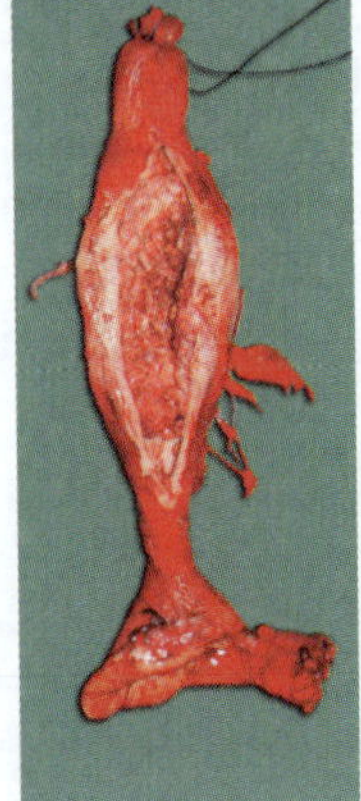

Fig. 40.41: Opened specimen showing extensive ulceration and nodularity—minimum 10 cm clearance for oesophageal cancer is important. Hence, THE is better than Ivor Lewis operation to get this length. (*Courtesy:* Dr Basavananda Hartimath, Associate Professor, Department of Surgery, KMC, Manipal)

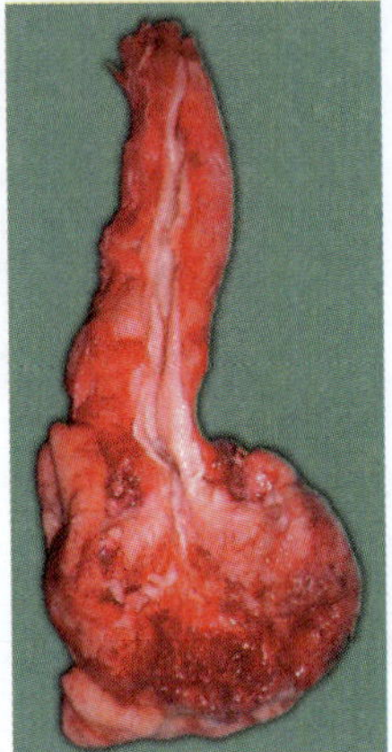

Carcinoma lower end of oesophagus—without opening the thorax by mobilisation from above and below, the oesophagus with the growth can be removed.

Fig. 40.42: Transhiatal (Orringer) total oesophagectomy. (*Courtesy:* Dr Sachidanand, Associate Professor, Karnataka Institute of Medical Sciences, Hubli, Karnataka)

Comments: Transhiatal oesophagectomy is a very good alternative (almost as good as *en bloc*) to lower oesophageal and GE junction tumours. No specific attempt is made to remove lymph nodes. Patients tolerate the procedure very well. No mediastinal complications related to leak are seen because of anastomosis in the neck. It gives a reasonably good relief from dysphagia and survival. It is not blind oesophagectomy. With good retraction of the hiatus, mobilisation can be done under vision. It is not the type of operation that influences survival but rather the stage of the disease at the time of the operation is performed.
- Prophylactic vagal sparing THE is indicated in severe dysplasia and intramucosal lesions.

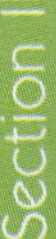

GASTRO-OESOPHAGEAL JUNCTION (GEJ) CANCERS

Definition: The TNM Classification of Malignant Tumors, 8th Edition, defines GEJ adenocarcinoma as adenocarcinoma with an epicenter within 5 cm of the GEJ and extending into the oesophagus. Smoking, obesity and consumption of red meat rich diet are important risk factors. GEJ tumours are classified as follows.

Siewert classification of GEJ tumours (Fig. 40.43)

Type I: It represents tumours arising from lower oesophagus which has changed to metaplastic columnar epithelium. They are oesophageal adenocarcinomas. Today, preoperative chemoradiotherapy has been considered as standard care for GE junction Type I tumours. Chemotherapeutic drugs used are:

- Cisplatin and paclitaxels—5 cycles
- Radiation—41.4–23 Gy fractions of 1.8 Gy each

This resulting in lower rate of lymph node positivity, good R–O resection rates and high chances of complete pathological response. They are treated like oesophageal cancer—total oesophagectomy

Type II: They are actually from GE junction and they are from stomach adenocarcinoma.

Type III: Gastric adenocarcinoma: They are treated like gastric cancer—gastrectomy.

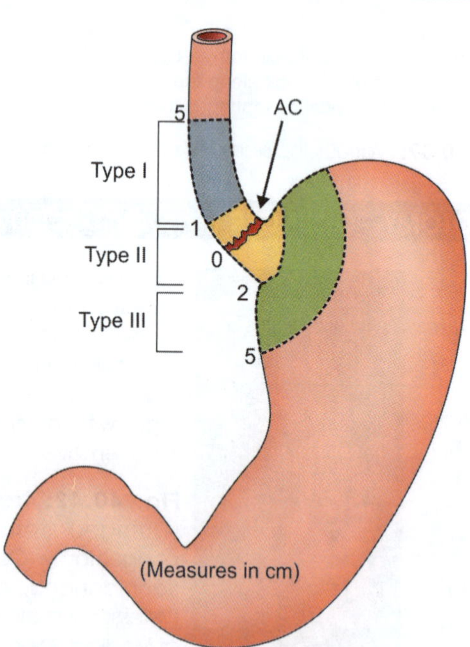

Fig. 40.43: Types of GE junction tumours

PALLIATIVE INTENT TREATMENT/PROCEDURES

- In spite of endoscopy and other investigations, the treatment of carcinoma oesophagus is palliative in more than 75% of cases, especially in our country. By the time the first symptom of dysphagia appears, it is too advanced. Also, the location of the tumour, adjacent structures in the mediastinum, widespread lymphatic drainage alters the overall prognosis to a very low percent of survival.
- A few considerations before treatment of carcinoma—since they often present at an advanced stage, 5-year survival is very low in the majority of cases. The following factors are considered for *palliative treatment*.

1. Comorbid conditions: Cardiac diseases, bad chest
2. Blood spread metastasis: Para-aortic lymph nodes
3. Contiguous organ: Trachea, aorta, pericardium invasion (CT scan)
4. Diagnostic laparoscopy: Peritoneal spread, omental nodules, ascites
5. CT scan or laparoscopic ultrasound: Lymph nodes metastasis: Para-aortic lymph nodes, supraclavicular lymph nodes

- Palliation is done to relieve dysphagia or to control bleeding lesions or for feeding purposes.
- Palliation to control pain.

1. **Intubation:** The choice of the intubation material is self-expanding metallic stent (SEMS, Key Box 40.17). Two types are available—covered and noncovered. The stent is deployed by endoscopy under fluoroscopic guidance. It is collapsed during insertion and once confirmed radiologically by position, it is expanded. Minimal dilatation of the oesophagus (8 mm) is required to place the stent (Figs 40.44 to 40.46). On the other hand, the plastic tubes which

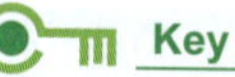 **Key Box 40.17**

SEMS

Self-expanding metallic stents (SEMS) are the best choice of stents in the palliation of malignant strictures and tracheo-oesophageal fistulae. Coated SEMS are now the device of choice for the management of tracheoesophageal fistulae.

They have 2 layers of superalloy monofilament wire with a layer of silicon between them. This prevents tumour growing within the lumen.

Although, SEMS placement is simple, inadequate insertion and positioning occurs. Complications can be dangerous too. However, in vast majority cases, it gives a best palliation.

Complications

- Severe chest pain is due to expansion of the stent
- Acute perforation rate reported in less than 1–2% of the cases.
- Bleeding is rare but can give rise to death by exsanguination.
- Recurrent dysphagia (10%).
- Occlusion of the stent by tumour (8%).

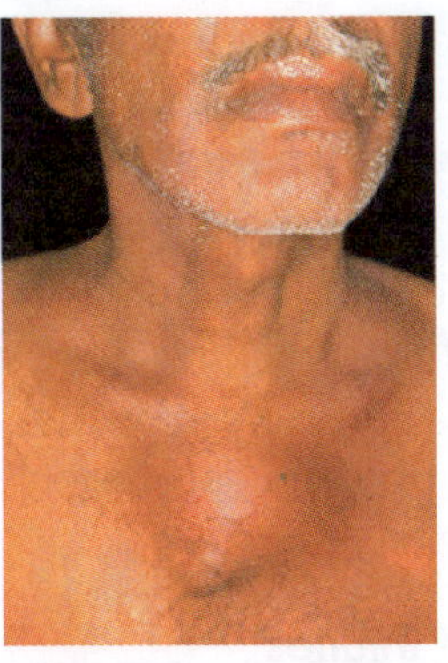

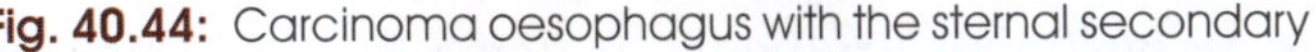

Fig. 40.44: Carcinoma oesophagus with the sternal secondary

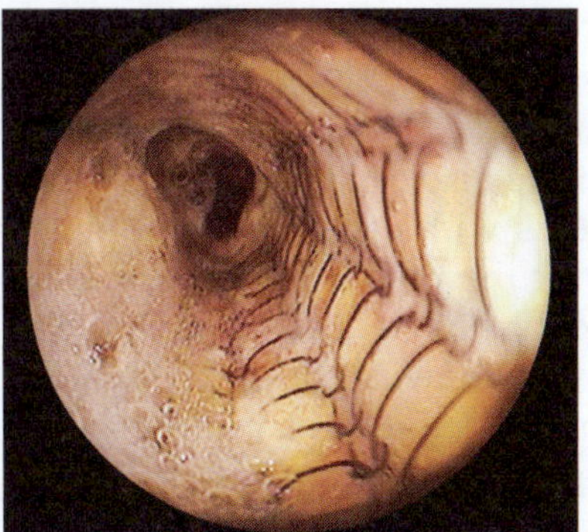

Fig. 40.45: Oesophageal stenting with metallic stent

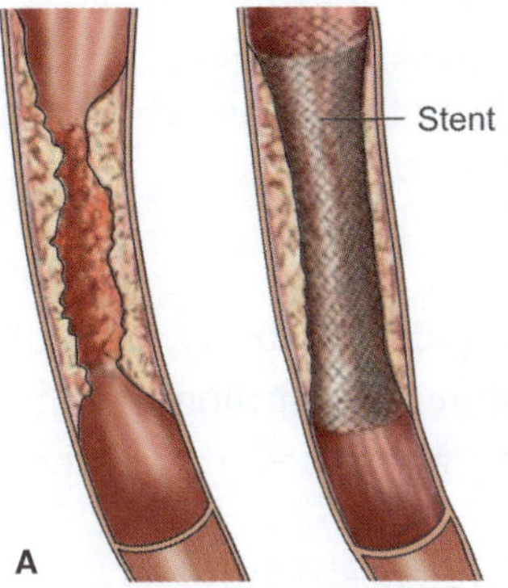

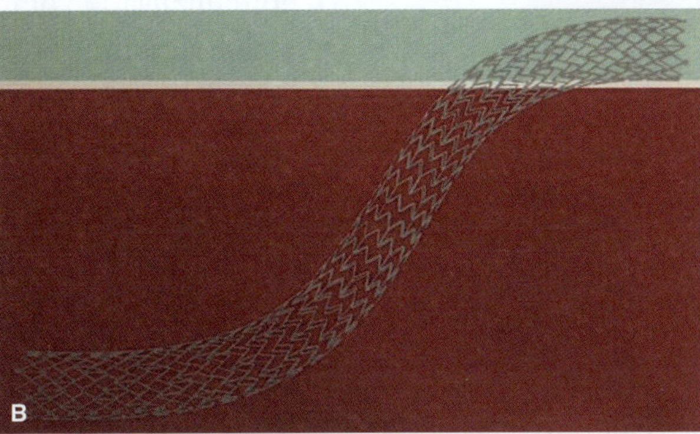

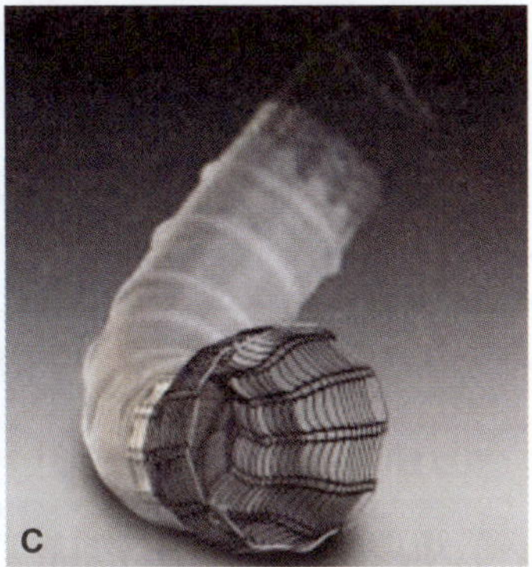

Figs 40.46A to C: Stent—SEMS (*Courtesy:* Dr Shirren Shetty, Head, Department of Gastroenterology, KMC, Manipal)

were used earlier, required more than 8 mm dilatation and there was always a risk of perforation. If the patient is expected to survive beyond 3 months, SEM stent can be considered. Complications include aspiration, feeling of tightness in the chest, bleeding, food blockage, etc.

- This is the choice in cases of tracheo-oesophageal fistula due to carcinoma oesophagus.

2. **Laser therapy:** Endoscopic laser treatment is used to core the tumour and widen the lumen to relieve dysphagia. Principle is thermal destruction of the tumour. The procedure has to be repeated. Laser used is Nd:YAG laser or diode laser. Infiltrative lesions are not suitable for laser treatment but exophytic lesions are ideal—less than 6 cm. Success rates are 80–90% in relieving dysphagia.
   - Perforation, fever, chest pain, fistula are complications.
3. **Photodynamic therapy:** It is used in early carcinomas—mucosal lesions wherein patients are not willing for surgical procedures including endoscopic mucosal resection. In this procedure, a photosensitiser (porfimer sodium) is given. It will be taken by dysplastic cells and malignant cells.
   - Perforation, fever, sunburn, pleural effusion are the complications.
4. **Radiotherapy, brachytherapy:** It is intraluminal radiation (RT) with short penetration distance 1500 cGy radiation is given. No systemic side effects. Palliative external beam radiation to doses of 50 to 60 Gy is successful in 50 to 70% of patients.
5. **Feeding gastrostomy or jejunostomy:** In very late advanced cases, where all other treatment feels.

Causes of Death in Carcinoma Oesophagus

- Cancer cachexia
- Complications such as bronchopleural fistula, aspiration pneumonia, haematemesis due to erosion of aorta, perforation of the growth and mediastinitis.

Summary of Treatment of Carcinoma Oesophagus

- Majority of oesophageal cancers are advanced at the time of diagnosis.
- 5-year survival rates after curative resections are around 10%.
- **The best results are obtained after surgery—radial oesophagectomy.** Curative resections are major surgeries and should be undertaken by an experienced surgeon. Curative resections can be attempted at all levels of carcinoma oesophagus (upper, middle and lower) provided vital structures are **not involved** (assessment by CT scan and endosonogram).

- **Chemoradiotherapy may cure the disease** in selected patients—these are squamous cell cancers.
- **Palliation:** Radiotherapy, chemotherapy, dilatation and stenting also can give palliation. As majority of the patients with carcinoma oesophagus have dysphagia, all the methods of palliation are aimed at relieving dysphagia. Endoscopy followed by dilatation using guidewire is a simple procedure with rate of complications such as perforation around 2–3%. However, the results are only for a few weeks. Self-expandable metal stents are regularly used nowadays as a palliation.
- **Endoscopic laser therapy** relieves obstruction and bleeding. It can be carried out as an outpatient treatment but needs multiple sittings.
- **Radiotherapy** alone has been tried for squamous cell carcinoma of the oesophagus—dose is 6,000 cG units. No survival advantage is seen with this method.
- **Combination chemotherapy** using cisplatin and 5-fluorouracil with radiotherapy has been tried in patients who are not fit for surgery. Paclitaxel achieves high response rate in metastatic oesophageal cancer and it also acts as a radiation sensitiser.
- **Endoscopic intraluminal brachytherapy** is used in, cases of recurrent tumour growing inside the lumen and causing obstruction.

Competency

SU28.6: Describe the clinical features, investigations and principles of management of corrosive strictures, oesphageal perforations, diverticulum (benign disorders).

CORROSIVE OESOPHAGEAL STRICTURE

These caustics are taken accidentally or in attempted suicide. The agents are sodium hydroxide, sulphuric acid, household bleach (Key Box 40.18).

- The acids affect acidic stomach mucosa.
- The squamous epithelium of oesophagus is relatively resistant to acids (also due to rapidity of flow of fluids).

Key Box 40.18

Causes of Stricture

1. Corrosive (caustic) injuries
2. Carcinoma
3. Columnar lined oesophagus—Barrett's oesophagus
4. Capsules of tetracycline group of antibiotics
5. C vitamins—potassium compounds
6. Chronic reflux due to GORD, results in **Schatzki ring**—a stricture at lower oesophagus at squamocolumnar junction. It is a circular ring consisting of fibrous tissue and cellular infiltrates.

- The alkali—sodium hydroxide affects oesophageal mucosa more than gastric mucosa. Alkali ingestion is more common than acid ingestion.
- Alkali ingestion is more devastating than acid.
- Alkali ingestion almost always leads to significant destruction of oesophagus.
- The corrosive injuries may involve oropharynx, larynx, oesophagus, stomach and sometimes intestines also.

Classification of Injuries

- **Superficial:** Erythema, oedema, blisters, etc. Re-epithelialisation of mucosa is complete by 6th week.
- **Deep:** Circumferential ulcers, produces scarring and contractures. Major injury of the stomach produces gastric outlet obstruction.

Clinical Features

- Severe pain, drooling of saliva, inability to swallow.
- Retrosternal burning, abdominal guarding and rigidity.
- Hoarseness, stridor, laryngeal oedema, if there is laryngeal injury.
- Dysphagia occurs later due to stricture.

Important Examinations in Corrosive Injury

- Examination of the oral cavity, chest and abdomen.
- Auscultation of the lungs
- Examination of upper airway
- Abdominal examination—guarding and rigidity of the abdomen indicate perforation.

Pearls of Wisdom

- What should not be done: Stomach wash or induced vomiting, as it will aggravate oesophageal injury or it may result in aspiration. No role for corticosteroids in cases of deep injuries or acid injuries.
- What should be done: Verification of the aetiologic agent and accurate assessment of depth and extent of injury.

Investigations

- Early endoscopy—within 12–24 hours—to grade the injury (*see* below ten commandments for detail).
- CT scan can reveal any perforation in the thorax or in the abdomen.

Treatment

Can be divided into acute and chronic cases. In acute cases, treatment depends upon the severity of the injury or burn.

Acute cases: Any surgical intervention should be done only in selected referral centres. Kindly follow the instructions given below.

Chronic cases present with **stricture** that need regular dilatation. This is ideally done after 6 weeks (the time for re-epithelialisation of oesophagus) (Figs 40.47 and 40.48 and Key Box 40.19).

- **Colonic pull-up** is the choice for impassable strictures, only after adequate nutrition is achieved through feeding jejunostomy.

Complications of Stricture

- **Development of malignancy** (3 to 5%)
- Progressive nutritional deficiency
- Recurrent respiratory tract infection.

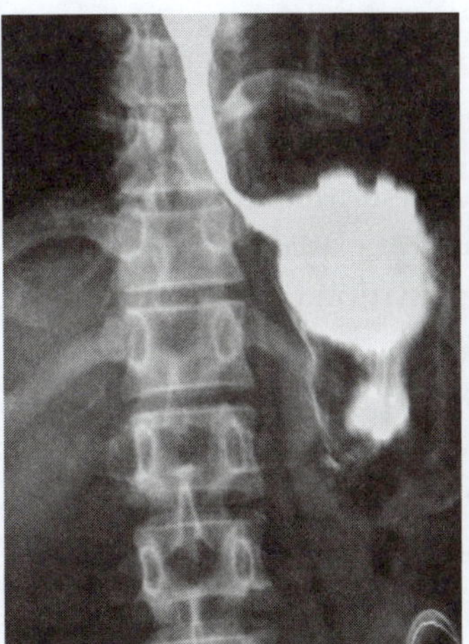
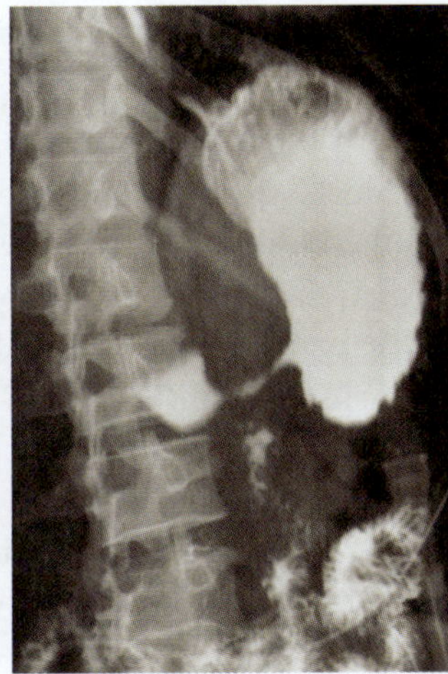

Figs 40.47 and 40.48: Corrosive strictures of lower end of oesophagus and pyloric antrum of stomach. Oesophageal stricture was dilated. However, antral stricture could not be dilated. Hence, he underwent vagotomy and gastrojejunostomy

Key Box 40.19

Dilatation of the Stricture

- Indicated in all cases of symptomatic oesophageal stricture.
- Peptic strictures, corrosive strictures, anastomotic strictures following oesophagogastric anastomosis in the neck after 'THE' or following oesophagogastrectomy for lower oesophageal cancer.
- Flexible oesophagoscopy is done and a guidewire is passed. The scope is withdrawn. Solid dilators of increasing diameter are passed over the guidewire.
- A stricture should be dilated to at least 16 mm in diameter to restore normal swallowing.
- Peptic strictures are easy to dilate as they are short.
- Beware of a GE junction stricture. It may be malignant. Once it is dilated, a growth may be seen. Take a biopsy.
- Pneumatic dilatation can also be used.

TEN COMMANDMENTS OF ACUTE CORROSIVE INJURY

1. Neutralisation of the ingested material
2. Alkalis are neutralised by half strength vinegar, citrus juices
3. Acids are neutralised by milk, egg white, antacids
4. Avoid emetics and sodium bicarbonates
5. Stabilise the patient and arrange upper GI scopy—classify the degree of injury.
6. **No burns:** Observe, small amount of clear fluids may be allowed orally
7. **First degree burns:** Observation for 48 hours. If he can swallow saliva, clear fluids can be started. Repeat endoscopies after a month, 3 or 6 months later to rule out stricture.
8. **Second degree burns:** Intravenous fluids, nil per oral, acid suppression, relieve airway obstruction, parenteral nutrition
9. Cervical oesophagostomy, staple the GE junction, feeding jejunostomy. 6 weeks later, gastric pull up and oesophagogastric anastomosis, in cases of perforation.
10. Call for senior surgeon's help

OESOPHAGEAL PERFORATIONS

- Oesophageal perforation is a serious, acute emergency carrying a very high mortality rate. Fortunately it is not common. There are many causes and are totally different from gastric or duodenal perforations.
- Instrumentation perforations are the most common cause of perforation.
- **Cervical oesophagus** is the most likely site of perforation.
- **Cricopharyngeal** region is the most common site.

Causes

- **Instrumentation:** Endoscopy, dilatation of strictures, injection sclerotherapy and laser treatment are the common causes.
- **Operative:** Thyroidectomy, vagotomy, spine surgery, mediastinoscopy.
- **Traumatic:** Caustic injury, sharp and blunt trauma.
- **Oesophageal diseases:** Carcinoma, Barrett's oesophagus.
- **Spontaneous rupture:** Boerhaave's syndrome.

Clinical Features

- **Severe pain in the neck,** chest or abdomen, stiffness of the neck depending upon the site of perforation.
- Haematemesis, dysphagia, dyspnoea, hypotension, **tachycardia, shock** and pleural effusion are the other features.

- **Mackler's triad:** Chest pain, vomiting and subcutaneous emphysema. It is present only in 10–15% of patients.
- **'Hamman's sign'** escape of air into the mediastinum resulting in "mediastinal crunch" which is produced by the heartbeating against air-filled tissues.

Investigations

- The investigation of choice is plain chest X-ray which can demonstrate **pneumomediastinum,** subcutaneous emphysema and mediastinal air fluid levels. When in doubt, **CT chest** is diagnostic.
- **Contrast swallow** can also be done.

Treatment Principles

- Infection is polymicrobial: Staphylococcus, Streptococcus, Pseudomonas and Bacteroides.
- **Early surgery** should be done within 24 hours. Closure of perforation and external drainage is the treatment.
- Perforation older than 24 hours—treated by temporary cervical oesophagostomy, ligation of oesophagus proximal to GE junction and feeding jejunostomy. After 6–8 weeks, oesophagectomy and gastric or colonic pull up is done.
- **Conservative treatment has risk of continuing leak,** sepsis and mediastinitis.

BAROTRAUMA—BOERHAAVE SYNDROME

Spontaneous Perforation

It occurs when a person vomits against a closed glottis.

Historical: First reported by Professor Hermann Boerhaave—a case of grand admiral who was a glutton and practising autoemesis.

Aetiopathogenesis

- Rupture is due to sudden rise in oesophageal pressure during vomiting, combined with negative intrathoracic pressure.
- Excessive eating as in bulimia/excessive alcohol has been thought to be responsible.
- It is a serious condition because of large volume of material realised under pressure.

Spontaneous Perforation of Oesophagus—Causes

- Vomiting—the most common causes
- Weightlifting
- Defecation
- Epilepsy
- Childbirth

Site of Perforation

- Posterolateral wall of the lower third of the oesophagus.
- Typically a middle-aged man after a bout of alcohol first vomits food contents followed by blood.
- He complains of lower thoracic pain—typically from 10 hours thoracic perforations.
- Pain in neck is due to cervical perforation.
- Tachycardia, tachypnoea, fever are present.
- **Hamman's sign is positive**.

Differential Diagnosis

- Myocardial infarction
- Acute pancreatitis.

Investigations

- Chest X-ray: Air in the mediastinum, air in the pleura, air in the peritoneum, pleural effusion
- CECT scan: It is the investigation of choice to detect the exact site of perforation
- Barium meal (Fig. 40.49).

Treatment Principles

- **Conservative:** It is indicated in small ruptures without any contaminations and they are contained rupture.
- **Endoscopic stent:** It is indicated in case of early cases without much contamination and delayed cases. It will help in presenting fistula formation.
- **Surgery:** Indicated in case of early perforations either open thoracotomy, repair or video-assisted thoracoscopic surgery (VATS) with reinforcement by using gastric fundus.

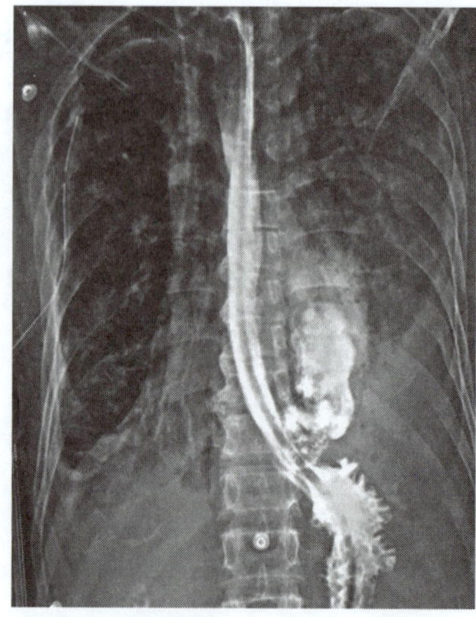

Fig. 40.49: Barium meal showing extravasation of barium—Boerhaave syndrome

DIVERTICULUM OF OESOPHAGUS

Types of Diverticulum

Table 40.8 describes types of diverticulum.

Cervical diverticulum (Fig. 40.50) is the commonest type of diverticulum which can present with regurgitation of meals, aspiration of food contents into the lungs or recurrent respiratory tract infections. It is treated by excision of the sac and repair of the defect along with cricopharyngeal myotomy—**posterior midline**.

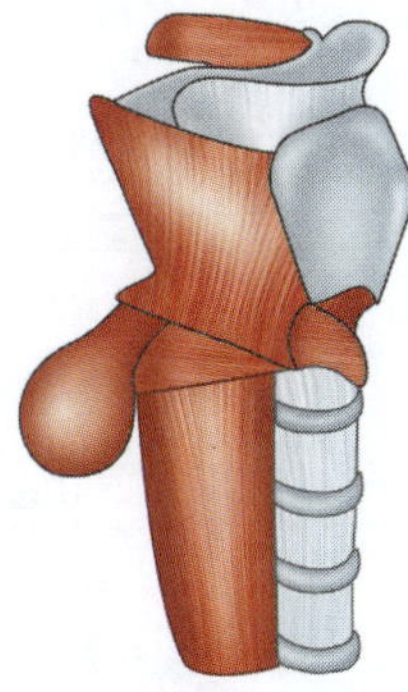

Fig. 40.50: Diverticulum

DIFFERENTIAL DIAGNOSIS OF DYSPHAGIA (Fig. 40.51)

I. Causes from outside (extraluminal) oesophagus
   1. Thyroid swellings
   2. Cardiomegaly
   3. Aortic aneurysm
   4. Mediastinal nodes: Tuberculosis, lymphoma or secondaries
   5. Rolling hiatus hernia

II. Causes in the wall of oesophagus (luminal)
   1. Oesophageal stricture
      - Corrosive acid poisoning
      - Tuberculous stricture
   2. Carcinoma oesophagus
   3. Oesophageal diverticulum
   4. Muscular spasm: Plummer-Vinson syndrome and achalasia cardia.
   5. Tetanus

III. Causes in the lumen of oesophagus
   1. Foreign body: Dentures, coins, etc.

History

1. **Acute dysphagia:** Common in children. Foreign bodies are common causes. Acute dysphagia with pain suggests tonsillitis or pharyngitis.

> *Pearls of Wisdom*
>
> In the absence of usual causes mentioned above, acute dysphagia in an old man may be a manifestation of vertebrobasilar insufficiency.

2. **Chronic dysphagia:** Stricture, achalasia, Plummer-Vinson syndrome and carcinomas produce chronic dysphagia. The increasing difficulty to swallow, first to solids and later to liquids is typical of carcinoma oesophagus (in achalasia cardia, it is the reverse).
3. **Age and sex:** Achalasia and Plummer-Vinson syndrome is common in females, carcinoma in men and foreign body in children.
4. **Change in voice** or even hoarseness with dysphagia suggests advanced laryngeal carcinoma.

> *Pearls of Wisdom*
>
> Dysphagia means difficulty in swallowing. Odynophagia means painful swallowing as in quinsy, retropharyngeal abscess, tonsillitis, etc.

RARE CAUSES OF DYSPHAGIA (RINGS, SLINGS AND WEBS)

1. **Vascular slings and pulmonary artery slings:** These occur due to developmental anomalies of great vessels causing dysphagia. More common is aortic arch anomaly wherein the right subclavian artery arising from the descending aorta travels behind oesophagus creating incomplete vascular ring to complete the course. Pulmonary artery sling is due to left pulmonary artery arising from right pulmonary artery causing anterior compression of oesophagus.
2. **Oesophageal ring (Schatzki's ring):** It is located at the squamocolumnar junction with oesophageal squamous epithelium above and columnar epithelium below. There is a concentric symmetrical narrowing with restricted distensibility of lower oesophagus. It presents as dysphagia and episodic aphagia. Diagnosis is by barium oesophagography.

Table 40.8 Types of diverticulum

Name	Situation	Aetiology
1. **Zenker's** diverticulum (**cervical** or pulsion)	Proximal to the upper oesophageal sphincter	Protrusion of oesophageal mucosa between cricopharyngeus muscle inferiorly and thyropharyngeus muscle superiorly
2. Epinephric diverticulum	Proximal to the lower oesophageal sphincter	It is due to some kind of motility disturbance, wherein protrusion occurs in the lower end
3. Parabronchial diverticulum	Midoesophagus	Tuberculosis, by causing enlargement of mediastinal nodes, fibrosis and adhesions produce traction on the oesophagus, which results in the diverticulum

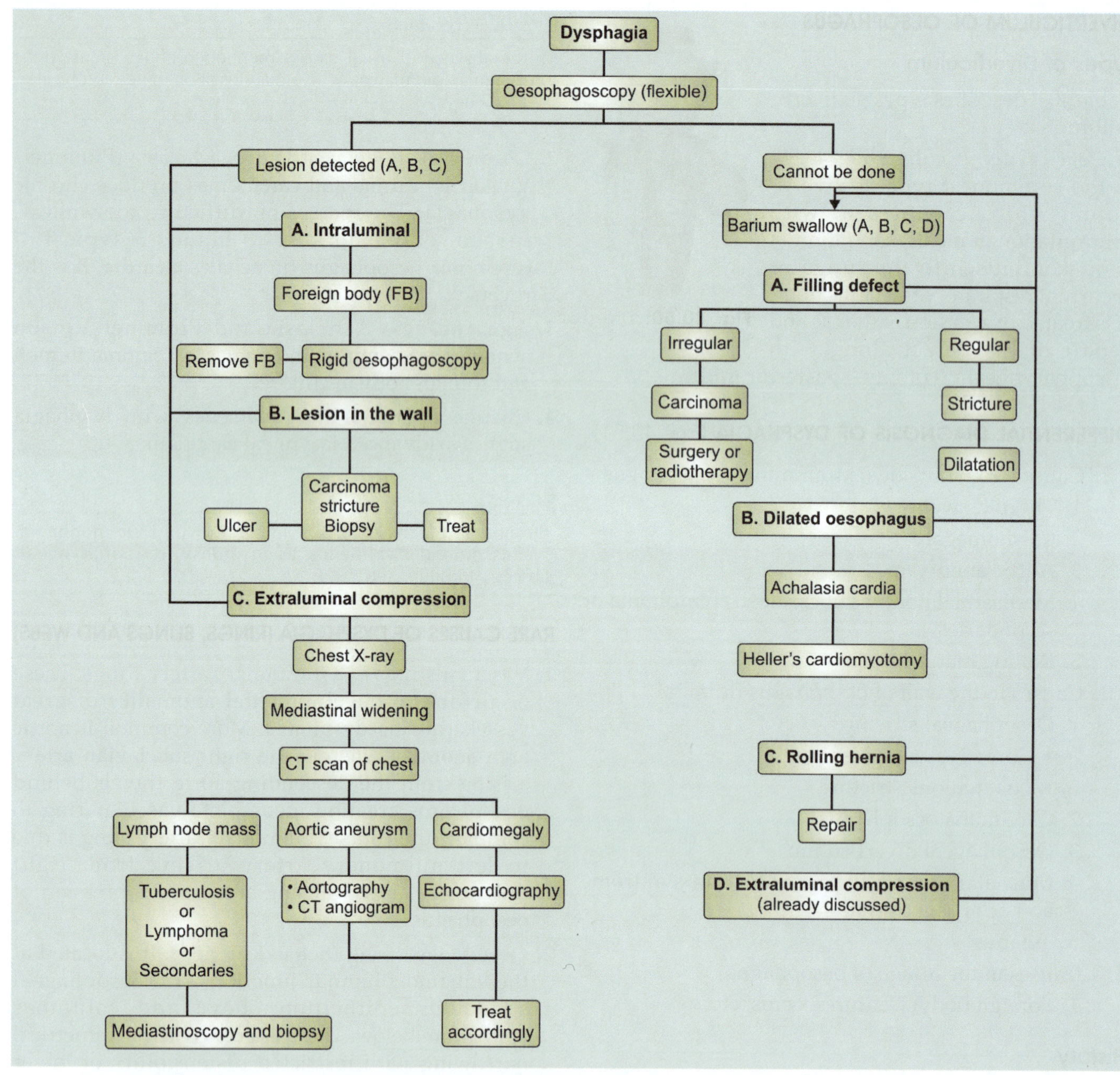

Fig. 40.51: Investigations of a case of dysphagia

It is treated by repeated bougie dilatation. The cause is obscure but there is strong association with reflux disease. Many rings are incidental findings in radiology. They do not have any symptoms.

3. **Webs:** Oesophageal webs are uncommon causes of dysphagia. They are treated by oesophageal dilatation. *Refer to* clinical notes.

Clinical Notes

- A 60-year-old agriculturist was referred to the department of ENT for dysphagia of 3–4 days duration. A registrar who saw the case did rigid oesophagoscopy under GA. The findings were normal. Later in the evening he was called to see this patient who had rigid abdomen. A general surgeon was consulted. He suspected a perforation. An X-ray abdomen (erect), however, was normal. A senior faculty surgeon was consulted who examined the case properly and gave a correct diagnosis. It was a case of tetanus with mild trismus. The patient had injured his left thumb a few days back. The anaesthesiologist acknowledged later that there was some difficulty in opening the patients mouth during endotracheal intubation.
- Occasionally, patients undergo gastroscopy for dysphagia which will be normal only to realise later that what he is having is a stroke!!!

Table 40.9 Diaphragmatic hiatus (Fig. 40.52)

Hiatus	Location	Structures passing through
1. Aortic hiatus (median arcuate ligament)	Posteriorly opposite 12th thoracic vertebra	Aorta, thoracic duct, azygos vein
2. Oesophageal hiatus (formed by right crus)	Anterior at the level of 10th thoracic vertebra 1 inch to the left side	Oesophagus, vagus nerves, oesophageal branches of left gastric artery, veins and lymphatics
3. Caval opening	Just to the right of the midline, opposite 8th thoracic vertebra	Inferior vena cava, right phrenic nerve

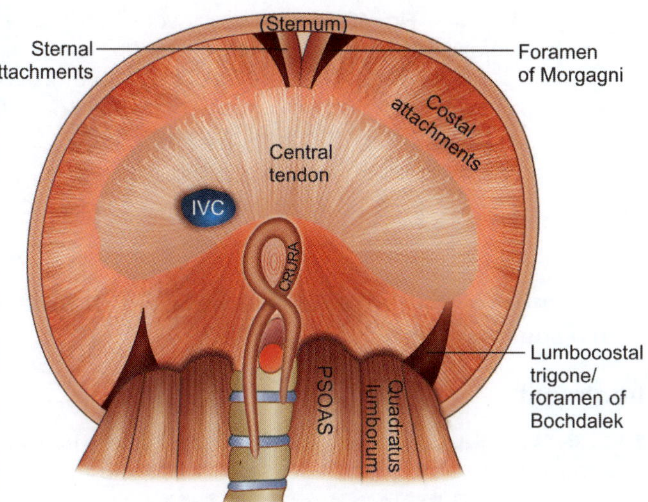

Fig. 40.52: Diaphragmatic hiatus

SURGICAL ANATOMY OF THE DIAPHRAGM

- The diaphragm is a dome-shaped thin sheet of muscle which separates the thoracic cavity from the abdominal cavity.
- It is derived from the innermost layer of the muscles of the body. Hence, it arises in continuity with transversus abdominis fibres from within the costal margins.
- It has a right and left dome with a central tendon (Table 40.9).

Attachments

- Anteriorly: Lower sternum
- Laterally: Costal margin
- Posteriorly (crura): First three lumbar vertebrae.

Nerve Supply

The muscles of the dome on its abdominal surface is supplied by phrenic nerve (C4). The crura are supplied by the lower intercostal nerves.

Blood Supply

Lower five intercostal arteries, subcostal arteries, and right and left phrenic arteries supply diaphragm.

DIAPHRAGMATIC HERNIA

Development of Diaphragm

The diaphragm develops from—muscle and its associated connective tissue, central tendon develops from three sources: The septum transversum, the pleuroperitoneal folds, and the somites. Two important parts of the muscle of the diaphragm are—costal and crural. The costal diaphragm is a thin domed sheet of muscle composed of a radially arranged myofibers extending laterally from the ribs and medially to a central tendon. The crural part of diaphragm is more posterior and thicker. It is attached to the vertebrae. Here we find the hiatus of oesophagus and aorta. The muscles and fibres of both the costal and crural muscles insert into the central tendon medially. The central tendon is located at the apex of the domed diaphragm. Caudally, it attaches to the liver via the falciform and coronary ligaments. Maldevelopment of the septum transversum results in diaphragmatic hernia.

Types of Diaphragmatic Hernia

It is of two types: Congenital and acquired.

- Majority of congenital hernias present shortly after birth. However, a few cases present late to the hospital, and most of such children are treated for recurrent respiratory tract infection elsewhere, without a proper diagnosis. 80% of congenital diaphragmatic hernias occur on the **left side.**
- The acquired diaphragmatic hernias are very often (almost always) due to road traffic accidents or due to stab injuries of the abdomen. They are discussed in blunt abdominal trauma.

Sites of Congenital Diaphragmatic Hernia

1. **Hernia through the foramen of Bochdalek:** This is the most common diaphragmatic hernia in children. These hernias occur through the persistence of the pleuroperitoneal canals. The defect is posterior. It occurs due to failure of closure of diaphragm posteriorly during development. Respiratory distress, shift of mediastinum and scaphoid abdomen clinch the diagnosis (Fig. 40.53). It can also occur in adults. Incidence is one in 5000 persons.

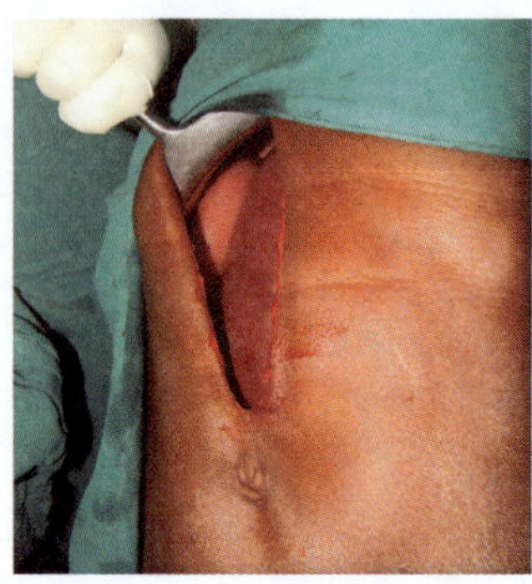

Fig. 40.53: Bochdalek hernia showing intestine above the liver as soon as laparotomy is done. The defect was two fingers (5 cm) in diameter. Non-absorbable sutures were used to close the defect (*Courtesy:* Dr Balakrishna Shetty, Surgeon, Chinmaya Hospital, Kundapur)

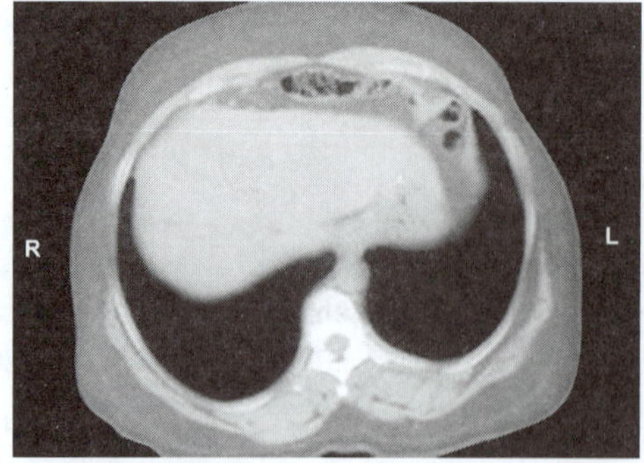

Fig. 40.54: Morgagni hernia—CT scan showing intestine (colon within the thorax). (*Courtesy:* Dr Srinivas Pai, Dr Nitin Nagpal, Dr Rohith Jain, Department of Surgery, KMC, Manipal)

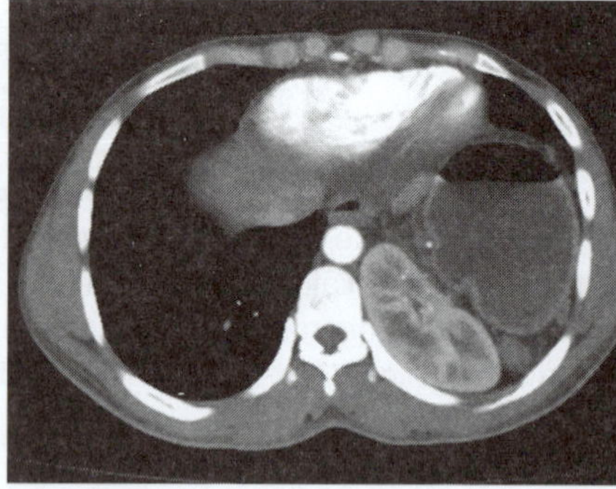

Fig. 40.55: CT chest reveled left Kidney is in the thorax with colon and stomach. Contents were reduced, eventration repaired with prolene mesh. (*Courtesy:* Dr Vijayendra, Dr Kalyan Reddy, Dr V. Vivek, KMC Manipal)

2. **Hernia through the foramen of Morgagni (parasternal hernia):** Failure of fusion of few fibres from going to xyphoid process with fibres from several costochondral arches result in a defect which is muscle free—it is called foramen of Moragani—both right and left. The defects are anterior (Fig. 40.54). These hernias present in late childhood or in adult life with features of partial (subacute) intestinal obstruction, pain in the right hypochondrium or tightness in the chest (Fig. 40.54). This is because majority of them contain transverse colon.

Pearls of Wisdom

Anterior diaphragmatic defect—foramen of Morgagni: Posterior (posterolateral) diaphragmatic defect foramen of Bochdalek.

3. **Herniation through the central tendon:**
   - This can affect the right or the left apex of the cupola or the central portion. The contents may be fundus of the stomach on the left side and a portion of the liver on the right side.
   - These cases are very often diagnosed accidentally by routine chest radiograph.
4. **Eventration:** Due to paralysis or atrophy of the muscle fibres, one or both hemidiaphragms are weak and they are elevated in position. Truly speaking, this is not a hernia, but signs and symptoms are almost like other types of hernia.

Diagnosis

- Chest radiograph: Gas and fluid level is within the chest. Left dome of the diaphragm can be elevated as you see in Fig. 40.55.
- The thin rim of the diaphragm, as seen in a plain radiograph, is broken or shows a defect.
- CT chest and abdomen is the gold standard investigation (Fig. 40.56A and B).

Treatment

- The repair of the defect is done by using non-absorbable sutures. If the defect is more than 20 m, might is used to close the defect.

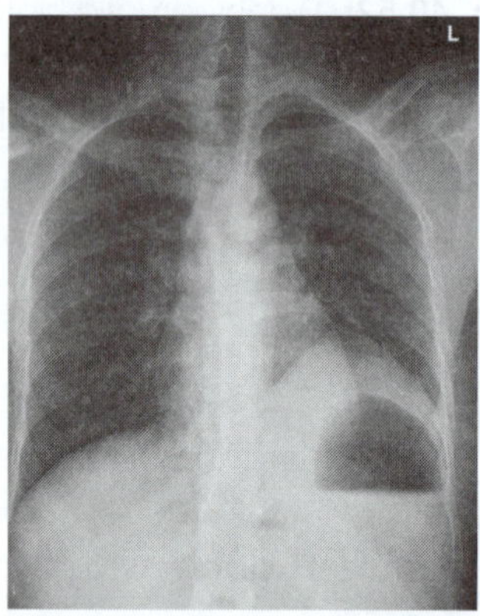

Fig. 40.56A: Left dome is elevated—fundic air bubble is separated. In fact this patient had spleen in that area

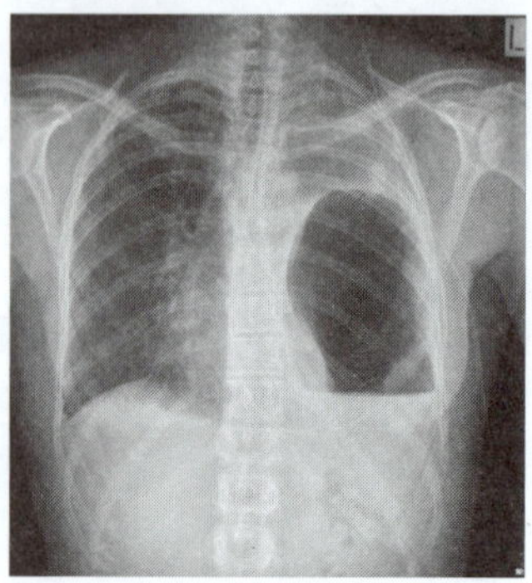

Fig. 40.56B: Left diaphragmatic hernia. (*Courtesy:* Dr Santhosh John Abraham, Cheif Surgeon, Director, Lourdhe Hospital, Cochin)

- Eventration of the diaphragm is repaired by placating the redundant diaphragm. A mesh can be used to reinforce the defect.

TRACHEO-OESOPHAGEAL FISTULA

Types

In majority of the cases (85%), lower end of the oesophagus communicates with the trachea and upper end is blind.

Associated Anomalies (Key Box 40.20, VACTER)

Clinical Features

- Continuous pouring of saliva from the mouth in the newborn baby is a diagnostic feature.
- Newborn baby regurgitates all feeds.
- Aspiration, cough and cyanosis are other features.
- It is commonly associated with maternal hydramnios (50%).

Key Box 40.20

Associated Anomalies

V : Vertebral defects
A : Anorectal malformation
C : Cardiac defect (PDA/VSD)
TE : Tracheo-oesophageal fistula
R : Radial hypoplasia and renal agenesis

- TOF should be recognised and diagnosed within 24 hours of birth—by introducing a red rubber catheter.

Management

- Right thoracotomy, ligation of TOF and primary anastomosis of oesophageal ends.
- Feeding gastrostomy and oesophagostomy in type III fistula.
- In difficult cases, where there is a long atretic segment, colonic or gastric transposition is required.

Complications

Pneumonia, reflux, dysphagia, anastomotic leak.

Multiple Choice Questions

1. Following are disorders of the pharyngooesophageal junction *except*:

A. Stroke
B. Myasthenia
C. Cricopharyngeal achalasia
D. Nutcracker oesophagus

2. Following are true for oesophageal lymphatics *except*:

A. Extensive lymphatic plexus in the submucosa
B. They are classified as perioesophageal, paraoesophageal and lateral oesophageal lymph nodes
C. Presence of coeliac nodes indicate inoperability
D. Longitudinal lymphatics are 6 times less than transverse

3. Which one of the following is highest percentage of premalignant condition, for carcinoma oesophagus?

A. Tylosis B. Lye strictures
C. Achalasia D. Oesophagus

4. Factors for adenocarcinoma oesophagus are following *except*:

A. Barrett's oesophagus B. Obesity
C. Reflux oesophagitis D. Oesophageal web

5. Factors for development of reflux disease of oesophagus include the following *except*:

A. Obesity
B. Absence of intra-abdominal length of oesophagus
C. Helicobacter pylori infection
D. Defective angle of His

6. Clinical features of reflux disease of oesophagus include the following *except*:

A. Heartburn B. Vomiting
C. Epigastric pain D. Regurgitation

7. Gold standard for the treatment of reflux disease is:

A. Barium meal
B. Oesophagoscopy
C. 24-hour pH monitoring
D. Endosonogram

8. The most effective drugs for reflux disease are:

A. Alginates
B. Antacids
C. H_2 receptor antagonists
D. Proton pump inhibitors

9. The most effective curative treatment for carcinoma oesophagus is:
   A. Radiotherapy
   B. Oesophagectomy
   C. Photodynamic therapy
   D. Chemotherapy

10. Following are features of Barrett's oesophagus *except*:
   A. 3 cm or more of columnar epithelium
   B. Cardiac metaplasia
   C. Development of squamous cell carcinoma
   D. Presence of mucus secreting goblet cells (intestinal metaplasia)

11. Which of the following conditions predisposes to volvulus of the stomach?
   A. Sliding hernia
   B. Para-oesophageal hernia
   C. Following gastrojejunostomy
   D. Wide hiatus

12. Following are true for PET scan *except*:
   A. Drug used is oral fluorosodeoxycholic acid
   B. Combining PET with CT is better for diagnosis
   C. Can be used after chemotherapy to see the response of the tumour
   D. High metabolic activity—glycolytic pathway

13. Following are true for transhiatal oesophagectomy *except*:
   A. Thoracotomy is a must for completion of the procedure
   B. Anastomosis is in the neck
   C. Ideal for lower oesophageal cancers
   D. Upper oesophagus mobilisation is blind

14. About achalasia cardia following are true *except*:
   A. It affects lower oesophageal end
   B. It is due to loss of inhibitory neurons
   C. Dilated oesophagus above contain normal ganglion cells
   D. In vigorous achalasia normal ganglion cells are present

15. About treatment of achalasia cardia following are true *except*:
   A. Balloon dilatation is ideal for patients above the age of 45 years
   B. Botulinum toxin injection gives the permanent relief from dysphagia
   C. Sublingual nifedipine can relieve symptoms
   D. Myotomy with anterior fundoplication is a good surgical procedure

16. Schatzki's ring is associated with:
   A. Proximal oesophagus B. Carcinoma oesophagus
   C. Reflux oesophagitis D. Congenital ring

17. For normal swallowing stricture should be dilated to at least:
   A. 12 mm diameter B. 14 mm diameter
   C. 16 mm diameter D. 18 mm diameter

18. Following are true for Mallory-Weiss syndrome *except*:
   A. The vertical split occurs in the lower end of oesophagus in majority of cases
   B. Surgery is rarely required
   C. Endoscopic sclerotherapy is very useful treatment
   D. More often it is a mucosal tear than rupture

19. For the diagnosis of intraperitoneal metastasis, which is the ideal investigation?
   A. Ultrasound B. CT scan
   C. MRI D. Diagnostic laparoscopy

20. Following are true about Heller's cardiomyotomy *except*:
   A. It is best done by laparoscopic method
   B. Many surgeons add fundoplication
   C. Myotomy should be more in length in the stomach side than oesophagus
   D. Reflux is a major complication

21. Most accurate method for the diagnosis of T stage for oesophageal cancer is by:
   A. Upper gastroduodenal scopy
   B. Barium swallow
   C. CT scan
   D. Endosonogram

22. The typical defect in Bochdalek hernia is:
   A. Posterior B. Posterolateral
   C. Anterior D. Anterolateral

Answers

1. D	**2.** D	**3.** A	**4.** D	**5.** C	**6.** B	**7.** B	**8.** D	**9.** B	**10.** C
11. B	**12.** A	**13.** A	**14.** C	**15.** B	**16.** C	**17.** C	**18.** A	**19.** D	**20.** C
21. D	**22.** B								

CHAPTER

41

Stomach and Duodenum

- Surgical anatomy
- Gastric physiology
- *H. pylori* infection
- Gastritis
- Peptic ulcer disease
- Acute complications of peptic ulcer
- Chronic complications of peptic ulcer
- Carcinoma stomach
- Gastrointestinal stromal tumours (GISTs)
- Gastric lymphoma
- Complications of gastrectomy
- Acute dilatation of stomach
- Volvulus of the stomach
- Bezoars
- Idiopathic hypertrophic pyloric stenosis
- Chronic duodenal ileus
- Duodenal anatomy and obstruction

Introduction

The oesophagus continues from the oesophagogastric (OG) junction as a muscular tube—the stomach.

Competency

SU28.7: Describe applied anatomy and physiology of stomach.

SURGICAL ANATOMY

Fundus

Part of the stomach which projects upwards and lies in contact with the left dome of diaphragm. It is usually full of gas.

Significance

- To identify the side (right or left) of the body in a plain X-ray abdomen.
- In achalasia cardia, fundic air bubble is absent.
- Fundic **'Wrap'** is used in hiatus hernia.
- During mobilisation of the fundus as in splenectomy or other upper gastric surgery, short gastric arteries need to be divided. If ligatures are too close to the stomach near the fundus, gastric fistula may occur due to **necrosis of the stomach**.
- GISTs (gastrointestinal stromal tumours) are common in fundus.

Body

Extends from fundus to *incisura angularis*. It has a lesser curvature and a greater curvature.

Significance

- Ability to have a large meal is due to receptive relaxation of the body of the stomach.
- Greater curvature is located at the level of umbilicus.
- Classical gastrojejunostomy (GJ), anterior or posterior, involves using body of the stomach.
- Posteriorly, it is related to the lesser sac and pancreas. Carcinoma of the body may infiltrate pancreas—necessitates careful dissection to separate from pancreas (sometimes not resectable).

Pyloric Antrum

It extends from incisura till pylorus. Pylorus is thicker than the rest of the stomach. It is a sphincter of circular muscle fibres. Its canal is usually closed.

Significance (Table 41.1)

- Pyloric antrum is a common site for gastritis, ulcer and carcinoma.

Table 41.1 Anatomy and surgical significance

2 Orifices	**Recognition**	**Pathology**	**Result**
• Pyloric orifice	Recognised by prepyloric vein of Mayo	Incompetence causes duodeno-gastric reflux	Biliary gastritis
• Cardiac orifice	Lower end of oesophagus	Incompetence causes acid reflux into lower end of oesophagus	Barrett's oesophagus
2 Curvatures			
• Lesser curvature	Concave lesser omentum is attached to it	Site of benign gastric ulcer	Hour-glass contracture
• Greater curvature	Convex greater omentum is attached to it	Site of carcinomatous ulcer	Carcinoma stomach
Part	**Common pathology**	**Commonly used for**	**Nature of the condition**
• Fundus	GIST	Fundic wrap	Hiatus hernia
• Body	Carcinoma	Gastrojejunostomy	Erosive gastritis
• Pylorus	Pyloric stenosis, carcinoma	Pyloric myotomy in idiopathic pyloric stenosis	Pyloric stenosis

- Incompetence of pyloric sphincter results in severe duodenogastric reflux.
- It is in close contact with the head of pancreas. During gastrectomy, extreme care has to be taken to mobilise the antrum to avoid bleeding in the pancreatic head region.

Greater Omentum

It lies in contact with transverse colon and gastrocolic omentum (Fig. 41.1 and Key Box 41.1). This has to be divided from transverse colon during gastrectomy which is done for carcinoma or ulcer.

Lesser Omentum

- The lesser omentum is a double-layered structure.
- It is suspended between the lesser curvature of the stomach and the proximal 0.5 inch (2 cm) of the first part of the duodenum inferiorly and the porta hepatis and the fissure of the ligamentum venosum superiorly.

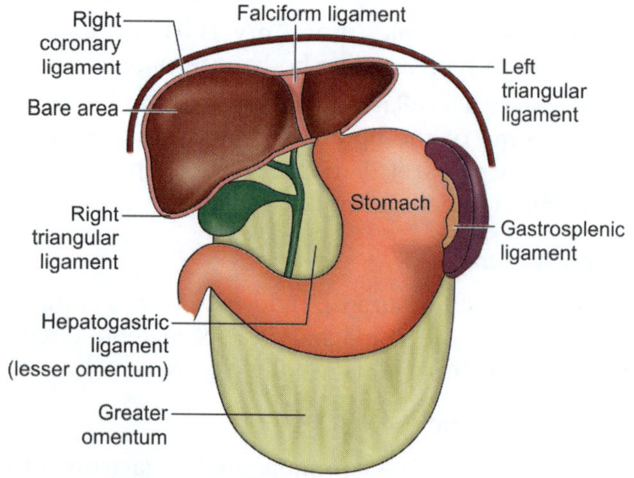

Fig. 41.1: Stomach, omentum and ligaments

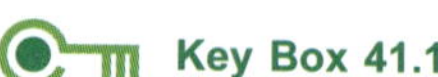
Key Box 41.1

Greater Omentum is a Friend and Sometimes Enemy of the Patient and the Surgeon

- The greater omentum is the **policeman** of the peritoneal cavity. It exhibits protective action in inflammatory processes and perforations.
- **Omentoplasty** (omental wrapping of anastomosis) may decrease the occurrence of anastomotic leakage when oesophagogastric anastomosis is performed for cancer of oesophagus or as in closure of duodenal perforation.
- It has many **important applications** and can be used in colorectal surgery, reconstruction of the irradiated pharyngeal wound and packing of bleeding liver wounds.
- It was used to **treat peripheral vascular disease** such as TAO wherein direct arterial surgery was not possible.
- It becomes an enemy when involved with metastasis or directly by malignant neoplastic process from ovary or colorectal cancer. Omentum is one of the common sites of involvement in tuberculosis also. Omentum itself can act like a **band** and can cause intestinal obstruction.

The lesser omentum is divided into two ligaments:

1. **Hepatogastric**
2. **Hepatoduodenal:** Located within the lesser omentum are the **hepatic triad**, branches of the anterior vagus nerve, some lymph nodes, and the right and left gastric arteries.

Vagus Nerves

- The left and right vagus nerves descend parallel to the oesophagus and form oesophageal vagal plexus between the level of the tracheal bifurcation and level of the diaphragm.

- From this plexus, two vagal trunks, anterior and posterior, form and pass through the oesophageal hiatus of the diaphragm **(mnemonic LARP: Left trunk—anterior gastric wall; right trunk—posterior gastric wall).**

Blood Supply of the Stomach (Fig. 41.2)

It is mainly supplied by coeliac trunk and its branches:

1. **Left gastric artery** is a direct branch of coeliac trunk. It ascends up to oesophageal hiatus and turns to the right along the lesser curvature of stomach. It branches and anastomoses with branches of right gastric artery and supplies anterior and posterior wall of the stomach. There is true anastomosis between branches of left gastric artery and branches from other arteries.
2. **Right gastric artery** is a branch of hepatic artery which comes from coeliac trunk. It also supplies lesser curvature and body of stomach, along with left gastric artery.
3. **Left gastroepiploic artery** arises from splenic artery and supplies greater curvature of stomach and anastomoses with right gastroepiploic artery.
4. **Right gastroepiploic artery** is a branch of gastroduodenal artery, which is a branch of hepatic artery.
5. **Short gastric arteries** are the branches of splenic artery. They supply the fundus of the stomach. They are also called *vasa braevia*.

Venous Drainage

- Veins run with the corresponding arteries.
- Right and left gastric veins drain into the portal vein directly.
- Right gastroepiploic vein joins superior mesenteric vein.
- Left gastroepiploic vein and *vasa braevia* join splenic vein.

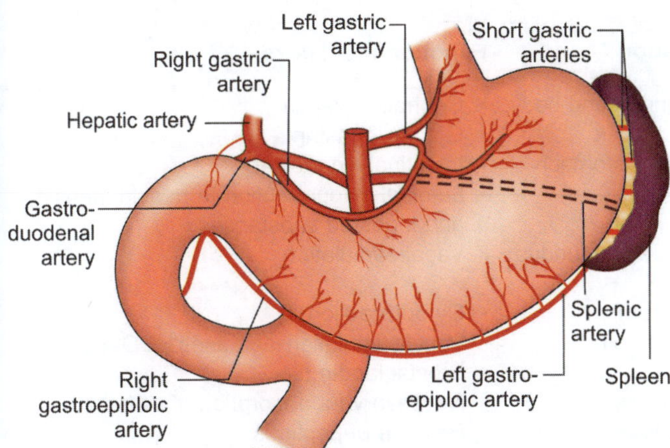

Fig. 41.2: Blood supply of the stomach arteries

- Prepyloric vein of Mayo is a useful guide to the junction between stomach and duodenum.

Surgical Importance

- Because of extensive anastomoses of blood vessels (extramural and intramural collateral vessels), stomach can survive with right gastric and right gastroepiploic arteries only. Thus stomach can be used to replace the entire oesophagus after oesophagectomy—gastric pull up.
- The order of ligation of blood vessels in gastrectomy is as follows: Left gastroepiploic, right gastroepiploic, right gastric (then stomach is divided) and lastly, left gastric arteries.
- Gastroduodenal artery, a branch of hepatic artery runs behind first part of duodenum and divides into right gastroepiploic artery and superior pancreatico-duodenal artery.
- It is this artery which bleeds when a posterior duodenal ulcer erodes into it.

Lymphatic Drainage (Fig. 41.3)

It is an important pathway for spread of carcinoma of the stomach. The spread occurs both by emboli and permeation.

1. Right gastric nodes/suprapyloric nodes mainly drain the pyloric antrum.
2. Subpyloric nodes/gastroepiploic nodes (right) drain the greater curvature of stomach and pyloric antrum.
3. Left gastroepiploic nodes (splenic nodes) drain the upper portion of stomach, mainly the fundus (carcinoma of fundus).
4. Left gastric (superior gastric) nodes drain the lesser curvature and body of the stomach (anterior and posterior wall).

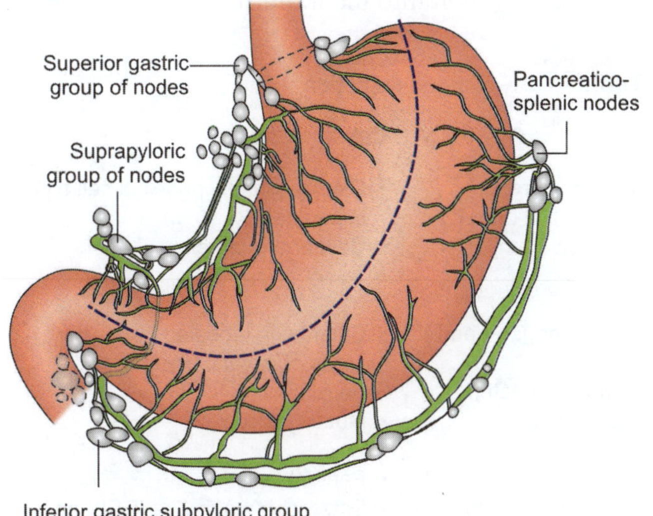

Fig. 41.3: Lymphatic drainage of the stomach

5. Coeliac nodes receive lymph from the entire foregut (including stomach) and drain directly into the *cisterna chyli* and the thoracic duct. Later, mediastinal nodes and left supraclavicular nodes (**Virchow nodes**) are involved. **Lymphatic zones are discussed under carcinoma stomach.**

Lymphatics of the Stomach

The lymphatics of the stomach are formed from two networks: Intrinsic and extrinsic.

Intrinsic network: The submucosal lymphatic plexus is perhaps the richest in anastomoses.

- Upward invasive spread of gastric cancer to the oesophagus is common but downward mucosal or submucosal invasion of the duodenum is not common.
- Hence, gastrectomy with distal oesophagectomy is done for carcinoma of the proximal stomach.

Extrinsic network: The extrinsic lymphatic vessels of the stomach follow the gastric veins.

- They drain to perigastric lymph nodes, which in turn drain to the lymph nodes located at the coeliac axis.
  1. **The superior gastric group** drains lymph from the upper lesser curvature into the left gastric and paracardiac nodes.
  2. **The suprapyloric group** of nodes drains the antral segment on the lesser curvature of the stomach into the right suprapancreatic nodes.
  3. **The pancreaticosplenic group** of nodes drains lymph high on the greater curvature into the left gastroepiploic and splenic nodes.
  4. **The inferior gastric and subpyloric group** of nodes drains lymph along the right gastroepiploic vascular pedicle.
- All four zones of lymph nodes drain into the coeliac group and then into the thoracic duct.

GASTRIC PHYSIOLOGY

Hypergastrinaemia

Various causes of surgical interest are given in Key Box 41.2.

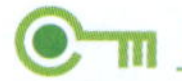
Key Box 41.2

Causes of Hypergastrinaemia

Ulcerogenic causes	Non-ulcerogenic causes
❍ Antral G cell hyperplasia or hyperfunction	❍ Antisecretory agents (PPIs)
❍ Retained excluded antrum	❍ Atrophic gastritis
❍ Zollinger-Ellison syndrome	❍ Pernicious anaemia
❍ Gastric outlet obstruction	❍ Acid-reducing procedure (vagotomy)
❍ Short-gut syndrome	❍ *Helicobacter pylori* infection
❍ Chronic renal failure	

Gastric Acid Secretion (Table 41.2)

- Gastric acid secretion by the parietal cells is regulated by three local stimuli: 1. Acetylcholine, 2. Gastrin, 3. Histamine.
- These three stimuli account for basal and stimulated gastric acid secretion.
- **Acetylcholine is the principal neurotransmitter** modulating acid secretion and is released from the vagus and parasympathetic ganglion cells.
- Vagal fibres innervate not only parietal cells but also G cells and enterochromaffin-like (ECL) cells to modulate release of their peptides.
- **Gastrin has hormonal effects on the parietal cell** and stimulates histamine release.
- **Histamine has paracrine-like effects** on the **parietal cell**. Its release from ECL cells plays a central role in the regulation of acid secretion by the parietal cell.

Table 41.2 Gastric secretion

	Cells	Location	Function/mediators
1. Acid secretion 150–160 mEq/L	• Oxyntic glands, principal cell type is parietal	• Fundus and body	• Cephalic—vagus • Gastric—gastrin • Intestinal—not clear
2. Mucus	• Columnar epithelium	• Entire stomach	• Luminal cytoprotection from acid, pepsin and ingested substances
3. Pepsinogen I and II	• Chief cells—located in deeper areas of oxyntic gland	• Body and fundus	• Vagal stimulation
4. Mucus, gastrin	• Antrum	• Antrum	• Cytoprotection
5. Bicarbonate	• Mucus cells	• Stomach	• Vagal stimulation increases HCO_3^- secretion • Prostaglandin E_2
6. Intrinsic factor	• Parietal cells	• Fundus	• Necessary for absorption of vitamin B_{12}
7. Peptides, histamine	• Enterochromaffin like (ECL) cells • D cells (delta)	• Fundus • Antrum	• Release of peptides • Somatostatin inhibits acid secretion

Ingestion of a meal stimulates vagal fibres to release acetylcholine ***(cephalic phase)***. Binding of acetylcholine to parietal cell and G cell results in the release of histamine, hydrochloric acid and gastrin, respectively.

Acetylcholine also inhibits somatostatin release by inhibiting ECL.

- Following a meal, G cells are also stimulated to release gastrin, which interacts with receptors located on ECL cells and parietal cells to cause the release of histamine somatostatin from D cells decreases histamine release and gastrin release from ECL cells and G cells, respectively. In addition, somatostatin inhibits parietal cell acid secretion (not shown). The principal stimulus for activation of D cells is **antral luminal acidification** (not shown).
- As depicted, somatostatin exerts inhibitory actions on gastric acid secretion.
- Release of **somatostatin from antral D cells** is stimulated in the presence of intraluminal acid to a pH of 3 or less.
- After its release, somatostatin inhibits gastrin release through paracrine effects and also modifies histamine release from ECL cells.
- In some patients with peptic ulcer disease (PUD), this negative feedback response is defective.
- Consequently, the precise state of acid secretion by the parietal cell is dependent on the overall influence of the positive and negative stimuli (Fig. 41.4).

Functions of Gastric Acid

Key Box 41.3 describes the functions of gastric acid.

Gastric Emptying

Vagus not only increases secretion but also increases motility of the stomach. Vagotomy produces decreased gastric motility. Decreased gastric motility or atony is

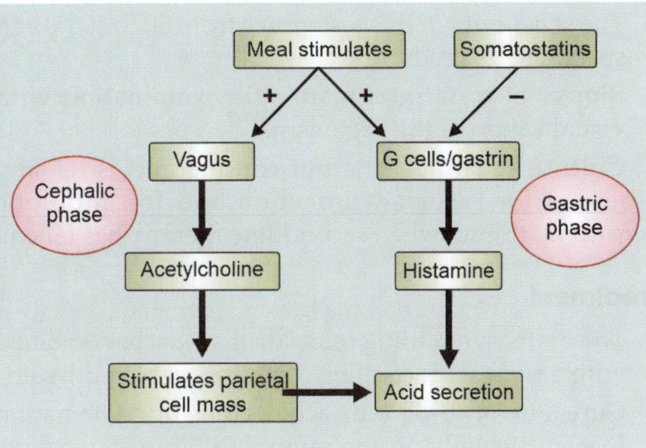

Fig. 41.4: Physiology of acid secretion

Key Box 41.3

Functions of Gastric Acid

- Gastric acid plays a critical role in the digestion of a meal.
- It is required to convert pepsinogen into pepsin, which is necessary for hydrolysis of proteins into polypeptides.
- Gastric acid also elicits the release of secretin from the duodenum, which results in pancreatic bicarbonate secretion.
- In addition, gastric acid functions to limit colonisation of the upper GI tract with bacteria.

called gastroparesis. It can be seen in patients who are taking narcotic drugs, severe anorexia, diabetes, etc. Following Whipple's pancreaticoduodenectomy, gastric motility is also affected. erythromycin helps in gastric emptying. Refer Key Box 41.4 for other details.

Key Box 41.4

Promotility Agents that Accelerate Gastric Emptying

Drug	Mechanism
Metoclopramide	Dopamine antagonist
Domperidone	Dopamine antagonist
Erythromycin	Motilin agonist
Bethanechol	Cholinergic agonist
Neostigmine	Cholinergic agonist

HELICOBACTER PYLORI INFECTION

- It is now established that 90% of duodenal ulcers and 75% of gastric ulcers are associated with *H. pylori* infection.
- **Warren and Marshall** were the first to identify and isolate the organism, originally referred to as ***Campylobacter pyloridis.***
- The organism is a **spiral or helical gram-negative rod** with **4 to 6 flagella** and resides in gastric-type epithelium within or beneath the mucus layer, which protects it from both acid and antibiotics.
- Its shape and flagella aid its movement through the mucus layer, and it produces a variety of enzymes that help it adapt to a hostile environment.
- Most notably, it is one of **the most potent producers of urease among any bacteria yet described.**
- This enzyme is capable of **splitting urea into ammonia and bicarbonate,** creating an alkaline microenvironment in the setting of an acidic gastric milieu, which facilitates establishing a diagnosis of this organism by various laboratory tests.

- The organism is microaerophilic, and the optimal temperature for isolation is 35 to 37°C, with growth occurring after 2 to 5 days.
- Interestingly, *H. pylori* **can only live in gastric epithelium** because only gastric epithelium expresses specific adherence receptors *in vivo* that can be recognized by the organism. Thus, it can also be found in **heterotopic gastric mucosa in proximal oesophagus** and **Barrett's oesophagus,** in gastric metaplasia in the duodenum and Meckel's diverticulum, and in heterotopic gastric mucosa in the rectum.
- **The mechanism responsible for *H. pylori*-induced GI injury** are not very clear but three potential mechanisms have been proposed:
  1. Production of toxic products to cause local tissue injury
  2. Induction of a local mucosal immune response
  3. Increased gastrin levels with a resultant increase in acid secretion.

Locally Produced Toxic Mediators

1. Urease activity, i.e. ammonia
2. Cytotoxins
3. Mucinase that degrades mucus and glycoproteins.
4. Phospholipases that damage epithelial cells and mucus cells.
5. Platelet-activating factor, which is known to cause mucosal injury.

Mediators of *Helicobacter Pylori*-induced Injury (Key Box 41.5)

- Most *H. pylori* strains express—**vacuolating cytotoxin.**
- **The VacA exotoxin** causes the release of cytochrome c from mitochondria and induces apoptosis.
- *H. pylori* infection is accompanied by an **abnormal T cell response** which may be partially responsible for the long-term persistence of *H. pylori* infection.

Diagnosis (Table 41.3)

H. pylori infection can be diagnosed by both noninvasive and invasive means.

I. Non-Invasive Methods

- They are **urea breath test, serology, and detection of antigen in stool samples**.
- The urea breath test is based on production of urease by *H. pylori* in the gastric mucosa.
- ^{14}C-labelled urea is ingested and ^{14}C-labelled CO_2 is produced and excreted in the breath.
- This test has a sensitivity and specificity of greater than 90% and indicates ongoing infection.

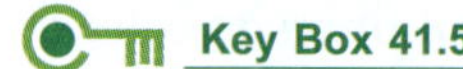

Key Box 41.5

Mechanism of *Helicobacter Pylori*-induced Injury—Summary

Helical gram-negative rod

Enzyme produced is urease, which splits urea. Resulting bicarbonate creates alkaline environment. Another enzyme mucinase degrades mucus.

Lives only in gastric epithelium

Injury is due to:
- Toxins such as **vacuolating cytotoxin**
- Increased gastrin levels
- Phospholipases
- Platelet-activating factor
- Increased immunoglobulin response (host response)

Cytotoxins

Other factors
- Local tissue injury
- Local ischaemia

Remember as **HELICO**

- The urea breath test is useful for initial diagnosis of infection and for follow-up after eradication therapy.

II. Invasive Methods

- The patient should undergo endoscopic diagnosis and it is indicated in following situations.
  - Individuals more than 50 years of age
  - Those with significant symptoms including gastrointestinal bleeding
  - Anaemia
  - Weight loss.
- During endoscopy, antral biopsies can be obtained and the organism cultured in agar containing both urea and a pH-sensitive colorimetric agent.
- *H. pylori* hydrolysis of urea causes a diagnostic change in colour.
- The sensitivity of this test varies from 80 to 100% and specificity exceeds 90%.
- Biopsy also permits histologic examination with visualisation of the organism.

Culture of *H. pylori* is not routine and is usually reserved for recurrent infection and for antibiotic sensitivity testing when second-line therapy has failed.

Treatment

- To be effective, antimicrobial drugs must be combined with gastric acid secretion inhibitors or bismuth salts.
- Cure rates of 80–85% are achieved using combination therapy, usually proton pump inhibitors, ranitidine, or bismuth citrate with two antibiotics.

Table 41.3 Test for *Helicobacter pylori*

Test	Indication	Advantages	Disadvantages
1. **Serologic test**	When the patient has not received treatment for *H. pylori* infection, test of choice is serological test	Non-invasive; sensitivity of >80%, specificity of about 90%	Does not confirm eradication, because serologic positivity remains for indefinite period after microbiologic cure
2. **Urea breath test:** Based on ability to hydrolyse urea	This test is to confirm cure of *H. pylori* infection, but no sooner than 4 weeks after completion of therapy	Simple; sensitivity and specificity of 90 to 99%	False-negatives possible, if testing is done too soon after treatment for *H. pylori* infection. Small radiation exposure with 14C method, cost and availability are disadvantages
3. **Histologic test** is done by staining with silver, Giemsa, etc.	Presence of *H. pylori* in biopsy material taken during endoscopy establishes the diagnosis	Sensitivity of 80 to 100%, specificity of >95%; Giemsa stain has sensitivity of >95% and specificity of 99%	Requires laboratory facilities and experience; when haematoxylin-eosin stain is nondiagnostic, other stains have to be used
4. **Rapid urease test**	Simplest method. However, endoscopy is required	Simple; rapid (once biopsy specimen has been obtained); sensitivity of 80 to 95%, specificity of 95 to 100%	Invasive; false-negatives possible, if testing is done too soon after treatment with proton pump inhibitors, antimicrobials or bismuth compounds
5. **Culture** (not routinely done)	When antimicrobial resistance is suspected after many drug failures	Allows determination of antibiotic susceptibility. Sensitivity is 80% and specificity is 100%	Time-consuming; expensive; usually not necessary unless resistance is suspected

- The most common antibiotics used are **clarithromycin, amoxicillin, and metronidazole or tinidazole.**
- Metronidazole has been a mainstay of *H. pylori* treatment.
- Eradication therapy with a proton pump inhibitor, metronidazole, and amoxicillin decreases the prevalence of metronidazole-resistant *H. pylori* strains.

Different Regimens

Bismuth triple therapy

Bismuth, 2 tablets four times daily + Metronidazole, 250 mg three times daily + Tetracycline, 500 mg four times daily.

PPI triple therapy

PPI twice daily + Amoxicillin, 1000 mg two times daily + Clarithromycin, 500 mg two times daily or metronidazole, 500 mg two times daily.

Quadruple therapy

PPI twice daily + Bismuth, 2 tablets four times daily + Metronidazole, 250 mg three times daily + Tetracycline, 500 mg four times daily.

Complications of *Helicobacter Pylori* Infection

1. Chronic duodenal ulcer
2. Gastric carcinoma
3. Gastro-oesophageal reflux disease
4. Barrett's oesophagus
5. Chronic gastritis
6. Gastric maltoma
7. Oesophageal cancer
8. Idiopathic thrombocytopenic purpura.

GASTRITIS

- Various forms of gastritis have been depicted in Table 41.4.
- Type B gastritis and erosive gastritis are common.
- Endoscopy and biopsy are the key investigations in all forms of gastritis.
- The treatment depends upon the type of gastritis.
- Rarer forms of gastritis include granulomatous gastritis, lymphocytic gastritis, etc.

NONULCERATIVE DYSPEPSIA

- Dyspepsia is characterised by symptoms related to upper abdominal viscera. Symptoms may include abdominal pain, bloating, indigestion, nausea and heart burn. Heart burn as a single symptom suggests gastro-oesophageal reflux disease and excludes the diagnosis of dyspepsia.
- Nonulcerative dyspepsia is considered when no anatomic or biochemical abnormality is discovered to explain the patient's symptoms.

Table 41.4 Gastritis

Type A	Type B	Reflux	Erosive
• Autoimmune—antibodies to parietal cell	• *H. pylori* associated	• After cholecystectomy, gastric surgery	• It occurs due to NSAID
• Fundus and body are affected	• Antrum is affected	• Antrum is affected	• It affects entire stomach
• Atrophy of parietal cell mass. Hence, hypochlorhydria and decreased intrinsic factor	• Predisposes to peptic ulcer disease	• Usually does not give rise to peptic ulcer disease	• It occurs due to defective gastric mucosal barrier
• Hypochlorhydria stimulates antral gastrin. Predisposes to development of gastric cancer	• Can give rise to intestinal metaplasia, dysplasia and predisposes to development of gastric cancer	• Treated by prokinetic agents or bile chelating agents	• Treated by H_2 blockers or proton pump inhibitors

- After *H. pylori* infection, ingestion of nonsteroidal anti-inflammatory drugs (NSAIDs) is the most common cause of nonulcerative dyspepsia and PUD.
- *H. pylori* infection is always associated with histologic gastritis which is absent in cases of nonulcerative dyspepsia.
- Hence *H. pylori* eradication therapy is not recommended in the treatment of nonulcerative dyspepsia.
- For surgeons, the importance of nonulcerative dyspepsia relates to its place in the differential diagnosis of epigastric pain. There is no role for surgery in the treatment of this disorder.
- Some of these patients, who have been diagnosed as nonulcerative dyspepsia, may have gallstones or oesophageal reflux disease. Hence, abdominal ultrasound and oesophageal manometry are required to rule out these diseases.
- Before we start discussion on peptic ulcer disease, we will discuss nonulcerative dyspepsia (commonly mistaken as peptic ulcer disease) and Zollinger-Ellison syndrome which is one of the rare causes of peptic ulceration. Oesophagogastroduodenoscopy should be done in all the patients with nonulcerative dyspepsia followed by biopsy from stomach to rule out *H. pylori* infection. One important cause of peptic ulcer disease—Zollinger-Ellison syndrome is being discussed first.

ZOLLINGER-ELLISON SYNDROME

Introduction

- Zollinger-Ellison syndrome (ZES) is a **clinical triad consisting of gastric acid hypersecretion, severe PUD, and non-islet cell tumours of the pancreas.**
- The tumours are known to produce gastrin and are referred to as gastrinomas (Fig. 41.5).
- These tumours are usually localised to the head of the pancreas, duodenal wall or regional lymph nodes. The majority (90%) of gastrinomas are thought to arise in gastrinoma triangle, also known as Passaro's triangle.
- About one-half of these gastric tumours are multiple and two-thirds are malignant.

Association with MEN

About one-fourth are associated with **multiple endocrine neoplasia syndrome (MEN 1)**. Other tumours in MEN 1 are pituitary adenoma and parathyroid adenoma.

Pathophysiology

Pathophysiologic features of ZES that distinguish it from duodenal ulcer are present and are all explained either by the actions of **gastrin to stimulate gastric acid secretion** and **mucosal growth** or by the action of other associated hormones in the MEN 1 syndrome.

Clinical Features

- Abdominal pain and PUD are the hallmarks of the syndrome and typically occur in more than 80% of patients.
- About one-half of patients have diarrhoea secondary to increased gastric acid secretion.

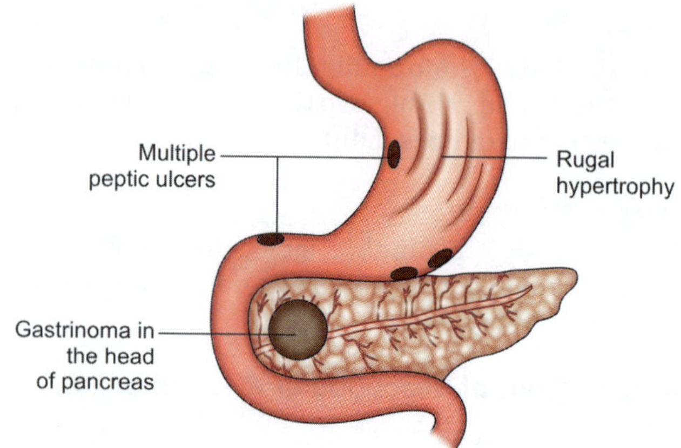

Fig. 41.5: Pictorial representation of gastrinoma (refer to page 645 also)

- Weight loss and steatorrhoea also occur secondary to decreased duodenal and jejunal pH and inactivation of lipase.
- Oesophagitis from gastro-oesophageal reflux is also common.

Investigations

I. Endoscopy

- **Demonstrates prominent gastric rugal folds, reflecting the trophic effect of hypergastrinaemia on the gastric fundus in addition to evidence of PUD.**
- Gastrinoma and ZES are always considered and ruled out in patients who have:
  1. Recurrent or intractable PUD despite eradication of *H. pylori* and appropriate antisecretory therapy.
  2. Multiple or atypically located ulcers.
  3. PUD associated with significant diarrhoea.
  4. PUD associated with symptoms of MEN 1 such as hyperparathyroidism or kindred of MEN 1.
  5. Large gastric rugae on endoscopy.
  6. **In those patients with other pancreatic endocrine tumours.**
  7. Patients undergoing elective surgical intervention for PUD have the possibility of gastrinoma included in their preoperative evaluation.

II. Serum Gastrin Levels

Most patients with gastrinoma have **elevated fasting levels (>200 pg/ml), and values greater than 1000 pg/ml may be diagnostic.**

III. The Secretin Test

- It is the most sensitive and specific provocative test for gastrinoma and aids in the differentiation between gastrinomas and other causes of ulcerogenic hypergastrinaemia.
- Secretin (2 mg/kg) is administered intravenously and serum gastrin samples are measured before and after secretin administration at 5-minute interval for 30 minutes.
- An increase in serum gastrin of greater than 200 pg/ml above basal levels is specific for gastrinoma.

Treatment

- Acid suppression therapy with a proton pump inhibitor.
- Localisation of the gastrinoma is performed before operative intervention is made.
- **Noninvasive methods** include computed tomography (CT) scanning, MRI, endoscopic ultrasound, and ^{111}In-octreotide scintigraphy (somatostatin receptor imaging).
- In patients with **resectable gastrinomas**, surgical resection is performed that includes tumour resection from the duodenum, pancreas and regional lymph nodes.
- **Total gastrectomy is rarely indicated** and is reserved for patients who are noncompliant with acid suppression therapy or when the tumour cannot be localised.

Competency

SU28.9: Describe and discuss the aetiology, the clinical features, investigations and principles of management of peptic ulcer disease.

PEPTIC ULCER DISEASE

Definition

Acid peptic digestion of the alimentary mucosa resulting in an ulcer is called peptic ulcer disease (PUD). The corrosive effects of acid with proteolytic effect of pepsin are responsible for PUD. Duodenum and stomach are the common sites of peptic ulcer disease. Rarely, they can occur in the jejunum and in Meckel's diverticulum when it contains ectopic gastric mucosa.

Types of Peptic Ulcer

I. Depending on the Site

A. **Chronic duodenal ulcer:** Typically occurs in the first inch of the first part of the duodenum.

B. **Chronic gastric ulcer:** Occurs in the lesser curvature adjacent to acid secreting parietal cell mass.

C. **Combined:** Gastric ulcer type II—Zollinger-Ellison syndrome

D. **Anastomotic ulcer**

II. Depending on the Duration

A. Chronic peptic ulcer, and B. Acute peptic ulcer.

CHRONIC DUODENAL ULCER (CDU)

Hyperacidity is the chief cause of duodenal ulcer. **No acid, no ulcer** still holds good for CDU.

1. **Neurological causes:** Stimulation of vagus increases secretion of acids. This is brought about by **anxiety, worry, hurry and curry**.
2. **Nonsteroidal anti-inflammatory drugs:** They are responsible for gastric ulcer rather than duodenal ulcer by altering mucosal defence.
3. **Genetic causes:** Family history of duodenal ulcer may be present in a few cases which suggests a genetic cause. Patients with blood group **'O'** are more prone, for the development of CDU because of **increased parietal cell population.**

4. **Food habits:** Spicy food, diet poor in vitamins, smoking and alcohol, alone or in combination precipitate the development of chronic duodenal ulcer.
5. **Bacteriological causes** (Fig. 41.6): ***Helicobacter pylori***, a spirochaetal bacterium, has been demonstrated in the submucosa of the antrum and duodenum, from the biopsies of the ulcer. **It increases pH levels by splitting urea and releasing ammonia.** Rise in pH results in proliferation of bacteria. This is the most important cause of chronic duodenal ulcer today.
6. **Endocrinal causes**
   - Zollinger-Ellison syndrome is a non-β cell tumour of the pancreas with hypergastrinaemia.
   - Hyperparathyroidism causes increased levels of calcium which stimulates the parietal cell mass resulting in hyperacidity.

Pathophysiology of Duodenal Ulcer

- Duodenal ulcer is a disease of multiple aetiologies.
- The only absolute requirements are acid and pepsin secretion in combination with either infection with *H. pylori* or ingestion of NSAIDs.
- **Duodenal ulcer patients have an increase in mean parietal cell number thus they secrete more acid,** whereas gastric ulcer patients do not have.

CHRONIC GASTRIC ULCER

- In majority of the patients, there is no **hyperacidity**. Many patients have hypoacidity, or normoacidity.
- Ulcer occurs due to a defective gastric mucosal barrier. This barrier is a coat of thick mucus which is impermeable to pepsin (Key Box 41.6).

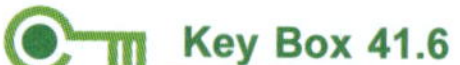

Key Box 41.6

Some Conditions that may Predispose to Gastric Ulceration

- Age older than 40, sex (female to male ratio of 2:1)
- Ingestion of barrier-breaking drugs such as aspirin or nonsteroidal anti-inflammatory drugs (NSAIDs)
- Abnormalities in acid and pepsin secretion
- Gastric stasis through delayed gastric emptying
- Coexisting duodenal ulcer
- Duodenal gastric reflux of bile
- Gastritis, and infection with *H. pylori*
- Chronic alcohol intake, smoking
- Long-term corticosteroid therapy
- Intra-arterial chemotherapy

- Prostaglandins, normally present in the gastric mucosa, do not allow back diffusion of hydrogen ions from the lumen.
- Nonsteroidal anti-inflammatory drugs inhibit the production of prostaglandins causing a loss of protective activity.
- This can also be damaged by smoking, spicy food, alcohol and reflux of bile into the stomach.

Classification (Johnson) Types of Chronic Gastric Ulcer (Figs 41.7 to 41.11)

I. Acute Superficial: Single or Multiple (Erosions)

II. Chronic

Type 1: Primary gastric ulcer on the lesser curvature in the antrum near the junction of oxyntic cells and central mucosa.

Type 2: Gastric ulcer with duodenal ulcer.

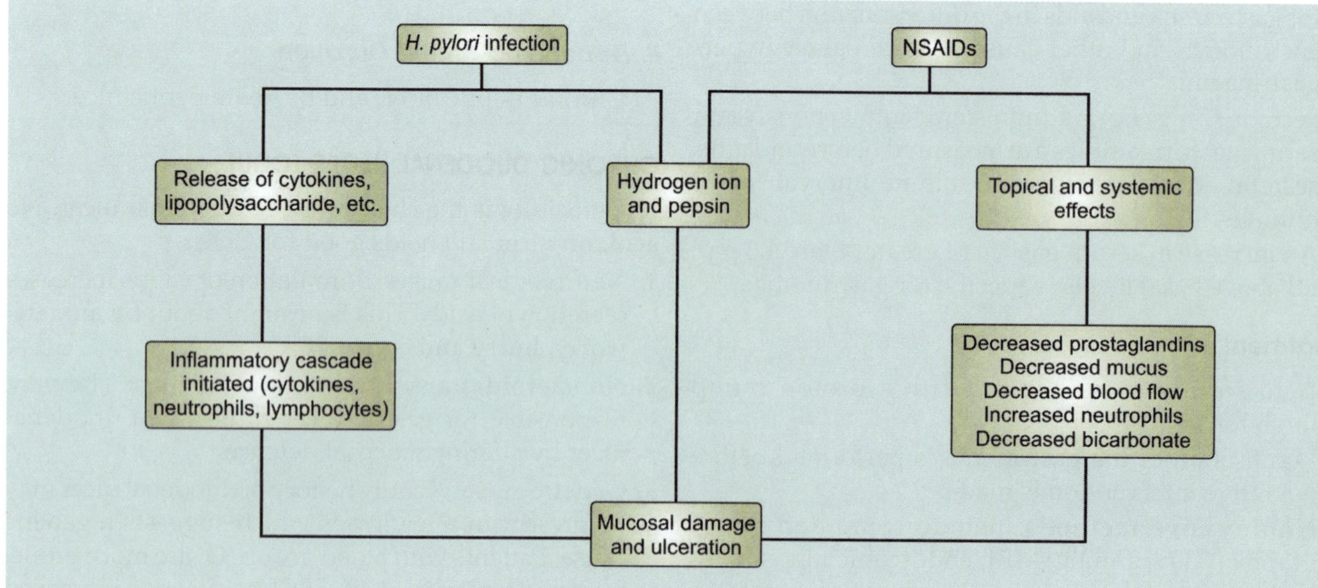

Fig. 41.6: Peptic ulceration

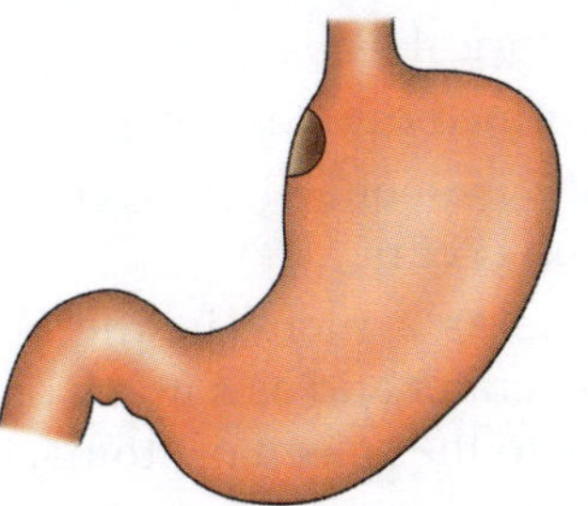
Fig. 41.7: Gastric ulcer—Type 1

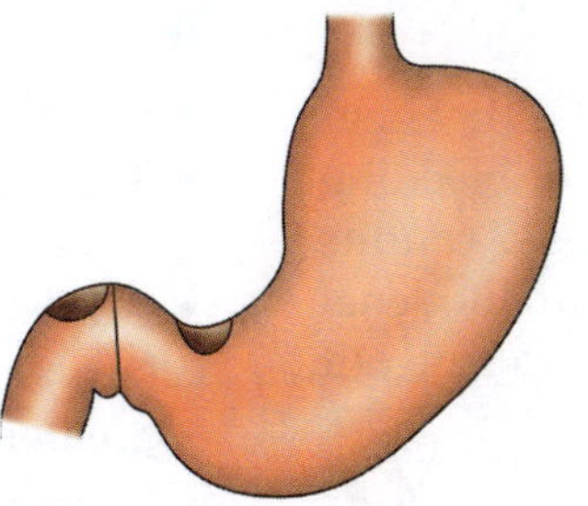
Fig. 41.8: Gastric ulcer—Type 2

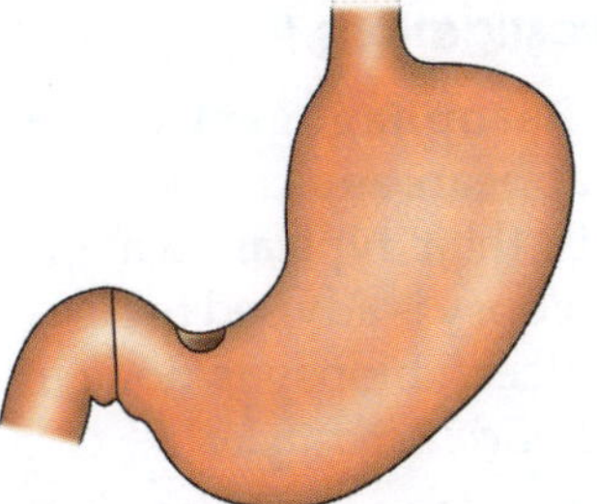
Fig. 41.9: Gastric ulcer—Type 3

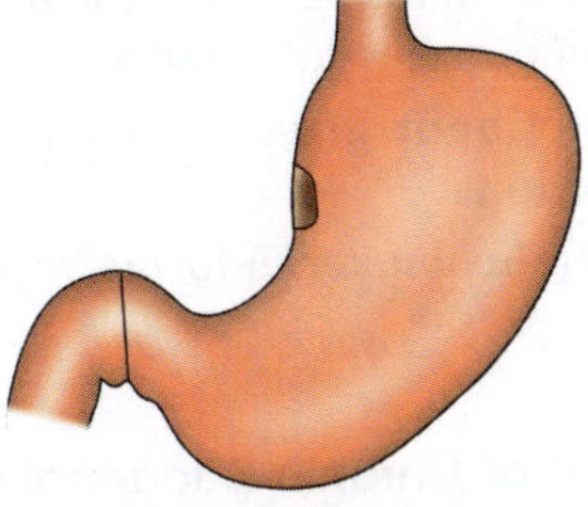
Fig. 41.10: Gastric ulcer—Type 4

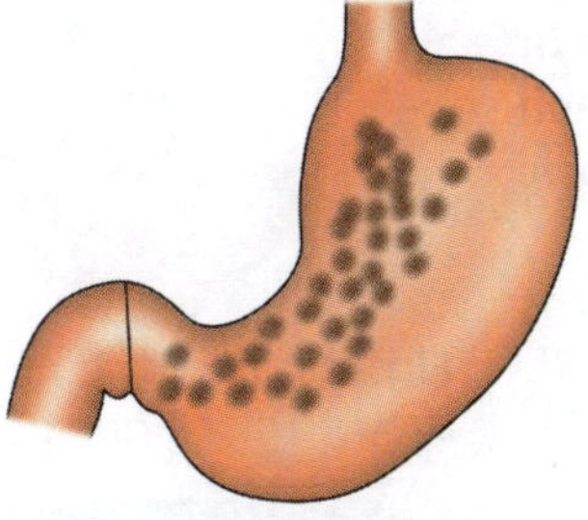
Fig. 41.11: NSAID-induced gastric ulcer—Type 5

Type 3: Prepyloric or channel ulcer.

Type 4: High gastric ulcer (cardia, proximal stomach) <2 cm from gastro-oesophageal junction.

Type 5: NSAID-induced gastric ulcers.

Pearls of Wisdom

Types 2, and 3 gastric ulcers are to be treated like duodenal ulcer because they are associated with hyperacidity.

Giant gastric ulcers: These are important because they are more prone for perforation and malignancy. Incidence may vary from 10 to 20 cm. **Refer Key Box 41.7.**

Key Box 41.7

Giant Gastric Ulcer

- Diameter >2 cm
- Typically, lesser curvature at incisura angularis
- Incidence of malignancy—10%
- High chances of perforation and bleeding
- Medical treatment heals majority of cases (80%)
- Re-endoscopy biopsy is a must to look for healing and also to rule out malignancy
- Gastrectomy including ulcer bed. Add vagotomy for type 2 and type 3 gastric ulcers

Clinical Features (Table 41.5)

Table 41.5 Classification of clinical features

	Chronic duodenal ulcer	Chronic gastric ulcer
1. Incidence	Common	Less common
2. Site	1st inch of 1st part of duodenum	The lesser curvature or prepyloric region
3. Pain	It is due to the acid irritating the ulcer (hunger pain). It is relieved on taking food. After 1–2 hours of food, the pain becomes severe. It is burning in nature with retrosternal radiation (heartburn) and increased salivation (water brash)	Pain occurs on taking food and it is relieved by induced vomiting. Pain is of burning nature as in duodenal ulcer
4. Vomiting	Never occurs in duodenal ulcer till the patient develops pyloric stenosis	Frequent and it occurs immediately after patient takes food
5. Weight	Weight gain	Weight loss
6. Periodicity	Common	Less
7. Haematemesis and melaena ratio	40:60	60:40
8. Incidence of malignancy	Never becomes malignant	0.5–5% (2%)
9. On examination	Tenderness in the right hypochondrium	Tenderness in the epigastrium

Investigations (Figs 41.12 to 41.21)

1. **Oesophagogastroduodenoscopy (OGD):** Ulcer appears as a crater with/without slough or bleeding in their typical locations. In gastric ulcers, routine biopsy is advised to rule out malignancy. In duodenal ulcers, biopsy is done in recurrent cases to rule out *Helicobacter pylori*.
   - In long-standing duodenal ulcers, there may be narrowing of the pylorus, with stasis of food in the stomach suggestive of pyloric stenosis.
   - Other uses of OGD is given in Key Box 41.8.

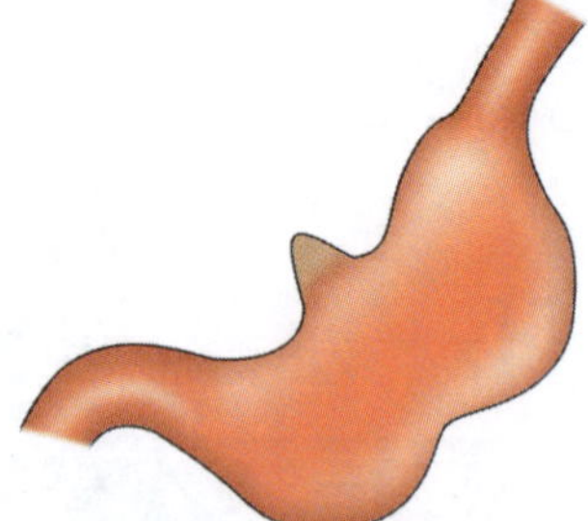

Fig. 41.12: Barium study showing niche and notch

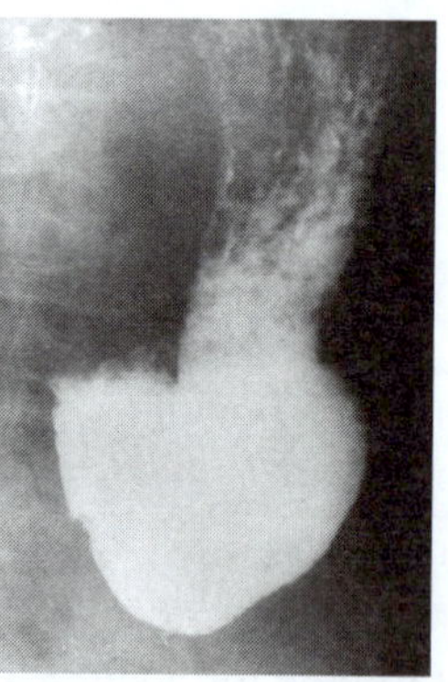

Fig. 41.13: Gastric outlet obstruction. Barium meal can detect dilated stomach

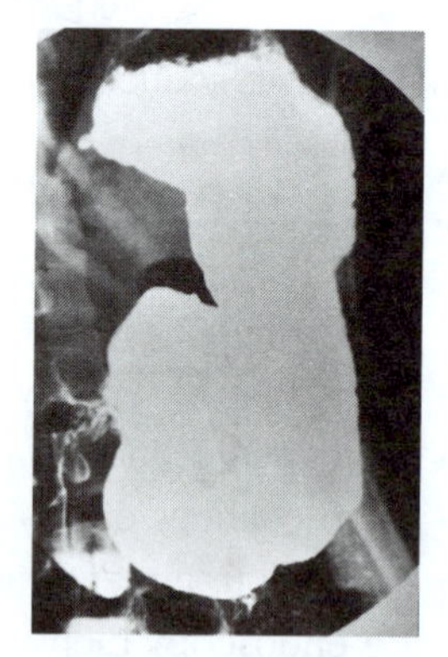

Fig. 41.14: Hugely dilated J-shaped stomach

Key Box 41.8

Oesophagogastroduodenoscopy(OGD)

Diagnostic (Figs 41.14 to 41.20)
- Peptic ulcers—acute and chronic
- Gastritis
- Carcinoma stomach
- Oesophageal varices, ulcers, oesophagitis
- Biopsy to rule out *H. pylori* infection
- Brush cytology and biology, yield is better

Therapeutic
- Injection of adrenaline into the bleeding vessel
- Variceal injection
- Snaring of polyps
- Electrocoagulation of bleeders
- Endoscopic cystogastrostomy
- Foreign body removal
- Percutaneous endoscopic gastrostomy (PEG)
- Endoscopic mucosal resection for early carcinoma stomach

2. **Barium meal study** (historical—obsolete now)
   - **Duodenal ulcer:** Deformed duodenal cap.
   - **Trifoliate deformity** is seen when secondary duodenal diverticulum occurs.
   - **Gastric ulcer** appears as a niche in the lesser curvature due to ulcer crater and as a notch on the greater curvature due to the spasm of stomach.
   - In general, benign ulcers are smoother, more regular, with rounded edges and a flat, smooth ulcer base. In malignancy, the mass protrudes into the lumen or has folds surrounding ulcer crater.
   - To detect **hour glass stomach** and **gastric outlet obstruction**.
3. **Test for *Helicobacter pylori*** (already discussed).

Treatment

A. Treatment of Chronic Duodenal Ulcer (CDU)

Aim is to decrease the pain because of its severity (by reducing acidity) and to prevent relapses (Key Box 41.9).

Key Box 41.9

Aims of the Treatment
- To relieve symptoms
- To heal the ulcer
- To prevent recurrence
- To prevent complications

I. Medical Line of Management

- **Pantoprazole in a dose of 40 mg/day for 4 weeks has become the first line of treatment for chronic duodenal ulcer.** Other drugs are esomeprazole: 40 mg/day, lansoprazole: 30 mg/day,
- Lifestyle modification: Stop smoking, decrease alcohol, avoid spicy food, minimize coffee.
- Discontinue aspirin or NSAIDs and other gastric irritants.
- **Eradication therapy if biopsy is proved for helicobacter pylori.**

II. Surgical Line of Management

Surgery: Indications for surgery is given in Key Box 41.10.

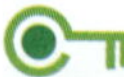 **Key Box 41.10**

Indications for Surgery
1. Frequent relapses, *H. pylori* negative
2. Complications of duodenal ulcer:
   - Gastric outlet obstruction
   - Haemorrhage

ENDOSCOPIC PICTURES

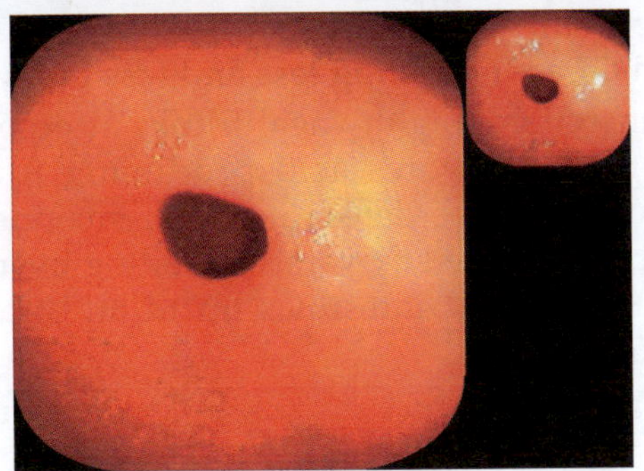
Fig. 41.15: Normal pyloric opening

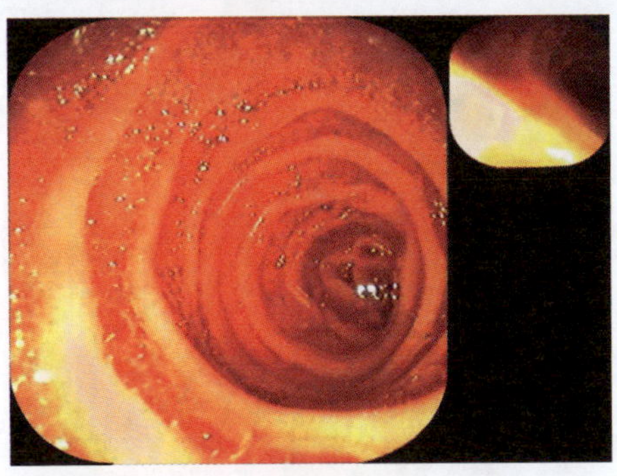
Fig. 41.16: Normal 2nd part duodenum

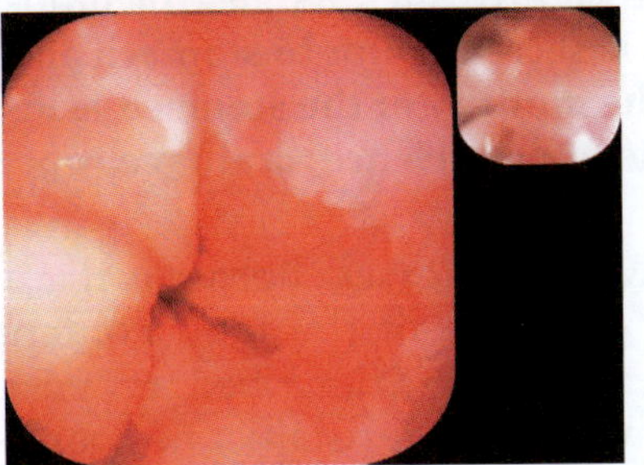
Fig. 41.17: Normal squamocolumnar junction—Z line

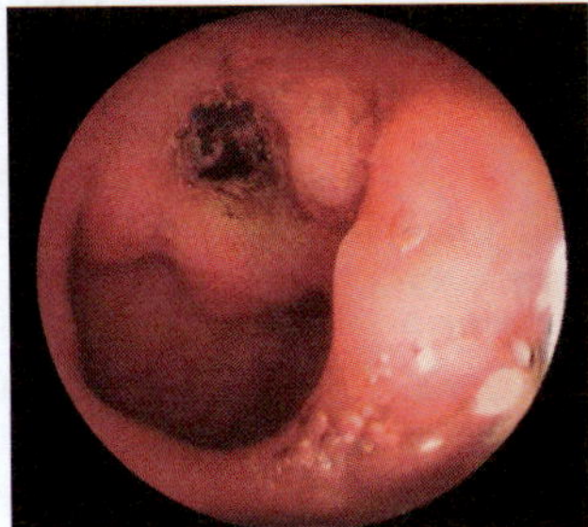
Fig. 41.18: OGD showing bleeding duodenal ulcer

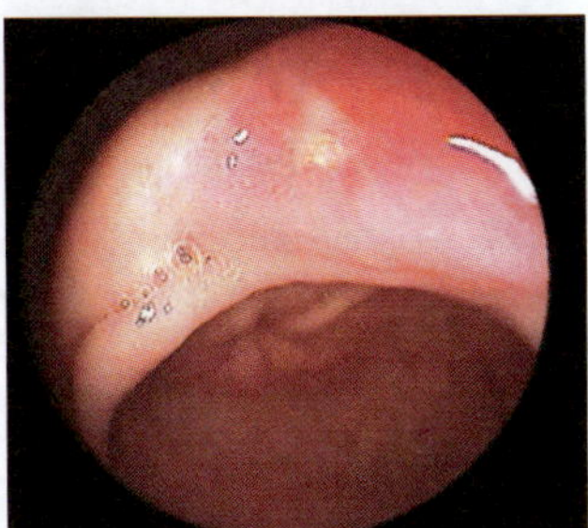
Fig. 41.19: OGD showing chronic gastric ulcer

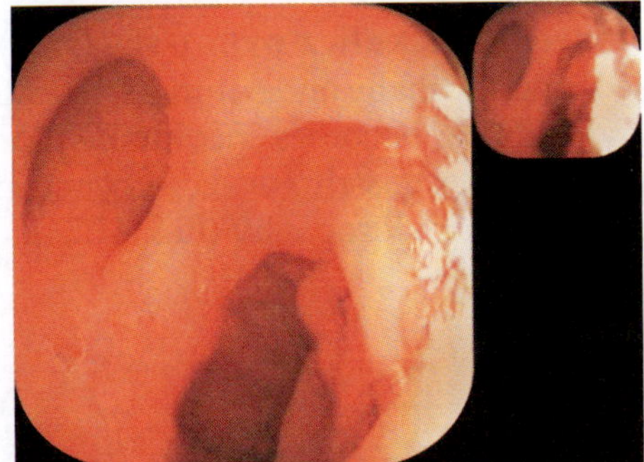
Fig. 41.20: OGD showing bleeding duodenal ulcer and diverticulum due to ulcer

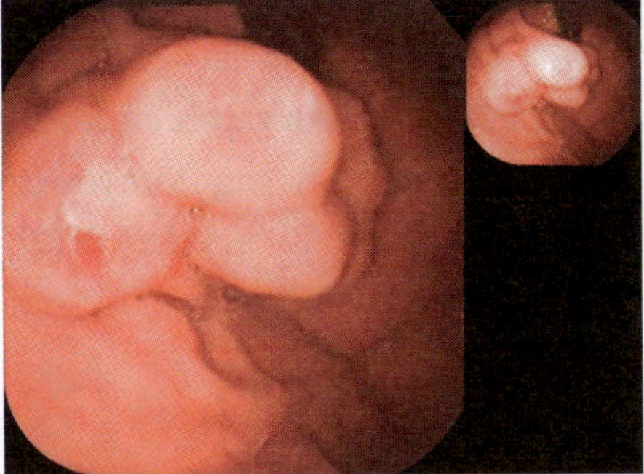
Fig. 41.21: Large gastric varices—this patient also had duodenal ulcer

(*Courtesy:* Prof Ganesh Pai, Head of the Department, Gastroenterology, KMC, Manipal)

1. **Highly selective vagotomy (HSV):** It is also called PCV (parietal cell vagotomy) or PGV (proximal gastric vagotomy) (Fig. 41.22).
   - In this operation, **vagi are not divided at the trunks**. Both anterior and posterior vagi are identified, isolated and preserved. Their branches which run along the lesser curvature are isolated. They are anterior and posterior greater gastric nerves of Latarjet. The branches of the nerves of Latarjet supplying parietal cell mass are divided. Hence, it is called parietal cell vagotomy. The terminal fibres of the nerve of Latarjet which supply pylorus are preserved (5–7 cm of 'Crow foot').

Advantages of HSV

1. More physiological, with **minimal disturbances.**
2. No drainage procedure is required because pyloric functions are preserved.
3. Nerve supply to gallbladder and liver is not disturbed.
4. No diarrhoea as that can occur in 5–8% of cases of truncal vagotomy which can be morbid.

Pearls of Wisdom

It is important to note that experience of many surgeons today with HSV is 'minimum'. Hence, it is safe to do 'vagotomy and gastrojejunostomy (GJ)'.

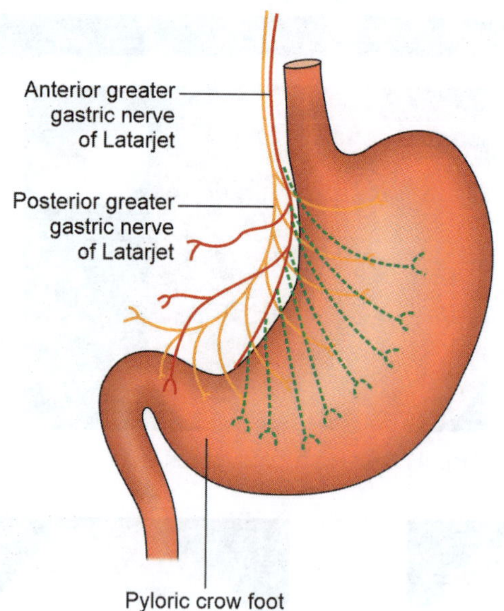

Fig. 41.22: Highly selective vagotomy—pyloric crow foot is preserved. Hence, drainage procedure is not required

Disadvantages of HSV

- This is not the procedure for prepyloric ulcer as there is a high recurrence rate.
- Complicated procedure—needs an experienced surgeon.
- Recurrence rate: 10–15%
- Rare chance of lesser curvature necrosis.

2. **Total truncal abdominal vagotomy with gastrojejunostomy of Mayo** (Fig. 41.23) **or pyloroplasty**

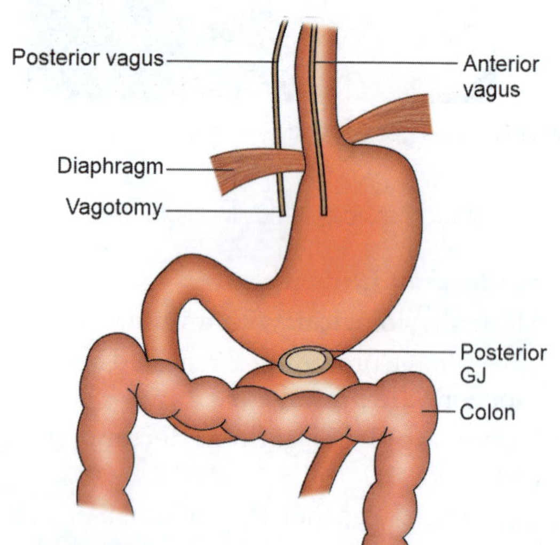

Fig. 41.23: Posterior GJ **(Mayo)**[1] with vagotomy—motility of the stomach is lost after vagotomy. Hence, drainage procedure (GJ in this picture) is required (vagus is secretomotor of the stomach)

- This is the most popular and most commonly done operation for peptic ulcer disease. However, it is important to realise that **indications for vagotomy and GJ are becoming less and less today**.
- Transection of both vagal trunks at oesophageal hiatus denervates acid producing fundus of stomach. It also denervates the remainder of the viscera supplied by vagus including liver, biliary tree, pancreas, intestines up to mid-transverse colon.

Procedure

- **Anterior and posterior trunks of the vagus are divided** just below the diaphragm followed by a drainage procedure such as gastrojejunostomy (GJ). **Vagus is secretomotor to stomach and after vagotomy the motility of the stomach is lost and gastric stasis occurs. Hence, drainage procedure is done.**
- Posterior GJ is preferred because it gives a dependent drainage of the food contents by gravity. Classically, it is described as "posterior, vertical, retrocolic, isoperistaltic, no loop (short loop), no tension, GJ of Mayo **(PVRING)**".
- Alternatively, pyloroplasty is preferred by a few surgeons instead of GJ.
- In **Heinecke-Mickulicz pyloroplasty,** pylorus is incised longitudinally and sutured vertically. Thus, the pyloric ring becomes incompetent and wide open. Bile reflux gastritis and diarrhoea are major problems after pyloroplasty (Fig. 41.24).

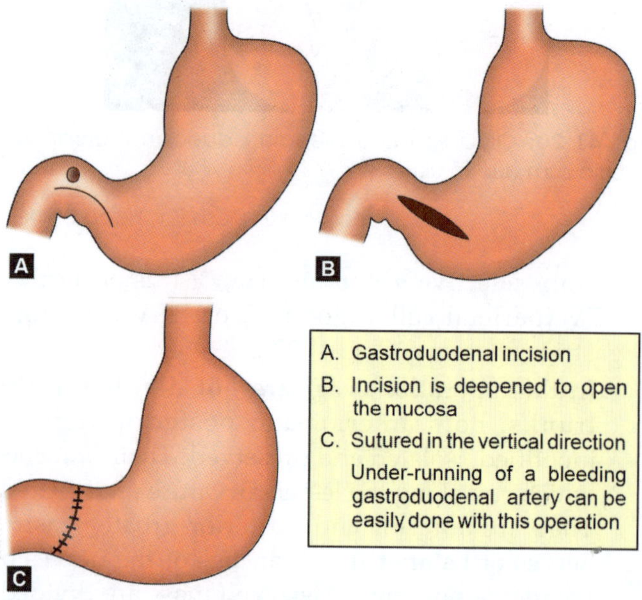

Figs 41.24A to C: Steps of Heinecke-Mickulicz pyloroplasty

[1]About Mayo—Mayo's scissors, Mayo's forceps, Mayo's GJ, Mayo's vein, Mayo's umbilical hernia repair to be remembered.

- **Finney pyloroplasty** is another procedure wherein inverted U-type of incision is given involving distal stomach and duodenum and a gastroduodenal stoma is created. This type of pyloroplasty is indicated when duodenum is dilated (Fig. 41.25).

3. **Vagotomy and antrectomy** (Fig. 41.26): By removing the vagal stimuli and the antral gastrin, the entire stimulus to acid secretion is lost. Hence, it carries the **least recurrence rate (1%)** but carries 3–4% mortality rate. Not done routinely.

B. Treatment of Chronic Gastric Ulcer

- Aim: Healing of the ulcer and relief of symptoms.
- Frequent biopsy is done to rule out malignancy.

I. **Medical line of treatment** can be given for duodenal ulcer, in the form of ranitidine or omeprazole. Cigarette smoking should be stopped. Drugs such as NSAID and aspirin are to be avoided. If an ulcer persists after 6 weeks, the aim is to eradicate *H. pylori* **provided malignancy is ruled out.**

II. **Surgery** is indicated in case of gastric ulcer persisting in spite of medical treatment.

1. **Billroth I partial gastrectomy** (Fig. 41.27): Partial gastrectomy is done including removal of the ulcer followed by gastroduodenal anastomosis. It has the least recurrence rate of less than 1% but mortality rate is around 1–2%.
2. **Billroth II gastrectomy** (Fig. 41.28): It is indicated when the gastric ulcer is located on the lesser curvature. Here the gastrectomy is done below the ulcer and remnant of the stomach is anastomosed to a jejunal loop (gastrojejunal anastomosis). This is also described as Polya gastrectomy.
3. **HSV with excision of the ulcer** can be done, if the experience of surgeon is good.

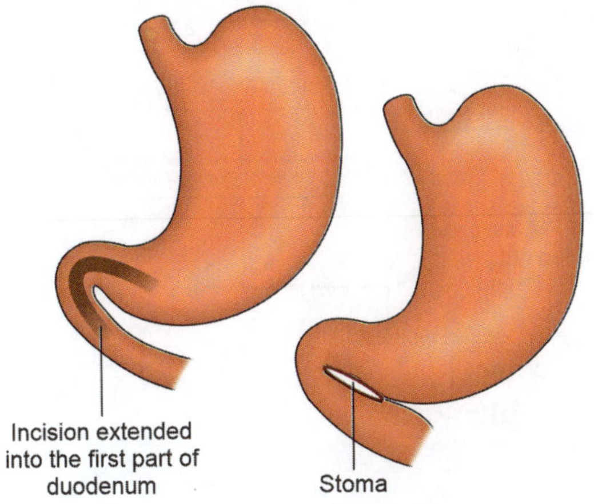

Fig. 41.25: Finney pyloroplasty

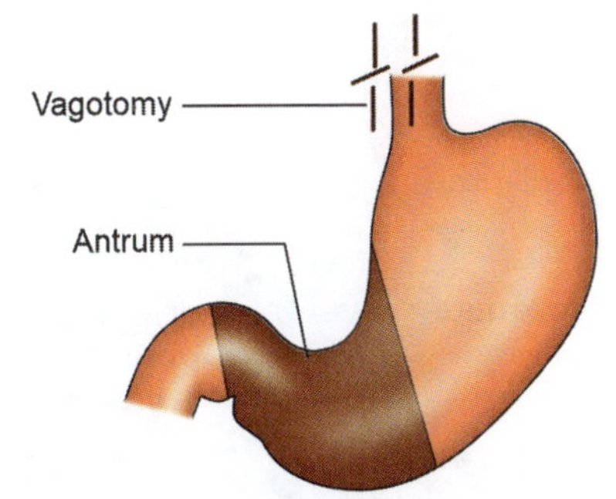

Fig. 41.26: Vagotomy with antrectomy

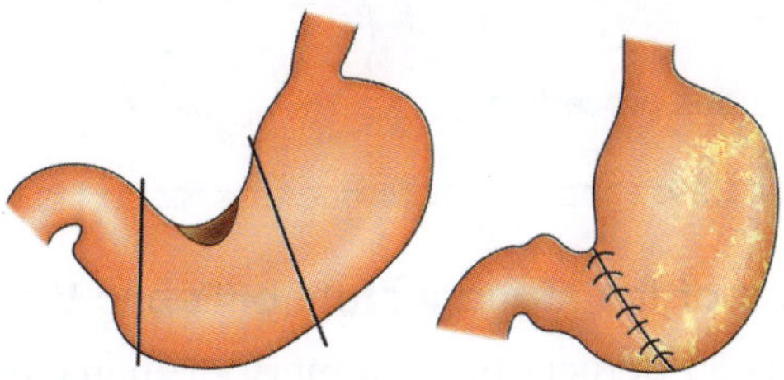

Fig. 41.27: Billroth I gastrectomy followed by gastroduodenal anastomosis

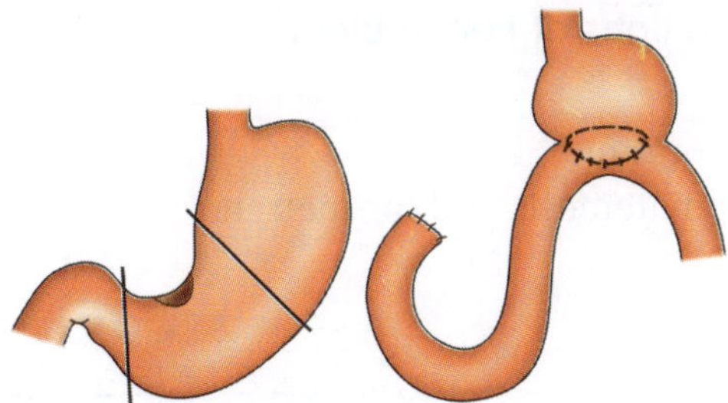

Fig. 41.28: Billroth II gastrectomy followed by gastrojejunal anastomosis

TYPE 4 GASTRIC ULCERS

- The type 4 gastric ulcer presents a difficult management problem.
- The surgical treatment depends on the ulcer size, distance from the GE junction and the degree of surrounding inflammation.
- Whenever possible, the ulcer should be excised.
- The most aggressive approach is to perform a gastrectomy that includes a small portion of the oesophageal wall and the ulcer followed by a Rouxen-Y oesophagogastrojejunostomy to restore intestinal continuity.
- For type 4 gastric ulcers that are located 2 to 5 cm from the gastroesophageal junction, a distal gastrectomy with a vertical extension of the resection to include **the lesser curvature with the ulcer can be performed (i.e. Pauchet procedure).** After resection, bowel continuity is restored with an end-to-end gastroduodenostomy.
- **The Csendes procedure may be useful in stable patients or the Kelling-Madlener operation in unstable ones** (Fig. 41.29).

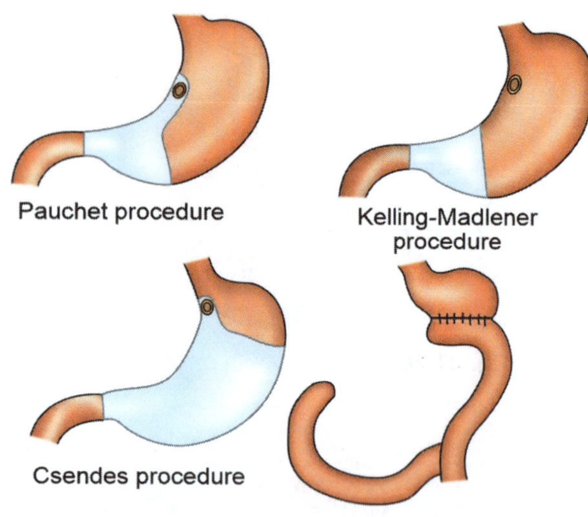

Fig. 41.29: Other types of resections for gastric ulcer

Summary of the Management of Peptic Ulcer

Figure 41.30 depicts the summary of management of peptic ulcer.

Complications of Peptic Ulcer

A. Acute

- Perforation
- Haematemesis and/or melaena

B. Subacute—residual abscess

C. Chronic

- Gastric outlet obstruction (pyloric stenosis)
- Teapot deformity
- Hour glass contracture of the stomach
- Penetration into the pancreas
- Carcinoma of stomach.

ACUTE COMPLICATIONS OF PEPTIC ULCER

PERFORATED PEPTIC ULCER

Introduction

- More common in males. The ratio is 8–10 men to 1 woman in India.
- **Anterior duodenal ulcer perforates and posterior duodenal ulcer bleeds.** An ulcer on the posterior wall of the stomach can perforate into the lesser sac.
- Usually, patients with a **long history of peptic ulcer**, suddenly complain of feeling something that has given way in their abdomen. It may be precipitated by excessive smoking, alcohol, drugs, etc. Rarely a **'silent' ulcer** can also perforate (especially those patients treated with cortisone).

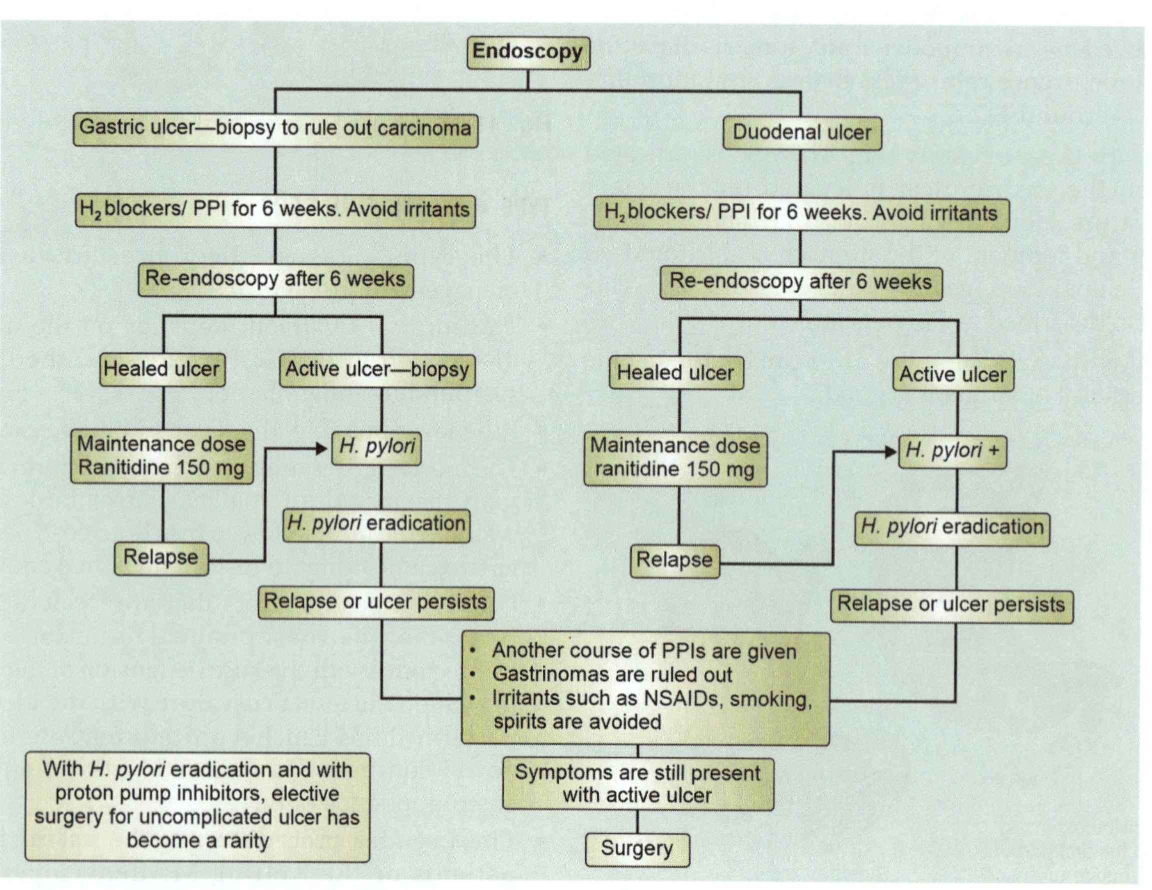

Fig. 41.30: Management of peptic ulcer

- Patients taking NSAIDs (often elderly) can present less dramatically.
- **Two factors** are associated with most perforated peptic ulcers: Chronic use of NSAIDs and *Helicobacter pylori* infection.
- Patients with ***H. pylori* infection** and perforated peptic ulcers tend to be **younger, with a male preponderance** and more prolonged period of dyspepsia. However, NSAIDs category of patients are elderly with equal proportion of both sexes being affected.
- Perforated peptic ulcers have a mortality rate of 5–10%.
- Perforated gastric ulcers in the elderly have 10–20% mortality rate.
- Golden time to operate is within 6 hours.

Stages of Duodenal Ulcer Perforation

1. Stage of Chemical Peritonitis

- Immediately after the perforation, gastric and duodenal contents leak into the peritoneal cavity and produce severe agonising pain in the right hypochondrium. It is mainly HCl which produces pain.
- There may be an episode of coffee-ground vomitus, followed by melaena later.
- The pulse rate increases. The patient is pale and anxious.
- Blood pressure may be normal in the initial few hours.
- *Per* abdomen, there is guarding and rigidity of the abdominal wall.
- Rebound tenderness is present all over the abdomen. This sign is called **Blumberg's sign**.
- On percussion, liver dullness is obliterated because of collection of free air (gas) under the right dome of diaphragm. This stage is seen for about 2–4 hours from the time of perforation.
- Bowel sounds are usually absent.

2. Stages of Reaction

- The peritoneum reacts to the chemical irritants by secreting peritoneal fluid. As a result of this, HCl and bile are diluted by the peritoneal secretions (reaction of peritoneum to the insult) resulting in an **improvement of symptoms**. Hence, it is also called **stage of dilution or stage of illusion.** This stage lasts for 3–6 hours. However, the signs are worse. Pulse is feeble, more than 120/min, hypotension persists, dehydration due to loss of fluid into peritoneal cavity, shifting dullness is present, abdominal distension is due to fluid and paralytic ileus.[1]
- Bowel sounds are absent and guarding and rigidity are worsened.

3. Stage of Bacterial Peritonitis

- The peritoneal contents get contaminated with gram-negative organisms resulting in bacterial peritonitis (the organisms are from the intestine itself and not from the peritoneum).
- The patient becomes severely ill, dehydrated, toxic with drawn in cheeks. The tongue is dry and coated but with bright eyes (**Hippocratic facies,** Fig. 41.31).
- Features of hypovolaemic and septicaemic shock such as feeble thready pulse, cold peripheries, shallow respiration, high grade fever and persistent hypotension are present. Gross abdominal distension, guarding, rigidity, abdominal tenderness all over suggest generalised peritonitis.

Investigation of Perforated Duodenal Ulcer

- Complete blood picture and electrolyte study. Immediate correction with ringer lactate o be started.
- Plain X-ray chest or abdomen (Fig. 41.32) in **erect position** shows collection of free gas under the right dome of diaphragm, in majority of cases. If patient is unable to stand, left lateral decubitus films are taken (Fig. 41.33). It can show signs such as appearance of gas on both sides of the bowel wall (**Rigler's sign**). Large volume of free gas resulting in a large round black area (**Football sign**).
- When in doubt, request a CT scan with contrast which can demonstrate pneumoperitoneum, fluid in the abdomen, site of perforation and some surprises also.

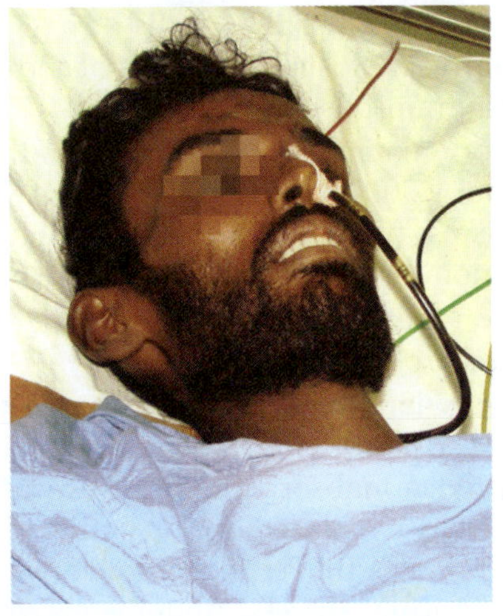

Fig. 41.31: Peritonitis—Hippocratic facies—sunken eyes, jaundice due to sepsis, nasogastric tube showing altered blood

[1]It resembles a strike by employees paralysing the work of a factory in response to an insult.

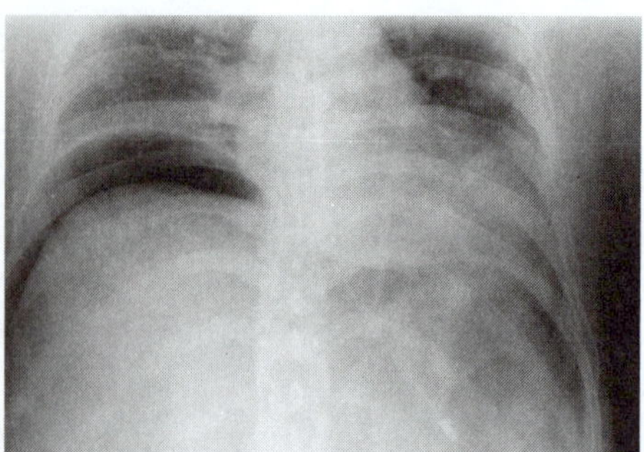

Fig. 41.32: Plain X-ray abdomen erect showing collection of free gas under the right dome of the diaphragm

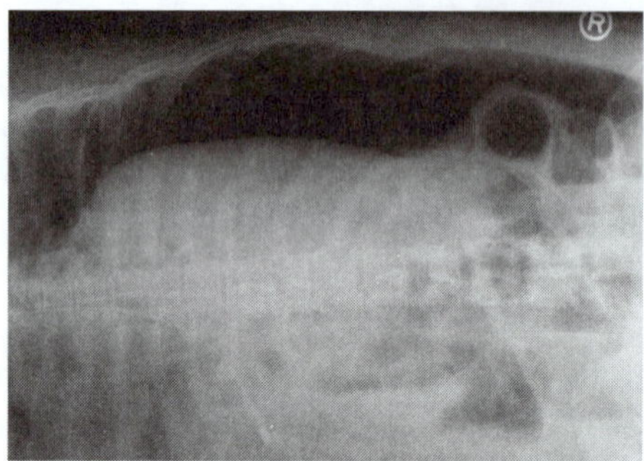

Fig. 41.33: Plain X-ray abdomen lateral decubitus showing collection of free gas under the abdominal wall

Treatment (ABCDEF)[1]

A **A**spiration of stomach contents with Ryle's tube to reduce further contamination and to decrease biliary and pancreatic juice.

B **B**lood grouping and cross-matching may be necessary for surgery.

C **C**harts: Temperature, pulse, BP, respiration, urinary output (urinary bladder is catheterised using a Foley's catheter).

D **D**rugs:

- Injection cephalosporins 1 g IV stat and 12th hourly against gram-positive organisms.
- Injection gentamicin 60–80 mg IV, 8th hourly or amikacin 700 mg stat against gram-negative organisms. (Check creatinine—if high dose need to be monitored or other drug has to be chosen.)
- Injection metronidazole 500 mg IV, 8th hourly to treat anaerobic organisms.

E **E**xploratory laparotomy is done through a midline incision. The perforation is identified and closed with interrupted nonabsorbable silk sutures, which is strengthened by **placement of pedicled omentum** (Fig. 41.34A and B). Peritoneal toilet/wash is given to avoid residual abscess. Abdomen is closed with a drain which is removed after 3–5 days. If it is a large gastric ulcer, it is better to do a gastrectomy, if condition of the patient permits.

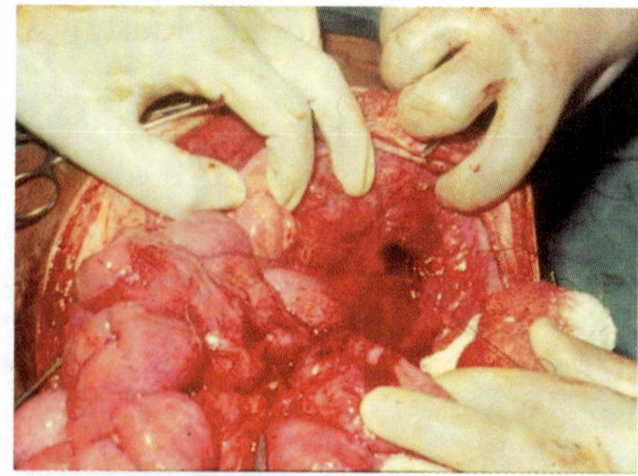

Fig. 41.34A: Duodenal ulcer perforation—closure

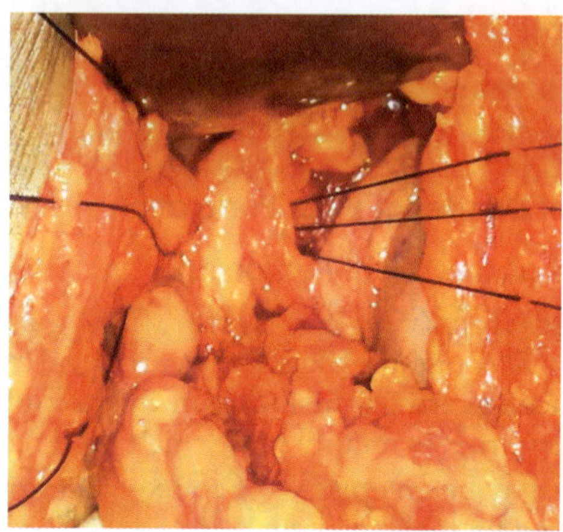

Fig. 41.34B: Pedicled omentum is used here

- Vagotomy and GJ is not done at this stage as the general condition of the patient is very poor and there is peritoneal sepsis.
- Postoperatively, the patient is put on anti-ulcer drugs. An endoscopy is done after 2 months. If the ulcer persists, it may be worthwhile giving a course of *H. pylori eradication treatment. Inspite of this treatment, if symptoms and ulcer persists* it is likely to be a chronic ulcer and an elective operation such as vagotomy and GJ is done. However, it should be remembered that *H. pylori* eradication and simple suturing cures vast majority of acute ulcers.

F **F**luids are given preoperatively to treat dehydration and postoperatively for 3–4 days till the paralytic ileus settles down (soft abdomen and bowel sounds present).

Early Cases of Perforation

It can also be managed by laparoscopic closure of perforation with peritoneal drainage. In fact, a thorough wash is really possible with a laparoscope.

[1]Students should remember that ABCDEF are the basic principles of treatment of any acute abdomen. In majority of cases of acute abdomen, these principles can be applied with minor modifications.

Subacute

Perforation with abscess. Some patients present late to the hospital with features of sealed perforation.

Non-operative Treatment of Perforated Duodenal Ulcer

- Initial steps of ABCD remain the same. There are few indications for non-operative line of treatment for perforated duodenal ulcer:
  A. Patients who are not fit for surgery due to severe comorbidities
  B. CECT shows no leak or no extravasation of the dye.
  C. Small perforation with no signs of peritonitis
- However, following precautions should be taken during non-operative treatment.
  1. **R**adiologically undetected leak
  2. **Repeated clinical examination**
  3. **R**epeated blood investigations
  4. **R**espiratory and renal support
  5. **R**esources for monitoring
  6. **R**eadiness to operate

  Observe **6 Rs**.

HAEMORRHAGE FROM PEPTIC ULCER

- Haemorrhage from peptic ulcer can be chronic which causes anaemia, or acute, resulting in massive haematemesis and melaena.
- It is the **posterior duodenal ulcer which commonly bleeds**, because it erodes into the gastroduodenal artery which runs posterior to the duodenum. A gastric ulcer on the lesser curvature erodes into one of the branches of left or right gastric artery.

Precipitating Factors for Haemorrhage

- **Chronicity**, results in destruction of the layers of the stomach, exposing the vessel.
- Sudden, severe acid peptic digestion brought about by **irritants** such as alcohol, drugs, etc.
- **Atherosclerosis:** Sclerotic artery does not contract, resulting in massive haemorrhage.

Characteristics of Individuals at an Increased Risk of Developing Acute GI Bleeding

- Increased age
- Male sex
- Cardiovascular disease
- Diabetes mellitus and renal disease
- Increased number of medications
- Oral anticoagulant use

Clinical Features of Bleeding Peptic Ulcer

- Previous history of abdominal pain of peptic ulcer disease.
- History of haematemesis or melaena (black tarry stools), one or more attacks.
- There may be features of haemorrhagic shock such as feeble, thready pulse, hypotension, syncope.
  - Oliguria, due to inadequate renal perfusion.
  - Brainstem hypoxia results in change in rate and depth of respiration.
  - There may not be any abdominal signs. However, due to accumulation of blood in the intestines and stomach, mild distension may be present.

  Perforation produces abdominal signs and haemorrhage produces systemic signs.

BLEAD Risk Classification

The following are some of the factors associated with increased morbidity and mortality (Key Box 41.11).

Key Box 41.11

BLEAD Risk Classification

- **BL**ood pressure low
- **E**levated prothrombin time
- **A**ltered mental status
- **D**ysfunction—myocardial, renal, comorbid disease

Forrest classification of endoscopic appearance of bleeding ulcers

Type	Description
Ia	Spurting, bleeding
Ib	Nonspurting, active bleeding
IIa	Visible vessel
IIb	Nonbleeding ulcer with overlying clot
IIc	Ulcer with haematin—covered (black) base
III	Clean ulcer base

As previously mentioned, endoscopy provides the opportunity not only for diagnosis but also for therapy.

Management

- Emergency upper OGD is done to confirm the diagnosis. If the source cannot be detected due to large clots or massive bleeding, it can be repeated a few hours after a stomach wash and blood transfusion.
- Emergency upper OGD should be done within 12–24 hours of bleeding depending upon condition of the patient.
- Resuscitation is more important than an urgent endoscopy.
- Since elderly patients cannot tolerate shock well, decision to control bleeding surgically must be taken early.

I. Conservative Line of Management

1. Emergency replacement of blood, after initial resuscitation with a plasma expander.
2. Ryle's tube is passed and cold saline stomach wash is given to produce vasoconstriction.
3. Cold antacids are given every 2nd hourly, about 10–20 ml.
4. IV ranitidine 50 mg, 8th hourly or IV pantoprazole 40 mg is given to reduce acidity.
   - Majority of cases respond to conservative line of management within 48 hours.

II. Nonsurgical Treatment

1. **Laser coagulation**
   - It can arrest the bleeding without direct tissue contact. Nd:YAG laser has been used more commonly because it can penetrate tissue more deeply compared to argon laser which penetrates very superficial tissues. The success rate of laser coagulation is around 80%.
2. **Sclerotherapy** (Key Boxes 41.12 and 41.13)
   - Epinephrine (1:10,000) arrests bleeding by vasoconstriction
   - 2% ethanolamine, a sclerosant, causes dehydration and shrinkage of surrounding tissues.
   - It also produces inflammation and thrombosis of the bleeding vessel (Fig. 41.35).
   - This is the most popular method. The success rate is around 80–90%. It is a cheap and easy treatment.
3. **Haemoclip application** (Fig. 41.36)
4. **Bipolar electrocoagulation**—failure rate is 50%.
   - Surgical eradication of *H. pylori* prevents rebleeding.

Key Box 41.12

Endotherapy

- Bipolar electrocoagulation—failure rate—50%
- Inj. sclerotherapy—failure rate—20%
- Haemoclip application

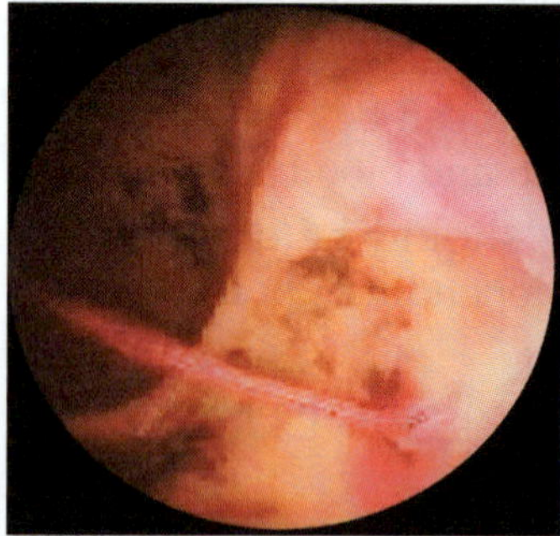

Fig. 41.35: Bleeding vessel

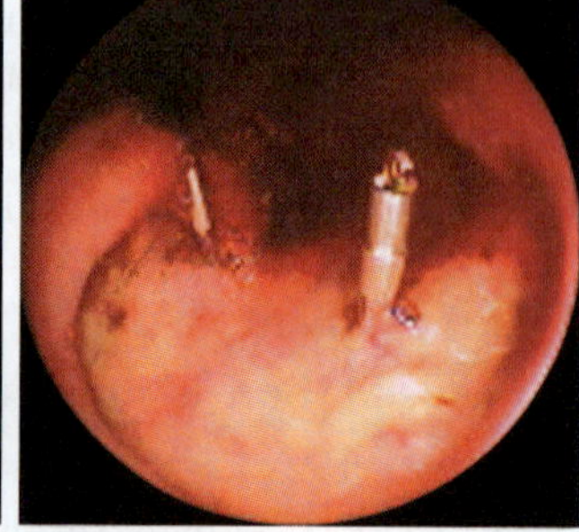

Fig. 41.36: Haemoclip applied

III. Surgical Control of Bleeding Peptic Ulcer

(Key Boxes 41.13 and 41.14)

Key Box 41.13

Endoscopic Prognostic Factors

- Visible level: 40–60% rebleeding ulcer >2 cm
- Adherent clot: 20% rebleeding
- Flat pigmented spot: 10% rebleeding
- Clean ulcer base: Rarely bleeding

Key Box 41.14

Role of Surgery

- Explore when endotherapy fails
- Explore when rebleeding occurs in the elderly
- Explore an unstable patient
- Gastroduodenotomy, under-running of ulcer base for CDU and partial gastrectomy for gastric ulcer

Indications

1. Failure of endoscopic haemostasis—prognostic factors are given below.
2. Rebleeding in the hospital (rebleeding is more common in gastric ulcer patients).
3. Bleeding requiring transfusion of more than 2000 ml blood in 24 hours (6 units).
4. Elderly patients with rebleeding.
5. Massive haemorrhage leading to shock or cardiovascular instability.
6. Recurrent haemorrhage requiring hospitalisation.

Types of Surgery

1. *Surgery for bleeding duodenal ulcer*

- Laparotomy and **anterior gastroduodenotomy.**
- Visualise the bleeding ulcer in the first part of duodenum.
- **Under-running** of the ulcer base by direct suture or 4 quadrant ligation of gastroduodenal artery by using nonabsorbable sutures (Fig. 41.37).

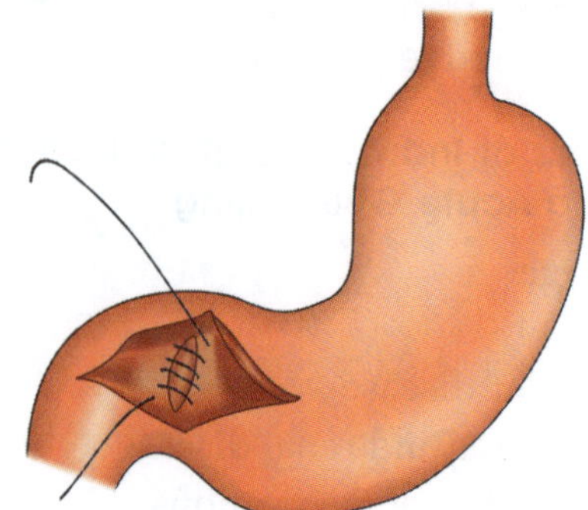

Fig. 41.37: Under-running of the duodenal ulcer

- **Gastroduodenotomy incision is converted into a pyloroplasty** followed by vagotomy which completes the treatment.

2. *Surgery for bleeding gastric ulcer (benign)*

- Laparotomy, gastrotomy and visualise the bleeding ulcer.
- Under-running of the ulcer base. There are chances of rebleeding with this method.
- **Partial gastrectomy** is the best treatment provided general condition of the patient is good (Figs 41.38 and 41.39). Otherwise, local excision of the ulcer, vagotomy followed by GJ or pyloroplasty can also be done.
- Haemostatic methods currently employed include thermotherapy (heater probe, multipolar or bipolar electrocoagulation) as well as injection of ethanol or epinephrine solutions.
- When the bleeding is controlled, long-term medical therapy includes antisecretory agents, usually in the form of a proton pump inhibitor, in addition to testing for *H. pylori* with treatment, if positive.
- If *H. pylori* is present, documentation of eradication should be performed after therapy.

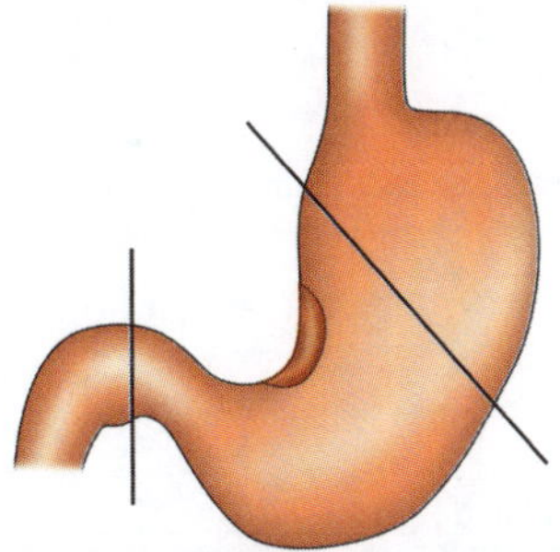

Fig. 41.38: Partial gastrectomy for gastric ulcer

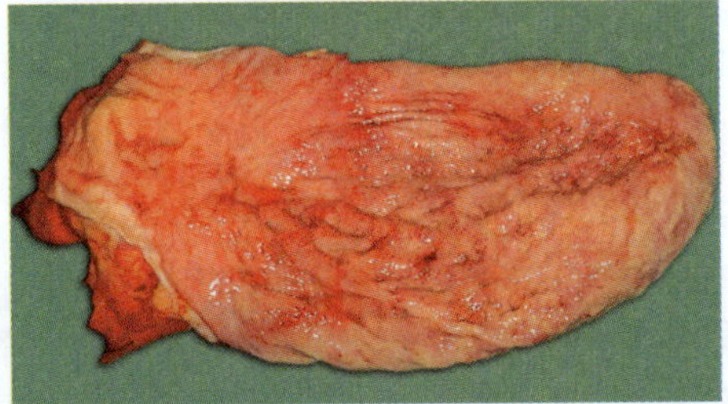

Fig. 41.39: Partial gastrectomy for bleeding gastric ulcer

DIFFERENTIAL DIAGNOSIS OF HAEMATEMESIS (UPPER GI TRACT BLEEDING)

- 80% bleeding is from upper GI tract.
- Almost 20% is from lower GI tract (colon).
- 1% from small intestines.
- Bleeding proximal to ligament of Treitz.
- Haematemesis refers to vomiting of fresh red blood. Melaenemesis refers to vomiting of dark altered blood. However, both are included under upper GI tract bleeding. Small bowel, even though is a midgut structure, some of its lesions can produce haematemesis. Hence, they are also included under this heading.

Causes (Fig. 41.40)

1. **Oesophageal causes**
   - Reflux oesophagitis
   - Mallory-Weiss syndrome
   - Oesophageal varices
   - Cancer of oesophagus, leiomyoma oesophagus
2. **Gastric causes**
   - Gastric ulcer
   - Gastric varices
   - Acute erosive gastritis
   - Gastric cancer
   - Stromal tumours—**GIST**
   - Lymphoma
   - Arteriovenous malformation
   - Gastric polyp
   - Dieulafoy vascular malformation
   - Gastric antral vascular ectasia (GAVE)
3. **Duodenal causes**
   - Duodenal ulcer
   - Arteriovenous malformation
   - Duodenal carcinoma
   - Aortoduodenal fistula diverticulae
   - Polyps

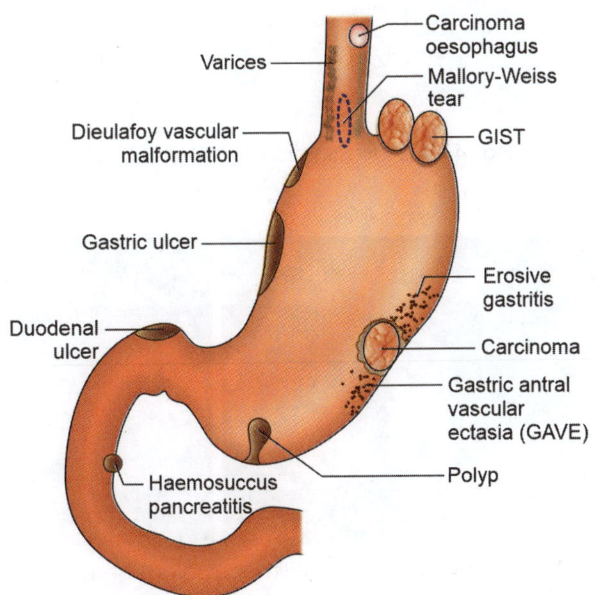

Fig. 41.40: Various causes of haematemesis

4. Other rare causes

- Purpura
- Haemophilia
- Haemobilia
- Pseudoaneurysms due to acute pancreatitis.

Pearls of Wisdom

Acute erosive gastritis, chronic peptic ulcer and oesophageal varices constitute almost 90% of the cases.

Initial Assessment

Table 41.6 describes the initial assessment of upper GI tract bleeding. Two 16 gauze cannulae are put for resuscitation in the emergency department. Patient should be stabilized first with Ringer lactate, blood transfusion and when he is stable, endoscopy is done.

Investigations (Fig. 41.41)

- **Fibreoptic endoscopy** should be done on an emergency basis within 6 to 36 hours of admission. It can diagnose variceal bleeding, erosive gastritis, bleeding peptic ulcer, carcinoma stomach, etc.
- Only when endoscopy cannot yield any diagnosis, selective coeliac angiography should be done which can detect uncommon causes such as angiodysplasia of the stomach or bleeding from a rolling hernia, etc. Barium study is done to rule out intestinal causes in less urgent cases.
- **Isotope studies:** Intravenous injection of **^{99m}Tc pertechnetate** can demonstrate hypertrophic gastric like mucosa in **Meckel's diverticulum**.
- **CT angiogram is the gold standard** investigation when haemobilia or haemosuccus pancreatitis is suspected (Figs 41.42 to 41.44).

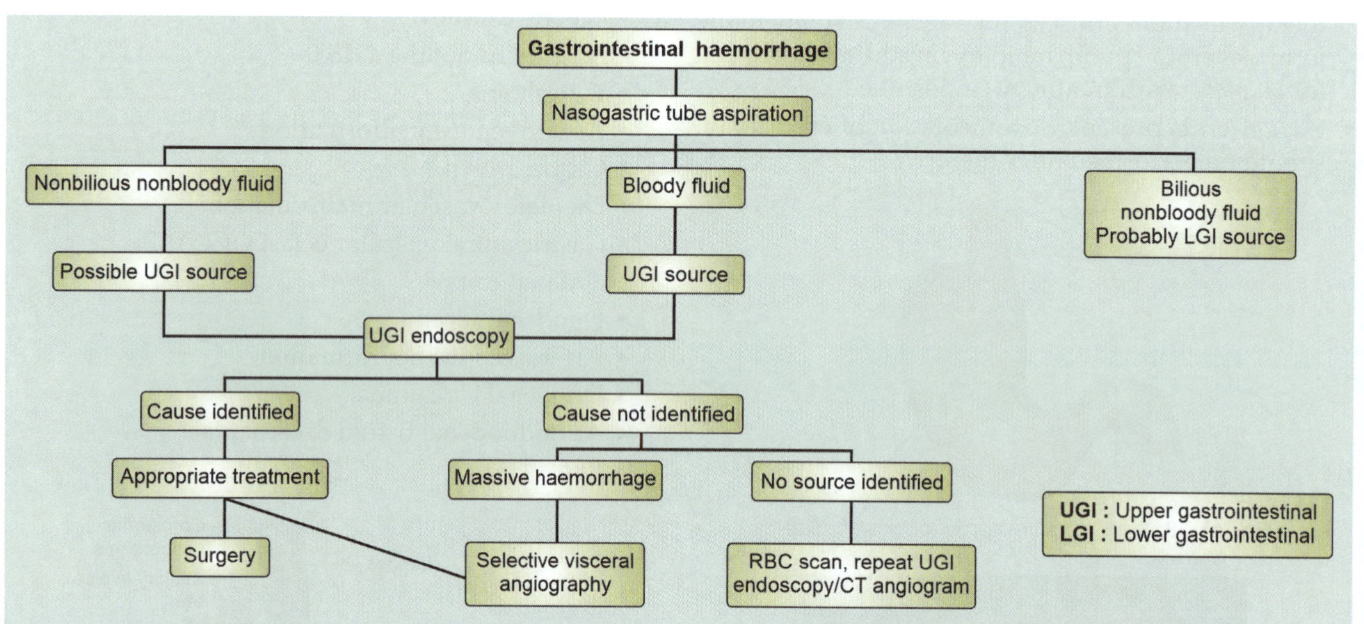

Fig. 41.41: Investigation algorithm of UGI bleeding (*Courtesy:* Dr Sibacis Bisoi, Asst Professor, KMC, Manipal)

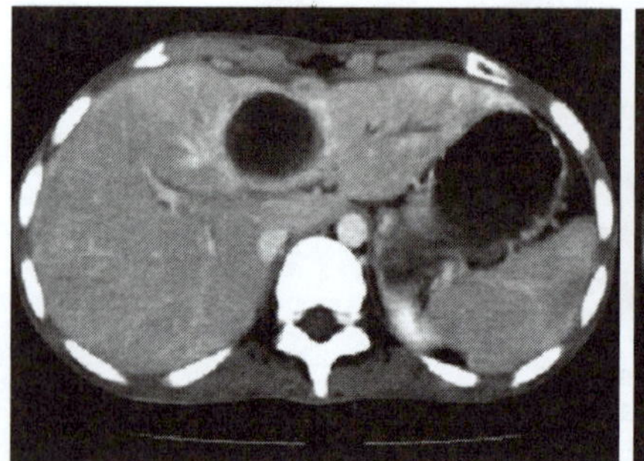

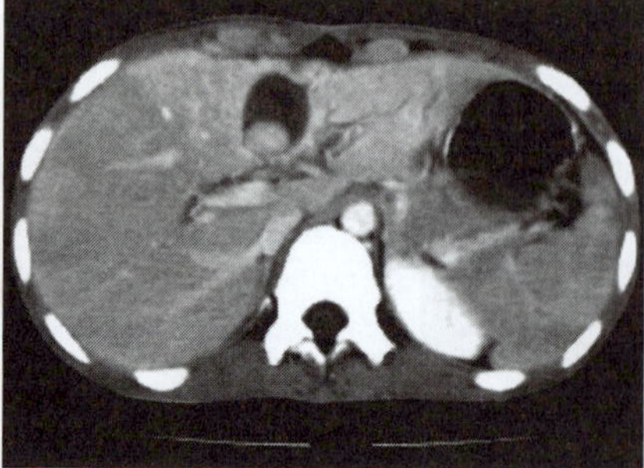

Figs 41.42 and 41.43: CT hepatic angiogram demonstrating extravasation of dye into a pseudoaneurysm of a branch of middle hepatic artery and thrombus—case of haemobilia

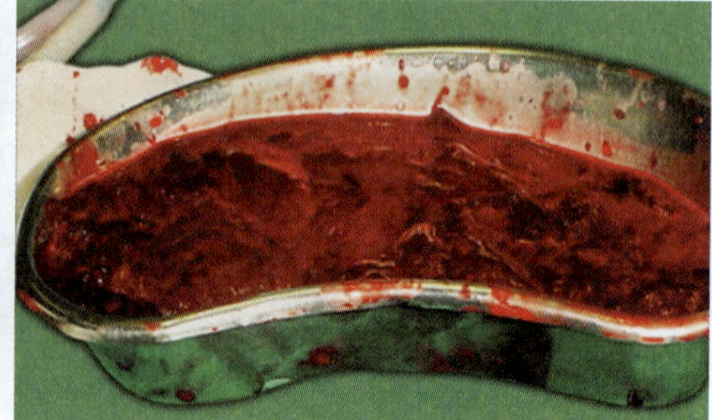

Fig. 41.44: Massive haematemesis in this patient of haemobilia

Table 41.6 Initial assessment

History	Probable causes
1. Abuse of drugs and alcohol	Acute erosive gastritis
Previous abdominal pain	Chronic peptic ulcer
H/o jaundice, liver cell failure	Oesophageal varices
Anaemia, loss of weight, loss of appetite	Carcinoma stomach
Violent vomiting—haematemesis	Mallory-Weiss syndrome
2. General physical examination	
• Testicular atrophy, gynaecomastia	• Cirrhosis of the liver
• Palpable left supraclavicular node	• Carcinoma stomach
• Arthritis—multiple joint involvement	• Acute erosive gastritis (use of NSAID)
• Purpuric spots (Fig. 41.45)	• Bleeding tendencies
3. Abdominal examination	
• Palpable spleen, ascites	• Portal hypertension
• Palpable stomach mass	• Carcinoma stomach
• Tenderness in the epigastrium	• Peptic ulcer disease
4. Assessment of haemorrhage	
Massive haemorrhage (more than 1,000 ml of blood)	Portal hypertension, acute erosive gastritis, chronic peptic ulcer
Moderate haemorrhage (500–1000 ml of blood)	Chronic peptic ulcer
Mild haemorrhage (less than 500 ml of blood)	Other causes

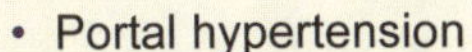

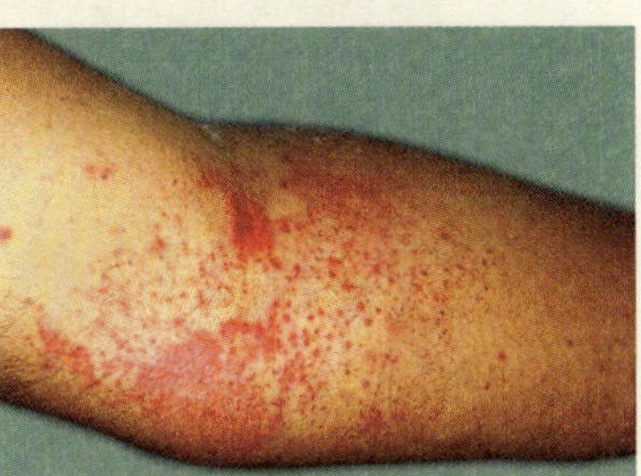

Fig. 41.45: Purpuric spots

CAUSES OF UPPER GI TRACT BLEEDING (Figs 41.46 to 41.51)

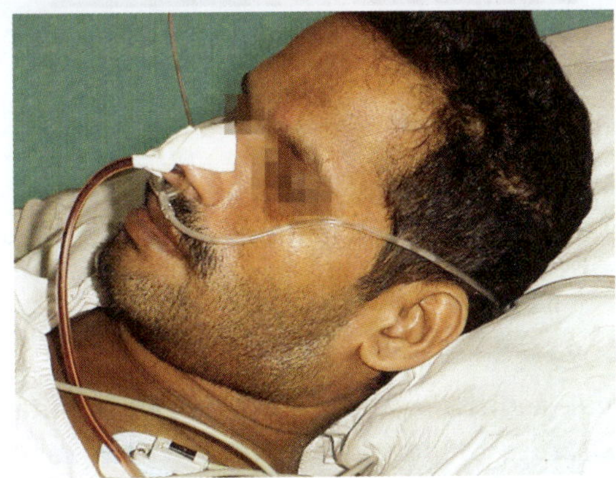

Fig. 41.46: Chronic duodenal ulcer with massive UGI bleeding. Diagnostic use of nasogastric tube is to detect active bleeding

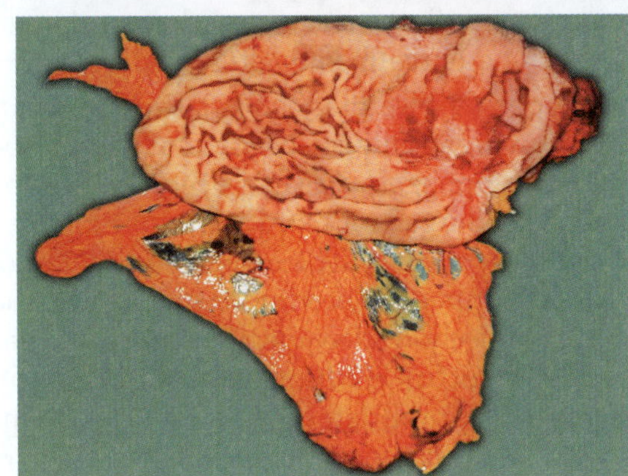

Fig. 41.47: Subtotal gastrectomy specimen showing bleeding gastric ulcer

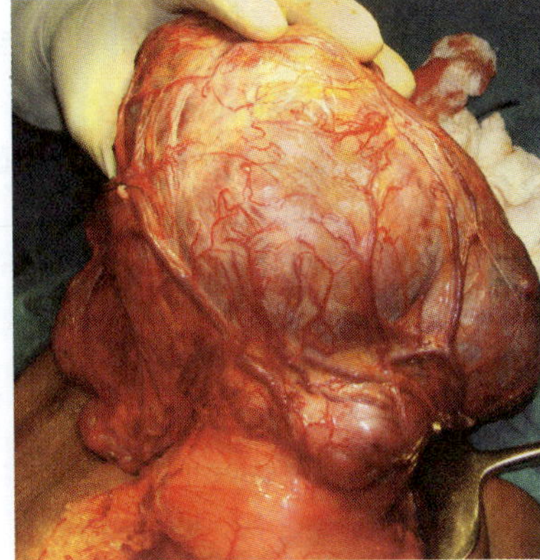

Fig. 41.48: Upper GI bleeding due to GIST of stomach

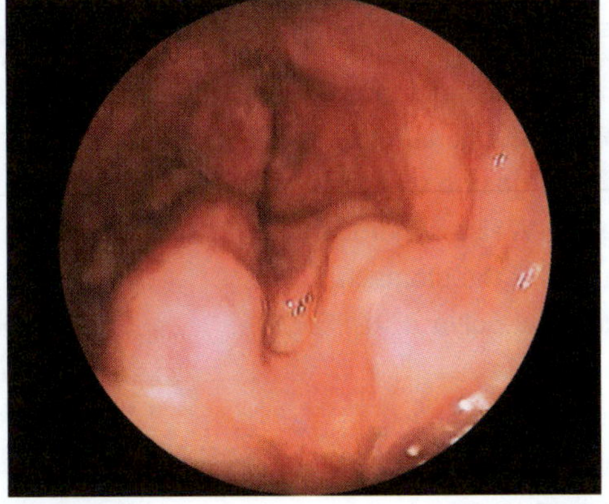

Fig. 41.49: Grade III oesophageal varices with bleeding

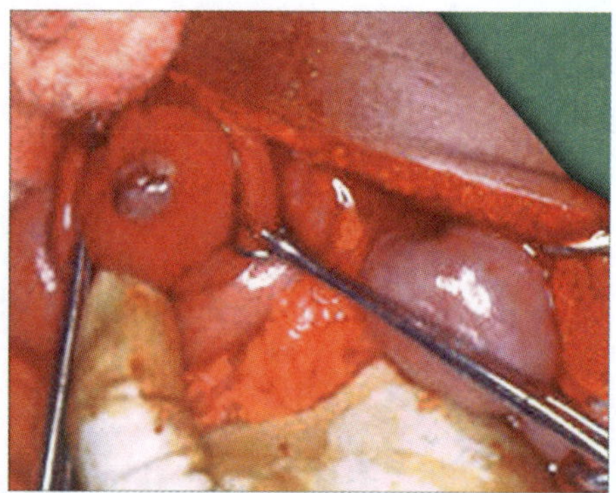

Fig. 41.50: Dieulafoy vascular malformation

Treatment

Initial management is to treat the shock in the line discussed for peptic ulcer haemorrhage.

Indications for Surgery

1. Elderly patients with rebleed in the hospital
2. Rarity of blood groups
3. Spurting vessel in an endoscopy

Surgery

- Surgical management of individual case has been discussed along with the concerned chapter. However, summary of the treatment is discussed in Table 41.7.
- Thus, upper GI bleeding can occur due to various causes. However, acute erosive gastritis, chronic peptic ulcer and oesophageal varices are the three important causes of bleeding. Endoscopy is the investigation for the diagnosis of upper GI bleeding (Fig. 41.52). Today, most of the upper GI bleeding is managed either in the form of injection sclerotherapy, laser coagulation, or with powerful H2 blockers or proton pump inhibitors. In appropriate cases, surgery is definitely indicated. Some common conditions which give rise to haematemesis are discussed in the following pages.

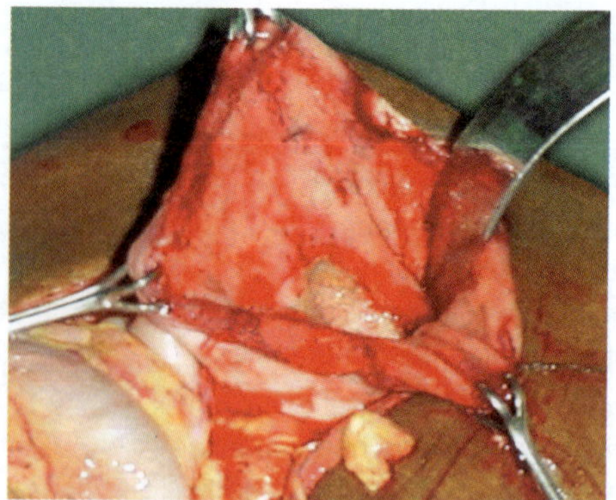

Fig. 41.51: Giant gastric ulcer with bleeding

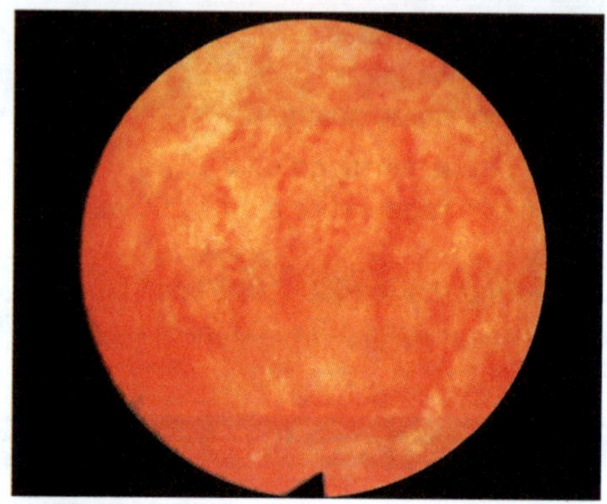

Fig. 41.52: Endoscopy showing erosions

ACUTE PEPTIC ULCER

They are also called acute erosive gastritis/acute stress ulcers/acute steroidal ulcers and **acute gastric mucosal lesions (AGML)**.

Aetiology

- Drugs—aspirin, analgin, steroids, phenylbutazone.
- Any stress or acute infection which results in sepsis.

Table 41.7 Surgery for haematemesis

Causes	Conservative ⟶ Failure ⟶	Surgical method
1. Acute erosive gastritis	Yes	Rarely—gastrectomy
2. Chronic duodenal ulcer	Yes	Vagotomy, under-running, pyloroplasty
3. Chronic gastric ulcer	Yes	Partial gastrectomy
4. Mallory-Weiss syndrome	Yes	Suturing of the tear
5. Cancer of the stomach	No	Gastrectomy
6. Duodenal polyp	Endoscopic snaring	Surgery, if endoscopic facility not available
7. Haemobilia	Yes, therapeutic embolisation	Ligation of feeding vessel
8. Variceal bleeding	Yes, sclerotherapy	Devascularisation
9. Haemosuccus pancreatitis	Yes, therapeutic embolisation	Ligation of pseudoaneurysm
10. Dieulafoy lesion	Yes, injection sclerotherapy	Wide excision

- Following tetanus
- After burns, they are called **'Curling's ulcer'.**
- After head injury or neurosurgical operations, they are called **'Cushing's ulcer'.**
- Following **hypotension** and shock, there is **hypoperfusion,** which results in **mucosal ischaemia** and acute stress ulcers. Example: Myocardial infarction, trauma, sepsis.
- Excessive consumption of spirits and smoking.
- Respiratory failure can also produce acute erosions.

Pathology

There is a diffuse mucosal damage and disruption of gastric mucosal barrier. Reflux of bile also may be a precipitating factor. This results in acute erosions when they are 1 to 2 mm or acute ulcers when they are 1 to 2 cm in size, shallow and well-demarcated. The entire stomach is involved by these ulcers.

Clinical Features

- Dyspepsia due to minor bleeding.
- Haematemesis—sometimes massive, fresh bleeding can produce hypotension and shock.
- Acute abdominal pain due to acute erosions or perforation of an acute ulcer.
- In ICU: **Drop in blood pressure,** nasogastric aspirate of blood and/or melaena.

Diagnosis

Emergency endoscopy to confirm diagnosis and to rule out other causes of upper GI tract bleeding.

Treatment of Acute Peptic Ulcers with Bleeding

1. **Admission in intensive care unit (ICU)** (Key Box 41.15).
2. **Ryle's tube** to be introduced first and empty the stomach. It helps in reducing vomiting and sometimes aspiration of gastric contents into the lungs also. Ice cold water or saline stomach wash (vasoconstriction) reduces bleeding.
3. **Regular antacids** 20–30 ml, 2nd hourly, preferably cold antacids.
4. **Replacement of blood** specifically coagulation factors.
5. **Injection ranitidine** 50 mg IV, 8th hourly or **pantoprazole 20 mg IV**. Majority of cases respond to conservative line of treatment.
6. **Endotherapy:** If there is solitary bleeding site.
7. **Surgery:** With modern investigations and their therapeutic role in addition to good ICU care, availability of blood and nursing care, almost all cases of erosive gastritis can be managed without surgery. In spite of above treatment, if the condition deteriorates, a total gastrectomy or a subtotal gastrectomy may be necessary (very, very rare) as a life-saving measure.

Key Box 41.15

Very Important Measures in ICU

- Correct coagulopathy
- Improve oxygenation
- Blood transfusion
- Control sepsis

MALLORY-WEISS SYNDROME

Aetiopathogenesis (Key Box 41.16)

- It occurs due to a tear in the gastric mucosa near the oesophagogastric (OG) junction.
- Also called partial thickness mucosal rupture.
- In Boerhaave syndrome, all layers are involved in a tear.

Key Box 41.16

Conditions wherein Mallory-Weiss Tear is Seen

- **S**pirit or alcohol
- **I**nfarction—myocardial
- **I**nfection—cholecystitis
- **P**ancreatitis
- **R**enal failure
- **T**umour—pregnancy

Remember as **SPIRIT**

Clinical Features (Fig. 41.53)

- The patient is usually a middle-aged male who, after consumption of alcohol, vomits the food contents first. During the course of vomiting because of straining and retching, a tear develops near the oesophagocardiac junction. Hence, the **second vomitus contains blood.**
- Sometimes, the bleeding can be so massive to produce hypotension and shock. In 90% of cases, the bleeding stops spontaneously.

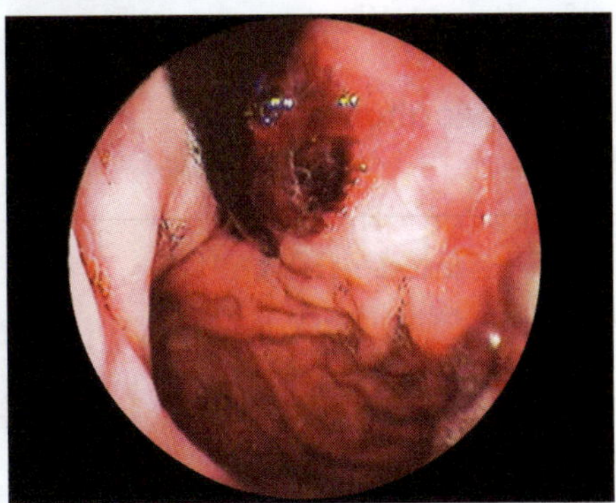

Fig. 41.53: Mallory-Weiss tear—with the endotherapy bleeding stopped (*Courtesy:* Dr Filipe Alvares, Gastroenterologist, KMC, Manipal)

Treatment

- Urgent resuscitation of haemorrhagic shock.
- Endoscopy to confirm the diagnosis—tear is seen in the lesser curvature.
- Ryle's tube aspiration for 48–72 hours.
- Endotherapy—injection adrenaline 1:10,000 dilution is effective. If not, haemoclipping can be done.
- Multipolar electric coagulation
- When all other measures fail, **gastrotomy** (opening in the stomach) and under-running is necessary with 2–0 silk sutures.

DIEULAFOY VASCULAR MALFORMATION

- In this condition, an unusually large artery runs in the submucosa which lies in close contact with mucous membrane (Fig. 41.54).
- Mucosal erosion precipitates the bleeding.
- In more than 80% cases, bleeding occurs within 6 to 8 cm from OG junction, at the lesser curvature.
- Endoscopy and endotherapy should be tried and if necessary, repeated also.
- Sudden, massive, painless, recurrent haematemesis with hypotension is the presenting feature.
- Angiography to confirm the bleeding lesion and gelfoam embolisation must be tried first.
- Failure to achieve control of the bleeding—**gastrotomy and wide excision** of the lesion should be done.

GASTRIC ANTRAL VASCULAR ECTASIA (GAVE)

- It is an uncommon cause of chronic GI bleeding resulting in iron deficiency anaemia.
- It is also called **watermelon stomach** because of the presence of long red streaky area which are present in the stomach resembling a watermelon (Key Box 41.17).

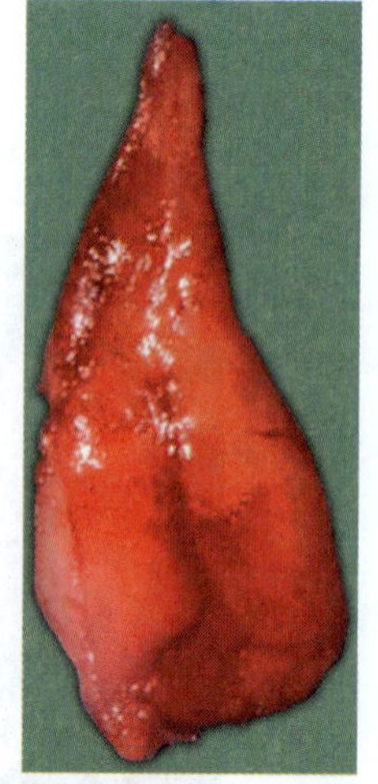

Fig. 41.54: Dieulafoy vascular malformation—excised

Subacute Complication of Peptic Ulcer

A small perforation of peptic ulcer which is sealed off by omentum may result in a residual abscess in one of the subphrenic spaces. It responds to conservative treatment. Otherwise, percutaneous drainage can be done with ultrasonographic guidance.

Key Box 41.17

Watermelon Stomach (Gastric Antral Vascular Ectasia)

- **W**omen in their 50s are commonly affected
- **A**ntrum is commonly involved
- **T**IPSS (*see* page 608) in patients with portal hypertension
- **E**ctasia of antral vessels gives rise to UGI bleeding
- **R**ed parallel stripes on the mucosal fold are characteristic
- **M**ucosal fibromuscular hyperplasia and hyalinisation are present
- **E**ndoscopy is the investigation of choice
- **L**iver disease in 25% patients—cirrhotic men
- **O**ther diseases—autoimmune connective tissue disorder may be associated with this—also *Helicobacter pylori*
- **N**o control of bleeding—antrectomy may be required

Remember as **WATERMELON**

CHRONIC COMPLICATIONS OF PEPTIC ULCER

I. GASTRIC OUTLET OBSTRUCTION

Earlier it was called pyloric stenosis. However, gastric outlet obstruction is a better word. Chronic cicatrisation of a duodenal ulcer or juxtapyloric ulcer results in narrowing of pyloric antrum which is described as pyloric stenosis. In India, pyloric stenosis is more common in South Indian patients, who usually present with a long history of duodenal ulcer and a recent history of vomiting (Key Box 41.18).

Symptoms

- Classical **hunger pain** of duodenal ulcer disappears. It may be replaced by a dull aching pain because of gastric distension. Colicky pain is due to hyperperistalsis of stomach.
- **Vomiting** is profuse, projectile, persistent, foul-smelling (because of stasis) and nonbilious.
- There may be **distension of upper abdomen** with epigastric fullness.

Key Box 41.18

Pyloric Stenosis

- Pyloric stenosis in CDU—**Misnomer**
- Stenosis is very often found in the **first part of duodenum**
- In cases of pyloric channel ulcer, true pyloric stenosis occurs
- Metabolic changes, such as paradoxical aciduria (Fig. 41.55), are usually seen in patients with ulcer, **not in carcinoma** because of relative achlorhydria in the latter

Signs

1. **Visible gastric peristalsis (VGP):** Stomach that you see
   - It is a wave of contraction of the stomach which starts in the left hypochondrium, runs across the umbilicus and ends in the right hypochondrium. These contractions can be felt—**stomach that you feel**. Presence of VGP is diagnostic of pyloric stenosis (right to left peristalsis is seen in left-sided obstructive colonic tumours). **If VGP is not seen, it can be made prominent by:**
     - Asking the patient to drink at least 500–1000 ml of water (it is difficult. Try and see!).
     - Stimulating the abdomen by flicking movement.
2. **Succussion splash**
   - Should be done on 'fasting' stomach. This test should be done before asking the patient to drink water.
   - In pyloric stenosis, there is always residual fluid in the stomach, which gives a splashing sound that can be heard with/without stethoscope—**stomach that you hear.**

Pearls of Wisdom

Thus, the stomach which is seen, felt and heard is diagnostic of pyloric stenosis.

3. **Auscultopercussion test/auscultoscraping test** to find out the greater curvature of the stomach.

   Procedure: Keep the "bell" of stethoscope in the centre of epigastrium (ask the patient to hold the bell of stethoscope) and percuss radially. Percussion over the stomach gives a dull note because of presence of fluid. When the note changes, it indicates the greater curvature of stomach. Mark it on the abdomen (instead of percussion, scraping can be done with finger nail). A line joining 3 or 4 such marks outlines the greater curvature of stomach.

Saline load test: 700 ml of normal saline is infused into stomach over a period of 3 to 5 minutes through a nasogastric tube and is clamped. If a volume more than 350 ml can be aspirated after 30 minutes, it indicates obstruction.

Electrolyte Changes in Gastric Outlet Obstruction

- Hypochloraemic alkalosis
- Hyponatraemia
- Hypokalaemia
- Paradoxical aciduria (Fig. 41.55)

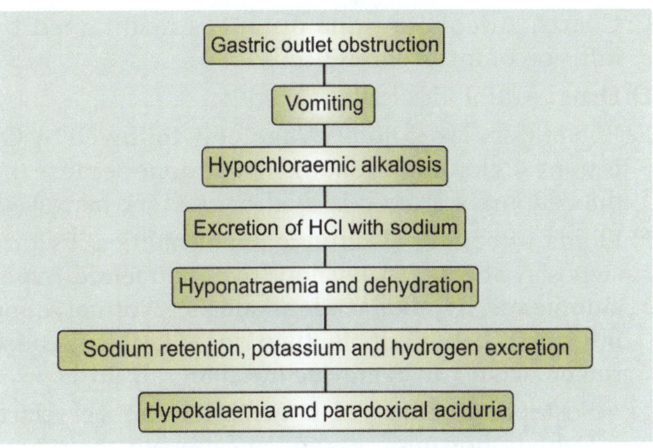

Fig. 41.55: Pathogenesis of paradoxical aciduria

Investigations

1. **Barium meal X-ray**
   - **Hugely dilated stomach (large and low stomach).**

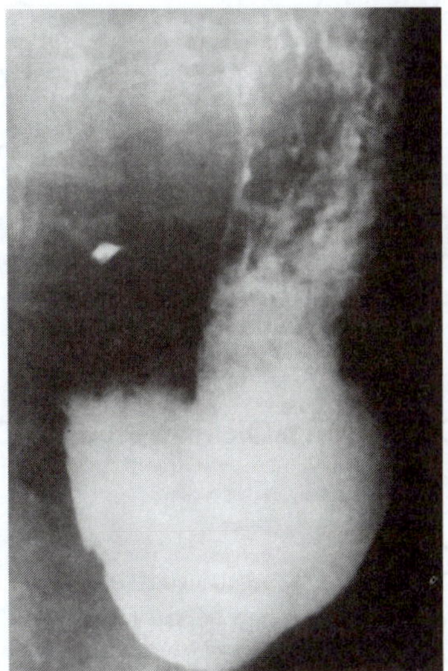

Fig. 41.56: Barium meal showing dilated J shaped stomach with mosaic appearance

   - Barium does not enter the duodenum. Barium mixed with food residue can give rise to ***mosaic appearance***. Delay in evacuation (on repeat X-ray) of barium into the duodenum is seen (Fig. 41.56).
2. **Gastroscopy**
   - The scope will not enter the duodenum. Stomach is full of foul-smelling food residue.
   - Gastroscopy is also done to rule out carcinoma of the stomach.
3. **Electrolyte study (*vide infra*)**

Treatment (ABCDEF)

A: Aspiration with Ryle's tube—good stomach wash, twice a day is given to keep the stomach empty. Saline is used as it decreases oedema of the stomach wall. Stomach wash should be given for at least 3–5 days before surgery.

B: Blood is arranged for surgery. Blood may be required preoperatively to treat anaemia.

C: Charts: Adequate urine output is maintained by infusion of intravenous fluids.

D: Drug: Antibiotics for surgery.

E: Exploratory laparotomy: **Vagotomy followed by GJ is done.** Pyloroplasty should not be done because the duodenum is scarred, cicatrised, fibrosed and narrowed.

F: Fluids to correct electrolyte abnormalities. Pyloric stenosis patients can develop **"hyponatraemic, hypochloraemic, hypokalaemic alkalosis"**. Normal saline infusion is better initially than ringer lactate because ringer lactate can aggravate metabolic alkalosis.

- Postoperatively these patients recover very fast. Dehydration improves and nutritionally they show dramatic improvement. Even the gastric tone may return after a few years.

Differential Diagnosis of Gastric Outlet Obstruction

- There are two important causes for gastric outlet obstruction have been given in Table 41.8. However, duodenum obstruction in the second part or third part by malignancies, annular pancreas or lymph nodal masses may give rise to persistent vomiting but usually it is bilious.

II. TEA-POT DEFORMITY OR HANDBAG STOMACH (Fig. 41.57)

- A long-standing lesser curve gastric ulcer causes shortening of the lesser curvature due to fibrosis. Such stomach resembles a tea-pot. As a result of this, the pylorus becomes nondependent. Hence, stasis occurs.
- **Treatment:** Partial gastrectomy followed by Billroth I anastomosis.

III. HOURGLASS CONTRACTURE (Fig. 41.58)

- When a saddle-shaped ulcer in the lesser curvature gets cicatrised, it involves both surfaces of the stomach resulting in conversion of stomach into two compartments.

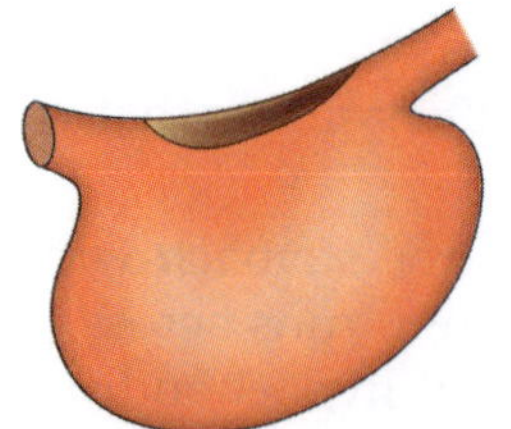

Fig. 41.57: Tea-pot deformity

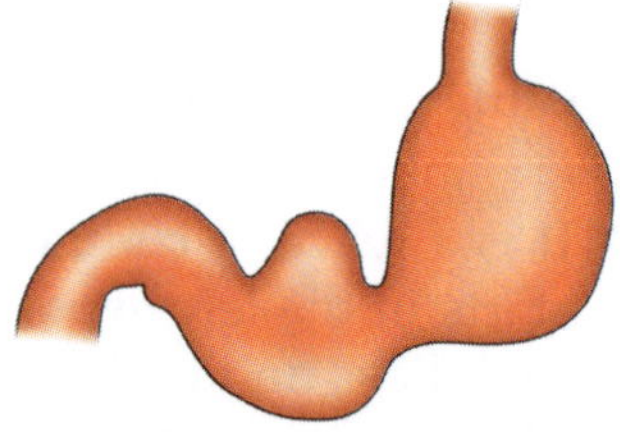

Fig. 41.58: Hourglass contracture of the stomach

- Features of stasis such as fullness, distension and persistent vomiting are present.
- Females are affected more often.
- Weight loss is present. Appetite is decreased.
- It is treated by **Billroth I partial gastrectomy** with removal of 2nd pouch.

IV. PENETRATION INTO PANCREAS

Posterior gastric ulcer can penetrate into pancreas, resulting in severe referred pain to the back resembling pancreatic pathology. However, this type of pain is relieved on lying down.

Competency

SU28.9: Describe and discuss the aetiology, the clinical features, investigations and principles of management of carcinoma stomach.

CARCINOMA STOMACH

Introduction

- Carcinoma stomach is more common (2 times) in men compared to women.
- Rare below 40. Average age is 63 years.

Table 41.8 Differential diagnosis of pyloric stenosis

	Cicatrised chronic duodenal ulcer	Carcinoma pyloric antrum
1. Age	20–40 years	>40–50 years
2. Duration of the symptoms	Long duration of abdominal pain and recent history of vomiting	Pain is usually absent, but vomiting is a feature. Symptoms are of short duration
3. Appetite	Decreased because of vomiting	Severe loss of appetite
4. Weight loss	Present	Significant
5. Anaemia	Not a feature	Present
6. Mass	Not palpable	Hard, irregular mass is palpable

- The palpable mass is the deciding clinical factor (sign). Other differences cannot truly differentiate between the two conditions. Rarely, carcinoma of the stomach is also seen in young patients at the age of 20. In congenital hypertrophic pyloric stenosis, the mass is palpable (*see* page 593).

- Worldwide, it is the fourth most common cancer and second leading cancer of death.
- North Eastern part of India, the district of Aizawl in the state of Mizoram has recorded the highest incidence in the country as per NCRP 2013 (64.2/100,000 population). The highest incidence of gastric cancer in Mizoram has been attributed to smoking local cigarettes like maizol and Taibur-tobacco smoke infused water. This is followed by a Southern Indian state, namely Tamil Nadu, where the incidence is 12.2/100,000 population in men.
- Incidence of proximal gastric carcinoma is increased—may be due to obesity and in rich socioeconomic status patients (Key Box 41.19).
- Carcinoma distal stomach is more commonly associated with *H. pylori*.
- Proximal carcinomas are more advanced at the time of presentation than distal carcinomas.
- D2 gastrectomy is currently the recommended surgical choice for cases of resectable advanced disease.
- The 5-year overall survival for resectable GC is approximately 20 to 30% worldwide, but it is 70% in Japan and in other eastern countries.

Key Box 41.19

Carcinoma Proximal Stomach (Cardia)

- Incidence is increasing. Obesity and high socio-economic group
- More aggressive
- Thin muscularis mucosa. Hence, submucosal invasion is seen early
- Diagnosis may also get delayed as endoscopy needs technical expertise
- Signet ring carcinoma is common here
- Surgical resection involves oesophageal anastomosis which is technically demanding. Leak rates are high
- Hence, prognosis is poor

Sites: Pyloric antrum is the commonest site. Refer Fig. 41.59 for sites and percentage of occurrence.

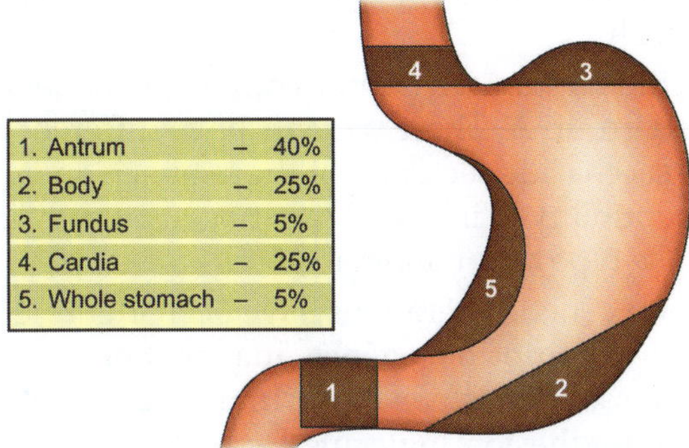

Fig. 41.59: Site and incidence of gastric cancer

Risk Factors for Carcinoma Stomach

(Fig. 41.60 and Key Box 41.20)

1. Environmental and Dietary Factors

- The incidence is increased in persons who consume red meat, cabbage, spices, spirits, salt-fish (Key Box 41.20).
- Smoked salmon fish was responsible for increased incidence of carcinoma stomach in Japanese population. Probably, it is related to release of polycyclic hydrocarbons and aromatic amino acids. Smoking, spicy food and alcohol consumed over a period of many years produce chronic gastritis which may change into carcinoma of stomach.

Pearls of Wisdom

WHO recommends increased consumption of fruits and vegetables. Vitamin C is an antioxidant which is a protective agent. Ascorbic acid prevents conversion of nitrates to nitrites.

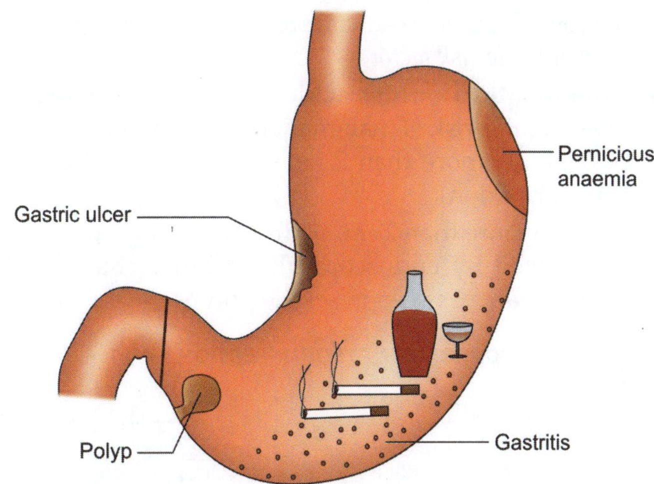

Fig. 41.60: Risk factors for carcinoma stomach

Key Box 41.20

Food Products which may be Carcinogenic

- Smoked food
- Spirits
- Smoking
- Salted food—salt based preservatives and lack of refrigeration
- Soil
- Diet low in carbohydrate
- Animal protein
- Rich fatty food
- High in complex carbohydrates
- *H. pylori* in contaminated water

2. Precancerous Conditions

a. **Atrophic gastritis:** This may be due to smoking, spicy food, continuous ingestion of drugs, reflux of bile into the stomach, etc.

b. **Pernicious anaemia:** Patients have increased risk (four to six times) of development of carcinoma when compared to general population. It causes atrophic gastritis and precipitates carcinoma of fundus of the stomach. Lesions are polypoidal and multicentric

c. Patients with **hypogammaglobulinaemia** (50-fold increase) are at high-risk.

d. ***H. pylori* infection** results in atrophic gastritis, followed by the intestinal type of gastric mucosa, metaplasia and then dysplasia. Eventually, it leads to **intestinal type of gastric cancer** (Figs 41.61 and 41.62). *H. pylori* can also cause proliferation of gastric cancer cells and decrease secretion of vitamin C. Cytotoxin associated gene A (Cag A) is associated with increased risk.

- Also both **type A** and **type B** gastritis can predispose to carcinoma stomach. Type A—proximal stomach, type B—distal stomach. *It is an important modifiable risk factor.*

e. **Adenomatous polyps** which occur in the antrum have highest risk of malignant transformation (larger polyps, i.e. more than 2 cm—10 to 20% malignant transformation).

- Polyp more than 2 cm, pedunculated polyp can be removed by endoscopically. Higher chances of malignancy is seen in sessile polyps.

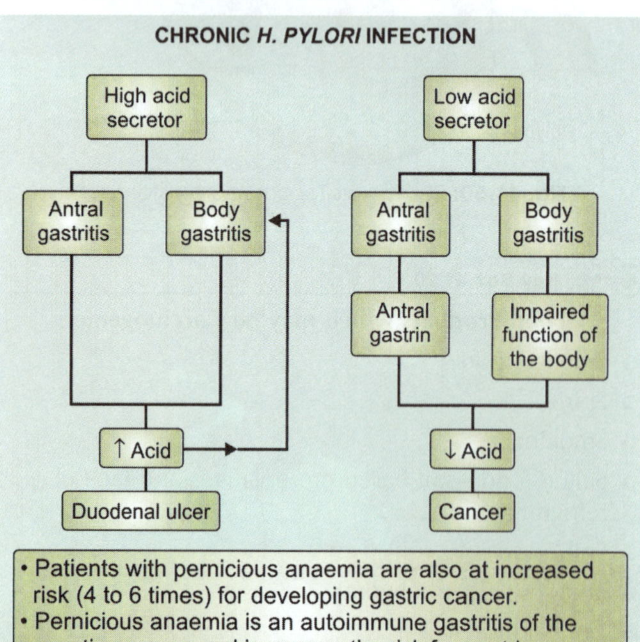

Fig. 41.61: *H. pylori* and pathogenesis of duodenal ulcer and carcinoma stomach

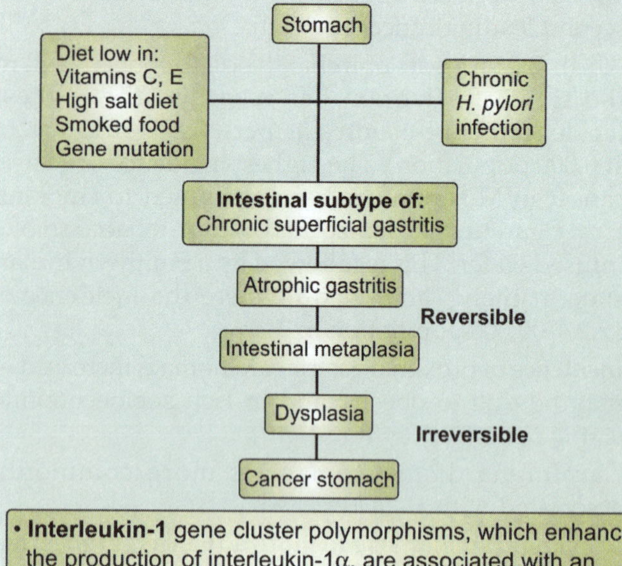

Fig. 41.62: Aetiopathogenesis of carcinoma stomach

f. **Menetrier's disease** is a protein-losing enteropathy, along with giant hypertrophy of gastric mucosal folds. It is a precancerous condition.

g. **Gastric ulcer (benign):** Incidence of malignancy is 2% (0.5 to 5%). Carcinoma arising in a gastric ulcer is called *"Ulcer Cancer of the Stomach"*.

h. **Previous GJ or gastric resection** predisposes to development of carcinoma of the stomach after a period of 15–20 years. Such a carcinoma is described as stump carcinoma. Pathogenesis is related to development of atrophic gastritis, achlorhydria and duodenogastric bile reflux.

3. Genetic and Familial Factors (Key Box 41.21)

- Carcinoma stomach can run in families. However, only 10% of patients give family history of carcinoma stomach.
- Carcinoma stomach is more common in patients with blood group A. These patients have different mucopolysaccharide secretion in the stomach and greater susceptibility to ingested carcinogens. They develop diffuse type of carcinoma.
- Several genetic alterations have been identified such as activation of oncogenes, inactivation of tumour suppressor genes p53 and p16, reduction or loss in the cell adhesion molecule E-cadherin (met proto-oncogene).

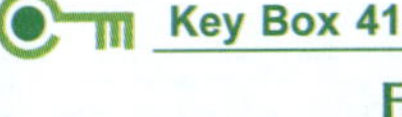

Key Box 41.21

Familial Gastric Cancer

- Only 10% of patients give family history of carcinoma stomach
- Associated with mutation of E-cadherin gene
- Bonaparte (Napoleon) appears to have this gene
- It is also called hereditary diffuse gastric cancer (HDGC)
- Diagnosis is made when carcinoma is detected below the age of 40 years
- E-cadherin mutation results in lifetime risk of gastric cancer by 60–90%.
- Hence prophylactic gastrectomy is recommended
- Familial diffuse gastric cancer (FGC)—at least 3 relatives in 2 generations are affected, one of them before 50 years of age.
- Hereditary nonpolyposis colon cancer carries—10% risk of gastric cancer

- Mutation of E-cadherin gene causes hereditary diffuse gastric cancer. Defective DNA mismatch repair (MLH1 or MSH2 mutation) causes Lynch syndrome. They have increased risk of gastric and colon cancer.

Gross Types

1. **Cauliflower**-like growth with friable tissue. This variety can give rise to melaena or bleeding causing anaemia.
2. **Infiltrative** type of lesion (diffuse) with dense submucosal fibrosis which converts the stomach into a small contracted, functionless stomach—**linitis plastica** or **leather bottle stomach.** Mucosa may appear normal.
3. **Ulcerative** variety, with classical everted edges with central slough.
4. **Ulcer cancer** refers to carcinoma arising in a pre-existing gastric ulcer. In this variety, complete destruction of the muscle coat is present.
5. **Colloid carcinoma:** In this condition, malignant cells are separated by colloid material. This is the type which is common in women and gives rise to Krukenberg's tumour—bilateral, bulky ovarian metastasis common in premenopausal women (signet ring carcinoma produces this).

Pathology

- Ninety-five percent of all malignant gastric neoplasms are adenocarcinomas.
- The Lauren system separates gastric adenocarcinoma into intestinal or diffuse types based on histology (Key Box 41.22).

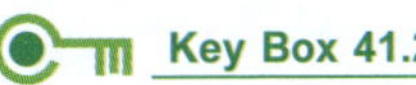

Key Box 41.22

Lauren Classification System

Intestinal	Diffuse
Environmental	Familial, blood type A
Gastric atrophy, intestinal metaplasia	Does not arise in gastritis
Men > women	Women > men
Higher incidence with age	Younger age group
Gland formation present	Poorly differentiated, signet ring cells, no gland formation
Haematogenous spread	Transmural/lymphatic spread
Microsatellite instability	
APC gene mutations	Decreased E-cadherin
p53, p16 inactivation	*p53, p16* inactivation

- Other histologic types include squamous cell carcinoma, adenoacanthoma, carcinoid tumours, GI stromal tumours, and lymphoma.

EARLY GASTRIC CANCER (Key Box 41.23)

- Early gastric cancer is defined as adenocarcinoma limited to the mucosa and submucosa of the stomach, regardless of lymph node status.
- The entity is common in Japan, where gastric cancer is the number one cause of cancer death, and where aggressive surveillance programs have been established.
- Approximately 10% of patients with early gastric cancer will have lymph node metastasis.
- Approximately 70% of early gastric cancers are well differentiated and 30% are poorly differentiated.
- The overall cure rate with adequate gastric resection and lymphadenectomy is 95%.
- In some Japanese centres, 50% of the gastric cancers treated are early gastric cancers.
- In the US, less than 20% of resected gastric adenocarcinomas are early gastric cancers.

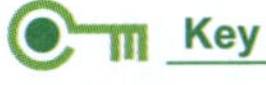

Key Box 41.23

Early Gastric Cancer (Japanese Classification)

Type I	Exophytic lesion extending into the gastric lumen
Type II	Superficial variant
IIA	Elevated lesions with a height no more than the thickness of the adjacent mucosa
IIB	Flat lesions
IIC	Depressed lesions with an eroded but not deeply ulcerated appearance
Type III	Excavated lesions that may extend into the muscularis propria without invasion of this layer by actual cancer cells

ADVANCED GASTRIC CANCER

It refers to involvement of muscularis mucosa and/or serosa with or without involvement of lymph nodes.

- The **Borrmann classification system** was developed in 1926 and remains useful today for the description of endoscopic findings (Fig. 41.63).
- The Borrmann system divides gastric carcinoma into five types depending on the lesion's **macroscopic** appearance.
  - **Type 1** represents polypoid or fungating lesions
  - **Type 2** ulcerating lesions surrounded by elevated borders
  - **Type 3** ulcerating lesions with infiltration into the gastric wall
  - **Type 4** diffusely infiltrating lesions
  - **Type 5** lesions that do not fit into any of the other categories.
- ***Linitis plastica*** is the term to describe type 4 carcinoma when it involves the entire stomach (Key Box 41.24 and Figs 41.64 to 41.66).
- The original histologic classification system was developed by Borders in 1942.
- Borders classified gastric carcinomas according to the degree of cellular differentiation, independent of morphology, and ranged from 1 (well-differentiated) to 4 (anaplastic).

WHO CLASSIFICATION: Five Main Categories

1. Adenocarcinoma 95%

- Papillary, tubular
- Mucinous
- Signet ring

2. Adenosquamous cell carcinoma

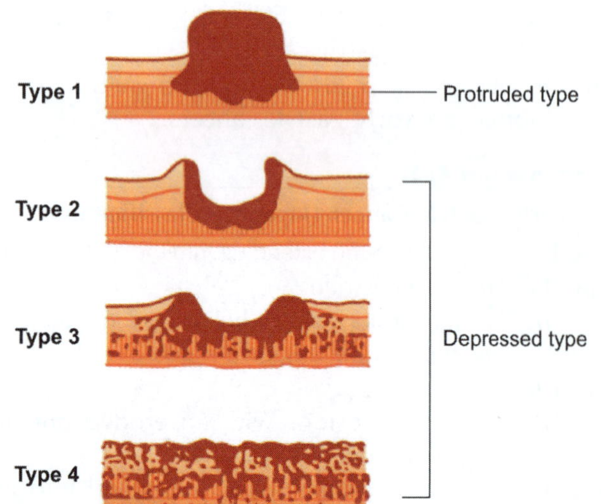

Fig. 41.63: Borrmann's classification (*refer to* advanced gastric cancer macroscopic type)

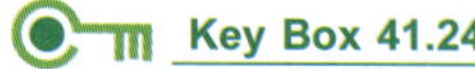 Key Box 41.24

The Diffuse Form of Gastric Adenocarcinoma—Linitis Plastica

- **Poorly differentiated**
- Lacks gland formation
- Composed of **signet ring** cells
- Consists of tiny clusters of small uniform cells
- Tends to spread submucosally
- Has less inflammatory infiltration
- **Metastases occur early**
- Intraperitoneal metastases are frequent
- Route of spread is generally by transmural extension and through lymphatic invasion
- Does not generally arise in the setting of prior gastritis
- **More common in women**
- Affects a slightly younger age group
- Association with blood type A and familial occurrences, suggesting a **genetic aetiology**
- The prognosis is less favourable for patients with diffuse-subtype histology.

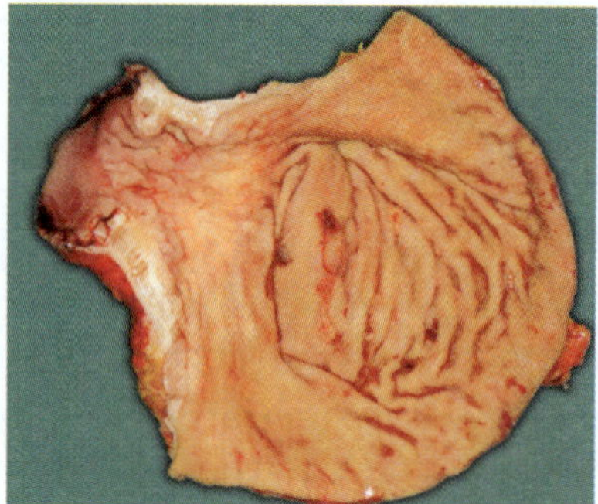

Fig. 41.64: Localised linitis plastica

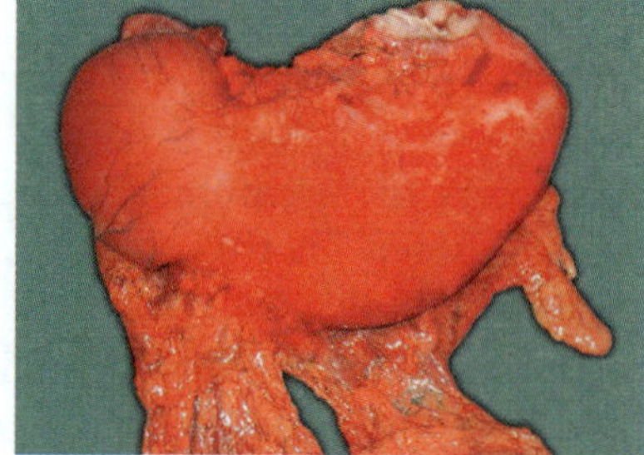

Fig. 41.65: Diffuse variety of carcinoma stomach

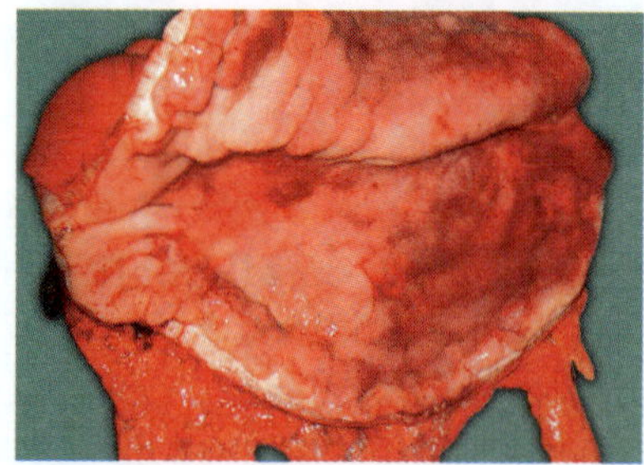

Fig. 41.66: Linitis plastica—opened specimen

3. Squamous cell carcinoma
4. Undifferentiated carcinoma
5. Unclassified carcinoma

Clinical Features of Carcinoma Stomach (SOLID)[1]

- Very often patients would have vague symptoms—early satiety, flatulence, discomfort, pain in the upper abdomen.
- Early satiety is due to decreased distensibility of the stomach (Fig. 41.67).
- Anaemia is due to many factors (Key Box 41.25).

S Silent: Growth is silent but manifests as secondaries in the liver, ascites, Virchow's node, rectovesical deposits, (Blumer's shelf), umbilical nodule (Sister Mary Joseph's nodule), left axillary nodes (Irish nodes), palpable ovarian mass (Krukenberg tumour) (Figs 41.67 to 41.72).

O Obstruction at pylorus (pyloric antrum) producing pyloric obstruction with features of vomiting with/without blood. Visible gastric peristalsis can also be present. Obstruction at cardio-oesophageal junction produces dysphagia.

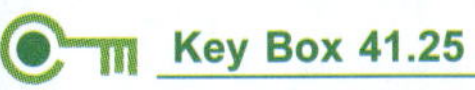

Key Box 41.25

Anaemia in Carcinoma Stomach

- This is one of the common presentations. Often patients get investigated for anaemia by the physician only to discover carcinoma stomach.
- Achlorhydria results in poor conversion of ferrous to ferric which causes anaemia.
- 15% of patients may also develop haematemesis as in ulcerative lesions or proliferative lesions. GI blood loss also accounts for anaemia.
- Early satiety, loss of appetite and poor intake also contribute to anaemia (minor role).
- 40% of carcinoma stomach patients have anaemia.

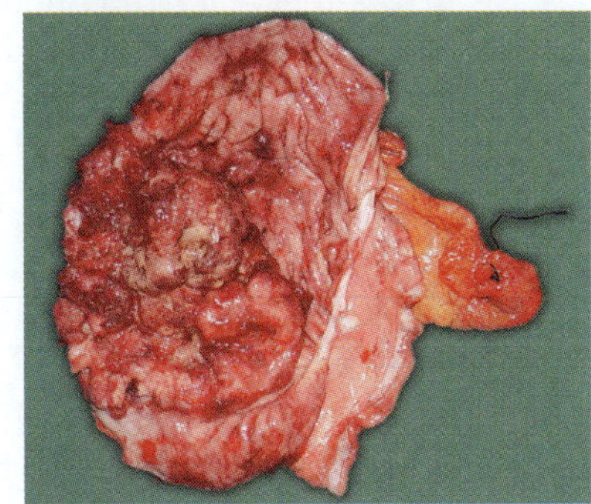

Fig. 41.67: Carcinoma stomach large ulcerative lesion with involvement of serosa

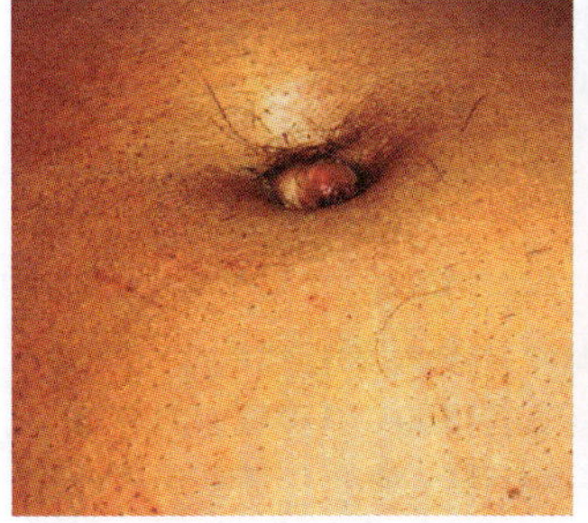

Fig. 41.68: Umbilical nodule—popularly called Sister Mary Joseph's nodule

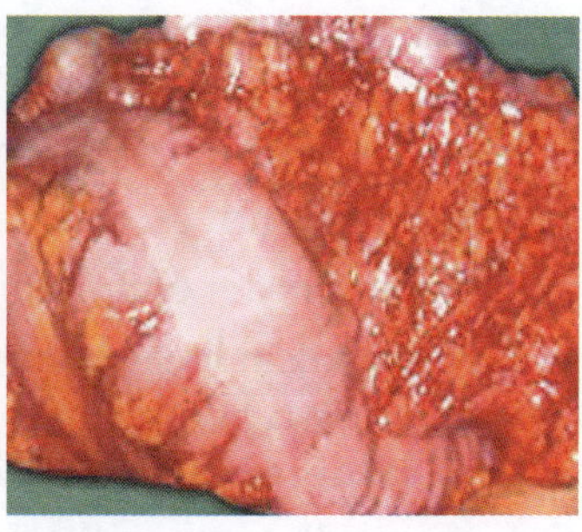

Fig. 41.69: Carcinoma stomach with nodules in the greater omentum

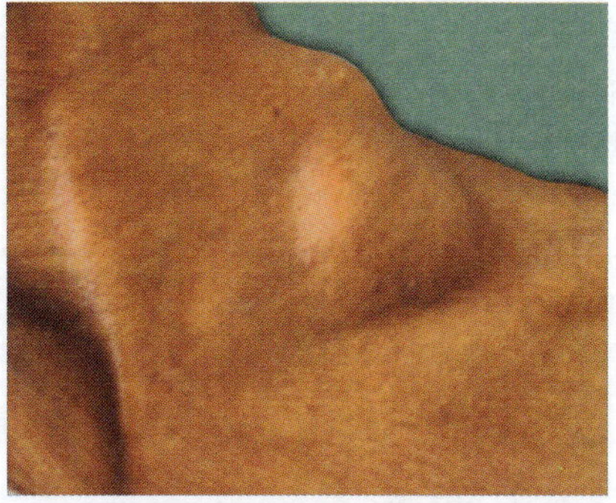

Fig. 41.70: Large supraclavicular nodes

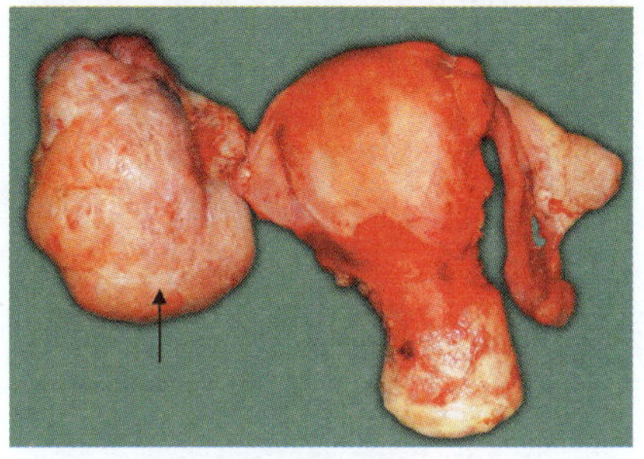

Fig. 41.71: Krukenberg tumours

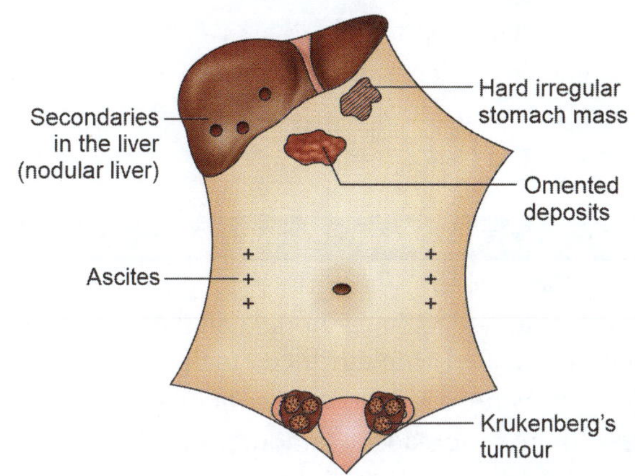

Fig. 41.72: Diagrammatic representation of secondaries in carcinoma stomach

[1]If you remember **SOLID**, you will get solid marks.

L Lump in the abdomen which is hard and irregular. Clinically, stomach mass is differentiated from liver mass by features mentioned below.

1. Stomach moves with respiration.
2. Upper border of the stomach mass can be made out.
3. Anatomical location of the mass: Right hypochondrium in a pyloric mass, epigastrium and left hypochondrium in a mass arising from body of the stomach.
4. Knee elbow position: The mass falls forwards, unless fixed.
5. The mass may have intrinsic mobility.

I Insidious in onset: Anaemia, anorexia and asthenia of short duration.

D Dyspepsia in a man over the age of 40: Carcinoma stomach should be ruled out. Early gastric cancer presents as dyspepsia.

Nonmetastatic conditions such as thrombophlebitis (Trousseau's sign) and deep venous thrombosis can occur due to change in thrombotic and haemostatic mechanisms.

Strong Suspicion of Carcinoma Stomach

- New onset dyspepsia in men >50 years of age
- Unexplained anaemia
- Unintentional weight loss
- GI bleeding
- Iron deficiency anaemia
- Progressive dysphagia

Clinical Signs of Inoperability

- Ascites
- Secondaries in the liver
- Para-aortic lymph nodes
- Krukenberg tumours
- Sister Mary Joseph nodule
- Blummer shelf deposits
- Supraclavicular nodes—Virchow node
- Irish node

Sister Marry Joseph Nodule

- Sister Mary Joseph—head nurse to William Mayo
- Was first to notice that a 'nodule' in the umbilicus was often associated with advanced malignancy
- Presents as firm, red, nontender nodule
- Results from spread of tumour within the falciform ligament
- 90% of tumours are adenocarcinomas
- Commonest primaries are stomach and ovary
- Primary tumour is almost invariably inoperable

Paraneoplastic Manifestations

- Sudden appearance of diffuse seborrhoeic keratoses (sign of Leser-Trélat) or acanthosis nigricans—velvety and darkly pigmented patches on skin folds.
- Hypercoagulable states (Trousseau's syndrome)
- Polyarteritis nodosa

Staging

Refer TNM staging. New clinical stage includes prognostic groups, cTNM, postneoadjuvant therapy pathologic stage groupings, ypTNM—new prognostic information change to anatomic boundary for staging carcinoma at oesophagogastric junction and changes to pathologic stage grouping. Refer NCCN guidelines for more details.

TNM STAGING AJCC 8th Edition

AJCC	TNM staging
Primary tumour (T)	
TX	Primary tumour cannot be assessed
T0	No evidence of primary tumour
Tis	Carcinoma *in situ*. Intraepithelial tumour without invasion of the lamina propria
T1	Tumour invades lamina propria, muscularis mucosa or submucosa
T1a	Tumour invades lamina propria or muscularis mucosa
T1b	Tumour invades submucosa
T2	Tumour invades muscularis propria
T3	Tumour penetrates subserosal connective tissue without invasion of serosa or adjacent structures
T4	Tumour invades serosa (visceral peritoneum) or adjacent structures
T4a	Tumour invades serosa (visceral peritoneum)
T4b	Tumour invades adjacent structures
Regional lymph nodes (N)	
NX	Regional lymph nodes (S) cannot be assessed
N0	No regional lymph node metastasis($)
N1	Metastasis in 1–2 regional lymph nodes
N2	Metastasis in 3–6 regional lymph nodes
N3	Metastasis in 7 or more regional lymph nodes
N3a	Metastasis in 7 to 15 regional lymph nodes
N3b	Metastasis in 16 or more regional lymph nodes
Distant metastasis (M)	
M0	No distant metastasis
M1	Distant metastasis
Histologic grade (G)	
GX	Grade cannot be assessed
G1	Well-differentiated
G2	Moderately differentiated
G3	Poorly differentiated
G4	Undifferentiated

Spread

1. **Penetration of gastric serosa:** This is the most important prognostic indicator. When serosa is NOT penetrated, 50% survive for 5 years after resection. When serosa is penetrated, this figure drops to 20%. Once serosa is involved, adjacent organs such as liver, pancreas, spleen, omentum, transverse colon get involved. **Endoscopic ultrasound** is the best investigation to detect the layers involvement in carcinoma of the stomach.
2. **Lymphatic spread:** More than 400 lymph nodes have been identified. Lymph node involvement is a poor prognostic indicator. 4 lymphatic zones have been described.
   - **Zone 1:** In the gastrocolic omentum along the right gastroepiploic vessels. This drains the pyloric antrum and lower half of greater curvature.
   - **Zone 2:** It lies in the gastrocolic omentum and gastrosplenic ligament along the left gastroepiploic vessels. This drains upper half of the greater curvature.
   - **Zone 3:** It lies in the lesser omentum draining proximal two-thirds of the stomach. From here, lymph drains into perioesophageal lymph nodes.
   - **Zone 4:** It is from distal portion of the lesser curve and pylorus along hepatic artery and right gastric artery into para-aortic nodes.
   - Lymph nodes have been given separate numbers. They are discussed under resections.
3. **Hematogenous spread:** Most common sites are liver and lungs. It produces extensive secondaries. They are signs of inoperability.
4. **Transcoelomic spread** results in ascites, Krukenberg tumour—bilateral bulky ovarian deposits and rectovesical deposits **(Blumer's shelf)**.

Investigations

1. **Complete blood picture:** 20% of early gastric cancer patients have iron deficiency (microcytic, hypochromic) anaemia. Preoperative blood transfusion may be necessary before endoscopy.
2. **Blood** sugars, ECG and Echo, renal function, liver function are assessed and ECOG score is given so that whether these patients can undergo radical surgery/preoperative–neoadjuvant chemotherapy/radiotherapy can be given or not. Preoperative optimization is done by normalizing blood sugars or renal functions or cardiac functions so as to get the best results.
3. **Flexible oesophagogastroduodenoscopy** (Figs 41.73 to 41.76)
   - Diagnosis of malignancy by ulcerated lesion with elevated edges, obliterated gastric rugae.

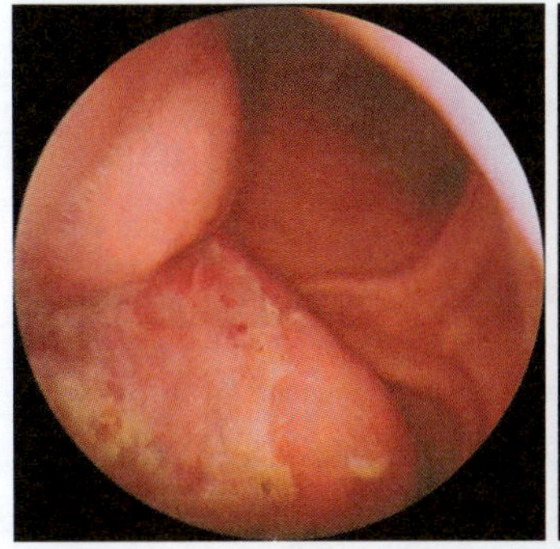

Fig. 41.73: Endoscopy showing superficial ulceration

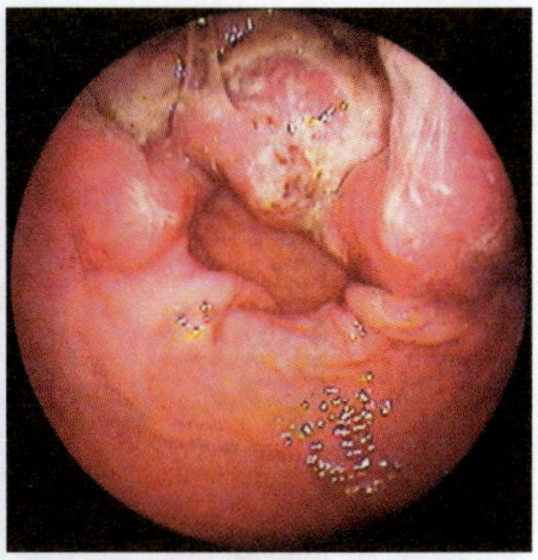

Fig. 41.74: Endoscopy showing ulceroproliferative growth

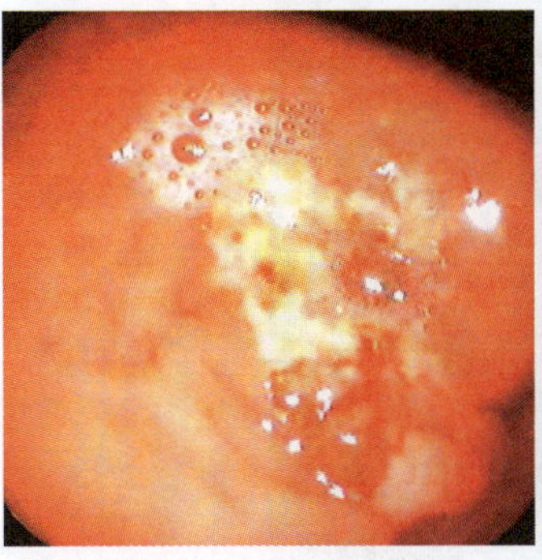

Fig. 41.75: Friable granular tissue—antral carcinoma

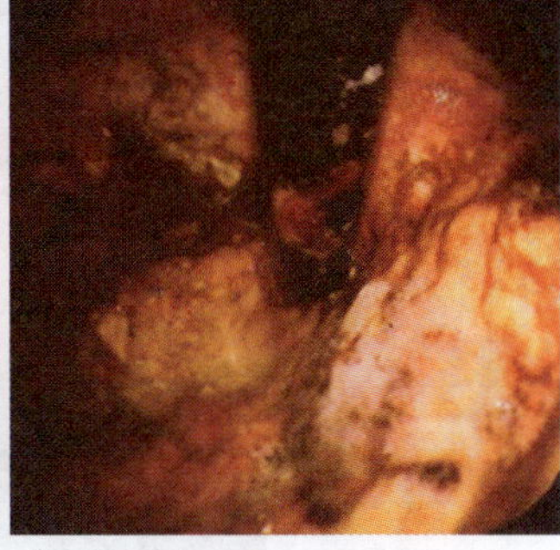

Fig. 41.76: Fundal carcinoma detected by J manoeuvre in endoscopy

   - To know the extent of the lesion
   - To confirm the diagnosis
   - To take multiple biopsy—6 to 8 pieces
   - Also, to aid brush cytology

   Biopsy is sent not only for histopathology but also for immune histochemistry. *Overexpression of HER-2 neu receptors is found in about 13 to 20% of gastric cancers.*
4. **Ultrasound of the abdomen**
   - To rule out secondaries in the liver.
   - To look for enlarged coeliac nodes.
   - Can detect ascites-guided fluid tap and cell cytology.
   - To detect Krukenberg tumour (pelvic CT).
   - Useful in detecting metastatic disease.
5. **CECT of the abdomen, pelvis and chest should be done** (Figs 41.77 and 41.78)
   - It is superior to ultrasound because it is objective and more specific.
   - Respectability—specially infiltration into pancreas, large fixed nodes at origin of left gastric artery retroperitoneal structures are better appreciated.
   - However, detection of peritoneal disease sensibility is only around 30–35%.
6. **Endoscopic ultrasonography** can detect advanced tumours in 80% of patients. Overall staging accuracy

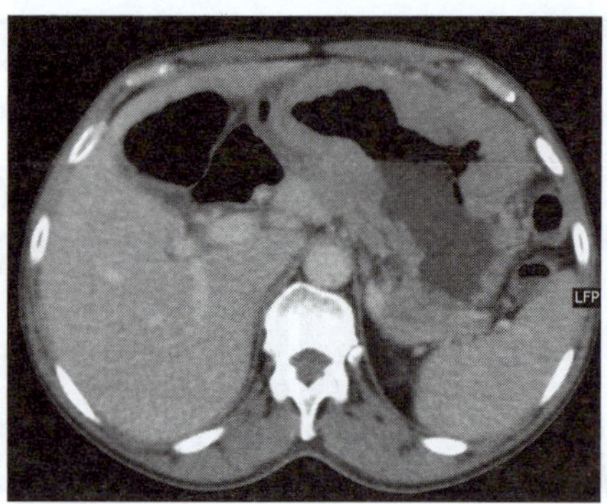

Fig. 41.77: CECT scan showing carcinoma body of the stomach—coronal section

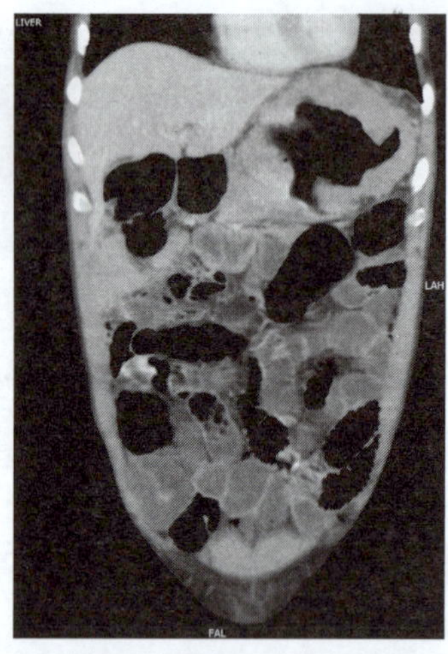

Fig. 41.78: CECT scan showing carcinoma for the body of stomach—sagittal section

is about 75%, however, it has significant limitations for staging mucosal disease. To know the T status—layers of the stomach involvement, it is the most sensitive and ideal investigation.

7. **Laparoscopy:** CT cannot detect liver or peritoneal metastasis (small <5 mm) and small lymph nodes. Laparoscopy is an ideal investigation. Almost 20 to 30% of so-called operable cases become inoperable. Laparoscopic peritoneal lavage for cytology is best test.
8. **Role of PET scan**
   - PET scanning is not routinely used in staging gastric cancer.
   - Gastric cancers have low avidity for 18F-fluoro-2-deoxyglucose.
   - In advanced cases, before doing a resection for controlling the locoregional disease, PET scan is done to rule out metastatic disease.
9. **CEA:** Carcinoembryonic antigen is elevated in about 60–70% patients. It indicates extensive spread of the disease. Also CA 19-9 (carbohydrate antigen) and alpha-fetoprotein can be done.
10. **Barium meal** has become obsolete (Fig. 41.79).

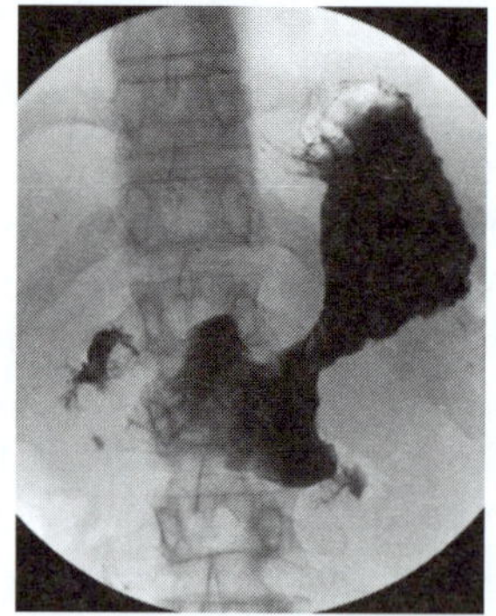

Fig. 41.79: Hourglass contracture of the stomach caused by carcinoma

Histopathology

It is an adenocarcinoma of the stomach. There are basically two types of gastric carcinomas as per **Lauren's classification.**

1. **Diffuse is more common in young, females and carries poor prognosis.** The leather-bottle stomach or linitis plastica is poorly differentiated with anaplastic cells. Signet-ring cell carcinoma and other poorly cohesive carcinomas are under diffuse variety as per WHO classification.
2. **Intestinal is more common in elderly males.** It shows areas of intestinal metaplasia. It has better prognosis. Papillary adenocarcinoma, tubular adenocarcinoma and mucinous adenocarcinoma are subtypes as per WHO classification.
   - There are so many other varieties which are grouped under indeterminate type (WHO classification). Few of them are mixed, e.g. adenosquamous, carcinoma with lymphoid type, etc.
3. HER-2 neu receptors to be checked by immunohistochemistry.

TREATMENT OF CARCINOMA STOMACH

- **Surgery is the main modality of the treatment.** Adjuvant chemotherapy has been found to be beneficial in a few patients only.
- Operable means cure is possible by doing radical surgery.
- Resectable means the growth can be removed.
- Inoperable means there are no chances of cure but growth may be resectable.

Signs of Inoperability at Surgery

- Growth infiltrating into pancreas, engulfing pedicle of left gastric vessels to pancreas or posterior abdominal wall.
- Rectovesical deposits, due to peritoneal seedings which are felt during per rectal examination.

- Enlarged, fixed coeliac nodes, para-aortic nodes.
- Ascites, peritoneal deposits.

Types of Resection

- Curative resection (R0) should be done whenever possible. Minimum 5 cm margin is required proximally. If serosa is involved, it qualifies for T3/T4 and not for curative resection
- Stage IA: Regionally confined disease should undergo primary surgical R-0 resection—radical subtotal gastrectomy.
- Stage T1a: Endoscopic resection for tumours less than 2 cm—curative.
- Stage II and III: Neoadjuvant therapy followed by radical resection. Curative but about 20%.
- Stage IV or inoperable patient with vomiting, if facilities are available, endoscopic stenting can be offered. Majority of these patients succumb to the disease by 3-6 months. Gastrojejunostomy is also another option provided some part of body of the stomach is healthy to consider anastomosis.
- Stage IV patient with bleeding, if fit for surgery: Palliative gastrectomy can be done to remove a fungating, ulcerative, bleeding mass. It gives better palliation.

Terminology

- Japanese Research Society for gastric cancer advocates very aggressive resection including lymphadenectomy (Fig. 41.80). Hence, more details of lymph node station are given in Table 41.9. However, the rest of the cancer research groups were not able to produce the same results as the Japanese.
- D1 resection refers to the removal of primary group of nodes such as nodes along the lesser and greater curvature, and juxtapyloric nodes. If tumour and N1

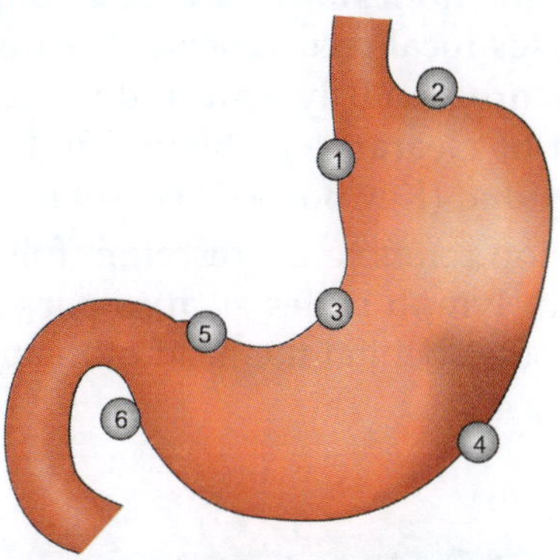

Fig. 41.80: Perigastric nodes: (1) Right pericardial; (2) left pericardial; (3) lesser curvature; (4) greater curvature; (5) suprapyloric; (6) infrapyloric

Table 41.9 Grouping of regional lymph nodes

Lymph node station (number)	Description	Location of primary tumour in the stomach: Upper third	Middle third	Lower third
1	Right paracardial	1	1	2
2	Left paracardial	1	3	M
3	Lesser curvature	1	1	1
4	Short gastric	1	3	M
4	Left gastroepiploic	1	1	3
4	Right gastroepiploic	2	1	1
5	Suprapyloric	3	1	1
6	Infrapyloric	3	1	1
7	Left gastric artery	2	2	2
8	Anterior common hepatic	2	2	2
8	Posterior common hepatic	3	3	3
9	**Coeliac artery**	2	2	2
10	**Splenic hilum**	2	3	M
11	Proximal splenic	2	2	2
11	Distal splenic	2	3	M
12	Hepatoduodenal	3	2	2
13	**Retropancreatic**	M	3	3
14	Superior mesenteric vein	M	3	2
14	Superior mesenteric artery	M	M	M
15	Middle colic (mesocolon)	M	M	M
16	Aortic hiatus (para-aortic)	3	M	M
17	Around lower oesophagus	–	–	–
18	Supradiaphragmatic	–	–	–

Numbers 1–3: Group number   M = Lymph nodes regarded as distant metastasis

nodes (group 1) resected = D1 gastrectomy. **This will become curative resection when lymph nodes are clinically not enlarged (N0) but they are removed** (Fig. 41.81).

- D2 resection refers to the removal of lymph nodes such as left gastric, common hepatic, splenic, retropancreatic nodes, etc. If tumour and N2 nodes (group 2) resected = D2 gastrectomy.

  This will become curative resection when lymph nodes are clinically enlarged (N1). So one step higher lymph nodes are cleared. Carcinoma stomach often causes local recurrence at the tumour site or in the locoregional lymph nodes. So aggressive approach of clearance of lymph nodes have been recommended (Key Box 41.26 and Fig. 41.82).
- D3 resection refers to D2 resection followed by the removal of lymph nodes such as para-aortic, porta hepatis nodes, behind the head of the pancreas, etc. (not done).

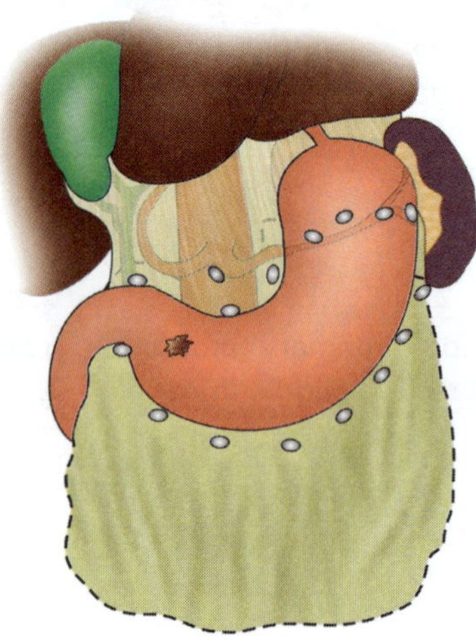

Fig. 41.81: Extent of D1 resection of tumour in distal one-third of stomach

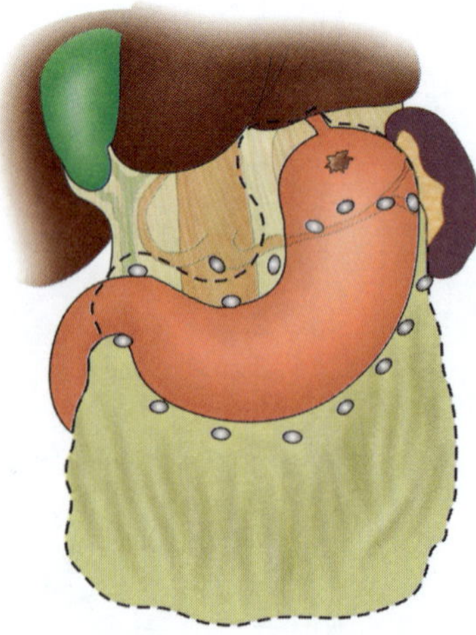

Fig. 41.82: D2 resection of tumours of the proximal third of stomach

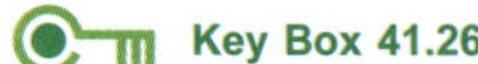

Key Box 41.26

Pathological Basis for D2 Dissection

- Gastric cancer has a great propensity to spread through the rich plexus of lymphatics of the stomach to local or regional lymph nodes. Hence, the need to remove stomach and lymph nodes.
- **Gastric cancer, unlike breast cancer, remains for a long time as a locoregional disease.**
- It is striking too, that when gastric cancer recurs it often does so locoregionally rather than more wide-spread dissemination.
- It is very rare for gastric cancer to recur 5 years after surgery, whereas for breast cancer, disseminated micrometastases continue to take their toll some 10–20 years after surgery.

Curative Resections

A. Gastrectomy and B. Endoscopic mucosal resections.

The term R status was first described by Hermanek in 1994 and is used to describe the tumour status after resection (Key Box 41.27). If no disease is identified in the lymph nodes, N0 nomenclature is used.

A. *Gastrectomy:* The extent of the gastrectomy (Figs 41.83 to 41.88) is site-dependent and focuses on complete removal of the gastric carcinoma with preferably a 5 cm margin from the gross edge of the tumour. Clearly, anatomic limitations influence this margin because in antral lesions close to or involving the pylorus, only a limited portion of the duodenum can be removed. In patients with a distal lesion, essentially a distal subtotal gastrectomy is performed regardless of T stage.

- **For proximal gastric cancers (fundic),** total gastrectomy is required.
- **For midbody or more extensive lesions**, total gastrectomy is required.
- **For more distal lesions,** a subtotal gastrectomy is the preferred approach.

Key Box 41.27

R-Resections

- R0 describes a microscopically margin-negative resection, in which no gross or microscopic tumour remains in the tumour bed.
- R1 indicates removal of all macroscopic disease but microscopic margins are positive for tumour.
- R2 indicates gross residual disease. Since the extent of resection can influence survival, some authors include this R designation to complement the TNM system.
- Long-term survival can be expected only after a R0 resection; therefore, a significant effort should be made to avoid R1 or R2 resections.

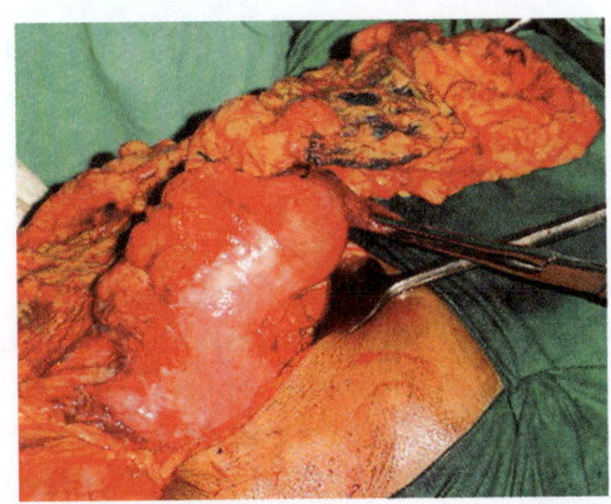

Fig. 41.83: Carcinoma stomach with involvement of serosa, endosonogram can detect this

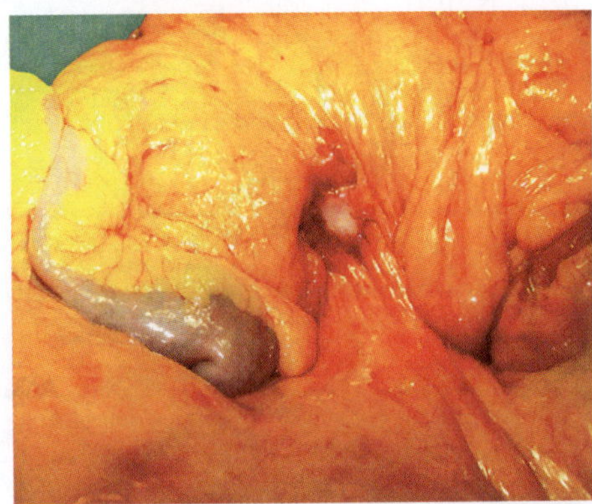

Fig. 41.84: Peritoneal metastasis from carcinoma stomach. Laparoscopy is the most ideal investigation to detect peritoneal metastasis

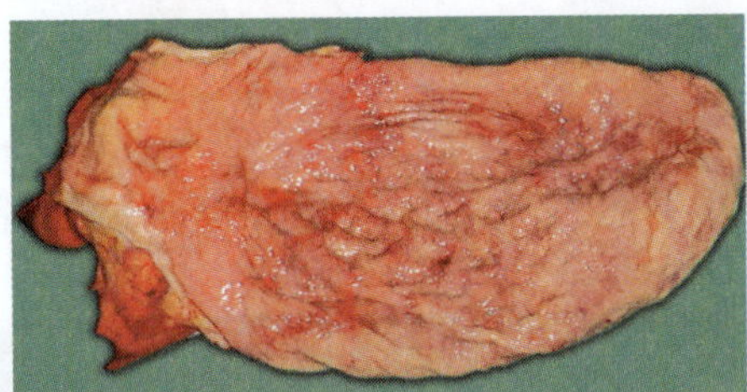

Fig. 41.85: Intestinal type—gland formation present, similar to adenocarcinoma colon—good prognosis

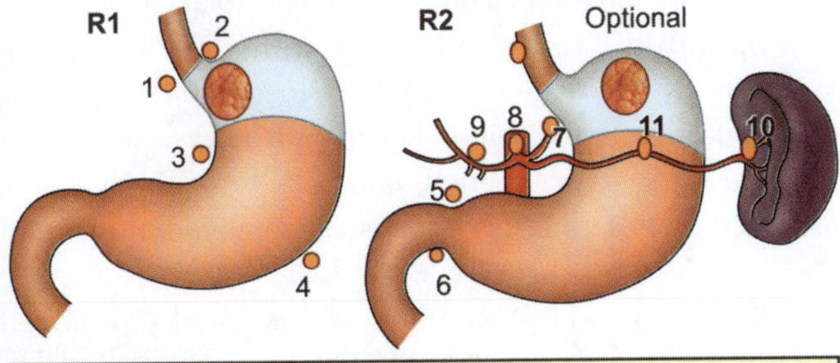
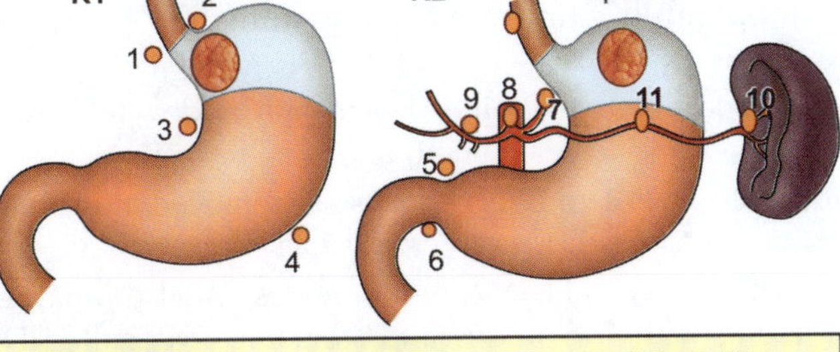

1. Right cardiac	5. Suprapyloric	10. Splenic hilar
2. Left cardiac	6. Infrapyloric	11. Splenic
3. Lesser curvature	7. Left gastric	
4. Greater curvature (and short gastric)	8. Hepatic	
	9. Coeliac	

Fig. 41.86: Proximal gastric cancer

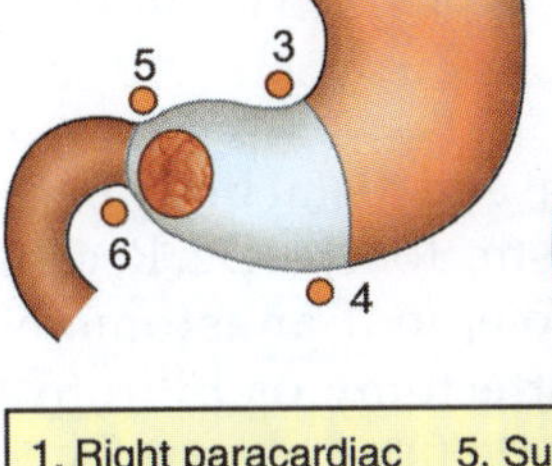

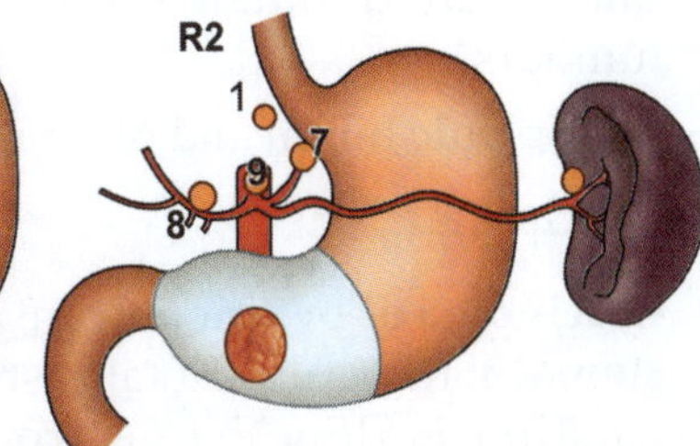

1. Right paracardiac	5. Suprapyloric	8. Hepatic
3. Lesser curvature	6. Infrapyloric	9. Coeliac
4. Greater curvature	7. Left gastric	

Fig. 41.87: Distal gastric cancer

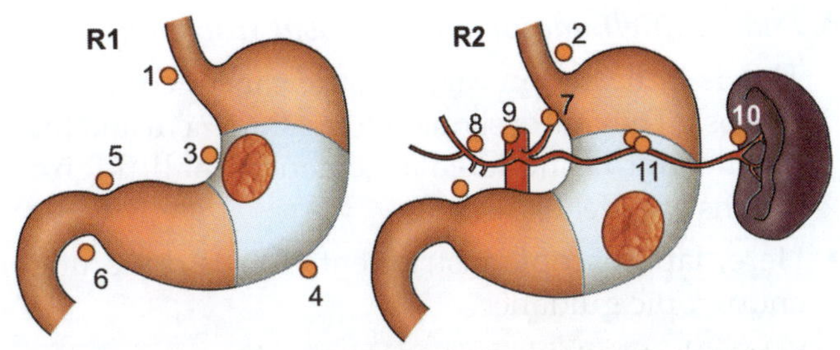

1. Right paracardiac	5. Suprapyloric	9. Coeliac
2. Left paracardiac	6. Infrapyloric	10. Splenic hilar
3. Lesser curvature	7. Left gastric	11. Splenic
4. Greater curvature	8. Hepatic	

Fig. 41.88: Mid-body gastric cancer

- **Extended organ resection** is reserved for patients with apparently node-negative T4 lesions, in which complete resection requires resection of the invaded portions of the diaphragm, pancreas, spleen, adrenal gland or colon.
- These patients usually are pretreated with chemotherapy.

Example:

Suregry: A standard D2 resection for gastric cancer involves:

1. Removing part or whole of the stomach.
2. The N1 (groups 1–6) and N2 (groups 7–11) lymph nodes. Minimum of 15 lymph nodes need to be removed. More centers are recommending more lymph nodes removal.
3. The greater and lesser omentum and omental bursa.
4. The spleen and tail of the pancreas are removed, if infiltrated by the tumours of the proximal stomach in order to remove groups 10 and 11 lymph nodes. All attempts should be made to preserve these structures but remove lymph nodes.

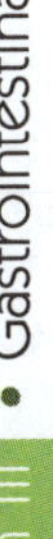

5. The hepatoduodenal nodes—level 12—in antral tumours.
7. The splenic hilum and other nodes—level 10, 11, 12.

Reconstruction

- **Carcinoma of pyloric antrum and distal body of the stomach:** Radical subtotal gastrectomy—D2. Reconstruction is done by gastrojejunal anastomosis. Popularly called Polya gastrectomy or Billroth II anastomosis (Figs 41.89 and 41.90).
- **Carcinoma of proximal stomach and diffuse carcinoma:** Radical oesophagogastrectomy (Figs 41.91 and 41.92): Removal of the entire stomach, lower end of oesophagus, with regional lymph nodes N2, followed by oesophagojejunal anastomosis.

B. *Endoscopic/Endoluminal mucosal resection*

- This is indicated in early gastric cancer confined to mucosa. The cancer should be less than 2 cm and there should not be node enlargement. Small, high up lesions are ideal.
- Here, laparoscopic instrumentation is done under endoscopic guidance.
- Stomach is suitable for endoluminal surgery because it can be distended, and contents are sterile.
- Ideally cancer should be elevated variety and well differentiated.
- Normal saline is injected into submucosal plane and lesion gets elevated.

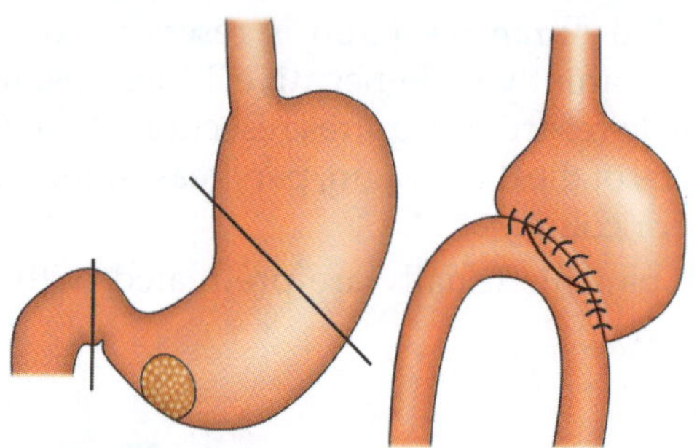

Figs 41.89 and 41.90: Radical subtotal gastrectomy with Billroth II anastomosis

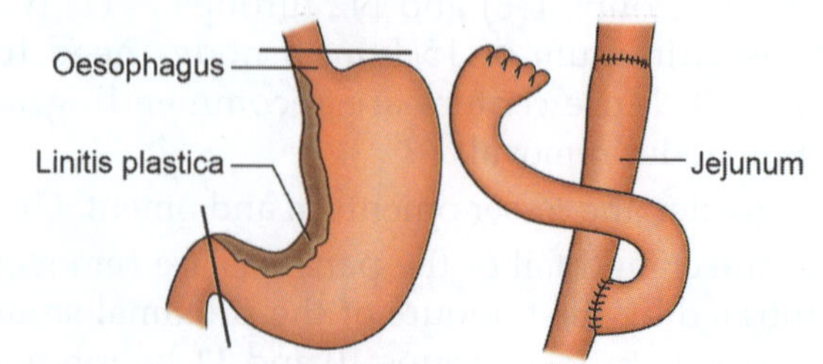

Figs 41.91 and 41.92: Radical total gastrectomy, with Roux-en-Y oesophagojejunostomy

- It is excised with 1 cm margin up to muscularis propria at a deeper plane.

Palliative Resections

1. Carcinoma pyloric antrum (inoperable): Palliative anterior GJ (Fig. 41.93) is done to relieve vomiting, by anastomosing a jejunal loop to the stomach in the prepyloric region. If posterior GJ is done, the growth may involve the GJ stoma early resulting in stomal obstruction. With anterior GJ, entero-enterostomy can be added to prevent bilious vomiting.
2. Palliative gastrectomy to get rid of ulcerated, necrotic or bleeding lesion.

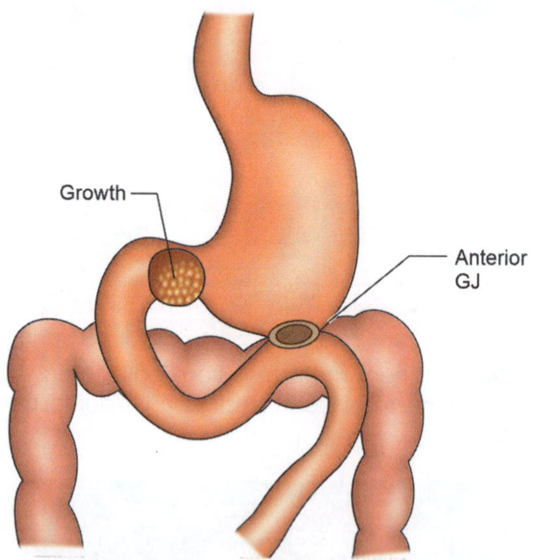

Fig. 41.93: Palliative anterior GJ

KEY POINTS ON SURGERY FOR CARCINOMA STOMACH

1. Carcinoma antrum and body—radical subtotal gastrectomy.
2. Carcinoma proximal stomach—radical total gastrectomy.
3. Inoperable carcinoma distal stomach—palliative anterior GJ.
4. Radical refers to removal of lymph nodes, fat, fascia greater and lesser omentum.
5. When level 1 to 6 (N1) nodes are removed along with stomach, it is D1 gastrectomy.
6. When level 7–11 (N2) lymph nodes are also removed along with 1–6 nodes and stomach, it is called D2 gastrectomy.
7. Early gastric cancer without lymph nodes can be treated with endoscopic mucosal resection or endoluminal gastric resection.
8. Palliative gastrectomy (subtotal) is worth considering in appropriate cases of obstruction/bleeding.

Role of Chemotherapy

A. The Adjuvant Treatment

Postoperative chemotherapy:

- Now it is understood that gastric cancers partially respond to chemotherapy—in about 30% of cases given at advanced stage (results are better than cancer colon). Injection 5-FU (fluorouracil) 500 mg IV daily for five days, every 28 days. It can be given by IV infusion or IV bolus over 15 minutes.
- **Mechanism of action:** It is an antimetabolite and acts by interfering with DNA synthesis. Side effects are myelosuppression, mucositis, excessive lacrimation, nausea, vomiting, etc.
- Combination of 5-FU with adriamycin, mitomycin and cisplatin has also been tried. However, toxicity is more with these drugs. FAM (5-fluorouracil, adriamycin and mitomycin C) and ECF (epirubicin, cisplatin and 5-FU) are popular agents.
- Intraperitoneal mitomycin and mitomycin C—impregnated charcoal have also been used (target the recurrence site—gastric bed).

Indications:

1. R0 resection (free margins): Any tumour greater than T2 including selected T2 cases should be considered for adjuvant therapy that includes 1 cycle of 5-FU+/− leucovorin OR capecitabine chemotherapy followed by 5-FU+/− leucovorin OR capecitabine based chemoradiation 3–4 more cycles of 5-FU+/− leucovorin OR capecitabine chemotherapy.
2. R1 (microscopic margin positive) and R2 (grossly positive margins) regardless of the TMN stage should receive chemoradiation followed by further cycles of adjuvant chemotherapy.
3. If the patient has received preoperative chemotherapy/chemoradiation then:
   A. Adjuvant treatment is usually recommended beyond T2N0M0 which is usually 5-FU+/− leucovorin OR capecitabine based.
   B. If patient has received ONLY preoperative chemotherapy and the resection was R1/R2, then postoperative chemoradiation is advised.

B. Neoadjuvant Chemoradiation

It is advised in medically fit unresectable—locally advanced diseases which generally includes concurrent 5-FU/capecitabine-based chemotherapy.

- Chemotherapy alone may also be used as a neoadjuvant modality.
- Recommended radiotherapy dose is 45–50.4 Gy (at 1.8 Gy/fraction).
- *Trastuzumab (Herceptin) can be used in metastatic or locally advanced gastric adenocarcinomas which are* **overexpressing HER-2 neu receptors** in about 13 to 20% of gastric cancers.

Role of Radiotherapy

External beam radiotherapy can also be used in metastatic cases as a part of palliation, especially when there is tumour bleed, gastric outlet obstruction due to the tumour pain. Dose for palliative radiotherapy is generally 30 Gy in 10 fractions over 2 weeks.

OTHER TUMOURS OF THE STOMACH

GASTROINTESTINAL STROMAL TUMOURS (GISTs)

- Previously named leiomyoma, leiomyosarcoma is called GIST today.
- In gastrointestinal tract, **stomach is the commonest** site of GIST.
- **Bleeding** is the commonest presentation. It occurs due to ulceration of mucosa which on endoscopy gives **appearance of cervix** (Fig. 41.94A and B).
- Larger tumours can present with dysphagia, weight loss, anaemia and palpable mass (Fig. 41.95).

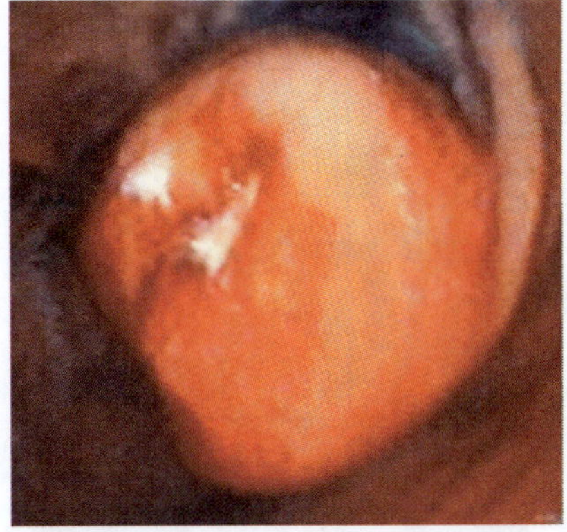

Fig. 41.94A: Bleeding ulcer of the stomach

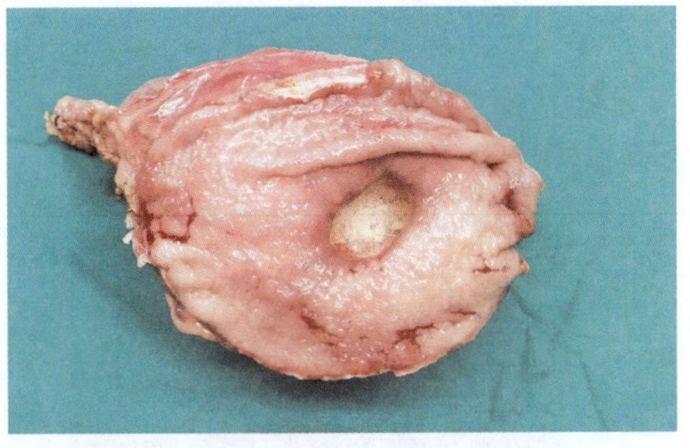

Fig. 41.94B: Wide excision specimen of GIST of the stomach showing ulcer crater. (*Courtesy:* Dr SS Prasad, Former Professor of Surgery, KMC Manipal)

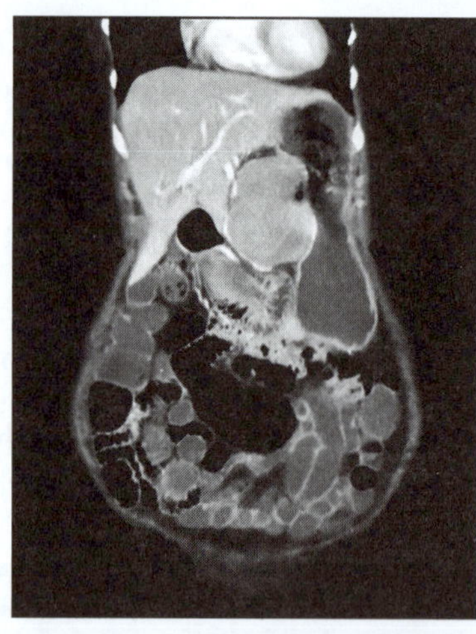

Fig. 41.95: Large GIST with air pocket. Torricelli-Bernoulli sign

- ***The diagnosis of malignancy is by greater mitotic figures.***
- **If mucosa is not ulcerated, 'biopsy on a biopsy'** or 'well biopsy' is necessary.
- Immunohistochemistry is mandatory for diagnosis—**C Kit gene amplification: It is the tumour marker of GIST.**
- CT scan is a useful investigation (Fig. 41.96).
- Resection is the best treatment (Fig. 41.97).

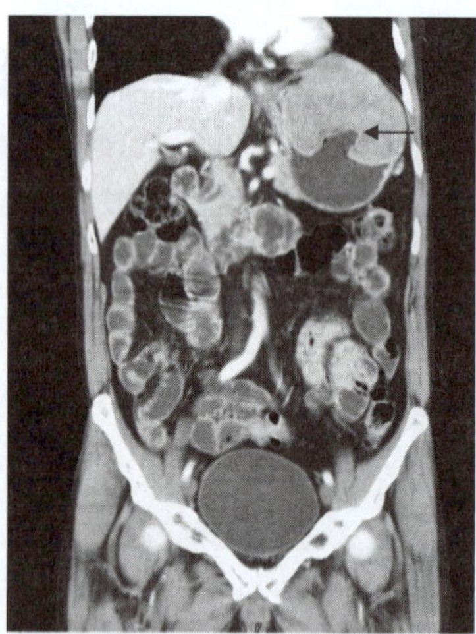

Fig. 41.96: CT GIST fundus

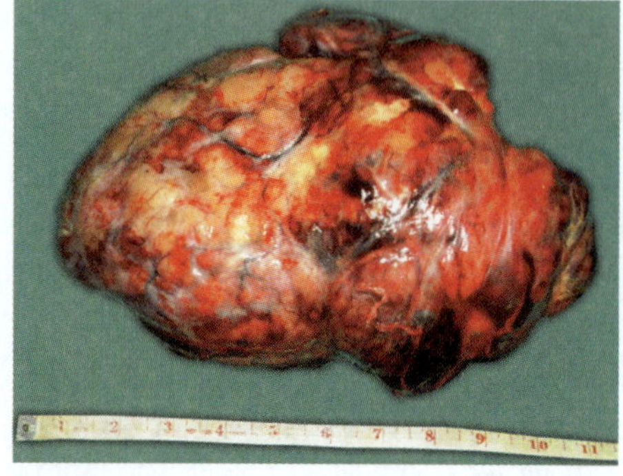

Fig. 41.97: GIST specimen

Chemotherapy for GIST

Capsule Imatinib 100 mg 4 capsules—to a total of 400 mg per day is given till toxicity appears or metastasis or residual tumour regresses (investigated by CT scan).

GASTRIC LYMPHOMA

- Incidence of primary gastric lymphoma is increasing.
- They are B cell derived from mucosa associated lymphoid tissue (**MALT**)—**MALTOMA**.
- Pain, weight loss, bleeding are common presentations.
- **6th decade** is the common age group.
- Endoscopic features are not specific but diffuse thickening with or without ulcerations may be seen.
- It is important to rule out **generalised process** by CT, ultrasound, bone marrow aspirate.
- Gastrectomy is the best treatment.
- Chemotherapy is better for systemic disease.

Pearls of Wisdom

Low-grade lymphoma associated with *H. pylori* infection may regress and totally disappear after eradication treatment for *H. pylori*.

COMPLICATIONS OF VAGOTOMY AND GJ

Can be classified as complications of vagotomy, complications of GJ and complications of gastrectomy.

1. Stasis of food in the stomach resulting in nausea, loss of appetite, distension of upper abdomen, foul eructation, etc.
2. Denervation of gallbladder can cause gallstones.
3. Postvagotomy **diarrhoea**—can be very troublesome at times (Key Box 41.28).
4. Vagotomy produces hypoacidity which allows bacterial proliferation. Nitrates are reduced to nitrites which are carcinogenic. Such a malignancy which develops at GJ site is called **stump carcinoma**.

Key Box 41.28

Causes of Diarrhoea

- Vagotomy results in removal of parasympathetic influence on the function of foregut and midgut.
- Fast gastric emptying occurring due to GJ or gastrectomy.
- Hypoacidity resulting in bacterial proliferation causing enteritis.
- Bile salts also play a role.

1. STOMAL OBSTRUCTION

It is due to oedema as in gastroduodenal anastomosis or nondependent drainage as in GJ. Sometimes, fat in the transverse mesocolon undergoes necrosis resulting in obstruction to the loops. Stomal obstruction also develops, if there is narrowing of the lumen. Treatment is conservative. Surgery may also be required later, after confirming obstruction by gastrografin studies.

2. RETROGRADE JEJUNOGASTRIC INTUSSUSCEPTION (Fig. 41.98)

It develops if efferent and afferent loops are not sutured properly. It can appear at any time after surgery.

Clinical Features

- Previous history of abdominal surgery (surgery done for peptic ulcer)
- Acute abdominal pain in upper abdomen
- Vomiting, sometimes blood stained
- **Palpable mass** in the upper abdomen.

Investigation

Barium meal X-ray shows filling defect in the stomach (Fig. 41.99). Sometimes, following a barium meal, intussusception is reduced.

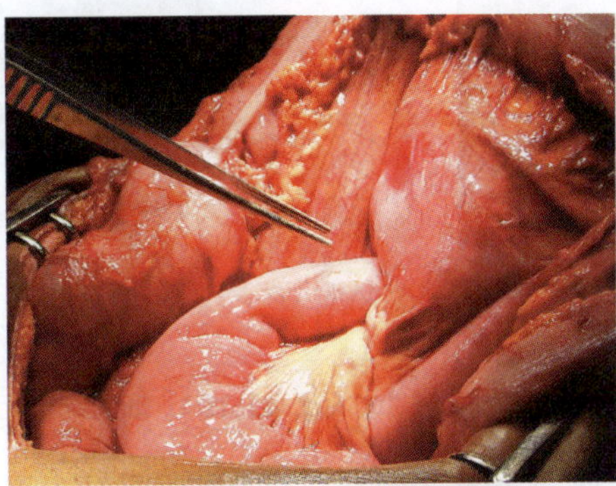

Fig. 41.98: Jejunogastric intussusception

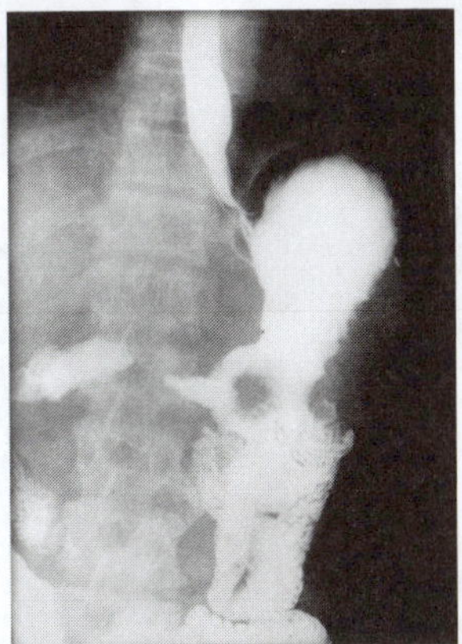

Fig. 41.99: Barium showing filling defect, in a patient who had undergone GJ

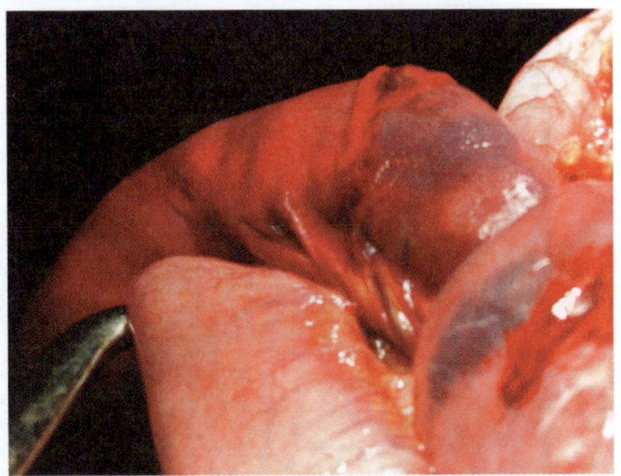

Fig. 41.100: Gangrene in jejunogastric intussusception

Treatment

Reduction of the intussusception and suturing of intestinal loops properly. If the loops are gangrenous, resection may be necessary (Fig. 41.100).

Complication

Gangrene of intestine.

3. GASTROJEJUNOCOLIC FISTULA

- It is a complication of GJ done for peptic ulcer, especially when vagotomy is not done or is incomplete.
- After a few years of GJ, a recurrent ulcer can develop at the stoma—GJ site.
- This recurrent ulcer slowly invades the adjacent structure such as the transverse colon resulting in gastrojejunocolic fistula.

Clinical Features

- Previous history of vagotomy and GJ.
- Foul eructation and foul vomiting due to colonic contents entering the stomach which is loaded with faecal matter and foul contents.
- Intense diarrhoea due to severe jejunitis brought about by colonic bacteria entering the jejunum.
- Rapid deterioration in health—loss of weight, loss of appetite, dehydration and emaciation.

Pearls of Wisdom

Diarrhoea is not due to food entering the colon. Contents of the colon enter the stomach and then jejunum resulting in jejunitis causing diarrhoea.

Diagnosis

Confirm by barium enema—barium entering the stomach (because of high pressure in the colon). Barium meal study should not be done (Fig. 41.101).

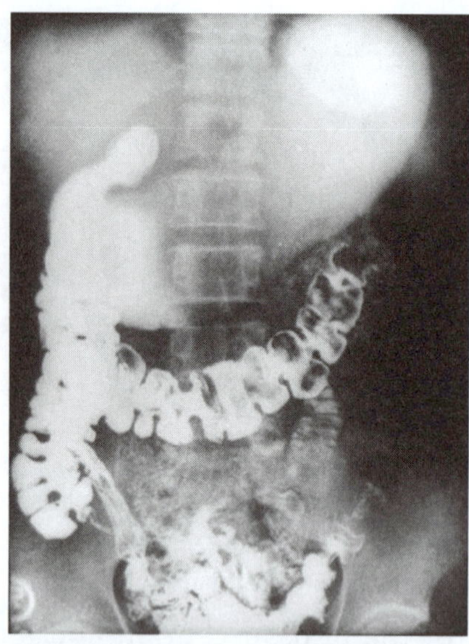

Fig. 41.101: Barium enema —barium entering into the stomach from colon (barium meal is not the investigation for gastrojejunocolic fistula)

Treatment

- Triple resection (Figs 41.102 to 41.104).
- Preoperative preparation is necessary in the form of blood transfusion, stomach wash, nutritional supplementation and correction of dehydration.
- Resection of portions of stomach, intestine and colon followed by end-to-end anastomosis.

4. STUMP CARCINOMA (Figs 41.105 to 41.107)

- It refers to carcinoma developing in the stomach after some surgery on the stomach. Classically, it happens after a gastrojejunostomy (GJ) Billroth II or after a pyloroplasty.
- It develops after 10 to 20 years of surgery.
- Reflux of bile, changes in the acidity due to vagotomy are a few factors that precipitate stump carcinoma. Metaplasia is due to enterogastric reflux and bacterial reduction of nitrates.

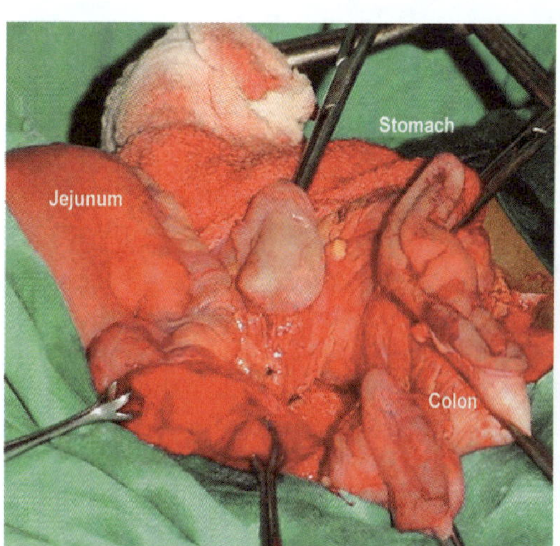

Fig. 41.102: Specimen of triple resection

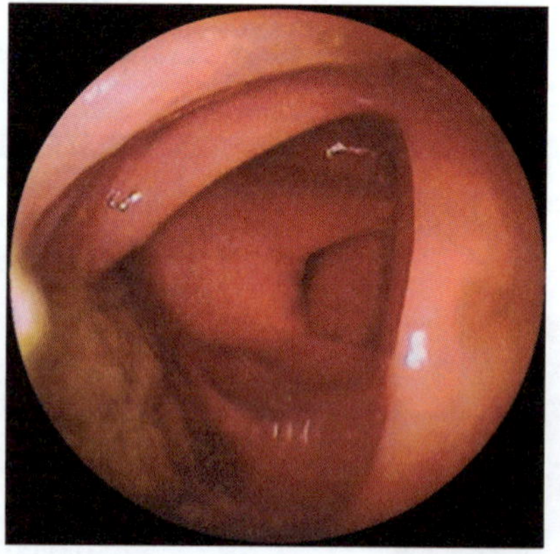

Fig. 41.103: Gastrojejunocolic fistula—gastroscopy shows faecal matter in the stomach, coming from colon (see the triangular folds of colon)

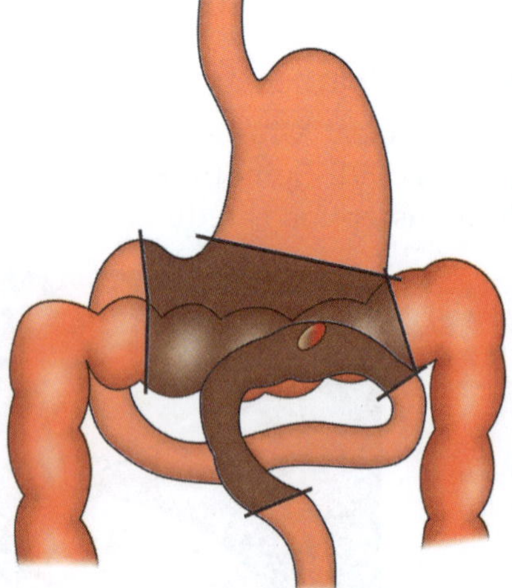

Fig. 41.104: Triple resection

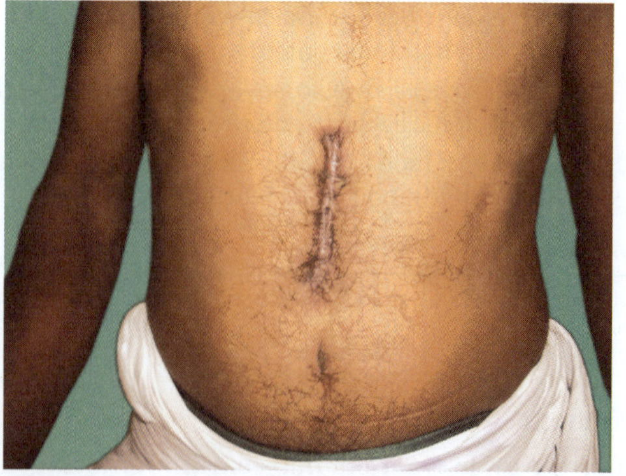

Fig. 41.105: GJ was done in this patient 20 years back. He came with stump carcinoma

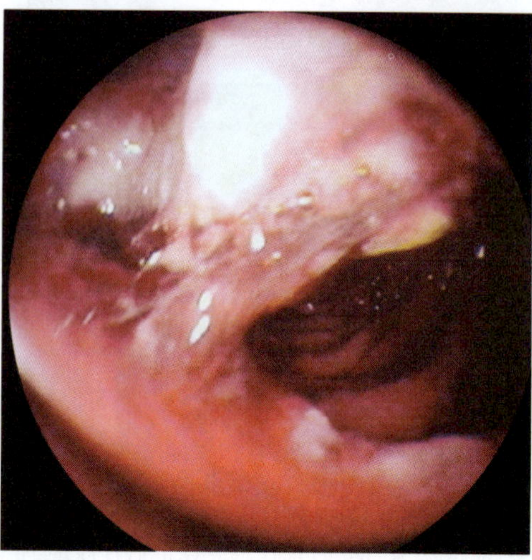

Fig. 41.106: Endoscopy showing stump carcinoma

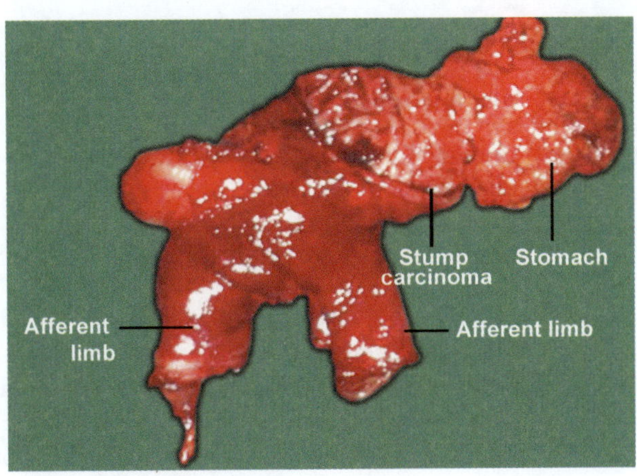

Fig. 41.107: Gastrectomy for stump carcinoma

- Clinical features include sudden loss of appetite, loss of weight with or without mass abdomen.
- Diagnosis is by endoscopy (Fig. 41.106).
- Treated by resection. However, many cases are advanced and they are inoperable.

5. GASTROILEOSTOMY (Fig. 41.108)

- It is an avoidable complication.
- Instead of the short loop—jejunum, ileum is anastomosed to the stomach.
- There will be severe uncontrolled diarrhoea, loss of weight and emaciation within a short period.
- Barium meal with fluoroscopy should be done which shows rapid flow of barium from stomach into the ileum.
- Laparotomy—undoing of gastroileostomy and fresh gastrojejunostomy should be done.

6. POSTCIBAL SYNDROMES

This syndrome complex results due to rapid emptying of stomach contents to the distal intestines resulting in various physiological changes such as vasomotor symptoms, hypoglycaemia, etc. They are of two types. Their comparison is given in Table 41.10.

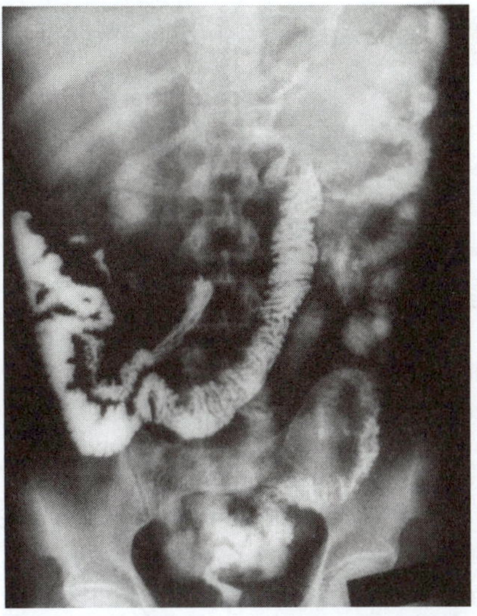

Fig. 41.108: Gastroileostomy—the biggest blunder a surgeon can do—it can be avoided by identifying the duodenojejunal flexure

Pearls of Wisdom

Alkaline reflux gastritis which develops after GJ should be differentiated from afferent loop syndrome (Table 41.11).

COMPLICATIONS OF GASTRECTOMY

1. NUTRITIONAL DISTURBANCES

- Vitamin B_{12} and calcium deficiency.
- Megaloblastic anaemia occurs late due to gastric mucosal atrophy.
- **Iron deficiency anaemia**, common after gastrectomy when duodenum is bypassed because of deficient iron absorption.

Table 41.10 Dumping syndrome—postcibal syndromes

	Early	Late
1. Onset	Increased emptying immediately after meals	One to two hours afterwards.
2. Causes	Rapid passage of food of high osmolarity from stomach into small intestine causes hypovolaemia. It is also due to loss of pyloric sphincter)	Initial hyperglycaemia causes increased release of insulin which is followed by hypoglycaemia.
3. Relief	Lying down	Glucose
4. Aggravating factors	More food, glucose, fullness	Exercise
5. Symptoms	Epigastric distension, sweating, diarrhoea	Tremors, fainting attacks (release of adrenaline)
6. Treatment	Small quantity, dry food. Over a period of time, symptoms settle down, less sugar content	Dietary adjustment of food
7. Incidence	More common (10%)	Less common (5%)

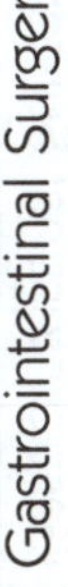

Table 41.11 Comparison of chronic afferent limb syndrome and alkaline reflux gastritis

	Chronic afferent limb syndrome	Alkaline reflux gastritis
• Pain	After meals	Unrelated to meals
• Vomitus	Bile	Bile and food
	Relieves pain	No changes in pain
	Projectile	Nonprojectile
• Occult bleeding	Rare	Common
• Cause	Limb obstruction—long loop	Enterogastric reflux (no obstruction)
• Treatment	Avoid a long loop at surgery	High fat, amino acid regimen
	Convert Billroth II to Billroth I	Proton pump inhibitors
	Roux-en-Y jejunostomy or	Ursodeoxycholic acid
	jejunojejunostomy	Jejunojejunostomy, converting Billroth II to Billroth
	(Braun modification of Billroth II)	I can be done

- **Diarrhoea** is due to vagotomy causing intestinal hurry or due to dumping.
- Due to poor nutrition, there is **weight loss** and they are susceptible for **pulmonary tuberculosis.**

2. DUODENAL FISTULA (duodenal blow out)

It is the leakage of duodenal contents to the exterior. It commonly occurs after surgery.

Causes

- After a partial gastrectomy/total gastrectomy, where the closure of duodenum was difficult.
- After closure of perforated duodenal ulcer, which gives way once again.
- Injuries to duodenum during right hemicolectomy, right nephrectomy, etc.

Precipitating Factors

- Faulty technique of closure of duodenal stump.
- Severely inflamed duodenum due to an active ulcer.
- If there is a distal obstruction, it increases tension in duodenal loop and may result in fistula.
- Ischaemia of duodenal stump.

Clinical Features

- Signs and symptoms develop usually after 4 to 5 days when oral fluids are commenced. These stimulate outpouring of biliary and pancreatic juices.
- Severe upper abdominal pain and guarding, rigidity, hypotension and shock-like features of biliary peritonitis develop, if there is no drainage tube.
- If drainage tube is kept in the first surgery, bile flows to the exterior. In such cases, signs of peritonitis are usually not present. However, severe electrolyte imbalance can occur (Fig. 41.109).

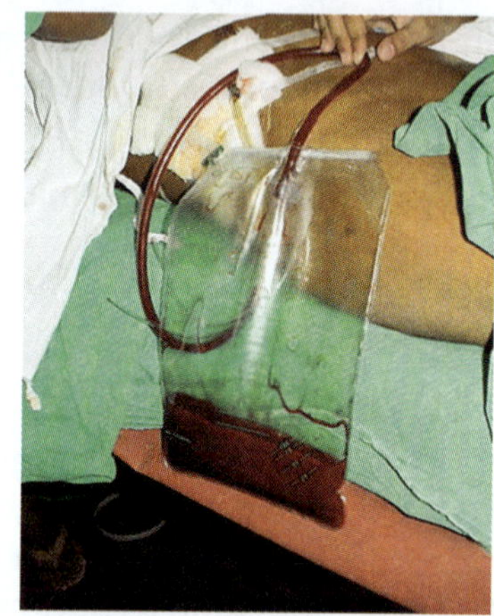

Fig. 41.109: Duodenal blow out following gastrectomy

Treatment

- Conservative treatment is successful in majority of the cases. Fistula heals in a few days, provided there is no distal obstruction. During this time hydration, electrolyte care is essential. Appropriate antibiotics are given.
- Surgical—if the fistula persists, laparotomy and closure of the fistula can be done by repairing with nonabsorbable sutures.

Complications

- Biliary peritonitis
- Septicaemia, if bile is not drained outside.
- Excoriation of abdominal skin can be prevented by zinc oxide application.
- Fluid and electrolyte imbalance.

3. RECURRENT ULCER

It can be true anastomotic ulcer (gastrojejunal, gastroduodenal or jejunal ulcer), or a gastric ulcer in the remnant, or recurrent ulcer following highly selective vagotomy (HSV).

Incidence

- 3% after Billroth II gastrectomy
- 5 to 8% after vagotomy and GJ
- 40% after gastrojejunostomy
- 10 to 12% following HSV.

Causes of Recurrent Ulcer (Fig. 41.110)

1. Incomplete vagotomy
2. GJ alone
3. Inadequate gastrectomy
4. Narrow stoma
5. Zollinger-Ellison syndrome
6. Hyperparathyroidism

Symptoms

- Appears within 1 to 2 years after the operation.
- Severe persistent pain, 'boring' type, which gets worse within a few minutes of taking food. The pain is felt on the left side of the abdomen, near the umbilical region and it passes downwards.

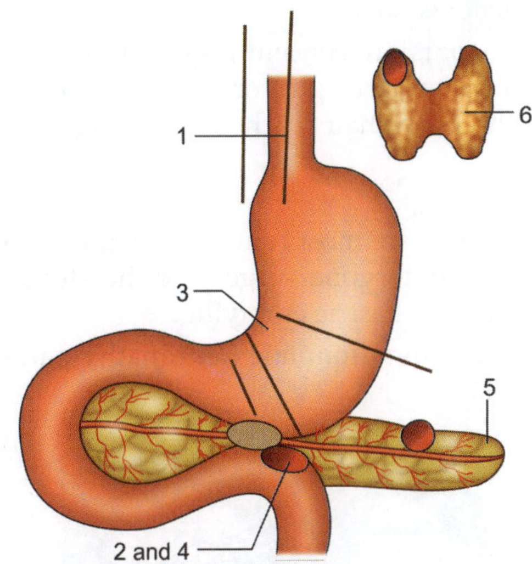

Fig. 41.110: Various causes of recurrent ulcer (see the text for numbers)

- The pain is felt in the lower left chest following antecolic anastomosis. It is not relieved by antacids or milk unlike peptic ulcer. Bleeding may manifest as haematemesis, melaena or anaemia. Perforation can occur, resulting in peritonitis.

Diagnosis

- Gastroscopy gives the correct diagnosis.
- Hypercalcaemia and hypergastrinaemia should be ruled out.

Management (Table 41.12)

- Conservative treatment with H_2 receptor blockers is nearly always effective but relapse occurs, if they are stopped. Smoking should be stopped.
- However, definitive surgery is indicated in appropriate cases.

ACUTE DILATATION OF STOMACH

Aetiopathogenesis

1. Can occur after any operation, particularly splenectomy and pelvic procedures.
2. It can occur following fracture femur, application of plaster of Paris, etc. Malnutrition, excessive distension of the stomach due to ventilation, aerophagia are other precipitating factors.

There is a **sudden loss of sympathetic tone** resulting in massive dilatation of stomach. Improper Ryle's tube aspiration and permitting intake of oral fluids too early before paralytic ileus settles down are additional factors.

Clinical Features

- History of surgery.
- **Hiccoughs**—due to irritation of under surface of the diaphragm, by the hugely distended stomach.
- Abdominal pain, vomiting, distension. Vomiting contains foul smelling dirty fluid and blood and is effortless.

Table 41.12 Management of recurrent ulcer

Type of first surgery		Corrective surgery
1. GJ alone	⟶	Vagotomy
2. Vagotomy + GJ (incomplete vagotomy)	⟶	Incomplete vagotomy is the cause. Usually posterior vagus is found and it has to be divided
3. Vagotomy + GJ (complete vagotomy)	⟶	Stoma is not adequate. Partial gastrectomy is the ideal treatment
4. Billroth partial gastrectomy	⟶	Vagotomy with or without revision gastrectomy
5. HSV	⟶	Vagotomy + partial gastrectomy

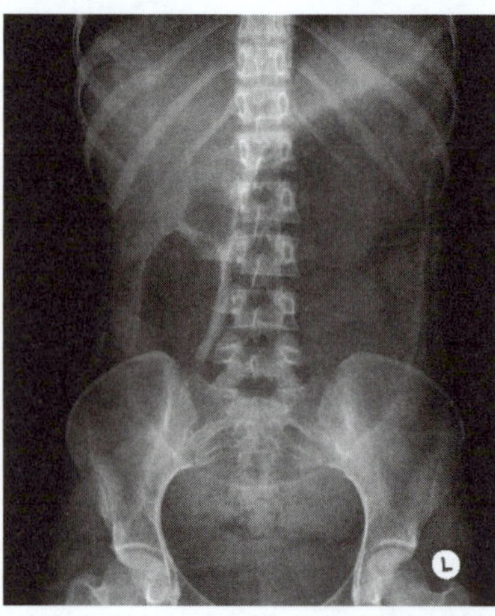

Fig. 41.111: Plain X-ray showing acute dilatation of the stomach. Ryle's tube insertion is a life-saving simple procedure in this condition

- Features of shock. In untreated cases, can lead to cardiovascular collapse.
- **Effortless vomiting** of litres of dark watery fluid is characteristic of this condition.

Treatment: Urgent resuscitation

- **Introduce a Ryle's tube and aspirate the stomach. It is the life-saving use of Ryle's tube** (Fig. 41.111).
- Rapid IV fluid replacement, with normal saline and dextrose saline. Both crystalloids and colloids may be necessary to treat the shock and electrolyte abnormalities.

Complications

- Pulmonary: In debilitated patients, aspiration may result in aspiration pneumonitis (Mendelson syndrome).
- It carries significant mortality.

VOLVULUS OF THE STOMACH

- It is a rare condition in which stomach rotates in a horizontal (organoaxial) and vertical (mesentericoaxial) direction resulting in an acute abdomen.
- Organoaxial is more common.
- Many times, volvulus is intermittent.
- In general, initially the colon moves upwards and later greater curvature of the stomach.
- There is associated eventration of the diaphragm which also precipitates this condition (in children, congenital).
- In adults, diaphragmatic defects are more commonly traumatic or paraoesophageal herniation.
- Clinical features include epigastric pain, fullness and tenderness.

Borchardt's Triad

1. Sudden, constant, severe upper abdominal pain
2. Recurrent retching with production of little vomitus
3. Inability to pass a nasogastric tube.

Diagnosis

- Plain X-ray abdomen/chest: Gas-filled viscus.
- Barium meal can demonstrate twisted stomach.
- Upper GI scopy.

Treatment

- Reduce the volvulus by dividing gastrocolic omentum
- Fix the greater curvature of the stomach to the duodenojejunal flexure or perform a GJ without stoma.
- Repair of eventration
- Fixing by tube gastrostomy can also be done.

BEZOARS

- Bezoars are collections of **nondigestible materials,** usually of vegetable origin (phytobezoar) but also of hair (trichobezoar).
- **Trichobezoars** are concentrations of hair, generally found in long-haired girls or women who often deny eating their own hair (trichophagy) (Fig. 41.112).

Causes

- **Phytobezoars** are most commonly found in patients who have undergone surgery of the stomach and have impaired gastric emptying.
- **Diabetics with autonomic neuropathy** patients are also at risk.

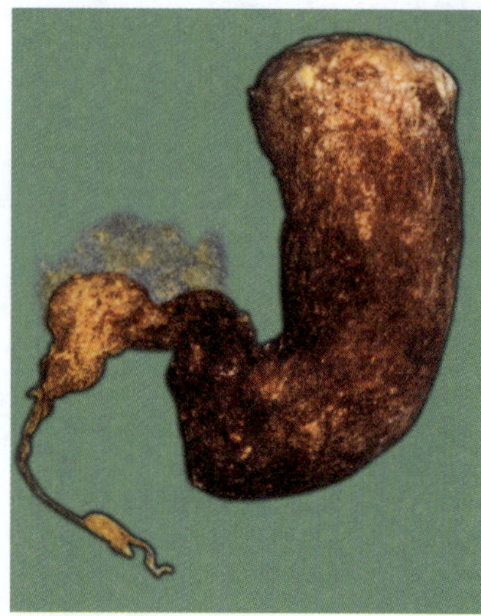

Fig. 41.112: Trichobezoar (*Courtesy:* Dr YV Krishna Rao, Professor of Surgery, Mamata Medical College and Hospital, Khammam, Andhra Pradesh)

Clinical Features and Diagnosis

- The symptoms of gastric bezoars include early satiety, weight loss, nausea, pain and vomiting due to **gastric outlet obstruction** with occasional gastric perforation and small bowel obstruction.
- **A large mass** may be palpable on physical examination and the diagnosis is confirmed by a barium examination or endoscopy.

Treatment

- **Papain:** Enzymatic therapy to attempt dissolution of the bezoar.
  - Papain found in Adolph's Meat Tenderizer (AMT) is given in a dose of one teaspoon in 150 to 300 ml water several times daily.
  - The sodium concentration in AMT is high, so hypernatraemia may occur.
- **Cellulase** has been used with some success.
- **Aggressive Ewald tube lavage or endoscopic fragmentation.**
- Failure of these therapies would necessitate surgical removal.

Pearls of Wisdom

Trichobezoars tend to form a cast of the stomach, with strands of hair having been observed as far distally as the transverse colon.

Competency

SU28.8: Describe and discuss the aetiology, the clinical features, investigations and principles of management of congenital hypertrophic pyloric stenosis.

IDIOPATHIC HYPERTROPHIC PYLORIC STENOSIS (IHPS)

Aetiopathogenesis

- In this condition, there is **hypertrophy** involving the pyloric antral **circular muscle fibres**. Duodenum is normal (Fig. 41.114).
- The lumen is so much narrowed as to give rise to pyloric obstruction.
- Familial history can be obtained in a few patients.
- Prenatal incoordination of muscles, lack of nitric oxide relaxation of smooth muscles may be some factors responsible for IHPS.
- Risk factors in babies include birth by preterm birth, cesarean section, bottle feeding, and being first born male.

Clinical Features

- **Incidence:** 1–2/1000 births. First born male child is affected very often. The child is normal at birth and the symptoms appear around 6–8 weeks.
- First symptom is **vomiting**. It is **projectile**, forcible, does not contain bile. A visible gastric peristalsis (VGP) can be seen especially when the mother feeds the child (Fig. 41.113).
- Loss of weight—dehydration.
- Constipation and oliguria are the features.
- *Per* abdomen—hypertrophied thickened pylorus can be felt as a mass in the right hypochondrium—'Olive like mass' (in adults with pyloric stenosis due to chronic duodenal ulcer, no mass is felt—Fig. 41.114).

Classic triad of IHPS is (projectile vomiting, palpable olive and visible peristalsis).

Ultrasound

- Long axis view of pylorus demonstrates 'cervix' sign.
- Short axis view of pylorus demonstrates 'target' sign.
- When muscle thickness is more than 7–15 mm size and pyloric canal length is 20–25 mm, it is diagnostic.

Treatment

- Correction of dehydration and electrolyte disturbance by intravenous half normal saline must always precede surgery.
- **Ramstedt's pyloromyotomy** is the surgical treatment (Figs 41.115 to 41.118).
- Laparotomy is done and an incision is made through the serosa. It then cuts through the circular muscle fibres till all the muscle fibres are divided and the mucosa bulges out.
- Avoid injury to the mucosa. If mucosa is opened, it is sutured and reinforced by using omentum.

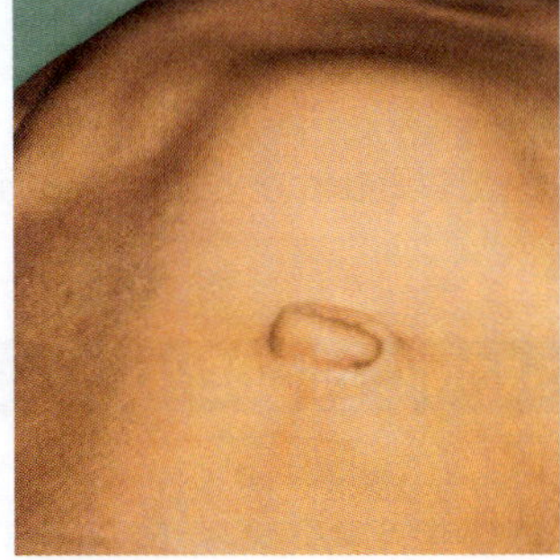

Fig. 41.113: Visible gastric peristalsis

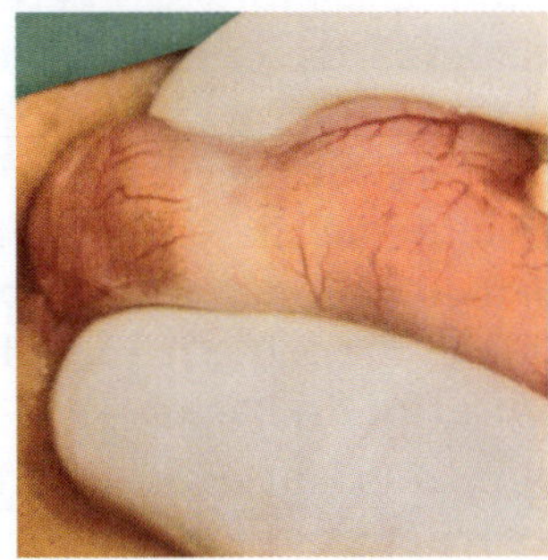

Fig. 41.114: Hypertrophied pylorus

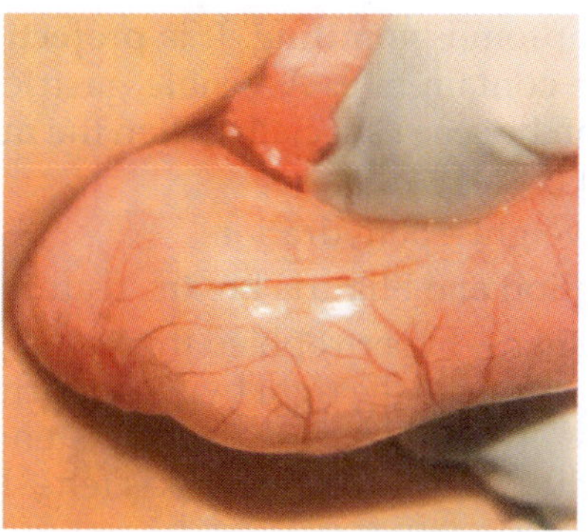

Fig. 41.115: Pyloromyotomy incision

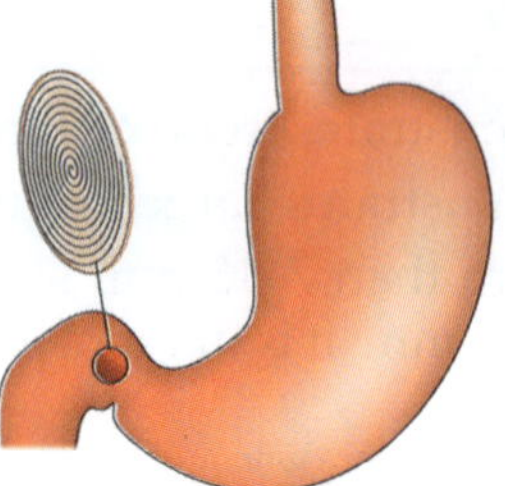

Fig. 41.116: Pyloric mass

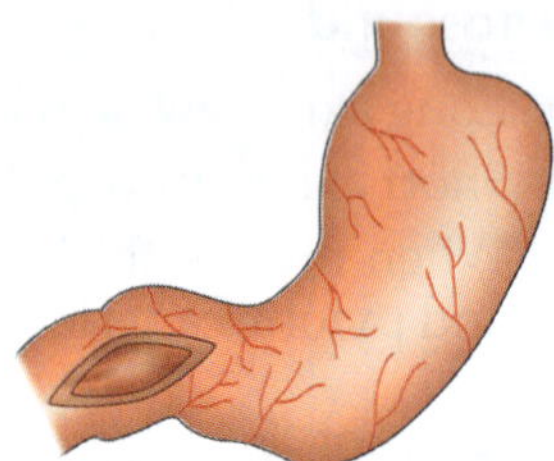

Fig. 41.117: Ramstedt's pyloromyotomy

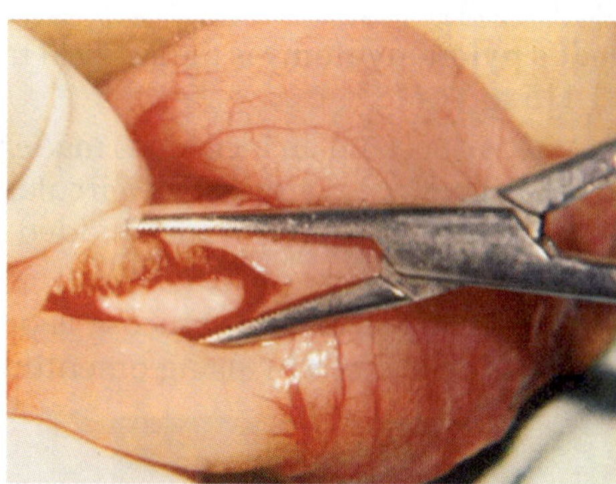

Fig. 41.118: Ramstedt's pyloromyotomy being done (*Courtesy:* Prof Vijaykumar, Head, Department of Paediatric Surgery, KMC, Manipal)

CHRONIC DUODENAL ILEUS

- It is also called superior mesenteric artery (SMA) syndrome, **Wilkie's disease or arteriomesenteric compression** (Figs 41.119 and 41.120). The third part of the duodenum is compressed between vertebral column and superior mesenteric vessels. Acute loss of fat and immobilisation with cast precipitates this disease. Hence, it is also called cast syndrome. Normal angle between superior mesenteric artery and aorta is 38–56°. Due to loss of fat or due to abnormal origin of the SMA, when the angle reduces to 6–25°, SMA syndrome occurs (for risk factor—*see* Key Box 41.29).
- In this condition, duodenum is dilated up to the 3rd part with obstruction to the 3rd or 4th part of duodenum (Fig. 41.119).

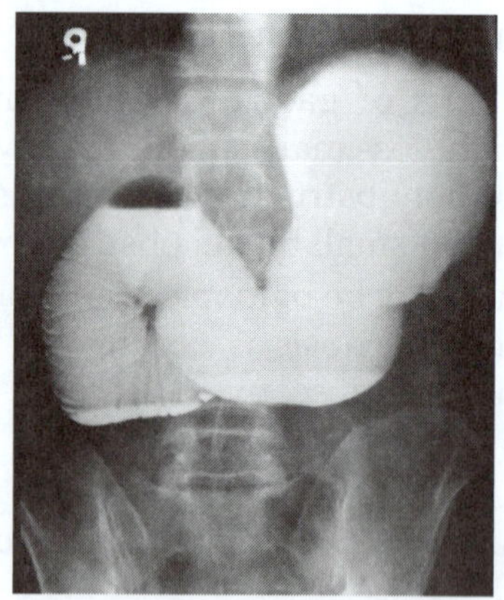

Fig. 41.119: Duodenal obstruction resulting in gross dilatation of duodenum—need for duodenojejunostomy than gastrojejunostomy in these cases

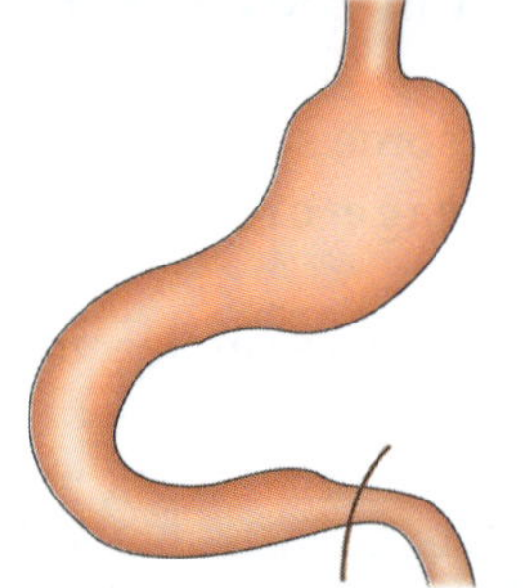

Fig. 41.120: Wilkie's disease—superior mesenteric artery syndrome

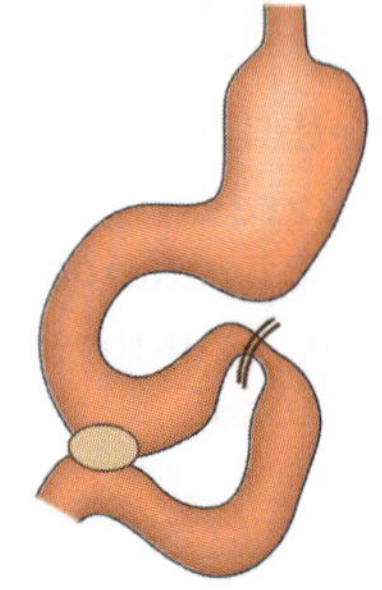

Fig. 41.121: Duodenojejunostomy

- Patients present with features of gastric outlet obstruction but vomitus contains bile—'Food Fear'.
- Abdominal pain is not severe as in intestinal obstruction but on careful questioning history of true nature of spasmodic pain is obtained.
- This condition is often misdiagnosed.
- Barium meal demonstrates the obstruction—dilated stomach and duodenum.
- Duodenojejunostomy is the treatment of choice (Fig. 41.121).

Key Box 41.29

Risk Factors for SMA Syndrome

- **A**sthenic and tall—thin and tall body build—aorto-mesenteric angle is narrow (congenital)
- **B**urns—prolonged bed rest → loss of weight
- **C**achexia, catabolic phases, cast application
- **D**uodenal insertion is high at ligament of Treitz
- **E**maciation, malnutrition
- **F**emales twice as susceptible
- **G**ut malrotation/poor motility of the gut
- **H**yperextension of spine. Lumbar lordosis

ABCDEFGH of SMA syndrome

IMAGES OF A 24-YEAR-OLD FEMALE WITH SMA SYNDROME

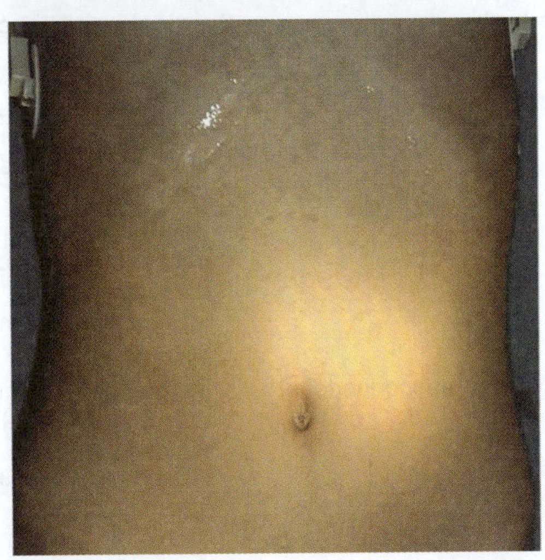

Fig. 41.122: A 24-year-old thin female patient presented with persistent bilious vomiting

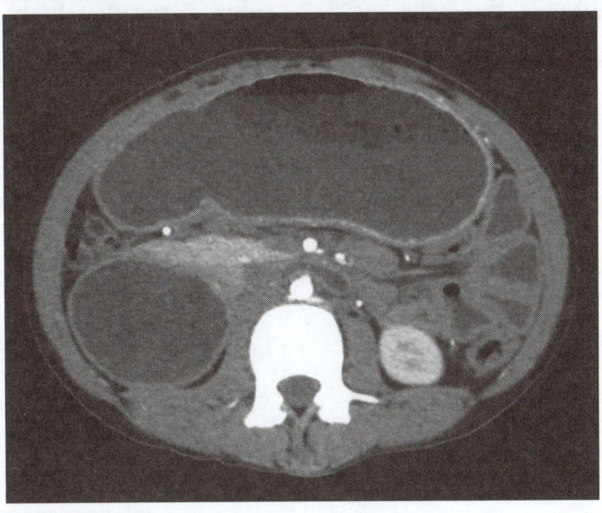

Fig. 41.123: CT scan revealed hugely dilated second part of the duodenum and stomach

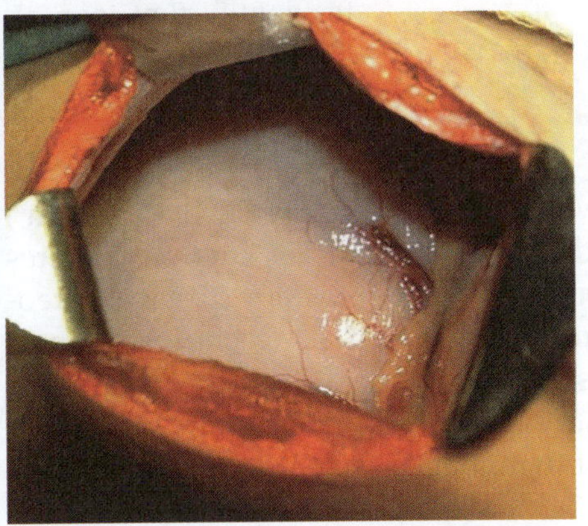

Fig. 41.124: At surgery, stomach was grossly distended with prominent vasculature

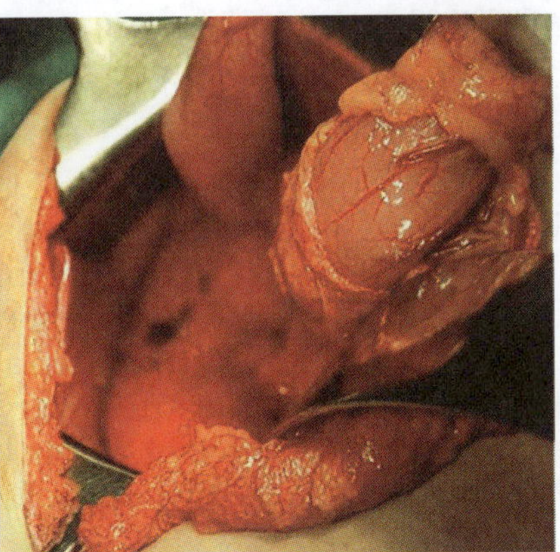

Fig. 41.125: You can see distended first and second part of the duodenum

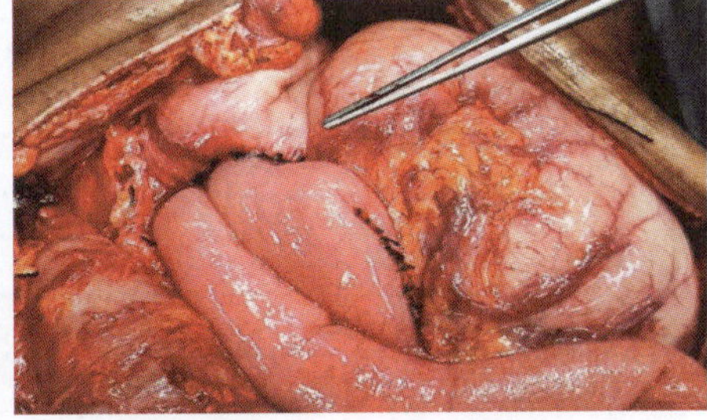

Fig. 41.126: Duodenojejunostomy is done in this patient (*Courtesy:* Dr SS Prasad, Dr Rajendra Benakatti, Dr Keerthan Kumar, Department of Surgery, KMC, Manipal)

Differential Diagnosis

1. **Pyloric stenosis:** In this condition, vomitus does not contain bile. Barium meal X-ray shows distended stomach. Duodenum is not seen.
2. **Annular pancreas:** Rarely, it can present in adults with obstruction to the second part of the duodenum. Vomitus may contain bile. Barium meal X-ray shows dilatation of the first part and also the second part of the duodenum.
3. **Tuberculosis of lymph nodes** can compress the 3rd part of the duodenum and can mimic Wilkie's disease.

What is nutcracker syndrome?[1]

DUODENAL ANATOMY AND OBSTRUCTION

- There are many causes of duodenal obstruction in children.
- In adults, important causes are given in Table 41.13.
  1st part: Postbulbar ulcer with stenosis.
  2nd part: Two causes:
  1. Annular pancreas in adults
  2. Carcinoma head of pancreas

  3rd part: Three causes:
  1. Carcinoma head of pancreas
  2. Arteriomesenteric compression
  3. Tuberculosis/metastatic nodes causing compression of the 3rd part of duodenum. Most common cause of duodenal obstruction in adults is carcinoma pancreas.

[1]Nutcracker syndrome is the entrapment of right renal vein between abdominal aorta and the SMA.

Table 41.13 Anatomy of duodenum and surgical importance

Parts	Development	Length	Relationships	Blood supply	Surgical importance
1st part	• Foregut	2 inches	• Gallbladder • Liver • Bile duct • Portal vein	• Superior pancreaticoduodenal • Supraduodenal artery of Wilkie	• Perforation of 1st part (causes peritonitis) • Injury to duodenum in laparoscopic cholecystectomy
2nd part	• Foregut above ampulla of Vater • Midgut below ampulla of Vater	3 inches	• Right lobe of liver transverse colon anteriorly and kidney, renal vessels posteriorly		• Perforation of 2nd part manifests late because it is retroperitoneal • Injury to duodenum in right hemicolectomy
3rd part	• Midgut	4 inches	• Retroperitoneal fixed • Anteriorly crossed by superior mesenteric vessels • Posteriorly related to inferior vena cava	• Inferior pancreaticoduodenal artery	• Careful separation of mesenteric vessels from duodenum during pancreaticoduodenectomy
4th part	• Midgut	1 inch	• Anteriorly by transverse colon • Superiorly body of pancreas	• Inferior pancreaticoduodenal artery	• 4th part continues as duodenojejunal (DJ) flexure. It is an important landmark to identify first loop of jejunum during gastrojejunostomy

4th part: Carcinoma pancreas (Fig. 41.127)

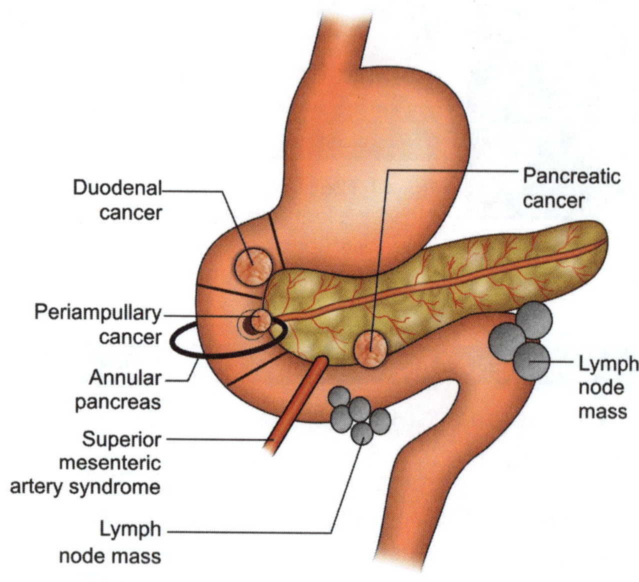

Fig. 41.127: Causes of duodenal obstruction

OBESITY, BARIATRIC AND METABOLIC SURGERY

Introduction

Obesity is a chronic, complex disease that negatively affects one's health. It is characterized by excess fat in the body, which occurs when calorie consumption is significantly higher than calorie expenditure. Body mass index (BMI), which is measured in kg/m^2, is used to classify patient's weight. Morbid obesity (BMI >35 kg/m^2) may be associated with comorbidities, such as diabetes mellitus, hypertension, coronary artery disease, osteoarthritis, sleep apnoea, etc., which reduce life expectancy. Bariatric surgery is often performed to reduce excess body weight and is known as metabolic surgery when primarily carried out to manage associated comorbidities.

Aetiology and Pathophysiology

The aetiology of obesity is multifactorial and occurs due to causes like a sedentary lifestyle, a familial tendency, environmental factors, psychosocial behaviour, a few medical conditions (e.g. Cushing's syndrome, hypothyroidism), and congenital diseases (e.g. Prader–Willi syndrome). An elevated BMI is associated with increased leptin levels. Obesity can affect any age and is becoming increasingly prevalent among children and adolescents. India has emerged as the third most obese nation after USA and China due to its socioeconomic changes. Obesity affects almost every organ of the body and causes many diseases that result in significant morbidity and mortality.

Management of Obesity

Medically treatable causes for obesity should be evaluated by appropriate tests. If no cause is established, a trial of diet and exercise with behavioural changes should be prescribed. If this also fails, bariatric surgery

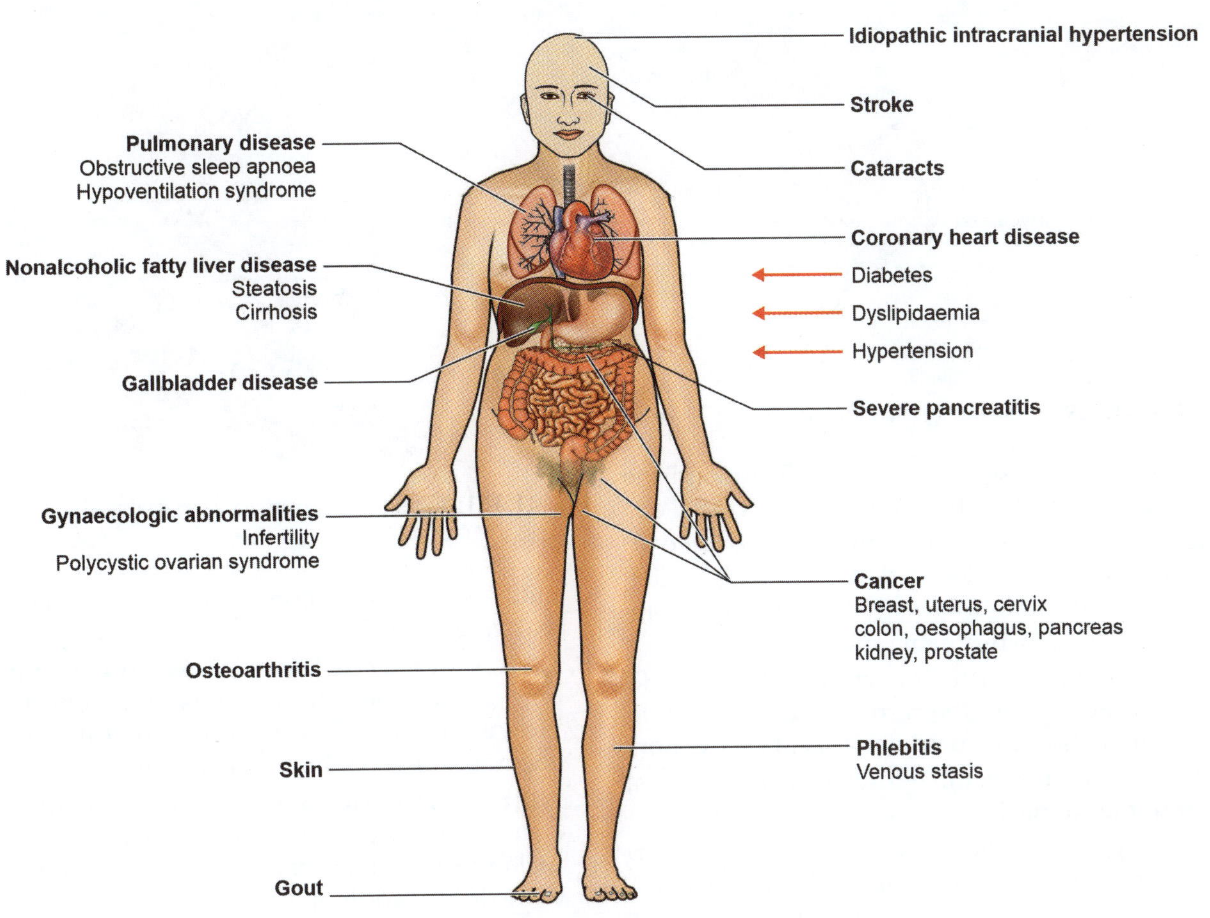

Fig. 41.128: Various problems caused by morbid obesity

should be considered after proper counselling. Patients with a BMI ≥35 kg/m^2 with comorbidities should be considered for surgery. Laparoscopic surgery is currently the standard of care, and robotic bariatric surgery is also sometimes adopted.

Types of Bariatric Surgery

1. Restrictive procedure, e.g. laparoscopic adjustable gastric banding (LAGB) and laparoscopic sleeve gastrectomy (LSG)—this largely restricts food intake.
2. Restrictive procedures with some malabsorption: Roux-en-Y gastric bypass (RYGB), one anastomosis gastric bypass or mini gastric bypass (OAGB or MGB)—this restricts food intake and causes some malabsorption.
3. Malabsorptive procedures with some restriction: Biliopancreatic diversion (BPD), duodenal switch (DS)—this causes severe malabsorption with less food restriction and is rarely performed in India.

Indications for Bariatric Surgery

1. BMI >40 kg/m^2 or BMI >35 kg/m^2 with associated medical comorbidity.
2. Failed dietary therapy with above BMI levels.
3. Psychiatrically stable without substance abuse.
4. Knowledgeable about the operation to be performed and its sequelae.
5. Motivated individual.
6. Age >18 years and <70 years.

Contraindications for Bariatric Surgery

I. **Medical:** Cirrhosis with portal hypertension, autoimmune connective tissue disorders, inflammatory bowel disease (IBD), chronic administration of steroids, poor fitness for general anaesthesia.

II. **Surgical:** Inability to ambulate, Prader–Willi syndrome (congenital obesity syndrome with severe hyperphagia, growth-hormone deficiency, hypogonadism, dysmorphic features, and cognitive impairment).

Details of Surgery

1. **Laparoscopic RYGB** (Fig. 41.129): Gastric bypass, which was first described by Mason and Ito in 1969, incorporates a loop of jejunum anastomosed to a proximal gastric pouch. However, loop gastric bypass may result in bile reflux. To overcome this disadvantage, RYGB was developed, and it has now become one of the most commonly performed bariatric surgeries.

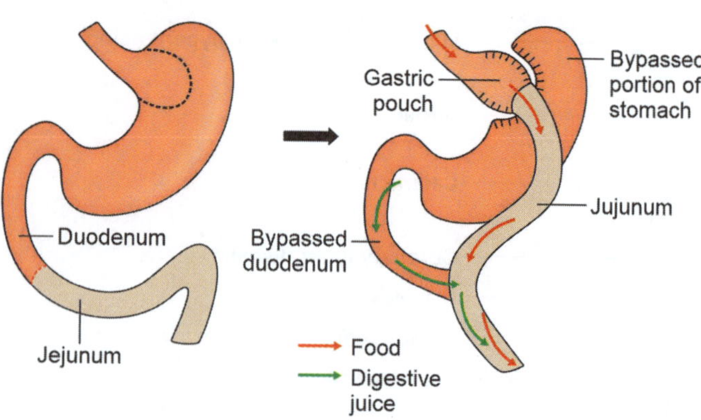

Fig. 41.129: Roux-en-Y gastric bypass (RYGB)

- The roux limb should be at least 75 cm, and the biliopancreatic limb should be 100–150 cm.
- Enteroenterostomy (jejunum) is performed to prevent stenosis or obstruction.
- All potential spaces for internal hernias should be closed using nonabsorbable sutures.
- A small proximal gastric pouch (15–20 ml) should be constructed from the cardia of the stomach to prevent dilation and to minimize acid production.
- The gastric pouch should be divided from the distal part of the stomach.

2. **Laparoscopic sleeve gastrectomy** (Fig. 41.130): It is widely practiced worldwide due to its simplicity. A narrow gastric sleeve is fashioned over a gastric calibration tube by stapling the stomach vertically, and the resected stomach is removed.
3. **One anastomosis gastric bypass or mini gastric bypass (OAGB or MGB)** (Fig. 41.131): This is a type of gastric bypass in which 150–200 cm of the jejunum is bypassed by anastomosing it to a long, narrow gastric pouch.

Complications of Bariatric Surgery

a. **Staple line/anastomotic leaks:** These may be lethal, if not recognized early. The leak rate is high in the initial period. More recent studies report anastomotic leak rates of 0.35–0.5%.

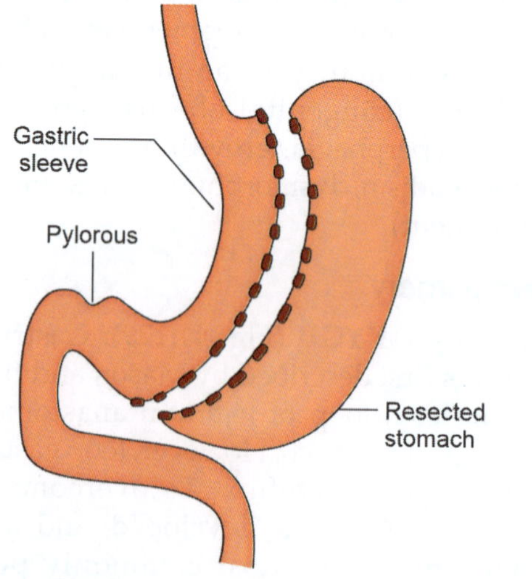

Fig. 41.130: Laparoscopic sleeve gastrectomy

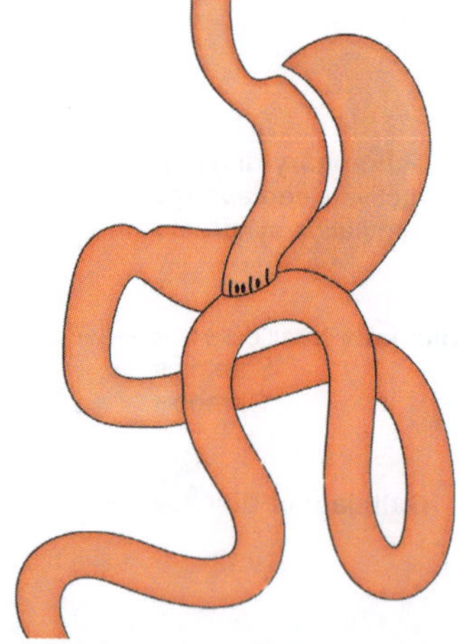

Fig. 41.131: One anastomosis gastric bypass or mini gastric bypass (OAGB or MGB)

b. **DVT (deep vein thrombosis) and pulmonary embolism:** Obese individuals are prone to DVT. However, this has become uncommon with chemoprophylaxis and early mobilization.

c. **Nutritional deficiency:** Various nutritional deficiencies may occur due to severe food restriction and malabsorption, if the patient is not taking the required daily dose of additional nutritional supplements and adequate proteins.

d. **Bowel obstruction after Roux-en-Y bypass:** It occurs due to the potential for internal hernias, which commonly occurs after laparoscopic RYGB and is estimated to be between 3 and 4.5%. Two potential locations: (A) Petersen's space: It is the space caused by the herniation of intestinal loops through the defect between the small bowel limbs, the transverse mesocolon, and the retroperitoneum after RYGB. (B) Jejunojejunostomy mesenteric defect.

e. **Marginal ulcer:** It occurs in 2–10% of cases who undergo gastric bypass surgery. It may lead to perforation, stricture formation, or gastric pouch outlet obstruction, which will require endoscopic dilation, if it not treated promptly.

Recent Advances

Certain endoscopic procedures, such as gastric balloon and endoscopic sleeve gastroplasty, are being tried to limit food intake. The use of appetite suppressants or drugs that limit food absorption cannot be taken for long time without adverse effects. Research is now directed towards the role of altering gut microbiota to manage obesity.

FURTHER READING

1. ASMBS Textbook of Bariatric Surgery.
2. www.theossi.com—Bariatric Surgery.

Multiple Choice Questions

1. **Regarding duodenum following are true *except*:**
   A. Lined by mucus-secreting columnar epithelium
   B. Brunner's glands are present
   C. Duodenum can produce cholecystokinin
   D. Duodenum will not secrete secretin

2. **Following are true regarding blood supply of the stomach *except*:**
   A. The fundus is supplied by left gastric artery
   B. Left gastric artery is a branch of coeliac axis
   C. Right gastroepiploic artery runs along greater curvature of the stomach
   D. Gastroduodenal artery is a branch of hepatic artery

3. **Duodenal ulcer commonly occurs in which part of duodenum?**
   A. First part
   B. Second part
   C. Third part
   D. Fourth part

4. **Following are true for *Helicobacter pylori* bacteria *except*:**
   A. It is spiral shaped
   B. It hydrolyses urea
   C. It can produce cytotoxins
   D. Mostly, it is associated with type A gastritis

5. **Following are true for duodenal ulcer *except*:**
   A. It occurs in the first part of the duodenum
   B. It may be associated with type B gastritis
   C. Smoking may precipitate development of ulcer
   D. It can erode branches of left gastric artery and result in massive bleeding

6. **Following are true for malignancy in a gastric ulcer *except*:**
   A. It occurs rarely
   B. Occurs in the lesser curvature of the stomach
   C. It produces a notch in barium studies
   D. Converging rugosity is lost

7. **Most important cause of duodenal stump leakage after Billroth II gastrectomy is:**
   A. Efferent loop obstruction
   B. Oedema of the stump
   C. Kinking of the afferent loop
   D. Fat necrosis

8. **About truncal vagotomy which one of the following is not correct?**
   A. Decreases acid secretion
   B. Decreases parasympathetic activity
   C. Increases gallstones
   D. Increases constipation

9. **More accurate investigation for the diagnosis of the perforated duodenal ulcer is:**
   A. Ultrasound of the abdomen
   B. Plain X-ray abdomen erect position
   C. Plain X-ray chest
   D. CT imaging

10. **Treatment of the perforated duodenal ulcer include following *except*:**
   A. Suturing the ulcer in transverse direction
   B. Truncal vagotomy
   C. Peritoneal toilet
   D. Omental patch

11. **The most common site of bleeding from peptic ulcer is:**
   A. Lesser curvature of the stomach
   B. Greater curvature of the stomach
   C. First part of the duodenum
   D. Fundus of the stomach

12. **Following are true with Dieulafoy's lesion *except*:**
   A. It is an arteriovenous malformation
   B. It is one of the causes of occult bleeding
   C. Local excision is the choice of treatment
   D. The site is fundus of the stomach

13. **Which one of the following is the complication of gastrojejunostomy?**
   A. Gallstones B. Duodenal blow out
   C. Intussusception D. Diarrhoea

14. **Following are complications of vagotomy *except*:**
   A. Diarrhoea B. Gallstones
   C. Achlorhydria D. Carcinoma stomach

15. **Hypochloraemic alkalosis in pyloric stenosis is treated by:**
   A. Normal saline
   B. Ringer lactate
   C. Isotonic saline with potassium
   D. Double strength saline

16. *H. pylori* is an important factor for carcinoma stomach in which region?

A. Distal
B. Proximal
C. Body
D. Gastro-oesophageal junction

17. Which one of the following is not a risk factor for proximal carcinoma stomach?

A. Chronic gastric ulcer
B. *H. pylori* induced gastritis
C. Pernicious anaemia
D. Obesity

18. Which one of the following is not a feature of early gastric cancer?

A. Confined to mucosa
B. Confined to mucosa and submucosa
C. Confined to mucosa with lymph nodes
D. Involving muscularis

19. Following are features of gastrointestinal stromal tumours (GISTs) of the stomach *except*:

A. Stomach is the most common site of GIST
B. More than 5 cm size tumour is considered to have malignant potential
C. Wedge excision is the treatment of choice for small lesions
D. Always do lymphadenectomy with wedge excision

20. Which one of the following features is false for gastrointestinal stromal tumour (GIST)?

A. It is arising from mesenchymal tissue
B. Associated with tyrosine kinase C-kit oncogene
C. They are sensitive to tyrosine kinase antagonist imatinib
D. Lymph node spread is very common

21. All are true for hormone ghrelin *except*:

A. Produced by gastric antrum
B. It is a hunger hormone
C. It stimulates growth hormone
D. It is produced by oxyntic glands

22. About Roux-en-Y gastric bypass following are true *except*:

A. It is the most common procedure done now
B. It prevents bile reflux
C. It allows endoscopic examination of gastric fundus
D. Obilteration of Peterson's space is also a part of the procedure

Answers

1. D	**2.** A	**3.** A	**4.** D	**5.** D	**6.** C	**7.** C	**8.** D	**9.** D	**10.** B
11. C	**12.** D	**13.** C	**14.** D	**15.** C	**16.** A	**17.** B	**18.** D	**19.** D	**20.** D
21. A	**22.** C								

CHAPTER

42

Gallbladder and Pancreas

- Surgical anatomy
- Physiology
- Congenital anomalies
- Gallstones disease
- Acute cholecystitis
- Chronic cholecystitis
- Obstructive jaundice
- Stricture of CBD
- Sclerosing cholangitis
- Choledochal cyst
- Caroli's disease
- Chronic pancreatitis
- Cholangiocarcinoma
- Congenital biliary atresia
- Carcinoma of the gallbladder
- Carcinoma of pancreas
- Endocrine tumours
- Acute pancreatitis
- Pseudocyst
- Annular pancreas
- Ectopic pancreas
- Cystic fibrosis
- Pancreatic divisum
- Pancreatic fistula
- White bile
- Pancreatic ascites

INTRODUCTION

- One may wonder why gallbladder and pancreas are discussed together!! Yes, biliary tract (gallbladder is an important part of that) ends after joining with pancreatic duct by opening into 2nd part of duodenum.
- Gallstones, when they block/pass through ampulla of Vater, produce acute pancreatitis.
- An important surgical condition—surgical jaundice or obstructive jaundice can be discussed better only if you know gallbladder and pancreas.
- Any surgery involving sphincter of Oddi in the form of sphincteroplasty/or removal (as in Whipple's pancreaticoduodenectomy), the gallbladder does not function and hence it needs to be removed.
- Embryologically, liver, biliary tree, ventral pancreas, gallbladder—all developed from a diverticulum on the ventral aspect of the foregut of the embryo.
- And gallbladder will be palpable in most of the cases of periampullary/carcinoma head of the pancreas.

Competency

SU28.1: Describe the applied anatomy of biliary system. Describe the clinical features, investigations and principles of management of diseases of biliary system.

SURGICAL ANATOMY OF THE GALLBLADDER AND BILE DUCTS

Gallbladder is a pear- or globular-shaped organ present in the right hypochondrium on the inferior surface of the liver, situated in the gallbladder fossa. It is about 8–12 cm long.

- **Fundus:** It is the dilated portion of the gallbladder adherent to undersurface of liver from which it can be separated easily.
- **Neck:** The narrow angulated distal portion of the neck is called ***Hartmann's pouch***—common site where stones occur and tend to stay for a long time (also called infundibulum of gallbladder) (Fig. 42.1).

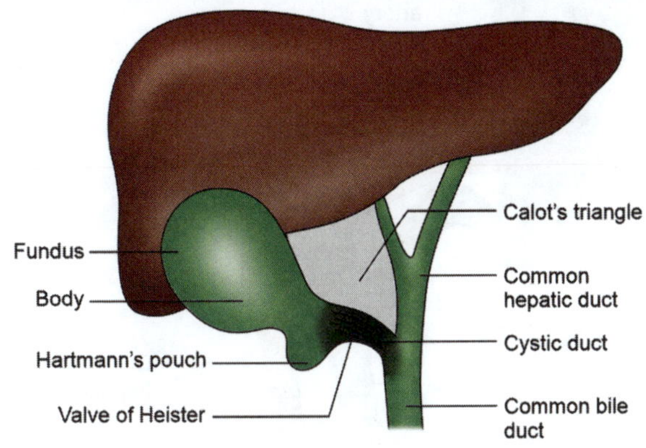

Fig. 42.1: Surgical anatomy of the gallbladder

- Gallbladder drains into the common bile duct (CBD) through ***cystic duct***, which is 3 cm long. It is lined by cuboidal epithelium. There are prominent mucosal folds within the cystic duct due to the presence of prominent circular muscle fibres underneath. Its lumen is usually 1–3 mm in diameter. Contraction of gallbladder produces a functional valve called ***valve of Heister*** which prevents the migration of stone into the CBD. The wall of cystic duct is surrounded by a sphincter structure called ***sphincter of Lutkens***. A spiral fold keeps cystic duct open for drainage of bile.

Cholecystohepatic Triangle or Calot's Triangle Boundaries

- **Lateral:** Cystic duct and gallbladder
- **Medial:** Common hepatic duct
- **Above:** Inferior surface of right lobe of the liver.

Calot's triangle is dissected free of all tissue except for the cystic duct and artery, and the base of the liver bed is exposed—**the critical view of safety—Strasberg et al.**

Contents

- Right hepatic artery and its branch, the cystic artery
- Cystic lymph node of Lund.

Blood Supply of Gallbladder

Cystic artery, a branch of right hepatic artery, arises behind the common bile duct. Soon, it branches out over the surface of gallbladder. ***Cystic artery is an end artery*** (Fig. 42.2). Multiple small veins from the surface of gallbladder join the liver surface. There is also a cystic vein, from the neck of gallbladder draining into portal vein directly. This explains early spread of gallbladder malignancy to the liver.

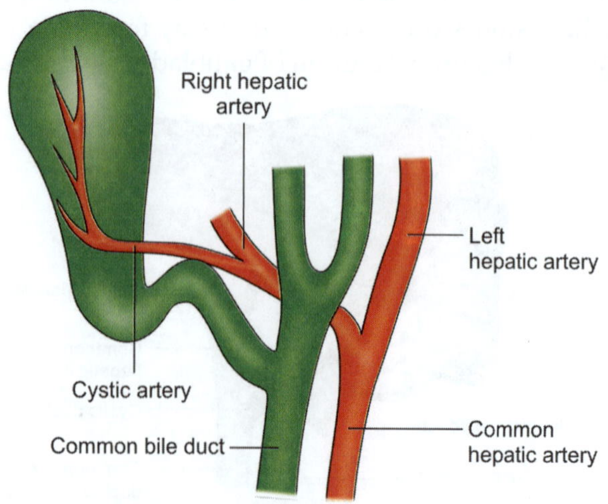

Fig. 42.2: Blood supply of the gallbladder

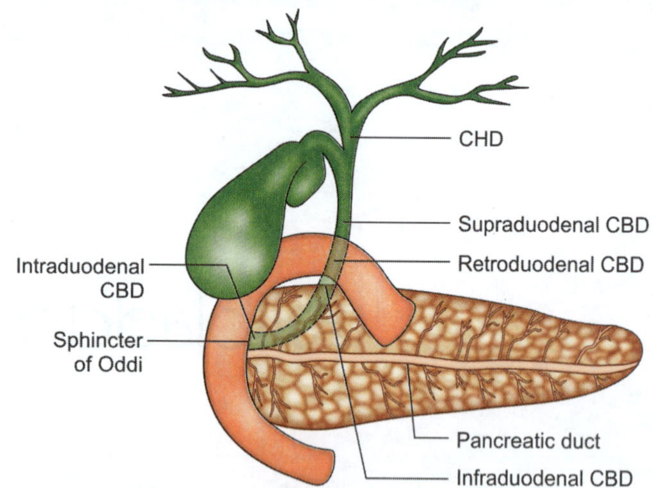

Fig. 42.3: Surgical anatomy of the bile ducts. Note how close gallbladder is to the duodenum (chances of injury in laparoscopic cholecystectomy)

Lymphatics

1. Subserosal and submucosal lymph nodes drain into ***cystic lymph node of Lund*** and from here they drain into nodes in the hilum of liver and coeliac nodes.
2. **Subserosal lymphatic vessels** of gallbladder are also connected to **subcapsular lymph channels** of liver, which accounts for frequent spread of carcinoma gallbladder to the liver.

Anatomy of the Bile Ducts

- **Common hepatic duct (CHD)** is formed by the union of right and left hepatic ducts. It is 3 cm long, receives cystic duct and continues as common bile duct (CBD).
- **Common bile duct** is about 8 cm long. It has four parts: Supraduodenal, retroduodenal, infraduodenal and intraduodenal. Along with pancreatic duct, it forms ampulla of Vater. Controlled by sphincter of Oddi, it ends by an opening into the second part of duodenum (Fig. 42.3).

PHYSIOLOGY

Functions of the Gallbladder

- **Reservoir for bile:** Bile excreted by the liver is stored in the gallbladder as total of about 500 to 1000 ml per day. At fasting, the tone of sphincter of Oddi is high. Food contents in the duodenum stimulates release of cholecystokinin, which causes gallbladder to contract.
- **Concentration:** Bile is 98% water. Due to active absorption of water, sodium chloride and bicarbonate, bile gets concentrated 5–10 times. Thus, a relative increase in bile salts, bile pigments, cholesterol and calcium occurs.

- **Mucus secretion:** It secretes about 20 ml mucus per day. Obstruction to the cystic duct causes mucocele of the gallbladder.

Bile

- Secreted from hepatocytes.
- pH is more than 7.0.
- 500–1000 ml/day, 98% is water.
- Concentrated in gallbladder because of absorption of water. Capacity of gallbladder is 40–50 ml.
- Fatty food stimulation releases cholecystokinin, which stimulates gallbladder to contract and at the same time, sphincter of Oddi to relax.
- It also has inorganic ions (more than plasma) and hence, severe electrolyte imbalance is seen in biliary fistula.
- Cholesterol, synthesised in the liver, gives rise to bile acids—cholic and chenodeoxycholic acids. They are metabolised in the colon to deoxycholic acid and lithocholic acids.
- Main function of bile acids in the bile is to maintain cholesterol in solution.

CONGENITAL ANOMALIES OF GALLBLADDER

Absence of gallbladder: Very rare; other variations include (Fig. 42.4):

A. **Floating gallbladder:** Results due to long mesentery. It is more vulnerable to torsion—a rare cause of recurrent upper abdominal pain. Such a gallbladder can be easily removed.

B. **Phrygian cap:** Cap which was worn by people of Phrygia (ancient Asian country, Mongolia). It is an anomaly connected with the fundus of the gallbladder.

C. **Double gallbladder:** The second one is always intrahepatic (rare).

D. **Absence of cystic duct:** Cholecystectomy becomes difficult. There are high chances of injury to the common bile duct.

E. **Low insertion of cystic duct:** Cystic duct opens into the common bile duct near the ampulla. This anomaly should be kept in mind when operating on cases of obstructive jaundice.

F. **An accessory or aberrant cholecystohepatic duct** is present in about 10% of the patients. It may be the cause of significant bile leakage after cholecystectomy. It is the segmental duct that joins biliary system outside the liver instead of within it.

G. Diverticulum of gallbladder

H. Cystic duct joining right hepatic duct

I. **Anomalies of blood supply**

1. Very, very tortuous hepatic artery: Caterpillar turn or Moynihan's hump. It runs in front of the origin of cystic duct.
2. Cystic artery is given anteriorly from right hepatic artery.

GALLSTONE DISEASE (CHOLELITHIASIS)

Aetiology

1. Metabolic Causes

- Cholesterol is produced from the liver, which gives rise to bile acids. Cholesterol is insoluble and it must be transported within the bile salt micelles and

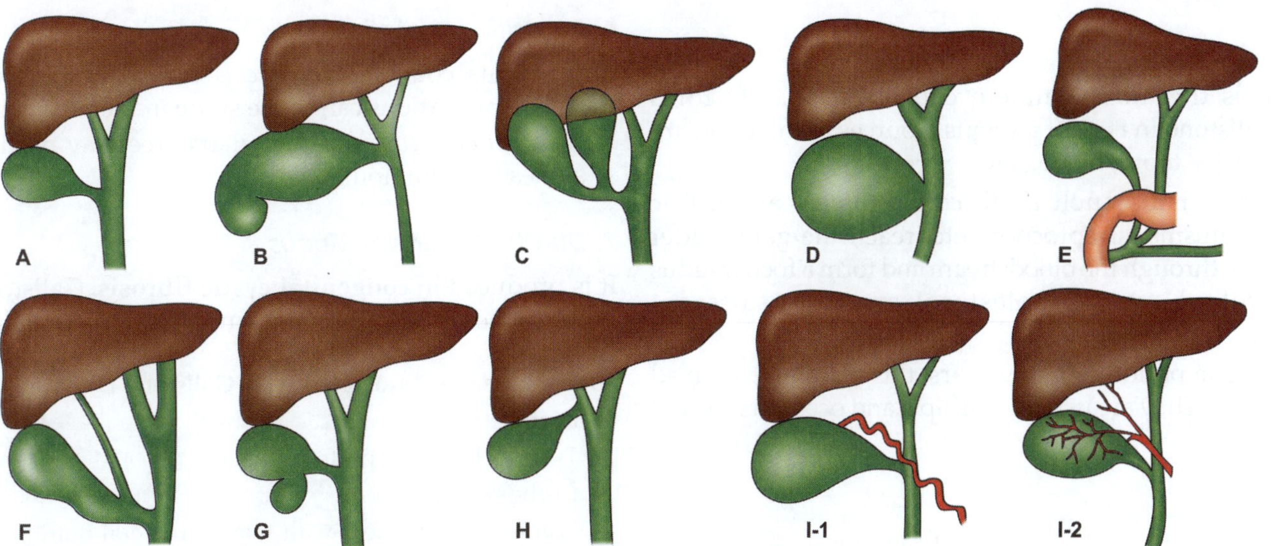

Fig. 42.4: Congenital anomalies of the gallbladder (see text A to I)

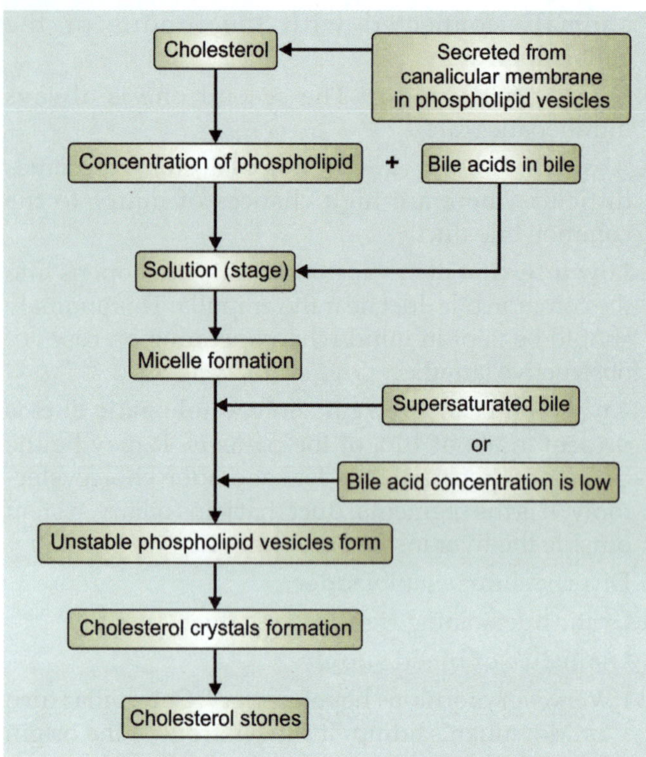

Fig. 42.5: Formation of cholesterol stones

phospholipid (lecithin) vesicles. Normal ratio of bile acids: cholesterol is 25:1 (Fig. 42.5).

- This ratio is necessary to maintain the cholesterol in liquid form by forming micelles. When the ratio drops down to 13:1 (which is called critical ratio), cholesterol crystals will nucleate and stones will form.
- Obesity, high calorie diet and medications which increase cholesterol secretion can result in stone formation.

2. Infection

- It is the most common cause responsible for a gallstone in 80% of patients. Sources of infection are tonsils, tooth, bowel, etc.
- Organisms such as *E. coli*, *Proteus*, anaerobic organisms, streptococci, etc. reach the gallbladder wall through the bloodstream and form a focus/nidus around which cholesterol and bile salts get precipitated.
- Over a period of many years, this results in a mixed stone. They are usually multiple and occur in infected bile.

Pearls of Wisdom

"A gallstone is a tomb stone erected in the memory of organisms within it".—Lord Moynihan

3. Bile Stasis and Decreased Bile Acid Pool

- Pregnancy, oestrogens, following vagotomy and prolonged total parenteral nutrition are associated with bile stasis.
- They are prone to mixed stones as a result of bile stasis (Key Box 42.1).

Key Box 42.1

Causes of Decreased Bile Acid Pool

1. Cirrhosis of liver—pigment stones
2. Gastrectomy
3. Ileal resection
4. Malabsorption
5. Obesity
6. Hypercholesterolaemia

4. Haemolytic Anaemia

- Examples: Hereditary spherocytosis, sickle cell anaemia.
- Bilirubin production is increased because of **increased breakdown of RBCs.** Since the production is more, they cannot conjugate with glucuronic acid, which is produced at normal levels.
- Such **unconjugated bilirubin** combines with calcium and is excreted in the biliary tree resulting in calcium bilirubinate stones (pigment stones) not only in the gallbladder but also in the entire ductal system.

5. Saint's Triad

Gallstones can occur along with two other conditions:
- Diverticulosis of colon
- Hiatus hernia

6. Parasitic Infestation

- In Oriental countries, *Clonorchis sinensis* (Chinese liver fluke) infestations can cause stone in the biliary tree.
- *Ascaris lumbricoides* in the biliary tree may produce stones the common bile duct.

7. Due to Abnormal Mucus

It is produced in **congenital cystic fibrosis.** Gallstones occur in these children due to impairment of bile flow.

Other Diseases Associated with Gallstone Disease

- Diabetes mellitus
- Type IV hyperlipoproteinaemia
- Cirrhosis of liver
- Fistulae on treatment with total parenteral nutrition
- Gastric surgery

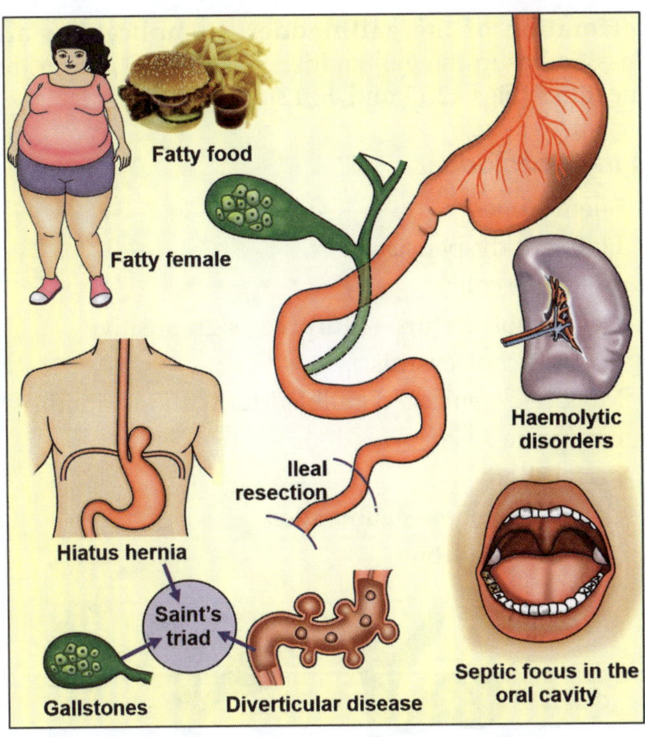

Fig. 42.6: A few risk factors for gallstone disease

8. Risk Factors for Gallstone Disease (Fig. 42.6)

- Female sex
- Obesity
- Maturity onset diabetes
- Age >40 years

Types of Gallstones (Figs 42.7 to 42.10)

1. Cholesterol stones

- **Constitutes about 10% of the gallstones.**
- Occur in patients with increased cholesterol levels.
- Fatty women are commonly affected.
- It is single, solitary, occurs in aseptic bile. Sometimes they can be multiple. Precipitation of cholesterol gives rise to stone.
- Such stones can be silent for many years. They are radiolucent.
- Pigment can also get precipitated along with cholesterol.

2. Brown pigment stones

- **Rare in gallbladder, occurs in bile duct.**
- Composed of calcium bilirubinate, calcium palmitate and calcium stearate + cholesterol.
- Occur due to bile stasis caused by foreign bodies, endoprosthesis, *Clonorchis sinensis* and *Ascaris lumbricoides.*

3. Mixed stones

- They constitute about 80% of gallstones.

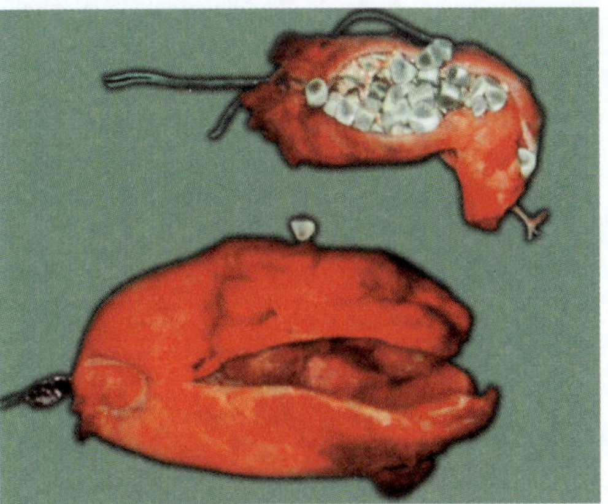

Fig. 42.7: Double GB with stones

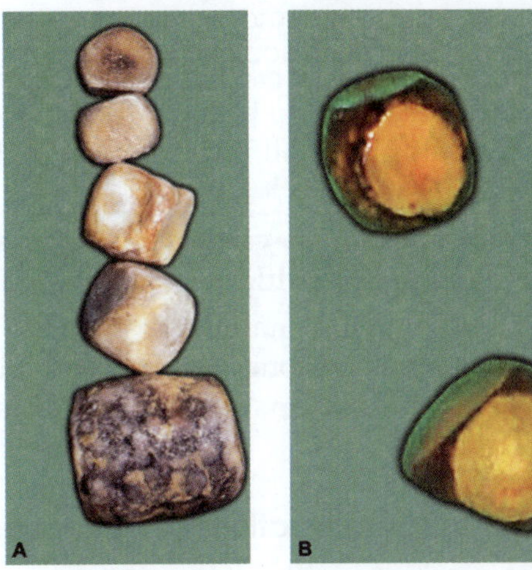

Fig. 42.8: Mixed stones—observe faceting—cause of gallstone colic

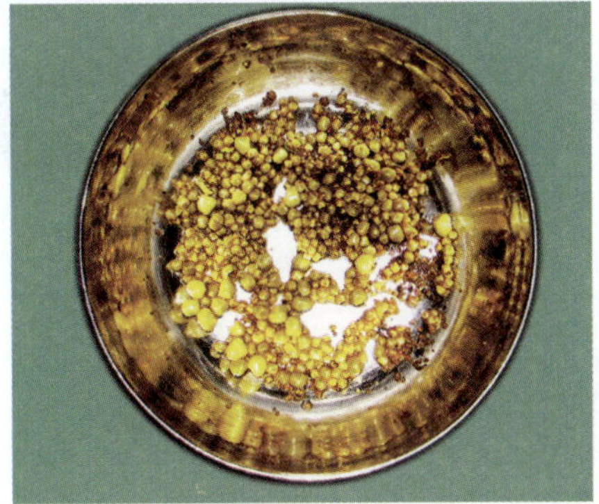

Fig. 42.9: Multiple 2 mm stones. This lady had 3 attacks of gallstone pancreatitis. Initially reported as sludge in the gallbladder

- They contain alternating layers of cholesterol and pigment with epithelial debris or vegetations, from infective organisms.
- They are multiple, small, faceted by mutual pressure.

4. Pigment stones

- They are found in 5 to 10% of patients.
- They are calcium bilirubinate stones.

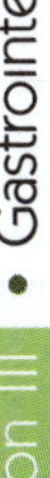

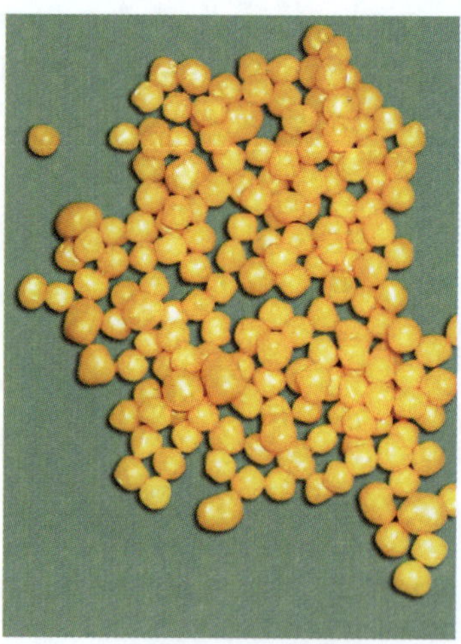

Fig. 42.10: Gallstones: Multiple small stones are responsible for obstructive jaundice by causing obstruction to CBD

- Commonly occur due to haemolysis. Hence, they are black, multiple, small, irregular concretions or sludge particles.
- For reasons not clear, **cirrhotic patients have increased incidence of black pigment stones.**
- Bacteria also have a major role to play in the formation of pigment stones. Patients with pigment stones have more sepsis than patients with cholesterol stones.

Clinical Features (Complications of Gallstones)

Clinical presentation of these patients vary from **dyspepsia** to severe forms such as **pancreatitis and perforation of the gallbladder.** Complications are classified as in the gallbladder, in the CBD and in the intestines (Figs 42.11 and 42.12).

In the Gallbladder

- Silent stones
- Flatulent dyspepsia
- Gallstone colic
- Acute cholecystitis—Murphy's sign positive
- Chronic cholecystitis
- Mucocele—enlarged gallbladder without jaundice
- Empyema
- Perforation
- Carcinoma of the gallbladder
- Mirizzi's syndrome

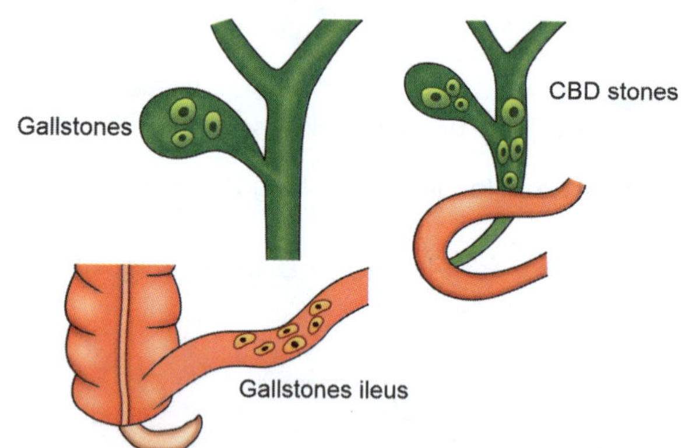

Fig. 42.11: Complications of gallstones

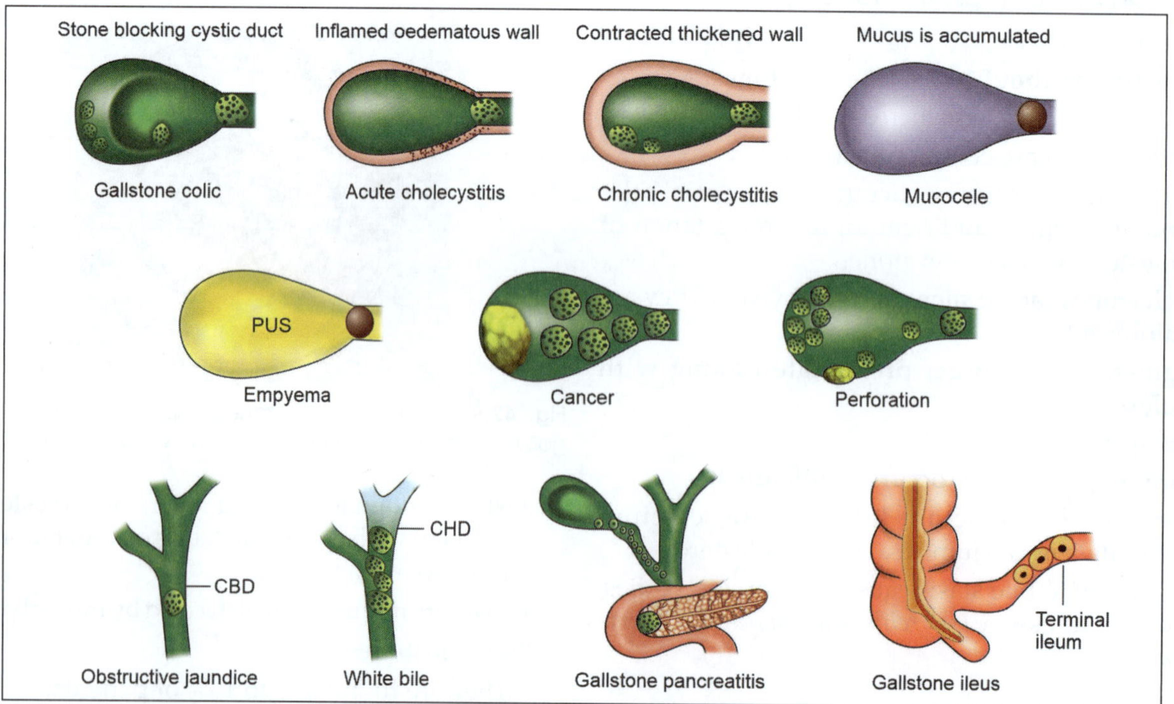

Fig. 42.12: Complications of gallstones. They are discussed in the subsequent pages

In the Bile Duct

- Obstructive jaundice
- Cholangitis
- White bile
- Acute pancreatitis

In the Intestine

Acute intestinal obstruction (gallstone ileus)

COMPLICATIONS IN THE GALLBLADDER

Silent Stones

- This is usually a single, silent, cholesterol stone which is symptomless.
- It is accidentally discovered, may be by an ultrasound or plain X-ray abdomen (since calcium content is low in a cholesterol stone, it is very rarely visible in a plain X-ray).
- This stone rarely causes obstructive jaundice.
- Hence, it is left alone without treatment.

Flatulent Dyspepsia

If an obese woman (fatty, fertile, flatulent, female in forties) complains of gaseous distention, intolerance to fatty food and discomfort in the abdomen, heartburn and belching, she probably has gallstones. These patients benefit from cholecystectomy.

Gallstone Colic

- It usually occurs at night wherein a stone tends to block the cystic duct or neck of gallbladder in the supine position.
- It is a severe colicky upper abdominal pain felt in the right hypochondrium, may shoot to the back or between shoulder blades. The pain is continuous and lasts for a few hours. Pain may radiate to chest also.
  - The pain is due to spasm of gallbladder.
  - It is associated with vomiting due to reflex pylorospasm, restlessness and sweating.
  - There is tenderness in the right hypochondrium.
- Pain may last for a few minutes to a few hours.
- **Differential diagnoses include:**
  - Chronic duodenal ulcer
  - Reflux oesophagitis (some causes can present as precordial chest pain)
  - Pancreatitis
  - Myocardial infarction

ACUTE CHOLECYSTITIS

Definition: Acute bacterial inflammation of the gallbladder with or without stone.

Types

- **Calculous:** Obstructive cholecystitis. It is the commonest variety. Calculi cause bile stasis.
- **Acalculous:** Nonobstructive cholecystitis. It is not uncommon and is seen in patients who are recovering from major illness (Key Box 42.2).
- **Acute emphysematous cholecystitis.**

Key Box 42.2

Acalculous Cholecystitis–Percutaneous Cholecystostomy

- In life-threatening situations with severe sepsis due to gallstones, percutaneous cholecystostomy seems to be a very good alternative to save the life of the patient.
- Indicated in acalculous cholecystitis in which the patient's condition is serious with sepsis with co-morbid conditions.
- Using ultrasound or CT guidance, a pigtail catheter can be inserted into the gallbladder, ideally trans-peritoneally.
- It is the treatment of choice for acalculous cholecystitis.
- 3–4 days later, when sepsis improves, laparoscopic/open cholecystectomy can be done.

Bacteriology of Acute Cholecystitis

- Majority of the cases of calculous cholecystitis are due to organisms such as *E. coli*, streptococci, *Salmonella*, *Klebsiella*, etc.
- Typhoid fever can also cause **typhoid cholecystitis** around 2nd week of infection (Key Box 42.3).
- *Clostridial* infection of the gallbladder produces acute cholecystitis with toxaemia.

Key Box 42.3

Typhoid Infection of the Gallbladder

- *Salmonella typhi* or *S. typhimurium* are the organisms.
- Acute cholecystitis can occur in the 2nd week of typhoid fever.
- Long-lasting infections—chronic cholecystitis can occur.
- Bacilli can be present in the bile for a long time.
- Obstruction by a pre-existing stone or any other cause.
- Necrosis of GB, ulceration, perforation can be dangerous.
- Local tenderness, on the right side of abdomen, guarding can occur.
- Antibiotics against *Salmonella* must be given.

Pathogenesis (Key Box 42.4)

- Acute calculous cholecystitis appears to be caused by obstruction to bile flow from gallbladder by stone or oedema formed as a result of local mucosal erosion and inflammation caused by stone. **Once mucosa is eroded, tissue planes are exposed to bile salts.** Toxic bile salts destroy cells by their detergent action leading to necrosis and perforation of gallbladder.
- At the same time, bacterial infection adds to the morbidity of acute cholecystitis. Positive bile cultures are found in 70% of cases of acute calculous cholecystitis.

Pathology

1. **Inflammation:** Entire gallbladder is inflamed, swollen and is friable. When the inflammatory exudate surrounding the gallbladder collects under the diaphragm, it results in pain radiating to the right shoulder (C3, C4) due to phrenic nerve irritation. It may undergo complete resolution with antibiotic therapy but such recurrent attacks are common at a later date.
2. **Perforation:** Extensive ulcerations of gallbladder may result in perforation with biliary peritonitis and carries a very high mortality rate. **Perforation** can occur when the stone is impacted in the **Hartmann's pouch**.
3. **Obstruction** to the neck of gallbladder results in **mucocele** or **pyocele** (empyema). Empyema of the gallbladder can occur in diabetic patients and is associated with high grade fever, chills, rigors and even septicaemia.
4. **Gangrene** of gallbladder can occur, if the blood vessels get thrombosed. All these features are more in an obstructive variety.
   - If there is clostridial infection as can occur in diabetics because of extensive gas production in biliary tree and associated toxicity, perforation is likely even without a stone.
5. **Jaundice** as in hereditary spherocytosis (Fig. 42.13).

Key Box 42.4

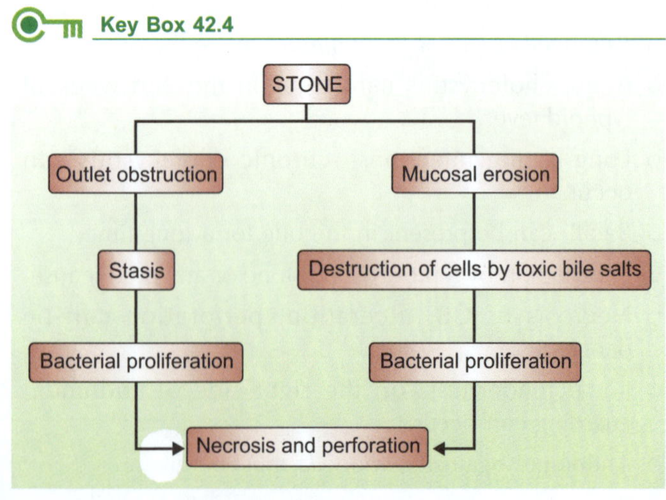

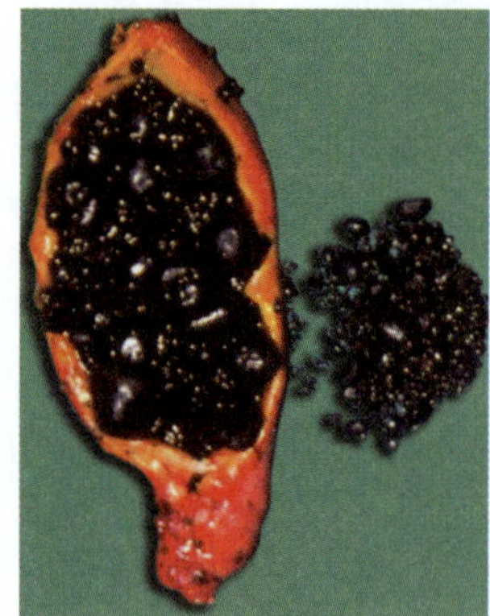

Fig. 42.13: Pigment stones—case of hereditary spherocytosis

Clinical Features

- A fatty, fertile, female is the typical victim who presents with severe upper abdominal pain. The pain is colicky in nature and more prolonged because of inflammation. Severe nausea and vomiting are present. In the initial phase, there is low grade fever, except in clostridial infection where there is high grade fever.
- Right shoulder pain is due to inflammatory exudate irritating under surface of the diaphragm (supplied by phrenic nerves C4–C5—shoulder region is supplied by supraclavicular nerves.

Pearls of Wisdom

You may be surprised to find a young boy, a girl or even a child with gallstones—suspect haemolytic anaemias.

Signs

1. *Murphy's sign*
   - Keep the fingers in the right hypochondrium and ask the patient to take a deep inspiration.
   - At the height of inspiration, there is a sudden catch in the inspiration.
   - It is due to inflamed gallbladder coming in contact with the abdominal wall under the fingers and producing pain. This is called **Murphy's sign positive**. It is a diagnostic sign of acute cholecystitis (Fig. 42.14).

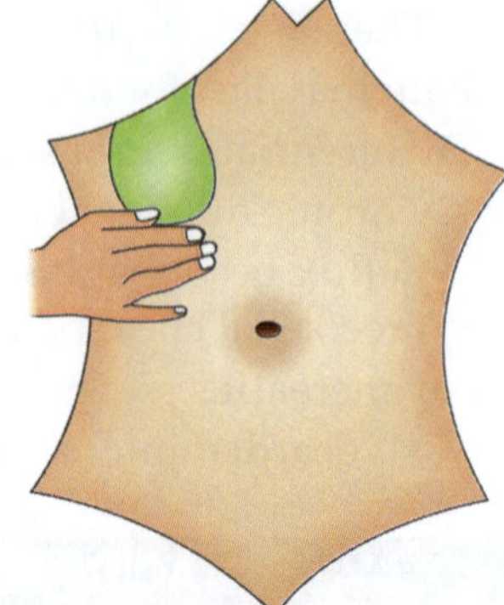

Fig. 42.14: Eliciting Murphy's sign

2. ***Boas' sign:*** An area of hyperaesthesia between 9th and 11th ribs posteriorly on the right side is a feature.
3. Upper abdominal **guarding, rigidity**.
4. **Vague mass** consisting of inflamed gallbladder, omentum, inflammatory exudate can be felt at times. Hence, even if a perforation occurs, generalised peritonitis is uncommon.

Differential Diagnosis (DD) (Fig. 42.15)

1. **Perforated peptic ulcer:** Severe sudden pain, severe tenderness in the right hypochondrium, guarding and rigidity caused by perforated peptic ulcer, can mimic acute cholecystitis. Obliteration of liver dullness, coffee ground vomitus, generalised guarding and rigidity clinches the diagnosis of perforated duodenal ulcer.
2. **Acute pancreatitis:** A severe pain in upper abdomen, tenderness in the right hypochondrium and epigastrium mimic cholecystitis. One should remember that pain of pancreatitis is more severe and classically radiates to back.
3. **High retrocaecal appendicitis:** Especially when appendix is in the subhepatic position. Once inflammatory fluid spreads in the general peritoneal cavity, there will be more difficulty in diagnosing clinically.
4. **Amoebic liver abscess:** Can also mimic very closely. It is more common in male alcoholics. Liver is enlarged and one can feel the round lower border of liver very closely. Liver will be extremely tender.
5. **Lobar pneumonia (basal):** It can give rise to referred pain in the right hypochondrium with guarding and rigidity.

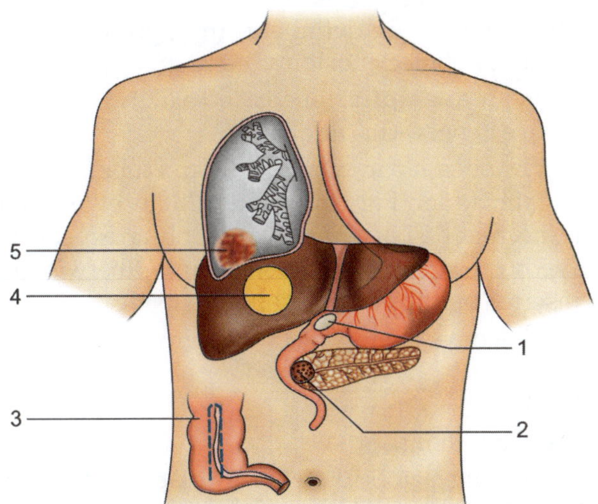

Fig. 42.15: Differential diagnosis of acute cholecystitis (see text)

Investigations

1. **Total WBC** count is always raised.
2. **Blood and urine sugar** estimation to rule out diabetes mellitus.
3. **Emergency ultrasonography** (Fig. 42.16)
   - To demonstrate stones, which cast **posterior acoustic shadow**.
   - Success rate is >95%.
   - It can demonstrate inflamed, thickened organ, in cases of acalculous cholecystitis.
   - More than 5–6 mm thickness of gallbladder suggests significant thickening.
   - Pericholecystic oedema may be present.
   - Demonstration of Murphy's sign, with the help of ultrasonography is possible which adds to the diagnosis.
   - Ultrasound can also measure gallbladder function by using ultrasonic dimensions of the gallbladder.
   - It can detect gallbladder polyps.
4. **Plain X-ray** abdomen erect position (Fig. 42.17)
   - Gallstones can be demonstrated in 10% of the patients as radio-opaque shadows in the right

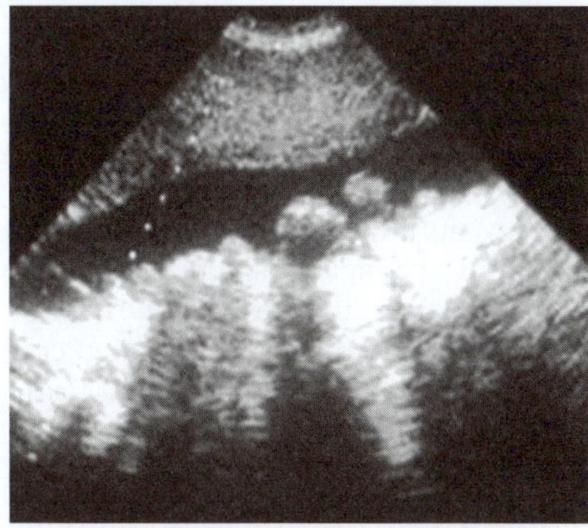

Fig. 42.16: Ultrasonography showing posterior acoustic shadows

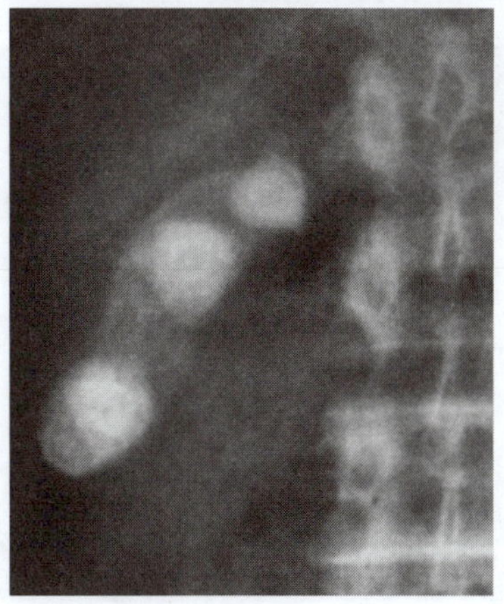

Fig. 42.17: Plain X-ray abdomen showing radio-opaque shadows

hypochondrium. In lateral view, the stone is seen in front of vertebral bodies.

- To rule out other causes such as perforated peptic ulcer (air under diaphragm).
- Rarely, it may show calcified gallbladder (porcelain gallbladder).

10% gallstones are radio-opaque, 90% gallstones are radiolucent. Centre of stones may contain radiolucent gas, either triradiate (**Mercedes-Benz sign**) or biradiate **(Sea Gull sign).**

5. **CT scan** (Fig. 42.18)
   - It is done when ultrasound findings are not clear
   - It not only diagnoses gallstones, but also detects other complications such as perforation, stones in the CBD, etc.
   - Renal halo sign is due to fluid around.
   - Obliteration of psoas shadow can be seen.
   - Air fluid level in duodenum are the features.

Treatment

I. Conservative Treatment (60 to 70%) Followed by Cholecystectomy

Basically there are two types of cholecystectomy—one is early cholecystectomy and other is elective cholecystectomy.

Elective cholecystectomy is followed by many surgeons because many patients are elderly often diabetic or may be having cardiac comorbidity. Also inflammation would have resulted in so-called frozen or difficult 'Calot's triangle' dissection. During surgery, dissection may result in injuries to CBD, hepatic artery, portal vein, etc. Hence, these are managed conservatively till pain inflammation settles down. Principles of conservative treatment are given below.

1. **Admission**
2. **Aspiration** with Ryle's tube: Aspiration of HCl decreases the stimulus to the secretion of bile. Spasm of gallbladder may come down.

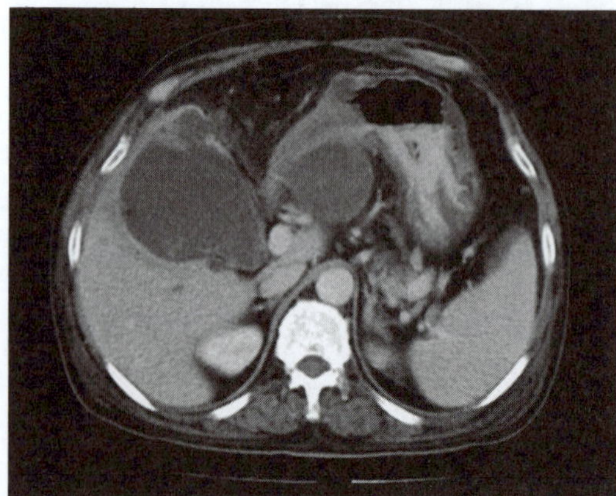

Fig. 42.18: Perforation of gallbladder

3. **Antispasmodics:** Injection tramadol 50 mg IV/IM is given and if necessary repeated.
4. **Antibiotics:** Broad spectrum antibiotics are given against gram +ve, gram –ve and anaerobic organisms. Cefazolin, cefuroxime or amikacin are the drugs of choice. The patient is kept nil orally for 2–3 days and during this time, IV fluids are given.

After 2–3 days, pain comes down, signs (tenderness) disappear and abdomen becomes soft. Ryle's tube is removed, clear oral fluid is given for 2–3 days followed by soft diet. After 6 weeks, the patient is advised to undergo elective cholecystectomy. Reason for conservative treatment is in majority of cases, inflammation will settle down.

II. Early Cholecystectomy

- Patients in the first group need two admissions, cost is increased and return to work is also delayed.
- Hence, if a surgeon is experienced and the set up is good, one can proceed to early cholecystectomy from 2nd day to 7th day.
- It has been proved that even though gallbladder is inflamed, complications are no way more than elective cholecystectomy in the hands of experienced surgeon while performing laparoscopic cholecystectomy.
- Thus, if a firm preoperative diagnosis is established and some of the comorbid conditions are corrected (diabetes, hypertension, etc.), surgery can be done safely. This is called early cholecystectomy done within 48 to 72 hours.

III. Emergency Cholecystostomy

- About 5% of cases of acute cholecystitis require emergency cholecystostomy.
- In these patients, high grade fever, sepsis, shock, high leukocyte count are the deciding factors.
- Acalculous cholecystitis and perforated gallbladder with peritonitis are definitely strong indications for emergency cholecystostomy.
- This is an attempt to decrease toxicity, fever and improve general condition.
- Either by open-laparoscopic method, a tube is inserted into gallbladder (Pig tail catheter/Malecot's) and the pus/necrotic tissue is drained out. Only an experienced surgeon can attempt cholecystectomy. Otherwise tube is inserted and fixed and brought outside.
- After 6–8 days later, cholecystectomy is done.

Prognosis

- Overall death rate is 3–5%.
- Contributing factors for death are diabetes, age above 60 years, cardiovascular or pulmonary disease.
- Uncontrolled sepsis, intra-abdominal abscess.

What is prophylactic cholecystectomy?

It means removal of gallbladder with stones without symptoms. It is indicated in:
- Congenital haemolytic anaemia
- Patients undergoing bariatric surgery
- Porcelain gallbladder

CHRONIC CHOLECYSTITIS

- Recurrent attacks of cholecystitis will convert the gallbladder into a fibrosed, nonfunctioning, contracted, shrunken, small gallbladder. Gallbladder wall is grossly thickened. Stones are invariably present. Such patients present with classical fatty food intolerance. Murphy's sign is positive.
- They are diagnosed by ultrasound which reveals a small, contracted gallbladder. Oral cholecystography (OCG) used to be done to know the function of the gallbladder earlier.

Treatment

Cholecystectomy (Fig. 42.19)

CHOLECYSTOSES

Definition

Uncommon group of conditions affecting gallbladder in which there are chronic inflammatory changes and hyperplasia of all tissue elements.

Types

1. **Cholesterolosis** (strawberry gallbladder): Aggregations of cholesterol crystals in the mucosa/submucosa. Yellow specks of cholesterol crystals are seen when gallbladder is opened (xanthogranulomatous) (Key Box 42.5 and Fig. 42.20).
2. **Cholesterol polyposis** (gallbladder polyp): Polypoidal projections of mucosa in the gallbladder. ***Polyp longer than 1 cm or change in size require surgery.***
3. **Cholecystitis glandularis proliferans:** Granulomatous thickening and hyperplasia of the gallbladder. All layers of gallbladder are thickened.
4. **Diverticulosis** of gallbladder.
5. Gallbladder wall with ***fistula.***

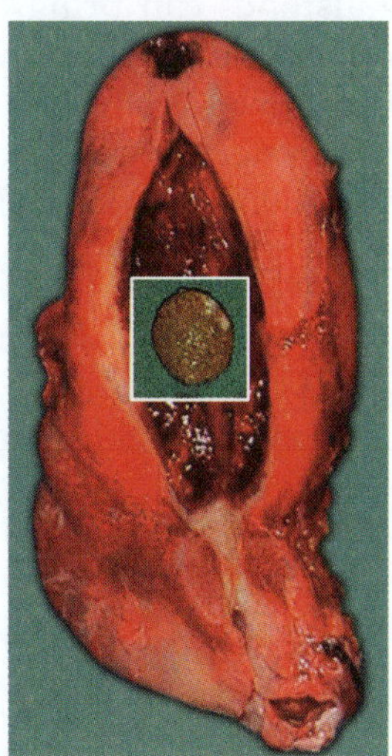

Fig. 42.19: Cholecystectomy specimen—observe thickened gallbladder wall

Key Box 42.5

Xanthogranulomatous Cholecystitis

- It is a pathological diagnosis.
- Gallbladder is chronically thickened, irregular with extension of yellow xanthogranulomatous inflammation to adjacent organs.
- It is thought to be due to bile penetrating gallbladder wall.

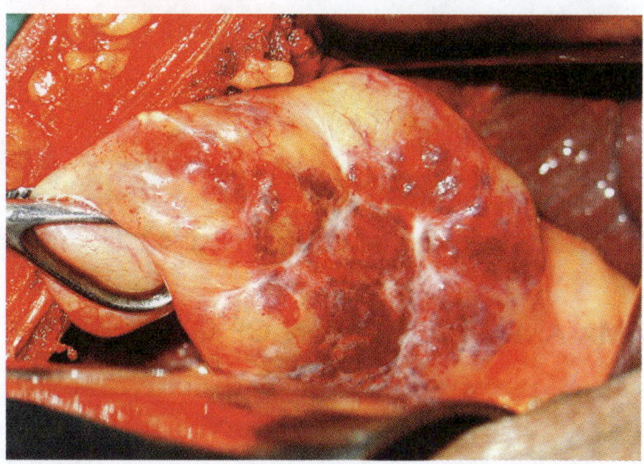

Fig. 42.20: Xanthogranulomatous cholecystitis at surgery

Clinical Features

Dyspepsia, upper abdominal discomfort, Murphy's sign is positive.

Management

Ultrasound to confirm the diagnosis followed by cholecystectomy.

MUCOCELE (Figs 42.21 and 42.22)

- It occurs when there is a stone blocking the cystic duct and the bile is not infected.
- As a result of obstruction, all the bile within the gallbladder is absorbed and is replaced by the mucus secreted from gallbladder epithelium.
- Clinically, it results in a soft, fluctuant, globular mass in the right hypochondrium which moves with respiration. It needs cholecystectomy.

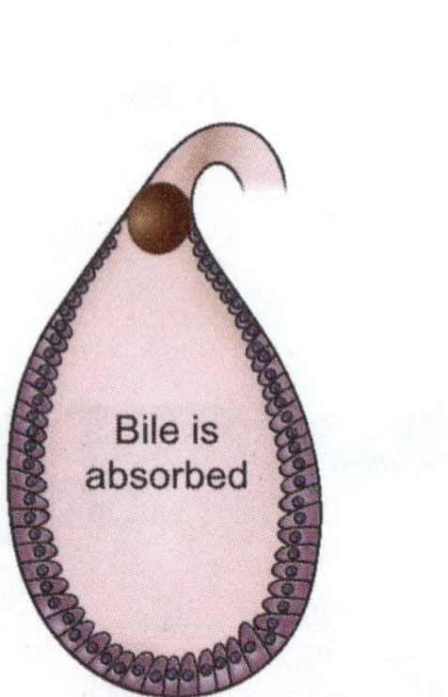

Fig. 42.21: Obstruction by stone

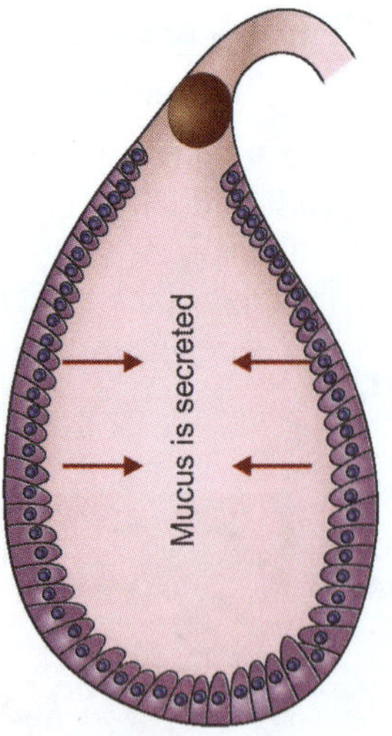

Fig. 42.22: Mucocele

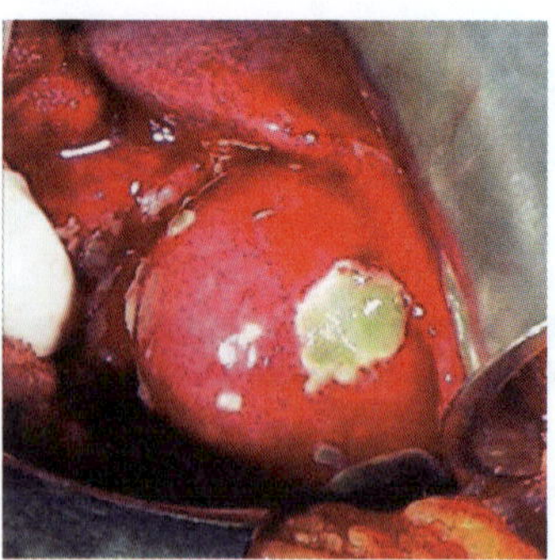
Fig. 42.23C: Gallbladder perforation at surgery

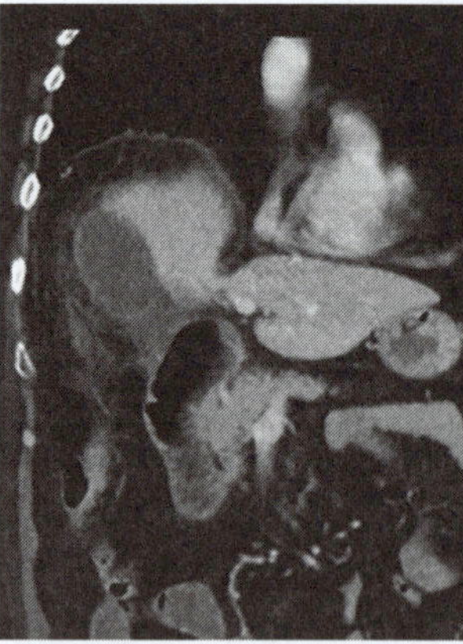
Fig. 42.23D: Acalculous cholecystitis—enlargd gallbladder with pericholecystitic oedema

EMPYEMA AND PERFORATION OF GALLBLADDER

- These are uncommon. Impacted stone, diabetes, virulent organisms precipitate pyocele and perforation.
- Patients present with high grade fever with chills and rigors, toxicity, high leucocyte count.
- Perforation can cause local abscess, if there are adhesions due to previous inflammation.
- Perforation into the general peritoneal cavity is rare but produces diffuse biliary peritonitis which has a high mortality rate.
- Urgent laparotomy, aggressive resuscitation, good antibiotic cover may help in reducing mortality. At laparotomy, removal of gallbladder is difficult. Hence, drainage of the pus and cholecystostomy with removal of gallstones can be done (Figs 42.23A to D).

Three types are (Fig. 42.24):

1. Localised perforation with pericholecystic abscess—managed by catheter drainage.
2. Free perforation into peritoneal cavity and peritonitis—urgent laparotomy drainage.
3. Hollow viscous perforation (duodenum).

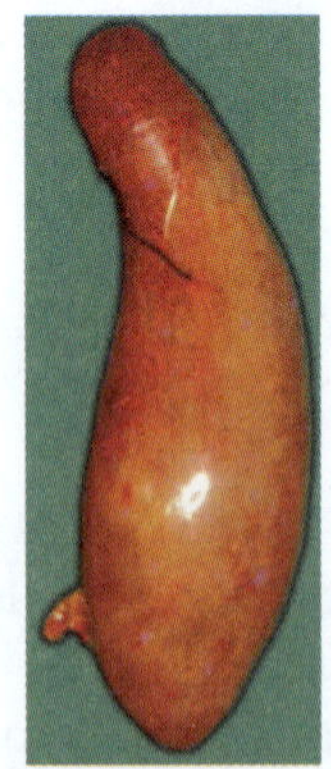
Fig. 42.23A: Empyema of gallbladder

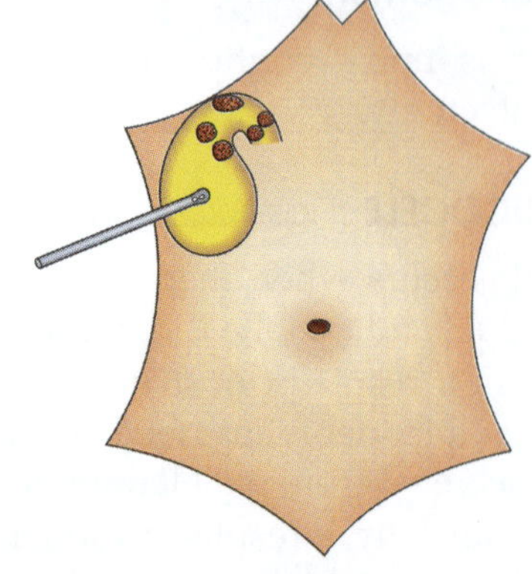
Fig. 42.23B: Percutaneous cholecystostomy for empyema of gallbladder

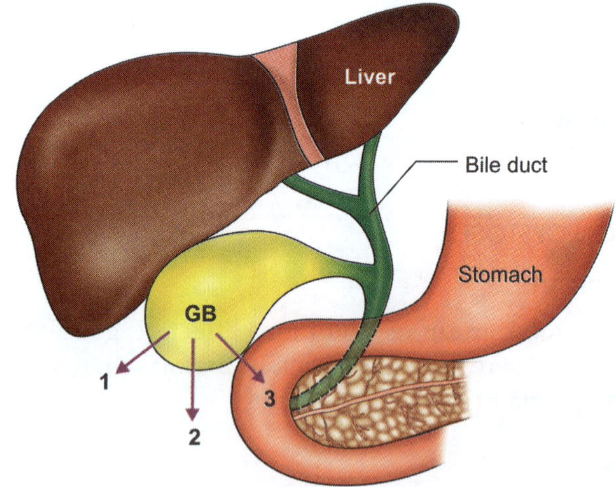

Fig. 42.24: Empyema of gallbladder—complications (see the text)

CARCINOMA OF GALLBLADDER (see page 638)

Long-standing gallstones can bring about squamous metaplasia of gallbladder epithelium and can cause carcinoma of gallbladder. However, the incidence is very low. Hence, routine cholecystectomy is not advised for silent gallstones. Porcelain gallbladder is a precancer condition.

Porcelain Gallbladder

- It occurs due to deposition of calcium carbonate in the gallbladder wall.
- Diagnosis can be made by plain X-ray of the abdomen.
- On ultrasound examination, calcification appears as hyperechoic semilunar structure with dense posterior acoustic shadowing.
- In case of difficulties, CECT can help to differentiate it from gallstones.
- Incidence of carcinoma gallbladder is around 1 to 5%.
- Prophylactic cholecystectomy is indicated.
- One should be ready to do hepatic resection, if required.

MIRIZZI SYNDROME (Figs 42.25 and 42.26)

Type I: Compression of CBD without lumen narrowing.

Type II: Compression of CBD with lumen narrowing.

Type III: Compression causing CBD wall necrosis.

Type IV: Stone ulcerating into CBD resulting in cholecystocholedochal fistula. It is treated by ERCP.

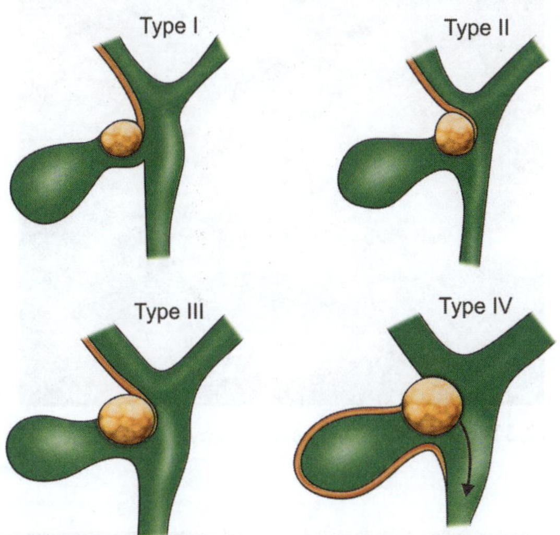

Fig. 42.25: Mirizzi syndrome

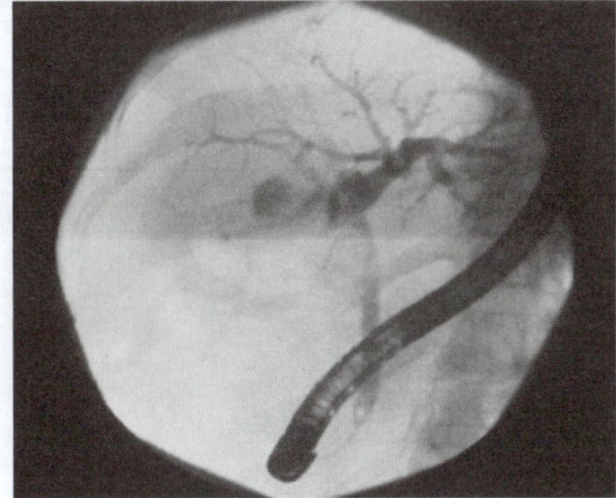

Fig. 42.26: ERCP showing Mirizzi syndrome

LAPAROSCOPIC CHOLECYSTECTOMY

It has become the most popular choice today. More than 95% of gallbladders can be removed through a laparoscope. Some principles and procedure of laparoscopic cholecystectomy are discussed below (Figs 42.27 and 42.32B).

Procedure

- 1 cm incision is made below the umbilicus, through which a pneumoperitoneum is maintained by CO_2 insufflation.
- Following this, a laparoscope is introduced and a camera is attached. Three small, 1 cm incisions are made in epigastrium and ½ cm in the right hypochondrium. These are used for suction, instrumentation, cauterisation, dissection, retraction purpose—dissection port.
- Gallbladder is mobilised by dissecting Calot's triangle by isolating cystic duct and cystic artery. Retraction of Hartman's pouch laterally opens up Calot's triangle (Fig. 42.28).
- Thus, it gives a view of liver bed and two structures—cystic artery and cystic duct. It is called critical view of Strasberg (Fig. 42.29).
- Cystic duct and cystic artery are clipped and gallbladder is removed using gallbladder-holding forceps and is brought outside through the epigastric port (Figs 42.30 to 42.32).
- Bleeding from liver is controlled using lasers/cautery.
- The procedure is done under general anaesthesia. It may take 1–3 hours depending upon the experience of the surgeon.

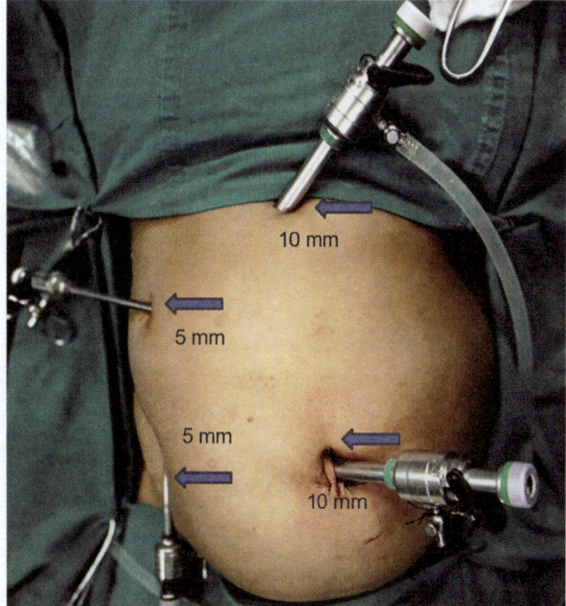

Fig. 42.27: Ports for laparoscopic cholecystectomy

Advantages

- Hospital stay is 1–2 days, recovery is very fast.
- Pain is minimal. Hence, mobilisation of the patient is much better and easy.
- It gives an acceptable and better cosmetic result.
- Complications such as adhesions and incisional hernia are rare.

Conversion to open when

- Very badly contracted, fibrosed gallbladder.
- Very difficult gallbladder—Calot's triangle anatomy is not defined well. Dissection may cause injury to the bile ducts and can cause stricture. **Partial cholecystectomy is a safe alternative.**

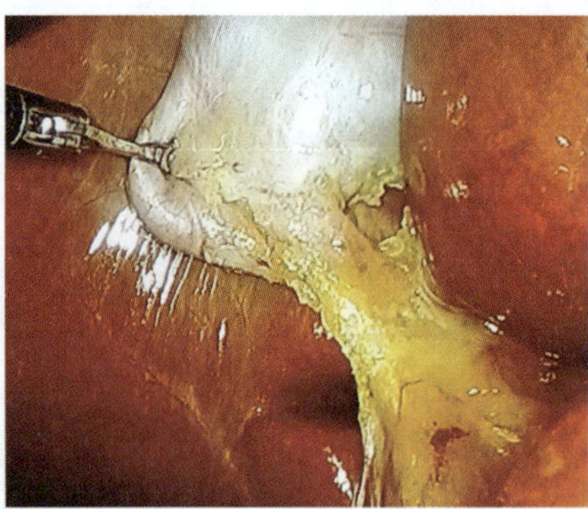

Fig. 42.28: First view of gallbladder once Hartman's pouch is retracted

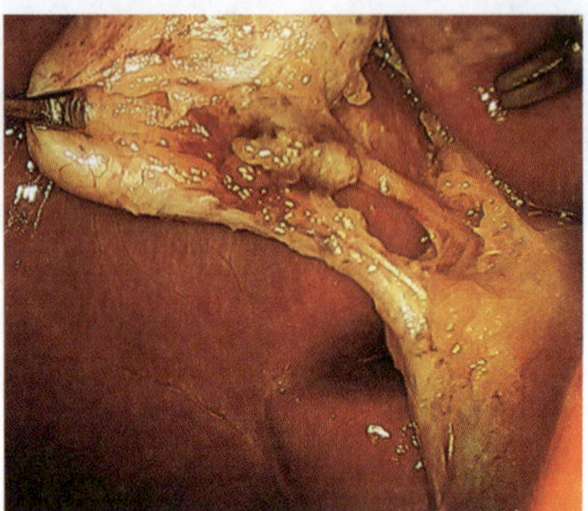

Fig. 42.29: Cystic artery and cystic ducts are seen—**critical view of safety** or **Strasberg** is achieved by dissecting the infundibulum off the liver bed, freeing it of all fatty tissue, both in its dorsal and ventral aspects

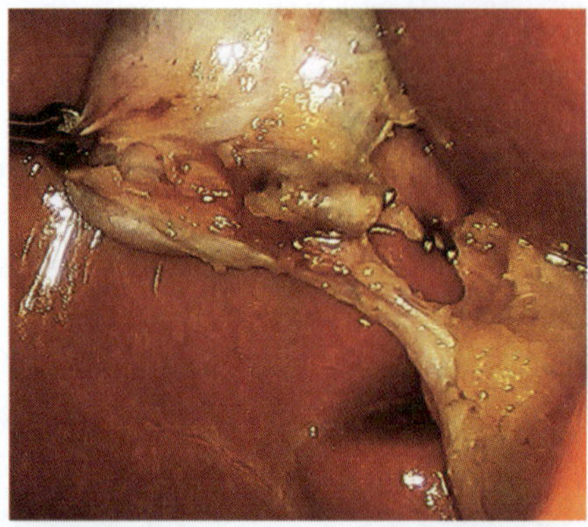

Fig. 42.30A: Cystic artery is ligated in 3 places

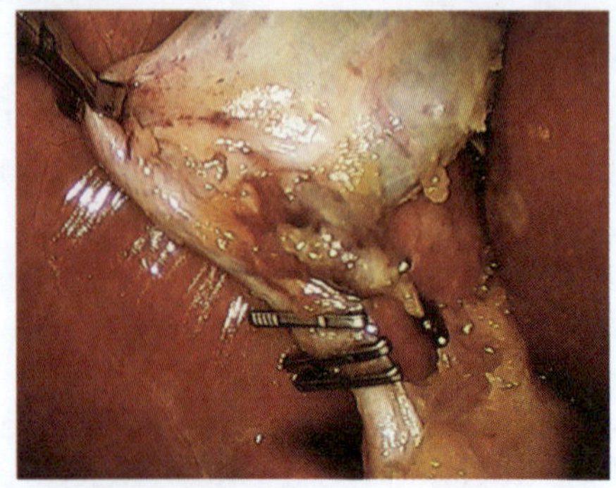

Fig. 42.30B: Cystic duct is clipped in 3 places

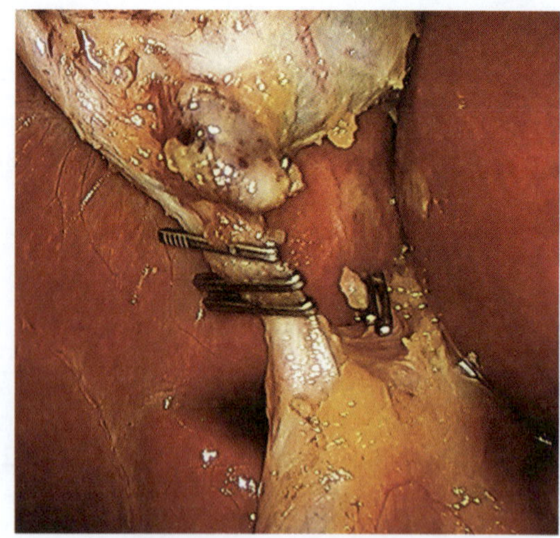

Fig. 42.31A: Cystic artery is divided

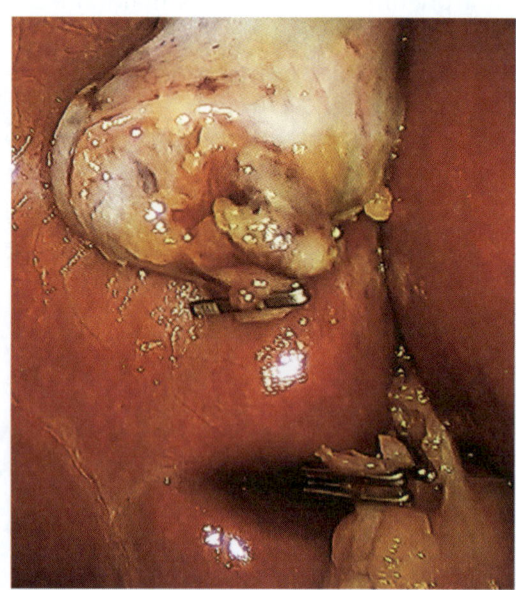

Fig. 42.31B: Both cystic artery and cystic duct are divided

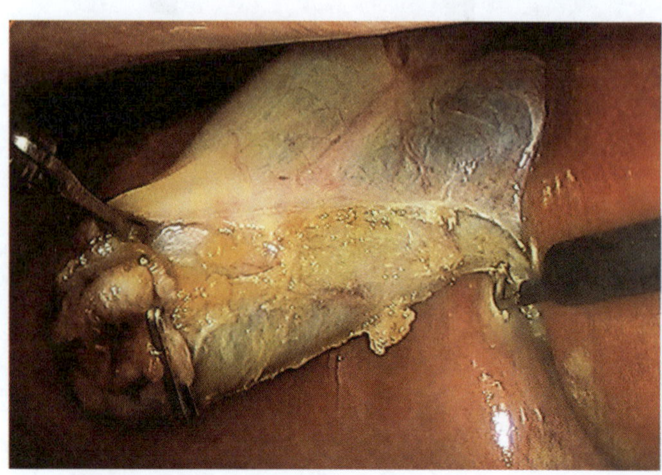

Fig. 42.32A: Gallbladder is dissected from liver bed

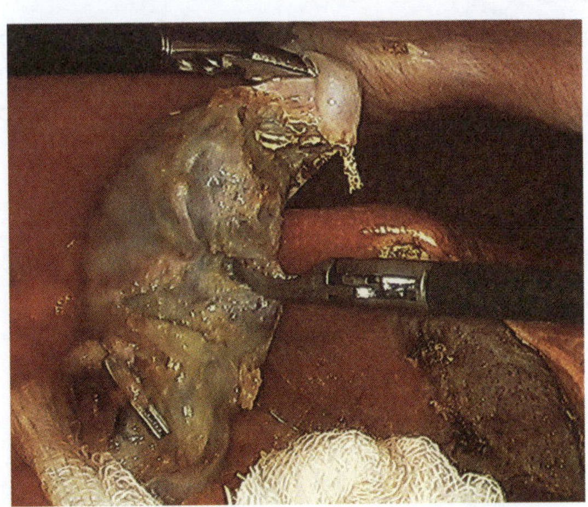

Fig. 42.32B: Gallbladder is completely dissected from the liver bed, placed in a bag and extracted

MEDICAL TREATMENT OF GALLSTONES

It is indicated for **pure cholesterol** stones only.

Patient Selection

- Patients with functioning gallbladder proven by OCG or scintigraphy.
- Young, thin, female patients.
- Tiny (<5 mm), translucent, floating stones.

Drawbacks

- Recurrence of stones once treatment is stopped.
- Lifelong maintenance is needed.
- After dissolution of the stones, lithotripsy or extracorporeal shock wave lithotripsy should be done.

Types of Medical Treatment

1. Oral Dissolution Treatment

- **Drugs used:** CDCA—chenodeoxycholic acid UDCA—ursodeoxycholic acid
- **Mechanism of action:** They inhibit HMG-CoA, a rate limiting step in the synthesis of cholesterol, thereby increasing the bile salt pool. UDCA also acts by decreasing cholesterol absorption in GIT.

2. Direct Contact Dissolution

MTBE—methyl tert-butyl ether is the drug which is given through a catheter placed in gallbladder percutaneously.

Drawbacks: Explosive and toxic, if it enters bile duct or duodenum.

Indications

- High-risk patients with symptomatic stones, refusing surgery.
- The patient must have patent cystic duct (proven by OCG/scintigraphy).

Side effects: Haemorrhage and catheter displacement.

Thus we have completed gallstones and their complications in the gallbladder. Now we will study the complication of gallstones in the common bile duct, mainly obstructive jaundice.

OBSTRUCTIVE JAUNDICE (SURGICAL JAUNDICE)

Definition

- Jaundice that occurs due to obstruction to the outflow of bile is called obstructive jaundice.
- Since these cases have to be managed by surgical intervention, it is also called surgical jaundice.
- However, haemolytic jaundice cases are not obstructive but a few are managed by splenectomy hence it is called as surgical jaundice.
- Before we start a detailed discussion of obstructive jaundice, we will study anatomy of the pancreas. This is an important long case in the university examination. For a better understanding of obstructive jaundice, **students are requested to understand various causes of obstructive jaundice which are given in the subsequent pages.**

Competency

SU24.2: Describe the anatomy of the pancreas. Describe the clinical features, principles of investigation, prognosis and management of pancreatic exocrine tumours.

SURGICAL ANATOMY OF THE PANCREAS

The pancreas is both endocrine and exocrine organ situated retroperitoneally behind the stomach. It is a soft and fleshy gland (pancreas—all flesh), extending from the duodenum on the right side to the spleen on the left side, the entire length being 6 inches (Fig. 42.33). It weighs approximately 80 g.

Parts

- The *head* lies within the C-loop of duodenum. The uncinate process projects from the left inferior portion of the head over which course the superior mesenteric vessels. There are 5–6 small thin veins connecting this portion of the head with superior mesenteric veins. These veins have to be carefully divided during pancreaticoduodenectomy. Superior mesenteric vein continues above as portal vein after joining the splenic vein. During pancreaticoduodenectomy for periampullary carcinoma, infiltration into the portal vein should be ruled out before any major structure is

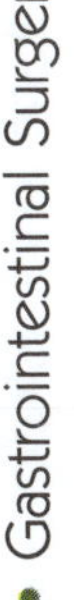

divided. This is done by inserting a finger between the portal vein and head of pancreas, both from above and below.

- The *neck* is about 2 cm and is related posteriorly to superior mesenteric vessels.
- *Body and tail:* The head and neck continue as body which is placed transversely. It slopes upwards across the aorta and ends as tail of the pancreas, which is enclosed within lienorenal ligament along with splenic vessels. A large cystadenoma arising from the tail of the pancreas can move with respiration because of its contact with the spleen.

BLOOD SUPPLY OF THE PANCREAS

Arterial Supply (Fig. 42.33)

- Splenic artery is the chief artery supplying the neck, body and the tail. Arteria pancreatica magna refers to one large branch of splenic artery.
- Superior and inferior pancreaticoduodenal arteries supply not only head of pancreas but also the adjacent duodenum. Thus, during any surgery which involves excision of the head, the C-loop of the duodenum is also removed. Thus, pancreaticoduodenectomy becomes a major surgery.

Venous Drainage

- Body, neck and tail drain into splenic vein by means of multiple small veins.

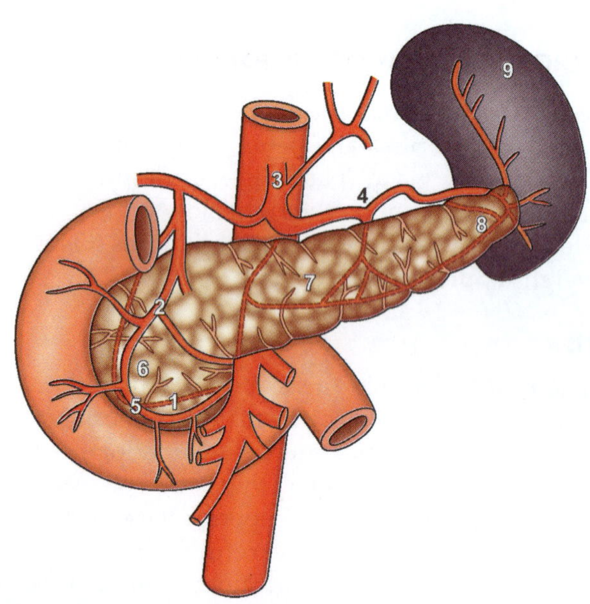

Fig. 42.33: Blood supply and parts of pancreas: (1) Uncinate process, (2) superior pancreaticoduodenal, (3) coeliac artery, (4) splenic artery, (5) inferior pancreaticoduodenal, (6) head of pancreas, (7) body of pancreas, (8) tail of pancreas, and (9) spleen

- The head is drained by superior pancreaticoduodenal vein which drains into portal vein and inferior pancreaticoduodenal vein drains into superior mesenteric vein.

Islets of Langerhans (Endocrine)

- 75% : β cells
- 20% : α cells
- 4% : δ cells

Pancreatic Duct

- The main pancreatic duct (duct of Wirsung), a tubular structure, drains entire pancreas from tail to the head. It joins the common bile duct and forms ampulla of Vater. This ampulla opens on the duodenal papilla (a nipple-like elevation) in the 2nd part of the duodenum. Normal diameter of pancreatic duct is 2–3 mm. When it is dilated more than 6–8 mm, as in chronic pancreatitis, longitudinal pancreatico-jejunostomy can be done.
- Accessory pancreatic duct of Santorini drains the uncinate process and lower portion of the head and opens into the duodenum 2 cm above the opening of the main duct. The two ducts communicate with each other at many sites.
- The main pancreatic duct is lined by columnar epithelium which becomes cuboidal in the ductules.

PANCREATIC JUICE

- Bicarbonate rich, protein rich, alkaline fluid
- 2.5 litres/day
- Rich in proteins—15 g of protein/day
- Thus acidic chyme in the duodenum is alkalinised by pancreatic juice.
- Protein is secreted by acinar cells, fluid and electrolytes by ductal cells.
- Secretions are stimulated by three phases:
  a. Cephalic phase is mediated by acetylcholine—10% of secretion
  b. Gastric phase—mediated by gastrin and vagus—15%
  c. Intestinal phase—75% release mediated by release of secretion from duodenal acidification and stimulated release of bile into 2nd part of duodenum following entry of fat and proteins.

A CASE OF OBSTRUCTIVE JAUNDICE

Choledocholithiasis and carcinoma head of pancreas/periampullary region are two important causes of obstructive jaundice. They constitute more than 90% of cases of obstructive jaundice treated surgically. Presence of jaundice, high-coloured urine, clay-coloured stools and itching gives the clue to the diagnosis. Palpable liver, palpable mass (cholangiocarcinoma, carcinoma head of pancreas) and palpable gallbladder (periampullary carcinoma) supports the diagnosis. Early diagnosis by imaging, endoscopy, ERCP, MRCP is possible. Since causes are many, they are treated accordingly. Relief of pain, relief of jaundice with or without resection (in malignancies) should be done early to prevent complications such as cholangitis, liver abscesses, septicaemia, renal failure and even death.

Aetiology (Fig. 42.34)

I. Causes in the Lumen

1. Stones in the common bile duct
2. Ova, cysts, ascaris worms
3. Hydatid cyst of the biliary tree
4. Stone in the pancreatic duct/CBD junction

II. Causes in the Wall

1. Periampullary carcinoma
2. Bile duct stricture
3. Stenosis of sphincter of Oddi (papillary stenosis)
4. Klatskin's tumour—carcinoma of the bile duct where right and left ducts join
5. Choledochal cyst
6. Post-laparoscopic cholecystectomy

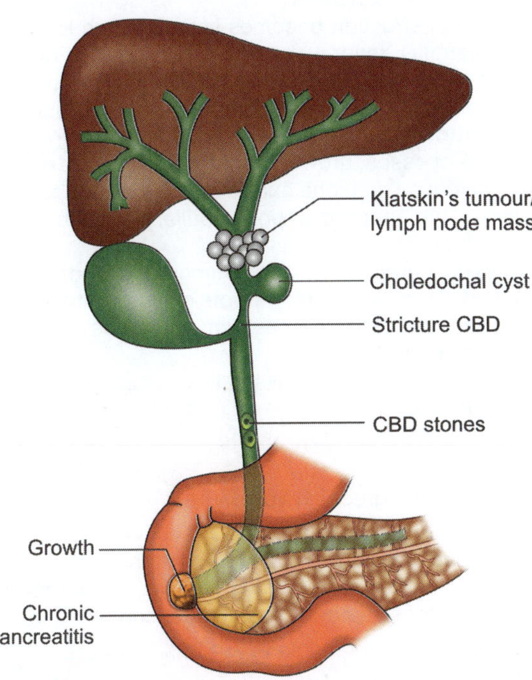

Fig. 42.34: Various causes of obstructive jaundice

III. Causes from Outside (due to Pressure)

1. Carcinoma head of pancreas
2. Chronic pancreatitis
3. Lymph nodes at the porta hepatis obstructing the biliary tree.

Clinical Features

First study to differentiate choledocholithiasis from carcinoma periampullary/head of pancreas (Table 42.1).

COURVOISIER'S LAW (Figs 42.35 and 42.36)

- In a jaundiced patient, if the gallbladder is palpably enlarged, it is not due to stones (Key Box 42.6). In case of stones, previous inflammation would have made gallbladder fibrotic and hence, will not be palpable.
- From clinical point of view, 90% of cases of obstructive jaundice are due to stones, periampullary carcinoma or carcinoma of the head of pancreas.

Key Box 42.6

Clinical Features of Gallbladder Mass

- Egg-shaped mass/pyriform shape
- Moves with respiration
- Tensely cystic, feels firm **(Murphy's point),** located in the right hypochondrium
- Superficially placed
- Intra-abdominal, intraperitoneal

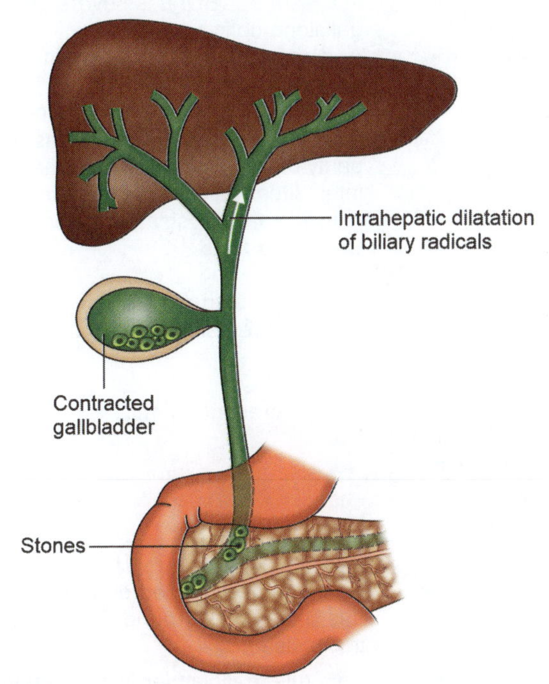

Fig. 42.35: Contracted thick gallbladder due to stones. Hence, not palpable

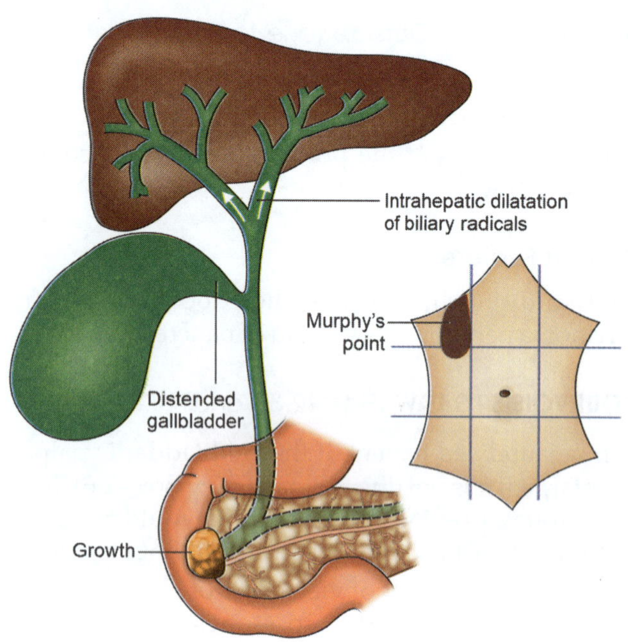

Fig. 42.36: Enlarged palpable gallbladder in cases of periampullary carcinoma

Exceptions to Courvoisier's Law

1. Double impaction: One stone in the CBD and one stone in the cystic duct. Gallbladder may be palpable in such cases.
2. Periampullary carcinoma in a patient who has undergone cholecystectomy.
3. Primary oriental cholangiohepatitis causing stones in the CBD (gallbladder is normal in these cases). These stones are called primary CBD stones.

Competency

SU28.12.2: Enumerate the causes, types, clinical features, investigations and management of a patient with cholelithiasis, and choledocholithiasis.

CHOLEDOCHOLITHIASIS (Table 42.1)

Types of CBD Stones

I. **Primary stones:** These stones are formed in the CBD or within intrahepatic ducts. They are multiple,

Table 42.1 Differences between stone in the CBD and periampullary carcinoma (Ca)/Ca head of pancreas

	Stone in the CBD	Carcinoma periampullary/head of pancreas
1. Age	30–50 years	50–70 years
2. Sex	More common in females	Equally common in both sexes
3. Duration of symptoms	Long duration	Short duration (1–3 months)
4. Symptoms		
Pain	It is due to a stone blocking the CBD resulting in spasm of CBD. It is severe colicky pain like gallstone colic	There may be some discomfort in abdomen but colicky pain is not a feature. Pain is relatively rare in carcinoma head of the pancreas
Fever	As a result of obstruction, multiplication of organisms results in fever	When obstruction becomes severe, there is bile stasis. Cholangitis, fever with chills and rigors can occur
Jaundice	Occurs due to obstruction. Once inflammation subsides, all these 3 symptoms are relieved partly but they occur after sometime. Hence, intermittent pain, intermittent fever, intermittent jaundice are classical of a stone in CBD—**Charcot's triad**	As a result of slow developing obstruction in periampullary region, jaundice is **persistent, progressive, painless, pruritic** In 5% of cases, growth may ulcerate into the duodenum. It can cause melaena and jaundice may temporarily subside. This happens in periampullary not in head of pancreas growth
Stools	Since the obstruction is never complete, clay-coloured stools are not commonly seen	Clay-coloured stools are common and when mixed with blood, it is called **silvery stools** or aluminium paint stools. This is called as Thomas' sign and it was first described by Heneage Ogilvie
Pruritus	May be present but mild	Severe—due to bile salts in the circulation
Loss of appetite	No	Significant
Loss of weight	No	Significant
5. Signs		
Jaundice	Deep yellow	Sometimes, greenish yellow
Anaemia	Absent	It is usually present
6. Per abdomen	Liver can be enlarged due to back pressure. It is smooth, with round border, firm in consistency	Liver can be enlarged due to back pressure. In such cases, it has smooth surface. If it is nodular, with sharp border, hard in consistency, it is due to secondaries in the liver
7. Gallbladder	As a rule, gallbladder is not palpable	Gallbladder is palpable in 70–75% of cases
8. Metastasis	No	Left supraclavicular node, ascites, etc. may be seen

Key Box 42.7

Primary CBD Stones

- Only 4–12% of all CBD stones.
- These stones do form primarily in common bile duct.
- Almost all primary CBD stones are pigment type (brown stones).
- Associated with bile duct stasis and infection (bacteria).
- Soft, easily crumble when manipulated.
- Associated with biliary stricture, papillary stenosis or sphincter of Oddi dysfunction.
- Mechanism; stasis—bacteria secrete bacterial glucuronidase which causes deconjugation of bilirubin diglucuronide. Bilirubin gets precipitated as calcium salt.

pigment stones or often mixed stones (Key Box 42.7). Various causes are:

- Infections of biliary tree and infestation—parasites such as clonorchiasis.
- Congenital—Caroli's disease or choledochal cyst.
- Biliary dyskinesia—defective pathophysiology of biliary tree.
- Other causes—diabetes, malnutrition.

II. **Secondary stones:** These stones originate from gallbladder and stay in CBD—usually supraduodenal portion—then get enlarged to attain large size over a period of time.

These stones can give rise to cholangitis.

Natural History of CBD Stones (Key Box 42.8)

Key Box 42.8

Natural History of CBD Stones

Symptom		*% of patients*
Asymptomatic	—	40%
Cholangitis	—	20%
Jaundice	—	20%
Biliary colic	—	15%
Pancreatitis	—	5%

Cholangitis

Bacterial infection of bile duct is called cholangitis.

Predominant Organisms

- *E. coli, Klebsiella, Pseudomonas,* enterococci, *Proteus.*
- Bacteroides and other anaerobes (*Clostridium perfringens*)

Important causes
- Choledocholithiasis
- Biliary stricture
- Neoplasm
- Less important causes are pseudocyst of pancreas, chronic pancreatitis stenosing sphincter of Oddi, biliary parasitic infections, etc.
- Post-ERCP, if stent cannot be passed as in obstructive jaundice cases.

Symptoms and Signs

- Biliary colic, jaundice and chills and rigors are called Charcot's triad.
- Tenderness may be present in the upper abdomen.

Investigations

- Leukocytosis, high bilirubin levels and alkaline phosphatase levels are diagnostic tests.
- Ultrasound, CT scans, ERCP are indicated to confirm/rule out the various causes.

Treatment

- Intravenous antibiotics
- Emergency endoscopic sphincterotomy, extraction of stones in choledocholithiasis, endoscopic stoning in cases of stenosis or stricture.
- Percutaneous transhepatic biliary drainage (PTBD) in high obstructions.
- Laparotomy—drainage of CBD—T-tube insertion.

Reynolds' Pentad of Acute Obstructive Cholangitis

A few cases of CBD stones present with serious problems of cholangitis described as Reynold's pentad

1. Persistent pain
2. Fever
3. Persistent jaundice
4. Shock
5. Altered mental status

INVESTIGATIONS IN OBSTRUCTIVE JAUNDICE

1. **Hb%** is low in malignancy.
2. **TC and DC** are increased in case of infections. High white cell counts suggest cholangitis and it becomes an indication for preoperative stenting in cases of carcinoma head/periampullary carcinoma. If cholangitis is due to CBD stones (more common), ERP followed by extraction of the stones with a stent is the initial definite treatment.
3. **BT, CT and PT** are altered in case of obstructive jaundice.

4. **Urine** for urobilinogen is negative in obstructive jaundice.
5. **Serum alkaline phosphatase:** Normal value 60–300 units/L. More than 500 units is suggestive of obstructive jaundice.
   - These are the enzymes which bring **hydrolysis** of phosphate esters in alkaline medium.
   - Sources of alkaline phosphatase include **liver, biliary tree**, bone, intestine, kidney.
   - Excretion is mainly through biliary tree (Key Box 42.9).
   - Segmental obstruction—bilirubin is LP.

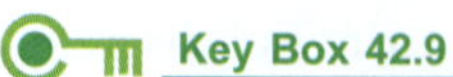

Key Box 42.9

Alkaline Phosphatase

- It is the product of epithelial cells of cholangioles—↑ levels are due to increased enzyme production.
- Intrahepatic cholestasis, cholangitis, and extrahepatic obstruction are the chief factors causing elevation.
- Focal lesions in the liver—single hepatic metastasis or liver abscess or a tumour can cause increased levels without jaundice.
- In cholangitis, bilirubin may be normal but alkaline phosphatase may be very high.
-

Gross elevation	**Mild elevation**
Obstructive jaundice, biliary cirrhosis, bone disease	Metastasis in the liver, hepatic abscess, hepatitis

6. **GGT:** Gamma-glutamyl transpeptidase.
7. **Abdominal ultrasound:** It is the **most useful, noninvasive, reliable and quick investigation for obstructive** jaundice. Dilated biliary radicles, both intrahepatic and extrahepatic, can be demonstrated (first clue in obstructive jaundice).
   - Gallstones can be diagnosed with their posterior acoustic shadow.
   - Mass lesion in the head region can be seen in cases of chronic pancreatitis or carcinoma head of the pancreas causing obstructive jaundice.
   - Ultrasound can detect multiple secondaries in the liver, thus, favouring the diagnosis of malignancy. However it is not an ideal investigation for CBD stones.
8. **CECT (contrast enhanced CT) scan:** A head mass of even 2–3 cm in size and portal vein infiltration can be demonstrated by CT scan. Obliteration of fat plane between the mass and superior mesenteric vessels can be demonstrated by CT scan which decides the operability of periampullary carcinoma or carcinoma head of the pancreas (Figs 42.37 to 42.40) relative contraindication.

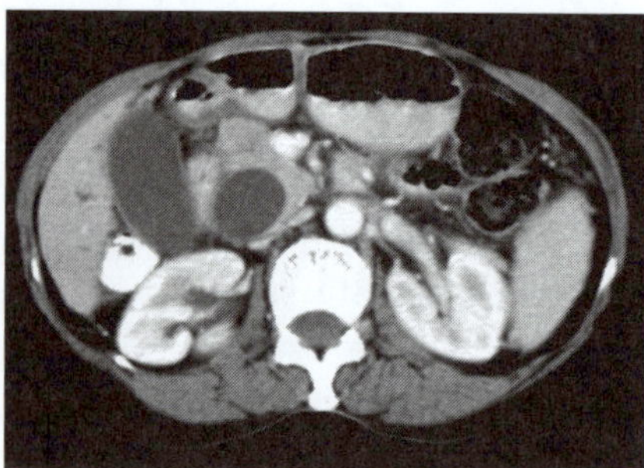

Fig. 42.37: CT scan showing hugely distended gallbladder and common bile duct—periampullary carcinoma. Growth was resectable. He underwent **Whipple's operation**

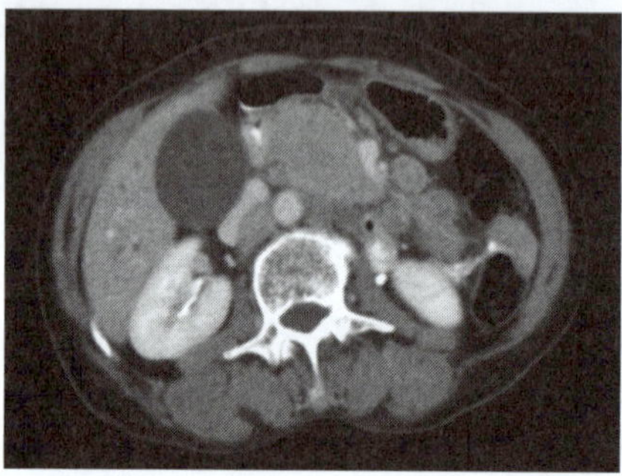

Fig. 42.38: Large 6 cm mass in the head of pancreas—patient not only had obstructive jaundice but also duodenal obstruction. He underwent **triple bypass**

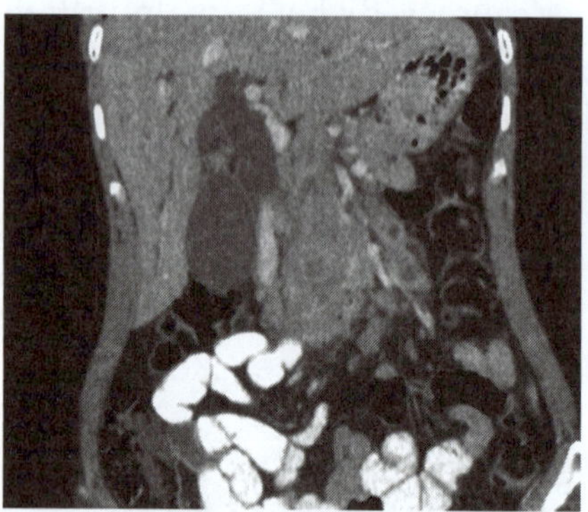

Fig. 42.39: 6 cm mass abutting mesenteric vessels and involving root of the mesentery. Such masses are usually nonresectable

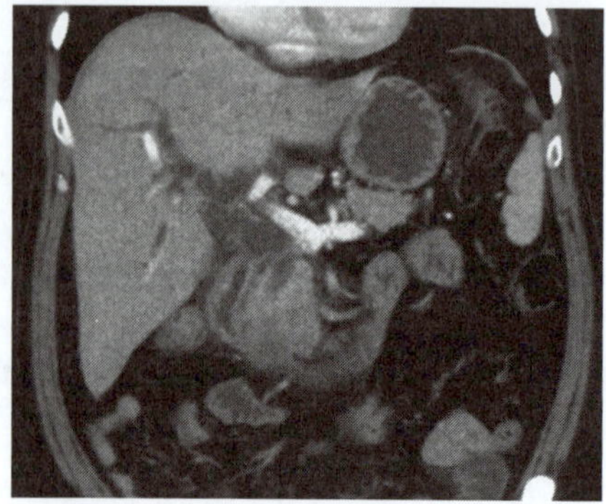

Fig. 42.40: Large head mass with obstructive jaundice with intrahepatic dilatation. When in doubt, diagnostic laparoscopy will help—to operate or palliate nonsurgically

Key Box 42.10

Complications of Percutaneous CT-Guided Biopsy of Head Mass

Death—rare
Enzymatic autodigestion
Abscess
Traumatic fistula
Haemorrhage
Remember as **DEATH**

- CT scan cannot differentiate head mass of carcinoma from chronic pancreatitis. (PET scan may differentiate.)
- CT scan can also detect coeliac nodes, presence of which is a contraindication for radical resections (Key Box 42.10).
- Take precautions against contrast-induced nephropathy.

9. **Endoscopy** is useful to diagnose a periampullary carcinoma which may be seen as an ulcerative lesion in the second part of the duodenum. Biopsy can also be taken which shows adenocarcinoma (Fig. 42.41). Please note if a lesion is detected such as growth, no stenting/or intervention (ERCP) is done. However, when bilirubin levels are very high and to improve general condition of the patient, as in cholangitis, temporary stenting can be done.
   - In case of obstructive jaundice due to stones, smooth bulge can be seen in the second part of the duodenum. In carcinoma, ulcerated lesion can be seen.
10. **MRI:** When CBD stones are suspected MRI is done. It is easy and no contrast is used. If stones are detected one can proceed with ERCP and basketting of stones (Figs 42.42 and 42.43).
11. **ERCP (endoscopic retrograde cholangiopancreatography)** (Figs 42.44 to 42.46).

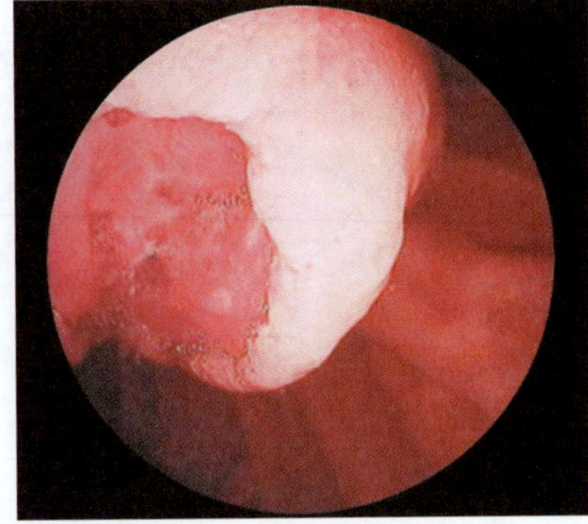

Fig. 42.41: Endoscopy showing growth in the periampullary region. These lesions are usually resectable

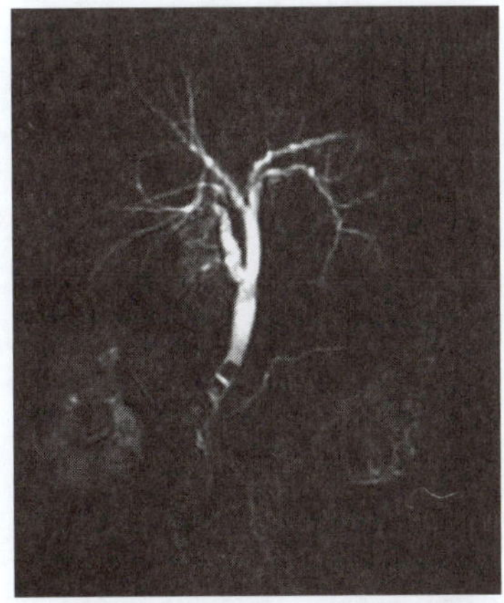

Fig. 42.42: MRI showing CBD stone

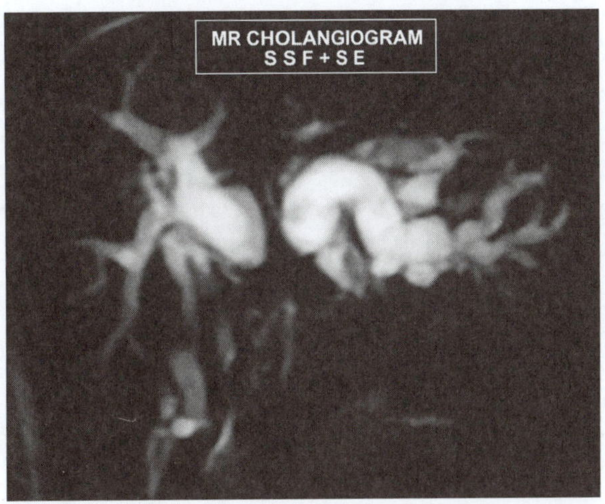

Fig. 42.43: MRC intrahepatic dilatation, another case of cholangiocarcinoma—biopsy is not possible with MRI. Brush cytology is possible while doing ERCP

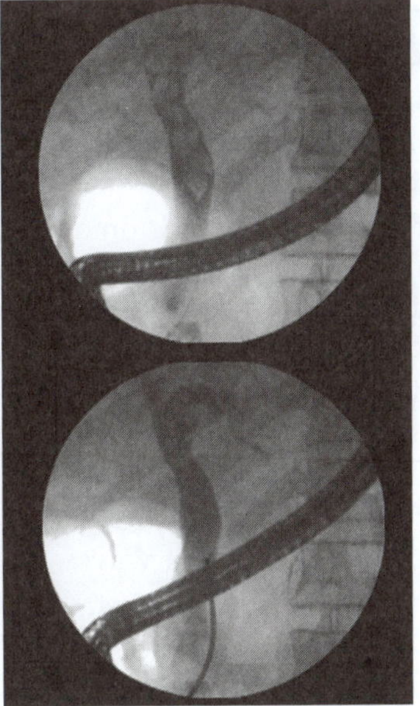

Fig. 42.44: ERCP showing stones in the CBD, stones are extracted and stent has been placed in the common bile duct

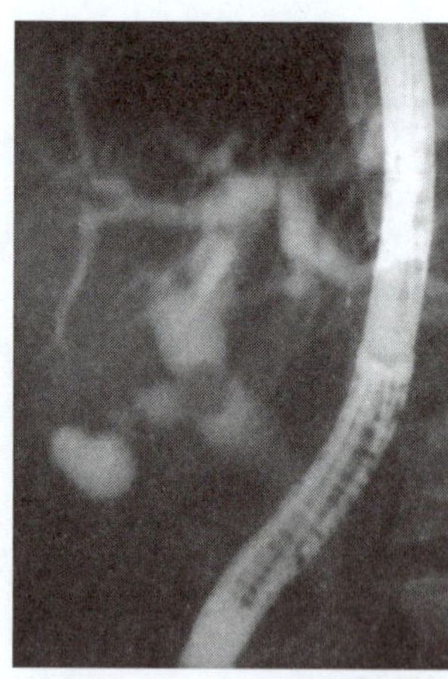

Fig. 42.45: ERCP showing stones in the CBD and contracted gallbladder

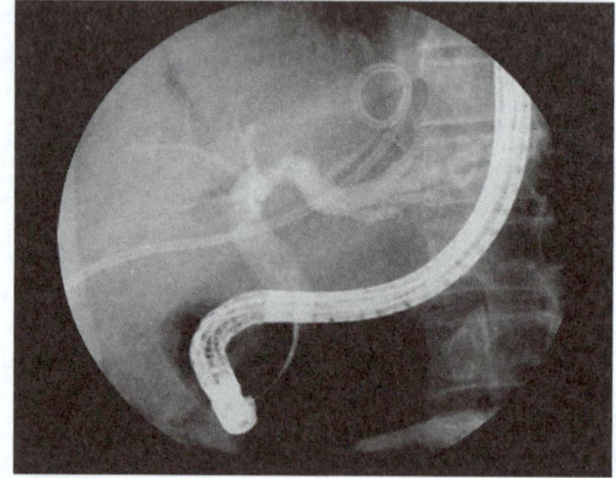

Fig. 42.46: ERCP basketting of stones followed by stent inserted into CBD

- With the help of a side viewing endoscope, ampulla of Vater is cannulated and a radio-opaque dye is injected.
- It fills up the biliary and pancreatic system.

Interpretation

- Stones appear as filling defects in the CBD or in the common hepatic duct (CHD) (Figs 42.44 to 42.46), which may be mobile (change position, if patient is moved).
- A periampullary carcinoma gives rise to an irregular filling defect or there may be total cut off in the flow of dye. (Done for cholangitis due to carcinoma cases.)
- Chronic pancreatitis may show the dilated duct and stones in the pancreatic duct—***'chain of lakes' appearance.***

Uses: If stones in the CBD are diagnosed, they can be treated in the following ways:

- Extraction by using a basket.
- Large stone can be crushed by using a lithotripter and can be extracted.
- Sphincterotomy (incision of sphincter of Oddi) can be done to facilitate extrusion of small stones.
- In patients with cholangitis with obstructive jaundice, stenting of common bile duct can be done to relieve obstruction. **Stent removal is necessary** at a later date.
- In selected patients with **biliary strictures**, stent is placed after ERCP to relieve obstructive jaundice (sometimes permanent in malignancies).
- In selected patients with **chronic pancreatitis**, pancreatic duct can be stented to relieve pain.

Pearls of Wisdom

ERCP and stenting is NOT indicated in operable cases of carcinoma periampullary/head of pancreas unless cholangitis is present.

Complications: Severe infection of biliary tree (cholangitis) and acute pancreatitis can occur in 1–2% of the patients. Hence, prophylactic antibiotics are given before the procedure.

12. **Endosonogram:** Endoscopy aided ultrasound can detect missed stones in the CBD. It can also detect pancreatic head mass, lymph nodes. Endosono-guided FNAC can also be done (Fig. 42.47).
13. **Percutaneous transhepatic cholangiography (PTC):** Using an ultrasound image-intensifier, a dilated biliary radicle is identified within the liver and a fine needle (Chiba needle[1]) is introduced into it. The stylet is then removed and a radio-opaque dye injected. Chiba needle is 15 cm long and 0.7 mm in diameter (Figs 42.48A and B, Key Box 42.11).

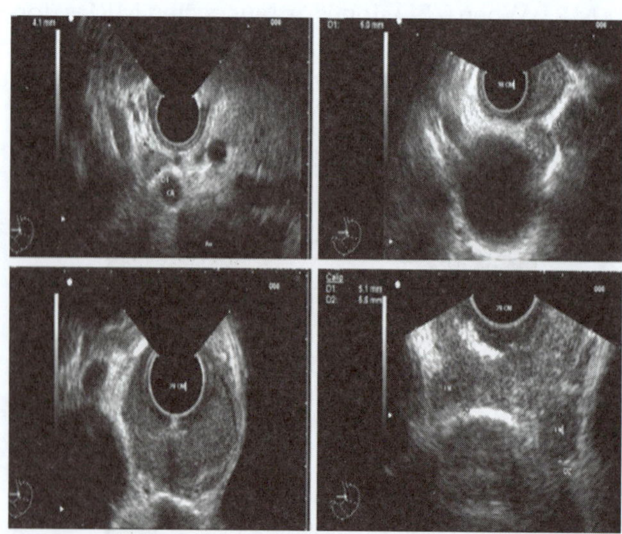

Fig. 42.47: Endosonography showing pancreatic tumour with celiac lymph nodes. (*Courtesy:* Dr Ganesh Pai, Head, Department of Medical Gastroenterology, KMC, Manipal)

[1]Chiba: It is the name of a university in Japan.

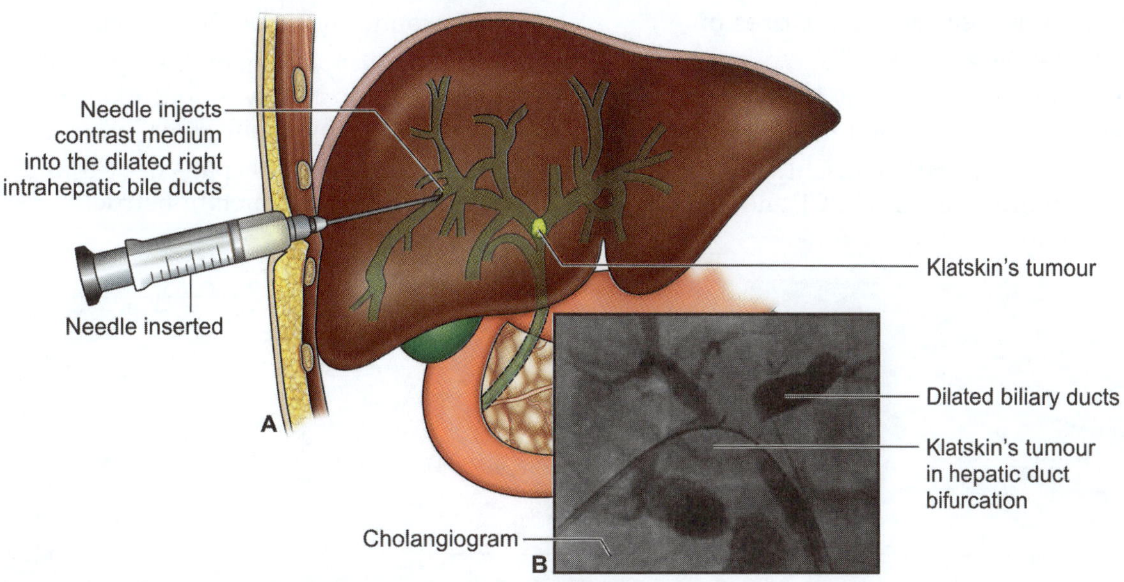

Figs 42.48A and B: (A) Percutaneous transhepatic cholangiography (PTC); (B) Dye had failed to fill-up the bifurcation of the common hepatic duct suggesting the obstruction (diagrammatic)

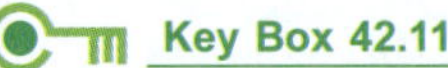
Key Box 42.11

Facts about PTC

1. In the diagnosis of high strictures, PTC is better than ERCP.
2. It can also be used in ERCP failure cases.
3. In the diagnosis of Klatskin's tumour, PTC is extremely useful. It can also delineate the dilated proximal duct, which helps in planning for a biliary-enteric anastomosis.
4. Catheter can be kept in the bile ducts to provide external drainage as in strictures or in inoperable malignancies with obstructive jaundice (Fig. 42.48C).

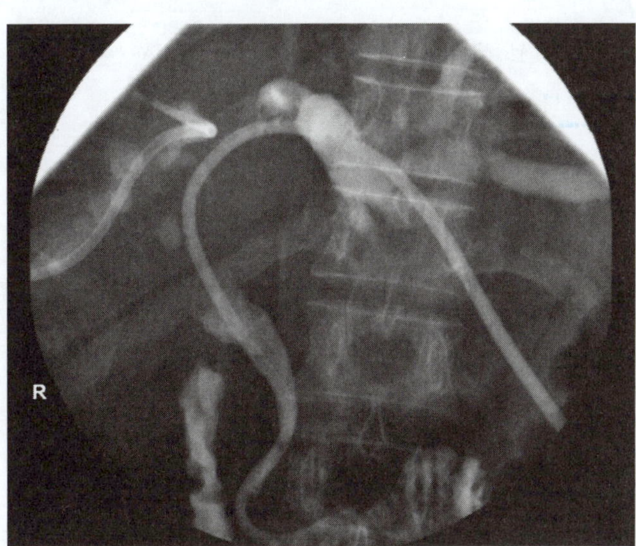

Fig. 42.48C: PTBD catheter inside CBD

Precautions

- BT, CT, PT should be normal. Otherwise, vitamin K injection 10 mg is given IV or SC for 3 days.
- If there is a bleeding tendency, this procedure should not be done.
- Broad-spectrum antibiotics are given before the procedure.

Complications

- Infection, cholangitis, septicaemia
- Biliary leak can be significant producing abdominal pain and guarding. Hence, PTC should be done just prior to the surgery.
- Haemorrhage

14. **Diagnostic laparoscopy**
    - It is used in many GI malignancies.
    - It can be aided by laparoscopic ultrasound.
    - It can complement the staging by CT, MRI, etc. It can improve prediction of resectability to about 98% accuracy.
    - It is a simple but invasive investigation, requires 3 ports.
    - Specially excellent to detect ***peritoneal metastasis*** (which cannot be picked by other tests) which is the sign of inoperability.
15. **CA 19–9:** Often head mass can be due to carcinoma/chronic pancreatitis. Biopsy is not mandatory. Clinical suspicion of a head mass may be treated with Whipple's pancreaticoduodenectomy. However, gross elevation of CA 19–9 (carbohydrate antigen) will suggest carcinoma.

Summary of the Investigations in Cases of Obstructive Jaundice (Fig. 42.49)

- CBP, LFT is done first to know the type of jaundice and to know the general condition of the patient.
- If ultrasound detects IHBR and CBD stones, no other investigations are necessary. ERCP and basketting of the stones is done.
- If ultrasound shows doubtful stones, CECT is done.
- If periampullary carcinoma is suspected, side viewing endoscopy and biopsy is done followed by CECT to detect signs of operability.
- In high (at the porta hepatis or at confluence of left and right hepatic ducts) obstructions—MRI and CECT are done.

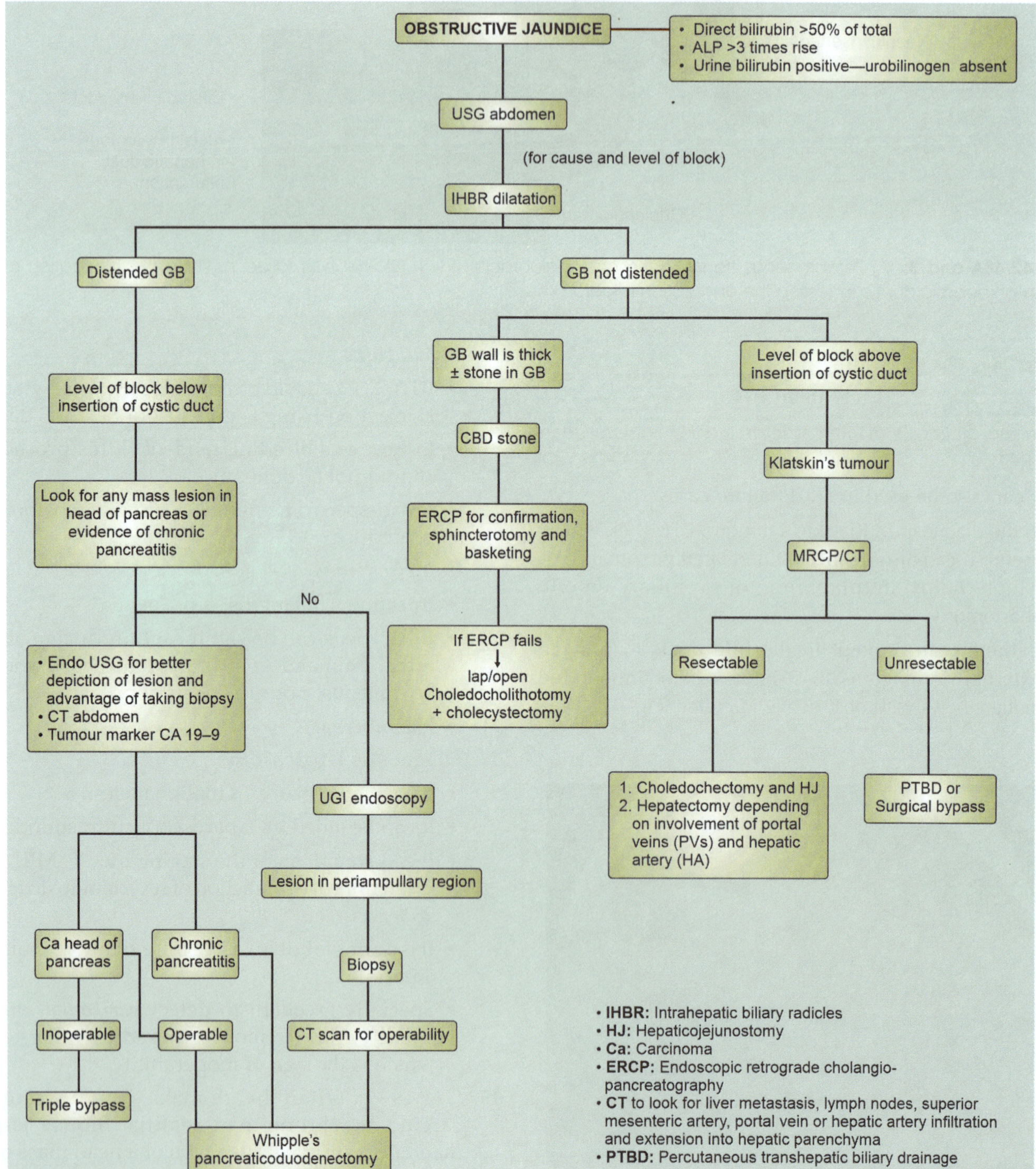

Fig. 42.49: Investigations and treatment of obstructive jaundice. (*Courtesy:* Dr Ankur Sharma, Asst Professor, Department of Surgery, KMC, Manipal)

TREATMENT OF OBSTRUCTIVE JAUNDICE

Preoperative Preparation

In all malignancies, Kernofsky criteria or ECOG criteria (page no. 681) of performance status is calculated and discussion is done with patient and relatives regarding the plan of treatment—surgery, complications, chemotherapy, etc. Discussion of the disease and the performance status should be discussed in tumour board once staging is done and appropriate treatment is done.

1. Correction of fluid and electrolyte status and adequate hydration before surgery for 2–3 days is essential, especially when patients have vomiting or have developed sepsis.

   Adequate hydration is done to improve the urinary output.
2. Injection vitamin K, 10 mg, subcutaneously or intravenously for 3 days is given to correct the prothrombin time. If prothrombin time is not corrected with this treatment, **fresh frozen plasma** should be given.
3. Broad-spectrum antibiotics are given before, during and after surgery.
4. Adequate blood transfusion to correct anaemia.

Treatment of CBD Stones

Once the diagnosis of CBD stones are confirmed by imaging, a few options are available depending upon expertise, facilities. They are given below.

1. ***Preoperative ERCP, sphincterotomy + extraction of stones followed by laparoscopic cholecystectomy:*** This method has become the choice today. Expertise and sophisticated equipment are necessary for this (Fig. 42.50).
2. *Cholecystectomy* is done first. This is followed by introduction of a cannula into the cystic duct and a radio-opaque dye is injected.
   - This is called **OTC** (**O**n **T**able **C**holangiography). If the dye goes freely into the duodenum without filling defect, it is a normal OTC. If there are filling defects in the CBD, it is explored.
   - **Precautions while doing OTC**
     - There should not be any air bubble in the syringe.
     - 5–10 ml of dye has to be injected.
     - Leakage of the dye should not occur.
     - OTC and CBD exploration can be done by laparoscopy only.
3. *Supraduodenal choledocholithotomy:* Some patients come after Lap. cholecystotomy and failed ERCP and basketting. They are managed by open method. Supraduodenal CBD is explored through an incision over the anterior wall and the stones are removed. Operating choledochoscope is passed into the common hepatic duct and its branches and the stones, if present, are removed. Closure of the CBD is done after inserting 'T-tube'. After 8–10 days, a T-tube cholangiography is done and if the dye goes freely into duodenum and no filling defect is seen in the CBD, the T-tube is removed by gentle traction. By 10–12 days, the track is well formed. Hence, even if minor leak occurs, bile flows outside without causing peritonitis (Key Box 42.12, Figs 42.51A and B).

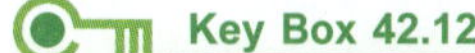

Key Box 42.12

Indications for Exploration of CBD

1. Ultrasound proven stones in CBD
2. OTC shows filling defect

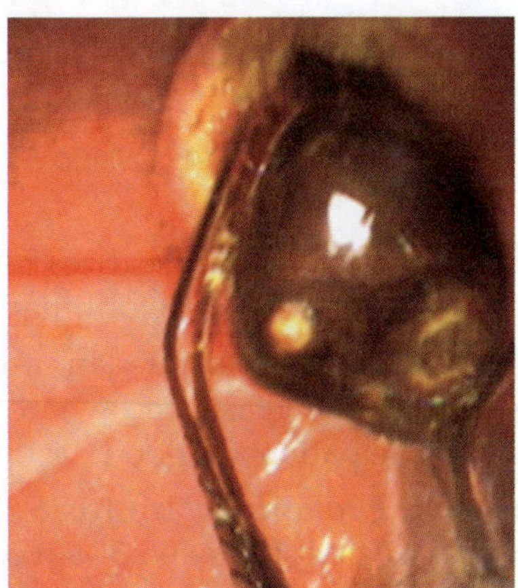

Fig. 42.50: Stone was removed through endoscopic papillotomy followed by basketing. There is a small risk of perforation and pancreatitis in these patients. Procedure is followed by a stent. (*Courtesy:* Dr Ganesh Pai, Prof and Head, Department of Medical Gastroenterology, KMC, Manipal)

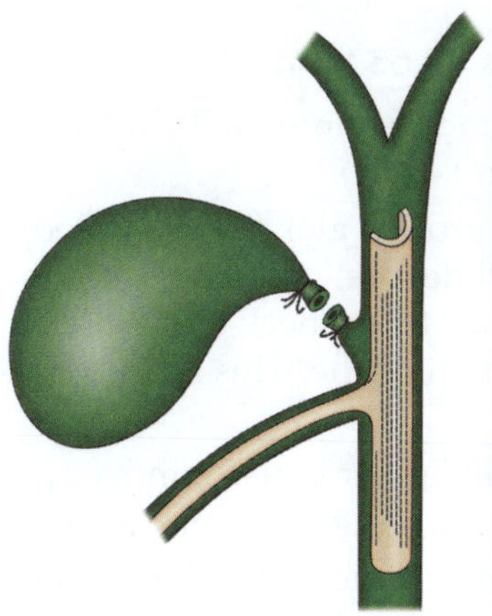

Fig. 42.51A: Cholecystectomy, CBD exploration followed by insertion of T-tube

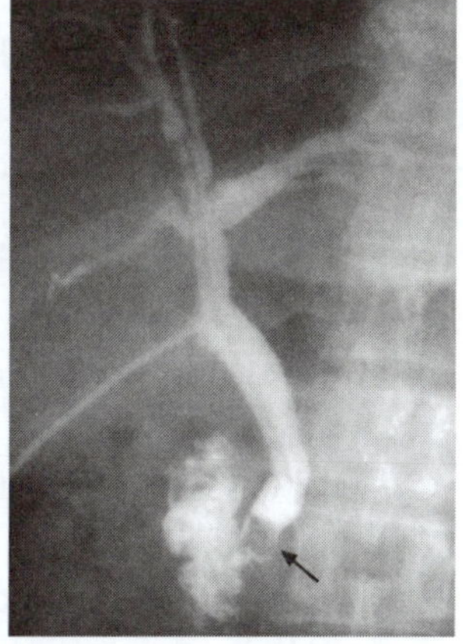

Fig. 42.51B: T-tube cholangiogram showing residual (retained) stone in the lower CBD—it was removed through endoscopic papillotomy and basketing

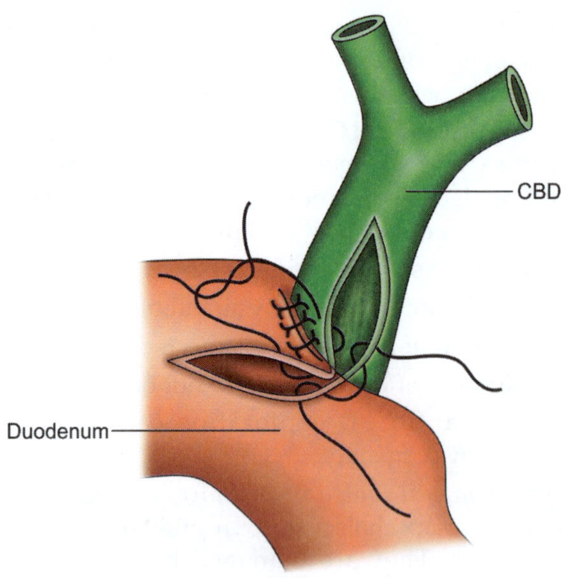

Fig. 42.52: Choledochoduodenostomy

4. ***Cholecystectomy + choledocholithotomy + choledochoduodenostomy:*** It can be done when CBD is dilated more than 1.5 cm in diameter and stoma should be at least 2–3 cm in size (Fig. 42.52). Indications are:
   - Recurrent stones in the CBD
   - Multiple intrahepatic stones (Caroli's disease)
   - Stricture of the lower CBD

   Advantages of choledochoduodenostomy
   - Biliary leak is negligible
   - There is no worry, even if there are retained stones in the CBD.
   - It is a permanent solution for stenosis, stricture or multiple intrahepatic stones.

TREATMENT OF PERIAMPULLARY CARCINOMA

I. Surgical Treatment (Figs 42.53 to 42.58)

1. **Radical pancreaticoduodenectomy—'Whipple's operation'** (Figs 42.53 and 42.54).
   - In this operation, the growth along with 'C' loop of duodenum up to DJ flexure, proximal jejunum, head of the pancreas up to the neck are removed and partial gastrectomy is done. This is followed by:
     - Lower CBD and gallbladder is also removed.
     - Pancreaticojejunal anastomosis (PJ), gastrojejunostomy (GJ) and choledochojejunostomy (CJ).

Pearls of Wisdom

Preoperative tissue diagnosis is NOT necessary with appropriate clinical and imaging findings, specially in head masses.

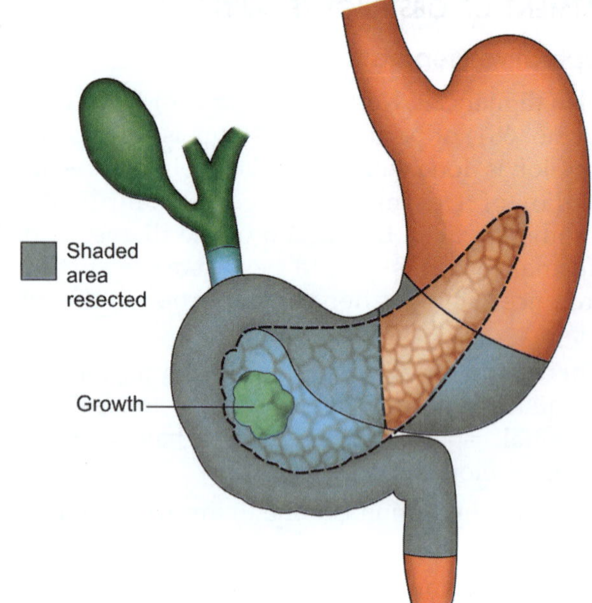

Fig. 42.53: Whipple's resection (diagrammatic)

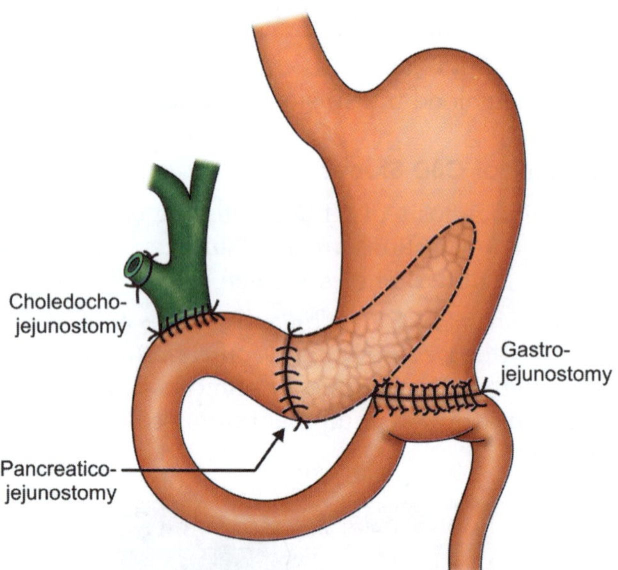

Fig. 42.54: Reconstruction following Whipple's operation

   - This is a major operation and carries 5–10% mortality due to pancreatic leakage or biliary leakage.
   - Whipple's operation is indicated in cases of mobile growth with no metastasis and where the general condition of the patients is good.
   - Patients with cholangitis are treated with preoperative CBD stent followed 3–4 weeks later by Whipple's procedure.

2. **Pylorus-preserving pancreaticoduodenectomy (PPPD) or Traverso-Longmire procedure:** In this operation, pylorus is preserved. Thus, gastric motility is not disturbed (Fig. 42.55).

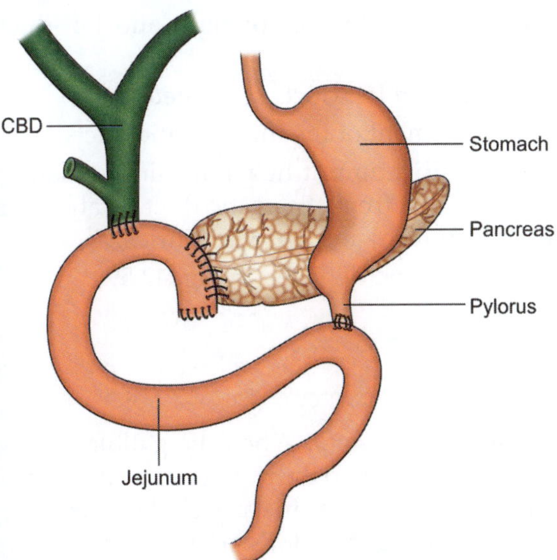

Fig. 42.55: Pylorus-preserving pancreatico-duodenectomy (PPPD)

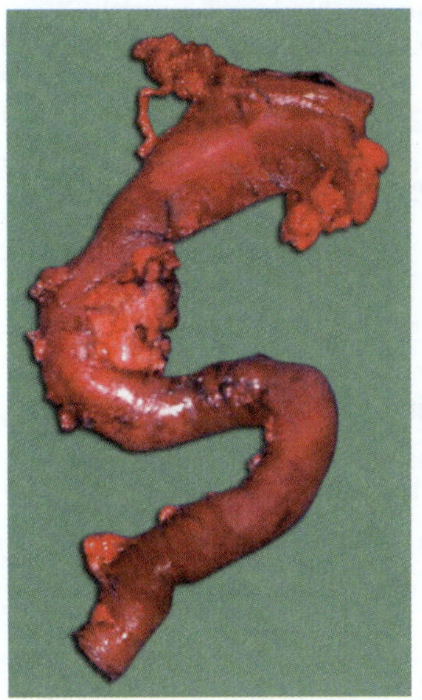

Fig. 42.56A: Whipple's resection specimen

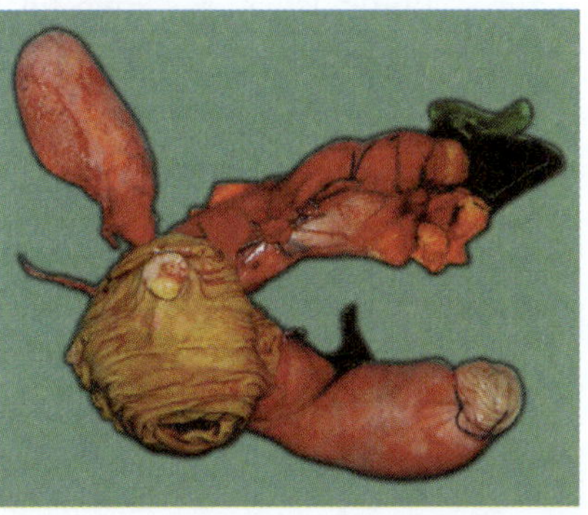

Fig. 42.56B: Whipple's specimen (*Courtesy:* Dr Satyanarayana N, Former Associate Professor, Yenepoya Medical College, Mangalore)

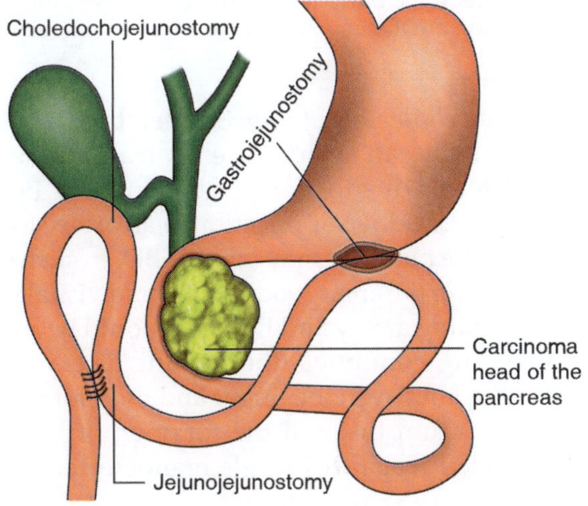

Fig. 42.57: Palliative triple bypass

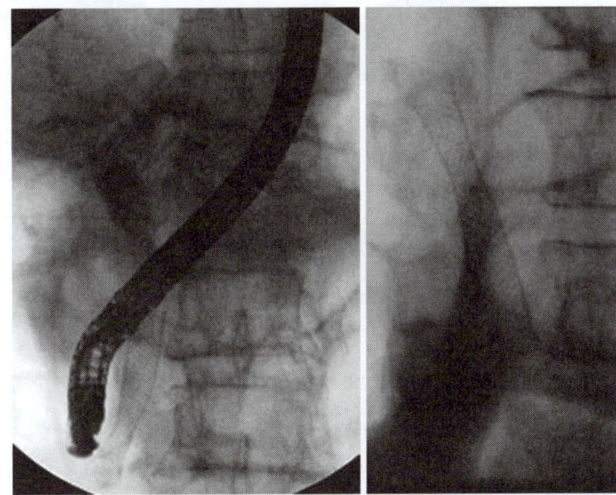

Fig. 42.58: Palliative stenting for carcinoma head of the pancreas

'TUNNEL OF LOVE'

During resectional surgery for pancreatic head and uncinate process tumours (Whipple's pancreaticoduodenectomy), after a preliminary search for metastases, a tunnel (the so-called tunnel of love) needs to be developed behind the neck of the pancreas and anterior to the underlying visceral vessels before concluding that the lesion can be resected. CBD is lifted gently by a tape and plane between CBD and portal vein is slowly developed by using a little finger from above. Another finger is inserted from below behind pancreas. Two should meet without any tissue.

3. Triple bypass: Cholecystojejunostomy + enterostomy + gastrojejunostomy

- This is a palliative surgery in which distended gallbladder is anastomosed to a long loop of jejunum (40 cm) to relieve jaundice. To prevent food particles entering into the gallbladder, enteroenterostomy is done (Fig. 42.50). Cholecystojejunostomy is easy to do compared to choledochojejunostomy.
- Most of the patients develop duodenal obstruction caused by the growth in the postoperative period. Hence, a palliative GJ is done at the same time.
- In the absence of duodenal obstruction, if surgeon thinks that patient may live longer, beyond 6 months, GJ is indicated (for a possible duodenal obstruction occurring later).

II. Nonsurgical Treatment

Very elderly patients (age criteria not clear) who are not fit candidates for surgery and patients who have metastasis can be treated by palliative stenting. However, results of a surgical bypass is superior to stenting. Also, the stent needs to be changed frequently.

OTHER CAUSES OF OBSTRUCTIVE JAUNDICE

Competency

SU28.12.4: Classify biliary strictures. Enumerate the causes, clinical features, investigations and management of biliary strictures.

STRICTURE OF THE CBD

- 80% of strictures occur following surgery on the biliary tree. They are called postoperative strictures. 20% are due to inflammatory pathology.
- It gives rise to slowly progressive, painless jaundice.
- Strictures account for 1–2% cases of obstructive jaundice.

Classification of bile duct injuries following laparoscopic cholecystectomy (Fig. 42.59)

1. **Bismuth classification:** Five types of bile duct injuries are recognosed based on the distance from the hilar structure—bile duct bifurcation, the level of injury, the involvement of bile duct bifurcation, and individual right sectoral duct.
   - ***Bismuth classification of postoperative stricture:***
     Type I: Low common bile duct; stump >2 cm
     Type II: Middle common hepatic duct, stump <2 cm
     Type III: Hilar—confluence of right and left duct intact
     Type IV: Right and left ducts separated
     Type V: Involvement of the intrahepatic ducts
2. **Strasberg classification:** It helps in differentiating small (bile leakage from the cystic duct or aberrant right sectoral branch) and serious injuries.
   Both these have been depicted in Fig. 42.59.

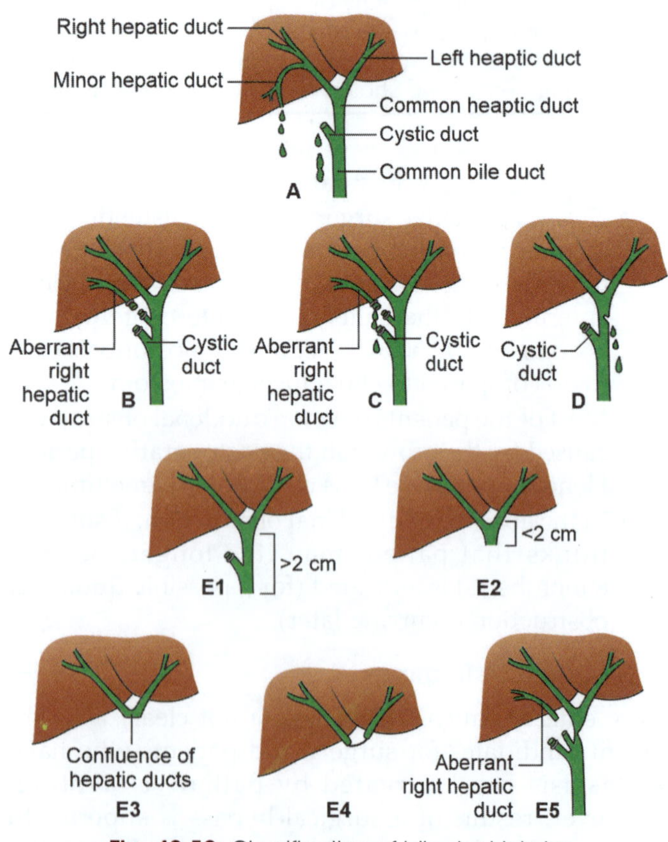

Fig. 42.59: Classification of bile duct injuries

Causes

1. Postoperative post-traumatic (Fig. 42.60)

- ***Difficult cholecystectomy:*** When the gallbladder is fibrosed, densely stuck to the right hepatic duct or to the common bile duct or as in early cholecystectomy due to oedema around Calot's triangle, injury can occur to the right hepatic duct or to the CBD or CHD resulting in stricture.

Pearls of Wisdom

Difficult cholecystectomy, dangerous cholecystectomy and faulty dissection are the important factors for postoperative bile duct strictures.

- ***Dangerous cholecystectomy:*** Sudden bleeding from cystic artery can occur due to traction on the gallbladder or due to lack of gentleness in ligating cystic artery. Sudden application of an artery forceps to control the bleeding may injure CBD. In such situations, packing the area, good suction and visualisation of the bleeding artery and ligation should be done. If the bleeding continues, the hepatic artery can be compressed between the finger and the thumb in the lesser omentum through the foramen of Winslow. This is called **Hogarth-Pringle manoeuvre**.

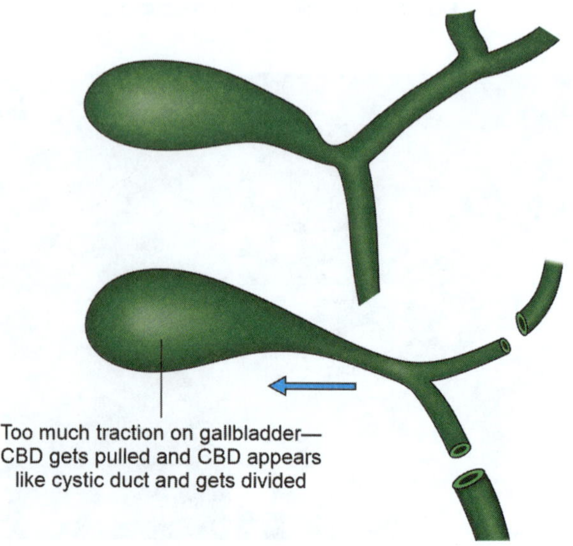

Fig. 42.60: Laparoscopy bile duct injury

- ***Dissection at fault:*** Ignorance of anomalies such as short cystic duct or too much traction on the gallbladder distorts CBD and predisposes to injury (Figs 42.61 and 42.62). It is the duty of the surgeon to show his assistants the Y junction which is formed by the cystic duct, common hepatic duct above and common bile duct below before dividing any structures in this area.

2. Post-inflammatory

Post-inflammatory strictures follow recurrent attacks of cholangitis due to:

- Stones in the CBD or CHD
- Parasites like *Ascaris lumbricoides* in the biliary tree or **Asiatic cholangiohepatitis** produced by Chinese liver fluke infestation (*Clonorchis sinensis*) (*see* page 640).
- Primary sclerosing cholangitis wherein the cause is not known.

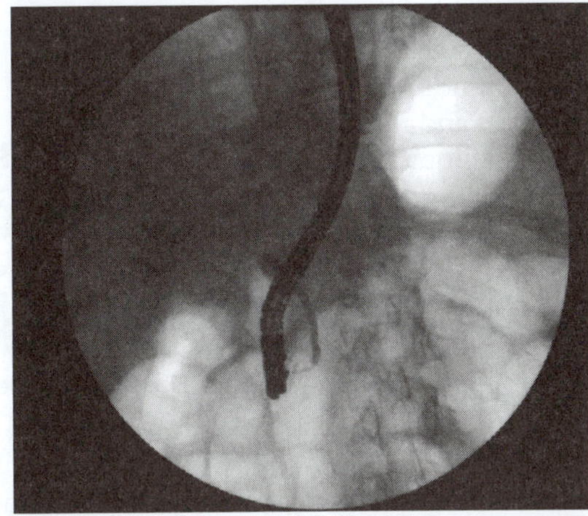

Fig. 42.61: ERCP showing complete transection of bile duct—type IV injury

3. Malignant strictures

Malignant strictures are due to cholangiocarcinoma.

Clinical features

- History of cholecystectomy in the past with or without profuse discharge of bile in the postoperative period.
- A slowly progressive, painless jaundice deepening day by day.
- Hepatomegaly due to back pressure.
- Recurrent cholangitis due to stasis of bile.

Investigations

- USG—to rule out residual stones in CBD, to demonstrate intrahepatic dilatation.
- ERCP or PTC may demonstrate a stricture in the CBD or CHD with proximal dilatation.
- T-tube cholangiography, if T-tube is in place.
- MRC is noninvasive and is better than PTC.

Treatment

- If it is due to laparoscopic clipping without transection of the CBD, it is better to re-explore and remove the clips and a T-tube or an endoscopic stent can be placed in the CBD (Fig. 42.63).
- Late cases can be managed by choledochojejunostomy or hepaticojejunostomy by anastomosing a loop of jejunum to the dilated portion above the stricture. However, the general condition of the patient should be improved before surgery (Figs 42.64 to 42.68).

Pearls of Wisdom

Prevention is better than treatment. Try to prevent bile duct injuries during laparoscopic cholecystectomy.

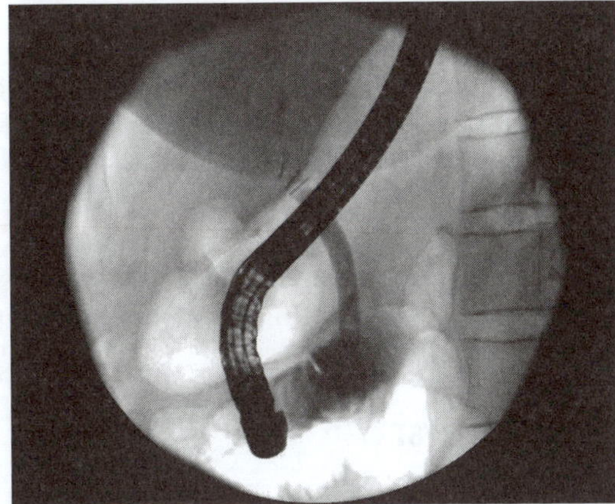

Fig. 42.62: CBD clipping—here, it was not transected. It was explored, clip removed and endoscopic stent was inserted

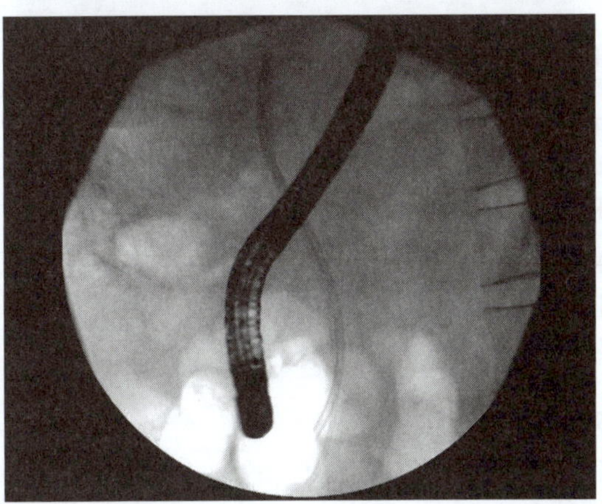

Fig. 42.63: Same patient as in Fig. 42.62. You can see the stent in the common hepatic duct. It was removed after 6 months

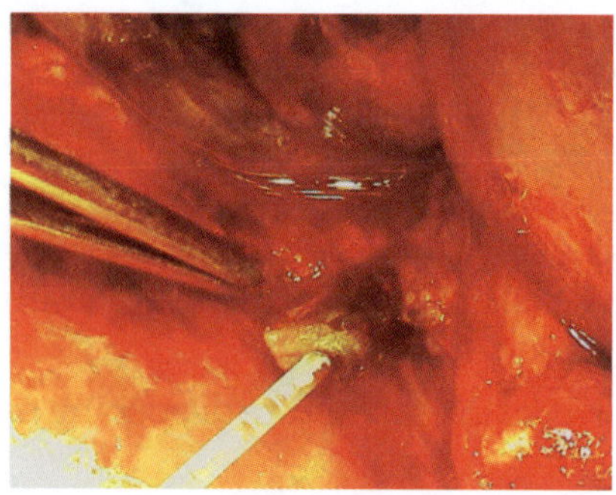

Fig. 42.64: Cut CHD—it was a difficult task to reach this area, it is trimmed for biliary enteric anastomosis

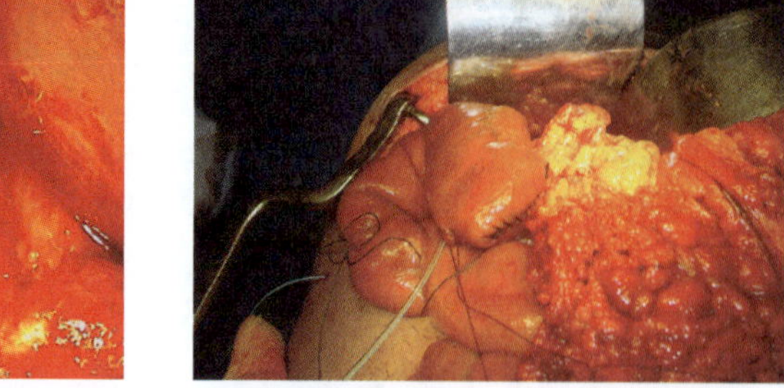

Fig. 42.65: Roux jejunal loop is prepared for hepaticojejunostomy

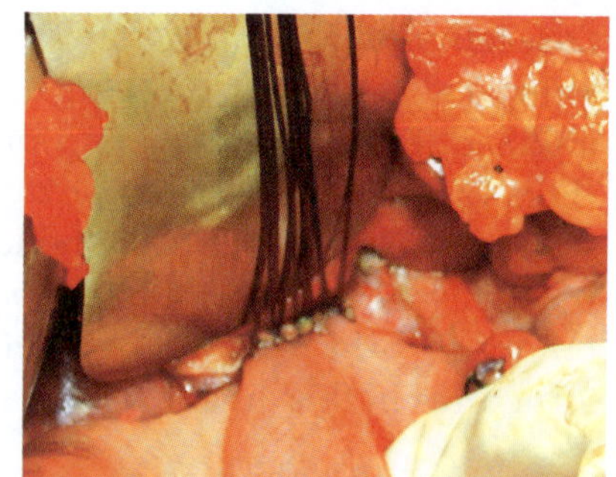

Fig. 42.66: Hepaticojejunostomy was done in another patient with type IV injury

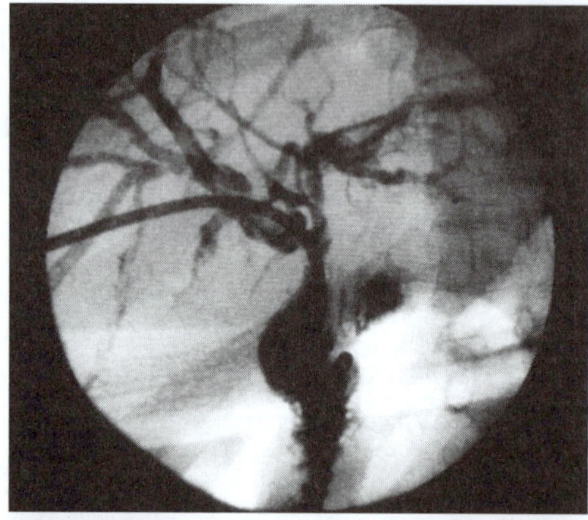

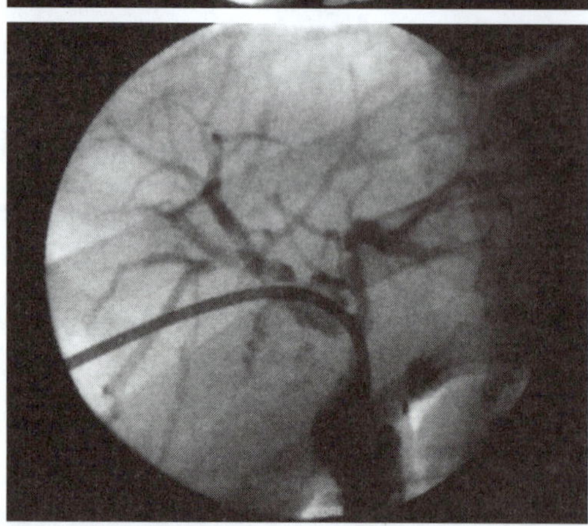

Figs 42.67 and 42.68: PTBD catheter was passed from above across strictured hepaticojejunostomy and dilatations were done in high strictures

SCLEROSING CHOLANGITIS

It is characterised by development of multiple strictures and dilatation of CBD with features of fibrous thickening of CBD.

Types

- **Primary:** No cause is found. However, it can be associated with conditions given in Key Box 42.13.
- **Secondary:** It is due to stones or injuries.

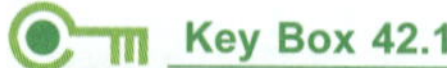

Key Box 42.13

Associated Conditions

- Ulcerative colitis
- Crohn's disease
- Graves' disease
- Sjögren's syndrome

Complications

Due to long-standing obstruction, biliary cirrhosis and cholangiocarcinoma can develop (Fig. 42.69).

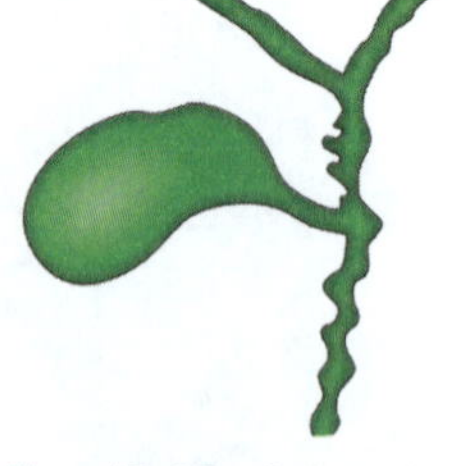

Fig. 42.69: Sclerosing cholangitis

Diagnosis

- **Ultrasound** can demonstrate intrahepatic dilatation.
- **MRCP** is a noninvasive investigation which can demonstrate multiple strictures and dilatation.
- **ERCP** is the investigation of choice which can demonstrate the strictures in the CBD and dilatation which is described as having a **beaded** appearance. However, the risk of suppurative cholangitis is present.

Treatment

- It is difficult.
- Stenting is the choice although stents may have to be replaced or changed, if blockage occurs or if infection sets in.

Competency

SU28.12.3: Describe the classification, etiopathogenesis, clinical features, investigations and management for different types of choledochal cyst.

CHOLEDOCHAL CYST

- It is a congenital cyst occurring in the CBD due to partial or complete weakness of the wall of the CBD.
- Majority of cases manifest by 1–2 years of age.

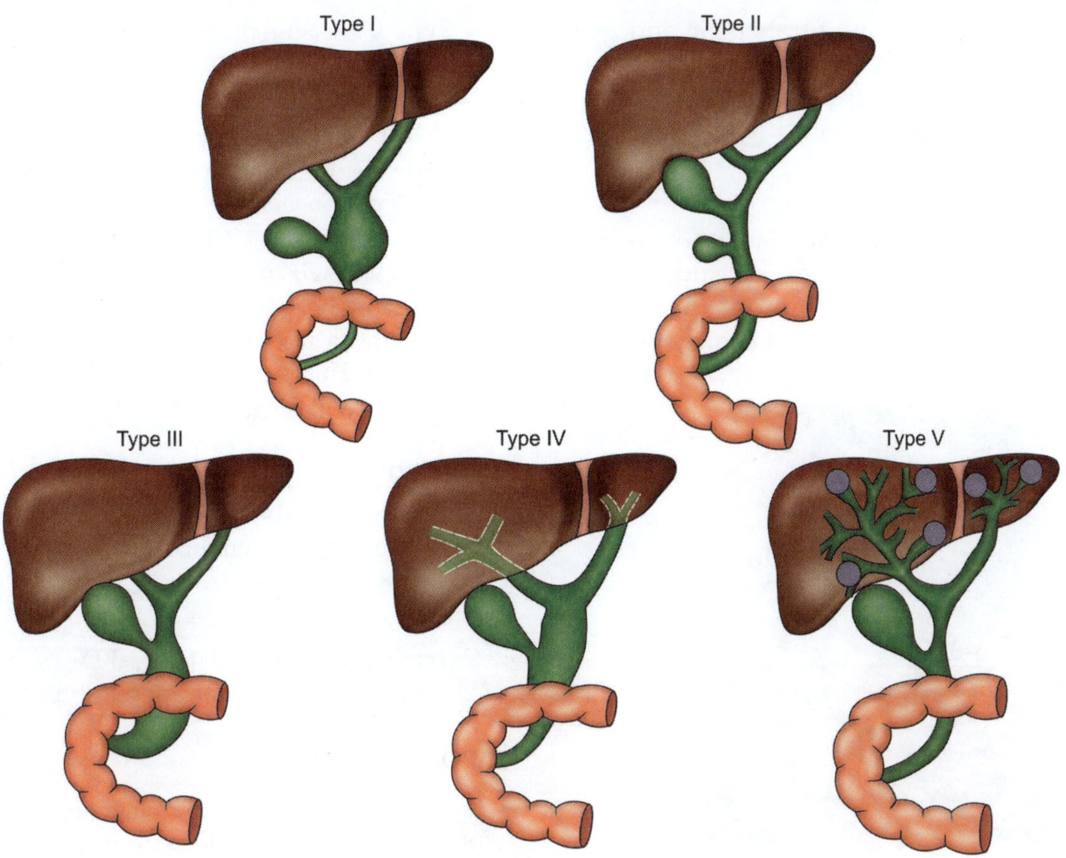

Fig. 42.70: Types of choledochal cysts

Classification (Fig. 42.70 and Key Box 42.14)

Recent advances: Type VI—cystic dilatation of cystic duct.

Clinical Features

- Age: Majority of cases manifest in children within 1–2 years of age. It can also present in adults.
- More common in **females**—4:1.
- **Abdominal distension** can be due to a large cyst. The cyst can be palpated per abdomen in the right hypochondrium.
- Slow progressive jaundice, recurrent attacks with abdominal pain and pyrexia.

Key Box 42.14

Todani Classification

Types

Type I:	Fusiform dilatation of CBD—commonest
Type II:	Lateral saccular diverticulum of the CBD
Type III:	Dilatation of intraduodenal segment of CBD (choledochocele)
Type IV:	Dilatation of CBD + intrahepatic biliary dilatation
Type V:	Multiple intrahepatic cysts—Caroli's disease

Investigations

1. **USG** will confirm presence of abnormal cyst. It is usually unilocular cyst.
2. **MRC:** It will define the relation between lower end of the bile duct and pancreatic duct to know basic anatomy (Fig. 42.71).

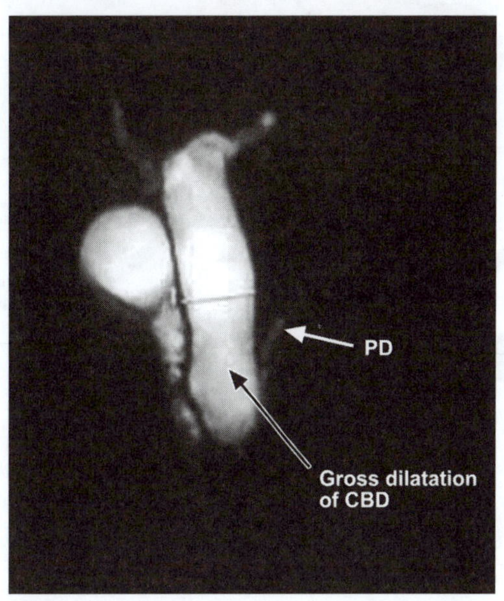

Fig. 42.71: MRC showing choledochal cyst

3. **CT** is also useful to know intrahepatic and extrahepatic dilatation.
4. **ERCP** may be done but it will not give any more information than MRC.

Treatment

- **This anomaly is premalignant.** Change to carcinoma is a well-recognised complication and it carries poor prognosis. **Hence, excision of the cyst and reconstruction is the treatment of choice** (Figs 42.72 to 42.74).

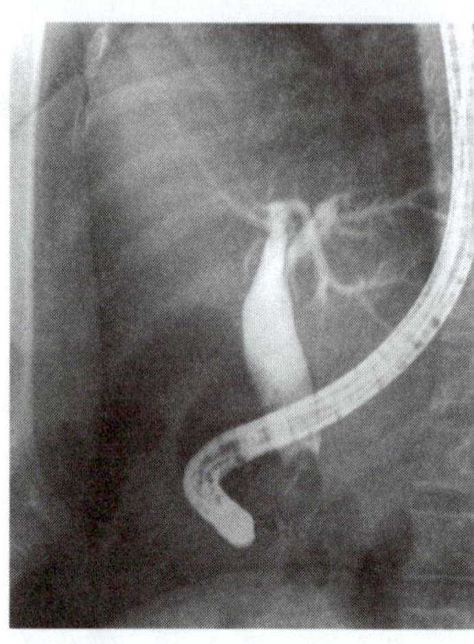

Fig. 42.72: ERCP showing choledochal cyst—type III treated by sphincterotomy

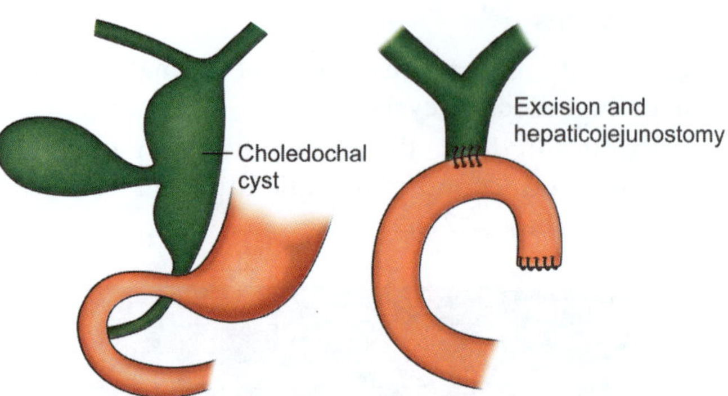

Fig. 42.73: Type I cyst

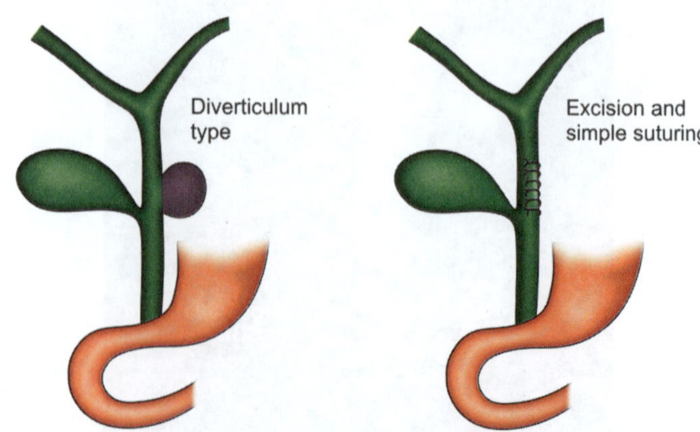

Fig. 42.74: Type II—excision and suturing

- **Type I:** Excision of the cyst followed by Roux-en-Y hepaticojejunostomy.
- **Type II:** Excision of the diverticulum with suturing of CBD.
- **Type III:** Endoscopic sphincterotomy is adequate (choledochocele).
- **Type IV:** They are difficult to treat. Due to recurrent cholangitis, if total excision is not possible due to adhesions between the cyst and portal vein, **posterior wall of the cyst can be left behind**, after removal of mucosa. This is described as **Lilly's technique**.
- **Type V** will be described later.

Complications

1. **Recurrent cholangitis** with high-grade fever, resulting in biliary cirrhosis.
2. **Rupture of the cyst** resulting in biliary peritonitis.
3. **CBD stones**
4. **Carcinoma in the cyst** (25–30% of cases). It is a cholangiocarcinoma common in types I and V.

CAROLI'S DISEASE

- It is a hereditary condition wherein there is dilatation of intrahepatic ducts with stenotic segments in between.
- Multiple, irregular saccular dilatations are characteristic.
- It is also an example of ***type V choledochal cyst.***
  Two types:
  1. **Simple:** Presents later with abdominal pain and sepsis.
  2. **Periportal:** It occurs in childhood, presents as recurrent cholangitis.
- Diagnosed by ultrasound and CT scan. MRI and ERCP are other investigations (Fig. 42.75).
- Associated lesions are given in Key Box 42.15.

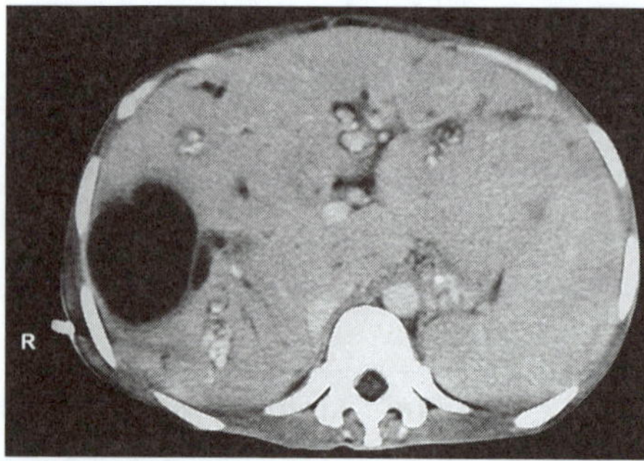

Fig. 42.75: Caroli's disease showing large cyst and intrahepatic dilatation

Key Box 42.15

Associated Lesions

- Congenital hepatic fibrosis
- Medullary sponge kidney
- Polycystic liver

Complications

- Cholangitis: It occurs due to constant obstruction.
- Stones: Obstruction and stasis precipitate stone formation.
- Biliary cirrhosis
- Cholangiocarcinoma

Treatment

- Hepatectomy (Fig. 42.76), liver transplantation.

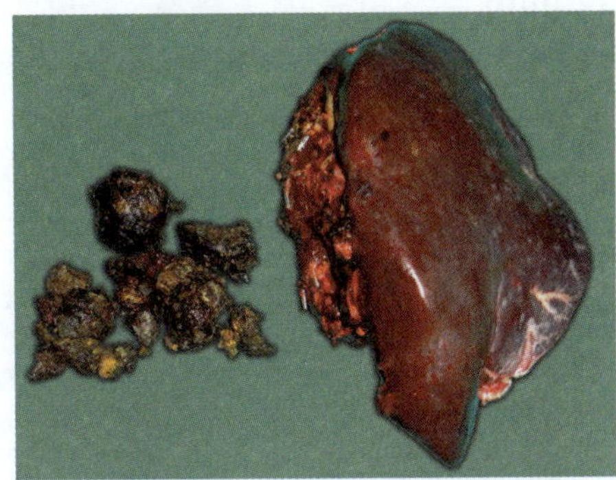

Fig. 42.76: Left lobectomy with extraction of stone—Caroli's disease. (*Courtesy:* Dr Nagaraj Palankar, Consultant, Manipal Hospital, Bangalore)

CHRONIC PANCREATITIS

Competency

SU24.1.3: Describe the types, etiopathogenesis, clinical features, investigations and management of chronic pancreatitis. Also the various surgical modalities available for treatment of chronic pancreatitis.

Definition

Diffuse inflammatory process of pancreas involving head, body and the tail resulting in permanent structural and functional damage to the pancreas.

Causes

1. **Alcohol:** High alcohol consumption is the most frequent cause. Alcohol stimulates pancreatic secretion rich in protein. This forms plugs in the pancreatic duct and results in stasis of secretion and stone formation. Alcohol also causes spasm of sphincter of Oddi.
2. **Idiopathic:** It is common in Kerala, and was thought to be due to **consumption of tapioca** (Fig. 42.77). It is also called Kerala pancreatitis or **tropical pancreatitis**. It is now thought to be due to malnutrition. It is also called **fibrocalculous pancreatic diabetes**.
3. **Hereditary pancreatitis:** It is a genetic disorder transmitted as a Mendelian-dominant trait.
4. **Cystic fibrosis:** Generalised dysfunction of exocrine glands causes secretions to precipitate in the lumen.

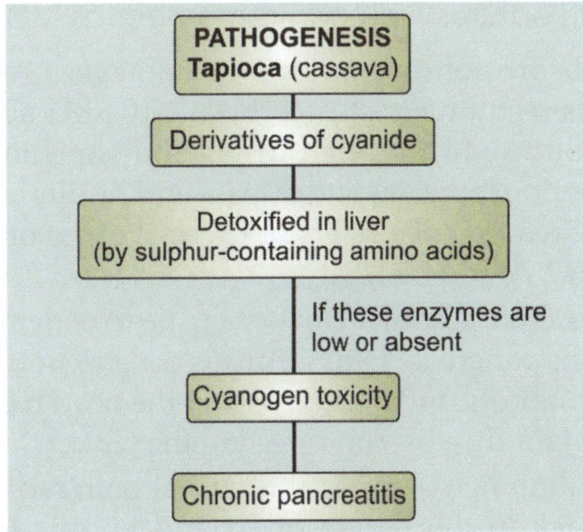

Fig. 42.77: Aetiopathogenesis of cassava pancreatitis

5. **Hyperparathyroidism** favours precipitation of calcium intraductally. It can also activate pancreatic enzymes.
6. **Autoimmune pancreatitis:** Diffuse enlargement of pancreas and narrowing of pancreatic duct is seen. Autoantibodies may be present. IgG4 is increased.
   - Multiple joint pains, salivary gland infections may give clue to the diagnosis.

Pathology

There is destruction of pancreas by ductal sclerosis, ductal strictures, glandular fibrosis and calcification, both intraductal and parenchymal (Fig. 42.78 and Key Box 42.16).

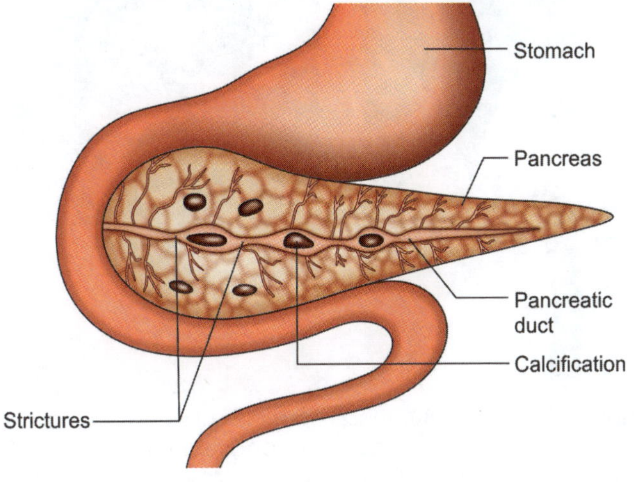

Fig. 42.78: Chronic pancreatitis showing pathological changes

Key Box 42.16

Chronic Pancreatitis Idiopathic Type

- Common in **warm** climates (Kerala)
- Common in **young age**
- High incidence of **diabetes**
- High incidence of **stones** in the duct
- Increased chances of **parenchymal calcification**
- Increased chances of **pancreatic cancer**

Clinical Features (you can remember as MOPED)

- **M**alabsorption occurs due to damage to exocrine glands resulting in steatorrhoea—10 to 15 stools per day, bulky, frothy, rich in fat, foul-smelling. Malabsorption indicates late disease and results in weight loss. Creatorrhoea refers to excessive loss of protein (Figs 42.79 and 42.80).
- **O**bstructive jaundice can occur due to oedema of the head of pancreas. Later, fibrous constriction of CBD due to fibrotic indurated mass in the head region can cause jaundice by compressing the CBD.
- **P**ain abdomen—upper abdominal pain radiating to the back in the region of L1 and L2 due to retroperitoneal inflammation (Key Box 42.17). Pain may be severe, sometimes radiating to both right and left sides. **The pain is due to multiple strictures in the pancreatic duct increasing the intraductal pressure.** It is relieved on stooping forward.
- **E**xploratory laparotomy—many cases are diagnosed at laparotomy where irregularity and hardness involving the entire pancreas are seen. Exploration is done for some other pathology.
- **D**iabetes—incidence of diabetes is about 10–20%. It should be suspected in diabetic patients with pain abdomen.

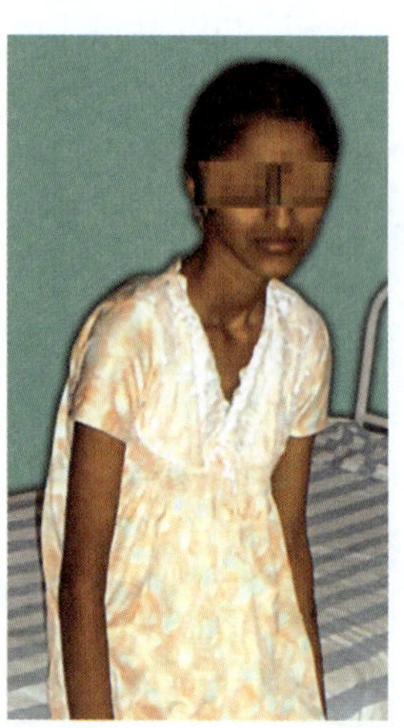

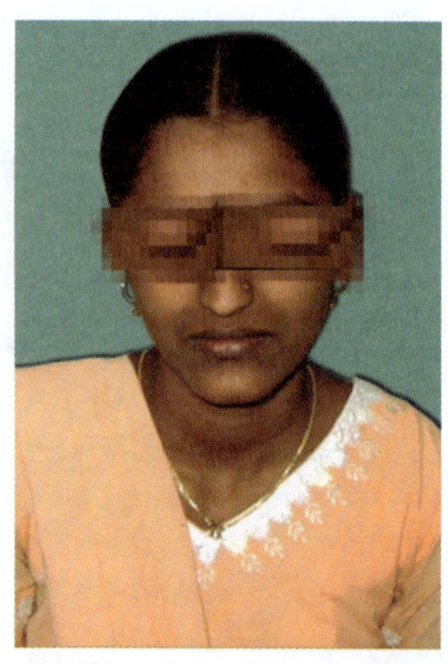

Figs 42.79 and 42.80: This 21-year-old girl was weighing 32 kg in 2006 when she underwent longitudinal pancreaticojejunostomy (LPJ) for failed medical treatment including stents. After 3 years, she has put on 22 kg weight

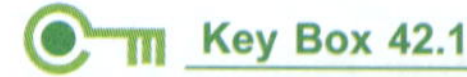

Key Box 42.17

Pain in Chronic Pancreatitis

- Parenchymal hypertension
- Perineural inflammation
- Ductal hypertension
- Pseudocyst formation
- Stenosis of bile duct

Investigations

- **Plain X-ray** abdomen can demonstrate stones in the pancreatic duct or parenchymal calcification (Fig. 42.81).
- **USG** can detect the stones, stricture, dilatation and associated cysts.
- **ERCP** (Fig. 42.82)
  - Ductal distension, ductal stricture
  - Dilated pancreatic duct (diameter of the normal duct is 2 mm)
  - Demonstration of stones—appear as regular filling defect.
- **CT scan:** It can reveal ductal anatomy, head mass, size and configuration of pancreas (Figs 42.83 and 42.84).

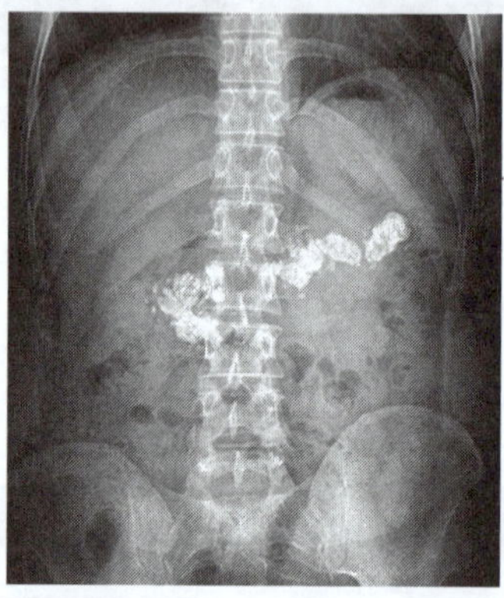

Fig. 42.81: Plain X-ray abdomen showing extensive calcification

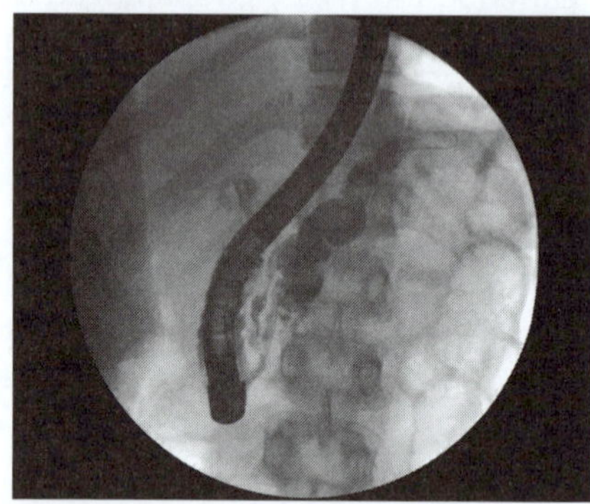

Fig. 42.82: ERCP showing dilated pancreatic duct—'chain of lakes' appearance

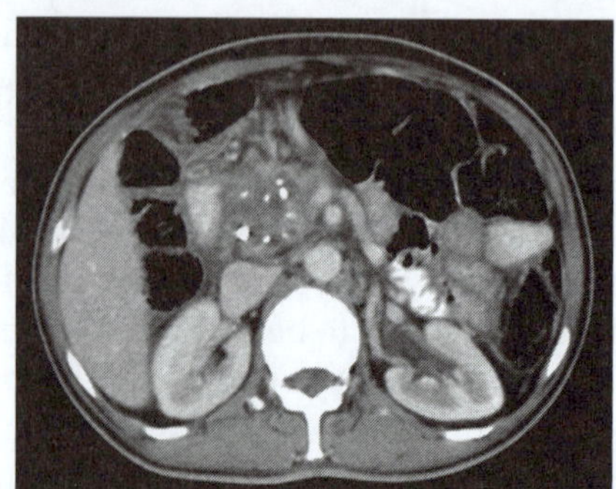

Fig. 42.83: CT scan showing chronic pancreatitis with head mass. This case should be treated with **head-coring** operation

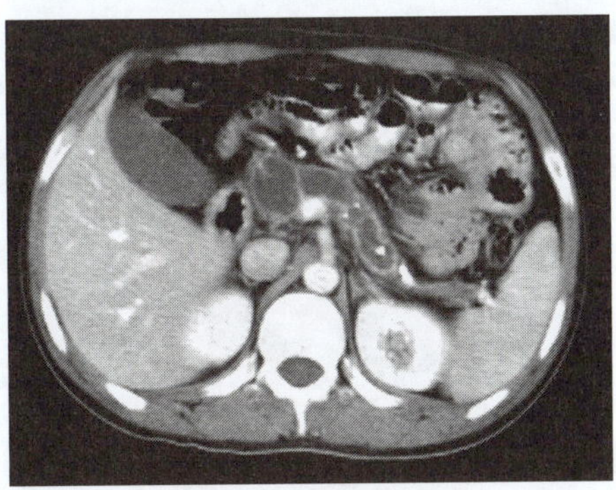

Fig. 42.84: CT shows dilated pancreatic duct of 10 mm in size with stones. ERCP is not required in such patients. This patient underwent LPJ

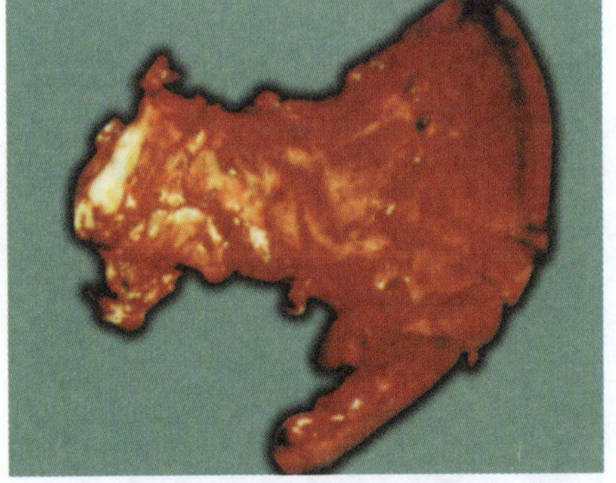

Fig. 42.85: Distal pancreatectomy. Chronic pancreatitis confined to tail of pancreas

Complications

- Obstructive jaundice due to a mass lesion in the head region
- Carcinoma of pancreas
- Pseudocysts
- Steroids in autoimmune pancreatitis

Treatment

I. Conservative

- Pain relief by analgesics, epidural analgesia, or splanchnic nerve block. Slow release opioid skin patches are useful.
- Supplement **pancreatic enzyme**—diet should be low in fat and **vitamin D** supplements should be given.
- Pancreatic enzymes not only help in treating exocrine insufficiency but they also denature CCK releasing peptide, thereby diminishing the release of CCK. Thus, pain is decreased. Six capsules of **pancreatin** are given.
- Control diabetes, stop alcohol consumption and tobacco smoking, antioxidants may help.

II. Surgery

Indications

- Unrelieved pain
- Suspicion of carcinoma
- Complications:
  - Ascites
  - Cysts
  - Abscesses
  - GI bleeding—left-sided, portal hypertension, pseudoaneurysm
  - Obstructive jaundice
  - Duodenal obstruction

Types of Surgery (Figs 42.85 to 42.91)

1. **Chronic pancreatitis involving tail of pancreas:** Distal pancreatectomy with removal of spleen.

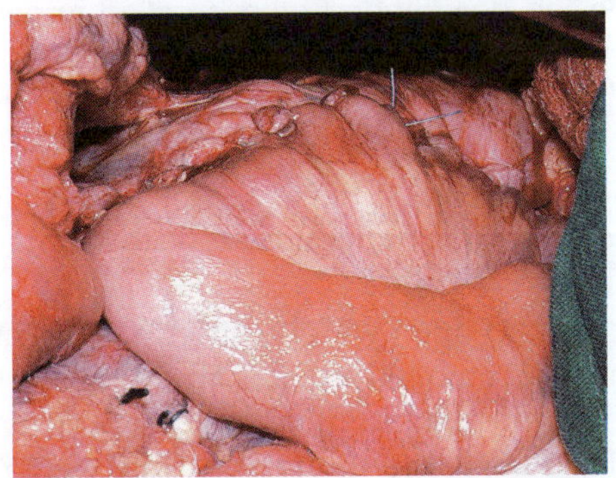

Fig. 42.86: Pancreaticojejunal anastomosis is being done

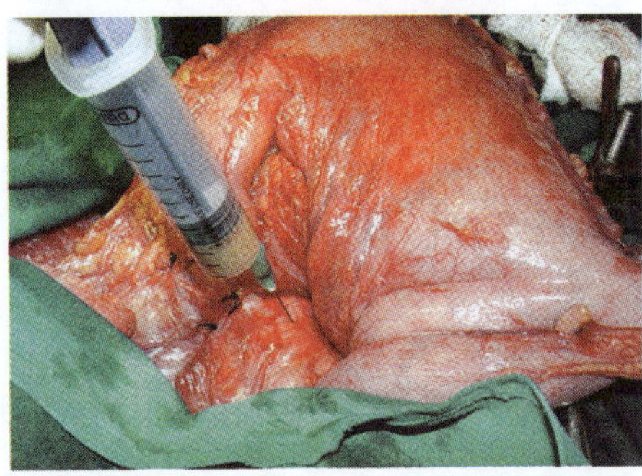

Fig. 42.87: Dilated duct is being aspirated to identify the duct followed by laying it open

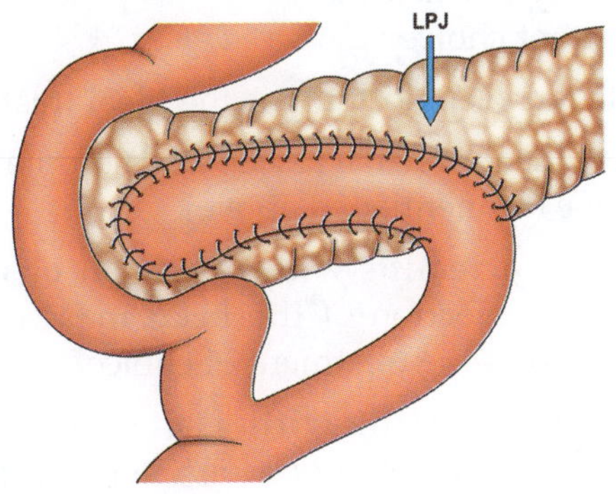

Fig. 42.88: Longitudinal pancreaticojejunostomy (diagrammatic)

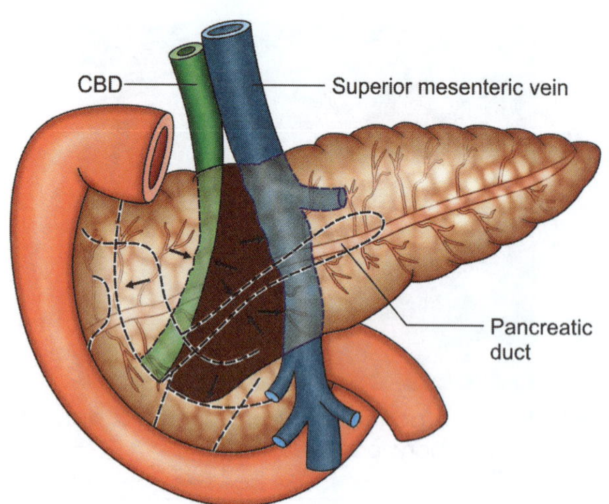

Fig. 42.89: The dark shaded area is called **pacemaker of chronic pancreatitis.** It should be removed in cases of head-coring operation. It is a triangle between lower CBD, pancreatic duct and superior mesenteric vessels

2. **Diffuse chronic pancreatitis with dilated (large duct) pancreatic duct**
   - Duct is laid open widely, strictures are cut open, stones are removed and it is anastomosed to a loop of jejunum—longitudinal pancreaticojejunostomy (LPJ)—**Puestow's operation** (Roux-en-Y jejunal segment). The duct should be at least 6 mm in diameter. Sutures hold very nicely because of fibrosis of pancreas. Pain relief is obtained in about 80% of the cases. Pancreatic fistula is a complication of this surgery. Majority of the fistulae close spontaneously.
   - This is a bypass procedure which preserve endocrine and exocrine functions.
3. **Chronic pancreatitis with a head mass:** In this situation, doubt arises whether it is malignancy or not. Even trucut biopsy and frozen section are not foolproof. Hence, pancreaticoduodenectomy is advised, provided experience of the surgeon is good and the mortality rate is less than 5%.
4. **Chronic pancreatitis with bile duct obstruction:** If malignancy is ruled out, a bypass procedure is the treatment of choice.
   - Choledochojejunostomy is the ideal treatment.
   - Pancreaticoduodenal resection (Whipple) can also be done (as mentioned above).
5. **Chronic pancreatitis with duodenal obstruction:** Here also, resection of the head mass or gastrojejunostomy is the treatment of choice.
6. **Chronic pancreatitis with ascites:** Treatment of choice is Puestow's operation (stenting may also relieve ascites).
7. **Resection:** A duodenum-preserving pancreatic head resection is called ***Hans Beger's procedure.*** Head-coring procedure is called ***Frey procedure*** (Figs 42.90 and 42.91 and Key Box 42.18).

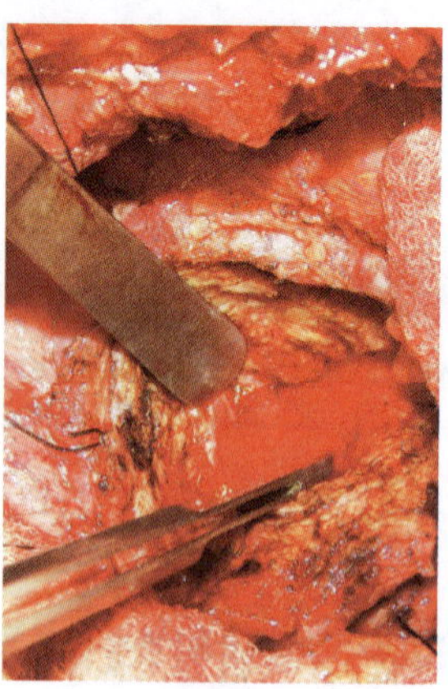

Fig. 42.90: Head-coring is completed. You can watch thin rim of pancreatic tissue all around

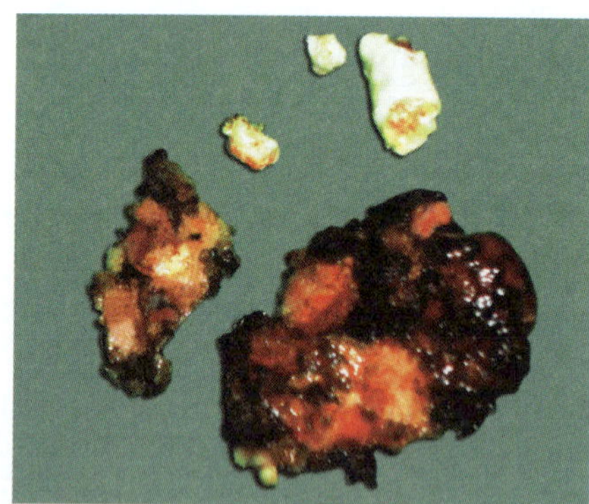

Fig. 42.91: Specimen of the portion of the head along with multiple stones

Key Box 42.18

Head-coring—Frey Procedure

- **Pathologic key** to recurrent pancreatitis is localised to pancreatic head. It is called **pacemaker**.
- It is located in the **crucial triangle** (*see* Fig. 42.89) which has to be excised.
- Pain and recurrent pancreatitis will decrease after Frey procedure.
- Surgery can be done with minimum blood loss.
- Try **avoiding injury to lower CBD**—if necessary, CBD can be opened and a sound can be introduced.

CHOLANGIOCARCINOMA—BILE DUCT CARCINOMA

Competency

SU28.12.5: Enumerate the types, etiopathogenesis, clinical features, investigations and management of cholangiocarcinoma.

Key Box 42.19

Risk Factors

Cholangitis—primary sclerosing
Colitis—ulcerative
Clonorchiasis
Choledochal cyst
Caroli's disease
Chemical carcinogens like thorium, nitrosamines, diosmin
Observe **6 Cs**

- Patients having **following diseases** have increased risk of developing cholangiocarcinoma (Key Box 42.19).
- It is an uncommon cause of obstructive jaundice.
- Elderly males >60 years are commonly affected.
- **Obstructive jaundice** is the presenting feature.
- Tender hepatomegaly is present due to congestion and may be due to cholangitis.
- **Gallbladder is not palpable** in cases of cholangiocarcinoma unlike in periampullary carcinomas.
- Cholangiocarcinoma at the bifurcation of the hepatic duct is called **Klatskin's tumour.**

Types

1. Perihilar is the most common, Klatskin's tumour comes under this.
2. Intrahepatic (10%)
3. Distal (CHD-CBD) 25%

Management

- Abdominal ultrasound, CT scan, ERCP will help in localising the site of obstruction (Figs 42.92 and 42.93). ERCP and stenting the CBD is indicated in inoperable cases. However, MRI is better.
- Treatment is difficult because most of the lesions are high up in the hilar region infiltrating the liver, portal vein, etc. Resection and hepaticojejunostomy or endoscopic stent placement are the treatment modalities available.
- Resection involves liver for hilar growth and for lower end growth.

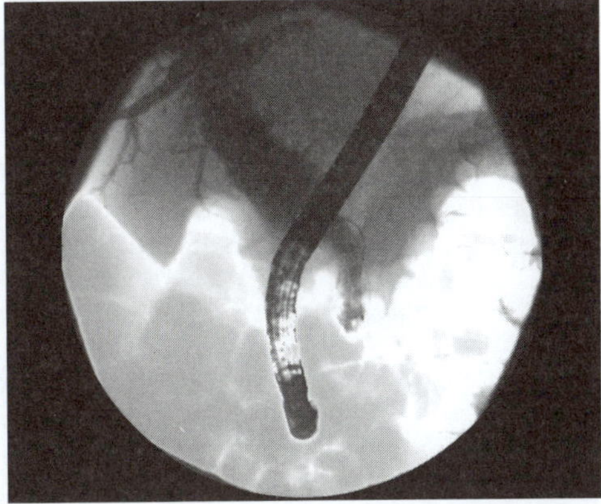

Figs 42.92: ERCP showing cholangiocarcinoma

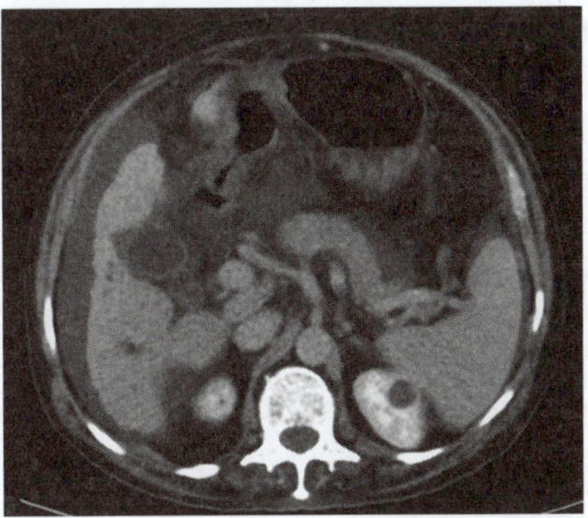

Fig. 42.93: CT scan showing extensive cholagiocarcinoma with ascites

CONGENITAL BILIARY ATRESIA

Aetiopathogenesis

A disease of unknown aetiology, though rare, is fatal. Viral aetiology and defective embryogenesis have been blamed for the development of biliary atresia.

Types (Fig. 42.94)

- Type I: Common bile duct is involved.
- Type II: Common hepatic duct is involved.
- Type III: Atresia of right and left hepatic ducts.

Clinical Features

- It presents as jaundice at birth or in the neonatal period.
- Due to absence of bile in the gut, meconium is not bile-stained. Hence, stools are pale.
- Gradually, due to backpressure, liver enlarges.
- Enlargement of the spleen may follow, if there is development of portal hypertension.
- Steatorrhoea, pruritus and clubbing are the other features.

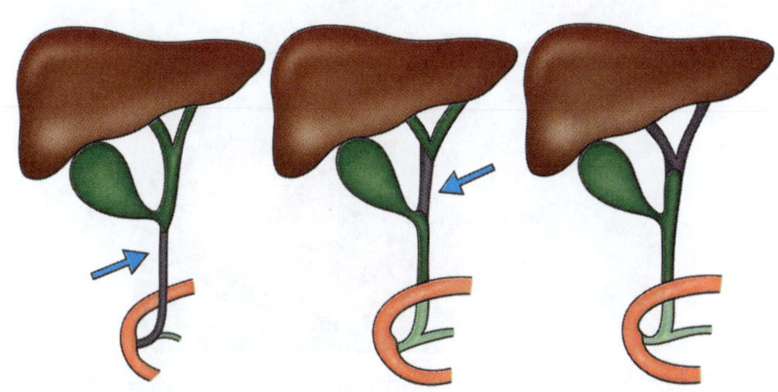

Fig. 42.94: Congenital biliary atresia—types I, II and III

Treatment

- **Surgical drainage of bile** is the only available treatment provided patent bile duct or radicle is seen. Anastomosis of Roux-en-Y loop of jejunum to the dilated bile duct or sometimes excision of bile duct tissue up to the liver capsule should be done followed by Roux-en-Y anastomosis. This is called **Kasai's portoenterostomy**.
- **Liver transplantation** is the choice when there is atresia of the intrahepatic duct.

Complications

1. Recurrent cholangitis giving rise to hepatic fibrosis.
2. Biliary cirrhosis and portal hypertension.

CARCINOMA OF GALLBLADDER

Incidence: It is common in North Eastern India. Occurs in elderly patients in their sixties/seventies.

Aetiology

- **Gallstones:** 80–90% of gallbladder cancers are associated with gallstones. Calcification of gallbladder is associated with carcinoma gallbladder. Porcelain gallbladder is a precancerous condition. Incidence of malignancy may range from 1 to 5% of cases.
- **Chemicals:** High incidence of gallbladder and biliary cancer is noted in people who work in rubber industries.
- **Gallbladder polyp** (Fig. 42.95)
- **Dietary:** Adulterated mustard oil for cooking is found to precipitate carcinoma gallbladder.

Pathology

- 85% of cases. It is usually adenocarcinoma. Undifferentiated carcinoma and squamous cell carcinoma may also occur. The tumour is most commonly nodular, infiltrates the entire gallbladder and adjacent tissues.
- Three types of adenocarcinomas have been identified: Nonpapillary adenocarcinoma, papillary adenocarcinoma and mucinous adenocarcinoma. Majority are nonpapillary adenocarcinoma.

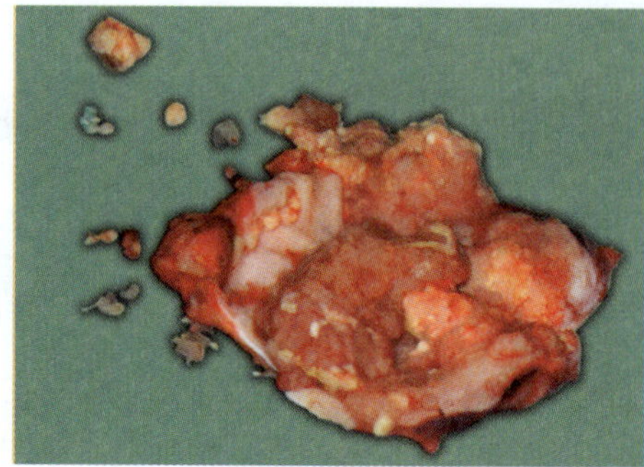

Fig. 42.95: You can see extensive carcinomatous polypoid lesions inside the gallbladder

Clinical Features

- Significant weight loss, jaundice and mass in the right upper quadrant are common presentations. Clinically, it is palpable as a hard irregular mass.
- A few cases can present as chronic cholecystitis with a mass or acute cholecystitis. Ultrasonography may diagnose as stones and they are subjected to cholecystectomy. During surgery or postoperatively, the diagnosis gets confirmed.
- Obstructive jaundice, bleeding, ascites are late features.

Staging

TNM STAGING Gallbladder cancer

Tumour (T)

TX	Primary tumor cannot be assessed
T0	No evidence of primary tumor
Tis	Carcinoma *in situ*
T1	Tumor invades lamina propria or muscular layer
T1a	Tumour invades lamina propria
T1b	Tumour invades muscular layer
T2a	Tumour invades the perimuscular connective tissue on the peritoneal side without involving the serosa
T2b	Tumour invades the perimuscular connective tissue on the peritoneal side without involving the liver
T3	Tumour perforates the serosa (visceral peritoneum) and/or directly invades the liver and/or one other adjacent organ or structure, such as the stomach, duodenum, colon, pancreas, omentum, or extrahepatic bile ducts
T4	Tumour invades main portal vein or hepatic artery or invades at least two extrahepatic organs or structures

Metastases (M)

M0	No distant spread
M1	Distant spread

Nodes (N)

Nx	Regional lymph nodes cannot be assessed
N0	Regional lymph node metastasis
N1	Metastases to 1–3 lymph nodes
N2	Metastases to >4 lymph nodes

Staging

Stage 0—Tis, N0, M0
Stage I—T1, N0, M0
Stage IIA—T2a, N0, M0
Stage IIB—T2b, N0, M0
Stage IIIA—T3, N0, M0
Stage IIIB—T1 to T3, N1, M0
Stage IVA—T4, N0 or N1, M0
Stage IVB—Any T, N2, M0; Any T, any N, M1

Note: Stage I is Localised; Stages II to IV B are unresectable

Investigations

- CA 19–9 is elevated in 80% patients.
- Ultrasonography and endosonography are very useful investigations. Ultrasonography-guided FNAC can be done for histological diagnosis in suspected cases of gallbladder mass.
- CT scan is useful for staging—lymph nodes metastasis in the liver (Fig. 42.96).
- ERCP, if there is obstructive jaundice to localise the exact site and nature of obstruction.
- Diagnostic laparoscopy. If peritoneal metastasis is present, it is not worth resecting.
- MRCP can be done. It visualises bile duct better than CT scan.

Treatment

- If gallbladder cancer is found at cholecystectomy and if **mucosa alone is involved**, then cholecystectomy is sufficient.
- If gallbladder wall is involved, then extended cholecystectomy is done (Fig. 42.97 and Key Box 42.20).
- Radiation has very small benefits.
- Chemotherapy also has been tried. 5-FU, mitomycin C, doxorubicin are the drugs used.

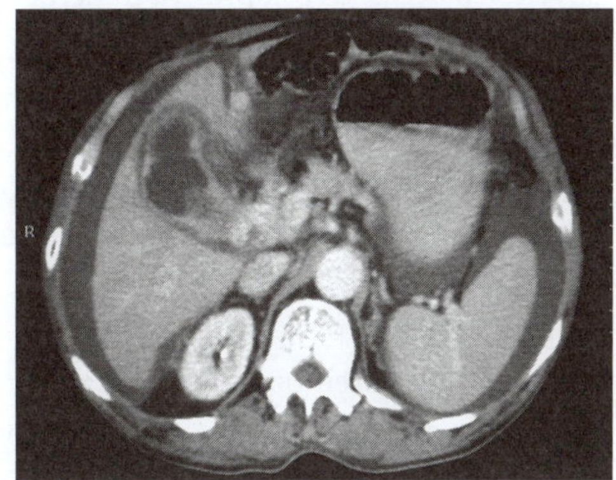

Fig. 42.96A: Advanced case of carcinoma gallbladder with ascites and liver infiltration

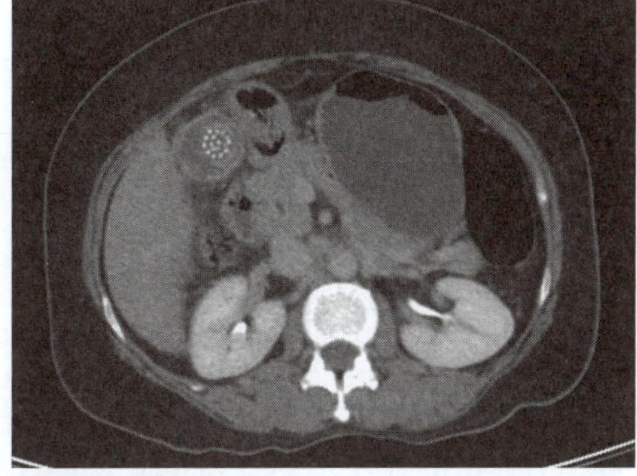

Fig. 42.96B: Gallstones with carcinoma gallbladder

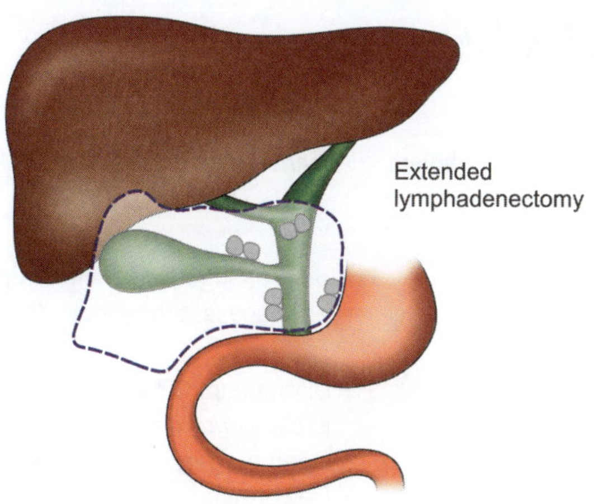

Fig. 42.97: Extended lymphadenectomy

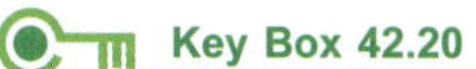 **Key Box 42.20**

Extended Cholecystectomy

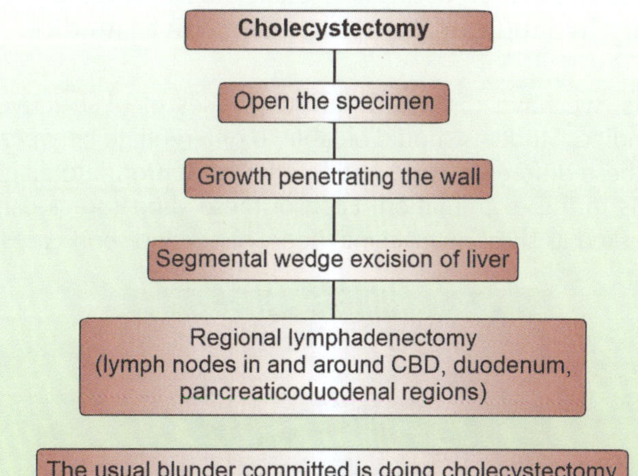

Prognosis

In general, five-year survival is very poor (Key Box 42.21). Aggressive surgery and complete clearance give best result (Fig. 42.97).

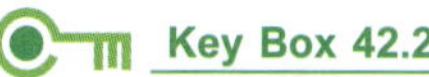 **Key Box 42.21**

Gallbladder Cancer is the Worst, Why?

- Biologically very aggressive cancer (unlike basal cell cancer, carcinoma colon, etc.)
- High incidence of lymphatic spread
- Easily spreads into liver by direct infiltration
- Spreads by blood, neural, intraperitoneal routes
- Intraductal extension into CBD causes obstructive jaundice
- Infiltration into stomach, colon, duodenum and liver can occur because of its location
- Radiation and chemotherapy is rarely of any benefit

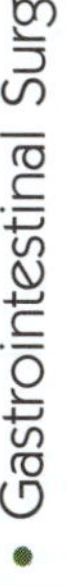

Table 42.2 Parasitic infestation of the biliary tract

	Biliary ascariasis	Clonorchiasis	Biliary hydatid
1. Causative organism	*Ascaris lumbricoides* (Fig. 42.98)	*Clonorchis sinensis*	*Echinococcus granulosus*
2. Route of entry	Ampulla of Vater	Ampulla of Vater	Rupture of hydatid cyst of liver into biliary tree
3. Complications	Stricture, suppurative cholangitis, liver abscess, empyema	Biliary pain, stone cholangitis, block, cirrhosis, bile duct carcinogenic	Obstructive jaundice, cholangitis
4. Management	• Ultrasound, CT scan • ERCP—worm can be extracted • Open surgery • Deworming	• Ultrasound, CT scan • Cholecystectomy and T-tube drainage • Choledochojejunostomy for a better drainage	• Ultrasound • ERCP, sphincterotomy, stent • Appropriate surgery

Rare or Uncommon Causes of Obstructive Jaundice

(Table 42.2 and Fig. 42.98)

Parasites such as ascariasis, *Clonorchiasis sinensis* and biliary hydatid can give rise to obstructive jaundice.

Thus, we have discussed various causes of obstructive jaundice. Students should be able to differentiate between all these different causes and to offer an appropriate diagnosis in the examination. Each of these short topics can be asked as short notes in the theory paper and short cases.

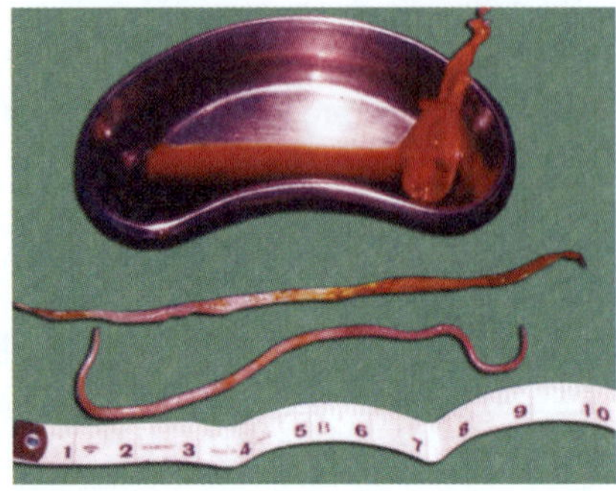

Fig. 42.98: Ascariasis of the biliary duct. (*Courtesy:* Dr CG Narasimhan, Consultant Surgeon, Mysore)

CARCINOMA OF PANCREAS

Introduction

- 70% of the cases occur in the head of the pancreas including periampullary region.
- 30% occur in the body and the tail.
- 70% of cases are adenocarcinoma of duct cell origin.
- It is 4th leading cause of death due to cancer in males, after lung, colon, prostate.

Aetiology

- **Chronic tropical pancreatitis** and hereditary pancreatitis are associated with pancreatic cancer—such malignancies can be multifocal.
- **Haemochromatosis** produces extensive calcification of pancreas. It is also a precancerous condition.
- **Diabetes:** Diabetic patients are 10 times more vulnerable to develop carcinoma of pancreas.
- **Other possible aetiological factors**
  - *Alcohol and smoking:* It is related to tobacco specific nitrosamines (including smokeless tobacco).
  - *Westernisation of diet:* Fatty food, rich in animal proteins can cause pancreatic cancer.
  - *Industrial carcinogens:* B11-naphthylamine, benzidine, gasoline are the possible agents.

Pathology

- Periampullary refers to carcinoma arising from ampulla of Vater, the duodenal mucosa or the lower end of the common bile duct.
- Microscopically, the types are:
  1. **Mucus-**secreting carcinoma of ductal origin.
  2. **Nonmucus-**secreting carcinoma of acinar origin.
  3. **Anaplastic** carcinomas are poorly differentiated and tend to arise from the body of the pancreas.
  4. **Cystadenocarcinomas** are rare, slow-growing and tend to attain a large size.

Clinical Features

- Periampullary and carcinoma head of pancreas present as obstructive jaundice (discussed already). Discussion here is on carcinoma body and tail of pancreas.
- Microscopically, the tumour shows malignant cells with a variable degree of differentiation, mitotic figures, etc. Not only it invades vessels and lymphatics, but also perineural spread occurs fast which explains backache (Key Box 42.22).

Key Box 42.22

Carcinoma of Pancreas—Pathology

- More than 80% are **ductal adenocarcinomas**
- **Solid and scirrhous** tumours by nature
- Plenty of **neoplastic tubular** glands are seen
- **Desmoplastic** reaction is extensive (feels hard)
- Infiltrates locally—spreads along nerve sheaths, lymphatics and into blood vessels
- Being retroperitoneal in location, **manifests late, spreads fast and carries poor prognosis**

Symptoms

- Severe pain radiating to the back in the region of L1 and L2. It is due to infiltration of retroperitoneal nerve plexuses or pancreatic duct obstruction.
- Pain is so severe, often patient requests for narcotic analgesics.
- Gross weight loss in 3–6 months.
- Anorexia, asthenia and generalised weakness.
- Jaundice cannot occur in carcinoma body and tail of pancreas unless there are secondaries in liver or lymph nodes at porta hepatis.
- Symptoms of vomiting suggest duodenal obstruction.
- **Trousseau's sign**[1] (thrombophlebitis migrans):
  - Migrating thrombophlebitis of the legs can occur in visceral malignancies particularly from carcinoma of pancreas, rarely carcinoma stomach, colon, etc.
  - It is supposedly due to sluggish blood flow resulting in thrombus formation.
  - It is superficial and affects the leg veins, such as long saphenous vein.

Pearls of Wisdom

Sudden development of diabetes mellitus is an early manifestation of carcinoma pancreas in 25% of patients.

Signs

- **Anaemia** may be present as in any other malignancy.
- **Jaundice** is not a feature. Left supraclavicular node may be palpable.
- **Per abdomen findings** (Table 42.3): Majority of these cases are advanced, fixed and are felt as a mass in the upper abdomen.

I. Characteristics of a pancreatic mass

- It is situated on the left side involving left hypochondrium, umbilical region and epigastrium.
- It does not move with respiration because it is retroperitoneal.

Table 42.3 Differences between pancreatic mass and stomach mass

Carcinoma body of the pancreas	Carcinoma stomach
1. Pain radiating to the back is the presenting feature	Vomiting, dyspepsia is present. Pain is not a feature
2. Haematemesis is not a feature	Haematemesis is a common feature
3. The mass does not move with respiration	Usually moves with respiration
4. Mobility is not a feature	Mobility is present
5. Knee elbow test—the mass does not fall forwards	Stomach mass falls forward (intraperitoneal), unless it is fixed
6. Retroperitoneal organ	Intraperitoneal
7. Percussion: Resonant note is obtained because of stomach anterior to it	Impaired note because of growth in the stomach

- It does not fall forwards in knee elbow position.
- Can get above the swelling.
- On percussion, it gives a resonant note because of anterior position of stomach.

II. Features of carcinoma

- It is common in elderly, male patients smokers.
- Hard, irregular, fixed lump.
- Significant weight loss +.

III. Evidence of metastasis: Secondaries in the liver, ascites, rectovesical deposits.

Differential Diagnosis

1. **Carcinoma stomach** infiltrating the pancreas
   - Such mass may not be mobile. It does not move with respiration because it is fixed to pancreas.
   - These patients will have vomiting first followed by backache at a later date.
2. **Carcinoma transverse colon**
   - Produces constipation and bleeding per rectum. Vertical mobility may be present.
   - Right to left peristalsis may be present.
3. **Para-aortic lymph node mass** may be due to: Intra-abdominal malignancies, lymphoma, testicular tumour, etc.

Investigations

I. Investigations for periampullary carcinoma and carcinoma of head of pancreas (discussed before).

II. **Investigations for carcinoma of body and tail** (discussed here)

[1]**Trousseau's sign** is also found in Buerger's disease

1. **USG:** First investigation of choice
   - Rules out calculous obstruction
   - Can detect a mass as small as 2 cm
   - Intraoperative ultrasound can be used to take a biopsy.
2. **Contrast-enhanced CT scan** (Figs 42.99 and 42.100)
   - Retroperitoneal invasion
   - Lymph node enlargement
   - Invasion of hepatic artery, superior mesenteric artery, ascites, liver metastasis—unresectable.
   - Infiltration of portal vein which makes it inoperable
   - In more than 70% of cases, pancreatic duct is dilated and in more than 60% of cases bile duct is dilated.

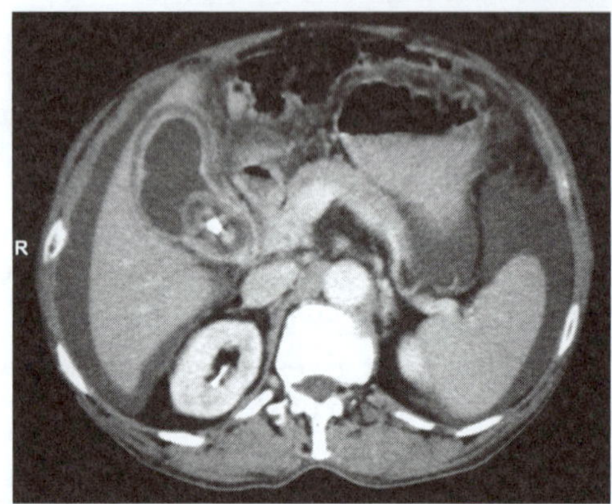

Fig. 42.99: Carcinoma body of the pancreas with para-aortic nodes and ascites

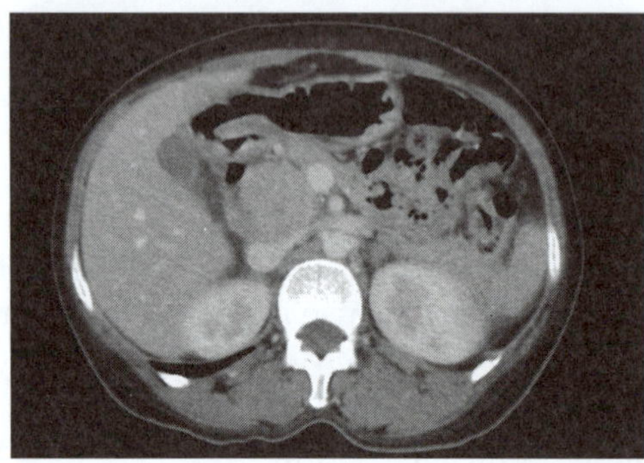

Fig. 42.100: Large mass in the head and body of pancreas

   - When both these ducts are dilated, it is most likely pancreatic cancer.
   - CT-guided aspiration biopsy is indicated for lesions to start neoadjuvant chemotherapy/RT (infiltrative lesions).
3. **ERCP** is indicated in the absence of a mass. Findings can be stenosis/obstruction.
4. **Carbohydrate antigen CA 19–9:** These are glycoproteins which are elaborated by malignancies. ***It is a tumour marker of pancreas to monitor carcinoma pancreas.*** Increased in 75% of patients with carcinoma pancreas and 10% of the patients in benign disease of pancreas, liver and bile ducts. Hence, it is not a diagnostic investigation. However, very high values suggest malignancy even when histology is inconclusive.

Treatment

I. Periampullary carcinoma—Whipple's operation

II. Carcinoma of body and tail

A. If the tumour is very small and diagnosed very early, they are ideally treated with **total pancreatectomy with removal of involved lymph nodes.**

B. Many cases are diagnosed late. They are inoperable either due to fixity to portal vein or due to metastasis. Hence, there is no role for curative surgery. For the confirmation of diagnosis, transabdominal USG-guided fine needle aspiration cytology can be done. Surgery is not indicated in such cases; only palliative treatment can be offered. Prognosis is very poor.

- **Palliative radiotherapy:** 4000–6000 cGy units can be given. Response rate is 5–10%. It reduces size of the tumour and **some pain relief is obtained** (Table 42.4).
- Palliative treatment is an important aspect of carcinoma pancreas even though such patients succumb to the disease within 3 to 6 months. Palliation is mainly to relieve pain.

Table 42.4 Palliation for carcinoma pancreas—3 chief symptoms

Pain	Jaundice	Duodenal obstruction
• Sustained release oral narcotic drugs—morphine sulphate • Celiac plexus nerve block (pain is due to invasion of retroperitoneal nerve trunks) • Intraoperative celiac plexus block by injecting 50% alcohol directly into tissues along side of aorta • Palliative RT and gemcitabine—survival improved by 1–2 months	• Stenting—recurrent obstruction and cholangitis chances are decreased • Choledochojejunostomy, cholecysto-jejunostomy (if cystic duct enters CBD well above the growth) • Surgical bypass has increased mortality and morbidity initially	• Occurs in 20% of patients • Posterior dependent GJ is preferable—indicated in cases of symptoms such as vomiting

TRUE CYSTIC PANCREATIC NEOPLASMS (CPNs)

- These are uncommon tumours present predominantly in women (Key Box 42.23).
- Other rare tumours are cystadenocarcinoma, acinar cell cystadenocarcinoma, etc.

Key Box 42.23

True Cystic Pancreatic Neoplasms (CPNs)

A. Serous cystadenoma: Benign
- Common in women, located in head of pancreas. They account for 30% of all CPNs. They can be observed, if asymptomatic.

B. Mucinous cystic neoplasms (MCNs)
- More common in women
- More often found in body and tail
- More incidence than serous (40%)
- Considered premalignant
- Do not communicate with ductal system
- Lesions more than 2 cm need to be resected

C. Intraductal papillary mucinous tumours (IPMTs) (Figs 42.103 and 42.104)
- Slightly more common in males
- Communicates with duct
- Incidence is about 25%
- High malignant potential
- More common in head involving ampulla of Vater
- Treated by Whipple's resection

- These tumours can be confused with pseudocyst of the pancreas. Hence, they should be differentiated at surgery (Figs 42.101 and 42.102). Otherwise, gross blunders can take place (Table 42.5).
- Serous and mucinous are important. They are discussed in Table 42.6.

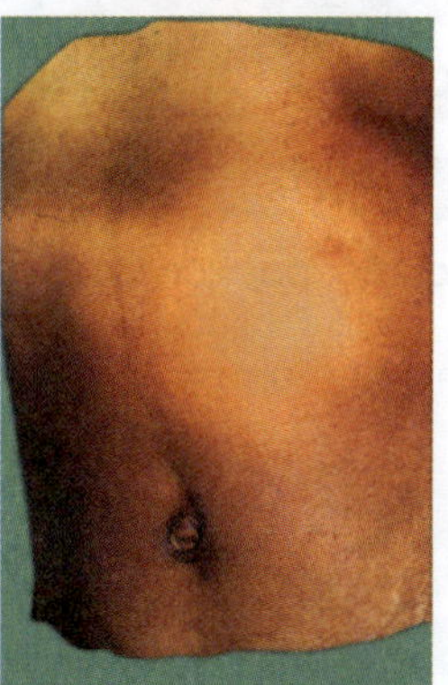

Fig. 42.101: Cystadenoma of the pancreas

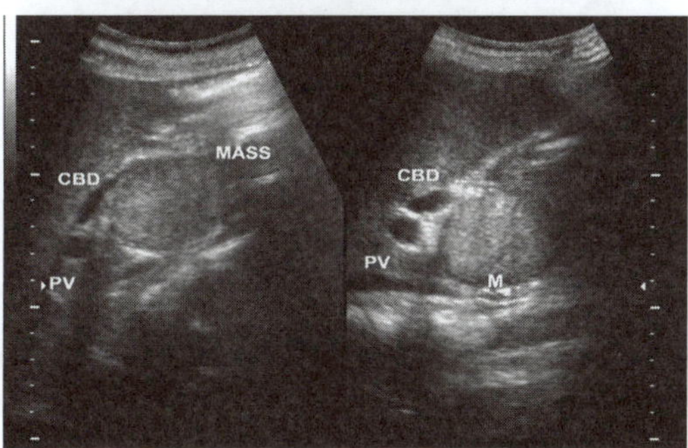

Fig. 42.102: Ultrasound showing cystic mass in the body of pancreas

Table 42.5 Differences between cystic neoplasm and pseudocyst

	Cystic neoplasm	Pseudocyst
1. History of pancreatitis	Absent	Present
2. Imaging	May demonstrate *solid component*	Usually absent
3. ERCP	Mucin egress from bulging papilla in cases of IPMTs	No
4. Mucin content of fluid	Present	Absent
5. CEA in fluid	Increased in mucinous cystic neoplasms	Absent
6. CA 19–9	Increased in malignant cystic neoplasms	Not elevated
7. Percutaneous wall biopsy	Epithelial lining can be present	No epithelial lining

Table 42.6 Cystic neoplasms

	Serous	Mucinous
• Gender	• No prediction	• More common in women
• Nature	• Multiple cysts are present	• More often multilocular
• Cut surface	• Microcystic adenomas with cut surface appearance of a sponge	• Macrocystic adenomas with smooth lining with papillary projections
• CT scan	• CT may show cysts with calcification	• Septal on CT scan is characteristic
• Nature of fluid	• Cystic spaces contain serous fluid	• Cystic spaces contain mucus
• Lining epithelium	• Lining is by cuboidal epithelium	• Lining is tall columnar and goblet cells
• Malignant potential	• No malignant potential	• Most of them turn into cystadenocarcinoma

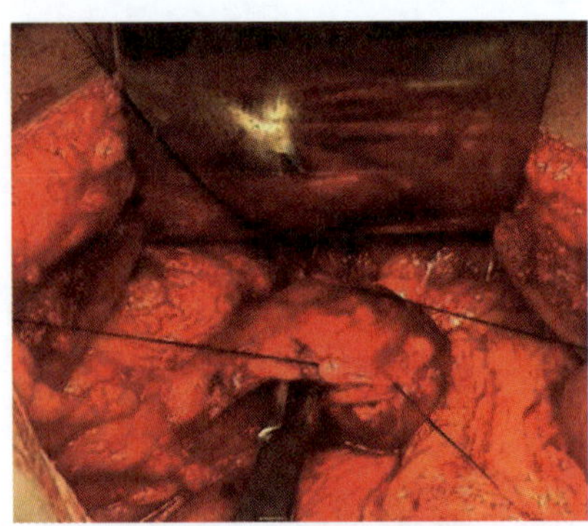

Fig. 42.103: Intraductal papillary mucinous tumour (IPMT) at surgery. (*Courtesy:* Dr SS Prasad, Dr Sunilkrishna, Dr Rajendra Benakatti, Department of Surgery, KMC, Manipal)

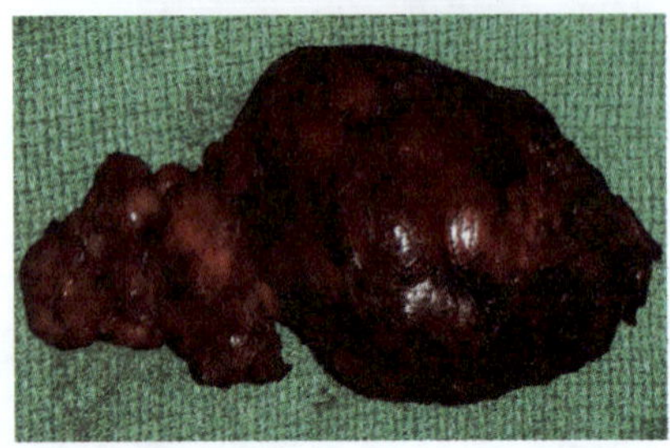

Fig. 42.104: Distal pancreatectomy specimen: Intraductal papillary mucinous tumour (IPMT) at surgery. (*Courtesy:* Dr SS Prasad, Dr Sunilkrishna, Dr Rajendra benakatti, Department of Surgery, KMC, Manipal)

ENDOCRINE TUMOURS OF THE PANCREAS

Competency

SU24.3: Describe the principles of investigation and management of pancreatic endocrine tumors.

These tumours are members of APUDOMA arising from APUD (**A**mine **P**recursor **U**ptake **D**ecarboxylation) cells. They are neuroectodermal in origin. Accordingly, following tumours can occur (Table 42.7A).

Types

- **Sporadic:** Usually occurs as a single tumour.
- **Familial:** Occur with other adenomas as in multiple endocrine neoplasia syndrome—**MEN Type I:** Pituitary, parathyroid, pancreatic adenoma.

INSULINOMA (β-CELL TUMOUR)

- Most common functioning islet cell tumour.
- Majority of the insulinomas occur in the tail and body of pancreas and majority of them are benign, one-third are malignant and one-third are multiple.
- It can be a single adenoma, can be due to diffuse hyperplasia or due to carcinoma.
- **Clinical features are that of hypoglycaemia** (Key Box 42.24 for other causes of hypoglycaemia).
- In early stages, it can mimic a duodenal ulcer. Due to hypoglycaemia, hunger pain develops and a tendency to ask for food is present.
- As it becomes severe, giddiness, dizziness, syncopal attacks, blurring of vision and diplopia can occur.
- Late stages—epilepsy, semiconsciousness and coma.

Key Box 42.24

Persistent Hypoglycaemia—Causes

- Insulinoma
- Hepatoma
- Hepatocellular damage
- Hypopituitarism
- Addison's disease
- Large mesenchymal tumour

Whipple's Triad of Insulinoma

1. Attack of hypoglycaemia in morning hours, in the fasting state.
2. Symptoms are relieved on taking glucose.
3. Blood sugar in the fasting state is less than 45 mg% during the attack.

Clinical Notes

The author remembers a case of recurrent epilepsy getting admitted to the department of neurology. He was found to have hypoglycaemia and was diagnosed as insulinoma only during the 4th admission. A 3 cm benign insulinoma was enucleated from the pancreas. The patient is asymptomatic till date.

Table 42.7A Summary of islet cells

Islet cells	Active agent	Syndrome	Presentation
Alpha	Glucagon	Glucagonoma	Hyperglycaemia
Beta	Insulin	Insulinoma	Hypoglycaemia
Delta	Somatostatin	Somatostatinoma	—
G	Gastrin	Gastrinoma	Hyperacidity

Investigations

1. **Serum insulin** levels done by immunoassay method are found to be very high. Proinsulin levels and C-peptide level are also very high.
2. Persistent hypoglycaemia—blood sugar level of less than 50 mg/dl relieved by glucose is suggestive of insulinoma.
3. **USG and CT scan** of abdomen can demonstrate the tumour, if it is more than 2 cm. (Intraoperative ultrasound is a useful test.)
4. Selective angiography will demonstrate tumour blush as majority of them are very vascular.

Treatment

- Enucleation is the treatment of choice.
- Resection of the tumour and if necessary distal pancreatectomy can also be done in selected patients.
- Diazoxide is given to suppress insulin release.
- For inoperable islet cell carcinoma, streptozocin is the best chemotherapeutic agents.

Insulinoma—interesting most

- The most common functioning islet cell tumour of pancreas
- Mostly are single (75%)
- Mostly multiple in 'MEN' syndromes
- Mostly benign (70%)
- Mostly occur in tail and body of pancreas
- Mostly present as bizarre behaviour confusing type due to hypoglycaemia
- Most useful diagnostic test—very high (disproportional) levels of insulin during fasting hypoglycaemia
- The most important test to localise the tumour before surgery is CT/MRI
- The most important test to localise at surgery is intra-operative ultrasound
- Mostly they can be enucleated when occur in the head
- Most insulinomas are small, less than 2 cm

GASTRINOMA (ZOLLINGER-ELLISON SYNDROME)

Two types are recognised.

- **Type I (rare):** These have antral G cell hyperplasia, wherein gastrin is stored. Hypergastrinaemia with chronic peptic ulceration is a feature. Pancreas is normal.
- **Type II: May be due to an ulcerogenic,** non-β-islet cell tumour or sometimes diffuse hyperplasia of the islet cells. Tumour secretes gastrin and is usually found in the tail of the pancreas. 50% of them are malignant.
  - Intractable peptic ulceration, hypergastrinaemia with massive acid hypersecretion of up to 500 ml/hr can occur.
  - Diarrhoea, steatorrhoea and hypokalaemia occur due to acid irritating the small bowel activity (Key Box 42.25).

Site

It commonly occurs in the gastrinoma triangle also called Passaro's triangle. Following three points form **Passaro's triangle.**

1. Junction of the cystic duct with the common bile duct (Fig. 42.105).
2. Junction between head and neck of pancreas.
3. Junction between second and third parts of the duodenum.

Diagnosis

1. **Endoscopy** will show prominent mucosal folds and large amount of acid in the stomach.
2. **Serum gastrin** is increased above normal levels (normal value <150 ng/dl).
3. **CT scan and arteriography** may localise the tumour.

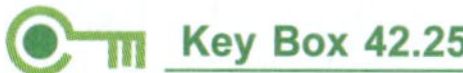
Key Box 42.25

Gastrinoma should be Suspected in Following Situations

1. **Unusual ulcer:** Peptic ulcer not responding to intensive medical treatment.
2. **Unusual recurrence:** Multiple recurrences in spite of the treatment.
3. **Unusual number:** Multiple ulcers scattered in the GIT.
4. **Unusual sites:** Ulcers present in the 2nd part of duodenum, an ulcer just distal to the ligament of Treitz.
5. **Unusual age:** Sudden development of an ulcer in a young boy or in a very elderly patient.

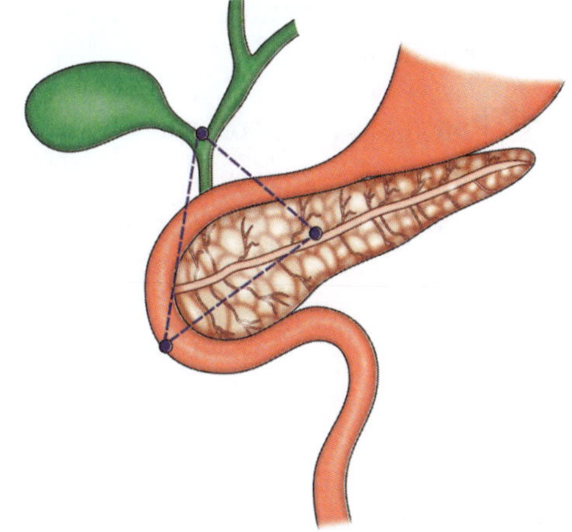

Fig. 42.105: Passaro's triangle of gastrinoma. (*Courtesy:* Dr Vidushi, Undergraduate student, KMC, Manipal)

Treatment

1. **Type I:** Partial gastrectomy to remove G cells-bearing area.
2. **Type II:** If the tumour is small, removal of the tumour can be done (enucleation).
3. If the **tumour is large**, omeprazole 20 mg twice a day or somatostatin derivatives have been used to control acidity. Total gastrectomy is the last resort, if gastrinoma is not found.

GLUCAGONOMA

- It arises from **alpha cells** producing glucagon. Around 90% are in the body and tail.
- Clinically, it presents with **extensive necrolytic migratory erythematous rashes.** Rashes occur due to low amino acid levels due to gluconeogenesis brought about by glucagon. Rashes involve legs and perineum.
- Age range is 20–70 years.
- This is common in women.
- **Mild diabetes**, weight loss, diarrhoea are the other features.
- Glucagon levels are increased in serum diagnostic.
- Localisation is by elective arteriography and CT scan.
- **Treatment is enucleation.**

Treatment Principles of Glucagonoma

- Correction of malnutrition by TPN (total parenteral nutrition).
- Treatment with somatostatin analogues.
- Enucleation is easy, if it is in the head.
- Considerable palliation, even if subtotal removal is achieved.
- Low dose heparin—before and after surgery—because of high risk of DVT—pulmonary embolism.
- Streptozocin and dacarbazine are the most effective chemotherapeutic agents.

Thus, endocrine tumours of the pancreas are rare but when they occur, they can present with varying clinical manifestations which confuse a clinician. A high index of suspicion is necessary. They may be benign but can be fatal, if left untreated.

ACUTE PANCREATITIS

Competency

SU28.1: Describe the clinical features, principles of investigation, prognosis and management of pancreatitis.

Definition

It is defined as acute nonbacterial inflammatory condition caused by activation, interstitial liberation and autodigestion of pancreas presenting as acute abdominal pain.

- *Acute pancreatitis stings like a scorpion (produces severe pain).*
- *Acute pancreatitis drinks like a fish (produces dehydration).*
- *Acute pancreatitis eats like a wolf (pancreatic necrosis).*
- *Acute pancreatitis burrows like a rodent (produces fistula).*
- *Acute pancreatitis kills like a leopard (life-threatening).*

Classifications

1. Marseille's classification
2. Modified Atlanta classification

1. Marseille's Classification

1. Acute pancreatitis
2. Acute relapsing pancreatitis
   - In both these conditions, pancreas returns back to normal.
3. Chronic pancreatitis
4. Chronic relapsing pancreatitis
   - In both these conditions, there is always permanent damage to the pancreas.

2. Modified Atlanta Classification

The latest classification which is used is given in Tables 42.7B and C.

Table 42.7B Pancreatic and peripancreatic collections

Collection	Time after onset of pain (wk)	Pancreatitis subcategory	Location	Imaging features
APFC	≤4	IEP	Extrapancreatic	Homogeneous, fluid attenuation, conforms to retroperitoneal structures, no wall
ANC	≤4	Necrotizing pancreatitis	Intra- and/or extra-pancreatic	Inhomogeneous, nonliquefied components, no wall
Pseudocyst	>4	IEP	Extrapancreatic	Homogeneous, fluid filled, circumscribed, encapsulated with wall
WON	>4	Necrotizing pancreatitis	Intra- and/or extra-pancreatic	Inhomogeneous, nonliquefied components, encapsulated

Table 42.7C Modified Atlanta classification

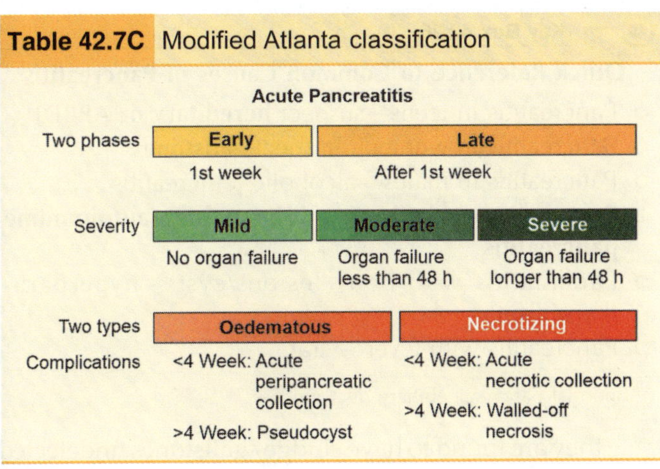

Acute Pancreatitis			
Two phases	Early 1st week	Late After 1st week	
Severity	Mild No organ failure	Moderate Organ failure less than 48 h	Severe Organ failure longer than 48 h
Two types	Oedematous	Necrotizing	
Complications	<4 Week: Acute peripancreatic collection >4 Week: Pseudocyst	<4 Week: Acute necrotic collection >4 Week: Walled-off necrosis	

Aetiology (Figs 42.106 to 42.108)

1. **Alcohol abuse (40 to 50%):** It is the **major cause of acute pancreatitis** in **our country** and is seen in about 50% of the cases. Alcohol stimulates pancreatic secretions rich in protein, forms protein plugs and results in obstruction to the pancreatic duct. Alcohol stimulates trypsinogen. It causes spasm of sphincter of Oddi. It also has **direct toxic effect on the pancreas**. Tobacco smoking contributes to its effects.
2. **Biliary tract disease:** Stone in the biliary tree (gallstone pancreatitis) is the major cause of acute pancreatitis in the Western world (40%). In our country, it may be responsible for pancreatitis in about 20–30% of patients.
3. **Collagen vascular disorders:** Autoimmune disease, such as polyarteritis nodosa, can be a causative factor in acute pancreatitis.
4. **Drugs:** Corticosteroids, tetracycline, oestrogens, azathioprine, valproic acid and diuretics can cause pancreatitis.
5. **Endoscopic procedures:** Sphincterotomy, cannulation of CBD or pancreatic duct, or basketing of stones from CBD can precipitate acute pancreatitis by duct disruption and enzyme extravasation.
6. **Familial or genetic** factors have been blamed for acute pancreatitis. Hereditary pancreatitis may be due to mutation of cationic trypsinogen gene. Symptoms begin in early childhood.
7. **Hyperparathyroidism** causing hypercalcaemia may stimulate pancreatic juices and can cause pancreatitis. It also facilitates precipitation of calcium in the ducts.

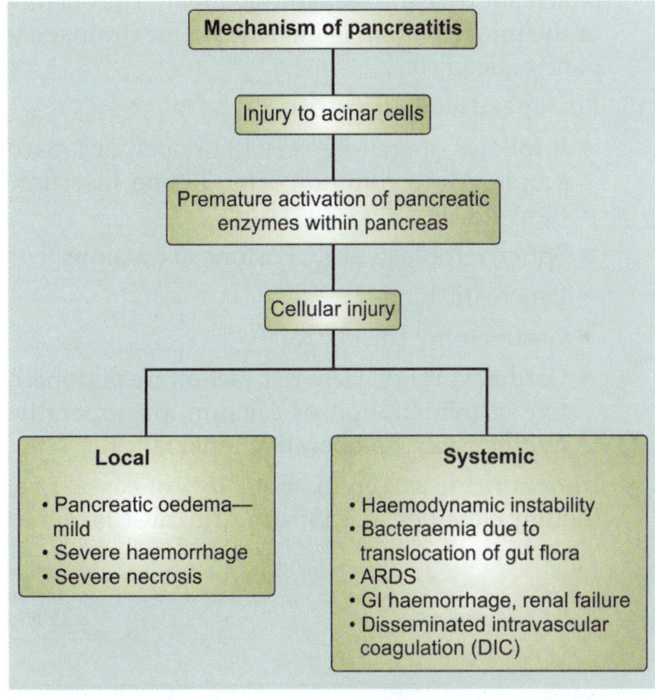

Fig. 42.106: Pathogenesis of tissue damage (see text)

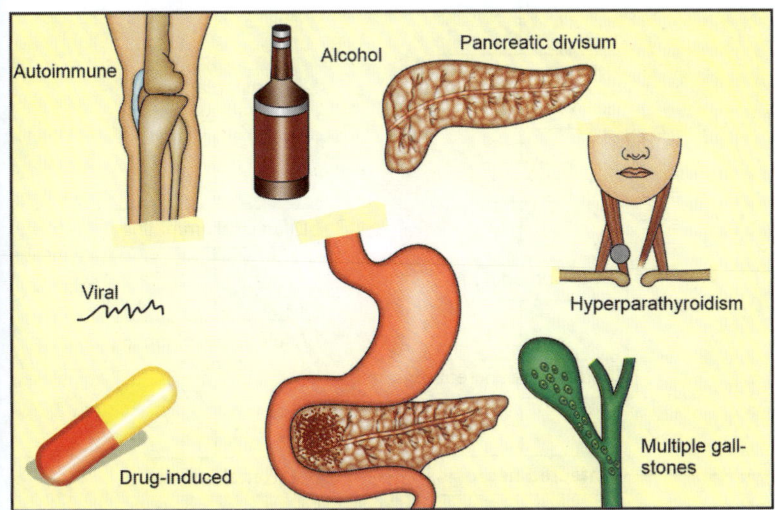

Fig. 42.107: A few causes of acute pancreatitis

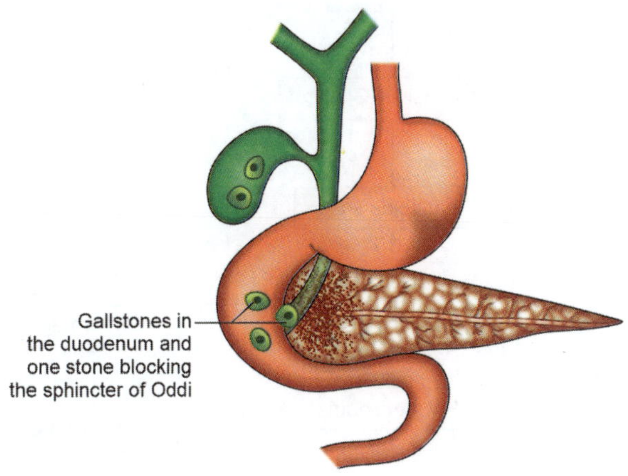

Fig. 42.108: Gallstone pancreatitis (diagrammatic)

8. **Hyperlipidaemia** (>1000 mg/dl of triglycerides) can also cause pancreatitis. Dietary control can cure pancreatitis.
9. **Hypothermia** and **hypotension** can cause ischaemia to the pancreas resulting in acute pancreatitis.
10. **Injury to the pancreas** either postoperative or following penetrating injury can result in pancreatitis.
11. **Infection:** Viruses such as *Mumps* and *Coxsackie* can cause pancreatitis. Scorpion sting can also cause pancreatitic abnormality.
12. **Ductal:** Around 20%. Some of them are due to pancreatic divisum seen during ERCP. The opening of the minor papilla is inadequate for drainage of pancreatic juice.
13. **Postoperative pancreatitis**
    - It follows operations on CBD—open or laparoscopic. More common after T-tube insertions (now it is less).
    - Sphincteroplasty, ERCP, stone extractions
    - Pancreatic biopsy
    - Gastrectomy (distal/total)
    - Cardiac surgery. Here risk factors are perioperative administration of calcium, postoperative hypotension, preoperative renal failure.
14. **Idiopathic:** It is seen in about 15% of cases. Even though, classified as idiopathic (no cause is found), they are found to have sludge/gallstones undetected by ultrasound examination (Key Box 42.26).

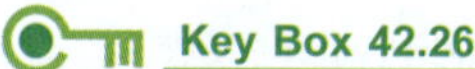

Key Box 42.26

Quick Reference to Common Causes of Pancreatitis

- Pancreatitis in teens—suspect **hereditary or APBDJ**[1]
- Pancreatitis in women—suspect **gallstones**
- Pancreatitis in males—alcoholic pancreatitis
- Pancreatitis with **fleeting joint pains—autoimmune pancreatitis**
- Pancreatitis with bony lesions/cysts—**hyperparathyroidism**
- Pancreatitis with fever—viral

[1]Abnormal pancreaticobiliary duct junction

Pathogenesis (Fig. 42.109)

- Autodigestion is the final common pathway leading to pancreatitis, a few theories have been explained as possible factors for autogenesis.
  1. **Obstruction/secretion:** Recurrent attacks of pancreatitis as in chronic cases can be due to multiple strictures, stasis, resulting in autodigestion.
  2. **Common channel theory:** In about 90% of cases, bile duct and pancreatic duct converge into ampulla of Vater. However, only in 10% of cases, they have common channel.
     Reflux of bile into pancreas has been blamed for 'gallstone pancreatitis'. However, strong evidence is lacking.

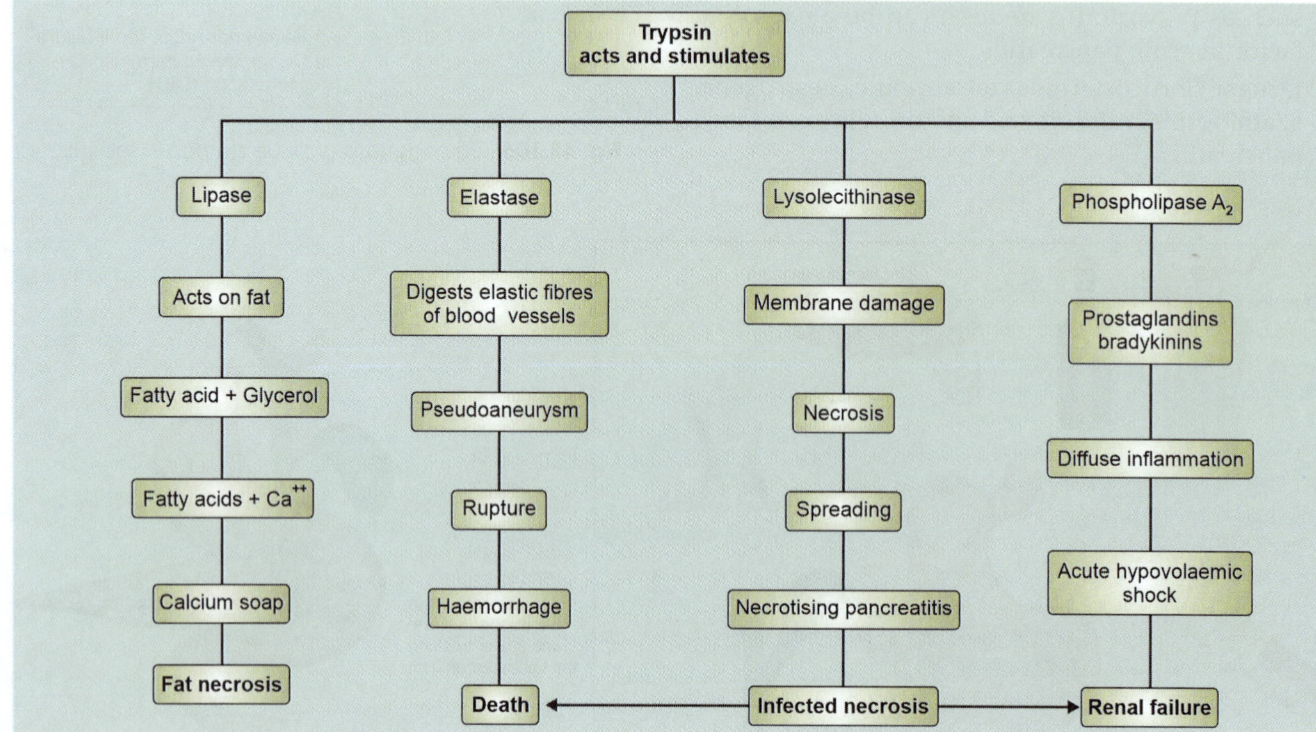

Fig. 42.109: Activation of trypsinogen to trypsin—pathogenesis of pancreatitis

3. **Duodenal reflux:** Activation of enzymes takes place in the duodenum through action of enterokinase. Hence, it is postulated that duodenal reflux is one of the causes of acute pancreatitis.
4. **Back diffusion:** Back diffusion of pancreatic enzymes through the ductal epithelium is a possible factor, when damaged by alcohol/bile acids, etc.
5. **Systemic sepsis:** Organ failure
   - ARDS, renal failure
   - Endotoxins originate from bacteria.

- Acute pancreatitis is an **autodigestion** following activation of trypsinogen. This is brought about by various agents mentioned above.
- It may also be due to reflux of bile into the pancreas.
- Trypsinogen is converted into trypsin. It acts and stimulates:

1. **Lipase:** Lipase splits the fat into fatty acids and glycerol. Fatty acids combine with calcium to form calcium soap. This is represented as fat necrosis seen in the omentum, subsynovial pockets of knee joint, etc. This also explains hypocalcaemia and tetany seen in acute pancreatitis.
2. **Elastase:** It digests the elastic fibres of the blood vessels resulting in rupture and haemorrhage into the peritoneal cavity.
3. **Lysolecithinase:** This is derived from the bile. It produces extensive tissue necrosis resulting in destruction of pancreas.
4. **Prostaglandins, bradykinins, kallikrein, etc.:** These are the inflammatory mediators. They produce profound hypotension, shock and collapse, due to loss of fluid in the retroperitoneum (III space loss).
5. **Extensive necrosis of pancreas:** It produces **MDF** (**m**yocardial **d**epressant **f**actor) which depresses ventricular contraction resulting in cardiac failure. Ultimate result is the development of **multiorgan failure**.

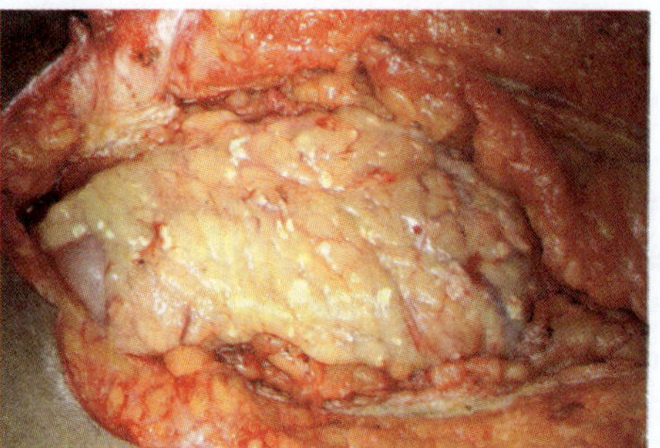

Fig. 42.110: Fat necrosis in the omentum

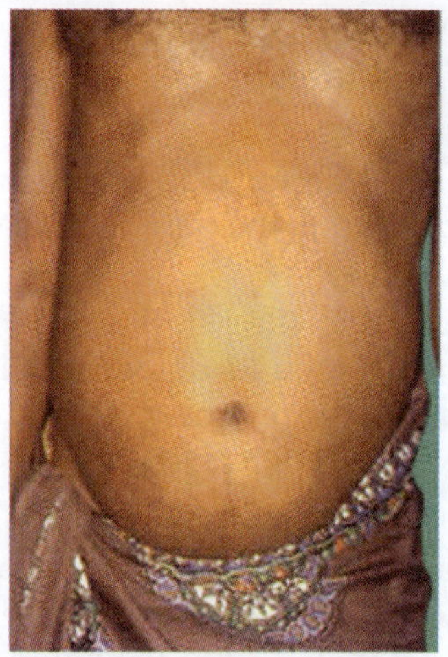

Fig. 42.111: Abdominal distension is due to paralytic ileus in the early stages. It can also be due to pancreatic ascites

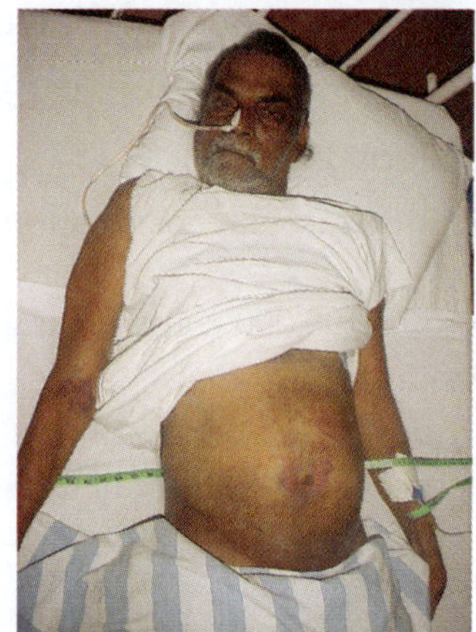

Fig. 42.112: Cullen's sign—discolouration around the umbilicus

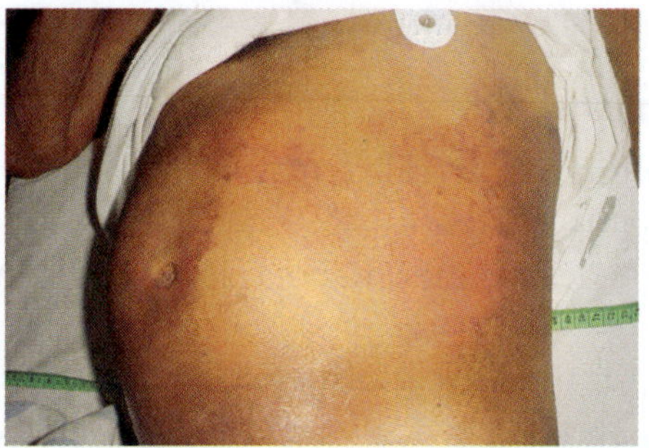

Fig. 42.113: Grey Turner's sign—discolouration in the flanks

Clinical Features (Figs 42.110 to 42.113)

Symptoms

- Severe upper abdominal epigastric pain radiating to the back increases over a period of hours—illimitable agony is a characteristic feature. It is partially relieved on stooping and bending forwards (Mohammedan Prayer sign). A meal or alcohol triggers the pain.
- Vomiting—frequent and effortless due to reflex pylorospasm.
- Fever—low grade.
- Haematemesis and melaena can occur due to necrosis of duodenum. It is a poor prognostic sign.

Signs

- **Febrile,** tachypnoeic patient in agony.
- **Cyanosis**—improper perfusion of lungs.
- **Faint jaundice** due to oedema of the head of the pancreas.
- **Features of shock**—feeble pulse, tachycardia, hypotension, cold extremities.
- **Abdominal findings**
  - Tenderness in epigastrium
  - Upper abdominal guarding and rigidity
  - Distension of the abdomen
  - Mass in epigastrium
  - Muscle guarding
  - Abdominal distension due to either accumulation of blood or fluid in the peritoneal cavity or due to paralytic ileus.
- **Cullen's sign** (Fig. 42.112): Bluish ecchymotic discolouration seen around umbilicus (first described for ruptured ectopic pregnancy).
- **Grey Turner's sign** (Fig. 42.113)
  - Bluish discolouration in the flanks
  - Both these signs are due to peripancreatic and retroperitoneal haemorrhage and seepage of blood along fascial planes, into the anterior abdominal wall and spread through falciform ligament.
- **Evidence of respiratory signs:** Tachypnoea, dullness, effusion, crepitations, rhonchi (pulmonary oedema, ARDS).

Systemic Complications

A. Disseminated intravascular coagulation as evidenced by:
- Platelet count <100,000 cells/cumm
- Fibrinogen <1 g/l
- Fibrin split products >80 µg/dl

B. Metabolic disturbance (serum calcium <7.5 mg/dl)

Local Complications

- Necrosis
- Abscess
- Pseudocyst

Investigations

1. **Haemogram (CBP):** Hb% may be low due to haemorrhagic pancreatitis.
   - Total count is raised above 15,000 cells/mm^3 due to inflammation.
2. **Blood for urea, creatinine** to rule out renal failure.
3. **Serum amylase** (widely used test) (Key Box 42.27).
   - Normal levels are 40–80 Somogyi units.

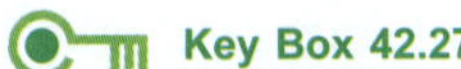

Key Box 42.27

Increased Amylase Levels—Seen in

- Acute pancreatitis and its complications
- Parotitis
- Afferent loop obstruction
- Spasm of sphincter of Oddi
- Biliary peritonitis—duodenal injuries
- Mesenteric infarction
- Ruptured ectopic gestation

- Values around 400 are suggestive and values more than 1000 Somogyi units are diagnostic of acute pancreatitis.
- It is increased in the first 24–48 hours and returns to normal within 3–4 days (Key Box 42.27).
- Persistent high level of amylase in acute pancreatitis indicates:
  - Unresolving inflammation
  - Recurrent attacks of pancreatitis
  - Complications—pseudocyst, pancreatic abscess
  - **Serum lipase levels—more specific** but difficult to measure. Lipase is only **secreted by pancreas.**

Pearls of Wisdom

Lipase levels tend to be higher in alcoholic pancreatitis and amylase levels are higher in gallstone pancreatitis.

4. **Blood and urine sugar estimation:** Glycosuria is present in almost 100% of patients.
5. **Serum calcium levels:** Hypocalcaemia is seen, due to hypoalbuminaemia or fat necrosis.
6. **Total proteins** are usually low, especially albumin.
7. **Plain X-ray abdomen (erect position)** (Fig. 42.114)
   - **Calcification suggests chronic pancreatitis.**
   - To rule out perforation of peptic ulcer.

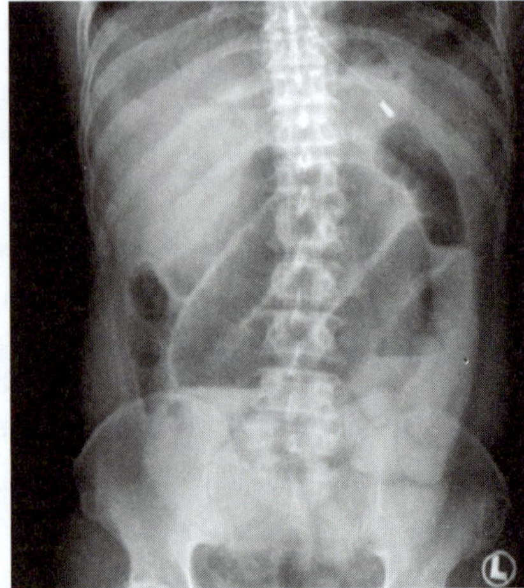

Fig. 42.114: Plain X-ray abdomen erect showing dilated jejunal loop due to paralytic ileus—sentinel loop sign

- **Sentinel loop sign**—one dilated jejunal loop of intestine which is seen in the region of pancreas.
- **Colon 'cut-off' sign** refers to mild distension of transverse colon with collapsed descending colon.

8. **Abdominal ultrasound**—can demonstrate oedematous pancreas, fluid in the abdomen or biliary tract disease.
9. **Contrast enhanced CT scan** of abdomen is done after 3–5 days in patients who fail to respond to conservative treatment. **If CT scan demonstrates infected necrosis, an urgent CT-guided FNAC is done and Gram stain is sent. If Gram stain is positive, it has to be treated urgently** (Figs 42.115 and 42.116).

Indications for CT scan in acute pancreatitis

- Patients with severe pancreatitis
- When the diagnosis is in doubt
- Patients with organ failure
- Patients with sepsis
- Localised complications such as pseudocyst, pseudoaneurysms
- Clinical deterioration

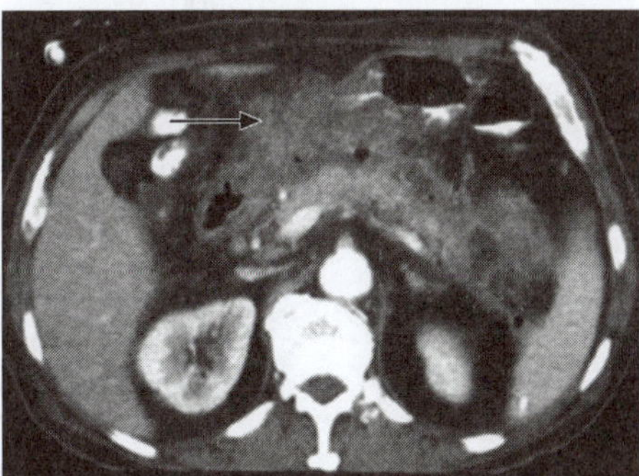

Fig. 42.115: Contrast enhanced CT (CECT) scan is the gold standard investigation in cases of acute pancreatitis. Useful after 7 days change to 4 days of acute pancreatitis. This photograph shows extensive necrosis. CT scan also helps in detecting pseudocysts, abscesses, presence of gallstones or any other unsuspected pathology in the abdomen. Modern thinking is to wait for 4–6 weeks for separation of necrosis before surgical necrosectomy

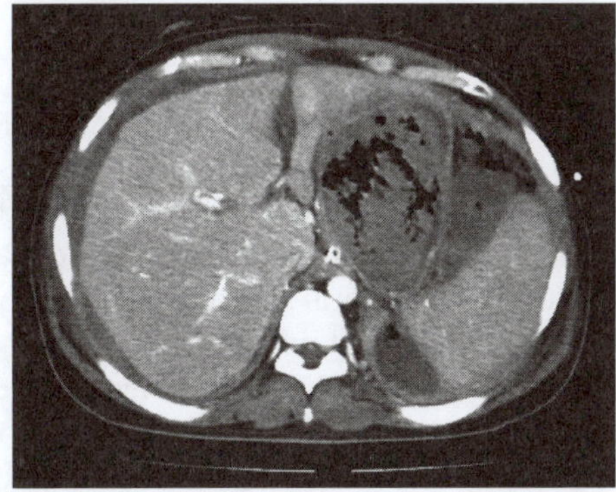

Fig. 42.116: CT scan showing infected necrosis with air pockets inside necrosis

Prognostic Indicators/Criteria for Acute Pancreatitis

There are several scoring systems available, a few important ones have been given below. Atlanta's Criteria for Acute Pancreatitis is applied for organ failure. Ranson score is applied for severity prediction and Balthazar score is applied for CT severity index.

Atlanta's criteria for acute pancreatitis

Organ failure as defined

- Shock (systolic blood pressure <90 mmHg)
- Pulmonary insufficiency (PaO_2 <60 mmHg)
- Renal failure (creatinine level >2 mg/dl after fluid resuscitation)
- GI bleeding (>500 ml/24 hr)

Balthazar-Ranson criteria for severity or computed tomography severity index (CTSI)

CT Grade	Score	Necrosis	Score	SI
A	0	None	0	0
B	1	One-third	2	1
C	2	One-half	4	4
D	3	>One-half	6	7
E	4			20

A = normal

B = focal or diffuse enlargement of the pancreas

C = intrinsic pancreatic abnormalities associated with haziness and streaky densities representing inflammatory changes in the peripancreatic fat

D = single, ill-defined fluid collection;

E = two or more multiple fluid collections

CTSI, 0–3, mortality 3% morbidity 8%

CTSI, 4–6, mortality 6%, morbidity 35%

CTSI, 7–10, mortality 17%, morbidity 92%

Severe pancreatitis is defined by the presence of any evidence of organ failure or a local complication.

Management

- Almost always conservative. However, a few scoring systems have been followed (Table 42.8).

Pearls of Wisdom

Early aggressive fluid replacement is the key in the management of acute pancreatitis.

- Even though management principles of any acute abdomen includes 'nil per oral' so as to give rest to the part, in cases of pancreatitis it has been divided broadly into three categories. It is desirable to know the treatment followed for these categories. It has been given in Table 42.9 and Fig. 42.117.

Table 42.8 Prognostic indicators/severity predictors

Ranson score	Glasgow Scale
On admission	
Age >55 years	Age >55 years
WBC count >16 × 10^9/l	WBC count >15 × 10^9/l
Blood glucose >10 mmol/l	Blood glucose >10 mmol/l
LDH >350 units/l	Serum urea >16 mmol/l
AST >250 Sigma Frankel unit/unit	PaO_2 <60 mmHg
After 48 hours	**Within 48 hours**
Increase in blood urea nitrogen levels >5 mg%	Serum calcium <2 mmol/l
Drop in haematocrit >10%	Serum albumin <32 g/l
Arterial oxygen saturation (PaO_2 <60 mmHg)	LDH >600 units/l
Serum calcium <8 mg/dl	AST/ALT >600 units/l
Base deficit >4 mmol/l	***Disease is classified as severe when three or more factors are present.***
Fluid sequestration >6 l	

Table 42.9 Management principles of acute pancreatitis

	Acute oedematous (mild—80%)	Necrotising pancreatitis (sterile necrosis—10%)	Infected necrosis (very severe—5%)
Admission	Acute ward with monitoring of vitals	Intensive care unit	Intensive care unit
IV fluids/ hypotension	**Early correction of hypotension,** hypovolaemia—crystalloids	IV fluids and inotropic* support may be required	May require inotropes and vasopressors for a long period
Blood transfusion	Rarely required	May be required	Definitely required
Antibiotics	No antibiotics	Early antibiotic prophylaxis is required	Broad spectrum antibiotics—imipenem, ciprofloxacin, metronidazole, etc.
Oral/nutrition	Oral fluids, soft diet by 3–4 days, once pain and ileus settle down	If pain is still present even after 4 days, nasojejunal feeding to be done	Enteral feeding/nasojejunal feeding. If calories are not sufficient, total parenteral nutrition is required
Hypomagnesaemia/ hypocalcaemia	Usually will not be a problem	Correction is required	Correction is required
Oxygen	By nasal cannula/face mask may be required	Early ARDS—ventilatory support	Ventilatory support may be required
Role of surgery/ natural course	Majority of patients will not require surgery. If gallstones are impacted at sphincter of Oddi, endoscopic basketing and laparoscopic cholecystectomy should be done	By 10–15 days, may resolve completely or may develop into pseudocyst or infected necrosis which require surgery	Ideal time to operate is after 4 weeks when necrosis is demarcated well. Initial percutaneous CT guided or laparoscopic retroperitoneal aspiration (step up approach) followed by necrosectomy

*Drug of choice in septic shock to treat hypotension and hypoperfusion is fluid boluses of crystalloids and norepinephrine

- Those of you who find it difficult can remember at least a few fundamentals of managing acute pancreatitis. They are given in the form of simple headlines: **ABCDEF.**

A: Aspiration with Ryle's tube, to give rest to the pancreas in cases of vomiting (may be for one or two days).

B: Blood transfusion if Hb% is low, or albumin and amino acids if proteins are low.

C: Charts—increasing pulse, increasing temperature indicates pancreatic necrosis which requires different care.

D: Drugs and fluids: Drug of choice in acute necrotizing pancreatitis is injection imipenem. Dose is 1 g intravenous infusion twice or thrice daily. It is given to reduce further damage to pancreatic and peripancreatic infections or to prevent progression to infected necrosis and multiorgan failure. Narcotic analgesics also can be given if pain is severe. Choice of fluid is Ringers' lactate . It is given at the rate of 125–150 ml/hr. Blood urea nitrogen (BUN) and creatinine should be used as markers to predict intravascular volume depletion and correction. Fluid resuscitation should be instituted early in cases of pancreatitis because of third space loss resulting in severe hypovolaemic shock. Hypovolaemia is due to endothelial cell damage and increase permeability.

E: Exploratory laparotomy (Key Box 42.28) is done when patient is **not improving** or when there is a complication of pancreatitis such as pancreatic fistula or necrosis. With the advent of wonderful imaging techniques, surgical intervention is rarely being done in the initial phase of acute pancreatitis. With conservative treatment, majority will return back to normal by 3–5 days. Those who develop complications are dealt separately. Details are given later.

Key Box 42.28

Indications for Surgery in Acute Pancreatitis

- Infected necrosis
- Pancreatic abscess
- Complications such as massive bleeding not responding to conservative treatment
- Cholangitis not responding to treatment

F: Fluid should be given early. Rapid infusion of 3–4 litres of Ringer lactate is used to treat hypovolaemic shock. Plasma or albumin may also be given.

- Factors predicting severe pancreatitis (Key Box 42.29).

Key Box 42.29

Identification of Severe Pancreatitis

- Age : >70 years
- Obesity : BMI >30 kg/m^2
- Pleural effusion : Present
- CT necrosis : >50
- CT severity index : CTSI
- Persistent : Organ failure

Pearls of Wisdom

In cases of infected necrosis proved by CT-guided FNAC and Gram stain, necrosectomy should be done. Ideal time is 4–6 wks. First do percutaneous aspiration/drainage.

Details of the important aspects of treatment of acute pancreatitis are given below. Refer Fig. 42.117.

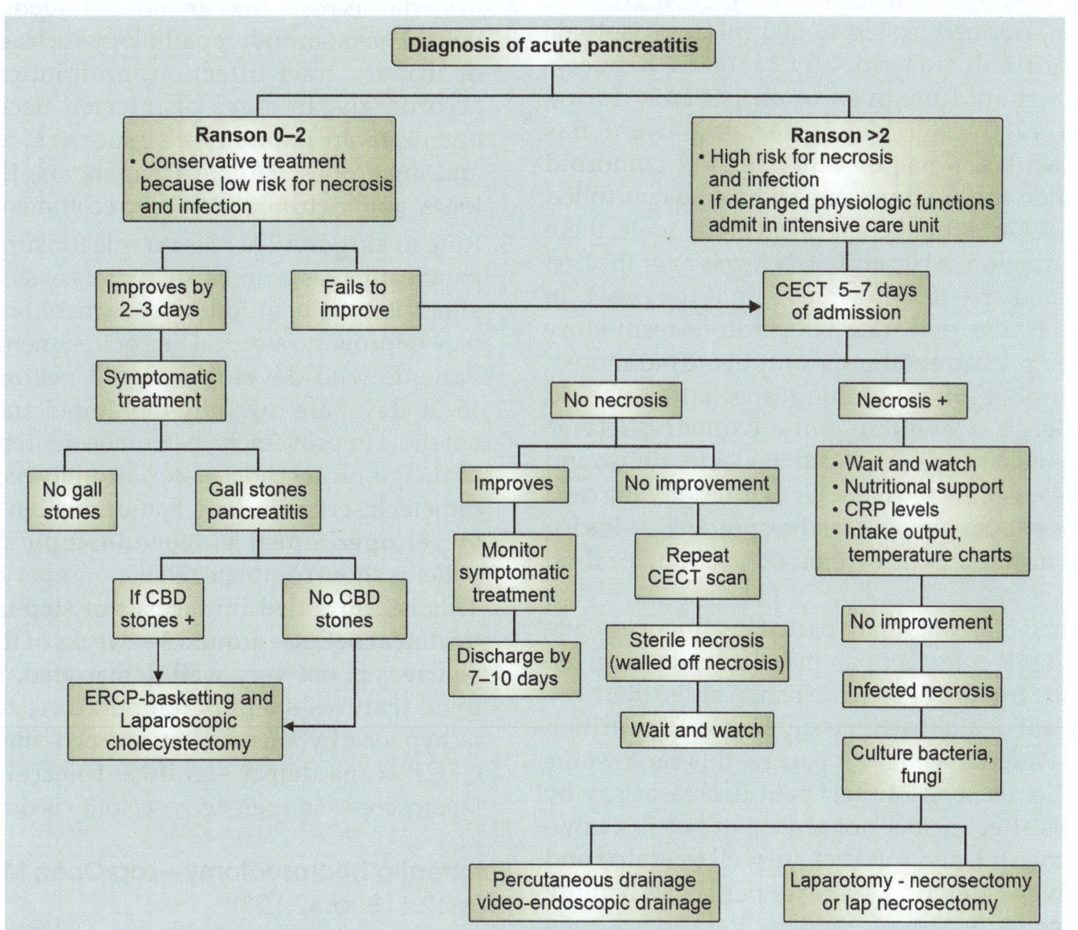

Fig. 42.117: Treatment of acute pancreatitis. (*Courtesy:* Dr SS Prasad, Dr L Ramachandra, Dr Kshama Hegde, Professor of Surgery, KMC, Manipal)

1. **Admission:** All patients with acute pancreatitis should be admitted and basic charts such as temperature, breathing, pulse, blood pressure intake output abdominal girth are monitored. Those patients with frequent vomiting, require nasogastric tube insertion for aspiration. Make a note of intake and output charts and accordingly fluid balance is maintained. Admission in ICU is recommended only in severe pancreatitis. Mild cases do not require oxygen supplementation. Early ARDS patients will require ventilator support and care in ICU.
2. **Pain relief:** It is very important because pain is severe, deep and penetrates to the back. NSAIDs (non-steroidal anti-inflammatory drugs) such as paracetamol, ibuprofen are started. If the pain relief is not happened, change over to powerful opioids, such as codeine. Still if pain persists, narcotic analgesics such as morphine or pethidine are recommended. Buprenorphine is better than pethidine because it is a long-acting analgesic and does not cause dependence. If pain is also due to stones in the CBD-gallstone pancreatitis, ERCP and extraction of stones is done.
3. **Fluid:** Fluid resuscitation in acute pancreatitis is an important step in resuscitation. Early aggressive hydration, defined as 250 to 500 ml/h of isotonic crystalloid solution (ideally lactated Ringer's solution), should be given to all patients during the first 12 to 24 h. However, if patient has cardiovascular, renal, or other related comorbid factors, then the fluid volume should be controlled or reduced. Once fluid replacement is adequate, there will be reduction in Hct and BUN levels over the first 24 h, particularly if they were high at the onset. In the same fashion, pulse rate, temperature, respiratory rate, blood pressure and urine output are monitored. Patients undergoing volume resuscitation should also undergo continuous pulse oximetry, receive supplemental oxygen as needed. Bedside ultrasound guided assessment of diameter of Inferior vena cava also helps in assessing the fluid response. Passive leg raising is a simple bedside method to check for fluid response.
4. **Nutrition:** It is an important part of treatment in acute pancreatitis. If enteral or parenteral nutrition is given early in the treatment of acute pancreatitis, there is a lower risk of death than if no supplemental nutrition is given. Patients with mild pancreatitis can resume an oral diet as soon as their pain decreases say by 2 to 3 days after an attack of acute pancreatitis. Low-residue, low-fat, and soft diet are well tolerated and can be given. Idea is to decrease peristalsis activity because some degree of paralytic ileus exists even after 2 or 4 days. Early refeeding also seems to result in a shorter hospital stay.

The enteral route is preferred over parenteral route because of following reasons:
- Intestinal mucosal barrier is maintained.
- Prevents the intestinal atrophy, if patients are kept NPO for long period.
- Intestinal atropy can promotes translocation of bacteria, thus sterile necrosis can turn to infective necrosis.
- Parenteral nutrition requires central IV catheters, thus the risk of infection of a catheter is present.
- Is less expensive.

A nasojejunal feeding tube is placed beyond the ligament of Treitz under radiological or endoscopic guidance. Reason being one can avoid stimulating the gastric phase of the digestive process. If one cannot insert nasojejunal tube, even nasogastric feeding should be initiated. Whenever nasogastric tube is inserted, the GE junction sphincter does not function well and there is also paralytic ileus. So, to avoid aspiration, head end of the patient should be elevated to about 30 degrees (Fig. 42.118A).

5. **Antibiotics:** In mild cases of acute pancreatitis and in sterile necrosis, they are not indicated. However, if patient has some other pathology such as respiratory or urinary tract infection, antibiotics are given accordingly. In cases of infected necrosis, usual organisms are gram-negative such as *E. coli, Klebsiella*, and anaerobes. Thus, carbapenems, fluoroquinolones, and metronidazole are recommended.
6. **Role of surgery:** There is no role for surgery in mild pancreatitis cases and also in cases of sterile necrosis after the treatment followed as mentioned above, if they improve no surgical line of treatment is required. Patients who develop infected necrosis (around 15–20 days) are carefully monitored and if they do not show improvement, percutaneous, retroperitoneal drainage of necrotic material, followed by pigtail catheter insertion is done. Same thing can also be done by **retroperitoneal videoendoscopic drainage**. If patients show complete relief, no surgery is required. **This is also called initial part of step-up approach treatment because around 3–4 weeks of time, necrotic pancreas is not very well demarcated.** However, if toxic features such as temperature, tachycardia, tachypnoea, hypotension, etc. are persisting and repeat CECT scans detect significant necrotic material, laparoscopic or open necrosectomy is done.

Pancreatic Necrosectomy—Lap/Open Method
(Figs 42.118 to 42.123)

- Ideally done 4–6 weeks later when sepsis is still present.
- CT-guided FNAC/bacterial culture is a must.

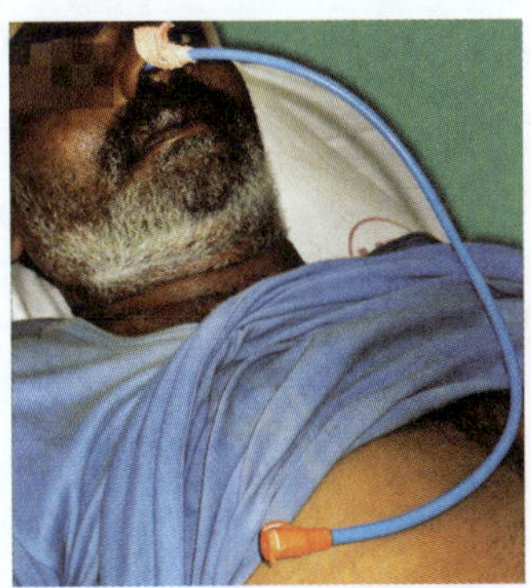

Fig. 42.118A: Acute necrotising pancreatitis. Patient had high temperature. Nasojejunal tube feeding is being done

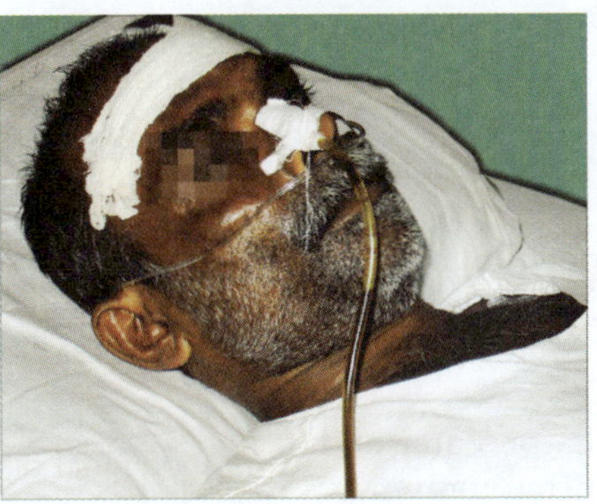

Fig. 42.118B: Acute necrotising pancreatitis with massive upper GI bleeding. Patient had high temperature, angiogram revealed pseudoaneurysm. He underwent therapeutic embolisation followed by necrosectomy

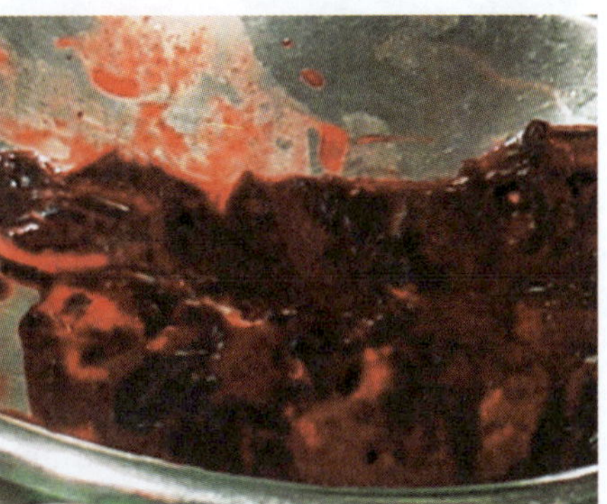

Fig. 42.119: Acute necrotising pancreatitis with massive upper GI bleeding. Patient had haematemesis of one litre of blood with clots

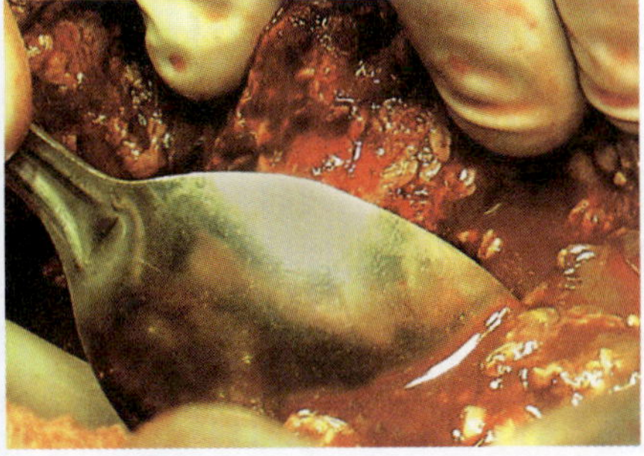

Fig. 42.120: You can see necrosectomy being done. It was done through lesser sac. Significant blood loss was present. Fingers are used to separate necrosis and it is removed with a spoon

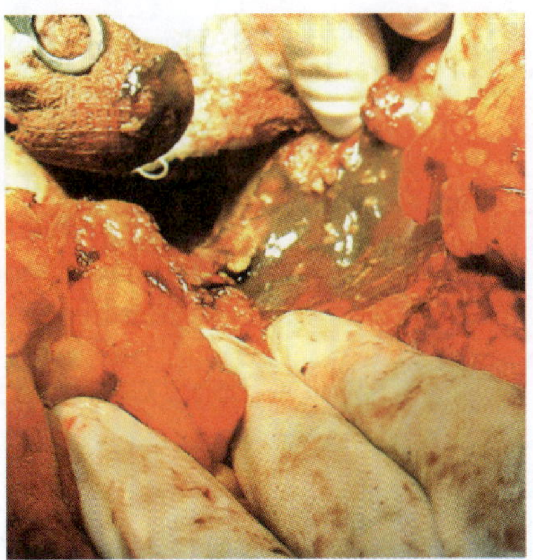

Fig. 42.121: After necrosectomy, pancreatic bed is washed with saline and tubes or sump drains are put so as to be able to irrigate in the postoperative period

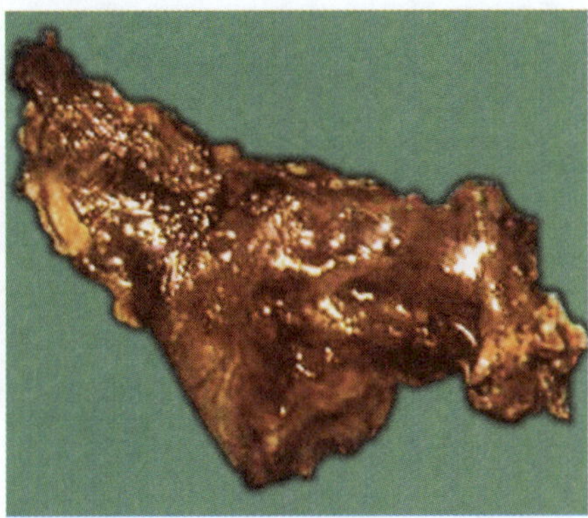

Fig. 42.122: Necrosectomy specimen

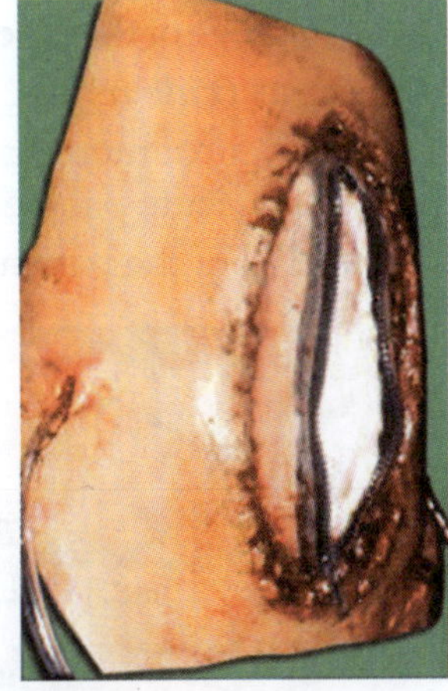

Fig. 42.123: After necrosectomy, it is better to perform zip laparotomy so that it can be opened any number of times for peritoneal toilet (*Courtesy:* Dr BH Ananda Rao, Prof and Head, Department of Surgery, Dr Siddhartha Bhandary and Dr Prashanth Shetty, Associate Professors, KMC, Manipal)

- A midline laparotomy is done.
- Lesser sac is entered.
- Thorough debridement of the dead tissue is done.
- All fluid and tissue should be sent for aerobic and anaerobic culture.
- Blunt dissection rather than sharp dissection is done to minimise bleeding.
- Antibiotics of choice should be carbapenems and quinolones.
- Ileostomy should be done for retrocolic necrosis.
- Cholecystectomy should be done for gallstone pancreatitis cases.
- Perfect haemostasis should be achieved using manual compression, sutures and ligatures.
- In cases of early necrosectomy, lesser sac is packed, reoperation done after 48 hours—zipper closure of the abdomen is used.

- Continuous lavage of the lesser sac and retroperitoneum is done.
- Other alternate methods are closed packing.
- Today all these cases are done through minimally invasive methods.
- Endoscopic necrosectomy, retroperitoneoscopic necrosectomy is also done.

Treatment of Gallstone Pancreatitis

If gallstone is obstructing the ampulla of Vater and causing pancreatitis, endoscopic sphincterotomy may be done within days. It has shown some benefit to the patients. After 2–3 weeks, once the jaundice subsides, cholecystectomy is recommended (Key Box 42.30).

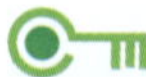 **Key Box 42.30**

Acute Pancreatitis

- Lipase is a more reliable test because it is more pancreas-specific and remains elevated for long after onset of symptom
- However, amylase is widely used

  It is not necessary to demonstrate CBD stone to prove the diagnosis of gallstone pancreatitis. Often stone has passed into duodenum

Complications of Acute Pancreatitis (Table 42.10)

Systemic Complications

1. **Shock**
   - Hypovolaemia and hypoperfusion are the major factors responsible for renal failure. Due to collection of large amount of fluid in the **third space**—peritoneal cavity, pleural cavity and extravascular space, shock occurs. Fluid replacement with blood or albumin should be done at appropriate time to treat the shock.
   - Electrolyte abnormalities should be corrected.

Table 42.10 Complications of acute pancreatitis

Local	General/systemic
Acute	***Systemic***
• Pancreatic necrosis (sterile)	• Pulmonary—ARDS
• Pancreatic necrosis (infected)	• Cardiac—shock, arrhythmias
• Pancreatic abscess	• Renal—renal failure
• Pancreatic ascites	• Gastro—ileus, intestinal colonic necrosis
Chronic	***General***
• Pancreatic pseudocyst	• Metabolic—hypercalcaemia, hypoglycaemia, hyperlipidaemia
• Peritoneal fluid collection	
• Pleural effusion	
• Pseudoaneurysm	• Haematological
• Partial/splenic vein thrombosis	

2. **Respiratory insufficiency:** Factors responsible for this are given in Key Box 42.31.

   Measurement of arterial blood gas values and administration of oxygen is enough in the initial stages. In late stages, pulmonary insufficiency needs to be treated with ventilatory support.

Key Box 42.31

Respiratory Failure

- Abdominal distension and elevation of diaphragm
- Intravascular coagulation in the lung
- Lecithin present in the pulmonary surfactant is altered due to lecithinase resulting in defective capillary alveolar exchange
- Defective ventilation caused due to pain
- Left-sided pleural effusion not responding to treatment

3. **Hypocalcaemia** needs to be treated with calcium IV. It is due to hypoalbuminaemia and due to calcium soap.
4. **Pleural effusion** is treated by pleural tap (ultrasound-guided), if it is symptomatic.
5. **ARDS, MODS:** Some mediators, such as phosphatase, damage alveolar membrane of lungs causing 'ARDS'. It manifests as respiratory failure.

Local Complications

1. **Pancreatic abscess** (Fig. 42.124)
   - It develops after 3–4 weeks of pancreatitis. Secondary infection in a pseudocyst results in pancreatic abscess. It usually points out on the left flank.
   - It has to be drained by CT-guided aspiration.
   - Laparoscopy may be necessary not only for the diagnosis but also as a therapeutic means for removal of necrotic pancreas.
   - Otherwise, open drainage of the abscess is required.
2. **Pseudocyst of pancreas** ***(vide infra)***
   - This complication is encountered after 2nd week following an attack of acute pancreatitis.
   - It is seen in about 20% of the patients.

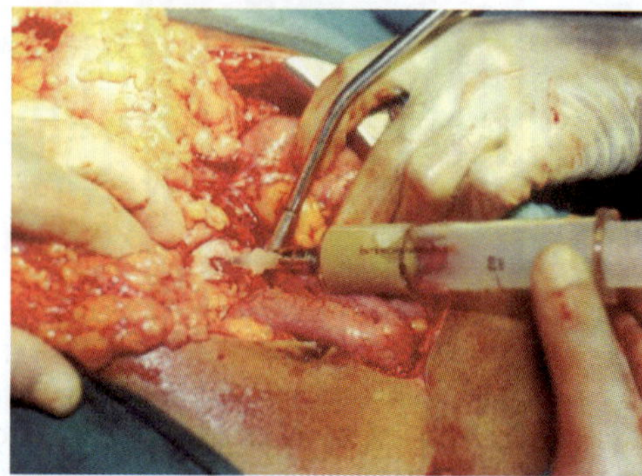

Fig. 42.124: Aspiration of pus from pancreatic abscess

3. **Perforation** of colon or stomach
4. **Pseudoaneurysm** resulting in massive upper gastrointestinal or lower gastrointestinal bleeding. Bleeding into the pancreatic duct is called **haemosuccus pancreaticus**.
    - This condition occurs due to enzymatic digestion of the blood vessels in the vicinity of pancreas. Thus splenic artery, gastroduodenal artery, etc. are commonly involved.
    - It has very high mortality. Prompt angiography followed by embolisation is the treatment.
    - Otherwise, laparotomy, ligation of pseudoaneurysm with or without intracystic ligation of the bleeders is the treatment (Figs 42.125 and 42.126).

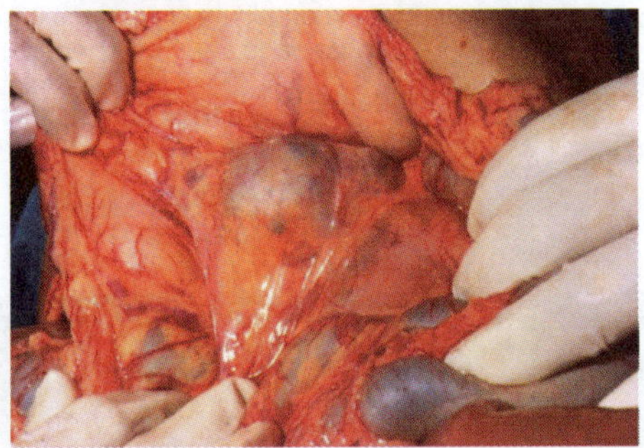

Fig. 42.125: Gastroduodenal pseudoaneurysm at surgery

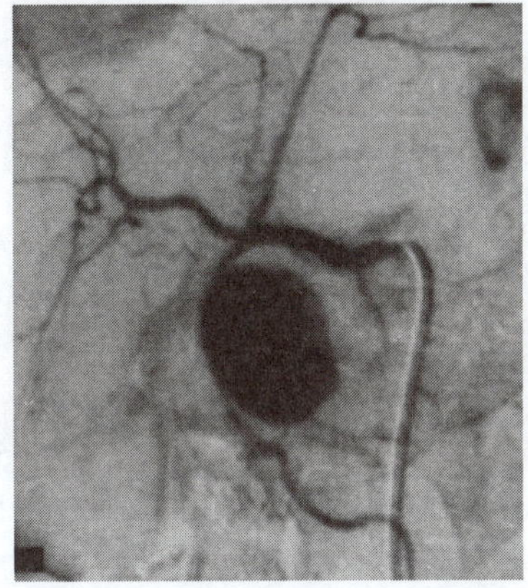

Fig. 42.126: Diagnosis by angiography

PSEUDOCYST OF PANCREAS

Definition

Collection of amylase-rich fluid in the lesser sac, due to pancreatic pathology. Fluid collection in the first 4 weeks is an acute fluid collection. After 4 weeks, it becomes an acute pseudocyst.

Pearls of Wisdom

It is called pseudocyst because it has no epithelial lining.

- Fluid is enclosed by a wall of fibrous granulation tissue and is called a pseudocyst.

Aetiology

1. Following an attack of **acute pancreatitis**, it usually appears after 4 weeks, as upper abdominal swelling.
2. **Blunt injury** of abdomen causing a ductal disruption wherein the pancreatic duct in the region of body is crushed against vertebral body results in a pseudocyst.
3. Some cause of **chronic pancreatitis** may be associated with pseudocyst.

Locations of Pseudocyst

1. Between stomach and transverse colon
2. Between stomach and liver
3. Behind or below the transverse colon

D'egidio Classification of Pseudocyst

Type I. Acute postnecrotic pseudocyst that occurs after **an episode of acute pancreatitis** and is associated with **normal duct anatomy** and rarely communicate with pancreatic duct.

Type II. Post-necrotic pseudocyst that occurs after an **episode of acute on chronic** pancreatitis and have a diseased but **not strictured** pancreatic duct and **there is communication between the duct and pseudocyst.**

Type III (also called retention cyst) **occurs in chronic pancreatitis,** uniformly associated with a duct stricture and a communication between duct and pseudocyst.

Clinical Features

1. Tensely cystic mass in the epigastrium, umbilical region or in left hypochondrium. Tensely cystic mass feels firm on palpation. Classically upper border of the mass is not felt.
2. Does not move with respiration because it is retroperitoneal in location.
3. It may have transverse mobility.
4. It does not fall forwards.
5. Percussion: It gives a **resonant note** because of stomach or intestine anterior to it.
6. **Transmitted pulsations** from aorta can be felt.
7. If a Ryle's tube is passed, it can be felt over the swelling. It is called **Baid sign**.
8. Depending upon the tension within the cyst, it can be tender or nontender.

Investigations

1. **USG/CT:** It can detect size, location of cyst and wall thickness. Confirm that there is no neoplasm of the pancreas before doing cystogastrostomy (Fig. 42.127).

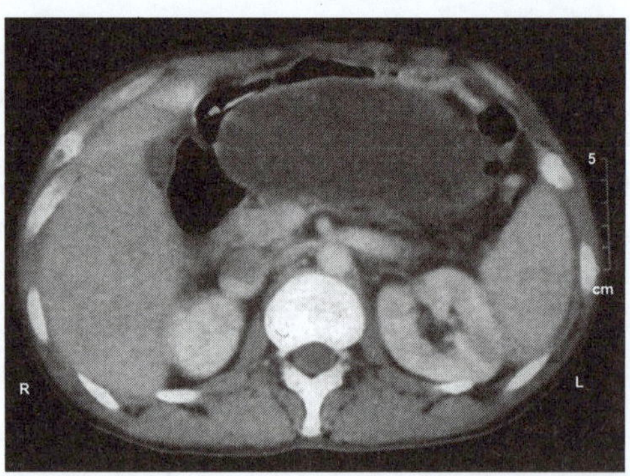

Fig. 42.127: CT scan: Classical pseudocyst pushing the stomach anteriorly—cystogastrostomy is ideal treatment

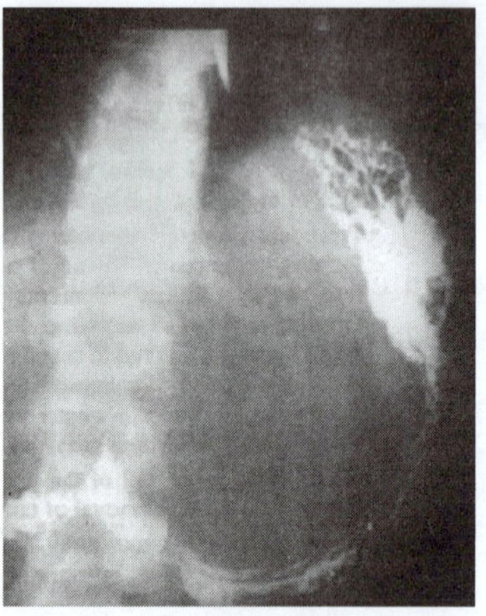

Fig. 42.128: Large pseudocyst behind the stomach demonstrated by barium meal

2. **Barium meal stomach:** In a lateral picture, the stomach is pushed anteriorly and increased vertebrogastric interval is seen (not done nowadays, Fig. 42.128).
3. **ERCP** may demonstrate communication of the cyst with the duct (routinely not done).

Treatment (Flowchart 42.1)

I. Conservative Line of Treatment

- Majority of the pseudocysts following acute pancreatitis resolve spontaneously within 3–4 weeks.
- Hence, regular ultrasound examination is done to observe the pseudocyst.

II. Surgery

Increase in size of cyst, severe pain, no response to conservative line of treatment are indications for surgery.

1. **Cystogastrostomy** (Figs 42.129 to 42.131)
   - *Indications:* Pseudocyst in relation to head and body of pancreas.
   - *Timing:* Surgery is done **after 6 weeks** because that is the time required for the wall to become fibrous.

Flowchart 42.1: Management of pseudocyst

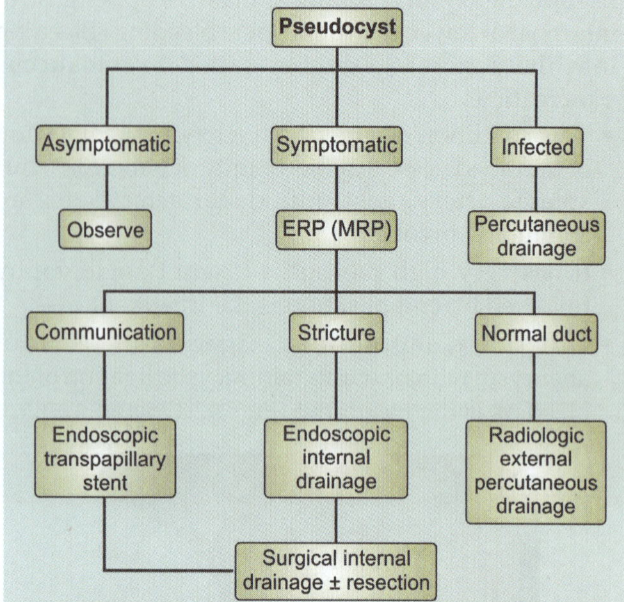

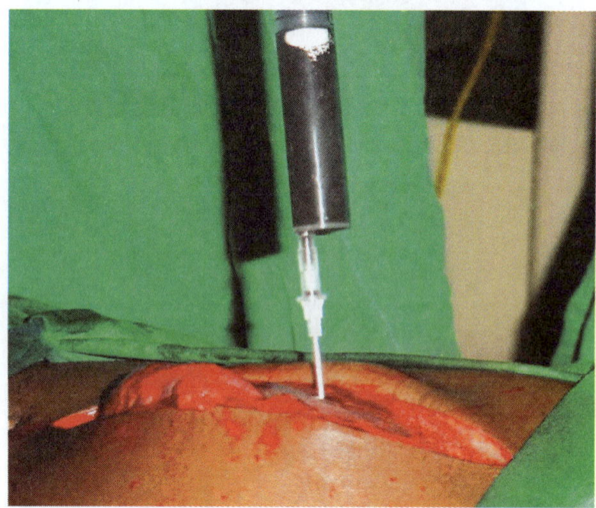

Fig. 42.129: Aspirated fluid is dark in colour, rich in enzymes—'engine oil' appearance

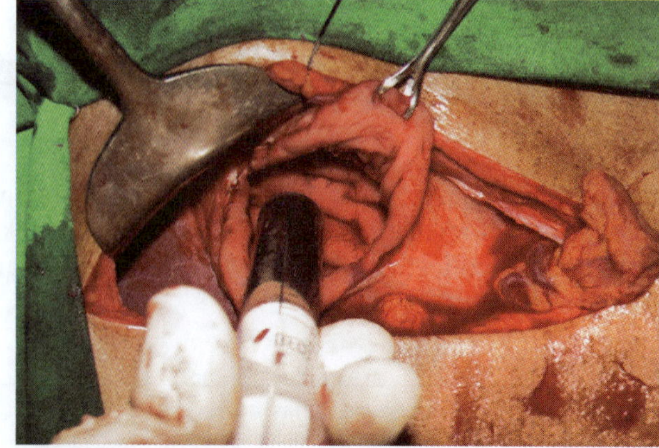

Fig. 42.130: Cystogastrostomy—anterior stomach wall is opened. Fluid is aspirated through the posterior stomach wall

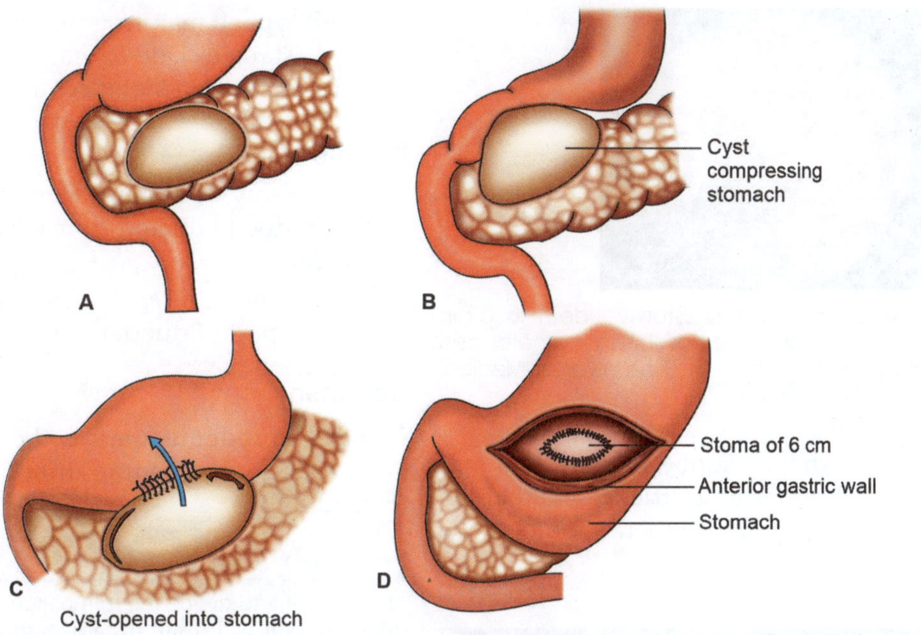

Figs 42.131A to D: Steps of cystogastrostomy. (*Courtesy:* Miss Vidushi, MBBS student, KMC, Manipal)

- *Size* of the cyst should be at least **6 cm**.
- *Procedure:* Anterior gastrostomy is done and an incision in the posterior wall of stomach opens into the cyst cavity. The contents are drained, opening is enlarged and cut end of stomach in posterior wall is sutured to cut edge of cyst wall. After one week, the cyst collapses. For reasons not known, the food does not enter the cyst cavity. **Size of cystogastrostomy stoma is about 6 cm. This procedure can also be done by endoscopic method.**

2. **Distal pancreatectomy:** Cyst confined to the tail of the pancreas is treated with removal of the tail and the cyst.
3. **Cystojejunostomy:** By using Roux-en-Y loop can be done, **for large cysts** by suturing jejunal loop to the cyst in the most dependent area (Figs 42.132 to 42.134).

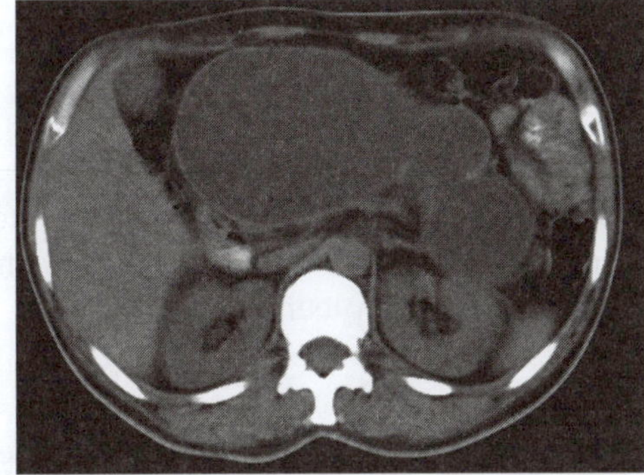

Fig. 42.132: CT scan showing large pseudocyst with multiple pockets. Cystojejunostomy is the ideal treatment

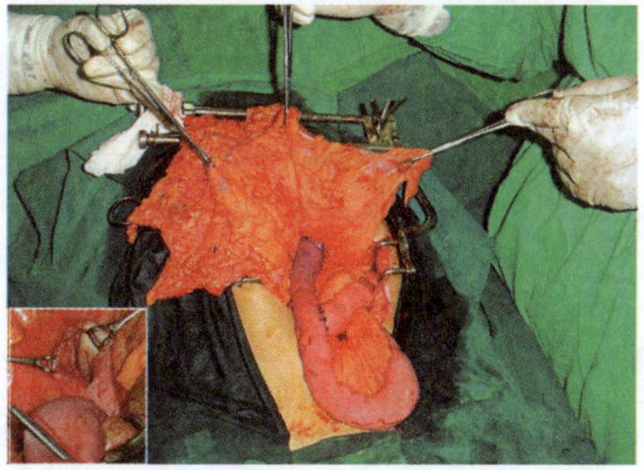

Fig. 42.133: Roux-en-Y cystojejunostomy at surgery, inset shows the opened cyst wall which is thick

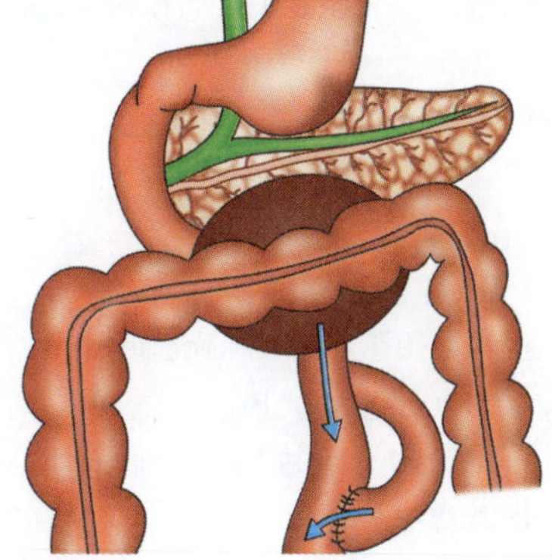

Fig. 42.134: Cystojejunostomy—diagrammatic representation

III. Endoscopic Drainage

This is easy, less invasive and ideal in draining acute pseudocysts. This procedure can also be repeated. However, chances of introducing infection are present. Endoscopic method of draining the pseudocysts is also being done for chronic cysts (Fig. 42.135). Few important

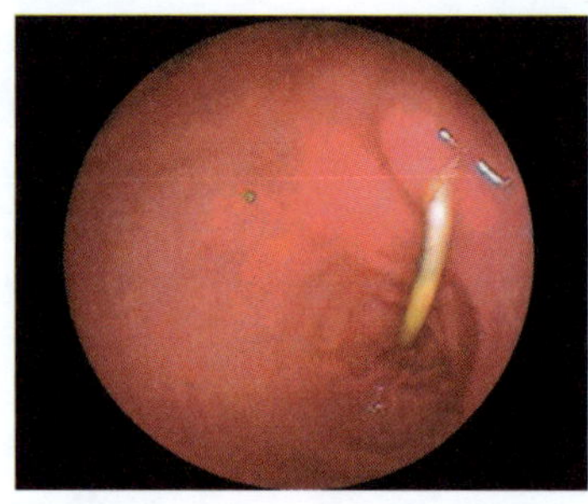

Fig. 42.135: Endoscopic cystogastrostomy—ideal to drain acute pseudocysts. After draining a nasobiliary catheter can be left in the cyst cavity. (*Courtesy:* Dr Filipe Alvares, Medical Gastroenterologist, KMC, Manipal)

points here are there should not be more than 3 mm gap between cyst and posterior gastric wall and at the site of incision in the posterior wall there should not be any varices.

CONGENITAL ANOMALIES OF THE PANCREAS

EMBRYOLOGICAL ANATOMY

- Pancreas is formed by fusion of ventral and dorsal buds. This will occur by 6 weeks. Malrotation of ventral bud causes annular pancreas.
- Ventral bud forms head and uncinate process.
- Ductal anomalies are given on page 662.

ANNULAR PANCREAS

It is a rare anomaly which occurs due to persistence of a portion of the ventral pancreatic anlage which fails to rotate. As a result of this, second part of the duodenum is surrounded by a thin rim of pancreatic tissue. Hence the name, annular pancreas (Key Box 42.32).

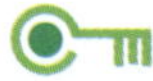 **Key Box 42.32**

Annular Pancreas

- Persistent ventral 'anlage'
- Neonatal or adult age
- Barium meal—obstruction to second part of duodenum
- Plain X-ray—'double bubble'
- Duodenoduodenostomy is the treatment
- Never divide the annulus

Associated Anomalies

Intrinsic duodenal atresia or stenosis.

Clinical Features

- **Neonatal type:** It manifests early in life. It produces symptoms of acute intestinal obstruction with vomiting and inability to take food.
- **Adult type:** It manifests after the age of 20. Vomiting is bile-stained. Due to stasis in the pyloric antrum, features of duodenal ulcer may be present.

Investigations

- **Plain X-ray abdomen:** Double bubble appearance occurs due to dilated stomach and dilated proximal duodenum.
- **Barium meal:** X-ray can demonstrate obstruction to second part of duodenum.

Treatment

Duodenoduodenostomy is the treatment of choice. Otherwise, duodenojejunostomy can be done (Fig. 42.136).

Pearls of Wisdom

It is tempting to divide the thin pancreatic rim. This should not be done as it will result in a pancreatic fistula.

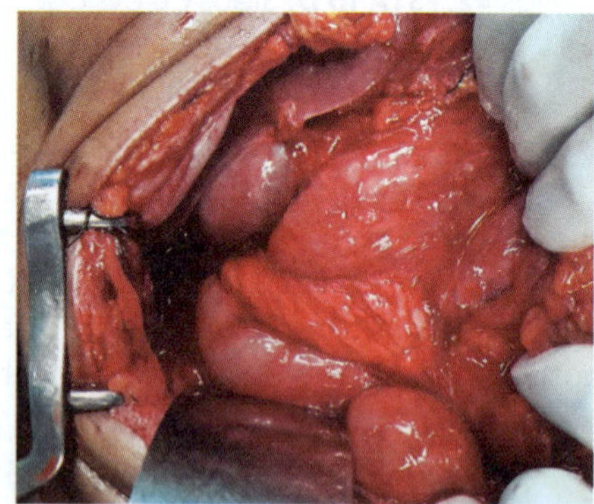

Fig. 42.136: Annular pancreas at surgery

Differential Diagnosis

- Pyloric stenosis
- Wilkie's disease (chronic duodenal ileus)

ECTOPIC PANCREAS

- This condition is not uncommon.
- Occasionally, at laparotomy for unrelated conditions, a soft to firm irregular tissue or nodule is found on the intestinal surface.
- Biopsy of this may come later as ectopic pancreas. Most of them are asymptomatic.
- It may be found in the submucosa of the stomach, duodenum, small intestines, Meckel's diverticulum or in the hilum of the spleen.

Complications

1. In the stomach: It may undergo cystic degeneration.
2. In the intestine: It can cause intussusception. Sometimes, it may be the source of gastrointestinal bleeding.

3. In the Meckel's diverticulum: Any of the complications mentioned above.

CONGENITAL CYSTIC FIBROSIS

- It is inherited as an autosomal recessive disorder.
- It is a generalised dysfunction of exocrine glands resulting in defective mucus secretion.
- Malabsorption due to pancreatic insufficiency is a feature.
- Pulmonary disease due to bronchiolitis occurs later (Key Box 42.33).

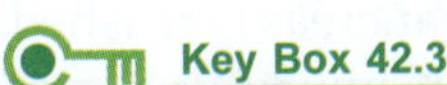
Key Box 42.33

Viscid Mucus—Conditions

- Meconium ileus
- Cystic fibrosis of pancreas
- Respiratory tract infection
- Increased Na^+ loss in the sweat

Pathology

The viscid mucin which is produced results in obstruction of the ducts and ductules. Stasis of pancreatic secretions, alveolar rupture due to increased pressure take place later. As a result of alveolar rupture, pancreatic enzymes leak outside resulting in pancreatitis.

Clinical Features

1. **At birth:** Meconium ileus or meconium peritonitis is an important manifestation of cystic fibrosis of pancreas.
2. **In infants**
   - Recurrent respiratory tract infection in the form of bronchiolitis and bronchiectasis results in cough with expectoration and dyspnoea.
   - Emaciation, steatorrhoea. Stools are pale and sticky.
3. **Older children:** Steatorrhoea, gross emaciation and wasting are the features. Due to poor nutritional status, cirrhosis of the liver with portal hypertension can be a feature.
4. **In adult:** Lucky survivors will suffer from gross wasting, diabetes, bronchiectasis, cirrhosis of the liver, sialoadenitis and choroiditis.

Investigations

- Normal contents of the electrolytes in the sweat: Na^+—70 mmol/l, Cl^-—60 mmol/l, K^+— 20 mmol/l.
- In these patients, sodium excretion may be three to four times more than normal.

Treatment (Only Symptomatic)

I. **Nutritional support**
   - Fat intake should be low, protein should be increased.
   - Pancreatic enzyme preparations (5 to 10 g) are given two to three times per day, to supplement pancreatic enzymes.

II. **Control infection:** Respiratory tract infection is treated with antibiotics, bronchodilators, mucolytic agents, etc.

III. **Role of surgery:** Indicated in meconium ileus to relieve intestinal obstruction.

PANCREATIC DIVISUM AND DUCTAL ANOMALIES

- Pancreatic divisum is the most common congenital abnormality of the pancreas. It is found in 5–10% of patients.
- It is caused by failure of fusion of the dorsal and ventral portions of the developing pancreas. In the majority of patients, this anomaly is of no clinical importance.
- In a certain subset of patients, however, estimated to be approximately 5–20%, pancreatic divisum is a clinically important cause of abdominal pain, acute recurrent pancreatitis or chronic pancreatitis.
- **The frequency of pancreatic divisum in patients with pancreatitis in recent studies is approximately 10%** (Key Box 42.34).

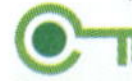
Key Box 42.34

Pancreatic Divisum

- It is one of the uncommon causes of acute pancreatitis.
- In 10% of patients. Majority of pancreas drains through duct of Santorini through lesser papilla.
- Outflow obstruction—treated by sphincteroplasty of minor papilla.

Pathophysiological Consequences

The cause of pancreatitis in this common anomaly is hypothesised to be caused by minor papillary insufficiency caused by papillary fibrosis and subsequent stenosis.

Diagnosis

- The diagnosis is established by ERCP.
- MRCP is a noninvasive and accurate method of establishing the diagnosis. However, a negative MRCP does not exclude the diagnosis of divisum as the concordance with ERCP ranges from 50% to more than 70%.
- The accuracy of the MRCP may be improved by administration of secretin.

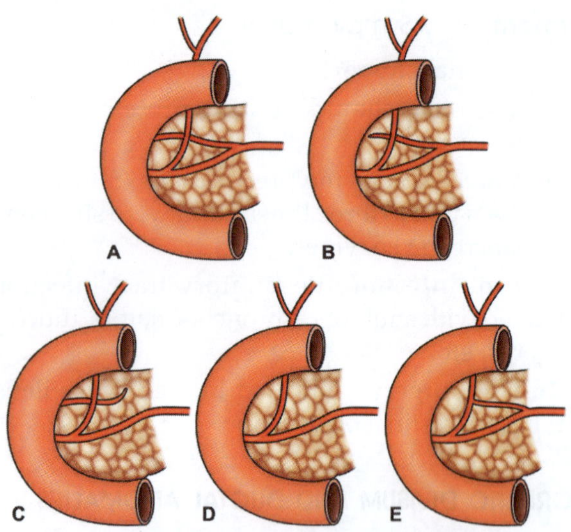

Figs 42.137A to E: Anomalies of pancreatic duct

Treatment

- In patients with minimal symptoms, treatment with pancreatic enzymes may reduce pancreatic secretion and hence, pain. Pain management referral may be necessary.
- Patients with acute pancreatitis are estimated to benefit from either surgical minor sphincteroplasty or endoscopic minor papillotomy.

A few anomalies of pancreatic duct are given below (Figs 42.137A to E).

A. Normal anatomy
B. Terminal end of accessory duct fibrosed
C. Blind ending of accessory duct
D. Absent accessory duct
E. Blind end of accessory duct with main duct communication.

MISCELLANEOUS

PANCREATIC FISTULA

Most common after **pancreatic trauma** (Fig. 42.138).

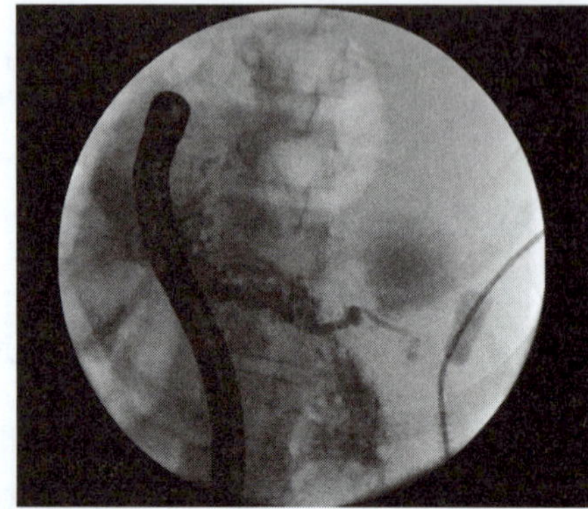

Fig. 42.138: Pancreatic fistula following acute pancreatitis

Causes

1. **External fistulae** occur due to operative injury to the pancreas or due to a pancreatic anastomotic leak.
   - Injury to the tail of pancreas during splenectomy or adrenalectomy.
   - Injury to the head and body during radical gastrectomy.
   - Pancreaticojejunostomy for chronic pancreatitis or following Whipple's operation can also give rise to fistula in the postoperative period.
   - External drainage of an infected pseudocyst.
2. **Internal fistulae:** It can occur following a blunt injury abdomen wherein the neck of the pancreas is crushed against lumbar spine resulting in injury. Internal fistulae can communicate with pleural space resulting in a pancreaticopleural fistula.

Clinical Presentation

- In many cases, the patients present with a discharge of straw-coloured fluid from the drain site in the postoperative period.
- Internal fistula can manifest in a totally unexpected manner, sometimes, as a case of pleural effusion.

Investigations

- **Amylase** levels in the pleural fluid, peritoneal fluid and in the discharge will be high.
- Abdominal ultrasound is done to rule out a pseudocyst of the pancreas.
- **ERCP:** It can demonstrate leakage of the dye from the pancreatic duct into the surrounding area or along the fistulous tract and proximal obstruction, if any.
- **CT fistulogram** can define the exact site of communication to pancreas. It can define the length of the fistula also.
- **CT angiogram** is indicated in cases of bleeding associated with pancreatic fistula.

Treatment

1. **Conservative treatment**
   - In majority of the cases following surgery, the fistulous discharge stops within one to three weeks of time. During this period, the skin is protected by application of zinc oxide cream. Electrolytes have to be checked frequently.
   - Injection octreotide in the dose of 50–100 mg, 8th hourly will help in decreasing fistula output by more than 80–90%.
2. **Stenting:** Endoscopy, ERCP followed by stenting can be tried, if successful, often fistula will heal. It is very useful in blunt abdominal trauma and pancreatic ductal disruption.

3. **Surgical treatment**
   - If the **fistula persists** in spite of conservative treatment, **fistulectomy** with removal of involved part of the pancreas and body or tail has to be done.
   - In very difficult cases (plastered abdomen) or in fistulas on the anterior abdominal side, **fistulogastrostomy** can also be done.
   - Pancreaticojejunostomy is another option.

Complications of Pancreatic Fistula

1. Secondary **infection**
2. **Massive bleeding:** It occurs due to digestion of elastin fibres of blood vessels resulting in pseudoaneurysms. Morbidity is high.
3. **Ramification** which means branching pattern of the fistula renders the surgery difficult.
4. **Bronchopancreatic fistula**—difficult to treat.

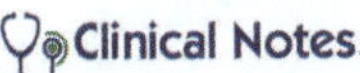

A patient was admitted to the hospital with acute breathlessness. He was found to have left-sided pleural effusion (massive). He had blunt injury abdomen 2 months back during which time laparotomy and closure of a proximal jejunal perforation had been done. There was no obvious sign of pancreatic injury. Aspiration of pleural fluid revealed high amylase. It was a case of pancreaticopleural fistula.

WHITE BILE

- It is a misnomer (Fig. 42.139)
- In long-standing cases of obstruction to the CBD, the bile in the CBD gets absorbed and is replaced by mucus secreted from the CBD.
- It is not white but straw coloured.
- It is not bile but is mucus.

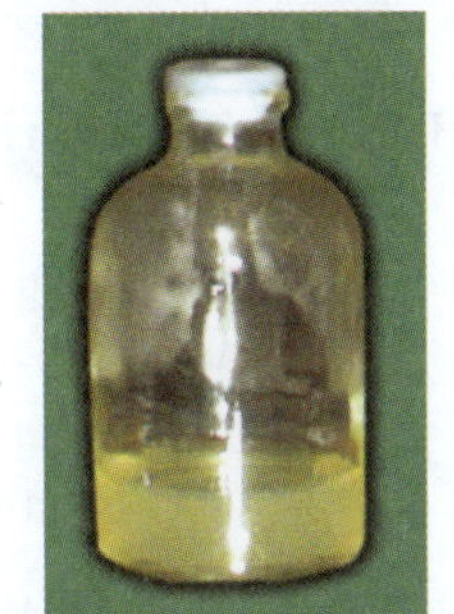

Fig. 42.139: White bile suggestive of severely impaired liver cell function

Significance

- It indicates a long-standing obstruction.
- It has to be relieved as an urgent procedure.
- White bile is seen in:
  - Long-standing stricture of the CBD
  - Due to the stones in CBD
  - Rarely, seen in periampullary carcinoma.

PANCREATIC ASCITES

Definition

- Accumulation of 'enzyme rich' pancreatic exudate in the peritoneal cavity is called pancreatic ascites.
- It is a protein-rich, noninfected fluid with protein levels greater than 25 g/L.

Causes

- Acute pancreatitis mainly alcoholic
- Chronic pancreatitis
- Trauma to pancreas
- Ruptured pseudocyst

Pathogenesis

- Disruption of ductal system of pancreas followed by spread of enzyme-rich fluid both anteriorly and posteriorly results in pancreatic ascites.
- Anterior rupture results in ascites.
- Posterior spread results in pleural effusion.

Clinical Features

- History suggestive of pancreatitis, gross abdominal distention.
- Shifting dullness
- Breathlessness—due to pleural effusion.

Investigations

- Serum amylase, may be elevated due to reabsorption across peritoneal membrane.
- Ultrasound/CT: It can detect fluid, pancreatic duct and guide aspiration.
- ERCP: May slow ductal communication.

Treatment

- Repeated **tapping**—follow with **albumin infusion.** Most of the cases are associated with hypoalbuminaemia (Fig. 42.140).
- Octreotide to decrease pancreatic secretion.
- Total parenteral nutrition
- ERCP—pancreatic duct stenting
- Surgical: If there is no response by 2–3 weeks, resection (for tail lesion) or drainage for body lesion is indicated.

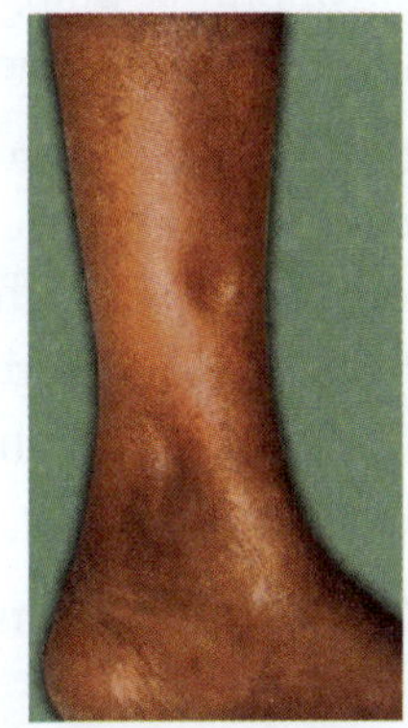

Fig. 42.140: Pedal oedema—severe hypoalbuminaemia

ISLET CELL TRANSPLANTATION

- This is emerging as a fine treatment for diabetes and chronic pancreatitis after pancreatectomy.
- Many patients have undergone islet cell transplantation with minimal complications (*see* Chapter 65).

Multiple Choice Questions

1. **Which of the following statements is false for pseudocyst of pancreas?**
   A. It occurs in lesser sac
   B. Cystogastrostomy is usually the treatment of choice
   C. Better to operate after 2 weeks
   D. It has no epithelial lining

2. **Which of the following is not the cause for gallstone formation?**
   A. Saint's triad B. Haemolytic anaemia
   C. Infection D. Gastrojejunostomy

3. **Gallbladder carcinoma has following features *except:***
   A. It is squamous cell carcinoma
   B. It does cause jaundice often
   C. It does not respond to radiation
   D. Prognosis is very poor

4. **Most ideal and quick method for the diagnosis of gallstones is by:**
   A. Endosonogram B. MRI scan
   C. CT scan D. Ultrasound

5. **Following is not the feature of acute cholecystitis:**
   A. It causes pain in the right hypochondrium
   B. If it perforates, gas under diaphragm is detected by percussion
   C. Shoulder pain can occur
   D. Acalculous cholecystitis is due to hypotension

6. **Following is the most important sign of acute cholecystitis:**
   A. Pain in the right shoulder
   B. Intercostal oedema and tenderness
   C. Positive Murphy's sign
   D. Hyperaesthesia of the abdominal wall

7. **Cystic duct joins supraduodenal CBD in what percentage of the cases?**
   A. 80% B. 90%
   C. 70% D. 95%

8. **Porcelain gallbladder has following features *except:***
   A. It is calcification of the gallbladder
   B. Plain X-ray is not very useful to detect this
   C. CT scan will detect this
   D. It may be associated with carcinoma gallbladder

9. **Which one of the following is true for choledochal cyst?**
   A. Acquired dilatation
   B. Not premalignant
   C. Type I cyst is the most common variety
   D. Does not cause pancreatitis

10. **Which one of the features is true in gallstone ileus?**
   A. Obstruction is in terminal ileum
   B. Stone reaches ileum via ampulla of Vater
   C. Obstruction and features of perforation of gallbladder are found
   D. Cholecystectomy and extraction of the stones by enterotomy is done

11. **Following are true for acalculous cholecystitis *except:***
   A. It can be seen in septic shock due to hypotension
   B. Some features of cholecystoses may also be found
   C. *Salmonella typhi* can also give rise to acute acalculous cholecystitis
   D. Rare to get chronic cholecystitis in Salmonella cholecystitis

12. **Following are indications for common bile duct exploration *except:***
   A. Palpable stones in the CBD
   B. Dilated common bile duct
   C. Jaundice
   D. Thickened common bile duct

13. **Following are risk factors for cholangiocarcinoma *except:***
   A. Choledochal cyst
   B. Caroli's disease
   C. Primary sclerosing cholangitis
   D. Biliary stricture

14. **Which one of the following is true for carcinoma gallbladder?**
   A. It is common in males
   B. Disease occurs around 5th decade
   C. Gallstone disease does not predispose to carcinoma gallbladder
   D. Majority are adenocarcinoma

15. **Caterpillar hump is an anomaly of what structure?**
   A. Cystic artery B. Hepatic artery
   C. Coeliac artery D. Gastroduodenal artery

16. **Portal veins is formed at:**
   A. Posterior to head of pancreas
   B. Posterior to body of pancreas
   C. Anterior to neck of pancreas
   D. Posterior to neck of pancreas

17. Following are true about anatomy of the pancreas *except:*
- A. 30% is by the head of pancreas
- B. 75% of islet cells are beta-cells producing insulin
- C. 80–90% pancreatic tissue is exocrine pancreatic tissue
- D. 5% of islet cells are A cells producing glucagon

18. To avoid spillage of cells after FNAC of the pancreatic head mass which is the best investigation?
- A. Endoscopic biopsy
- B. CT-guided biopsy
- C. MRI-guided biopsy
- D. Endosonographic biopsy

19. Which one of the following is true for pancreatic divisum?
- A. Dorsal pancreatic duct become accessory duct
- B. It does not cause pancreatitis
- C. MRCP is not an ideal investigation for diagnosis
- D. Endoscopic sphincterotomy has a definitive role

20. Following are true for annular pancreas, *except:*
- A. It is more prevalent in children with Down syndrome
- B. It surrounds 2nd part of duodenum
- C. Duodenal obstruction causes vomiting in neonate
- D. Gastrojejunostomy is the treatment of choice

21. The use of ultrasound in the diagnosis of acute pancreatitis is mainly to:
- A. Rule out perforation
- B. To look for oedematous pancreatitis
- C. To rule out gallstones
- D. To look for pancreatic stones

22. Role of CT scan in acute pancreatitis include following, *except:*
- A. To detect gallstones
- B. Diagnostic uncertainty
- C. To detect necrotizing pancreatitis
- D. To find out the localized complication

23. Following are features of acute pancreatitis, *except:*
- A. Shock
- B. Cullen's sign
- C. Grey Turner's sign
- D. Kehr sign

24. Which one of the following is not routinely recommended in severe pancreatitis?
- A. Aggressive fluid resuscitation
- B. Nasogastric feeding
- C. ICU monitoring with oxygenation
- D. Antibiotic prophylaxis

25. Which one of the following is true for pancreatic necrosectomy?
- A. Usually done within 2–3 weeks of acute attack of pancreatitis
- B. Gallstones, if present, should not be removed along with necrosectomy
- C. Blunt dissection is the best technique
- D. Feeding jejunostomy may not be useful

26. Sudden rise in platelet counts in acute pancreatitis suggests:
- A. Pancreatic fistula
- B. Bleeding
- C. Portal vein thrombosis
- D. Pancreatic necrosis

27. Following are true about pseudocyst fluid, *except:*
- A. Ultrasound can easily detect pseudocyst
- B. CEA levels are usually above 400 ng/ml
- C. High amylase levels
- D. Inflammatory cells in the aspirate

28. Following are true for tropical pancreatitis, *except:*
- A. Starts in young age
- B. High incidence of stone formation
- C. High incidence of diabetes mellitus
- D. Does not predispose to pancreatic cancer

29. The best surgical treatment for chronic pancreatitis with dilated duct is:
- A. Frey's operation
- B. Whipple's operation
- C. Longitudinal pancreaticojejunostomy
- D. Distal pancreatectomy

30. Following are the risk factors for carcinoma pancreas *except:*
- A. Cigarette smoking
- B. Hereditary pancreatitis
- C. Chronic pancreatitis
- D. Female sex

31. About porcelain gallbladder following is true:
- A. Requires conservative treatment
- B. It cannot be detected by ultrasound
- C. Prophylactic cholecystectomy is not indicated
- D. It is a precancerous condition

Answers

1. C	**2.** D	**3.** A	**4.** D	**5.** B	**6.** D	**7.** A	**8.** B	**9.** C	**10.** A
11. D	**12.** D	**13.** D	**14.** D	**15.** B	**16.** D	**17.** D	**18.** D	**19.** D	**20.** D
21. C	**22.** A	**23.** D	**24.** B	**25.** C	**26.** C	**27.** B	**28.** D	**29.** C	**30.** D
31. D									

CHAPTER

43

Liver

- Surgical anatomy
- Physiology
- Pyogenic abscess
- Amoebic abscess
- Hydatid cyst
- Other cystic diseases
- Benign tumours
- Hepatoma
- Secondaries in the liver
- Portal hypertension
- Ascites in portal hypertension
- Portal gastropathy
- Portal biliopathy
- Budd-Chiari syndrome
- Role of octreotide in surgery
- Liver transplantation
- Haemobilia

Competency

SU28.10.1: Describe the segmental anatomy of liver and the variations in vascular anatomy of liver.

SURGICAL ANATOMY OF THE LIVER

- Liver is located in the right hypochondrium extending into epigastrium and left hypochondrium.
- It weighs about 1,500 g—three quarters of it is the right lobe and rest is the left lobe (Figs 43.1 and 43.2).

Ligaments

- **Right triangular ligament** fixes the right lobe to the undersurface of the right dome of diaphragm. When this ligament is divided, right lobe can be mobilised and can be turned to left as during right hepatic lobectomy or to control bleeding from liver trauma.
- **Left triangular ligament** fixes the left lobe to the diaphragm in a similar fashion. For a complete vagotomy, when this ligament is divided, left lobe can be easily retracted—vagotomy becomes easy. This ligament also needs to be divided to get access to retrohepatic inferior vena cava.
- **Falciform ligament:** It is the remnant of umbilical vein. It runs from umbilicus to the liver dividing the liver into right and left lobes, passing into the interlobar fissure. Division of superior leaves of falciform ligament helps in exposing suprahepatic inferior vena cava (IVC).

Blood Supply

- 80% is derived from portal vein, 20% from hepatic artery.
- Right branch of hepatic artery supplies entire right lobe and left branch supplies the left lobe.
- Ligation of hepatic artery may not cause necrosis of liver in normal individuals. However, it can cause liver failure in cirrhotic patients (it was done in olden days to control secondaries in the liver), and in obstructive jaundice patients.

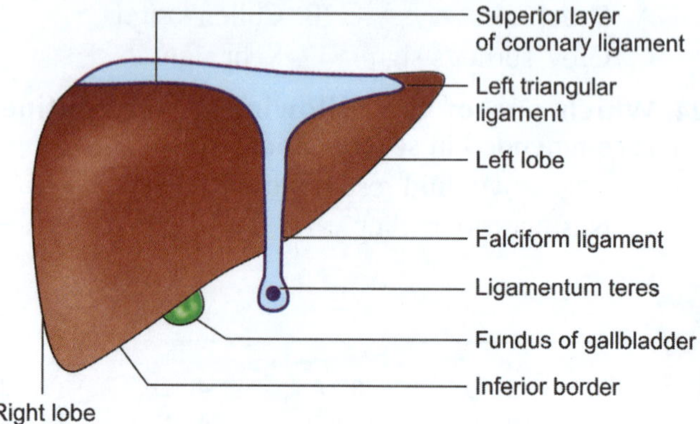

Fig. 43.1: Liver seen from the front

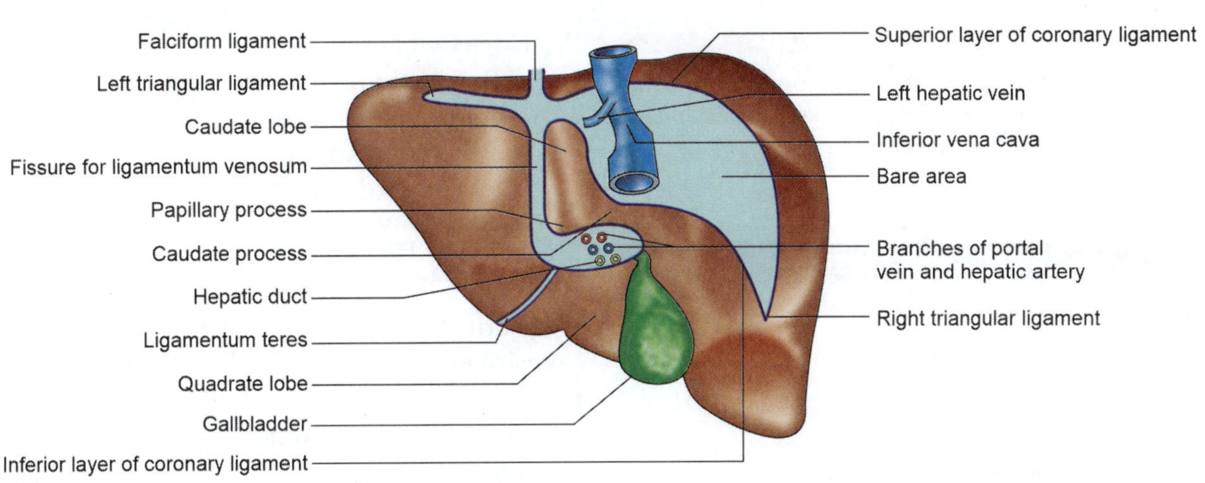

Fig. 43.2: Liver seen from behind and below

Venous Drainage of the Liver

- Major venous drainage is through 3 hepatic veins: Right, middle and left. They join the inferior vena cava (IVC) immediately below the diaphragm. *Right hepatic vein has a small extrahepatic course.* On the other hand, middle and left hepatic veins usually join within liver parenchyma.
- In fact, these three veins keep the liver suspended.

Lymphatics

- Superficial lobules: Subcapsular course to diaphragm or to suspensory ligament or posterior mediastinum.
- Deep lobules: Along IVC or portal vein into porta hepatis.

Hilum of the Liver

- This is also called **porta hepatis**. It has the most vital structures within it—hepatic artery, bile duct anteriorly and portal vein posteriorly.
- These structures are present within the free edge of lesser omentum—hepatoduodenal ligament.
- Within the hilum, these structures divide into right and left branches. Left bile duct has a **longer extrahepatic course** of approximately 2 cm. In CBD strictures, this can be used for **hepaticojejunostomy**.

Regeneration

- Liver has an excellent **capacity for regeneration** after partial resection.
- A factor released from **pancreas** is supposed to be responsible for this.

Hepatic Lobules

The ***functional unit*** of the liver is the hepatic lobule. Each hepatic lobule consists of sheets of liver cells, separated by hepatic sinusoids, venous channels which drain blood to central vein, a tributary of the hepatic vein from portal tracts that contain branches of the hepatic vein and portal vein.

PHYSIOLOGY (Table 43.1)

Table 43.1 Physiology of the liver

Functioning of the liver	Significance
• Principal site of synthesis of all proteins **except globulins**, which are produced in reticuloendothelial systems	• Hypoalbuminaemia in chronic liver disease
• **Glucose metabolism, glycolysis and gluconeogenesis**	• Persistent hypoglycaemia is a feature of fulminant hepatic failure (FHF), also seen in hepatoma
• Synthesis of **clotting factors**	• Bleeding tendencies in chronic liver disease
• Maintaining **core body temperature**	• Hypothermia in FHF
• Bilirubin formation	• Congenital hyperbilirubinaemia and other
• Drug and hormone metabolism	• Hepatitis due to drugs such as rifampicin and other anti-tuberculous drugs
• Monitoring pH and correcting **lactic acidosis**	• Severely impaired in FHF
• Removal of endotoxins and foreign antigens	• Severely impaired in FHF
• Urea formation from protein catabolism	• After portacaval shunt, endotoxins bypass the liver, results in encephalopathy

Competency

SU28.10.2: Enumerate the types, etiopathogenesis, clinical features, investigations and principles in management of liver abscess. Also difference between the types of liver abscesses.

PYOGENIC LIVER ABSCESS

Causes (Fig. 43.3)

I. Infection through the portal vein
- Acute appendicitis
- Acute diverticulitis (sigmoid)
- Acute amoebic colitis
- Acute bacillary dysentery
- Ulcerative colitis

II. Infection through the common bile duct (CBD)
- Stricture of the CBD
- Periampullary carcinoma resulting in stasis of the bile, precipitating infection (cholangitis)
- Recurrent cholangitis due to stone in the CBD
- ERCP

III. Infection through the hepatic artery
- Septicaemia and pyaemia
- Actinomycosis of faciocervical region

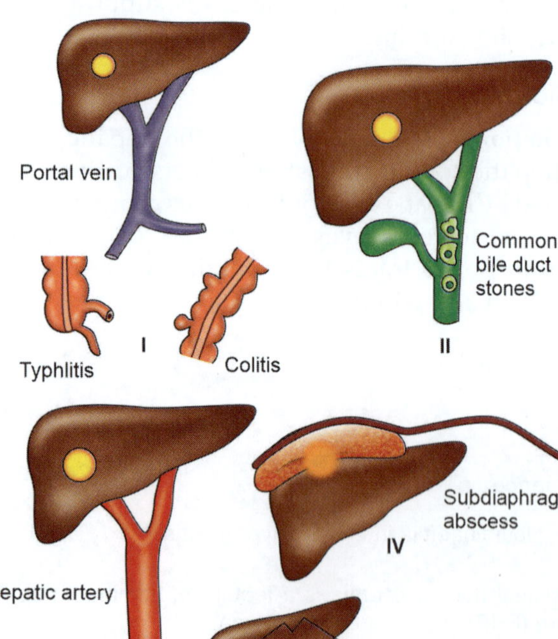

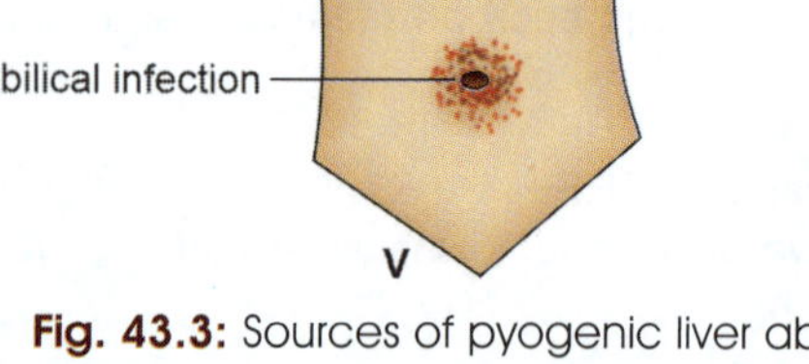

Fig. 43.3: Sources of pyogenic liver abscess

IV. Extension abscess
- Subdiaphragmatic abscess
- Empyema thoracis
- Penetrating injuries

V. Infection through umbilicus: Neonatal umbilical sepsis giving rise to pyaemia.

Certain Facts

- Majority of the infective bacteria are derived from gastrointestinal tract (Key Box 43.1).
- In majority of cases, it is **polymicrobial** infection.
- ***E. coli*** is the most common facultative organism.
- ***Bacteroides fragilis*** is the most common anaerobe.
- ***Candidal infection*** is increasing due to chemotherapy, especially for leukaemic patients.

Key Box 43.1

Bacteriology

1. Anaerobic bacteria	: 60% (*Bacteroides fragilis*)
2. Enteric gram –ve bacteria	
• *Escherichia coli*	: 40%
• *Klebsiella pneumoniae*	: 10–20%
• Others	: 4–40%
3. Gram +ve bacteria	
• *Staphylococcus aureus*	: 4–25%

Clinical Features

- Alcoholic males and debilitated men suffer more, probably because of poor immunity.
- Acute abscesses are usually multiple, chronic abscesses are single.
- Tender hepatomegaly, low grade or high grade pyrexia with abdominal discomfort are the main features.

Investigations

- **Total WBC count** is raised.
- **Stool routine examination:** Amoebic cysts, culture and sensitivity for typhoid bacilli.
- **Abdominal ultrasound** and ultrasound-guided aspiration establishes the diagnosis.
- When in doubt, CT scan can be done (Figs 43.4 and 43.5), followed by FNAC which draws frank pus. Pus is sent for Gram's stain, culture and sensitivity. CT also helps in the diagnosis of ***associated conditions such as diverticulitis of the colon.***
- Further investigations are directed towards the associated conditions. **Examples:**
  - **Chest X-ray:** Air under the diaphragm (perforation of hollow viscus) or diagnosis of empyema thoracis.

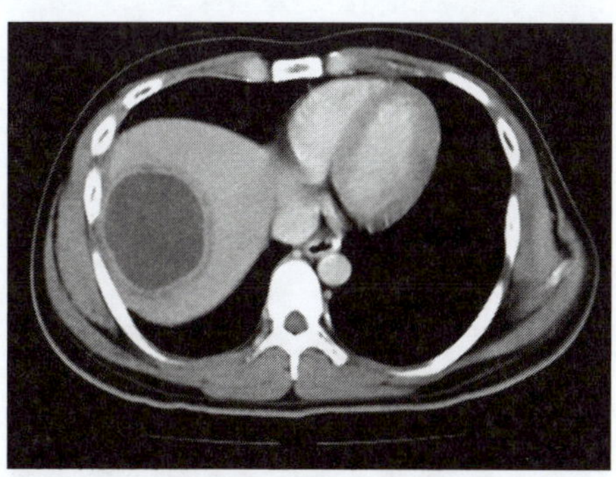

Fig. 43.4: CT scan showing hypodense lesion in the right lobe of liver suggestive of pyogenic liver abscess

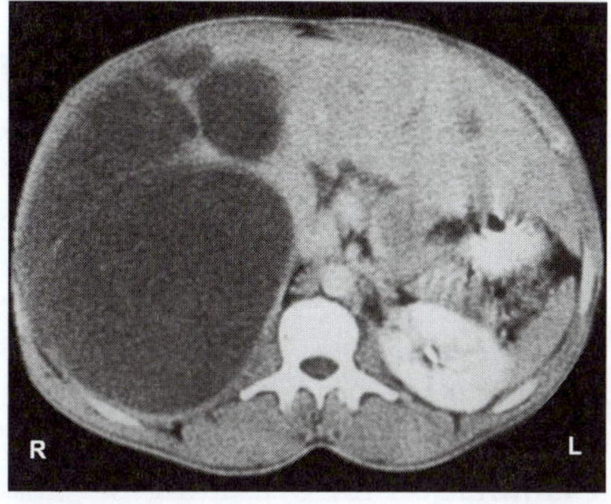

Fig. 43.5: CT scan showing multiple liver abscesses proved to be due to amoebiasis

Treatment

1. **Conservative:** Multiple small abscesses may respond to antibiotics. However, they have to be given for 4 to 6 weeks.
2. **Percutaneous drainage** (Key Box 43.2)

   Method
   - Ultrasound or CT-guided aspiration and drainage by using a pigtail catheter.
   - Irrigation of abscess cavity with saline.
3. **Open (surgical) method** (Key Box 43.3): Laparotomy is required mainly to treat the primary causes, e.g. appendicectomy, drainage of appendicular abscess. If liver shows a significant abscess, it is drained. Alternately, a pigtail catheter is introduced into the abscess cavity and brought outside through a separate opening. It helps to drain for a longer period of time.
4. Laparoscopic drainage can also be done.

Key Box 43.2

Percutaneous Drainage—Indications

- Superficial abscesses
- Abscess with no intra-abdominal pathology
- Abscess of unknown aetiology

Key Box 43.3

Open (Surgical) Method—Indications

- Abscess with intra-abdominal pathology
- Ascites
- Deep-seated abscess
- Multiple abscesses

AMOEBIC LIVER ABSCESS

It is also called **tropical abscess** (dysenteric abscess). It is the commonest extraintestinal manifestation of amoebiasis.

Aetiopathogenesis

- This disease is caused by ***Entamoeba histolytica.***
- It is almost always a complication of amoebic dysentery. This can occur in the acute stage or in the chronic carrier stage.
  - **Infection from the caecum** (typhlitis) spreads through the tributary of **superior mesenteric vein.**
  - **From sigmoid colon**, through the tributary of **inferior mesenteric vein** (Fig. 43.6).
- The right branch of the portal vein is in direct line with the portal vein. Hence, by ***streamline phenomenon*** organisms reach the right lobe more often than the left lobe. The right lobe is also much bigger than the left lobe.
- In the right lobe, it is the posterosuperior surface which gets involved because it is extraperitoneal ***(bare area of liver)***. It has no peritoneal covering.
- After reaching the liver, the organism causes destruction of hepatocytes by releasing powerful ***cytolytic enzymes*** resulting in ***liquefaction necrosis***. It also causes aseptic thrombosis of blood vessels resulting in necrosis of liver tissue.

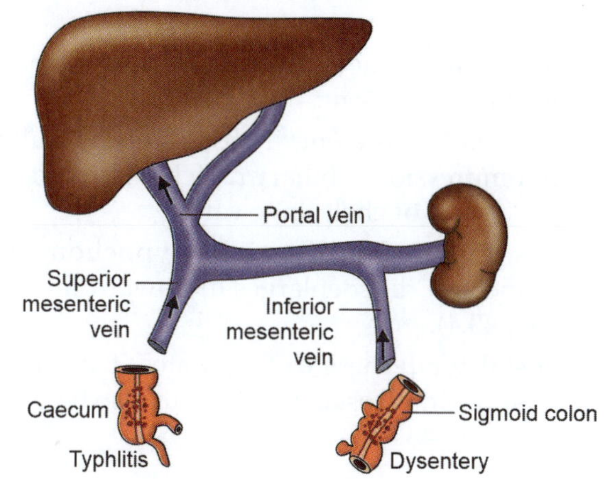

Fig. 43.6: Aetiopathogenesis of amoebic liver abscess

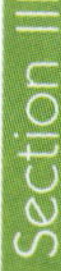

- At the same time, some RBCs[1] are also broken down. This causes ***anchovy sauce pus***, which is chocolate brown in colour, and is a mixture of broken down RBCs, hepatocytes, etc.
- **Green pus** is referred to pus mixed with bile, which is seen in a few patients.
- In majority of the cases, ***pus is sterile***. Secondary infection occurs in about 20 to 30% of the cases.
- Amoebae are rarely present in the pus but are present in the wall of the abscess cavity. The wall contains monocytes, plasma cells, lymphocytes and fibroblasts. Abscesses are multiple which fuse to form a single large abscess cavity in about 70% of the cases. Due to ***perihepatitis***, abscess gets fixed to the diaphragm resulting in immobility of the diaphragm. Liver abscess in the left lobe gets adhered to anterior abdominal wall.
- It is interesting to note that amoebic infection of gallbladder and bile does not occur because of ***deleterious effect of bile on amoebae***.

Clinical Features (Fig. 43.8A)

- **Male alcoholics** are commonly affected, in the age group of 20–40 years. It is eight times more common in men.
- Seen in patients with low socioeconomic status.
- Severe pain in the right hypochondrium is due to the enlarged liver. This stage is called stage of **amoebic hepatitis**. If USG is done, it may not demonstrate any abscesses but there may be many microabscesses. At this stage, there is low grade fever, weakness, anorexia, etc.
- High grade fever with chills and rigors develop if the stage proceeds to pyogenic liver abscess due to secondary bacterial infection of amoebic abscess.
- Thoracic symptoms such as nonproductive cough, pleurisy and right shoulder pain are common.

Signs

- Anaemia, emaciation, toxic look and an earthy complexion are present.
- Jaundice may be present, if abscesses are multiple, due to compression of biliary radicles. However, it is rare (15%). It is of cholestatic variety.
- Liver is enlarged in the right hypochondrium, tender and soft (liver enlarges in upward direction) (Key Box 43.4).
- **Intercostal tenderness** differentiates it from acute cholecystitis. Intercostal oedema can also be present (Figs 43.7 and 43.8A).

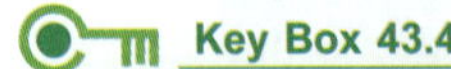
Key Box 43.4

Very Tender Liver

- Amoebic liver abscess
- Hepatoma
- Congestive cardiac failure

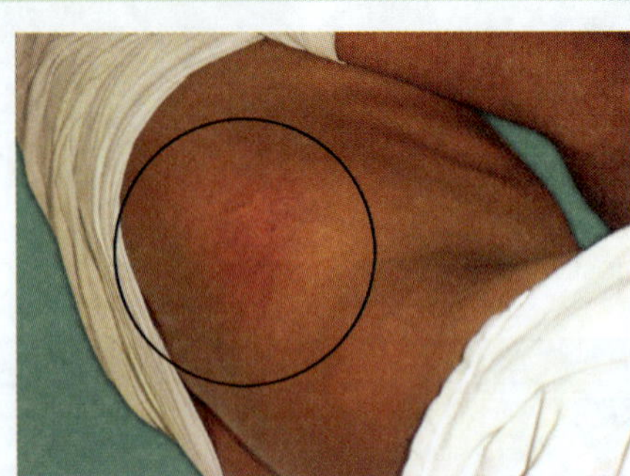

Fig. 43.7: Intercostal bulge and tenderness are important features of amoebic liver abscess of the liver—these signs are not seen in acute cholecystitis

Investigations

1. **Total WBC count** may be increased, if there is secondary infection.
2. **Stool examination** for ova and cysts of *Entamoeba histolytica* may be positive in 25% of cases.
3. **Serologic testing:** The indirect haemagglutination test is positive in 90–95% of patients with an amoebic abscess.
4. **Screening chest:** When the patient is asked to take a deep breath, right side of the diaphragm does not move due to inflammatory (**perihepatitis**) adhesions between liver and diaphragm. This is called **homolateral immobility of the diaphragm**. A small pleural effusion may also be present.
5. **Sigmoidoscopy** may demonstrate large, deep amoebic ulcers—**flask shaped**.
6. **Abdominal USG:** It is the investigation of choice.
   - To locate site of abscess and then to confirm diagnosis.
   - Ultrasound-guided needle aspiration can also be done and biopsy of abscess wall should be taken.
   - Multiple abscesses can be made out.
7. **CT scan** can demonstrate an abscess cavity as a low density zone surrounded by peripheral hypodense zone due to inflammatory reaction.

Treatment

It can be classified into:

I. Conservative
II. Ultrasound-guided aspiration and pigtail drainage
III. Surgery—drainage

[1]Absence of WBC is an important feature. Hence, regeneration of abscess cavity is complete without scarring.

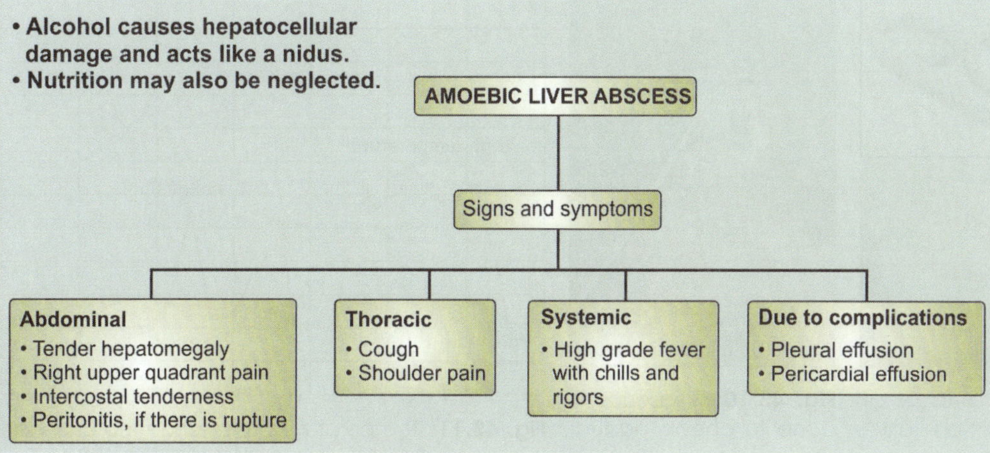

Fig. 43.8A: Clinical features

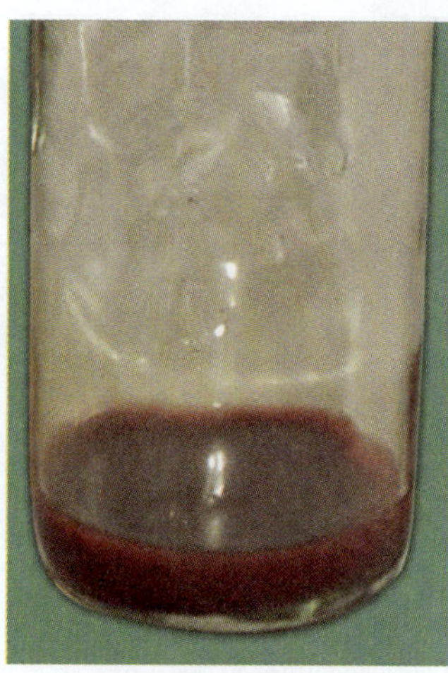

Fig. 43.8B: Anchovy sauce pus

I. Conservative Line of Management

- It is indicated in ***amoebic hepatitis***. Tab. ***metronidazole*** 400–800 mg 3 times a day is given for 14 days.

  The only recognisable side-effect is metallic taste.
- If the condition does not improve, injection ***emetine*** 1 mg/kg body weight to a total of 60 mg/day deep IM for a maximum of 6 days is given.

Side-effects and Precautions during Emetine Therapy

- Systolic BP should be at least 100 mmHg.
- ECG should be recorded before, during and after the therapy.
- Cardiotoxicity in the form of arrhythmias can occur.
- Absolute bed rest during treatment (because of these complications, it is not used nowadays).
- Adequate hydration, rest, analgesics to relieve the pain.

Improvement can be seen within one to two days in the form of disappearance of pain, fever and return of appetite.

II. US-guided Needle Aspiration/Pigtail Catheter Drainage (Key Box 43.5)

- It is indicated in cases of ***amoebic liver abscess***.
- Before it is aspirated, bleeding profile (BT, CT, PT) should be normal and injection vitamin K 10 mg, IM should be given for at least 3 days.
- US-guided aspiration is also the treatment of choice where ***metronidazole is contraindicated***, e.g. 1st trimester of pregnancy.
- It can be easily done under local anaesthesia.
- Can be repeated, if pus recollects. Typically, it is anchovy sauce pus. Aspiration is followed by insertion of pigtail catheter.

Key Box 43.5

Pigtail Catheter

- They are the catheter used to drain clear fluids from cavities such as pleural fluid, ascites, bile, etc.
- Different sizes are available 8 to 12 French
- Radio-opaque polyurethane catheter
- Length—20 or 30 cm
- Large oval holes in pigtail for maximum drainage
- Thus, maximum efficiency is when 'transudate' pleural effusion is drained, than empyema, haemothorax or anchovy sauce pus

- Before removal of the catheter do a repeat ultrasound to check for residual pus (Fig. 43.8B).

The clinical response to the aspiration may be observed as subsiding of fever (Figs 43.8B to 43.11).

Complications

1. Bleeding—rare
2. Incomplete aspiration results in leakage of pus and bile into peritoneal cavity which may produce peritonitis. Hence, prophylactic antibiotics need to be given before and after the procedure along with metronidazole therapy.

III. Surgery (Open Drainage) and Laparoscopic

Indications

1. Failure of US-guided needle aspiration.
2. Ruptured amoebic liver abscess with amoebic peritonitis.

Procedure

- Laparotomy is done first. Abscess cavity is identified. Contents are evacuated, a thorough peritoneal wash is given and a self-retaining **Malecot's catheter (any**

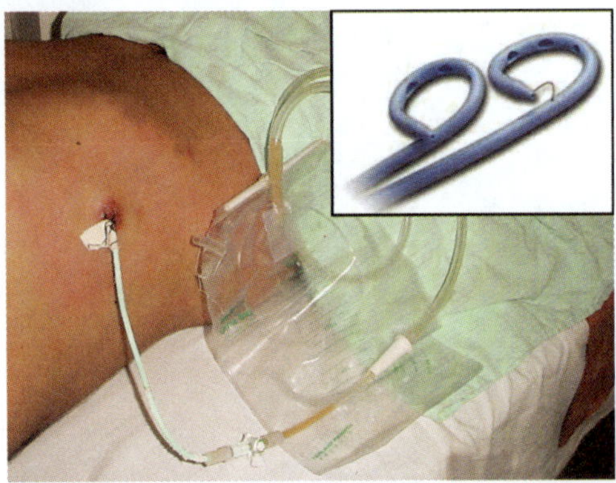

Fig. 43.9: Pigtail catheter drainage of amoebic liver abscess—it is a non-operative method of treatment

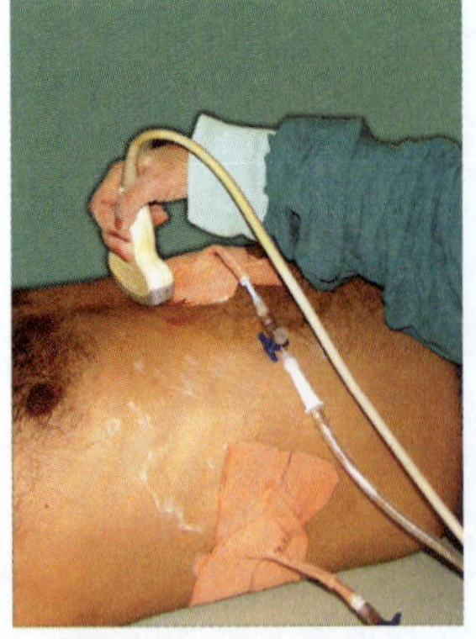

Fig. 43.10: Ultrasound is done to check residual abscess cavity

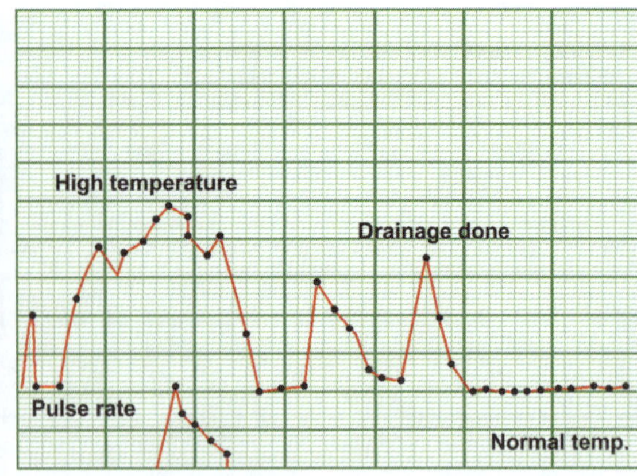

Fig. 43.11: Temperature chart—once the drainage is done, temperature comes back to normal

tube drain) is introduced into the abscess cavity, brought outside and connected to a bag.

- With the advent of metronidazole, **amoebiasis cutis is rarely seen**. Hence, catheter can be safely placed inside the cavity and brought out. Malecot's catheter is now being replaced by other tube drains.
- Postoperatively for 3–5 days, necrotic liver tissue, anchovy sauce pus and blood drain outside.
- Once the drainage becomes minimal, Malecot's catheter is pulled out.
- Same procedure can be done by laparoscopic method.

Complications of Amoebic Liver Abscess

- **Amoebic peritonitis**, resulting in acute abdomen with shock. It has to be treated like any peritonitis—laparotomy, drainage of pus and drain the abscess cavity to outside (possibility of ***amoebiasis cutis*** is still present but rare).
- Rupture into pleural space causing ***pleural effusion***.
- Rupture into the bronchus resulting in coughing out anchovy sauce (may be a natural cure)—***broncho-pleural fistula***.
- **Amoebic pericardial effusion** occurs due to rupture of left liver lobe abscess into pericardial space.

Competency

SU28.10.3: Enumerate the etiology, pathogenesis, clinical features, investigations and various approaches in management of hydatid cyst of liver.

HYDATID CYST OF THE LIVER

The disease is caused by *Echinococcus granulosus*, transmitted by dogs which are the chief mediators (host)

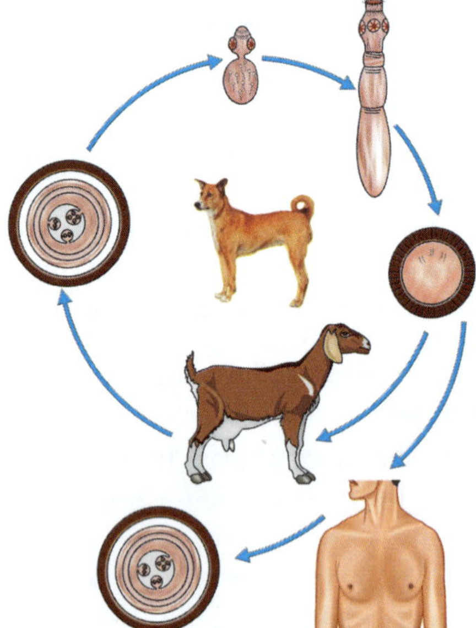

Fig. 43.12: Life cycle of hydatid cyst

and man is the intermediate host (Fig. 43.12). After swallowing the ova, they penetrate gastric mucosa[1], reach retroperitoneal structures, penetrate portal vein directly and then enter into liver. Having reached liver, the organisms grow and develop their own protective layer and form hydatid cyst.

Layers of Hydatid Cyst (Fig. 43.13)

1. **The adventitia (pseudocyst)[2]:** This is the fibrous layer derived from the liver tissue. It is the reaction of liver to the parasite. It is adherent to the liver and cannot be separated—pericyst.
2. **The ectocyst (laminated membrane):** It is white and elastic and is produced by endocyst. It is this layer which gets peeled off at surgery.

[1]Reason why hydatid ova do not produce lesions in the intestine.

[2]It is the protective coat given by the host to the ghost.

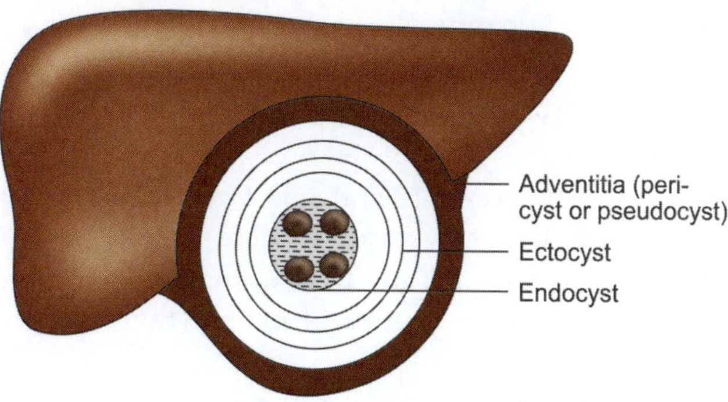

Fig. 43.13: Layers of hydatid cyst

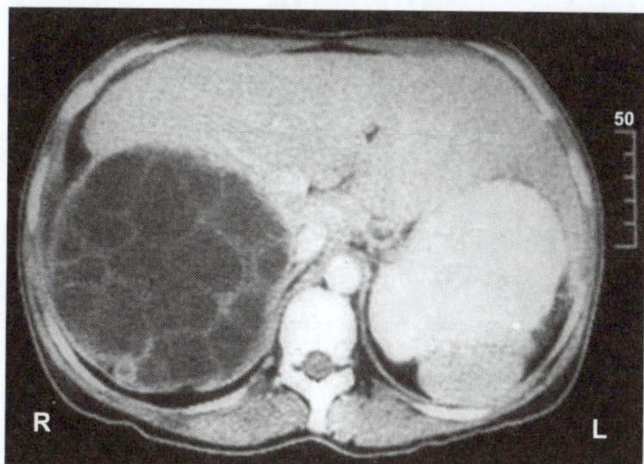

Fig. 43.14: CT scan of the liver showing classical cart wheel pattern—coronal section

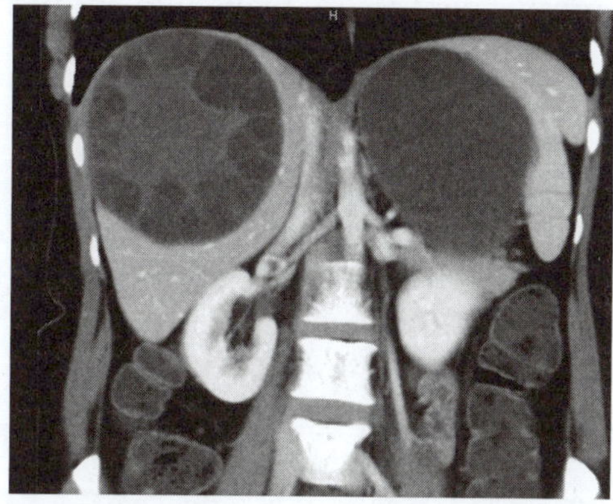

Fig. 43.15: CT scan of the liver showing classical cart wheel pattern—sagittal section

3. **The endocyst:** This is called germinal epithelium and it is the innermost part of hydatid cyst. It secretes hydatid fluid inside and ectocyst outside. Within the hydatid fluid, the 'brood capsules' develop within which the scolices of *Echinococcus granulosus* develop.

Clinical Features

- It can be silent—without any symptoms throughout life, accidentally discovered on routine examination.
- Dragging pain in the upper abdomen due to hepatomegaly.
- Liver is enlarged, has a smooth surface, round borders and is nontender.
- **Typical hydatid thrill** can be present on rare occasions. Hydatid thrill is demonstrated by 3-finger method. Keep 3 fingers over the liver, percuss over the middle finger and get the impulse by other 2 fingers (fluid thrill).
- Patient may present as an emergency with severe abdominal pain following minor trauma.
- May present as an emergency with features of anaphylatic shock without any obvious cause.

Gharbi Classification

Five types have been identified:

Type I: Pure cyst—clear fluid

Type II: Fluid and detached germinative epithelium

Type III: Fluid collection with septa

Type IV: Heterogenous cyst—hypo- or hyperechoic lesions

Type V: Calcified cyst and calcified wall.

Investigations

1. **USG** can detect the cyst, localise the cyst and is used for aspiration purposes (details later—PAIR).

   WHO—Informal working group of echinococcosis (WHO—IWGE) (USG classification)

   Group 1: Active group—cyst larger than 2 cm and often fertile

   Group 2: Transition group—cyst starting to degenerate because of host resistance or treatment; may contain viable protoscolices

   Group 3: Inactive group—degenerated partially or totally calcified cyst; unlikely to contain viable protoscolices
2. **Plain X-ray abdomen** may demonstrate **speckled** calcification.
3. **CT scan** may be necessary in selected cases (Figs 43.14 and 43.15). The cyst which is superficial and has reached surface, should be operated upon.
4. **ERCP** if there is obstructive jaundice—in such cases, a wide sphincterotomy should be given so as to allow free drainage of the hydatid contents into the duodenum.
5. **Casoni's intradermal test:** Sensitivity and specificity of this test is low and hence, **no longer used.**
6. ELISA and immunoelectrophoresis may point towards the diagnosis.

Treatment

It can be discussed under following headings.

I. Conservative

1. Calcified cysts are dead cysts. They are left alone.
2. Symptomless, small hydatid cyst can be left alone. Once symptomatic, or if the size is more than 5 cm, they may be treated.

II. Medical Treatment (Key Box 43.6)

- Albendazole 8 mg/kg or 400 mg BD is given for 21 days followed by drug holiday for 2 weeks.
  If no improvement occurs, maximum of 3 such cycles can be given.
- Watch for neutropenia

III. Surgery

There are different types of surgeries for hydatid disease of the liver which have been summarised below. Indications are given in Key Box 43.7.

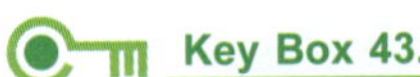
Key Box 43.6

Indications for Medical Treatment

- Disseminated hydatid cyst
- Inaccessible for surgery (deep seated, multiple, recurrent)
- Patient unfit for surgery
- Contamination of peritoneal cavity at surgery

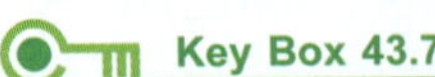
Key Box 43.7

Indications for Surgery

- Symptomatic cyst
- Asymptomatic patient with cyst >5 cm, noncalcified
- Infected cyst (Figs 43.20 and 43.21)

Principles of Surgery

1. **Laparotomy** and **isolation of the cyst** from peritoneal cavity by packs dipped in hypochlorite solution.
2. Aspirate the contents and inject **scolicidal agents** such as savlon or hypertonic saline (Key Box 43.8).
3. Incise the cyst, **peel off the laminated membrane** by using sponge-holding forceps (Figs 43.16 to 43.19).
4. An attempt to remove adventitial layer may result in bleeding. It need not be removed.
5. At surgery, all laminated membrane, endocyst has to be removed. Perfect haemostasis must be achieved. Any bile leak to be sutured. Postoperative significant bile leak is managed by ERCP stenting.

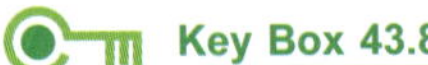
Key Box 43.8

Scolicidal Agents	Side-effects
Hypertonic saline	Hypernatraemia
Chlorhexidine	Acidosis
Alcohol (80%)	Cholangitis
Sodium hypochlorite	Hypernatraemia

Precautions

- Albendazole should be given before surgery.
- Avoid spillage into the peritoneal cavity to avoid peritoneal hydatid.
- **Injection hydrocortisone** 100 mg IV before, during and after surgery to avoid anaphylactic shock.

Different Types of Surgical Procedures

They have been summarised in Key Box 43.9. However, excision of the cyst leaving the adventitial layer is the most commonly performed surgery (Fig. 43.19).

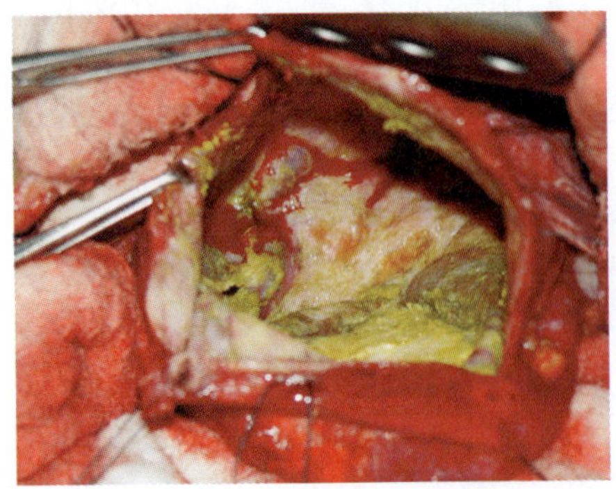

Fig. 43.16: Infected ruptured hydatid cyst—observe green colour due to biliary communication. In such cases, look for any bile lead and suture the opening of biliary duct branches

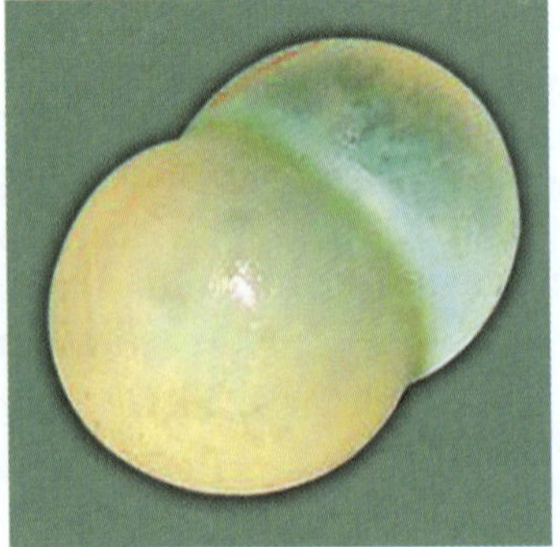

Fig. 43.17: Pearl-like daughter cysts (very precious!!)—Hydatid means dew drop in Latin and watery vesicle in Greek

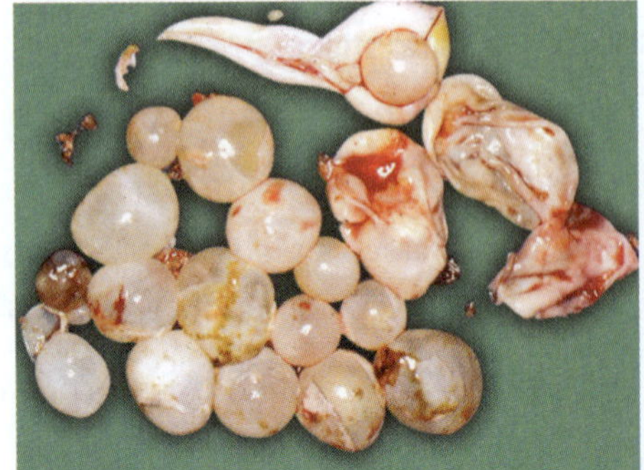

Fig. 43.18: Daughter cysts—it is important to clear all these to prevent recurrence. Please take care not to rupture them while removing

(*Courtesy:* Dr Geetha R, Dr Ankur Sharma, Dr Rajesh Nair, Department of Surgery, KMC, Manipal)

Key Box 43.9

Surgical Procedures

- **Excision:** It is the most commonly performed operation.
- **Cystopericystectomy:** Here, the cyst is excised in a plane outside adventitial layer. It results in excessive bleeding but it removes the cyst completely.
- **Capitonnage:** If omentum is not available for closing the cavity, redundant cyst wall can be infolded into the cyst cavity and sutured.
- **Hepatic resection** in good centres when there are proper indications.

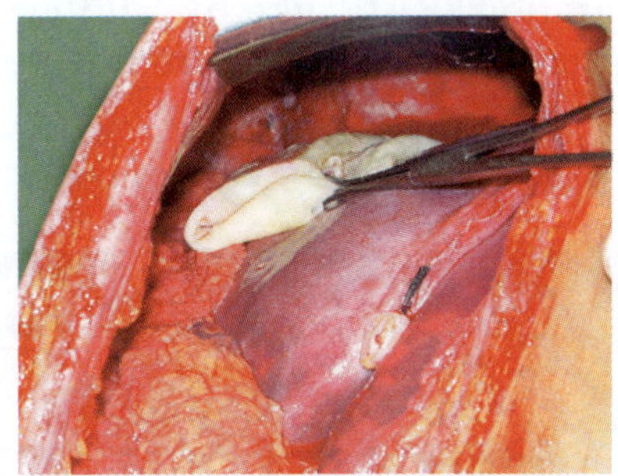

Fig. 43.19: Laminated membrane removed at surgery with sponge-holding forceps

IV. Percutaneous Drainage

- It is done after taking all necessary precautions/ equipment with all emergency drugs and with CT/ US guidance.
- It is also called **PAIR**—**P**uncture, **A**spiration, **I**njection and **R**easpiration.

Indications (Fig. 43.20A and B)

- Unilocular uncomplicated cyst
- Poor surgical candidate
- Previous multiple abdominal surgeries
- Relapse following surgery
- Management algorithm of hydatid cyst is given in Fig. 43.21.

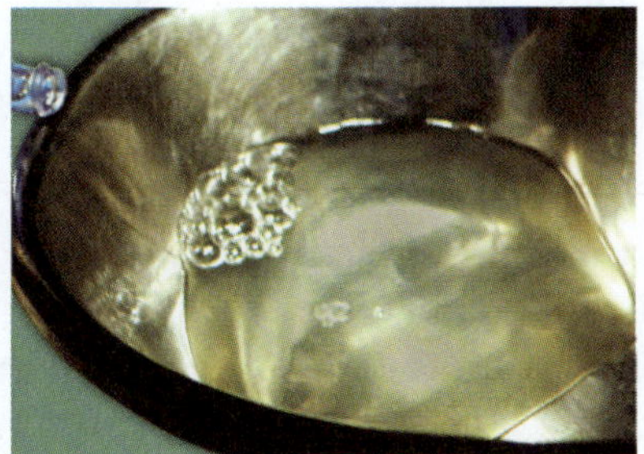

Fig. 43.20A: Clear fluid being aspirated as a part of PAIR treatment

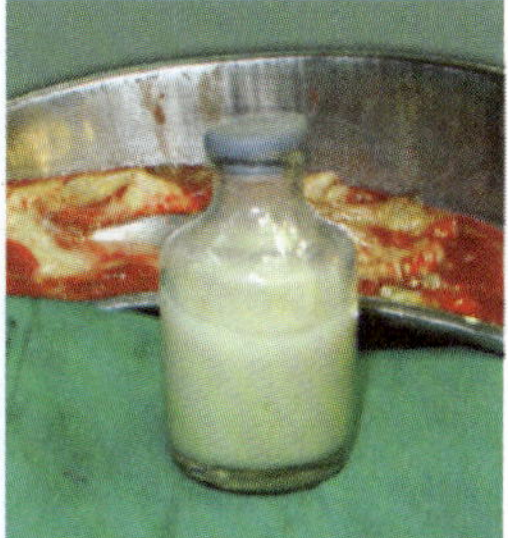

Fig. 43.20B: As the aspirated fluid was turbid, open drainage was done in this patient

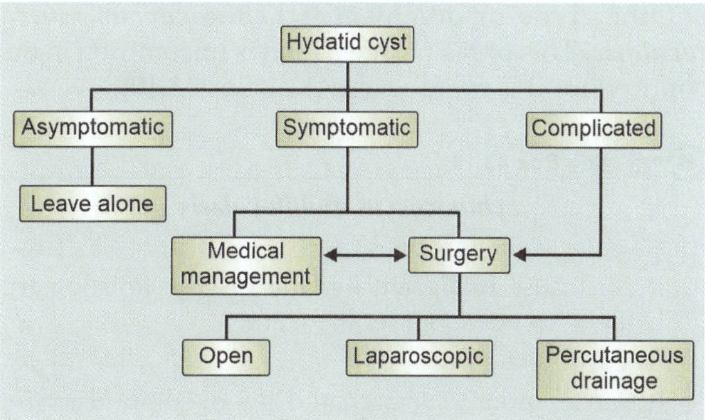

Fig. 43.21: Algorithm of management of hydatid cyst

Contraindications to PAIR

- Multiple septal divisions, communicating cysts
- Dead or inactive cysts, laparoscopic approach for these procedures are being done.

Summary of the treatment of hydatid cyst of the liver is given below (Fig. 43.21).

Complications of Hydatid Cyst

1. **Rupture** of the cyst into the peritoneal cavity can occur due to trauma (rare) and may result in anaphylactic shock. It should be treated accordingly with injection hydrocortisone and laparotomy.
   - Rupture can result in implantation of active cysts within peritoneal cavity and they grow within. Rupture through diaphragm can cause **empyema**. It can also rupture into biliary radicles and can cause obstructive jaundice.
2. **Jaundice** due to cysts within biliary tree or due to a large cyst compressing biliary ducts. ERCP followed by endoscopic removal of hydatid cysts from the common bile duct followed by sphincterotomy should be done.
3. **Suppuration** is rare due to the tough tunica adventitia.
4. **Calcification** of the cyst wall in long-standing cases (Fig. 43.22).

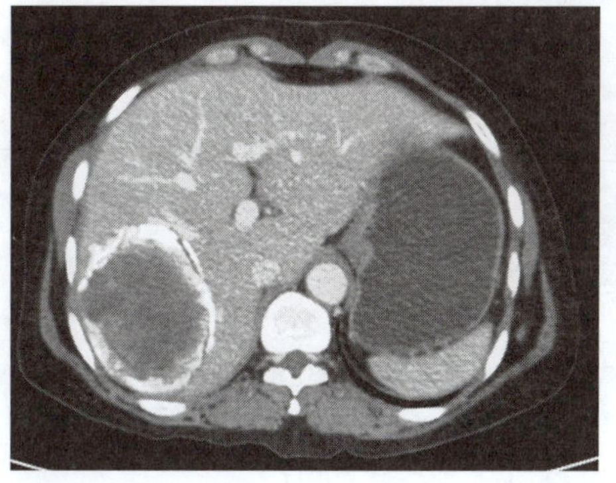

Fig. 43.22: CT of the liver—hydatid calcification

Other type of organism is ***Echinococcus multilocularis.*** This parasitic infestation is uncommon in our country but it is more severe (Key Box 43.10).

Key Box 43.10

Echinococcus multilocularis

- Alveolar echinococcosis
- It can cause **malignant hydatid disease** (misnomer). Difficult to treat. Hence, the name
- Needs resection
- It causes poorly demarcated honeycombed cystic specimen
- It infiltrates liver and invades vascular system

Competency

SU28.10.5: Enumerate the various benign neoplasms of the liver. The clinical presentation, investigations and principles of management of benign neoplasms of liver.

OTHER CYSTIC DISEASES

SIMPLE CYSTIC DISEASE

- When the cyst is thin walled, unilocular and regular it is usually a simple cyst (Fig. 43.23).
- The host response is usually not present (unlike hydatid cyst).
- Incidentally discovered by ultrasound examination.
- Clinically, if they are big, liver will be palpable with smooth surface and round borders. It is nontender.
- Asymptomatic cysts do not require any treatment.
- Ultrasound-guided aspiration, laparoscopic de-roofing and open surgical de-roofing are the methods of treating the cyst.
- Differential diagnosis includes hydatid cyst, polycystic disease.

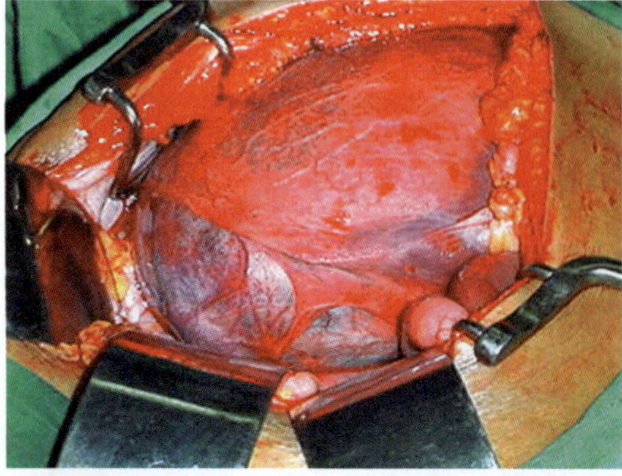

Fig. 43.23: Simple cyst at surgery. Observe the thin wall with slight bluish colour

POLYCYSTIC LIVER DISEASE

- Congenital abnormality.
- Cysts occur within liver, pancreas and kidney (principally).
- Cysts are asymptomatic.
- Cysts do not produce liver cell failure (unlike polycystic kidneys).
- Cyst haemorrhage may be the presenting feature with right hypochondriac pain mimicking cholecystitis.
- CT scan and ultrasound are investigations.
- Cyst aspiration (PAIR like hydatid cyst), decompression may rarely be required in large painful lesions (laparoscopic).

Observe 7 Cs of polycystic liver (Fig. 43.24).

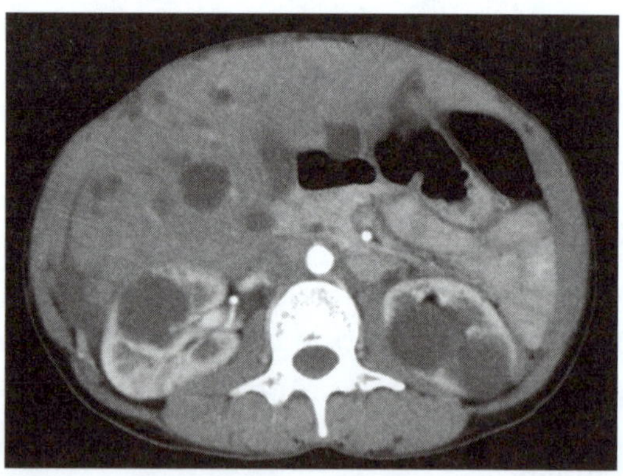

Fig. 43.24: CT scan showing polycystic liver and polycystic kidney

BENIGN TUMOURS OF THE LIVER

- These are not uncommon tumours.
- They are more frequently diagnosed now with frequent use of ultrasound. Majority of them are asymptomatic and do not require specific treatment.
- Their removal should be attempted only by an experienced surgeon. Hepatic adenoma and focal nodular hyperplasia are compared in Table 43.2.
- They have a rare potential for malignant change.

HAEMANGIOMA

- **Commonest benign tumour** of the liver.
- Majority (75%) occur in **women.**
- Most of them are **solitary, subcapsular,** occur in right lobe of liver.
- It may be associated with **cavernous haemangioma** at some other sites such as head and neck region. Clinically, it is difficult to diagnose as it presents as hepatomegaly.

Table 43.2 Comparison of hepatic adenoma and focal nodular hyperplasia

Hepatic adenomas	Focal nodular hyperplasia
• Occur in young women	• Occurs in young women
• Occur due to oral contraceptive pills (OCPs)	• Occurs due to oral contraceptive pills
• Usually **solitary**	• Can be **multiple**
• Haemorrhage, rupture, necrosis can occur	• Haemorrhage, rupture, necrosis do not occur
• Can undergo malignant change	• **Rarely, malignant** change can occur
• If it is due to OCPs, it can regress after discontinuing OCPs. Otherwise, adenomas need to be resected	• Generally does not regress
• Kupffer cells are **not present** in hepatic adenomas	• In addition to hepatocytes, it also contains Kupffer cells

- **Kasabach-Merritt syndrome: Thrombocytopenia and consumptive coagulopathy.**
- Sometimes it may cause cardiovascular failure due to sequestration of blood.
- Ultrasound/CT scan can diagnose their location, number (single or multiple) or presence of any other complications associated with that (thrombosis, infection). MRI is a better investigation.
- Haemangioma **bigger than 8 cm** have **chances of rupture.**

Treatment

1. **Transarterial embolisation (TAE)**
   - Indicated in large haemangiomas which are unresectable.
   - Large haemangiomas on the inferior surface of the liver are ideally suitable for the treatment (Figs 43.25 to 43.27).

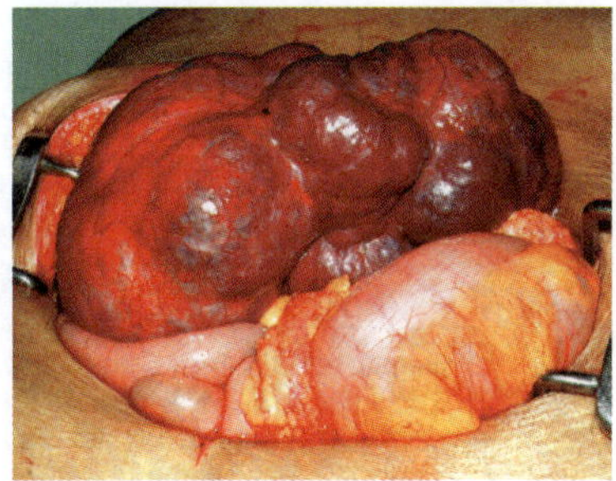

Fig. 43.25: Haemangioma arising from the inferior surface of the liver, is exposed at surgery

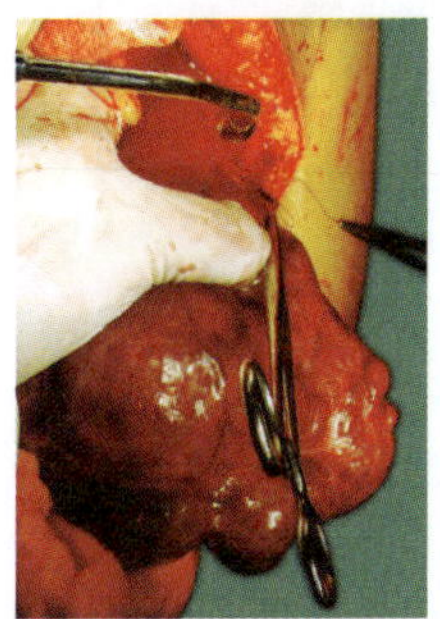

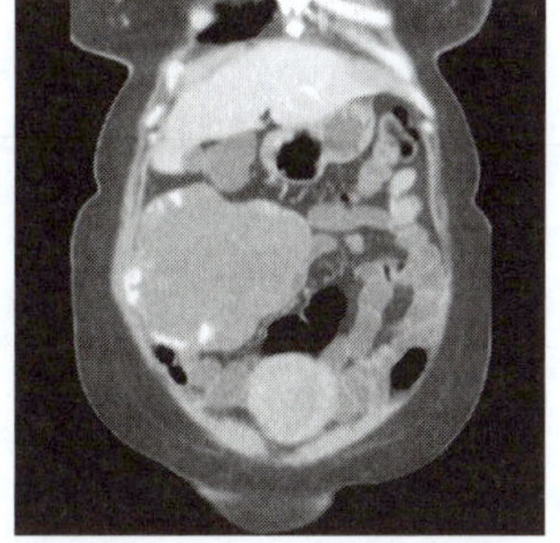

Figs 43.26 and 43.27: As it had a very narrow strip of the liver tissue, it was easily excised

   - Embolic materials
     (A) Temporary: Gel foam
     (B) Permanent: Steel coils, polyvinyl alcohol, isobutyl cyanoacrylate.
   - Polyvinyl alcohol particles 300–500 µm in size are used often.
2. They can be resected or can be enucleated.

Caution: Before putting a needle into the space occupying lesion in the liver, make sure it is **NOT a haemangioma**.

Differential Diagnosis

- Hepatoma, liver cysts, liver abscess.

Other benign tumours are **hepatic adenomas** and **focal nodular hyperplasia**.

PRIMARY LIVER CANCER—HEPATOMA OR HEPATOCELLULAR CARCINOMA (HCC)

- Before discussion on HCC, one has to have a knowledge about segmental anatomy of the liver, which forms the basis of hepatic resection.
- Even though the details about hepatic resection may not be required for undergraduate students, it is desirable to know about the segmental anatomy to have a better understanding about hepatic resection.

Competency

SU28.10.1: Describe the segmental anatomy of liver and the variations in vascular anatomy of liver.

SEGMENTAL ANATOMY OF THE LIVER

- The liver is divided into two lobes by the main portal fissure, which is also called **Cantlie's line**. This line extends from the gallbladder fossa to the left side of IVC and is inclined at an angle of 75° to the horizontal plane. The main portal fissure is a constant feature. Each lobe is equal in size.

- The **right portal fissure** divides the right lobe into an anteromedial and posterolateral sector. The right hepatic vein courses along this fissure. This fissure is inclined at an angle of 40° with the horizontal.
- The left portal fissure divides the left lobe into an anterior and posterior sector, and it is in this fissure that the left hepatic vein courses.
- The liver is further divided into segments, which represents the smallest anatomic unit of the organ. In the right lobe, each of the two sectors is divided into two segments: The anteromedial sector and posterolateral sector. The anteromedial sector is divided into segment V anteriorly and segment VIII posteriorly, while the posterolateral sector is divided into segment VI anteriorly and segment VII posteriorly.
- In the left lobe, the anterior sector is divided into segment IV (or quadrate lobe) and the segment III. The posterior sector is comprised of only one segment, segment II. The Spigelian lobe or segment I is considered as an ***autonomous*** segment. It is also labelled ***caudate lobe***.
- Each segment has its own identifiable portal vein, hepatic arterial supply, bile duct and hepatic veins. All these segments can be removed individually. However, segment I receives tributaries from both the right and left branches of portal vein and hepatic artery. ***However, hepatic venous drainage is independent and may terminate directly into IVC*** (Fig. 43.28).

Introduction

Hepatocellular carcinoma is uncommon in United States but more in Asians. It arises from hepatocytes. When it arises from biliary epithelial cells, it is intrahepatic cholangiocarcinoma. In neonates, it is hepatoblastoma as it resembles foetal liver.

Competency

SU28.10.6: Describe in detail the etiopathogenesis, premalignant conditions, clinical features, investigations, staging and treatment options available for treatment of hepatocellular carcinoma. Also types of hepatic resections.

Aetiology of HCC

1. **Hepatitis B virus (HBV):** High titres of hepatitis B surface antigen (HBsAg) was found in 50 to 60% of patients with HCC. Its incidence is higher in chronic carriers and it is increased, if patients consume alcohol, aflatoxin and tobacco.
2. **Hepatitis C virus (HCV):** HCV infection induces cirrhosis and increases the incidence of development of HCC.
3. **Hepatitis D:** It is another viral infection also called **delta hepatitis**. This virus requires hepatitis B virus (HBV) for replication. It can cause dangerous hepatitis—HCC.
4. **Cirrhosis:** It is a definite premalignant condition. A palpable hard liver in a cirrhotic patient suggests development of HCC. **It is the single most common risk factor for HCC.**
5. **Aflatoxin consumption** (a fungus found in infected butter yellow, bread) is responsible for increased incidence of HCC as in Mozambique.
6. **Oral contraceptive pills** are known to cause adenoma and there is a rare chance of adenoma turning into HCC.
7. **Other risk factors:** Heavy alcohol consumption, cigarette smoking, diabetes mellitus, haemochromatosis are the other factors responsible for HCC. ***Wilson's disease is rarely associated with increased risk of HCC.***

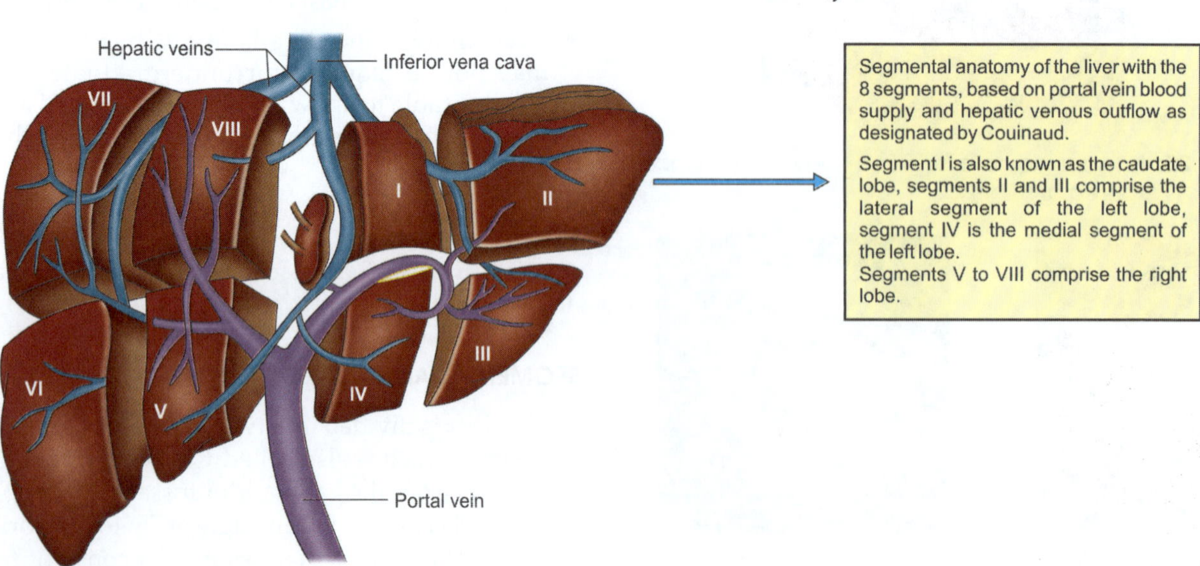

Fig. 43.28: Segmental anatomy of the liver

Pathology: It is a highly vascular tumour and fatal if left untreated. Few types and histological features are given below

Histologic variants of HCC

1. Fibrolamellar
2. Mixed hepatocellular cholangio-carcinoma cellular
3. Clear cell variant
4. Giant cell variant
5. Childhood HCC
6. Carcinosarcoma

*Refer to Table 43.3

Pathology: Histology types

- It is a highly vascular tumour with indistinct margin.
- **Hanging type:** It is attached to the liver by a small stalk—easily resected.
- **Pushing type:** A tumour pushing the blood vessels. It is also resectable.
- **Infiltrative type:** Difficult to resect because of infiltration into surrounding structures.
- Hence, in cirrhotic patients, resection is not advisable.

8. Hereditary tyrosinaemia is a metabolic disorder characterised by deficiency of enzyme fumaryl acetoacetate resulting in, accumulation of toxic tyrosine metabolites—can progress to HCC.
9. **Other causes:** Type I glycogen storage disease and familial polyposis coli alpha-1 antitrypsin deficiency, Budd-Chiari syndrome. It is 4 times more common in Asians and two times in Hispanics. Less common in Caucasians.

Clinical Features

- **Age group:** Highest incidence is found after 50 years of age. It is rarely seen in children also.
- **Sex:** ***Male alcoholics*** are commonly affected.

Pearls of Wisdom

Thus, almost 80% of the cases are due to underlying chronic hepatitis B and C virus infection.

- A *slow growing* mass in the right hypochondrium. It is the enlarged liver with an irregular surface and is hard in consistency. Evidence of cirrhosis may be present.
- It can be a ***rapidly growing*** neoplasm, highly vascular and clinically palpable as a soft to firm pulsatile mass with or without a bruit.
- Rapid development of ***anorexia, asthaenia, anaemia and loss of weight.***
- Jaundice is not common unless the tumour arises in a cirrhotic liver in hepatocellular failure.
- Worsening of portal hypertension.
- **Low grade pyrexia** is common. It is due to tumour necrosis.
- Liver being an important organ of metabolism, **hypoglycaemia** is found in 10% of the patients.
- Ascites
- **Triad of abdominal pain, weight loss and abdominal mass** is the most common clinical presentation.

Spread of Hepatoma

1. **Direct infiltration** of the neighbouring structures such as diaphragm results in hiccoughs due to irritation of phrenic nerve.
2. **Lymphatic spread:** Lymph nodes at the hilum (porta hepatis) are involved first. Later, mediastinal nodes and left supraclavicular nodes (Virchow's node) are involved.
3. **Blood spread** causes massive malignant pleural effusion by dislodgement of tumour emboli into inferior vena cava because of spread through the hepatic veins. Vertebral involvement follows soon.
4. **Haemoperitoneum** due to spread involving peritoneal surface or due to rupture of an enlarging hepatoma may occur.

Investigations

1. **CBP:** Hb% is usually low.
2. **Liver function tests** may show hepatocellular failure in the form of high bilirubin, low albumin and high globulin levels.

Table 43.3 Comparison of HCC and fibrolamellar carcinoma

	Hepatocellular carcinoma	**Fibrolamellar carcinoma**
1. Age (years)	50–60	20–30
2. Sex	More common in males	Equal in both sexes
3. Aetiology	Cirrhosis	Does not arise in a cirrhotic liver
4. Involvement of lobe	Right lobe	Left lobe
5. Gross pathology	Solitary or nodular, central necrosis is common	Solitary or nodular, central necrosis is not common
6. Microscopy	Basic structure is trabecular pattern with acidophilic cytoplasm and large nuclei	Deeply eosinophilic hepatocytes, fibrous stroma is arranged in the form of thin hyalinised bands in layers. Hence the name, **fibrolamellar**
7. Resectability rate	Less	More
8. Prognosis	Not good	Good

3. **Chest X-ray:** CT chest pulmonary metastasis
4. **Abdominal USG:** Findings:
   - Diffuse distortion of hepatic parenchyma and a well-circumscribed hyperechogenic mass suggests HCC.
   - **Mosaic pattern** of the tumour with thin halo and lateral shadows, **nodule in nodule pattern** with separating fibrous septa and **posterior echo enhancement**.
   - **Tumour thrombi** in portal vein, hepatic vein or IVC.
5. **Contrast enhanced CT of the abdomen[1]:** It appears as a hypodense mass with internal mosaic architecture in the early phase and hypodense lesion with enhanced fibrous capsule in late phase. Guided FNAC can be done to confirm the diagnosis. A small fear of tumour embolisation *via* portal venous radicles exists and is a complication. Enhancement in arterial phase and washout in delayed portovenous phase is diagnostic of HCC (Figs 43.29 and 43.30).

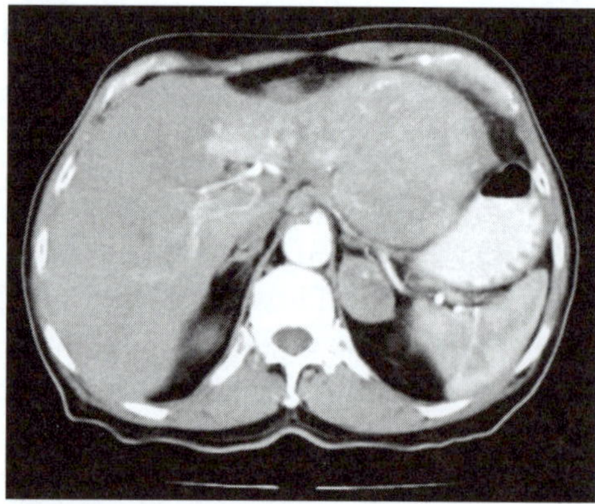

Fig. 43.29: CT scan showing a large hypodense mass lesion in the left lobe

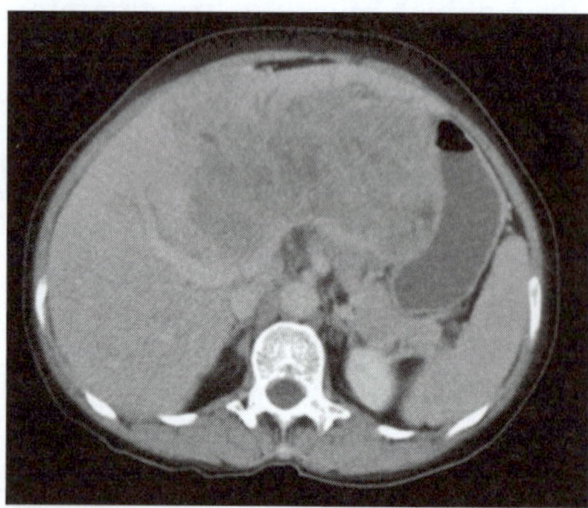

Fig. 43.30: CT scan showing a large hepatoma displacing the portal vein branches

6. **Alpha-fetoprotein**
   - It is a foetal antigen which disappears after birth. Hence, it is not measurable in normal persons.
   - Values above 20 ng/ml are suggestive of hepatoma.
   - Levels above 400 ng/ml in a cirrhotic patients with hypervascular mass larger than 2 cm in diameter is diagnostic.
   - α-fetoprotein levels indicate size of the tumour, invasion and even recurrence.
   - In patients who are not operated, levels reflect response to treatment (Key Box 43.11).
   - Values around 200 ng/ml is also seen with regenerating nodules.
   - 20 to 40% HCCs do not secrete LFP.
7. **Selective angiography:** It is done only if hepatic resection is planned. It can demonstrate a highly vascular tumour (tumour blush due to neovascularisation) or involvement of portal vein thrombus in the IVC. Hence, venous phase must be recorded. It can define arterial supply also.
8. **MRI:** It appears as a high intensity lesion (adenomatous hyperplasia as a low intensity lesion).
   - MRI is much more sensitive for diagnosis of 1–2 cm HCC.
9. **Liver biopsy for HCC:**
   - It is done only in unresectable cases or metastatic disease before starting other treatment such as chemotherapy, etc.
   - The images from contrast CT scan and MRI and raised levels of α-fetoprotein—almost always suggest HCC. Hence, biopsy is not done.
   - Also rises of haemoperitoneum and peritoneal implantation of tumour cells present.
   - Core-biopsy has increased risks of all the complications mentioned above.
   - With normal INR, fine needle aspiration can be done in selected cases (clinical trials) with minimal risk.

Key Box 43.11

Increased α-Fetoprotein Levels

1. **Hepatoma—hepatoblastoma**
2. Carcinoma stomach
3. Carcinoma pancreas
4. Embryonal cell carcinoma of testis

Not increased in fibrolamellar carcinoma

[1]Triple phase—precontrast, early vascular or arterial, portal phase and delayed phase—multislice spiral CT is the gold standard investigation for liver tumours. If clinical, radiological and biochemical features strongly suggest HCC, there is no need to prove histopathological diagnosis by FNAC.

Differential Diagnosis (Key Box 43.12)

- Secondaries in the liver—nodular surface and usually both lobes are enlarged.
- Polycystic disease of the liver.
- Hydatid cyst of the liver—smooth surface, round borders.

Refer TNM staging of liver cancer.

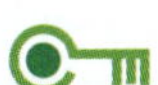 Key Box 43.12

Differential Diagnosis

- Fibrolamellar carcinoma
- Secondaries in the liver
- Haemangioma
- Focal nodular hyperplasia
- Polycystic liver

TNM STAGING — AJCC 8th edition–hepatocellular carcinoma

Primary tumour (T)

T1a Solitary tumour ≤2 cm with/without vascular invasion

T1b Solitary tumour >2 cm without vascular invasion

T2 Solitary tumour >2 cm with vascular invasion or multifocal tumours, note >5 cm

T3 Multiple tumours at least one of which is >5 cm

T4 Single tumour or multifocal tumours of any size involving a major branch of the portal vein or hepatic vein or tumour(s) with direct invasion of adjacent organs other than the gallbladder or with perforation of visceral peritoneum

Regional lymph nodes (N)

Nx Regional lymph nodes cannot be assessed

N0 No regional lymph node metastasis

N1 Regional lymph node metastasis

Distant metastasis (M)

M0 No distant metastasis

M1 Distant metastasis

Stage

Stage	T	N	M
Stage IA	T1a	N0	M0
Stage IB	T1b	N0	M0
Stage II	T2	N0	M0
Stage IIIA	T3	N0	M0
Stage IIIB	T4	N0	M0
Stage IVA	Any T	N1	M0
Stage IVB	Any T	Any N	M1

Prognosis

Prognosis of HCC depends upon not only any about stage of the disease but also about whether patient can withstand/tolerate surgery or not? As most of the patients have active hepatitis/cirrhosis, resection may carry very high mortality. Hence, the Eastern Cooperative Oncology Group (ECOG) have adopted a performance status which is called ECOG performances status as given below.

ECOG

0. Fully active, able to carry on all pre-disease performance without restriction.
1. Restricted in physically strenuous activity but ambulatory and able to carry out work of a light or sedentary nature, e.g. light house work, office work.
2. Ambulatory and capable of all self-care but unable to carry out any work activities. Up and about more than 50% of waking hours.
3. Capable of only limited self-care, confined to bed or chair more than 50% of waking hours.
4. Completely disabled. Cannot carry on any self-care. Totally confined to bed or chair.
5. Dead

CHILD-TURCOTTE-PUGH (CTP) SCORE

Classification of hepatocellular function in cirrhosis

Points	1 point each	2 points each	3 points each
• Bilirubin (μmol/L)	<34	34–50	>50
• Albumin (g/L)	>35	25–35	<25
• Ascites	None	Easily controlled	Poorly controlled
• Encephalopathy	None	Grade I–II	Grades III–IV
• INR	<1.7	1.7–2.2	>2.2
A—5–6 points C—10–15 points		B—7–9 points	

INR—international normalised ratio

Treatment of Hepatocellular Carcinoma

It can be classified under following headings.

1. **Resection** is the best possible treatment for hepatocellular carcinoma. Up to 3 segments of the liver can be resected. Rest of the liver will be enough to maintain life provided remaining liver is healthy/noncirrhotic (Flowcharts 43.1, 43.2 and Table 43.4).
   - Functional liver remnant (FLR) should be >20% of standardised total liver volume after resection.
   - The remnant liver should have vascular inflow, venous outflow, biliary drainage.
   - Two contiguous liver segments must be left behind (Figs 43.31 to 43.34).

Flowchart 43.1: Various segments for liver resection

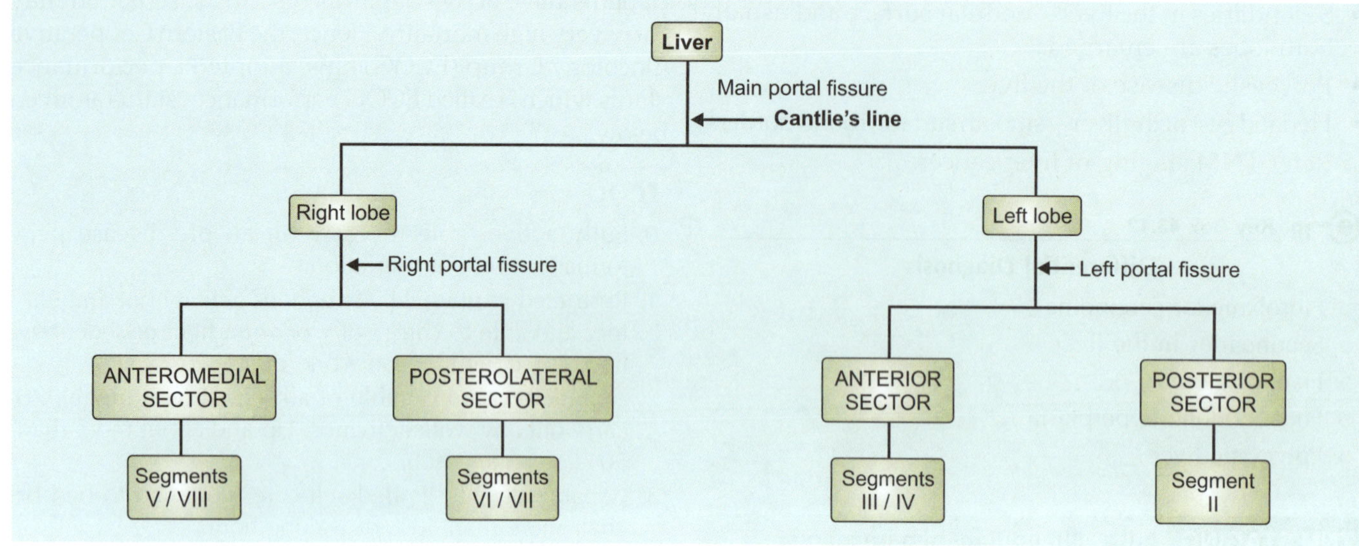

Flowchart 43.2: Treatment of HCC

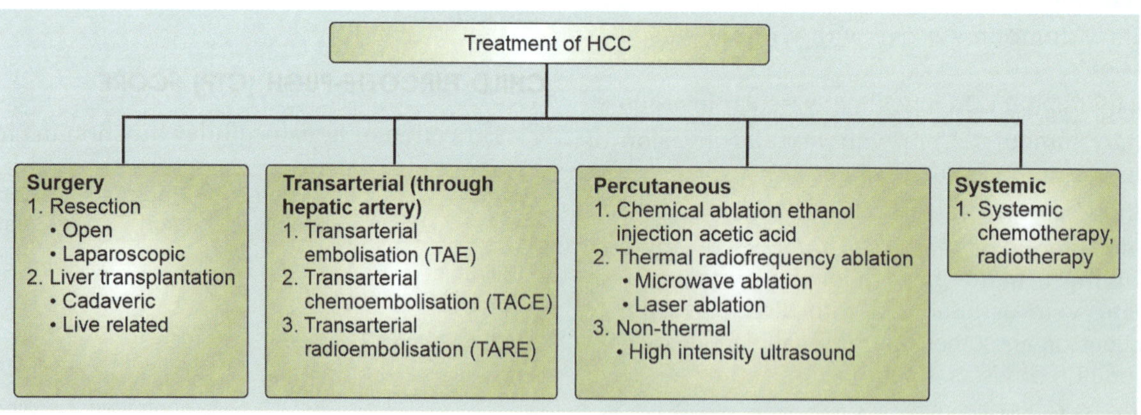

Table 43.4 Types of hepatic resections

Hepatic resection	Nomenclature
1. Resection along the main portal fissure, separating right and left lobes of the liver	• Right or left lobectomy
2. Resection of entire right lobe and the medial segment of left lobe	• Right extended lobectomy or trisegmentectomy
3. Removal of segments II and III	• Left lateral segmentectomy
4. Removal of a single segment	• Unisegmentectomy
5. Removal of 2 or more segments	• Plurisegmentectomy
6. Removal of segments VI and VII	• Right lateral sectorectomy
7. Removal of a small portion of liver, entirely within a single segment or transferring segmental plane	• Wedge resection

2. **Systemic chemotherapy** using intravenous doxorubicin has been tried with some success in the postoperative period. Intra-arterial 5-FU has also been tried.
3. **Transcatheter arterial embolisation (TAE):** By introducing gel foam into the branches of hepatic artery some amount of tumour necrosis occurs. This arterial embolisation is combined with chemotherapeutic agents such as doxorubicin, results are better because the tumour has prolonged exposure to the drug. This is called **transarterial chemoembolisation (TACE)**. This method is followed only as a palliative procedure.

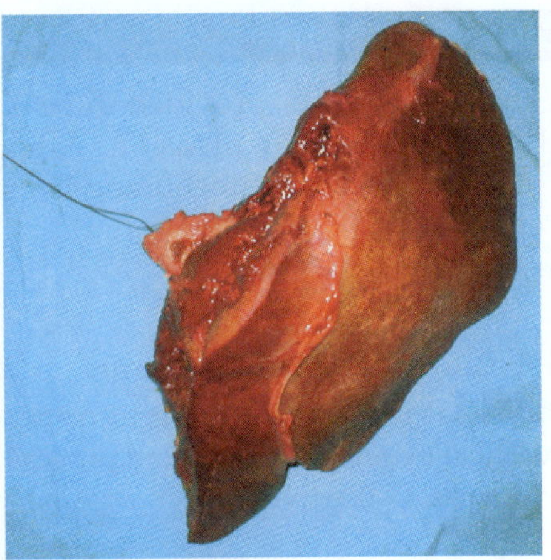

Fig. 43.31: Left lobectomy for cholangiocarcinoma. (*Courtesy:* Dr Ramesh Rajan, Associate Professor, Department of Surgical Gastroenterology, Trivandrum Medical College, Kerala)

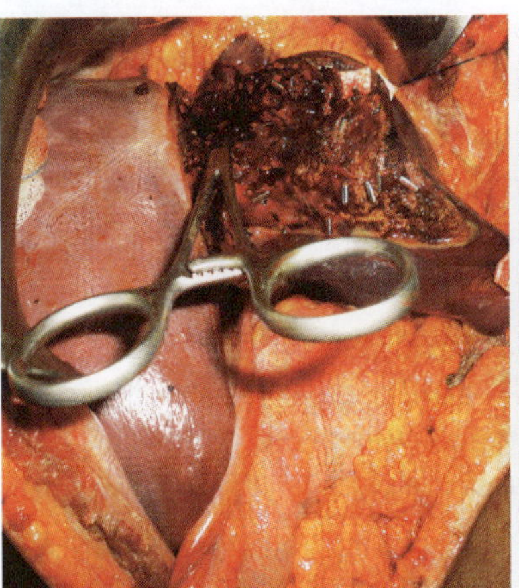

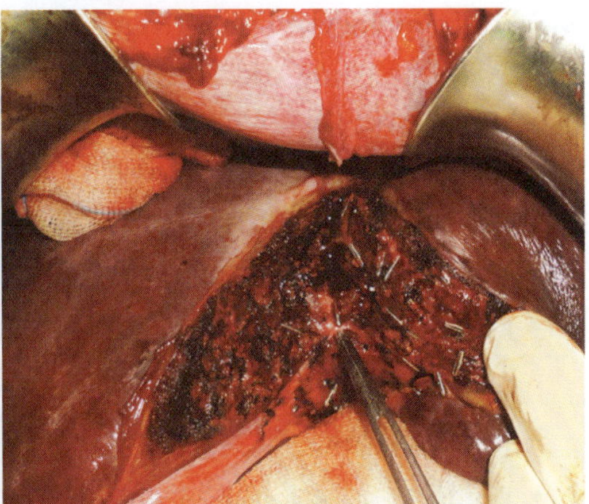

Figs 43.32 and 43.33: Liver resection for adenoma. (*Courtesy:* Dr Prasad Babu TLVD, Dr Ramcharan Thyagarajan, Dr Srikanth Gadiyaram, Prof Sadiq S Sikora, Department of GI Surgery, Manipal Hospital, Bengaluru, Karnataka)

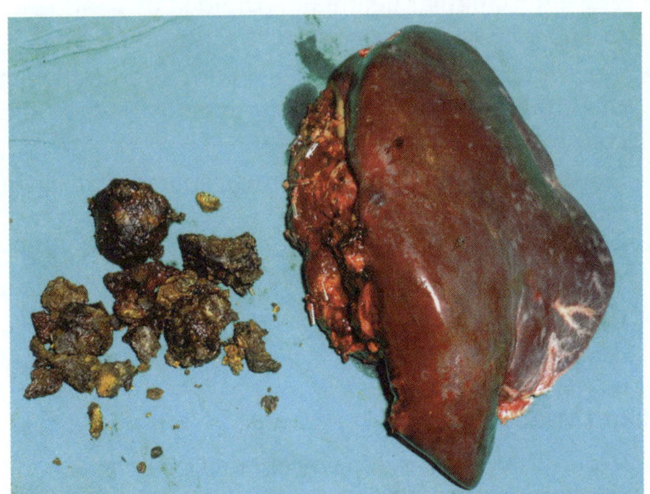

Fig. 43.34: Liver resection for Caroli's disease (*Courtesy:* Dr Nagaraj Palankar, Assistant Professor, Kasturba Hospital, Manipal)

- Basically they are used for unresectable HCC not suitable for other treatments.
- Most commonly used agents are doxorubicin, cisplatin and mitomycin.
- Contraindications are portal vein occlusion and poor liver function.

Embolising agents:

- Gel foam
- Chemotherapeutic agent (like doxorubicin) with or without lipiodol
- Side-effects are abdominal pain, liver abscess, acute pancreatitis, etc.
- As a definitive curative intent, TAE is not recommended, as there is no strong evidence.

Pearls of Wisdom

Lipiodol is derived from poppy seed oil. It is an iodinated ester. It is highly concentrated ester gets concentrated by hepatocytes. The contact time between tumour cells and chemotherapeutic agents is prolonged and it leads to cancer cell death.

4. Transarterial radioembolisation (TARE)

- It is another option for unresectable HCC.
- It is called internal radiation.
- Most commonly used radioactive material is Yttrium-90 (^{90}Y).
- It emits β-radiation.
- It is delivered through feeding vessels of the tumour.
- Thus, any tumour, any size, any nodules can be irradiated.
- Survival is prolonged with this treatment.
- Can be used in cirrhotic patients of poor liver function.
- It is indicated in advanced disease, portal vein thrombosis.
- Thus, later resection or transplant can be option.

5. Percutaneous ethanol ablation (PEA): It is cheaper and is a palliative treatment. Tumour less than 3 cm and nodules not more than 3 are candidates. It reduces the tumour size and decreases pain.

- Tumour necrosis occurs as a result of cellular dehydration denaturation of proteins and occlusion of small tumour vessels.
- It requires 4–6 sessions under ultrasound guidance with 2–10 ml alcohol injection.
- Injections are given on an outpatient basis. Easy to give because of the soft consistency of the tumour.

6. **Radiofrequency ablation (RFA)**
   - It is now being tried for inoperable tumours or patients who are not ideal candidates for surgery, as per Milan's criteria.

     Indications: Tumour deep in parenchyma, away from hilum and less than 3 cm.
   - Electrical energy (500 kHz) is delivered through a 18 G needle inserted under US or CT guidance through the skin into the tumour. In the following few months, the tumour is destroyed and the cells are killed.
   - The route of insertion of this needle can be percutaneous, laparoscopic or by open route.
   - There should not be any evidence of extrahepatic disease preoperatively or intraoperatively.
   - **Mode of actions:** Cytodestruction of the tumour. In one sitting 6–7 cm of necrosis zone can be achieved for a 5 cm tumour.
   - In most cases a tumour can be adequately treated in one session. The procedure can also be repeated. It is done under general anaesthesia.
   - It is better to avoid RFA when the tumour is in the hilar plate wherein portal vein and the hepatic arterial branches enter the liver. Damage to these structures and bile duct can occur.
   - Thus, RFA is considered for small HCCs, CP grade A cirrhotic patients who are not candidates for resection and it is to be considered as bridging procedure before transplantation.
7. **Injection octreotide**, an analogue of somatostatin, has been used in advanced cases. It has shown promising results in decreasing the size of the tumour. It also reduces the pain and discomfort. This is combined with chemotherapy such as gemcitabine and carboplatin. However, the treatment is costly and results are temporary.
8. **Sorafenib** is the drug of choice in advanced HCC and with good liver function.
   - It is a multi-tyrosine kinase inhibitor.
   - It promotes apoptosis and inhibits angiogenesis.
   - These agents because of their mode of action, inhibit cell proliferation and thus control growth and improve survival. It also inhibits vascular endothelial growth factors (VEGF).
   - Thus, it is indicated in management of advanced HCC with good systemic function.
   - **Side effects:** Fatigue, skin rashes, hand-foot syndrome, hypertension, hair loss, itching.

LIVER RESECTIONS

It should be the first choice in HCC, provided there is no extrahepatic disease or vascular invasion. After getting a negative margin, adequate functioning liver tissue should be present.

Incision

- Aim of the incision is to get adequate exposure.
- A transverse abdominal incision in the right upper quadrant with a vertical extension to xyphoid process gives excellent exposure to the liver.

Mobilisation of the Liver

- The key point is division of ligaments which are attached to it or which support the liver and suspend the liver.
- The falciform ligament is divided and followed along anterior surface of the liver.
- The left triangular ligament is divided by gentle pull on the left lobe of liver towards right side.
- The right triangular ligament is divided between diaphragm and right lobe of the liver by traction and countertraction.
- Lesser omentum is divided. Thus, separating the liver from stomach.
- Small multiple veins from the inferior surface of the liver join inferior vena cava. These should be divided.
- Last hepatic veins to be dissected and divided above renal veins.

Hilar Dissection

- Cholecystectomy is done by ligating cystic artery and cystic duct. The CBD is then exposed at the free edge of lesser omentum. A sling is applied around CBD to isolate it and gently traction is applied.
- This visualises the common hepatic artery.
- By dissection of common hepatic artery, its right and left branches are dissected out.
- Slings are applied to these arteries, portal vein is exposed. This facilitates freeing of portal vein by dividing lymphatic tissues joining portal vein.
- The congenital anomalies such as aberrant right hepatic artery and accessory left hepatic artery also should be looked for.
- CBD, CHD, left and right hepatic ducts are exposed at the hilum.

Division of the Parenchyma

- This requires ligation of artery or branch by 4/0 prolene, transfixation of the bile duct by 4/0 PDS and transfixation of portal vein with 4/0 prolene.

- Once the demarcation appears on the liver, parenchyma is divided by using diathermy.
- Cavitron ultrasonic surgical aspirator (CUSA) is the commonly used dissector for dividing liver parenchyma.
- Vessels and bile duct branches which are exposed are clipped or diathermised.
- Continue dissection till you reach hepatic veins/ branches. They are ligated or divided.

Segmental and Local Resection

- Since each segment (*see* segmental anatomy) carries its own arterial supply, venous drainage and bile drainage, resection can be done with 1 cm margin.
- In a few cases, hilar dissection may not be necessary.

Complications

- Intraoperative bleeding
- Biliary leakage
- Hepatic decompensation
- Ascites due to portal HTN, severing of lymphatics
- Infection

Competency

SU28.10.7: Enumerate the clinical features, investigations and management of various types of secondaries in the liver.

A CASE OF SECONDARIES IN THE LIVER

History

Details are shown in Table 43.5.

General Physical Examination

1. **Anaemia** — It is a common feature of most of the malignancies. Severe pallor may indicate carcinoma stomach or carcinoma colon.
2. **Jaundice** — Deep jaundice is obstructive in nature. Hence, periampullary carcinoma is likely.
3. **Bilateral pedal oedema** — Inferior vena caval obstruction due to enlarged liver.
4. **Spine tenderness** — Metastasis from breast, prostate, bronchus, kidney, etc.
5. **Absent testis in scrotum** — Probably seminoma arising from undescended testis.

Abdominal Examination

I. Criteria of Secondaries in the Liver

1. Both lobes are enlarged.
2. Lower border is sharp.
3. Surface is nodular.
4. Hard in consistency.
5. Umbilication refers to central necrosis in a nodule but is difficult to appreciate clinically.

II. Evidence of Primary

- **Example 1:** Secondaries in the liver from carcinoma stomach. A distinct stomach mass may be felt (Figs 43.35 and 43.36).
- **Example 2:** Secondaries in the liver from periampullary carcinoma. A palpable gallbladder gives clue to the diagnosis (Fig. 43.37).

Table 43.5 History taking

Complaint	Explanation
1. Dull-aching and continuous pain in the right hypochondrium of short duration (3–6 months)	Enlarged liver stretches the parietal capsule which is responsible for dull-aching pain
2. Loss of appetite, weakness, asthenia, malaise	Due to destruction of an important metabolic organ
3. Jaundice of a few days' duration, is mild, usually nonprogressive and is not associated with pruritus (hepatocellular variety)	By the time jaundice appears, it is late and enough liver tissue is damaged
4. H/o persistent vomiting with or without blood, with loss of appetite	It suggests that the primary may be in the stomach
5. H/o severe backache without jaundice, disturbing the sleep at night	Carcinoma body and tail of pancreas infiltrating retroperitoneal nerve plexuses
6. H/o jaundice first and associated with itching	Periampullary carcinoma
7. H/o constipation, bleeding per rectum	Primary may be in the colon or rectum
8. H/o previous surgery such as mastectomy	Probably primary is carcinoma of the breast
9. Amputation of toes or leg or wide excision of mole	Malignant melanoma is the likely cause

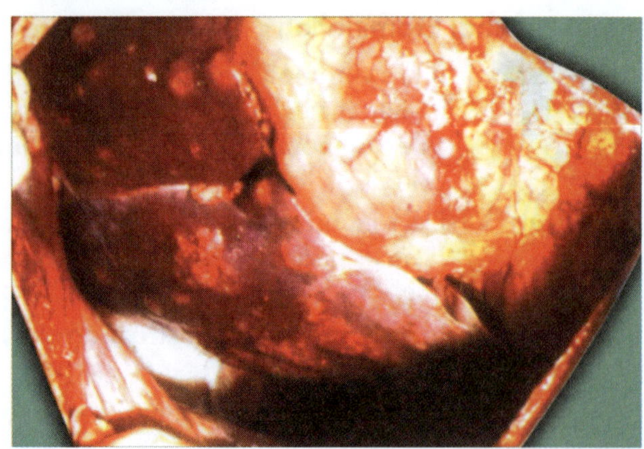

Fig. 43.35: Nodular liver with the stomach mass—stomach is the commonest site of primary

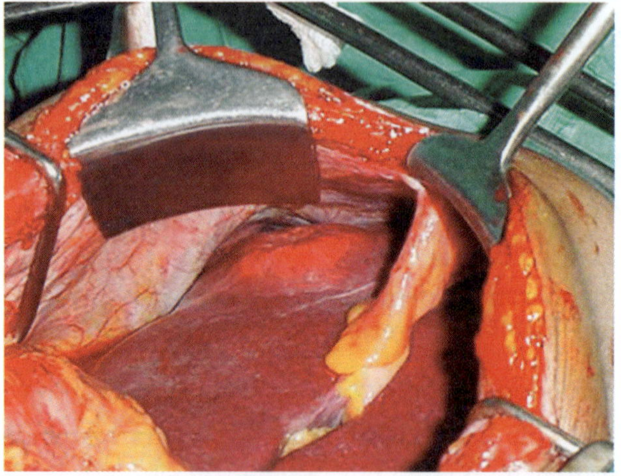

Fig. 43.36: Classical secondary in the liver with umbilication from carcinoma colon. However, it is impossible to appreciate it clinically

- **Example 3:** Secondaries in the liver from carcinoma colon or rectum. H/o bleeding per rectum with or without mass. Diagnosis is made by per rectal examination (Fig. 43.38).
- **Example 4:** Secondaries in the liver from seminoma testis. Many times, deep seated seminoma arising from undescended testis cannot be felt per abdomen.
- **Example 5:** Secondaries in the liver from malignant melanoma of foot or leg. Evidence of amputation with enlarged inguinal nodes is usually present (Fig. 43.39).

When there are massive secondaries in the liver and if you suspect melanoma—look for

1. Artificial eyeball
2. Missing toes
3. Amputated leg
4. Ulcerated pigmented anal canal
5. A surgical lesion which is erased
6. Wide excision and grafted site
7. Mastectomy scar
8. Laparotomy scar

Investigations[1]

They depend upon the type of primary which could be detected in a clinical examination. However, when the primary could not be found out, following investigations may have to be done.

1. **Upper gastrointestinal scopy and biopsy:** To detect a growth in the oesophagus or stomach.
2. **Sigmoidoscopy/colonoscopy:** To rule out carcinoma rectum and colon (melanoma of the anal canal).

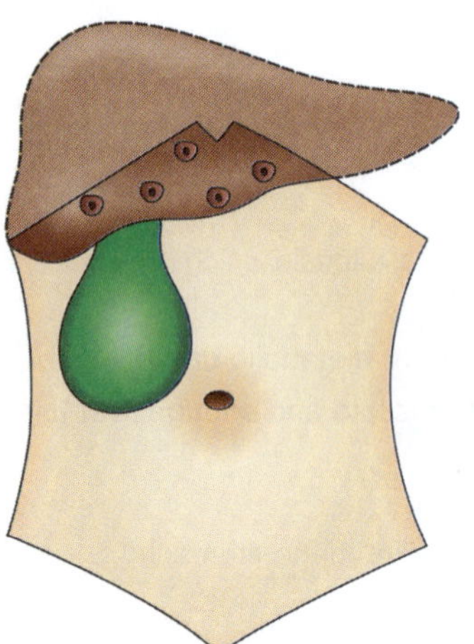

Fig. 43.37: Nodular liver with palpable gallbladder—carcinoma head of the pancreas

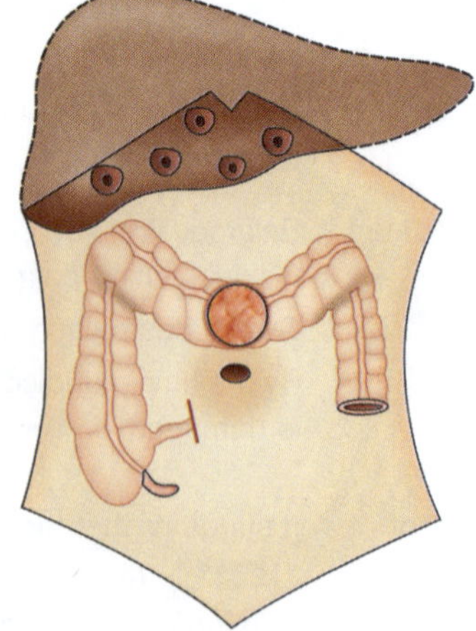

Fig. 43.38: Nodular liver in a case of carcinoma colon—not uncommon to find this

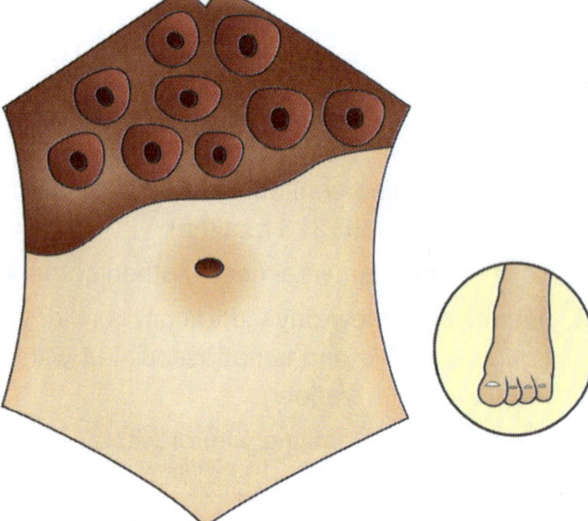

Fig. 43.39: Secondaries in the liver from melanoma—bulky liver with massive hepatomegaly. Note the missing toe

[1]It is important to prove the diagnosis by FNAC or laparoscopic biopsy because if it is neuroendocrinal in origin or is a carcinoid, patient can live a longer life with minimal morbidity.

3. **Abdominal ultrasound**
   - It can diagnose secondaries in the liver which can be hypo- or hyperechoic and multiple with normal hepatic parenchyma in between.
   - It can detect a carcinomatous growth in the periampullary region.
   - It can detect enlarged lymph nodes—portal, coeliac, para-aortic, etc.
   - It can detect deep seated testicular tumour arising from the testis.

   In spite of these investigations, if the primary cannot be detected, other investigations may have to be done such as bronchoscopy for bronchogenic carcinoma, acid phosphatase for carcinoma prostate or computed tomography (CT scan), etc.

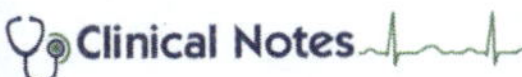

A 38-year-old lady came to the hospital with pain in the right hypochondrium. On examination, firm to hard nodular liver was palpable up to umbilicus. Before investigations, the treating doctor told the husband and relatives that she has secondaries in liver and she may not live for 6 months. 5 years later, she came to the hospital. What she was having was ***Polycystic Disease of Liver!!*** (Fig. 43.24)

4. **High quality CT scan** triple phase with IV and oral contrast medium provides actual assessment of the liver disease (decision of hepatectomy) and other pathology in the abdomen.
5. **FDG-PET:** 14-fluorodeoxyglucose positive emission tomography is used to stage the disease, to detect extrahepatic disease.
6. **Liver biopsy:** Laparoscopy and tissue diagnosis is a must, if primary cannot be detected. **Lymphoma, carcinoid tumours and metastatic neuroendocrinal tumours have better prognosis.**

Treatment

I. Surgery

In majority of the cases, treatment is only palliative aiming at relieving symptoms. The following are a few examples:

1. Carcinoma stomach with secondaries—palliative GJ, if vomiting is present.
2. Periampullary carcinoma with secondaries—triple bypass to relieve jaundice.
3. In cases of colonic cancer and carcinoid tumour, the primary can be resected because these primaries are slow growing and carry good prognosis. If metastasis is to one lobe of liver, hepatectomy can also be done.

II. Chemotherapy

- When the primary is detected to be in gastrointestinal tract, injection 5-FU can be given. The dosage is 500 mg IV for 5 days/28 days for five cycles.
- When the primary is detected outside the gastrointestinal tract, depending on the nature of the malignancy, appropriate chemotherapy is given (they are discussed in appropriate chapters).

III. Therapeutic Embolisation

- A catheter is placed in the hepatic artery and substances such as blood clot or gel foam are injected. They produce thrombosis of hepatic artery resulting in liver necrosis. Thus, liver regresses in size leading to decrease in pain.
- Gel foam is cheap and easy to manipulate. The effect is temporary.
- Autologous blood clot undergoes lysis within 12–24 hours. Hence, it is not ideal.
- Embolisation is an alternative to ligation of hepatic artery.
- Permanent embolising substances include savlon sponge, steel coils, bicrylate, etc.

Some Interesting Observations

(Key Boxes 43.13 to 43.16)

1. Secondaries in the liver from neuroendocrine tumours, carcinoid tumours and colorectal carcinoma have good prognosis.
2. Secondaries in the liver can appear many years after treatment of primary. One example being malignant melanoma of the choroid.
3. It is unusual and uncommon for secondaries to develop in a cirrhotic liver.
4. When metastasis appear in the liver from lung cancer, mostly bones, brain, adrenals would have been involved by metastasis, but it is not true/for colorectal cancer. **Often, liver metastasis for colorectal is the only visceral site of metastasis.**
5. More hepatic resections are done for colorectal metastasis than hepatocellular carcinoma.
6. Liver is the most common site of cancer recurrence after a complete resection.
7. Debulking and partial hepatectomy are indicated in metastasis from neuroendocrine tumours.

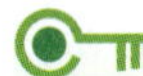

Key Box 43.13

Differential Diagnosis of Nodular Liver

- Secondaries and hepatoma—hard
- Polycystic disease and hydatid cyst—firm

Key Box 43.14

Common Causes of Secondaries in the Liver

- Carcinoma stomach
- Carcinoma rectum
- Malignant melanoma
- Carcinoma pancreas
- Carcinoma colon
- Testicular tumours

Key Box 43.15

Causes of Bulky Secondaries

- Malignant melanoma
- Carcinoid tumours
- Colloid carcinoma

Key Box 43.16

Special Types of Secondaries

- **Precocious** metastasis—before primary is suspected, e.g. carcinoid, rectal carcinoma
- **Synchronous** metastasis—primary and metastasis detected at the same time, e.g. carcinoma stomach
- **Metachronous** metastasis—metastasis appearing much later than treatment of primary, e.g. melanoma of the choroid

PORTAL HYPERTENSION

- When portal venous pressure is ***more than 10–12 mmHg or 20 cm of saline***, or more than 5 mm gradient between inferior vena cava and portal vein it is called portal hypertension.
- Despite high prevalence of varices in patients with cirrhosis, bleeding occurs in only 1/3rd of patients.
- 10–30% of upper GI bleed are due to rupture of varices due to cirrhosis.
- Variceal haemorrhage occurs in 25–35% of patients with cirrhosis.
- Up to 30% of initial bleeds are fatal and as many as 70% of survivors have recurrent bleeds after the first variceal bleed.

Anatomy of Portal Venous System (Key Box 43.17)

- Splenic vein after receiving inferior mesenteric vein, joins the superior mesenteric vein behind the neck of pancreas and forms the portal vein. It runs in the free edge of the lesser omentum covered by common bile duct.
- It is 6–8 cm in length in its extrahepatic course and divides at the porta hepatis into right and left branches. Rarely, two branches are given on the right side.
- ***Portal vein carries 75% of the blood supply to the liver.***

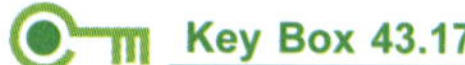

Key Box 43.17

Portal Vein

Portal vein is 6–8 cm in length

Occurs by confluence of superior mesenteric vein and splenic vein

Runs posterior to common bile duct

Two venous communications between coronary and azygos veins give rise to varices

Approximately, it supplies 75% of total blood flow to the liver

Ligament related to portal vein is hepatoduodenal

Valveless structure

Esophagogastric varices develop if there is portal hypertension

Increased portal pressure results in liver damage and bleeding

Normal pressure is 3–5 mmHg

Remember as **PORTAL VEIN**

Left gastric vein enters the portal vein on its anteromedial aspect just cephaloid to the margin of the pancreas. In 25% of cases, left gastric vein joins splenic vein.

Aetiology (Fig. 43.40)

I. Extrahepatic Portal Hypertension (Prehepatic)

1. **Splenic vein thrombosis:** It is also called as segmental or sinistral portal hypertension.
2. **Portal vein thrombosis:** It is secondary to umbilical vein sepsis in neonates (omphalitis). In adults, thrombosed portal vein is surrounded by a leash of vessels 'cavernoma'. Portal vein thrombosis can also occur due to carcinoma of the pancreas in elderly patients.

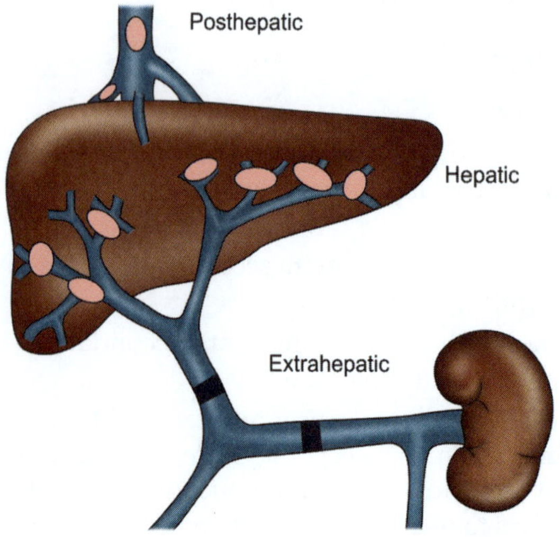

Fig. 43.40: Causes of portal hypertension

3. **Portal vein agenesis:** Extrahepatic portal hypertension is seen in 20–25% of cases and is common in female children. Liver function is normal in these cases.

II. Intrahepatic Portal Hypertension

It accounts for nearly 80% of cases.

1. **Cirrhosis of the liver:** The regenerating nodules compress the portal venous radicles within the liver. Liver function is very poor.
2. **Schistosomiasis:** Common in Egypt. *Schistosoma mansoni* and *S. japonicum* lay eggs within branches of portal vein and cause hepatic fibrosis resulting in portal hypertension.

III. Posthepatic Portal Hypertension

These are medical causes:

1. Tricuspid incompetence
2. Constrictive pericarditis
3. Budd-Chiari syndrome

Pathophysiology

As a result of obstruction to portal vein, in an attempt to reduce portal pressure, the normally present insignificant collaterals open up.[1] They become significant and result in development of portosystemic anastomosis.

- Even though, portosystemic shunts develop in many places, their important locations and clinical significance have been outlined in Table 43.6 and Fig. 43.41.

Table 43.6 Anastomosis between the portal and systemic venous system

Site	Portal tributaries	Systemic tributaries	Effect
1. Lower end of oesophagus	Branches of left gastric vein and short gastric vein	Branches from azygos vein	Oesophageal varices
2. Falciform ligament of liver (paraumbilical vein)	Veins which run in the falciform ligament	Anterior abdominal wall veins	Caput medusae*
3. Lower end of rectum	Superior haemorrhoidal vein	Inferior and middle haemorrhoidal vein	Piles (very rare), rectal varices
4. Retroperitoneum mesenteric veins	Branches of superior and inferior subdiaphragmatic veins	Retroperitoneal veins (silent)	Retroperitoneal varices

Note: Most often,veins which run in the falciform ligament are obliterated from birth. Hence, it is not commonly seen.

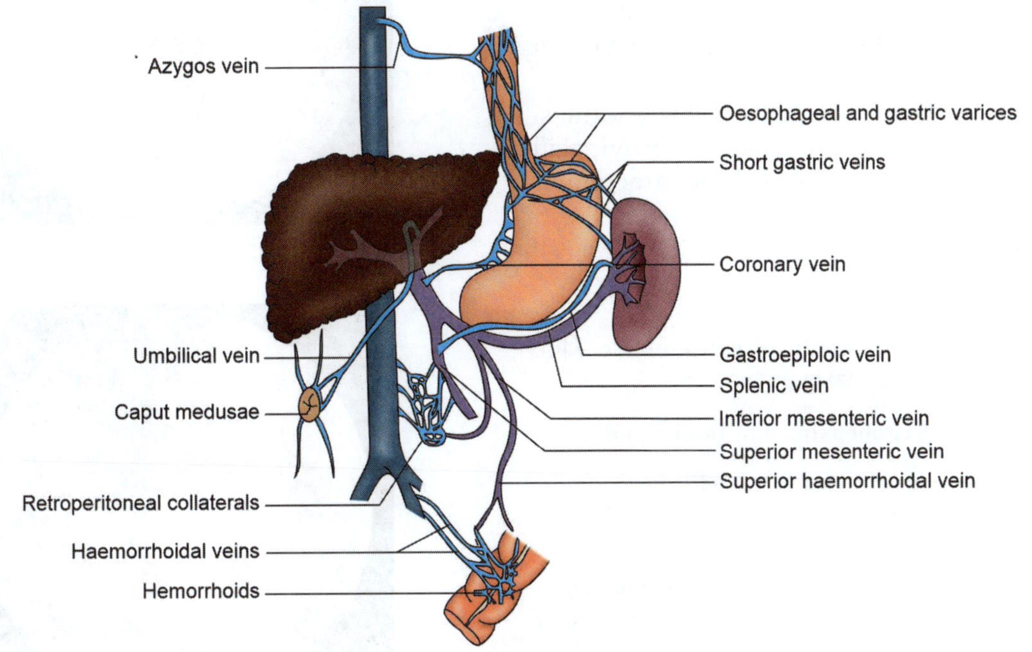

Fig. 43.41: Collaterals

[1] When the main highway is blocked, small insignificant roads become significant, is it not?

- The lower end of the oesophagus is one of the important areas giving rise to oesophageal varices. These varices rupture resulting in massive haematemesis.
- This is exactly the reason why every attempt at newer modality of treatment, medical or surgical, is aimed at controlling oesophageal varices.

Clinical Features (Table 43.7)

Bleeding gastroesophageal varices are one of the common causes of death among cirrhotic patients.

Prediction of Variceal Haemorrhage

1. **Physical factors:** Elastic properties of vessels, intravariceal and intraluminal pressure, and variceal wall tension are major factors.
2. **Continued alcohol use**
3. **Poor liver function**
4. **Hepatic venous pressure gradient (HVPG)**
   - HVPG = (wedged/occluded hepatic venous pressure)–(free hepatic venous pressure). **Normal gradient is 5 mmHg**. HVPG >12 mmHg indicates portal hypertension.

Investigations

1. **Complete blood picture**
   - Anaemia is usually present due to bleeding.
   - Peripheral smear to rule out hypersplenism—pancytopenia in the presence of normal bone marrow.
2. **Liver function tests**
   - Serum proteins: Total protein, albumin are low and albumin: globulin ratio is reversed in cirrhosis of the liver.
   - Enzymes SGOT (serum glutamic oxaloacetic transaminase) and SGPT (serum glutamic pyruvic acid transaminase) are increased in hepatocellular failure.
   - Serum bilirubin: Increased levels indicate liver cell failure.
   - Prothrombin time, bleeding time and clotting time must be checked before a liver biopsy is done.
   - **Liver biopsy** is done provided bleeding profile is normal. However, injection vitamin K 10 mg, IM is given for 3 to 5 days.
   - HBsAg serum hepatitis predisposes to cirrhosis of the liver.
   - Liver functions are usually normal in extrahepatic portal hypertension.
3. **Oesophagogastroduodenoscopy (OGD)**
   - To confirm oesophageal varices which appear as a bluish red longitudinal column in the lower end of the oesophagus. When they extend to the stomach, they are called gastric varices (Figs 43.42 to 43.44).
   - Cherry red spots indicate impending rupture.
   - Grading of varices (Key Box 43.18). Grading can also be done according to the size. Grade 1—small, straight oesophageal varices. Grade 2—enlarged, tortuous oesophageal varices occupying less than one-third of the lumen. Grade 3—large, coil-shaped oesophageal varices occupying more than one-third of the lumen of oesophagus.

Table 43.7 Clinical comparison of extrahepatic with intrahepatic portal hypertension

	Extrahepatic	Intrahepatic
1. Age	10–25 years	>40 years
2. H/o alcohol	Absent	Strongly positive
3. H/o jaundice	Absent	Present
4. Sex	More in females	More in males
5. Splenomegaly	Moderate to big	Mild to moderate
6. Ascites	Absent	Present
7. Liver cell failure	Absent	Present
8. Encephalopathy	Not a feature	It is common

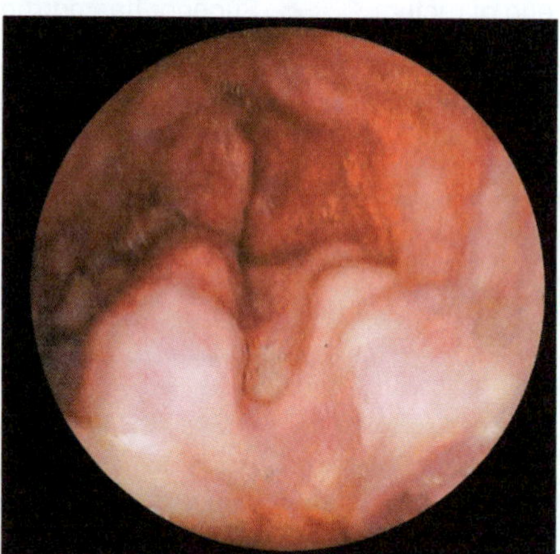

Fig. 43.42: Oesophageal varices

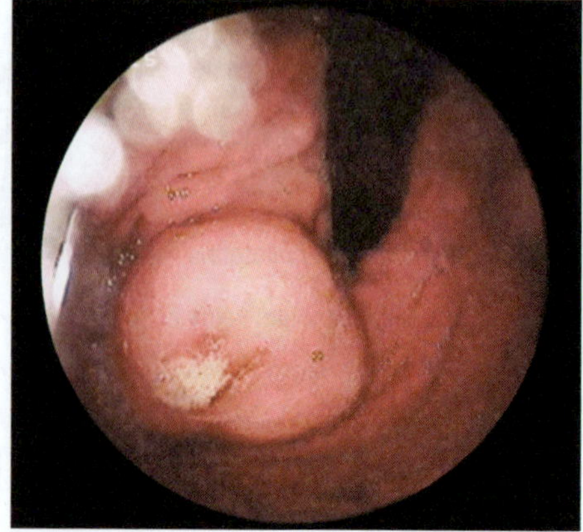

Fig. 43.43: Gastric varices

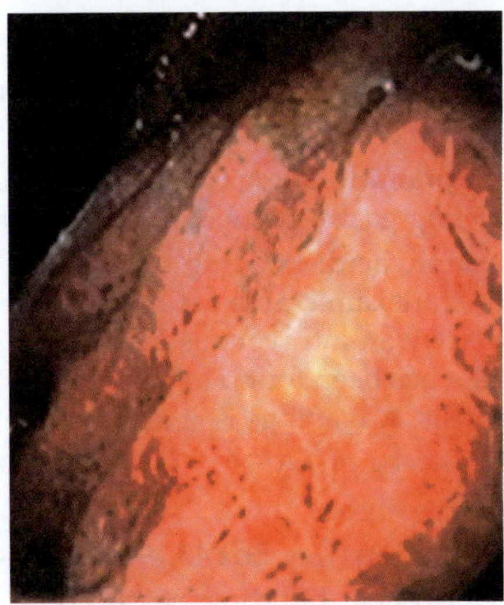

Fig. 43.44: Gastropathy

Key Box 43.18

Endoscopic Grading of Varices based on Varix Height at 2 cm from OG Junction

Grade	Bite width 1.7 mm forceps = 5 mm
1+	One-fourth bite width
2+	One-half bite width
3+	Three-fourths bite width
4+	One or more bite width(s)

Mathur's classification of gastric varices

Type 1: Oesophageal varices with lesser curvature varices

Type 2: Oesophageal varices with fundal varices (2a—subcardiac and 2b—diffuse fundal)

Type 3: Isolated fundal varix (3a—due to splenic vein thrombosis, 3b—due to generalized portal hypertension)

Type 4: Lesser curvature gastric varices with oesophageal varices with fundal varices

Type 5: Antral varices

4. **Ultrasonography:** To assess the nature of the liver (**cirrhosis**), to know the portal vein, portal cavernoma, splenic vein diameter, etc. It has become a valuable investigation today.

Causes of Rupture of Varices

- Variceal bleeding can occur even without any specific cause. The bleeding can be very minor in the form of occult blood in the stools to massive bleeding. Following hypothesis has been postulated for massive bleeding from varices.

  Eruptive theory: Due to increased intravariceal pressure.

  Erosive theory: Erosion of mucosa over the varices.

- Bleeding manifests as haematemesis or malaena. Haemodynamic instability is common.

Treatment of Portal Hypertension—Guidelines

I. Primary prophylaxis
II. Secondary prophylaxis
III. Acute variceal haemorrhage

I. Primary Prophylaxis (before Bleeding)

This is aimed at reducing portal pressure and consequently intravariceal pressure.

A. **Pharmacotherapy:** Drugs used are **nonselective β-blockers** alone (propranolol) or in combination with **isosorbide mononitrate.**
   - Reducing portal pressure by at least 20% or HVPG <1 mmHg is associated with significant protection against bleeding.
   - The dose of β-blocker is titrated to maintain heart rate around 55 beats/min or reducing by 25% from baseline rate.

B. **Endoscopic therapy: Endotherapy**
   - **Endoscopic band ligation** of varices is better than sclerotherapy. It is very effective and associated with less side-effects.
   - Indicated in patients **who do not tolerate β-blockers** and varices which are large and are associated with red wheal markings.

II. Secondary Prophylaxis

- It means prevention of rebleeding following acute variceal haemorrhage.
- The different forms of treatment and their success depends upon various criteria. The most popular of these is the modified Child's criteria (Table 43.8). Serum albumin, bilirubin, ascites, encephalopathy and prothrombin time are included under this criteria.

Table 43.8 Modified Child's criteria: Grade A = 5–6 points, Grade B = 7–9 points, Grade C = above 10 points

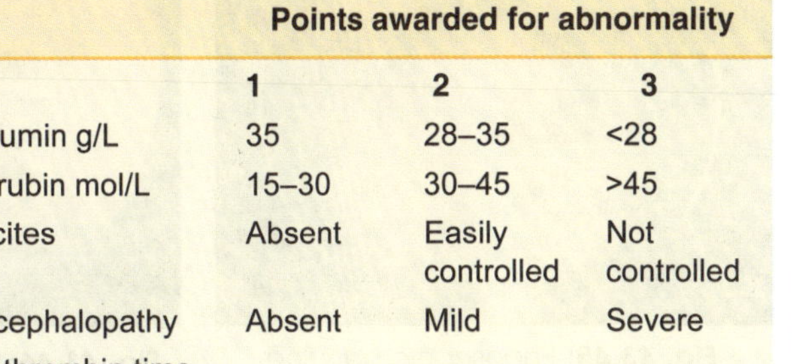

	Points awarded for abnormality		
	1	2	3
1. Albumin g/L	35	28–35	<28
2. Bilirubin mol/L	15–30	30–45	>45
3. Ascites	Absent	Easily controlled	Not controlled
4. Encephalopathy	Absent	Mild	Severe
5. Prothrombin time (in seconds)	1–4	4–6	Above 6

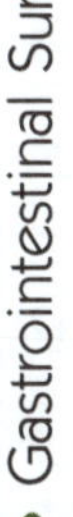

III. Treatment of Massive Bleeding from Varices

1. General measures

- Admission, hospitalisation, preferably in an intensive care unit, elevation of foot end of the bed to increase venous return. Proton pump inhibitors (PPI) are very effective in inhibiting acid secretion. However their role in portal hypertension has doubtful value because most of the cirrhosis patients have low acidity. Injection pantoprazole 40 mg can be given Iv is given 2 times/day.
- Intravenous cannulation or a venous cut down and replacement of fluid till blood is ready.
- Blood transfusion.

2. Measures to prevent encephalopathy

- Ryle's tube is introduced and stomach wash is given with ice-cold saline.
- Bowel wash is given to decrease blood from gut, to decrease ammonia and uric acid levels so as to prevent encephalopathy.
- Oral neomycin 1 g, 6th hourly as intestinal antiseptic.
- Oral lactulose 30 ml, 8th hourly is given. It also helps in decreasing encephalopathy.

3. Pharmacotherapy for variceal bleeding

- **Injection vasopressin,** 20 units in 200 ml of saline is given intravenously over a period of 20 minutes. This dose avoids coronary and peripheral vasoconstriction. By causing powerful splanchnic vasoconstriction, it decreases the blood flow to the varices and reduces bleeding in about 50% patients.
- **Injection somatostatin** 250 µg IV bolus followed by an infusion of 50 µg/h. It is very effective and has no side-effects. However, it is costly.
- **Injections octreotide** and **terlipressin** are preferred because of their long half-life. They act by producing splanchnic vasoconstriction. Thus, they decrease the portal pressure. Once started, they have to be continued for 2–5 days. Once bleeding stops, the varices are treated with **endotherapy** to prevent rebleeding.
- **Metoclopramide** 20 mg IV arrests the bleeding by constricting gastro-oesophageal sphincter.
- **Tranexamic acid:** Loading dose of 1 g of intravenous tranexamic acid for 10 min, immediately followed by an intravenous infusion of 3 g of TA over 24 h has been found to be useful in few cases of cirrhosis. Advantage is it decreases rebleeding. ***Total dose:*** 4 g of TA.

4. Endotherapy—types

A. Variceal banding (Key Box 43.19 and Fig. 43.45)

- Today, variceal banding has become the gold standard for oesophageal varices because of their efficiency in controlling the bleeding and less chances of complication.
- In 10% of the cases, rebleeding can occur.

B. Sclerotherapy (Key Box 43.20 and Fig. 43.46)

- 2% ethanolamine oleate or sodium tetradecyl sulphate (STD) is used, 3–5 ml into each varix **(intravariceal)** or 0.5 ml into the side of varices **(paravariceal).**

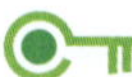
Key Box 43.19

Variceal Banding

Advantages

- Controls bleeding in 80–90% of cases
- Less rebleeding rates
- Easy
- Less risk of complication such as perforation or stricture

Disadvantage

- Costly

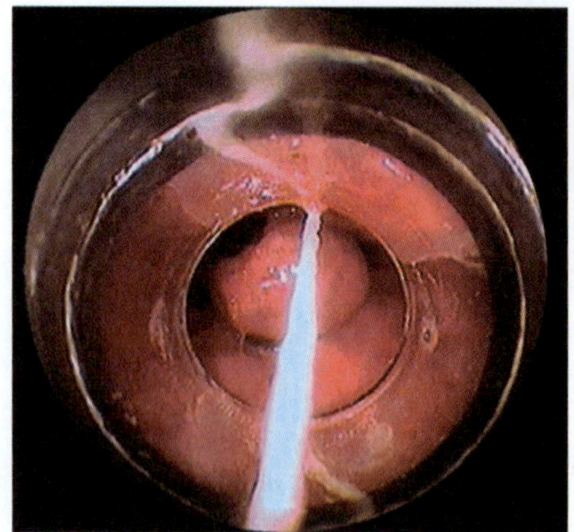

Fig. 43.45: Endoscopic banding

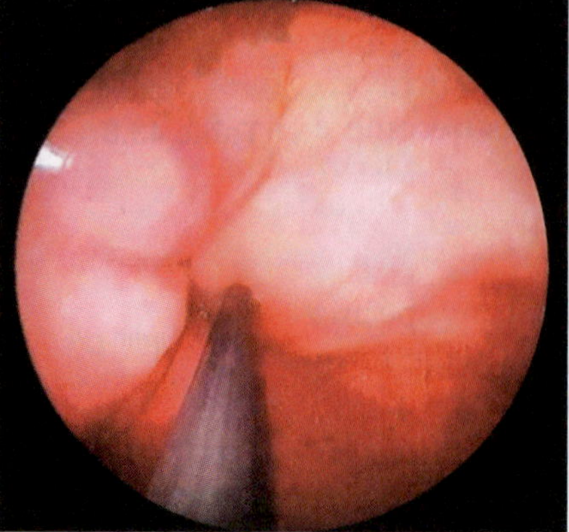

Fig. 43.46: Endoscopic sclerotherapy

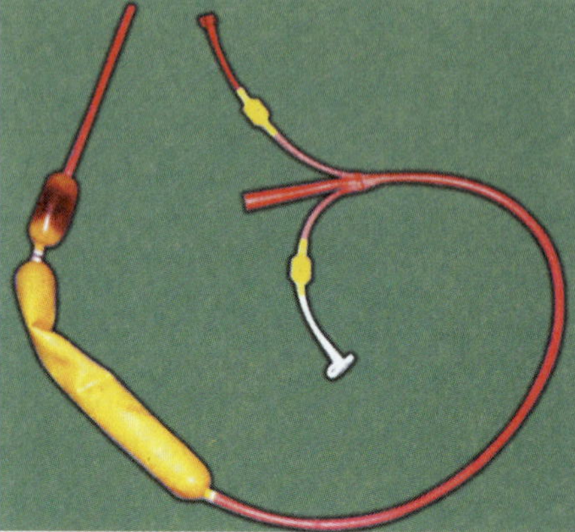

Fig. 43.47: Balloon tamponade

(*Courtesy:* Dr Filipe Alvares, Medical Gastroenterologist, KMC, Manipal)

Key Box 43.20

Sclerotherapy

Advantages
- Cheap
- Easy
- More commonly available

Disadvantages
- Complications such as perforation or stricture and massive bleeding can occur
- Higher rebleeding rates

- Bleeding can be controlled in about 80–90% of patients. If the bleeding continues, repeat injections can be given.
- If the bleeding continues in spite of the above measures, balloon tamponade is done.

Disadvantages of endoscopic sclerotherapy

1. Gastric varices cannot be managed by sclerotherapy.
2. Multiple oesophageal ulcers can develop at the injection site.
3. 10–20% of the patients develop low grade fever.
4. It can precipitate massive bleeding.
5. It can cause mediastinitis, left pleural effusion.
6. Chances of rebleeding are high. Hence, repeated injections are necessary.

C. Balloon tamponade (Figs 43.47 and 43.48)

- Balloon tamponade must be used as a **rescue procedure** and to bridge more definitive therapy in case of uncontrolled haemorrhage.
- Sengstaken's tube or its modification, the **Minnesota tube** is used. It acts directly by internal tamponade. It is passed through the nose. Gastric balloon is distended with up to 250–300 ml of air and oesophageal balloon with about 50–60 ml of air or to get a pressure of 20–30 mmHg. The tube cannot be kept in place for more than 12 to 24 hours as it can cause **pressure necrosis**. The method is reliable only in experienced hands.
- Recurrent bleeding is common after decompression.

D. TIPSS: Transjugular intrahepatic portosystemic stent shunt (Fig. 43.49)

- Consists of vascular placement of expandable metal stent across the tract created between hepatic vein and major branch of portal system.
- TIPSS helps a small group of patients (5 to 10%) who have refractory bleeding.

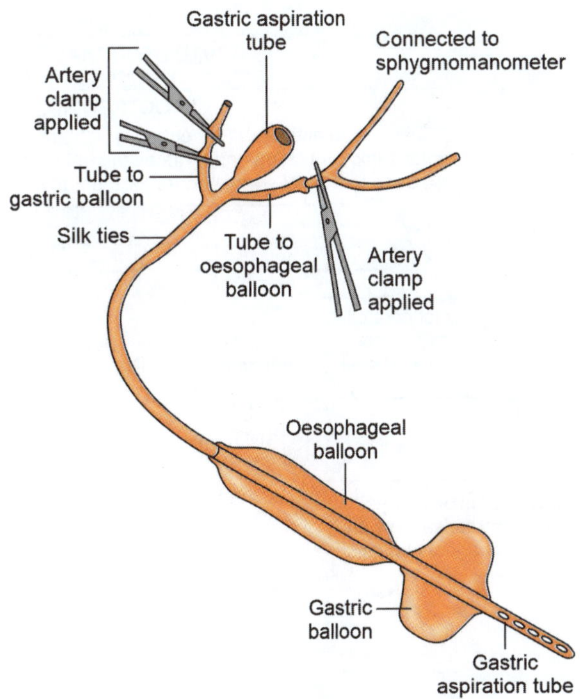

Fig. 43.48: Sengstaken tube sketch

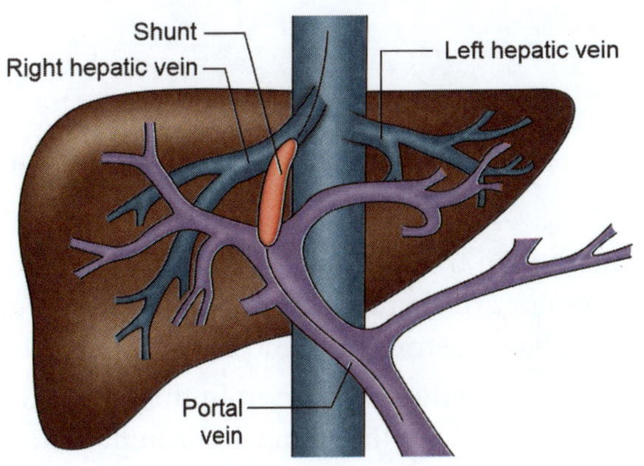

Fig. 43.49: TIPSS

- Low morbidity and mortality.
- Incidence of encephalopathy is similar to surgical shunts. Management of acute oesophageal variceal bleeding is shown in Fig. 43.50.

5. **Surgery:** It is of two types—devascularisation procedures and shunt procedures.

Pearls of Wisdom

Devascularisation procedures are aimed at reducing the pressure in the varices by disrupting the blood supply and shunt procedures are aimed at reducing portal pressure.

A. Devascularisation Procedures

1. Oesophageal transection

- It is done through left thoracoabdominal route called 'Milnes-Walker operation'.

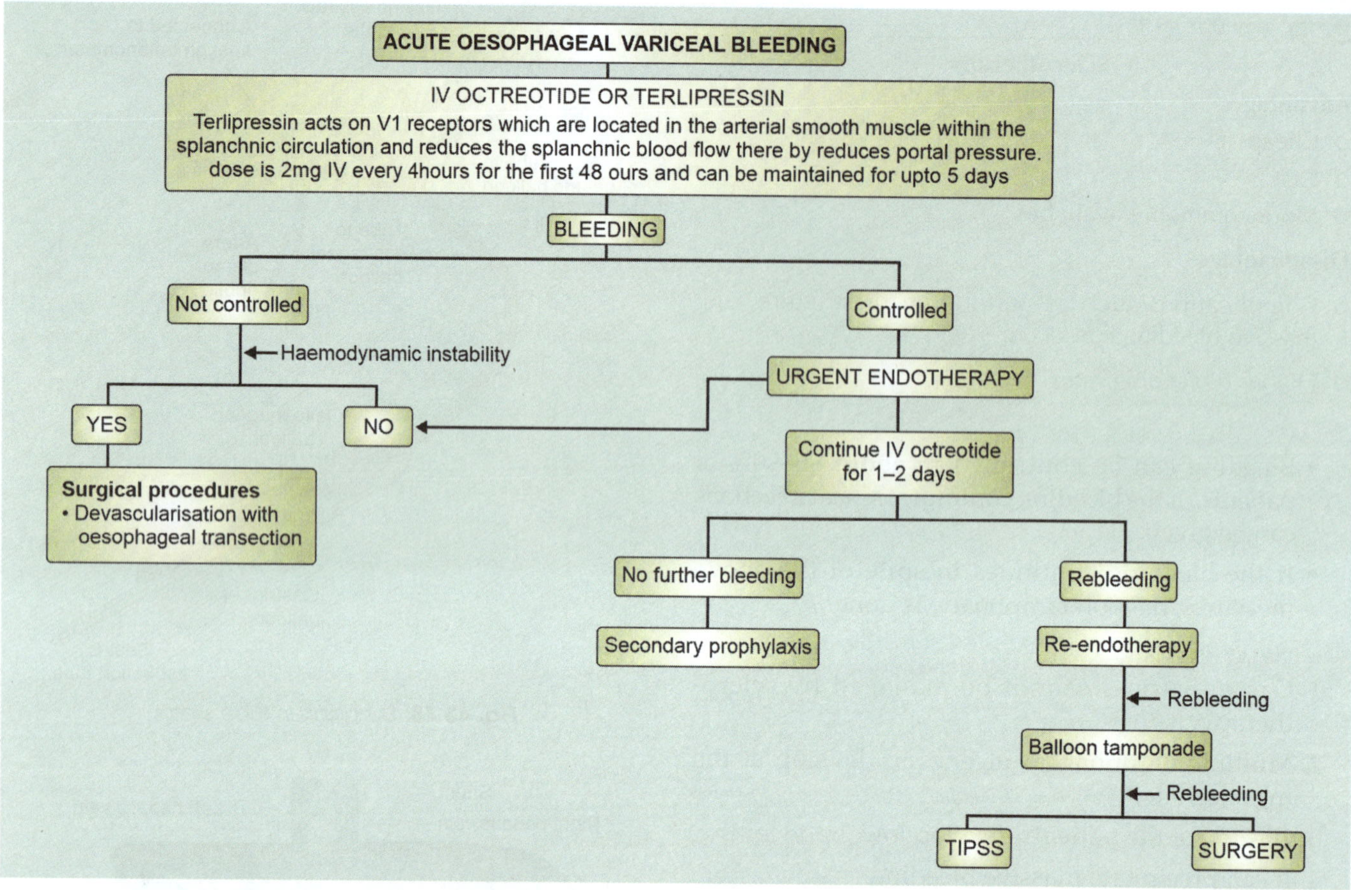

ACUTE OESOPHAGEAL VARICEAL BLEEDING

IV OCTREOTIDE OR TERLIPRESSIN
Terlipressin acts on V1 receptors which are located in the arterial smooth muscle within the splanchnic circulation and reduces the splanchnic blood flow there by reduces portal pressure. dose is 2mg IV every 4hours for the first 48 ours and can be maintained for upto 5 days

BLEEDING

- Not controlled
  - ← Haemodynamic instability
    - YES
      - **Surgical procedures**
        - Devascularisation with oesophageal transection
    - NO
- Controlled
  - URGENT ENDOTHERAPY (→ NO)
    - Continue IV octreotide for 1–2 days
      - No further bleeding
        - Secondary prophylaxis
      - Rebleeding
        - Re-endotherapy
        - ← Rebleeding
        - Balloon tamponade
        - ← Rebleeding
        - TIPSS / SURGERY

Fig. 43.50: Management of bleeding varices

- During the transection, varices are disconnected, bleeders are ligated or under-run, followed by oesophagogastric anastomosis.

2. **Gastric transection of Tanner:** In this operation the division is made in the stomach through abdominal route.
3. **Sugiura and Futagawa operation:** It is an extensive devascularisation procedure.

   Aim: To interrupt the intramural and submucosal veins.

   Procedure (Fig. 43.51): In this operation, the following procedures are done:
   - Splenectomy
   - Devascularisation of the greater curvature of the stomach and devascularisation of lesser curvature of the stomach as in highly selective vagotomy.
   - Oesophagogastric transection and suturing by using **EEA** (**E**nd-to-**E**nd **A**nastomosis) staplers. It is a major surgery. Mortality is around 10–15%. It is the most effective devascularisation.

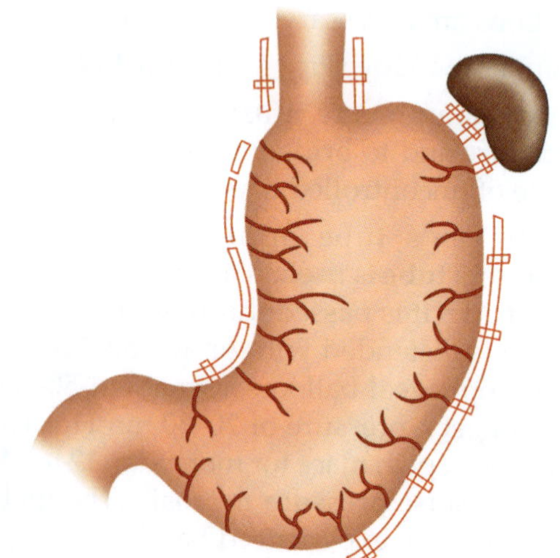

Fig. 43.51: Sugiura and Futagawa operation (splenectomy with devascularisation). Ideally done through thoracoabdominal incision

B. Portosystemic Shunt Procedures

Indications

1. Continuing variceal bleeding in spite of sclerotherapy wherein the general condition of the patient is good (Child's A, Child's B).

2. As an elective procedure in patients who had bleeding in the past.
3. The selection of shunt is based on the availability of a good vein. Jaundice, ascites and low albumin are contraindications for shunt surgery.

Types

1. **End-to-side portocaval shunt** (Fig. 43.52)
   - Portal vein is divided from the liver and the end is anastomosed to the side of inferior vena cava (IVC).
   - This controls the bleeding in 90–95% of patients but chances of encephalopathy is 30% because of sudden deprivation of liver blood supply.

   Indications: Cirrhosis of liver due to schistosomiasis, provided liver function is reasonably good.
2. **Side-to-side portocaval shunt:** Side of portal vein is anastomosed to side of inferior vena cava (Fig. 43.53).

   Advantage: Incidence of encephalopathy is 10%.

   Disadvantage: Control of bleeding is about 50–70%.
3. **Proximal splenorenal shunt** (Fig. 43.54): In this operation, spleen is removed. Then, proximal end of the splenic vein is sutured to the side of renal vein in the retroperitoneum. This is preferred in children.

   Proximal lienorenal shunt is probably the most useful shunt in patients of tropics as majority of them are EHPVO with some element of hypersplenism and having a good liver function. The proximal shunt includes splenectomy which cures hypersplenism too. These shunts are however difficult to perform but remain patent in about 90–95% in long term follow up.
4. **Distal splenorenal shunt (DSRS)—Warren's shunt** (Fig. 43.55)

   Indications
   - Extrahepatic portal hypertension with portal vein thrombosis, provided the splenic vein is dilated more than 1 cm.
   - It can also be done in cirrhosis of liver. Chances of encephalopathy is almost minimal after this procedure. In this operation, distal end of splenic vein is divided and sutured to the side of renal vein in the retroperitoneum. Postoperatively, ascites can occur due to extensive retroperitoneal dissection which damages lymphatics.
5. **Mesentericocaval shunt** (Figs 43.56 and 43.57)

   Indications
   1. Splenic vein is not dilated or thrombosed.
   2. Portal vein is thrombosed

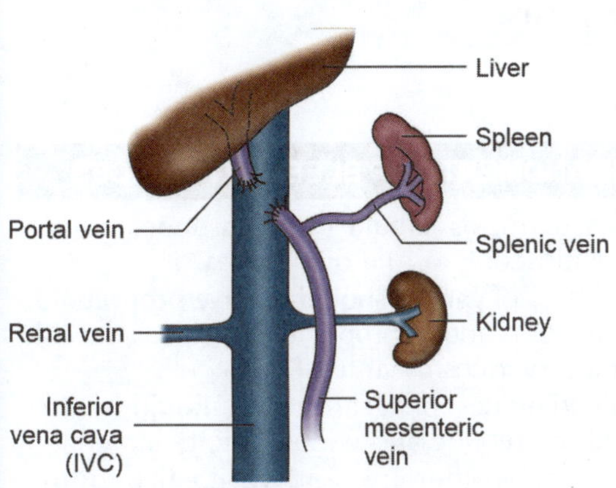

Fig. 43.52: End-to-side portocaval shunt

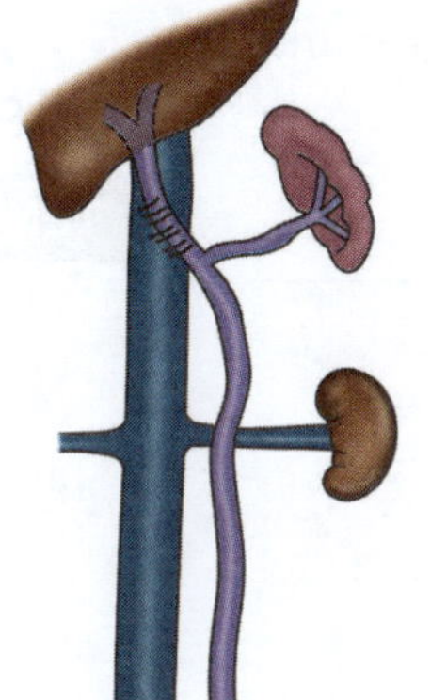

Fig. 43.53: Side-to-side portocaval shunt

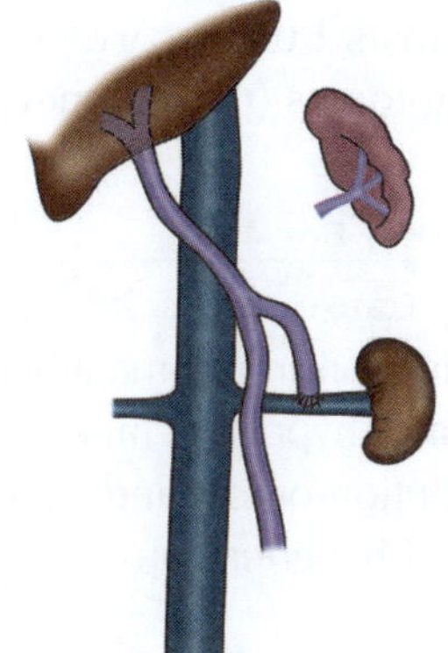

Fig. 43.54: Proximal splenorenal shunt

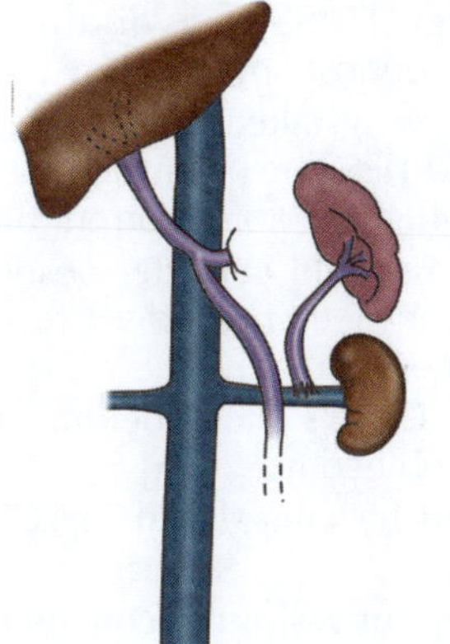

Fig. 43.55: Distal splenorenal shunt (DSRS)

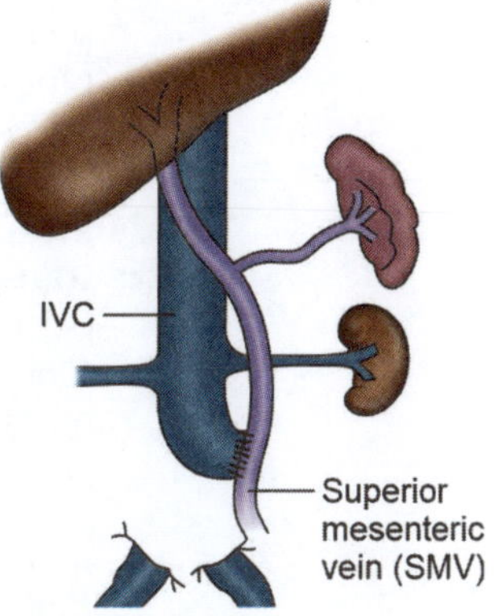

Fig. 43.56: Mesentericocaval shunt

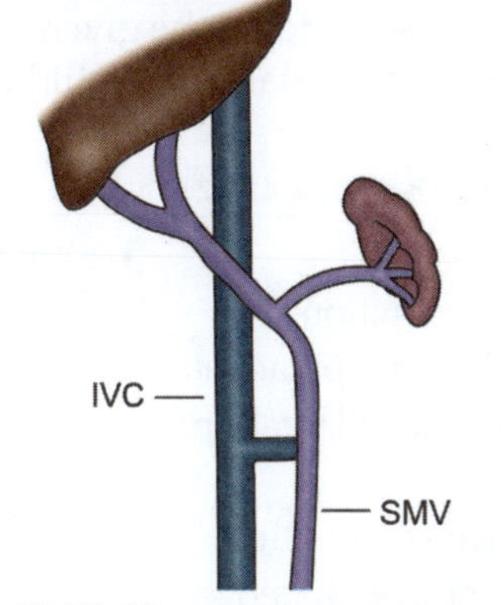

Fig. 43.57: Mesentericocaval shunt—H-graft

Procedure

- **The inferior vena cava is divided** and its proximal end is sutured to the side of superior mesenteric vein (SMV).
- Otherwise, a dacron graft can be placed between IVC and SMV. This is described as mesenterico-caval H-graft or jump graft.
- In children, IVC can be divided without fear of pedal oedema.

Shunt procedures have to be undertaken only by an experienced surgical gastroenterologist in an institution. These patients have to be carefully monitored in the postoperative period for possible blockage of shunt.

MISCELLANEOUS

CONTROL OF ASCITES IN PORTAL HYPERTENSION

- Ascites in portal hypertension is a slow, insidious accumulation of free peritoneal fluid, an occurrence in advanced liver disease (Key Box 43.21).
- It can be troublesome and refractory to commonly available treatment.
- Diagnosis is confirmed by ultrasound and aspiration.
- When there is a doubt regarding the diagnosis, **laparoscopy** is advisable which not only detects and confirms cirrhosis but also rules out other intra-abdominal pathologies (malignancy, tuberculosis, etc.).

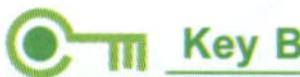 Key Box 43.21

Causes of Ascites in Portal Hypertension

- Reduction in plasma albumin
- Central hypovolaemia
- Retention of salt and water by kidneys
- Portal hypertension

Treatment (Key Box 43.22)

1. **Diuretics:** K^+ sparing diuretics such as spironolactone or frusemide can be given. However, hyponatraemia and hypokalaemia should be monitored.

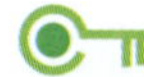 Key Box 43.22

Treatment

Salt restriction
Abdominal paracentesis
Liver transplantation
TIPSS
Intake of diuretics
SHunt—peritoneovenous
Remember as **SALTISH**

2. **Restriction of salt intake:** 20 mg/day is advised.
3. **Peritoneovenous shunt: Le Veen shunt**
   - Le Veen shunt is done by using a silastic tube to insert into ascites. It is then tunnelled subcutaneously to the neck and inserted under vision into internal jugular veins.
   - **Mode of action:** Ascitic fluid is drawn into systemic circulation with each respiration because of the presence of a one-way valve.

Complications

- Occlusion
- Displacement
- Infection

Other causes of hypoalbuminaemia are given in Key Box 43.23.

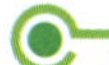 Key Box 43.23

Causes of Hypoalbuminaemia

Sepsis
Enteropathy—protein-losing
Poor nutrition—malnutrition
Syndrome—nephrotic
Injury—trauma
Sick Liver—chronic liver disease
Remember as **SEPSIS**

Miscellaneous

TEN COMMANDMENTS OF BLEEDING VARICES

1. All cases of cirrhosis **should undergo** upper gastrointestinal endoscopy to rule out varices.
2. Almost all cases of varices **should receive propranolol** prophylaxis. Propranolol prophylaxis reduces the risk of bleeding in varices by at least 10%.
3. Acutely bleeding oesophageal varices **should be first** treated with octreotide and endoscopic treatment.
4. Endoscopic sclerotherapy, and variceal banding **should be tried** in all patients with variceal bleeding. Banding is safer than sclerotherapy.
5. One should **consider TIPSS** if available, when pharmacotherapy and endoscopic therapy fail.
6. One should **consider Sengstaken-Blakemore** tube if endoscopic facilities and TIPSS are not available although it is associated with a high rate of recurrent bleeding.
7. Inexperienced surgeon **should consider oesophageal transection** to tide over bleeding varices resistant to octreotide and endoscopic treatment.
8. One **should consider Child's score** before planning measures to prevent rebleeding.
9. Surgical **shunts should be considered for Child's A and B** categories.
10. In **Child's C category, one should consider TIPSS followed by liver transplant.**

PORTAL HYPERTENSIVE GASTROPATHY

- Due to increased portal pressure and collaterals, vascular dilatation and ectasia occur in the stomach.
- Endoscopically they appear pink speckled with red mosaic-like pattern in the gastric mucosa.
- Lesions are diffuse (unlike GAVE—*see* page 570).
- They are responsible for about 3.5% of cases of upper GI bleeds and 15% in portal hypertension cases.
- They can present as acute bleeding with needs to be managed conservatively.
- Chronic bleeds present as anaemia.
- Propranolol is used to reduce portal pressure which in turn reduces bleeding.

PORTAL BILIOPATHY
(PSEUDOSCLEROSING CHOLANGITIS)

- It refers to bile duct changes due to portal hypertension.
- More common in extrahepatic portal hypertension.
- Portal cavernosa, ischaemic injury to the bile duct are the causes. Infection is also one of the causes.
- Changes in the bile duct include strictures and dilatation of both extra- and intrahepatic bile ducts secondary to varices encircling CBD and gallbladder wall. Choledocholithiasis is common.
- Can present with bile duct obstruction, cholangitis and bleeding into the CBD.
- Prolonged obstruction leads to secondary biliary cirrhosis.
- Investigation: U/S, CT scan, colour Doppler to image varices.
- Treatments: Endoscopic sphincterotomy, clear the CBD, stenting.
- Portosystemic shunt in failed endoscopic extraction of stone.

BUDD-CHIARI SYNDROME

It occurs due to obstruction to the hepatic vein.

Causes

1. Congenital: It is a potentially curable condition where in a web exists in the suprahepatic portion of inferior vena cava.
2. Clotting disorders—polycythaemia
3. Contraceptive pills
4. Cancerous infiltration of hepatic veins (hepatocellular carcinoma).
5. Crotalaria, a plant extract used in the tea.

Clinical Features

1. **Acute form** is dangerous, resulting in rapid enlargement of liver, severe abdominal pain, vomiting and hypotension.
2. **Chronic form** resembles cirrhosis: Hepatomegaly—firm, can be irregular, dilated veins over the abdominal wall. Bilateral pedal oedema which can be irritating, signs of liver cell failure are seen. Haematemesis occurs later.

Treatment

In congenital cases, if web can be proved by venacavography, it can be excised by transatrial meatotomy. However, in general, prognosis is very poor. Peritoneovenous shunt has to be considered as an alternate method to drain the ascitic fluid into one of the veins in the neck (internal jugular vein).

ROLE OF OCTREOTIDE IN SURGERY

1. **Variceal bleeding**
   - **Acute**—50 mg IV stat followed by 50 mg/h infusion for 120 hours.
   - Long-term **prophylaxis** is 100 mg s/c tds for 15 days.
2. **Pancreatic disorders**
   - ERCP-induced pancreatitis
   - Acute pancreatitis
   - Relapsing pancreatitis
   - Chronic pancreatitis
   - Pancreatic surgery—100 mg s/c 1 h prior to surgery and to continue 100 µg tds for 7 days.
3. **Bowel dysfunction—**AIDS-related diarrhoea, short bowel syndrome, dumping syndrome, chemotherapy-induced diarrhoea.
4. **Gastrointestinal fistulae.**
5. **Carcinoid and other neuroendocrine tumours.**
6. **Advanced malignancies:** Hepatocellular carcinoma, metastatic breast cancer, colonic cancer, pancreatic cancer.
7. **Acromegaly.**

LIVER TRANSPLANTATION

Details are given on page 1192.

Indications

- Decompensated cirrhosis: Chronic hepatitis C, primary biliary cirrhosis, etc.
- Acute fulminant hepatic failure (FHF): Causes are paracetamol overdosage, acute hepatitis B infection, Wilson's disease, drugs.

Signs and Symptoms of Decompensated Liver

- Hepatic encephalopathy
- Ascites
- Spontaneous bacterial peritonitis
- Hepatorenal syndrome
- Hyperbilirubinaemia, coagulopathy

Types

1. **Living donor transplant:** Easily available, no waiting period but potential risk to donor (normal person) is present.
2. **Cadaveric:** Preserving organ by hypothermia (Key Box 43.24)
   - Waiting period
   - No risk to donor
   - To be done within 12 hours, ideally within 6 hours.

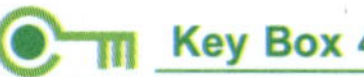
Key Box 43.24

Organ Preservation

- Hypothermia and by cold storage solutions
- University of Wisconsin solution is commonly used. It contains:
  – Lactobionate: Prevents intracellular swelling
  – Hydroxyethyl startch: Decreased interstitial oedema, decreased hypothermia-induced damage to cells.

Types of Liver Transplantation

- Partial hepatectomy: Usually right lobe (60% of total liver)
- Split liver transplant: Divide into two functioning units and transplant into two patients.

Procedure

- Mobilise the diseased liver and isolate vena cava, portal vein, hepatic artery and bile duct.
- Remove the diseased liver.
- Donor liver is transplanted and anastomosis of various structures done.

Complications

- Thrombosis of hepatic artery
- Thrombosis of portal vein
- Bile leak
- Nonfunctioning of hepatic allograft
- Infections

HAEMOBILIA

Definition

Bleeding from liver into the biliary tree. There is usually a **communication between a blood vessel and the bile duct** or any other part of the biliary tree.

- Accidental trauma
- Malignant liver disease
- Portal hypertension
- Percutaneous diagnostic and therapeutic procedures
- Vascular disease of hepatic artery
- Gallstones may get impacted, erode the hepatic artery and cause life-threatening haemobilia.

Clinical Features

- **Triad of Sandblom**—jaundice, pain and melaena
- Pain abdomen—colicky
- Obstructive jaundice
- Haematemesis or melaena

Investigation

LFT, USG abdomen, selective arteriography, upper GI endoscopy.

Treatment

- Selective arterial embolisation (angiographic, under fluoroscopic guidance)
- Blood transfusions and antibiotics to prevent cholangitis.

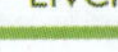

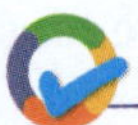

Multiple Choice Questions

1. **Which of the following statements is false about hepatic encephalopathy?**
   A. It is caused by ammonia
   B. Precipitated by sedatives
   C. Not precipitated by bleeding into gastrointestinal tract
   D. Precipitated by diuretics

2. **About hepatorenal syndrome following are true *except:***
   A. It can occur in sepsis
   B. Most of them have advanced liver disease
   C. It is associated with profuse intrarenal vasodilatation
   D. Orthotopic liver transplantation can reverse hepatorenal syndrome

3. **Which of the following is not the cause for over-production of bilirubin?**
   A. Total parenteral nutrition
   B. Haemolytic anaemias
   C. Blood transfusion
   D. Gilbert's syndrome

4. **Triad of Sandblom includes the following *except*:**
   A. Colicky abdominal pain
   B. Obstructive jaundice
   C. Haematemesis or melaena
   D. Sepsis

5. **The following are indications for percutaneous method for drainage of pyogenic liver abscess *except*:**
   A. Superficial abscesses
   B. Abscess with no intra-abdominal pathology
   C. Abscesses of unknown aetiology
   D. Multiple abscesses

6. **Very tender liver is a feature of the following *except*:**
   A. Secondaries in the liver
   B. Amoebic liver abscess
   C. Hepatoma
   D. Congestive cardiac failure

7. **A differentiating feature of amoebic liver abscess from acute cholecystitis is:**
   A. Intercostal tenderness
   B. Abdominal tenderness
   C. Guarding
   D. Fever

8. **The drug of choice for the treatment of amoebic liver abscess is:**
   A. Penicillin B. Gentamicin
   C. Metronidazole D. Cotrimoxazole

9. **The following are scolicidal agents *except*:**
   A. Hypertonic saline
   B. Chlorhexidine
   C. Sodium hypochlorite
   D. Hydroxyethyl starch

10. **Indications for PAIR in the treatment of hydatid cyst includes:**
   A. Relapse following surgery
   B. Multiple septal divisions
   C. Communicating cysts
   D. Dead or inactive cysts

11. **The following feature is true about *Echinococcus multilocularis* *except*:**
   A. Alveolar echinococcosis
   B. Causes malignancy
   C. Poorly demarcated honeycombed cystic lesion
   D. Infiltrates liver and invades vascular system

12. **A 65-year-old patient presents with the following: Serum bilirubin: 4 mg%, serum albumin: 1.8 mg%, INR: 2. He has gross ascites and is drowsy. What Child-Pugh Class does he belong to?**
   A. A B. B
   C. C D. D

13. **The following are features of polycystic liver disease *except*:**
   A. They are usually asymptomatic
   B. The cysts do not produce liver cell failure
   C. They are acquired
   D. Cysts also occur in kidneys and pancreas

14. **Which of the following is the commonest benign tumour of the liver?**
   A. Haemangioma
   B. Adenoma
   C. Focal nodular hyperplasia
   D. Hepatoma

15. **For purposes of hepatic resection, the liver can be divided into ______ number of segments.**
   A. 2 B. 4
   C. 6 D. 8

16. The main portal fissure is also called:

A. Cantlie's line
B. Murphy's line
C. Spigelian line
D. Macewan's line

17. The following conditions are associated with increased risk of hepatocellular carcinoma *except:*

A. Hepatitis B carrier state
B. Cirrhosis
C. Malignant hydatid cyst
D. Aflatoxin consumption

18. Up to ______ segments of the liver can be resected safely without the danger of hepatic failure provided rest of the liver is normal.

A. 2 B. 3
C. 4 D. 5

19. Transcatheter arterial embolisation is a good option in the treatment of hepatocellular carcinoma in following situation:

A. Serum bilirubin >3 mg%
B. Tumour thrombus in the main portal trunk
C. Early hepatocellular carcinoma
D. Inoperable tumours

20. Which of the following is true criteria for secondaries in the liver?

A. Single lobe enlargement
B. Rounded border
C. Soft in consistency
D. Nodular liver

21. Commonest gastrointestinal tract primary in a nodular liver secondaries is from:

A. Stomach B. Pancreas
C. Gallbladder D. Duodenum

22. Portal hypertension is defined as a portal venous pressure exceeding _____ mmHg.

A. 5 B. 10
C. 15 D. 20

23. Portal vein normally carries _______ % of blood supply to liver.

A. 25 B. 50
C. 75 D. 100

24. Causes of bulky secondaries include the following *except*:

A. Malignant melanoma
B. Carcinoid tumours
C. Colloid carcinoma rectum
D. Testicular tumours

25. Which of the following is true about the use of vasopressin in variceal bleeding?

A. 20 units is diluted in 200 ml of saline and given over 20 min
B. Causes coronary vasodilatation
C. Is a powerful inotrope
D. Is a splanchnic vasodilator and reduces pressure in the splanchnic vessels

26. Gastric transection of Tanner is an operation performed for:

A. Carcinoma stomach
B. Carcinoma pancreas
C. Portal hypertension
D. Hepatocellular carcinoma

27. About sorafenib following are true *except*:

A. It is tyrosine kinase inhibitor
B. It has anti-angiogenesis property
C. Vascular endothelial growth factor is inhibited by sorafenib
D. It is not a drug for hepatocellular carcinoma

Answers

1. D	**2.** C	**3.** A	**4.** D	**5.** D	**6.** A	**7.** A	**8.** C	**9.** D	**10.** A
11. B	**12.** C	**13.** C	**14.** A	**15.** D	**16.** A	**17.** C	**18.** B	**19.** D	**20.** D
21. A	**22.** C	**23.** C	**24.** D	**25.** A	**26.** C	**27.** D			

CHAPTER

44

Spleen

INTRODUCTION

Diseases of the spleen and causes of enlargement of the spleen are a great concern for physicians. Dozens of differential diagnoses of splenomegaly are being taught in medicine. However, a surgeon's role in the treatment of an enlarged spleen is minimal. However, it is he **who does this 'magic' of removing** the spleen within minutes and saves the life of a patient with a ruptured spleen. A surgeon plays a major role by **treating hypersplenism with splenectomy**. In this chapter, only topics related to surgeon's interest are dealt with. Other topics are mentioned briefly.

SURGICAL ANATOMY (Fig. 44.1)

Competency

SU28.11: Describe the applied anatomy of spleen.

The spleen is an anatomically small organ, hidden underneath the **9**th to **11**th ribs (dull note on percussion) measuring 1 × 3 × 5 inches and weighing about 7 oz (80–300 g). It lies in intimate contact with the undersurface of the diaphragm. This explains why a splenic abscess can rupture through the diaphragm causing empyema. When blood collects due to splenic injury, it irritates the diaphragm causing referred pain to the shoulder tip (**Kehr's sign**).

The **anterior border** is **notched** and is in contact with the stomach. It is enclosed by the **gastrocolic omentum**. The surgical importance of this is that when traction is applied on the stomach during vagotomy, a splenic capsular tear can occur, resulting in bleeding. The **two leaves** of gastrocolic omentum pass backwards in front of the kidney forming the **lienorenal ligament** (Fig. 44.2). This ligament is responsible for some part of the posterior fixation of the spleen. When this ligament is divided, the spleen can be brought to the surface of the wound during splenectomy.

The inferior part of the **hilum** of the spleen is (just) in contact with the **tail of the pancreas**. Often, during an emergency splenectomy, the tail of pancreas can get injured, resulting in a pancreatic fistula (Figs 44.2 and 44.3)

Splenic Parenchyma

- It is **highly vascular.**
- Splenic pulp has red pulp and white pulp.
- **Red pulp** is a honeycombed vascular space which is made up of cords of reticular cells and sinuses.
- **White pulp consists of lymphatic tissue** and lymphoid follicles containing lymphocytes, plasma cells and macrophages.

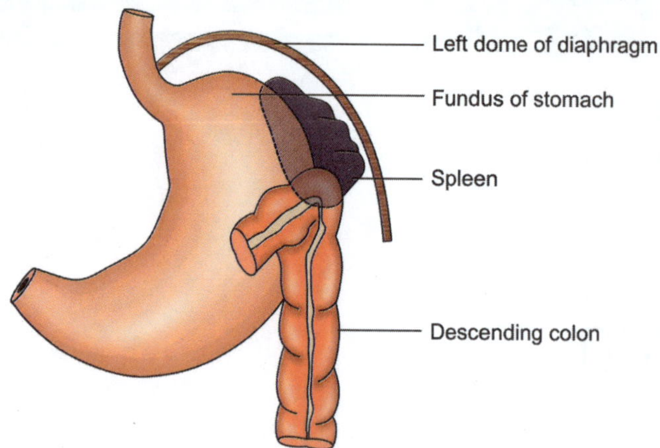

Fig. 44.1: Location of the spleen in relation to the fundus of the stomach and the diaphragm

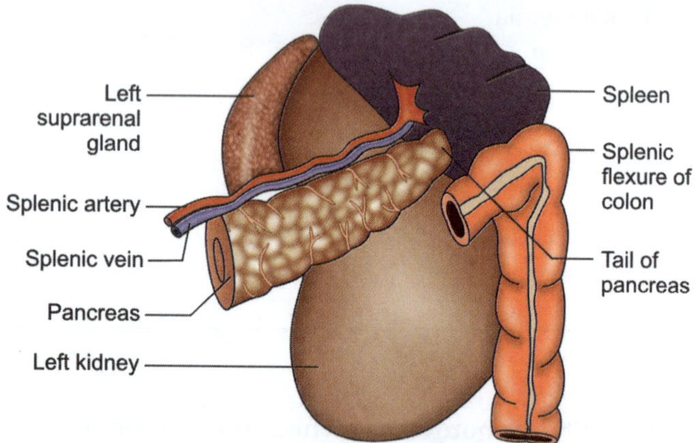

Fig. 44.2: Visceral relations of the spleen

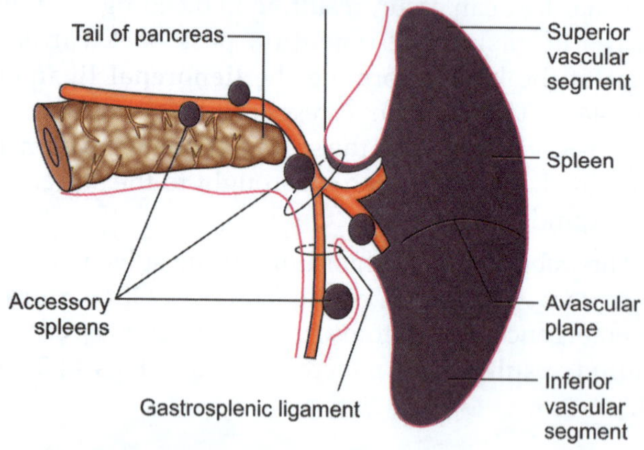

Lienorenal ligament containing tail of pancreas and splenic artery
Tail of pancreas
Superior vascular segment
Spleen
Accessory spleens
Avascular plane
Inferior vascular segment
Gastrosplenic ligament

Fig. 44.3: Peritoneal ligaments attached to the spleen and common sites of accessory spleen

Blood Supply

- **Arterial supply:** Splenic artery is a branch of celiac artery. At the hilum of the spleen, it divides into 4–5 trabecular arteries and then branches into central arteries. Central arteries pass through white pulp and give radial branches to periphery including distal red pulp. Anatomical knowledge of these branches helps when performing partial splenectomy for ruptured spleen. (The blood flow rate through spleen is about 300 ml/min.)
- Spleen has 3–7 segments and each has its own vascular supply. Splenic artery divides into larger superior artery and smaller inferior artery. ***Lacerations of the spleen parallel to segmental vessels*** result in minimal haemorrhage. Lacerations perpendicular to the segments result in significant haemorrhage.
- In children, splenic capsule is thick and more tolerant to damage. Hence majority of the children with blunt abdominal trauma to the spleen are managed by conservative/non-operative treatment.
- **Venous drainage:** Four to five branches of the vein join and form the splenic vein. This forms the portal vein by joining with superior mesenteric vein behind the 2nd part of the duodenum.

Lymphatic Drainage

The lymph drains into hilar nodes, then into retropancreatic nodes and finally into celiac nodes. Since it has intimate contact with the fundus of the stomach and tail of the pancreas, spleen also used to be removed (nowadays not done) along with the stomach and tail of the pancreas during radical gastrectomy and distal pancreatectomy.

FUNCTIONS OF THE SPLEEN

1. **Destruction:** The process of removal of abnormal aged, damaged red blood cells is called *culling*. *Culling*, the Greek word, implies sorting a collection of two groups: One that will be kept and the other that will be rejected. For example, spherocytes, in hereditary, spherocytosis are broken down in spleen. This happens in red pulp.
2. **Production:** Production of lymphocytes, monocytes and plasma cells. Lymphopoiesis continues throughout life. Lymphocytes take part in immune response of the body.
3. **Antibody production:** Spleen synthesises antibodies in its white pulp. It removes antibody-coated bacteria and antibody-coated blood cells via blood and lymph node circulation.
4. **Immune response:** White pulp is composed of Malpighian corpuscles. They are composed of B lymphocytes and T lymphocytes—which are in periarteriolar lymphoid sheaths (PALS). Thus white pulp plays a major role in active immune response through humoral and all mediated pathways.
5. **Reservoir of platelets:** It is a storehouse of platelets, which are released into circulation in an emergency

situation. Thus when spleen is enlarged, 80% of the platelets are sequestrated resulting in thrombocytopenia.

Pearls of Wisdom

Splenomegaly typically involves expansion of red pulp.

6. **Immune function:** It is the major site for synthesis of tuftsin, a peptide that stimulates phagocytic activity of leucocytes. Opsonins are antibodies produced by spleen against bacteria and fungi.
7. **Removal:** Heinz bodies, Howell-Jolly bodies, etc. are removed from RBCs. These cells are non-deformable intracellular substances.
8. **Erythrocyte production:** During foetal development, white and red blood cells production occur till 5th month of gestation. In adults, in case of myelofibrosis, erythopoiesis can occur.

CONGENITAL ABNORMALITIES

1. **Accessory spleens: Splenunculi:** They are found in about 10–20% of the population.
   - They can be found near the hilum of spleen, tail of pancreas, splenic ligaments or in the mesocolon.
   - In diseases of the spleen (haemolytic anaemia, thrombocytopenic purpura), all these accessory spleens have to be removed along with spleen.
2. **Splenic agenesis** is rare.
3. **Polysplenia** is rare. It occurs due to failure of splenic fusion.
4. **Wandering spleen** is due to loose ligaments. It is more vulnerable for torsion.
5. **Hamartoma:** Rare, small masses of 1 cm in diameter. It may be in lymphoid tissue also (Hamartoma = misfire).

RUPTURE OF THE SPLEEN

Competency

SU28.1.1: Describe the clinical features, investigations and principles of management of splenic injuries.

CAUSES

- **Blunt injury abdomen**
  - Injury to the left side of chest, left lower rib fractures, due to fall from a tree, road traffic accidents can be associated with splenic rupture.
  - Retroperitoneal haemorrhage, fracture spine and renal injuries may be associated with splenic injury.
- **Penetrating injuries** to the abdomen may cause **rupture of spleen**.
- **Spontaneous rupture** of the spleen is seen in malaria and infectious mononucleosis, rarely in sarcoidosis, haemolytic anaemia and leukaemia.
- **Iatrogenic:** Splenic capsule may be torn during surgical procedures such as vagotomy or gastrectomy due to traction on the stomach.

TYPES OF INJURIES

Most of these injuries are diagnosed by CT scan today (CT classification is given).

1. **Subcapsular haematoma:** A capsular tear or parenchymal tear results in subcapsular haematoma.
2. **Clean (incised wounds):** This can happen in sharp injuries, staal injuries (not common) or operative injuries.
3. **Lacerated wounds:** Often they are multiple as in blunt injuries abdomen.
4. **Hilar injuries** with **pedicle avulsion** are the most serious injuries. Need urgent laparotomy and ligation of bleeders and splenectomy. Otherwise, death will occur.
5. **Splenic injury** with other organs. Tail of pancreas, diaphragm, left kidney, left colon.

Splenic Injury CT Scan Grading (Fig. 44.4)

Grade I:	Nonexpanding subcapsular haematoma <10% surface area
	Nonbleeding capsular laceration with <2 cm deep parenchymal involvement.
Grade II:	Nonexpanding subcapsular haematoma 10–50% surface area.
	Nonexpanding intraparenchymal haematoma <2 cm diameter
	Bleeding capsular tear or parenchymal laceration 1–3 cm deep
Grade III:	Expanding subcapsular haematoma or intraparenchymal.
	Bleeding subcapsular. Haematoma or subcapsular haematoma >50% surface area
	Intraparenchymal haematoma >2 cm
	Parenchymal laceration >3 cm deep
Grade IV:	Ruptured intraparenchymal haematoma with active bleeding.
	Laceration involving segmental or renal vessel >25% spleen volume devascularised.
Grade V:	Completely shattered or avulsed spleen.
	Hilar laceration which devascularises entire spleen.

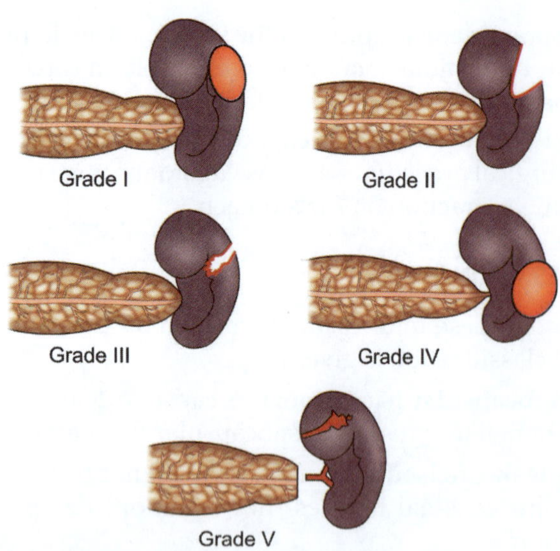

Fig. 44.4: Various grades of splenic injury

CLINICAL PRESENTATION

It can be divided into three groups:

1. **Tearing of splenic vessels:** Avulsion of splenic pedicle can result in severe haemorrhage and shock. Death can occur within a few minutes. Even in the best of the situations, death cannot be prevented often.
2. **A slow developing haemorrhagic shock** followed by recovery. Examination reveals evidence of intraperitoneal bleeding. This can occur due to a capsular tear or injury to the splenic parenchyma. Its clinical features are as follows:
   - Anaemia—pallor
   - Pulse—tachycardia, more than 100/min
   - BP—low/hypotension
   - Cold, clammy extremities
   - Abdominal distension
   - Paralytic ileus develops slowly
   - Guarding and rigidity
   - **Kehr's sign** is positive. Irritation of undersurface of the diaphragm by the blood causes irritation of phrenic nerve (C3, 4). Thus, this pain is referred to shoulder region (supraclavicular nerve C4).

Pearls of Wisdom

Kehr's sign can be elicited by elevation of the foot end of bed for about 10 minutes.

   - **Ballance's sign:** Blood in the vicinity of spleen is fresh blood which is coagulated and blood in the periphery is not coagulated. Hence, there will not be shifting dullness on the left side of the abdomen but can be present on the right side.
   - **Saegesser's splenic point of tenderness:** An area of tenderness on the left side between sternomastoid and scalenus medius (rare sign).
3. **Initial features of haemorrhagic shock, recovery and sudden haemorrhagic shock** after a few hours to a few days. It is due to the following reasons:
   - Greater omentum seals off a tear which gets reopened after some time. Time period is called **"latent period of Randet"**.
   - A subcapsular haematoma which had developed, ruptures after some time.
   - Associated injury to the tail of pancreas causes release of enzymes which digests the tissues at a later date. This variety is called "delayed type of shock" or delayed rupture of spleen.

Pearls of Wisdom

In polytrauma, if a hypotensive patient responds to intravenous fluids, it is a hypovolaemic shock. Head injury is rarely a cause of hypovolaemic shock.

COMPLICATIONS OF SPLENIC INJURIES

1. Haemorrhagic shock—if not treated—multiorgan failure results.
2. Disseminated intravascular coagulation due to massive bleeding and blood transfusion.
3. Injuries to the tail of pancreas—manifesting later as pancreatic ascites, pancreatic fistula or pseudocyst of pancreas.
4. Splenic artery pseudoaneurysm.
5. Splenic arteriovenous fistula.

INVESTIGATIONS

1. **Hb%** estimation, PCV (packed cell volume) estimation (however, in appropriate cases, it should be repeated at frequent intervals to detect continuing haemorrhage).
2. **Four quadrant tap/aspiration** by using a fine needle (23 gauge) demonstrates blood either fresh or old. However, diagnostic peritoneal lavage **(DPL)** is more reliable (*vide infra*).
3. **Emergency USG** can reveal a splenic tear, a subcapsular haematoma and can rule out other injuries. It is the most important investigation in suspected cases of splenic injury.
4. CT scan is more reliable. It should be used in cases of doubtful diagnosis and stable patients.[1] It also rules out hollow viscus perforation, pancreatic injuries, etc. (Fig. 44.5).

[1]Deaths have been reported in CT scan room, in unstable patients with haemoperitoneum.

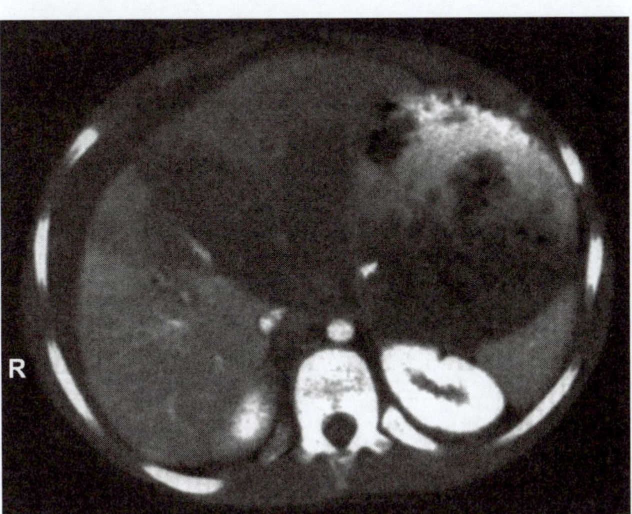

Fig. 44.5: CECT showing splenic and liver injuries

5. **Diagnostic peritoneal lavage (DPL):** It is indicated in blunt injury abdomen where there are **equivocal signs** or **doubtful signs** of peritonitis.
   - **Indications:**
     - Unconscious patient with polytrauma with signs of abdominal injury.
     - Unexplained shock
     - Associated spinal cord injury
   - **Procedure** (Fig. 44.6):
     - A 1 cm incision is made in the subumbilical region under local anaesthesia (LA) after emptying the bladder. The peritoneum is opened and a 12 or 14 Fr peritoneal dialysis catheter is introduced into the peritoneal cavity.
     - The skin is closed and 1000 ml normal saline is allowed to flow over 30 minutes.

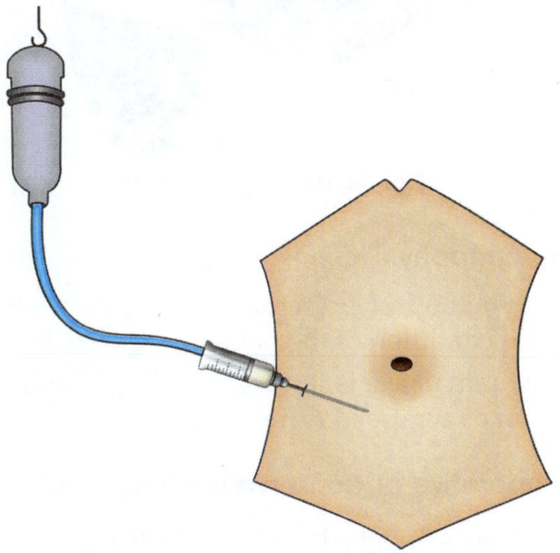
Fig. 44.6: Diagnostic peritoneal lavage

     - The patient is turned to the right and left sides and fluid is allowed to flow out.
   - **DPL is positive when:**
     1. Fresh blood of more than 20 ml is removed immediately after inserting dialysis catheter and it does not clot.
     2. RBC count 1,00,000/mm^3 or WBC >500/mm^3.
     3. Amylase level of over 175 units/dl.
     4. Bile, food or any other fresh contents.
     5. Gram stain is positive in the contents of lavage.
   - Diagnostic accuracy is around 95%. DPL is useful to rule out intestinal injury in addition to intra-peritoneal bleeding.

Pearls of Wisdom

DPL is more sensitive for mesenteric injury than CT scan. However, in early diagnosis of hollow viscus injuries, DPL is superior to CT scan. However, with the availability of ultrasound and CT scans, this investigation is rarely performed today.

6. **Plain X-ray abdomen**[1] erect **should not be done in an emergency situation** when patients are in shock. Findings of splenic trauma in plain X-ray abdomen are given here.
   - Splenic outline may not be seen clearly.
   - Fundic air bubble may be indented by the haematoma.
   - Psoas shadow is obliterated (KUB X-ray).
   - Evidence of fracture of lower ribs.
   - Evidence of fluid in the peritoneal cavity—**'ground glass' appearance**
   - Elevation of left dome of diaphragm.

TREATMENT (Key Box 44.1 and Fig. 44.7)

Key Box 44.1

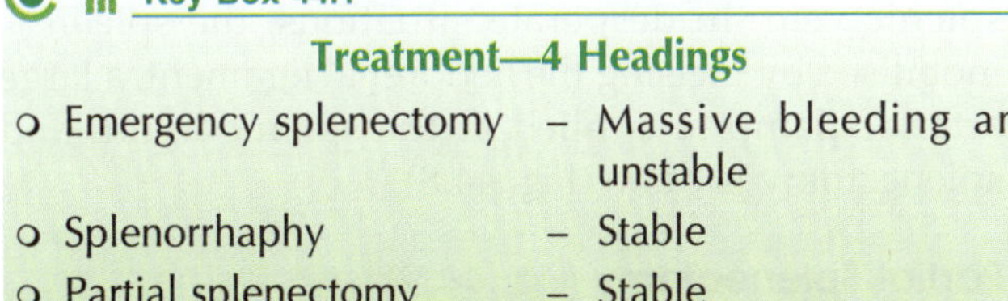

Treatment—4 Headings

Emergency splenectomy	– Massive bleeding and unstable
Splenorrhaphy	– Stable
Partial splenectomy	– Stable
Nonoperative	– Stable patient

1. Emergency Splenectomy

- Haemodynamic instability is the main indication for emergency splenectomy. Blood pressure less than 90 mmHg and heart rate more than 130 per minute is a clear indication for surgery.

  When there is active bleeding with hypotension due to large lacerations, emergency splenectomy is the

[1]Please do not make an unstable patient stand for the sake of X-ray. He may collapse due to hypotension.

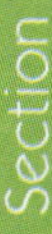

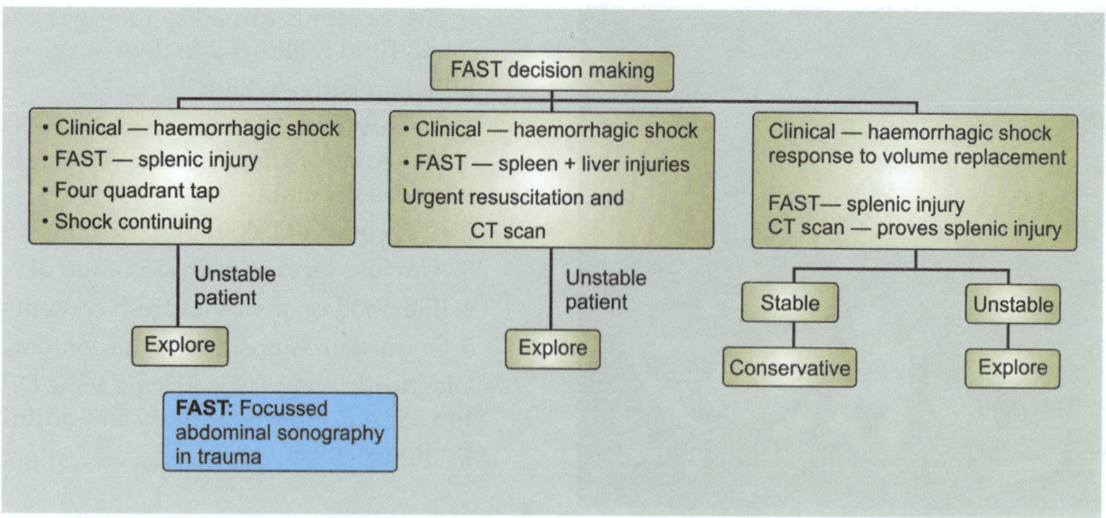

Fig. 44.7: Management of splenic rupture

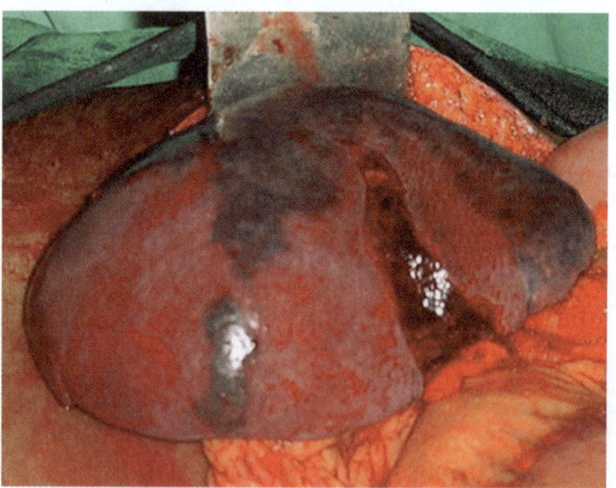

Fig. 44.8: Large laceration of the spleen

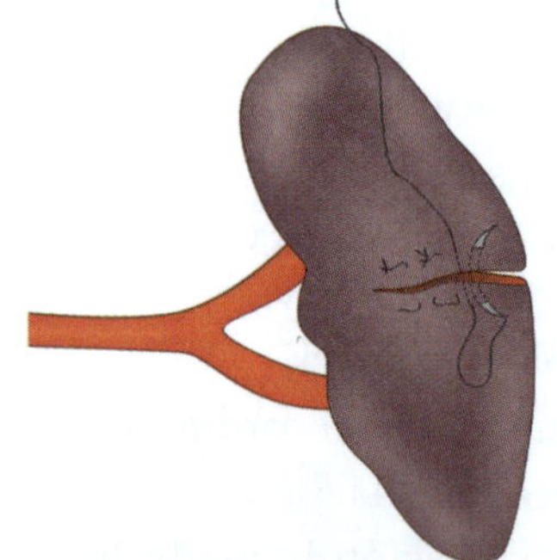

Fig. 44.9: Partial splenectomy

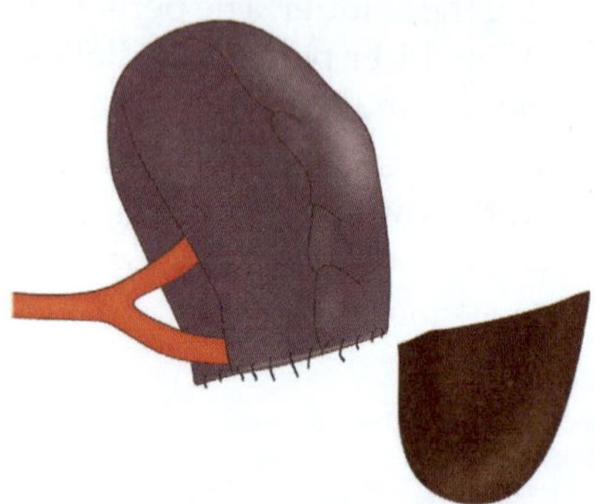

Fig. 44.10: Splenorrhaphy

treatment of choice since it is quick, easy to perform and can be life-saving. The splenic artery is ligated first at the upper border of pancreas followed by splenic vein. In desperate situations, the spleen is mobilised by incising the lienorenal ligament, a large arterial clamp is applied at the splenic hilum and splenectomy is done (Fig. 44.8).

2. Partial Splenectomy (Fig. 44.9)

- It can be done because the splenic artery gives an **upper polar branch and a lower polar branch** which again divides into 2 branches. Hence, when one of the branches of splenic artery is ligated, the bleeding stops and a partial splenectomy can be done comfortably.
- After splenectomy, the spleen can be cut into multiple pieces and can be implanted within the greater omentum. The spleen survives because of neovascularisation and functions like a spleen in the production of antibodies. This can be done in children.

3. Splenorrhaphy (Fig. 44.10)

- It is a method of preservation of spleen when the general condition of the patient is reasonably good.
- In this, a small tear is sutured by using chromic catgut and can be wrapped using greater omentum.

4. Nonoperative or Conservative Treatment

- It is safe in selected adult and paediatric patients with isolated splenic injuries.
- Small risk of delayed rupture should be explained to the patient (Key Box 44.2).

Key Box 44.2

Nonoperative Treatment Patient Selection

1. Haemodynamically stable patients after initial evaluation.
2. No other associated organ injuries which require laparotomy.
3. No extra-abdominal injuries which may preclude assessment of abdomen.
4. Facilities for emergency resuscitation, ultrasonography, CT scan should be available.
5. Patient must be willing for hospitalisation and close observation.
6. Regular monitoring by duty doctors, expert nursing staff who maintain hourly vital charts.

- Patients are admitted in intensive care unit. Serial monitoring of haemoglobin, total WBC counts are done. Abdominal girth and blood pressure are monitored. If there is any doubt of hypotension, exploration is done.
- While managing following patients, utmost care should be given with the non-operative treatment.
  1. Older patients above the age of 50
  2. Grade 3 and 4 injury
  3. More than 500 ml of blood detected by the CT scan
  4. Other solid organ injury (liver)
  5. Systemic vascular abnormalities, such as pseudoaneurysm or AV fistula, etc.

Pearls of Wisdom

If any vascular abnormalities are detected by CT scan, embolisation should be attempted first. In majority of the cases, bleeding will stop. If bleeding continues, they should be taken for splenectomy.

EARLY: COMPLICATIONS OF SPLENECTOMY

1. **Pancreatic injury (0–6%):** Treated by drain placement and measuring drain amylase. Usually, it is a minor discharge, generally settles over a few days.
2. **Vascular injury (2–3%):** Slippage of ligature (splenic artery), hilar dissection, capsular tear during retraction.

   Needs to be identified and sutured or coagulated or clamped.
3. **Injury to bowel:** Colon, stomach. These can be avoided with careful dissection techniques. During ligation of short gastric arteries too close to the stomach side, injury to the stomach can occur. It is repaired in two layers. Colonic injury can occur during dissection to separate the lower pole. It is also repaired in the similar manner.
4. **Diaphragmatic injury:** This can happen when adhesions are present between spleen and diaphragm due to perisplenitis or recurrent infarctions. Simple suturing is enough, if recognised.
5. **Splenosis:** This refers to multiple small implants of splenic tissue on the peritoneal surface following traumatic rupture of spleen. They can give rise to adhesions.
6. **Pulmonary:** These are common complications. Generally get unnoticed. It can range from minor cough to atelectasis to pneumonia and pleural effusion. Basal atelectasis is one of the common causes of postoperative fever.
7. **Paralytic ileus:** Treated by drip and suction.
8. **Haematemesis** can occur due to congestion of the gastric mucosa as a result of ligation of the short gastric vessels.
9. **Subphrenic abscess:** Not common. If it occurs, percutaneous drainage and antibiotics (Fig. 44.11).
10. **Wound problems:** Haematomas, seromas and wound infection.
11. **Thrombocytosis and thrombotic complications:** Sometimes it can be dangerous. They can present as abdominal pain and vomiting which is confused for incision pain, gastritis, etc. Ultrasound examination is a must. One of our patients had portal vein thrombosis which was managed by anticoagulants. Platelet count after splenectomy was 8 lakh/mm^3.

INDICATIONS FOR SPLENECTOMY

I. Always indicated

a. Primary splenic tumour
b. Hereditary spherocytosis

II. Usually indicated

a. Primary hypersplenism
b. Chronic ITP
c. Splenic vein thrombosis
d. Splenic abscess

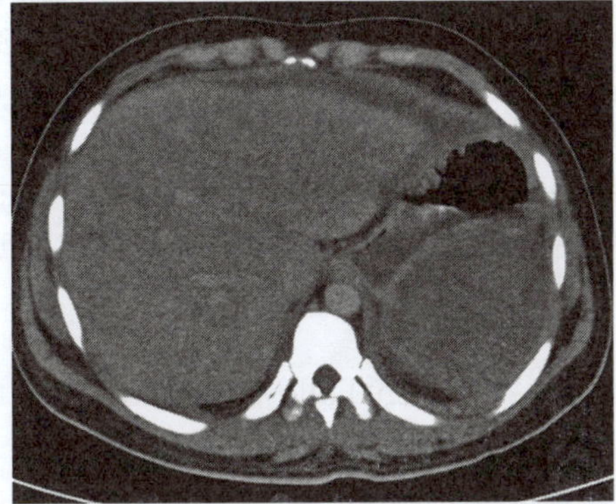

Fig. 44.11: Post-splenectomy large collection

III. Sometimes indicated

a. Splenic injury
b. Autoimmune haemolytic disease
c. Elliptocytosis haemolysis
d. Nonspherocytic congenital haemolytic anaemia
e. Hodgkin's disease with anaemia
f. Thrombotic thrombocytopenic purpura
g. Idiopathic myelofibrosis
h. Splenic artery aneurysm
i. Wiskott-Aldrich syndrome (Key Box 44.3)
j. Gaucher's disease

IV. Rarely indicated

a. Chronic leukaemia
b. Thalassaemia major
c. Sickle cell anaemia
d. Felty's syndrome
e. Hairy cell leukaemia

Key Box 44.3

Wiskott-Aldrich Syndrome

- X-linked disorder predominantly presents as features of thrombocytopenia such as epistaxis, bloody diarrhoea, petechiae in young age
- Combined 'B' and 'T' cell immunodeficiency causes eczema
- More incidence of malignancies
- Spleen destroys platelets count as low—20,000 or 40,000 cells/microlitre
- The best treatment is human leukocytic antigen (HLA) matched sibling bone marrow transplantation
- Otherwise—splenectomy and antibiotics are the treatment of choice

HAEMATOLOGICAL INDICATIONS FOR SPLENECTOMY

IDIOPATHIC THROMBOCYTOPENIC PURPURA (ITP)

- This condition occurs due to development of autoantibodies against patient's own platelets (Key Box 44.4).
- Normal levels of platelets are between 1,50,000 and 4,00,000 cells per mm^3.
- The spleen is probably responsible for sequestration of platelets and for production of antibodies.

Types

Type 1: Acute—children: Follows an acute infection and resolves spontaneously in about two months.

Type 2: Chronic—adults: Longer than six months. No cause is identified.

Key Box 44.4

Other Causes of Purpura

- ↓ Production: Cytotoxic drugs, aplastic anaemia.
- ↑ Consumption of platelets: DIC as in septicaemia.
- ↑ Destruction: SLE, infectious mononucleosis.
- ↑ Capillary fragility: Steroid-induced or Henoch-Schönlein purpura.

Clinical Features

- Condition is common in females, F : M :: 3 : 1.
- **Purpuric patches** (ecchymosis refers to skin discolouration due to extravasation of blood) are found on the buttocks and petechial haemorrhages (spots) are found on the limbs. These are **dependent areas** having high intravascular pressure (Figs 44.12 to 44.14).
- All types of haemorrhages are common and can be mild or moderate (Key Box 44.5).

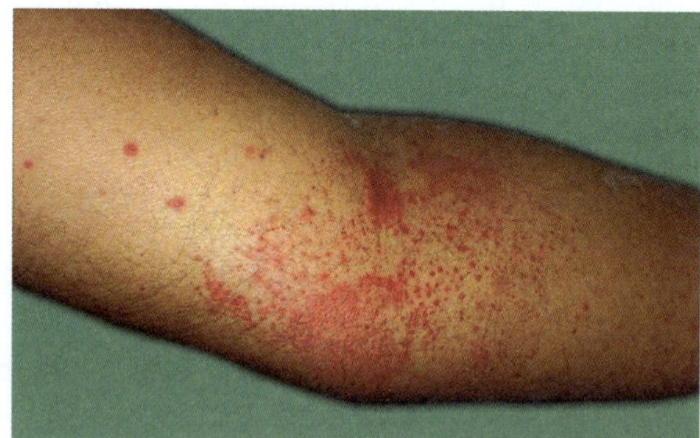

Fig. 44.12: Purpuric spots in the forearm

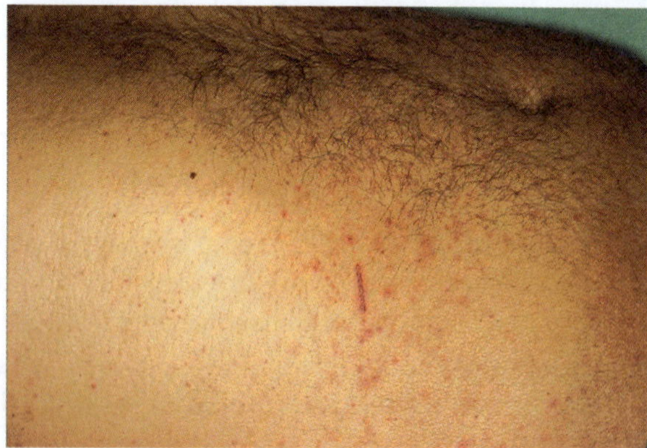

Fig. 44.13: Purpuric spots on the abdomen

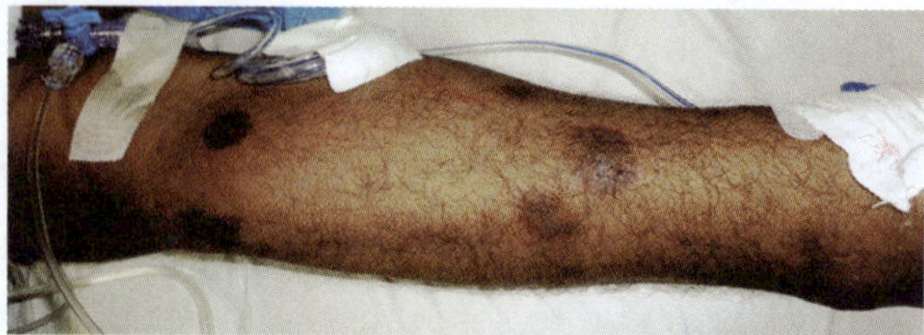

Fig. 44.14: Severe sepsis with thrombocytopenia

Key Box 44.5

Common Types of Haemorrhages

- Epistaxis
- Menorrhagia
- Haematemesis
- Bleeding gums
- Haemarthrosis
- Haematuria

- Intracranial haemorrhage is found in 1–2% of patients but it may be the cause of death.
- In 25% of cases, the spleen is just palpable (small size).
- **Hess tourniquet test:** More than 20 petechiae in a circle of 3 cm diameter in cubital fossa suggests purpura.

Pearls of Wisdom

If the spleen is big, it is not ITP.

Investigations

- Bleeding time is prolonged in purpura. Clotting and prothrombin times are normal.
- Platelet count is reduced.
- Bone marrow biopsy: Precursors of platelets (megakaryocytes) are increased.

Treatment

In Children

- Spontaneous regression occurs in majority of cases.
- Short course of corticosteroids is beneficial. Tablet prednisolone in the dose of 10 mg/day over a period of 6 weeks is given.

In Adults

Splenectomy is indicated in the following situations:

- ***When ITP has presented for more than 6–9 months.***
- ***When ITP has relapsed in spite of steroids,*** the patient is given a trial of prednisolone, 1 mg/kg/day. Platelet count rises within 7 days of starting steroids after which splenectomy can be done (Key Box 44.6).
- Also indicated, if a patient has two relapses on steroid therapy or if the platelet count is less.

Results

70–80% of patients respond permanently and do not require any further treatment. Counts rise above 1,00,000/mm^3 in 7 days. Even if counts are not raised, recurrent bleeding rarely occurs.

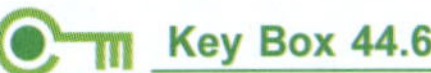

Key Box 44.6

Surgery in ITP

- Can be done even when platelets are as low as 10,000 cells/mm^3.
- **Diathermy** is used to open layers of the abdomen.
- **Ligate splenic artery first** at the upper border of pancreas after opening lesser sac.
- **Splenectomy is not difficult. Accessory spleen** (15–30%), if present, should be **removed.**
- Platelet transfusion may be required postoperatively, if there is bleeding.
- **Two-thirds** of patients will be **cured** by surgery.
- 15% will show improvement.
- Remaining will not benefit.

Haemolytic Anaemia

This type of anaemia results from an increased red cell destruction which occurs in the spleen. The lifespan of red blood cells is also shortened. Hence, irrespective of the cause of haemolytic anaemia, these cases can benefit from splenectomy. **Anaemia, jaundice** and **splenomegaly** are the triad of haemolytic anaemia.

Causes of Haemolytic Anaemia

1. Hereditary spherocytosis
2. Acquired autoimmune haemolytic anaemia
3. Thalassaemia
4. Sickle cell disease

HEREDITARY SPHEROCYTOSIS

This hereditary disorder is transmitted by either parent as Mendelian autosomal dominant. The disease is characterised by a **defect in cell wall protein of the red cell, namely spectrin,** which increases reflux of sodium into the cell. This causes the biconcave red cell to swell and become spherical. Hence, the name spherocytosis.

Consequences of Spherocytes in Circulation

1. The spherocyte is already weak. Adding onto this, there is a greater loss of membrane phospholipid which results in a delicate fragile spherocyte.
2. Because of the altered shape, **oxygen and energy requirements of RBCs increase which cannot be met by the spleen**. In the spleen, they are destroyed and release excessive haemoglobin which is converted into bilirubin.
   - The amount of bilirubin produced is increased and most of it is unconjugated. It gets attached to albumin as it is **lipid soluble** and, therefore, cannot be excreted in the urine. Hence, this type of jaundice is also known as acholuric jaundice.

Pearls of Wisdom

Most of this bilirubin is excreted in the biliary tree resulting in pigment stones in the biliary tree.

Clinical Features (Figs 44.15 to 44.18)

- Commonly seen in young children but can manifest in adults also.
- Seen equally in both sexes.
- History of recurrent attacks of jaundice can be elicited from childhood.
- Jaundice is mild, never deep, not associated with itching or bradycardia.

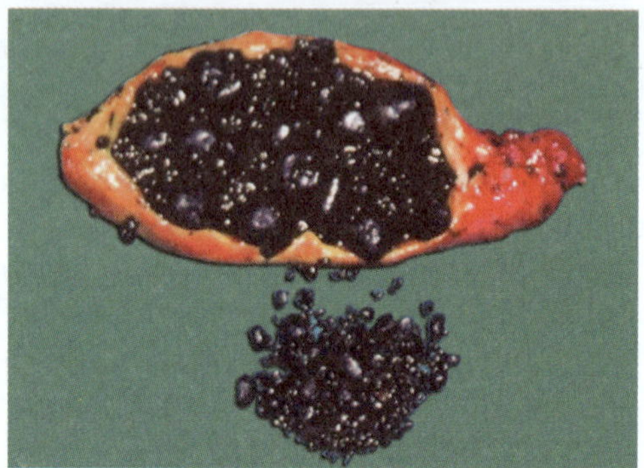

Fig. 44.15: Pigment stones

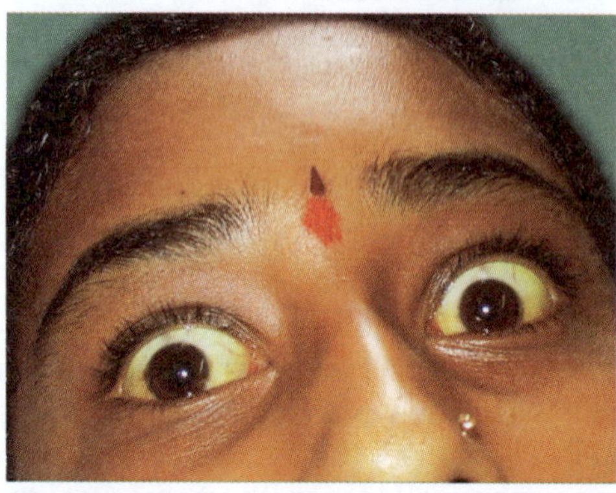

Fig. 44.16: Case of hereditary spherocytosis with faint jaundice in a 22-year-old girl

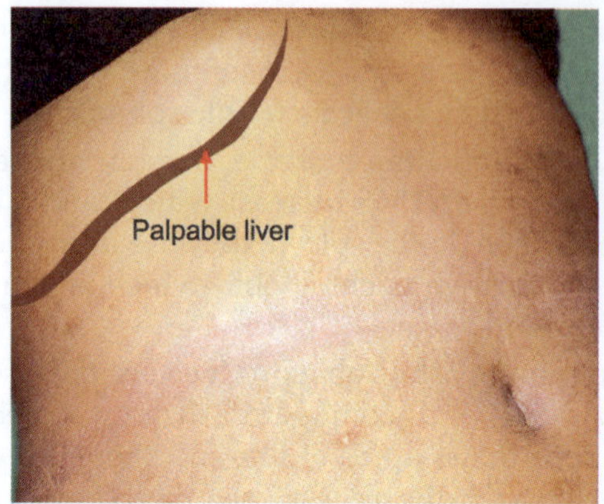

Fig. 44.17: She also had 2 cm enlarged liver and gallstones

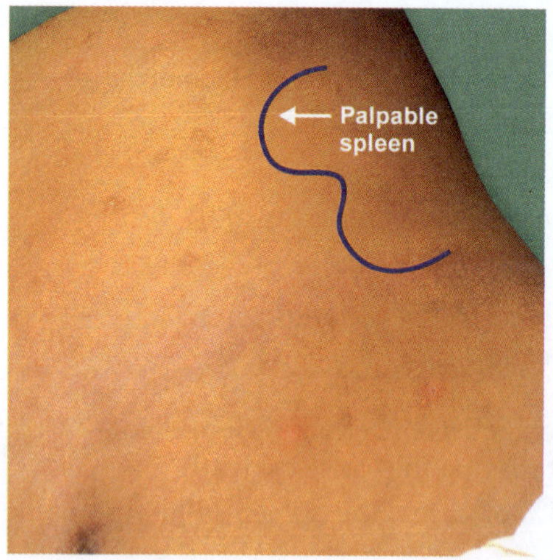

Fig. 44.18: Splenomegaly—its size was 5 cm

- **Pallor** is an important feature due to destruction of the red cells.
- **Acute haemolytic crisis:** It is precipitated by an acute infection or stress. Abdominal pain, nausea, vomiting, pyrexia and pallor are the features. The condition can be confused for an abdominal emergency. In severe cases, anaemia, thrombocytopenia, leukopaenia can occur.
- **Spleen is moderately enlarged.** The liver is also palpable in a few cases.
- In adults, **gallstone colic** and obstructive jaundice due to **CBD** stone can also complicate the disease process. Incidence of gallstone disease is around 50%. **It is common after the age of 10.**
- Leg ulcers may occur as a result of anaemia.

Pearls of Wisdom

Young, pale, jaundiced, fatigued child with gallstones—think of hereditary spherocytosis.

Investigations

1. **Peripheral smear: Spherocytes** are present.
2. **Reticulocyte count is increased (15–25%):** These are immature red cells which are discharged by the bone marrow due to loss of red cells.
3. **Coombs' test is negative:** Serum bilirubin is mildly elevated and most of it is unconjugated.
4. **Fragility test:** Normal red cell haemolysis occurs in **0.47%** saline solution. Here, it occurs at **0.6%** or even in weaker solution.
5. **Ultrasound** abdomen is done to rule out gallstones.

Treatment

Splenectomy is the treatment including removal of accessory spleen.

- Ideally, it should be done from the age of 6 to 10 years. Why after 6 years? The incidence of post-splenectomy sepsis is more when splenectomy is done within 6 years of age. Why before 10 years? After 10 years of age, the incidence of gallstone increases.

Splenectomy helps in the following ways (Figs 44.16 to 44.18)

1. By decreasing erythrocyte destruction, anaemia improves, thus avoiding blood transfusions.
2. Erythrocytes achieve normal lifespan. Hence, jaundice also disappears.
3. Leg ulcers heal quickly.
   - If gallstones are also found in these cases, laparoscopic splenectomy and cholecystectomy can be done in the same sitting.

Pearls of Wisdom

Hereditary elliptocytosis is also a genetic disorder wherein RBCs are oval in shape. It also responds to splenectomy.

ACQUIRED AUTOIMMUNE HAEMOLYTIC ANAEMIA

Due to an autoimmune reaction, the red cell surface is damaged and it gets destroyed in the splenic red pulp. Antibodies develop against red cell antigens. In 50% of cases, the cause is not known. The following are the probable causes:

- SLE, lymphoma, chronic lymphocytic leukaemia
- Drugs: Methyldopa, mefenamic acid
- Exposure to chemicals or infections

Clinical Features

- More common in females after 50 years of age.
- Splenomegaly, moderate in size.
- Gallstones are found in around 25% of the cases.

Investigations

- Anaemia is present.
- Spherocytes may be present because of damage to the red cell surface.
- Coombs' test is positive.

Treatment

- It is a self-limiting disorder. Reassurance plays an important role.
- **Corticosteroids:** A short course of prednisolone 60 mg/day is given.
- Splenectomy is done when steroid response is not satisfactory. ***80% of patients respond to splenectomy.***

THALASSAEMIA

It is also called Cooley's anaemia, Mediterranean anaemia, Heinz body haemolytic anaemia.

Aetiopathogenesis

- It is a hereditary disorder, transmitted as a **dominant trait.** It is characterised by a defect in haemoglobin peptide chain synthesis. Depending on type of peptide chain involvement, it is classified into α, β and γ. However, β-thalassaemia is more common. There is a decrease in haemoglobin and red cells will be destroyed prematurely due to intracellular precipitates **(Heinz bodies)**.
- When it is a heterozygous disorder, it is called beta-thalassaemia minor and when homozygous, it is called beta-thalassaemia major (Cooley's anaemia). **The abnormal gene is inherited from either or both the parents.**

Clinical Features

- Severe anaemia resulting in weakness, lethargy, leg ulcers, etc.
- Splenomegaly is mild to moderate in size. Sometimes, it is massive resulting in abdominal discomfort or may cause abdominal distension.
- Jaundice due to haemolysis. Liver can also be enlarged.
- To compensate for anaemia, bone marrow hyperplasia occurs resulting in bossing of skull and prominent malar bones. Thalassaemia major usually manifests in the first year of life.

Complications

1. **Haemosiderosis** (deposition of iron in tissues) of pancreas results in chronic pancreatitis and diabetes.
2. **Hepatic cirrhosis** due to liver haemosiderosis.
3. **Aplastic crisis** with severe life-threatening infections.
4. **Gallstones** occur in about 20% of cases.

Investigations

- Peripheral smear demonstrates microcytic hypochromic anaemia. Red cells are small, thin and are resistant to osmotic lysis.
- Haemoglobin electrophoresis reveals reduction or absent levels of haemoglobin A (HbA). There is a compensatory increase in foetal haemoglobin (HbF).

Treatment

- **Blood transfusion:** Multiple repeated transfusions may be necessary.

- **Surgical:** Splenectomy is indicated in a few cases who require multiple transfusions and patients with gross splenomegaly.

SICKLE CELL ANAEMIA OR SICKLE CELL DISEASE

This is a hereditary haemolytic disorder in which haemoglobin A is replaced by haemoglobin S (HbS). This results in crescent-shaped erythrocytes. This HbS molecule crystallises, if there is hypoxia, strenuous work or due to dehydration. As a result of this, red cells are distorted and elongated. Therefore, blood viscosity is increased, causing obstruction in the splenic circulation (Key Box 44.7).

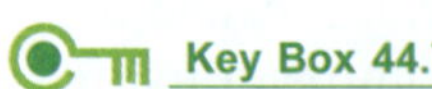

Key Box 44.7

Functional Abnormalities in Sickle Cell Anaemia

- Spleen sometimes acts as a large reservoir for red cells and the sickle cells are destroyed.
- Antibody production is decreased.
- Spleen's ability to filter *Streptococcus pneumoniae* is reduced.

Effect of HbS Blockage

- Splenic microinfarcts
- Splenomegaly or **autosplenectomy** due to repeated infarcts (Fig. 44.19).

Clinical Features

- The disease is very common in Africans. Most of the patients in India have high HbF levels which protect HbS. Hence, symptoms are not seen in the first few weeks.
- Abdominal pain is due to recurrent infarcts or due to gallstone in a few patients.
- Skin ulcers occur due to anaemia or hypoxia.

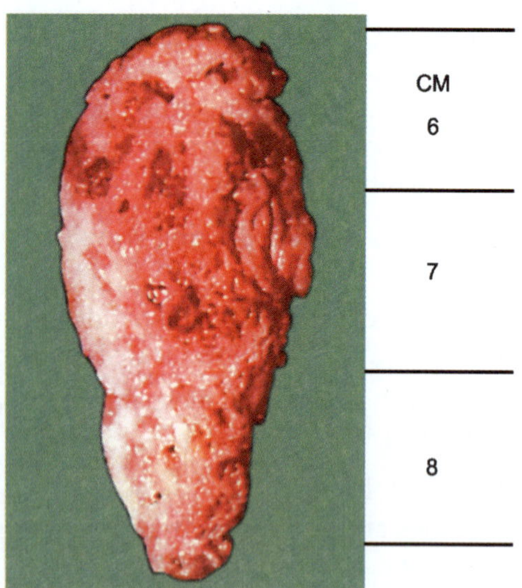

Fig. 44.19: Sickle cell anaemia—Nugget spleen (3 cm size). An example for autosplenectomy

Pearls of Wisdom

Microinfarction of carpal and tarsal bones resulting in bony pains is described as hand-foot syndrome.

Investigations

- Peripheral smear demonstrates sickle cell.
- Haemoglobin electrophoresis to identify the type of haemoglobin.

Treatment

- Folic acid supplements
- Splenectomy has a doubtful value. It is indicated only when excessive numbers of RBCs are sequestrated causing anaemia (Table 44.1 for comparison).

Complications

- Infarct of cerebrum resulting in hemiplegia.

Table 44.1 Summary of haemolytic anaemias

	Aetiology	Shape of RBC	Spleen	Investigation	Treatment
1. Hereditary spherocytosis	Increase in red cell permeability to sodium	Spherocyte	Large	Reticulocyte count	Splenectomy very beneficial
2. Autoimmune haemolytic anaemia	SLE, drugs	Spherocyte	Medium size	Coombs' test is positive	Steroids: Splenectomy in steroid failure cases
3. Thalassaemia (Cooley's anaemia)	Reduction of β-chain of haemoglobin	Small, thin and no shape	Moderate size	Resistance to osmotic lysis Electrophoresis HbA	Splenectomy for bulky spleen and in patients requiring frequent blood transfusion
4. Sickle cell	HbA is replaced by HbS	Sickle shape	Mild and later not palpable	Electrophoresis HbS	If hypersplenism +, splenectomy

- Mesenteric infarction resulting in gangrene of the bowel.
- Pulmonary infarction resulting in chest pain.

SPLENECTOMY FOR OTHER CONDITIONS

HYPERSPLENISM

It is defined as pancytopaenia in the presence of normal or hypercellular bone marrow. Following are the causes of hypersplenism:

It usually involves red pulp expansion. It must be remembered that in cirrhosis of the liver, 15% of patients develop hypersplenism. Anaemia and thrombocytopenia are mild. Rarely requires splenectomy (a few causes are given below):

- **Tropical splenomegaly** due to malaria, kala-azar or schistosomiasis, etc. Since these diseases are endemic in tropical countries, it is called tropical splenomegaly. Gross enlargement of the spleen and hypersplenism are indications for splenectomy in such cases.
- **Myeloproliferative disorders:** Splenectomy reduces need for transfusion and may relieve abdominal discomfort.
- **Portal hypertension:** Maximum benefit is in segmental portal hypertension with oesophagogastric varices (Fig. 44.20).
- **Genetic:** Gaucher's diseases.
- Neoplastic infiltration.
- **Inflammatory disease:** Sarcoidosis, lupus erythematosus.
- Chronic infections, such as tuberculosis, brucellosis and malaria.
- **Chronic** haemolytic diseases—spherocytosis, thalassaemia, glucose-6-phosphate dehydrogenase deficiency, elliptocytosis.

CYSTS OF THE SPLEEN (Figs 44.21 to 44.23)

- *Parasitic cyst* is rare. Typically, it is caused by echinococcal disease **(hydatid disease)**.
- *Traumatic cysts* are due to a haematoma giving rise to liquefaction. These are false cysts of the spleen.
- *Congenital cysts* can be due to a dermoid cyst, haemangioma or lymphangioma.
- *Better* save the spleen by deroofing cyst wall.

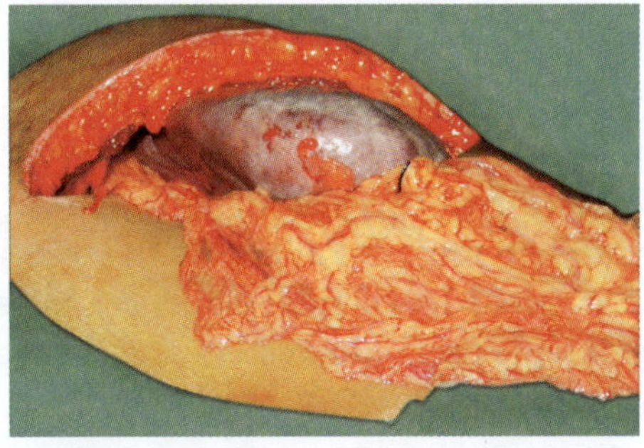

Fig. 44.20: Splenectomy done for left-sided portal hypertension due to splenic vein thrombosis

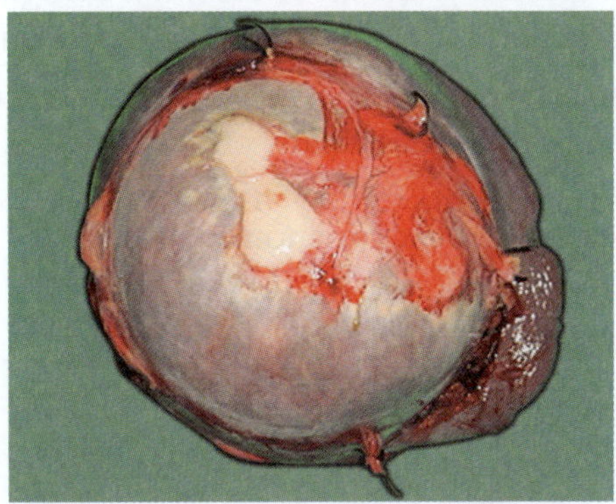

Fig. 44.21: Simple cyst of the spleen resulting in compression of the spleen—appearance like that of a ***globe***

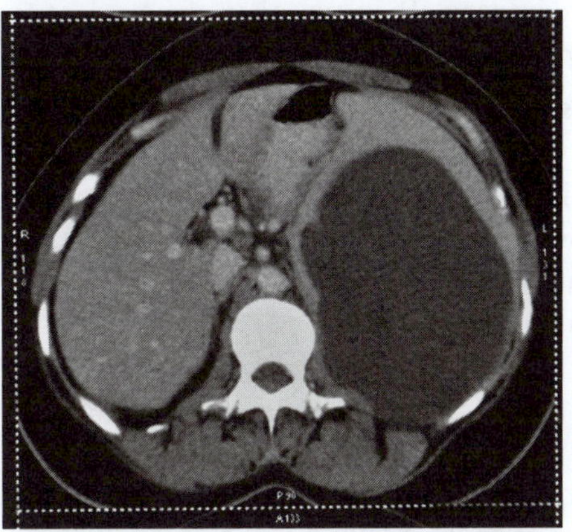

Fig. 44.22: Splenic cyst coronal view

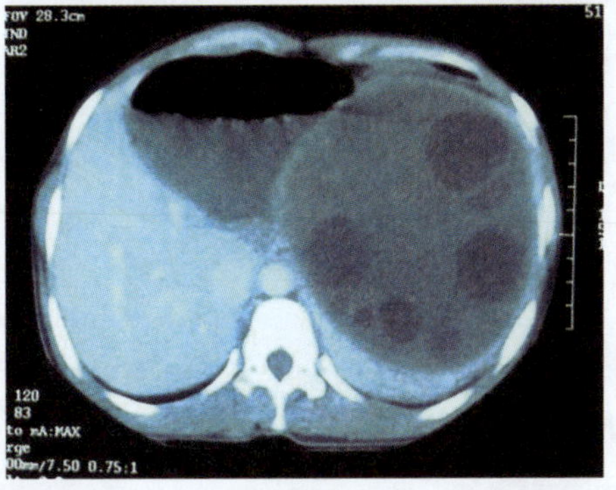

Fig. 44.23: Splenic hydatid cyst (*Courtesy:* Prof Dr Anandravi BN, Dr Balakrishna, Dr Dinesh, Dr Ravi, KR Hospital Mysore)

TUMOURS OF THE SPLEEN/NEOPLASMS

- Among neoplasms, **lymphoma** is the commonest cause of ***enlargement*** of spleen. Spleen used to be removed as a part of a staging laparotomy. Now, it is very rarely removed. Patients with **large spleen** of chronic myeloid leukaemia, Gaucher's disease and hairy cell leukaemia (details later) will also benefit from splenectomy.
- **Fibrosarcoma** and **angiosarcoma** are rare malignant tumours.
- **Haemangioma** is the ***most common benign tumour*** of the spleen. It may turn into haemangiosarcoma.
- **Spleen** is removed in oesophagogastrectomy or upper carcinoma stomach—only when it is directly infiltrated. Sometimes it happens in carcinoma tail of pancreas/splenic carcinoma.

OTHER INDICATIONS FOR SPLENECTOMY

(Figs 44.24 and 44.25)

- **Splenic abscess** can occur due to infected septic emboli from otitis, typhoid fever or due to thrombosis of splenic vein causing infarction followed later by infection (Key Box 44.8). **Tubercular abscess** of the spleen is rare. It is usually affected secondary to abdominal or pulmonary tuberculosis.
- **Felty's syndrome** refers to splenomegaly, neutropenia with rheumatoid arthritis. After splenectomy, leg ulcers heal quickly and neutropenia also improves. The patient may respond to steroids better and the incidence of recurrent infection becomes less (Fig. 44.26).

SPLENIC ARTERY ANEURYSM

It is an uncommon condition. More common in women, and some of them occur during *pregnancy*.

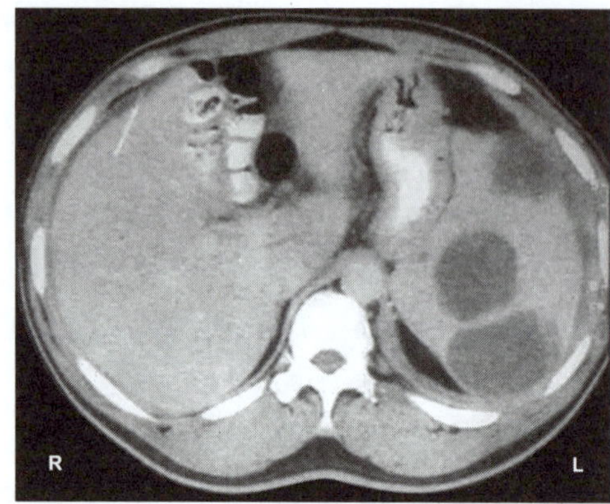

Fig. 44.24: CT scan showing multiple splenic abscesses

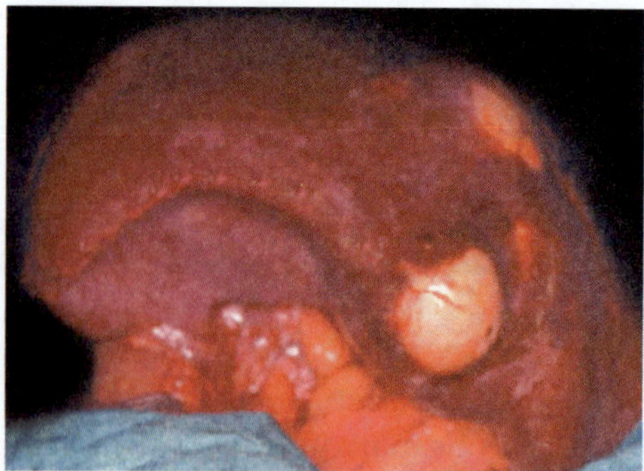

Fig. 44.25A: Same patient as in Fig. 44.24 with multiple abscesses in the spleen

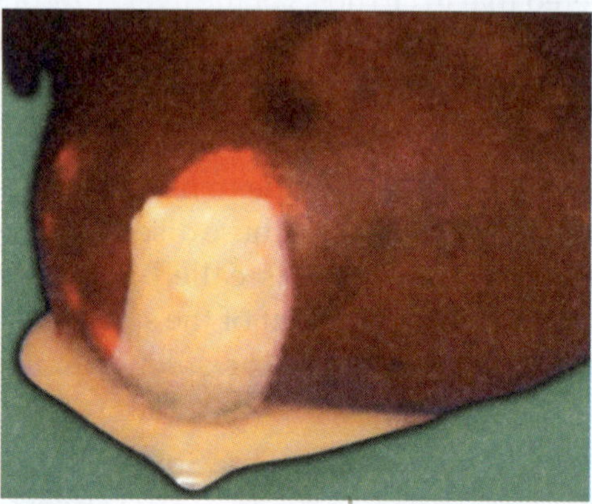

Fig. 44.25B: Incision of the abscess after splenectomy

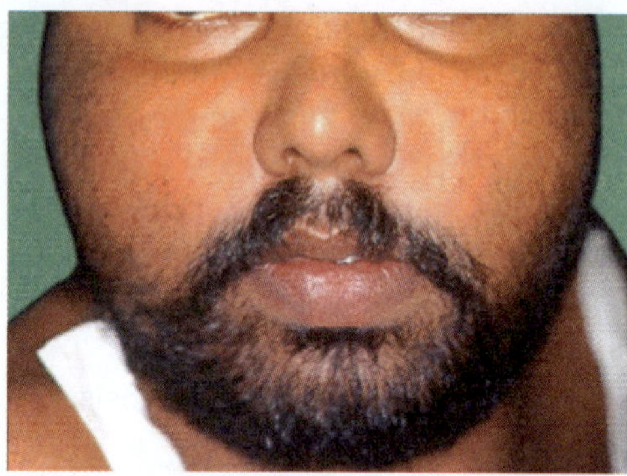

Fig. 44.26: Felty's syndrome. The patient had received steroids for one year. *See* the Cushingoid facies

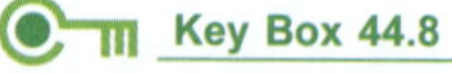

Key Box 44.8

Causes of Splenic Abscess

Salmonella infection
Paratyphi infection
Labour—puerperal sepsis
Ear infection—otitis
Necrosis of pancreas
Infection of bone—osteomyelitis
Chronic disease—tuberculosis

Remember as **SPLENIC**

Causes

- **Atherosclerosis:** Commonly seen in elderly patients.
- **Congenital:** Young patients. These patients may present for the first time during pregnancy with enlargement or rupture.
- **Acute pancreatitis:** Inflammatory process may give rise to pseudoaneurysm specially because of pancreatic necrosis.

Clinical Features

- Pain and vomiting—haematemesis
- Thrill or bruit
- Calcification in a routine X-ray
- Rupture and features of haemorrhagic shock.

Investigations (Figs 44.27 to 44.29)

- Ultrasound/CT scan
- Angiography

Treatment

- **Non-operative:** Embolisation of splenic artery (Fig. 44.30).
- **Operative:** Ligation of splenic artery at the upper border of pancreas after opening lesser sac followed by splenectomy.
- **Rupture:** Carries high mortality rate.

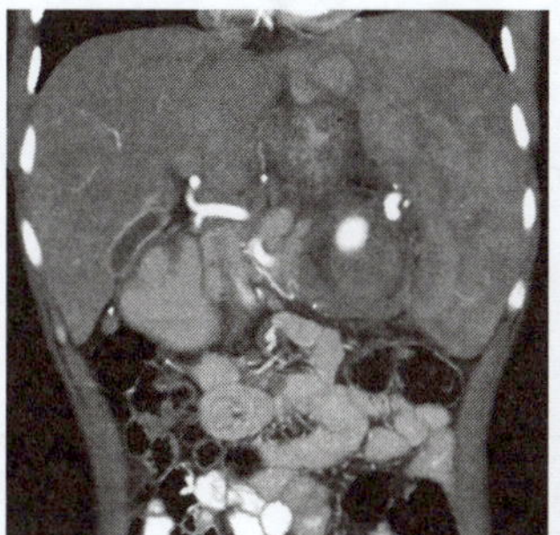
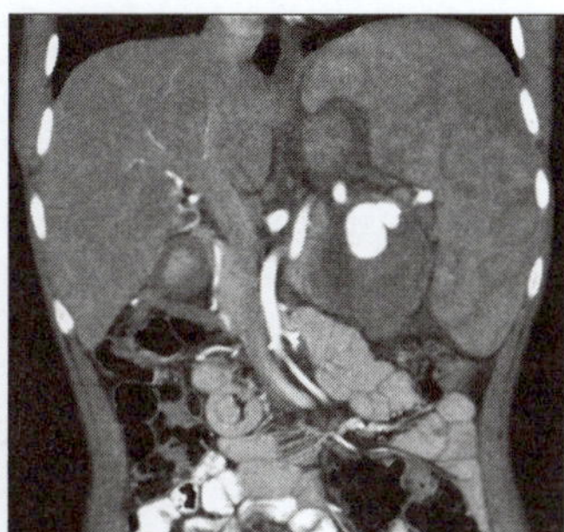
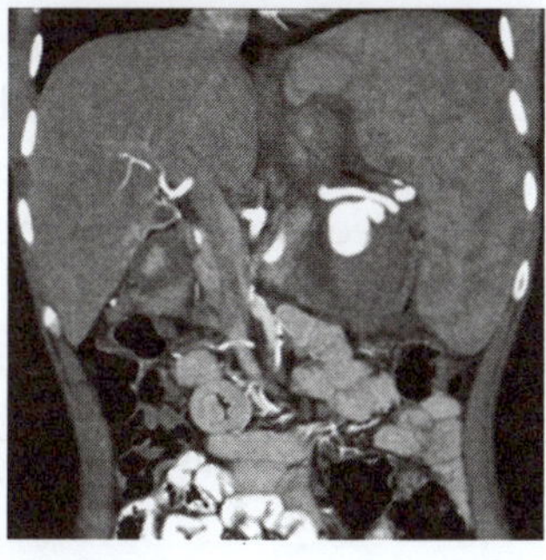

Figs 44.27 to 44.29: A 28-year-old man presented with pain abdomen. CT scan showed splenic artery aneurysm with haematoma and thrombus suggestive of ruptured splenic artery aneurysm. He also had splenomegaly and features of portal hypertension. He was alcoholic. He might have had pancreatitis and developed splenic artery aneurysm (*Courtesy:* Prof Sampath Kumar, Dr Basavaraj Patil, Dr Dinesh, Dr Pawan Kumar Addala, Department of Surgery, KMC, Manipal)

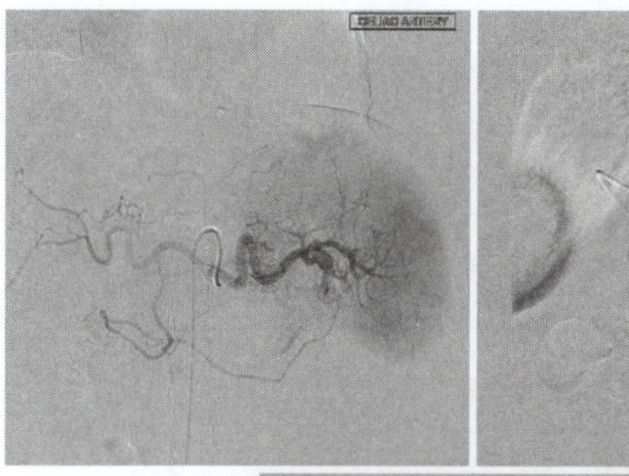
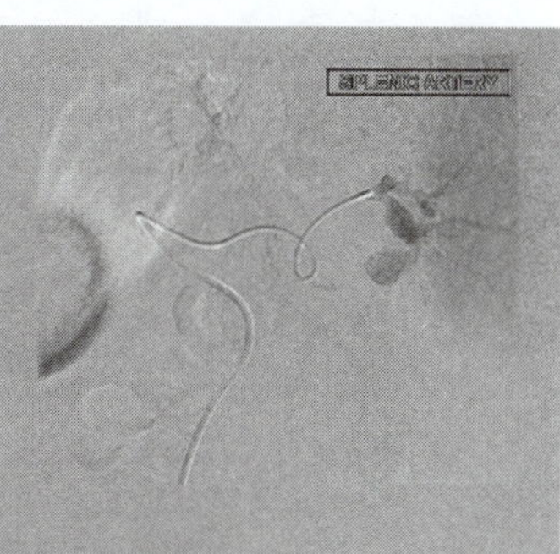
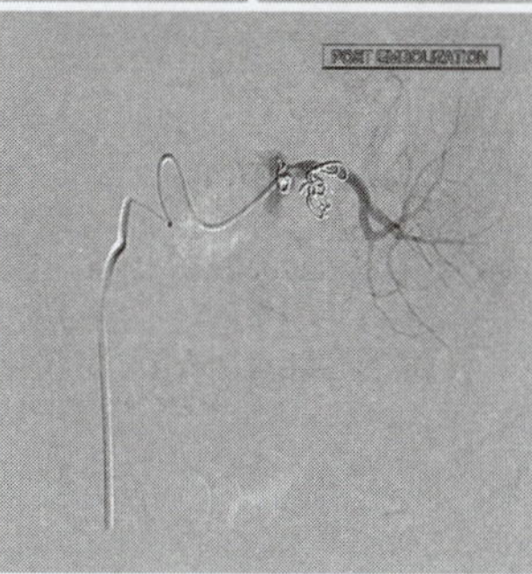

Fig. 44.30: Splenic artery embolisation. You can see reduction in the size of pseudoaneurysm in the last picture (*Courtesy:* Dr Rajgopal V, Dr Sunil Krishna, Dr Chitra Bhatt, KMC Manipal)

Clinical Notes

A 49-year-old female came with chief complaints of pain abdomen since 10 years, aggravated since 10 days. Pain is in the left hypochondriac region, epigastrium and radiating to back. Patient is a known patient with chronic pancreatitis treated many times. CT scan revealed chronic calcific pancreatitis with splenic artery pseudoaneurysm (2.5–3 cm). Angiogram revealed a pseudoaneurysm arising from main branch of splenic artery. Coiling of the pseudoaneurysm was done using 3 nester coils—one 5.0 cm × 3 cm and two 5 cm × 4 cm. After embolisation, the pseudoaneurysm decreased in size. Danger lies in rupture of pseudoaneurysm and massive bleeding.

HAIRY CELL LEUKAEMIA (HCL) (Fig. 44.31)

- The cells on a blood smear have an irregular outline due to the presence of filament-like cytoplasmic projections. Hence, the name **hairy cells**.
- HCL is a clonal proliferation of abnormal B cells (very rarely T cells).

Clinical Features

- Anaemia
- Recurrent infection
- Massive enlargement of spleen.

Investigations

- Blood counts are low. White cell count may be raised with circulating hairy cells.

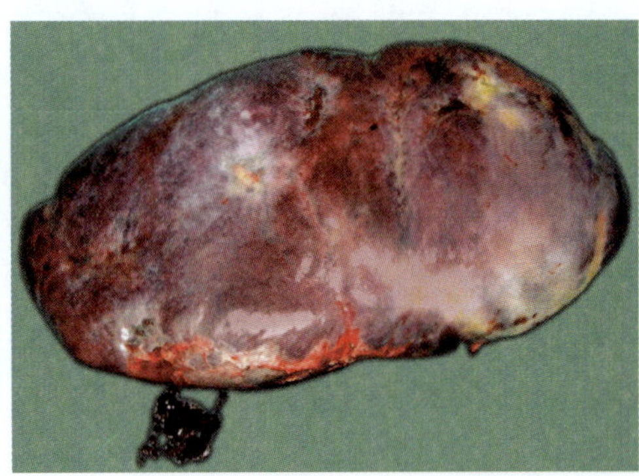

Fig. 44.31: Patient had pyrexia of unknown origin with pancytopaenia. Spleen was enlarged. Splenectomy was done and the biopsy report was non-Hodgkin's lymphoma

- Bone marrow has increased cellularity with characteristic infiltration by **hairy cells**.

Treatment

- Drug: 2-Chloradenosine acetate (2-CDA) has been beneficial. It can induce remission.
- Splenectomy is indicated in cases of diagnostic difficulties and in very large spleens.

OPSI

Competency

SU26.11: Describe the post-splenectomy sepsis—prophylaxis.

Definition

It is a generalized non-specific flu-like prodrome followed by rapid deterioration to serious full-blown fulminant septic shock within 24–48 hours of the onset. It is also called as Post splenectomy sepsis

Introduction

It is a medical emergency and if it not treated, cardiovascular collapse and death can occur. OPSI has high mortality rates. Fever, body ache, myalgia chills are a few features of OPSI.

Bacteriology and Pathogenesis

- The bacteria covered with a polysaccharide capsule are called as encapsulated bacteria. Streptococcus pneumoniae, Klebsiella, Hemophilus influenzae, Neisseria meningitidis, and Pseudomonas aeruginosa are examples.
- Normally, encapsulated pathogens are opsonized with antibodies. After that, phagocytosis takes place in the spleen by specialized macrophages. Thus, patients who had splenectomy are more prone to develop serious infection and sepsis.

Factors Precipitating OPSI

- Loss of splenic phagocytic function,
- Low levels of serum immunoglobulin levels,
- Low activity- suppression of lymphocyte sensitivity,
- Loss of functioning of opsonin

Prevention

- Educating patients including children and parents is also an important part of prevention of OPSI
- In all elective cases, vaccination should be given against S. pneumoniae, hemophilus influenzae type b, Neisseria meningitidis and influenza at least 2 weeks before surgery and annually.
- Daily antibiotics for at least 2 years after splenectomy should be given more so in children. In emergency cases, vaccines should be given as soon as possible.
- Any infections should be treated as emergency and by antibiotics.

Treatment

- Early diagnosis
- Early antibiotics
- Early aggressive resuscitation: Fluids, vasopressors, monitoring

Following are the recommendations; to avoid OPSI (Key Box 44.9).

I. Elective Splenectomy

- All children who undergo splenectomy before 5 years of age, should receive daily dose of penicillin until 10 years.
- *Haemophilus influenzae* type B vaccination for all irrespective of age and pneumococcal vaccine to be given (repeated once in 5 years).
- Meningococcal protection for only those who travel to high-risk areas.

Pearls of Wisdom

Vaccination should be given at least 2 weeks before elective splenectomy.

II. After Emergency Splenectomy

- Vaccines should be given as early as possible. However, protection is **not always** guaranteed.
- Daily dose of oral prophylaxis with penicillin, erythromycin or amoxycillin to all children till 10 years who undergo splenectomy before the age of 5.

Benefits of Splenectomy (Fig. 44.32)

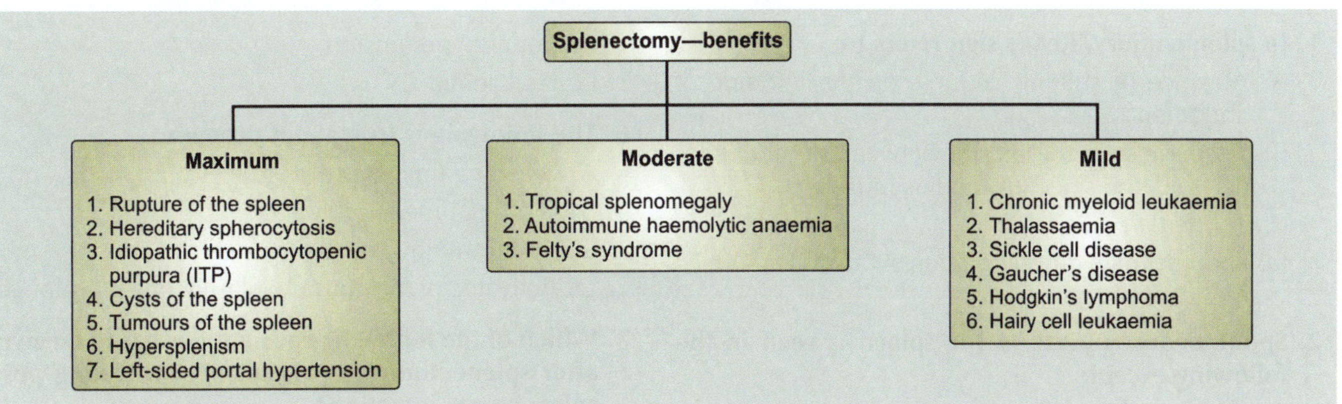

Fig. 44.32: Benefits of splenectomy

INTERESTING 'MOST COMMON' FOR SPLEEN

- Haemangioma is the most common benign tumour of the spleen.
- Lymphoma is the most common cause of enlargement of spleen (in India, malaria is the cause).
- It is the most common solid organ injured in blunt abdominal trauma.
- Most common cause for splenic rupture is blunt abdominal trauma.
- Most significant benefit of doing a splenectomy for hypersplenism is from segmental left-sided portal hypertension.
- Most commonly performed investigation for suspected splenic trauma is abdominal ultrasound.
- Most common malignancy affecting spleen is lymphoma.
- Most common complication of splenectomy is pulmonary complication.
- Most common neoplasm of spleen—lymphoma.
- Most common primary tumour of spleen—haemangioma.
- Most common primary malignant tumour of the spleen—haemangiosarcoma.
- Most common infection after splenectomy is by *Streptococcus pneumoniae*.
- Most common indication for splenectomy—splenic trauma.
- Most common indication for splenectomy in elective setting—ITP.

Multiple Choice Questions

1. In splenic injury, Kehr's sign refers to:
- A. Absence of shifting dullness on the left side of abdomen
- B. Tenderness on the left side between sternocleido-mastoid and scalenus medius muscle
- C. Tender left iliac fossa
- D. Shoulder pain due to irritation of the under-surface of the diaphragm

2. Spontaneous rupture of the spleen is seen in the following *except:*
- A. Idiopathic thrombocytopenic purpura
- B. Malaria
- C. Infectious mononucleosis
- D. Leukaemia

3. Diagnostic peritoneal lavage is said to be positive in all of the following *except*:
- A. Fresh blood >20 ml is aspirated after inserting dialysis catheter
- B. Gram stain is positive in the contents of the lavage
- C. RBC count >100,000 cells/cu mm
- D. Amylase level of 75 units/dl

4. The following is not true about nonoperative treatment in splenic trauma *except*:
- A. Hemodynamically stable patient
- B. Hollow viscus injury
- C. Close monitoring is available
- D. Hospitalisation is required

5. Big spleen is not a feature of:
- A. Malaria
- B. Idiopathic thrombocytopenic purpura
- C. Portal hypertension
- D. Leukaemia

6. The following is true about purpura:
- A. Bleeding time is prolonged
- B. Clotting time is prolonged
- C. Prothrombin time is prolonged
- D. Activated partial thromboplastin time is prolonged

7. Which of the following vaccinations has to be given after splenectomy to prevent overwhelming post-splenectomy infection?
- A. Measles vaccine
- B. Pneumococcal vaccine
- C. Hepatitis vaccine
- D. Varicella vaccine

8. The following is true about splenectomy in idiopathic thrombocytopenic purpura (ITP):
- A. Is required in all cases of ITP
- B. Must be done when platelet count is >100,000 cells/cu mm
- C. Accessory spleens, if present must be left behind
- D. Two-thirds of patients will be cured by surgery

9. The following is true about splenectomy for hereditary spherocytosis:
- A. Splenectomy should be done as a last resort
- B. Splenectomy must be done either before 6 years or after ten years of age
- C. Accessory spleen, if present must be left behind
- D. Jaundice disappears after splenectomy

10. The most common benign tumour of the spleen is:
- A. Haemangioma
- B. Lymphoma
- C. Tuberculoma
- D. Lipoma

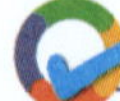

Answers

1. D **2.** A **3.** D **4.** B **5.** B **6.** A **7.** B **8.** D **9.** D **10.** A